The Hospital for
Sick Children

Handbook of Pediatrics

12th EDITION

The Hospital for Sick Children

Handbook of Pediatrics

EDITORS

Deborah Schonfeld, MDCM, FRCPC
Staff Physician, Division of Emergency
Medicine
Department of Pediatrics, The Hospital
for Sick Children
Assistant Professor, Faculty of Medicine,
University of Toronto

Shawna Silver, MD, FRCPC, PEng
Staff Physician, Division of Pediatric
Medicine
Department of Pediatrics, The Hospital
for Sick Children
Lecturer, Faculty of Medicine, University
of Toronto

Catherine Diskin, MB BCh BAO,
MSc, MRCPI
Pediatric Medicine Fellow
Department of Pediatrics, The Hospital
for Sick Children

Siobhán Neville, MB BCh BAO, MSc,
MRCPI, MRCPCH
Pediatric Medicine Fellow
Department of Pediatrics, The Hospital
for Sick Children

ELSEVIER

Elsevier
1600 John F. Kennedy Blvd.
Ste 1800
Philadelphia, PA 19103-2899

Notice

Practitioners and researchers must always rely on their own experience and knowledge in evaluating and using any information, methods, compounds or experiments described herein. Because of rapid advances in the medical sciences, in particular, independent verification of diagnoses and drug dosages should be made. To the fullest extent of the law, no responsibility is assumed by Elsevier, authors, editors or contributors for any injury and/or damage to persons or property as a matter of products liability, negligence or otherwise, or from any use or operation of any methods, products, instructions, or ideas contained in the material herein.

Previous edition published under title The HSC Handbook of Pediatrics

Library of Congress Control Number

Content Strategist: Marybeth Thiel
Content Development Specialist: Meredith Madeira
Publishing Services Manager: Deepthi Unni
Project Manager: Radjan Lourde Selvanadin
Design Direction: Patrick C. Ferguson

Printed in India

Last digit is the print number: 9 8 7 6 5 4 3 2 1

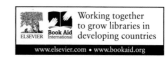

DEDICATION

To...
All the students, residents and fellows whom I have taught and have taught me, and to mom and dad—the most inspiring pediatricians I know.   **DS**

To...
All the children, families and colleagues from whom I have learned so much, and my family—you are truly gems.   **SS**

To...
Those that support me, family and friends.   **CD**

To...
My closest champions and confidantes, whose patience for me talking about this project knew no bounds.   **SN**

CONTENTS

FOREWORD TO THE 12TH EDITION

It is a privilege and a pleasure to write the foreword to the 12th edition of The Hospital for Sick Children Handbook of Pediatrics. Why do I regard this as a privilege and a pleasure?

It is a privilege to be associated with an iconic pediatric "bible" that has provided such value to so many generations of child health students and clinicians. The consistent excellence in presenting comprehensive state of the art, evidence-based, practical guidance has ensured that this handbook has not only endured into its 12th edition over more than 60 years since the 1st edition, but improved and reinvented itself with every new version. The Hospital for Sick Children, or SickKids as it is affectionately known, has been a world leader in the provision of clinical care and research in child health for over 140 years. Generations of learners have travelled from across the world to train here, and SickKids is famous for its leadership in teaching. There are currently 320 inpatient beds, 90,000 visits to our Emergency Department and 250,000 visits to our ambulatory clinics annually. Across the hospital we have close to 1000 clinical and research trainees. SickKids is the most research-intensive hospital in Canada and our Research Institute is a world leader in discovery and cutting-edge science. Of note is that this handbook has essentially been written by our residents and fellows, who are often the unsung heroes of the teaching hospital; long hours, hard work, and together with the nursing and support staff, provide the energy that keeps the hospital ticking and the patients cared for 24/7. Thanks also to the faculty chapter authors and especially to the Editors Drs. Shawna Silver and Debbie Schonfeld who have done an outstanding job, supervising the trainees, and diligently driving this process from concept to finish with great determination, talent and skill. Some of the brand new features include helpful practical chapters on Mental Health as well as Technology and Medical Complexity.

It is a pleasure to write this foreword because it is so much more fun than my relationship with the previous three editions. When I was a young innocent first year resident in 1990 I carried the 9th edition of this handbook around in the pocket of my neatly starched white coat. It was thick, heavy and had a serious red cover. I think I kept it under my pillow when I rarely had the opportunity to reach my on-call room for a brief nap. Toward the end of my residency it was replaced by the 10th edition, which was thinner, had a more soothing blue cover and was still seldom more than an arm's length away from me as I navigated the transition to my new role as junior faculty. The 11th edition which was published in 2009 was co-edited by myself and Dr. Anne Dipchand. It has a yellow cover with a bright picture of our hospital atrium, and was the first edition that had an electronic version, which was just becoming popular at the time. I remember very clearly just how much time and effort it took over the course of two years to coordinate and edit the excellent contributions of the one hundred trainee and faculty chapter authors. So honestly being invited to write this one page foreword and being able to pass the baton to Drs. Silver and Schonfeld and their team, is truly a pleasure!

I invite you to enjoy and benefit from the combined experience and wisdom that comes from 140 years in the child health business. I believe that regardless of your level of expertise and context, you will find advice and practical approaches that will be informative and useful. I salute not only all those who have contributed to this excellent 12th edition, but also all of you readers, who have dedicated your service to improving the health of children all over the world.

Jeremy Friedman, MBChB, FRCP, FAAP
Interim Pediatrician-in-Chief,
Hospital for Sick Children
Professor and Interim Chair,
Department of Pediatrics,
University of Toronto

Thank you for choosing this 12th edition of *The Hospital for Sick Children Handbook of Pediatrics*. Much like the pediatric healthcare practiced at The Hospital for Sick Children, this book is up-to-date, evidence-based, interdisciplinary and patient-focused in its approach.

Our intention as we undertook the unwieldy task of updating this handbook was to create a practical and applied resource for bedside teaching, study and practice. We hope this text will act as a valuable reference for medical students, residents, pediatricians, family doctors, emergency physicians, nurses and other practitioners who provide care to children—at The Hospital for Sick Children, throughout Canada and worldwide.

Content has been extensively revised throughout the handbook, reflecting current best practice. This edition has been reformatted, making it easier to read and navigate. Where possible, we have provided algorithmic approaches to clinical problems, ensuring the content is accessible and easy-to-use. We have added a new feature of "Pearls" and "Pitfalls" to each chapter, to highlight important clinical points and common mistakes or misconceptions. New chapters cover Mental Health, and Technology and Medical Complexity, reflecting emerging areas of importance in clinical practice.

We are extremely grateful to the chapter authors who have shared their expertise and wisdom. We hope that the 12th edition of *The Hospital for Sick Children Handbook of Pediatrics* will prove itself a worthy guide and companion to your study or practice of the care of infants, children and adolescents.

Deborah Schonfeld
Shawna Silver
Catherine Diskin
Siobhán Neville

ACKNOWLEDGMENTS

So many people have helped make the 12th edition of *The Hospital for Sick Children Handbook of Pediatrics* a reality. In particular, we would like to acknowledge Dr. Adelle Atkinson, the Director of Postgraduate Medical Education at The Hospital for Sick Children and Dr. Jeremy Friedman and Dr. Anne Dipchand, editors of the 11th edition of *The Hospital for Sick Children Handbook of Pediatrics* for their guidance, wise insight, and support. We are grateful to all of the authors and editors of the previous editions of *The Hospital for Sick Children Handbook of Pediatrics* for the opportunity to build on all of their outstanding work. Thank you to Erika Schippel, The Hospital for Sick Children Publishing Coordinator, for her ongoing help with the contracts and ensuring smooth communication with the publishers. Thank you to Dr. Brie Yama for her help in the early stages of content organization and development. Many thanks go to MaryBeth Thiel, Elsevier, for facilitating the process of a new edition. Special thanks go to our content development specialists and project managers at different stages, Meredith Madeira and Radjan Selvanadin, for being a tremendous source of advice and support throughout the production process. Finally, we would like to thank all of the chapter authors—both learners and staff—for their dedication and perseverance culminating in the 12th edition of *The Hospital for Sick Children Handbook of Pediatrics*.

Deborah Schonfeld
Shawna Silver
Catherine Diskin
Siobhán Neville

CHAPTER AUTHORS

Section I:
ACUTE CARE PEDIATRICS

1: Resuscitation
Melanie Bechard, BSc, MD
Fellow, Emergency Medicine (CHEO)
Andrew Helmers, MDCM, MHSc(c), MSc, FRCPC
Fellow, Critical Care Medicine
Lianne J. McLean, MB, BCh, BAO, MHI, FRCPC
Staff Physician, Emergency Medicine

2: Emergency Medicine
Marie-Pier Lirette, MBChB
Resident, Pediatrics
Maya Harel-Sterling, MD
Fellow, Emergency Medicine
Iwona Baran, MD, FRCPC
Staff Physician, Emergency Medicine
Suzanne Beno, MD, FRCPC, D(ABP)
Staff Physician, Emergency Medicine

3: Poisonings and Toxicology
Zamin Ladha, MD, MSc
Resident, Pediatrics
Elana Thau, MD
Fellow, Emergency Medicine
Savithiri Ratnapalan, MBBS, PhD, FRCP(UK), FRCP(C), FAAP
Staff Physician, Emergency Medicine and Clinical Pharmacology & Toxicology

4: Pain and Sedation
Tahira Daya, MD
Fellow, Emergency Medicine (University of Alberta)
Lisa Isaac, MD, FRCPC
Staff Anesthesiologist, Anesthesia and Pain Medicine

5: Procedures
Zachary Pancer, BPHE, MBBS
Fellow, Emergency Medicine
Meghan Gilley, MD, FRCPC
Fellow, Emergency Medicine
Jonathan Pirie, MD, MEd, FRCPC
Staff Physician, Emergency Medicine

Section II:
SUBSPECIALTY PEDIATRICS

6: Adolescent Medicine
Valene Singh, MD
Resident, Pediatrics
Samantha Martin, MD, FRCPC
Fellow, Adolescent Medicine
Alene Toulany, MD, MSc, FRCPC
Staff Physician, Adolescent Medicine

7: Allergy
Stephanie Erdle, MD
Fellow, Immunology and Allergy (BC Children's Hospital)
Melanie Conway, MD, FRCPC
Fellow, Immunology and Allergy
Adelle R. Atkinson, MD, FRCPC
Staff Physician, Immunology and Allergy

8: Cardiology
Michael D. Fridman, MD, FRCPC
Fellow, Cardiology
Jonathan Wong, BMBS, FRCPC, FAAP
Fellow, Cardiology
Koyelle Papneja, MD, FRCPC, FAAP
Fellow, Cardiology
Jennifer L. Russell, MD, FRCPC
Staff Physician, Cardiology

9: Child Maltreatment

Tanvi Agarwal, MD
Resident, Pediatrics
Rebecca Wang, MD
Resident, Pediatrics
Elodie April, MD
Fellow, Pediatric Medicine
Romy Cho, MD, FRCPC
Staff Physician, Pediatric Medicine
Jennifer Smith, BMBS, MSc, FRCPC
Staff Physician, Pediatric Medicine

10: Dentistry

Rodd Morgan, BDSc, DCD, FRACDS
Fellow, Dentistry
Jane Ho, DCD
Fellow, Dentistry
Shonna Masse, HBSc, DDS, FRCDC
Staff Dentist, Dentistry

11: Dermatology

Laura Morrissey, MD
Resident, Pediatrics
Kimberly Tantuco, MD
Fellow, Dermatology
Rebecca Levy, MD, FRCPC
Staff Physician, Dermatology

12: Development

Audrey Tilly-Gratton, MD
Resident, Pediatrics
Claire K. Nguyen, BNSc, MSc, LLB, MPH, MD
Fellow, Developmental Pediatrics
Jenna Doig, MD, FRCPC
Staff Physician, Developmental Pediatrics
Amber Makino, MD, BHSc, FRCPC
Staff Physician, Developmental Pediatrics

13: Diagnostic Imaging

Alisha Jamal, MD, MSc, FRCPC
Fellow, Emergency Medicine
Jeffrey Traubici, MD
Staff Radiologist, Diagnostic Imaging

14: Endocrinology

Joju Sowemimo, BSc, MD
Resident, Pediatrics
Julia Sorbara, MD, FRCPC
Fellow, Endocrinology
Jonathan D. Wasserman, MD, PhD
Staff Physician, Endocrinology

15: Fluids, Electrolytes, and Acid–Base

Laura Betcherman, MD
Resident, Pediatrics
Emma Ulrich, MD
Fellow, Nephrology
Katie Sullivan, MBChB
Fellow, Nephrology
Damien Noone, MB BCh BAO, MSc
Staff Physician, Nephrology

16: Gastroenterology and Hepatology

Ameilia Kellar, MD, MSc
Resident, Pediatrics
Eileen Crowley, MB BCh BAO, MRCPI, MSc
Fellow, Gastroenterology, Hepatology and Nutrition
Thomas Walters, MBBS, MSc, FRACP
Staff Physician, Gastroenterology, Hepatology and Nutrition

17: General Surgery

Jonathon Hagel, MD
Resident, Pediatrics
Justyna M. Wolinska, MD, FRCSC, MPH(c)
Staff Surgeon, General and Thoracic Surgery
Georges Azzie, MD, FRCSC
Staff Surgeon, General and Thoracic Surgery

18: Genetics and Teratology

Areej Mahjoub, MD
Resident, Neurology
Gregory Costain, MD, PhD
Resident, Medical Genetics and Genomics
Roberto Mendoza-Londono, MD, MS, FRCPC, FCCMG
Division Head, Clinical and Metabolic Genetics

19: Growth and Nutrition

Justin Lam, MD
Resident, Pediatrics

Laura Kinlin, MD, MPH, FRCPC
Fellow, Pediatric Medicine

Meta van den Heuvel, MD, PhD
Staff Physician, Pediatric Medicine

Mara Alexanian-Farr, MSc, RD
*Clinical Dietician, Infant and Toddler Growth
and Feeding*

Alisa Bar-Dayan, RD
Clinical Dietitian, Endocrinology

Jordan Beaulieu, RD
*Clinical Dietitian, Pediatric Medicine and
Complex Care*

Kelsey Gallagher, RD
*Clinical Dietitian, Endocrinology and
Rheumatology*

Daina Kalnins, MSc, RD
Director, Clinical Dietetics

Alissa Steinberg, RD
Clinical Dietitian, Endocrinology

Lori Tuira, RD
Clinical Dietician, Critical Care

Laura Vresk, MSc, RD
*Clinical Dietitian, Pediatric Medicine and
Complex Care*

Kellie Welch, BASc, RD
*Clinical Dietitian, Pediatric Medicine and
Respiratory Medicine*

Caroline Currie, RN, IBCLC
Lactation Specialist, Breastfeeding Program

Laura Mclean, BScN, IBCLC
Registered Nurse and Lactation Consultant

Samantha Sullivan, RN, IBCLC
Registered Nurse and Lactation Consultant

Ashley Graham, MScOT, MHM
*Occupational Therapist, Rehabilitation
Services*

20: Gynecology

Lauren Friedman, BHSc, MD
Resident, Pediatrics

Heather Millar, MIPH, MD, FRCSC
Staff Physician, Gynecology

Anjali Aggarwal, MD, MHSc, FRCSC
Staff Physician, Gynecology

21: Hematology

Adam Yan, MD
Resident, Pediatrics

Vanja Cabric, MD
Resident, Pediatrics

Soumitra Tole, MD, MSc, FRCPC
Fellow, Hematology/Oncology

Michaela Cada, MD, FRCPC, FAAP, MPH
Staff Physician, Hematology/Oncology

22: Immunology

Ori Scott, MD, FRCPC
Fellow, Immunology and Allergy

Amiirah Aujnarain, MSc, MD, FRCPC
Fellow, Immunology and Allergy

Vy Kim, MD, MScCH, FRCPC
Staff Physician, Immunology and Allergy

23: Immunoprophylaxis

Ana C. Blanchard, MDCM, MSc, FRCPC
Fellow, Infectious Diseases

Shama Sud, MD
Fellow, Immunology and Allergy

Shaun K. Morris, MD, MPH, FRCPC,
FAAP, DTM&H
Staff Physician, Infectious Diseases

24: Infectious Diseases

Ryan Giroux, MD
Resident, Pediatrics

Jennifer Tam, MD, MHPE, FRCPC
Fellow, Infectious Diseases

Ari Bitnun, MD, MSc, FRCPC
Staff Physician, Infectious Diseases

25: Mental Health

Gabrielle Salmers, MBBS
Fellow, Community Pediatrics

Daphne J. Korczak, MD, MSc, FRCPC
(peds), FRCPC (psych)
Staff Physician, Child and Adolescent Psychiatry

26: Metabolic Disease
Carsten Krueger, MD
Resident, Pediatrics
Resham Ejaz, MD
Resident, Clinical and Metabolic Genetics
Neal Sondheimer, MD, PhD
Staff Physician, Clinical and Metabolic Genetics

27: Neonatology
Amy Zipursky, MD
Resident, Pediatrics
Julia DiLabio, MD, MSc
Fellow, Neonatal-Perinatal Medicine
Tapas Kulkarni
MB BCh BAO, FRCPC
Fellow, Neonatal-Perinatal Medicine
Aideen Moore, MD, MHSc, FRCPC
Staff Physician, Neonatology

28: Nephrology and Urology
Magdalena Riedl, MD, PhD
Resident, Pediatrics
Mallory L. Downie, MD, FRCPC
Fellow, Nephrology
Anne Sophie Blais, MD, FRCSC
Fellow, Urology
Joana Dos Santos, MD, MHSc, FRCPC
Staff Medical Urologist, Urology
Seetha Radhakrishnan, MDCM, FRCPC,
MScCH
Staff Physician, Nephrology

29: Neurology and Neurosurgery
Djurdja Djordjevic, MD
Resident, Neurology
Nurin Chatur, MD
Resident, Neurology
Cristina Y. Go, MD
Staff Physician, Neurology

Abhaya Kulkarni, MD, PhD, FRCSC
Staff Surgeon, Neurosurgery
Liza Pulcine, MD, MSc, FRCPC
Staff Physician, Neurology

30: Oncology
Amy Lu, BHSc, MD
Resident, Pediatrics
Mohammed Al Nuaimi, BSc, MD,
FRCPC
Fellow, Hematology/Oncology
Reena Pabari, MSc, MD, FRCPC
Fellow, Hematology/Oncology
Sumit Gupta, MD, PhD, FRCPC
Staff Physician, Hematology/Oncology

31: Ophthalmology
Shelby Thompson, BSc, MD
Resident, Pediatrics
Asim Ali, MD, FRCSC
*Ophthalmologist-in-Chief, Ophthalmology and
Vision Sciences*

32: Orthopedics
Allyson Shorkey, MD
Resident, Pediatrics
Unni Narayanan, MBBS, MSc,
FRCSC
Staff Surgeon, Orthopedic Surgery

33: Otolaryngology
Talia Greenspoon, MD, HBA
Resident, Pediatrics
Sharon L. Cushing, MD, MSc, FRCSC
Staff Surgeon, Otolaryngology

34: Plastic Surgery
Laura Kaufman, MD
Resident, Pediatrics
Kristen M. Davidge, MD, MSc,
FRCSC
Staff Surgeon, Plastic Surgery

Note: All chapters were written by residents, fellows and staff of The Hospital for Sick Children. Chapter authors are affiliated with The Hospital for Sick Children unless otherwise noted.

Chapter Authors

COMMON ABBREVIATIONS

↑	increased
↓	decreased
>	greater than
≥	greater than or equal to
<	less than
≤	less than or equal to
AAP	American Academy of Pediatrics
ABC	airway, breathing, circulation
ABG	arterial blood gas
AD	autosomal dominant
ALP	alkaline phosphatase
ALT	alanine aminotransferase
ANA	antinuclear antibody
AP	anteroposterior
AR	autosomal recessive
AST	aspartate aminotransferase
AXR	abdominal x-ray
βHCG	beta human chorionic gonadotropin
BID	twice daily
BMI	body mass index
BP	blood pressure
BSA	body surface area
BUN	blood urea nitrogen
C&S	culture and sensitivity
Ca	calcium
CBC	complete blood count
CK	creatine kinase
Cl	chloride
cm	centimeter
CNS	central nervous system
CPS	Canadian Paediatric Society
Cr	creatinine
CRP	C-reactive protein
CSF	cerebrospinal fluid
CT	computed tomography
CVL	central venous line
CVS	cardiovascular system
CXR	chest x-ray
DBP	diastolic blood pressure
DDx	differential diagnosis
EBV	Epstein-Barr virus
ECG	electrocardiogram
EMLA	eutectic mixture of local anesthetic
ESR	erythrocyte sedimentation rate
ETT	endotracheal tube
f/u	follow-up

GAS	group A *Streptococcus*
GGT	gamma-glutamyltransferase
GI	gastrointestinal
GU	genitourinary
Hb	hemoglobin
HCO$_3$	bicarbonate
HIV	human immunodeficiency virus
HR	heart rate
Hx	history
I&D	incision and drainage
IBD	inflammatory bowel disease
ICP	intracranial pressure
ICU	intensive care unit
IM	intramuscular
INR	international normalized ratio
IQ	intelligence quotient
IV	intravenous
kg	kilogram
K	potassium
LDH	lactate dehydrogenase
LFTs	liver function tests
LP	lumbar puncture
m	meter
μ	micro-
M:F	male to female ratio
max	maximum
mcg	microgram
mg	milligram
Mg	magnesium
min.	minimum
mL	millilitre
mos	months
MRI	magnetic resonance imaging
MSK	musculoskeletal
Na	sodium
NaCl	sodium chloride
NAI	nonaccidental injury
NICU	neonatal intensive care unit
NPO	nil per os
NS	normal saline
NSAID	nonsteroidal antiinflammatory drug
O$_2$	oxygen
OR	operating room
PALS	Pediatric Advanced Life Support
PA	posteroanterior
PICC	peripherally inserted central catheter
PICU	pediatric intensive care unit
PIV	peripheral intravenous catheter
PO	per os (by mouth)
PO$_4$	phosphate
pRBCs	packed red blood cells
PRN (prn)	pro re nata (as needed)

PTH	parathyroid hormone
PTT	partial thromboplastin time
q	every (e.g., q4h—every 4 hours)
QHS	every night
QTc	corrected QT interval
RBC	red blood cell
RR	respiratory rate
SBP	systolic blood pressure
SC	subcutaneous
SL	sublingual
STI	sexually transmitted infection
tCO2	total carbon dioxide
TFI	total fluid intake
TID	three times daily
TORCH	congenital infections including toxoplasmosis, other agents, rubella, cytomegalovirus, herpes
TPN	total parenteral nutrition
TSH	thyroid stimulating hormone
URTI	upper respiratory tract infection
US	ultrasound
UTI	urinary tract infection
VBG	venous blood gas
WBC	white blood cell
XR	x-ray
yrs	years

Section I

Acute Care Pediatrics

Resuscitation

Melanie Bechard • Andrew Helmers • Lianne Mclean

COMMON ABBREVIATIONS

Also see page xviii for a list of other abbreviations used throughout this book

ABC	airway, breathing, circulation
ABG	arterial blood gas
APLS	advanced pediatric life support
BVM	bag-valve mask
CPAP	continuous positive airway pressure
CPR	cardiopulmonary resuscitation
ETT	endotracheal tube
FiO_2	fraction of inspired oxygen
FRC	functional residual capacity
LMA	laryngeal mask airway
PALS	Pediatric Advanced Life Support
PEA	pulseless electrical activity
PICU	pediatric intensive care unit
ROSC	return of spontaneous circulation
RSI	rapid sequence intubation
SVR	systemic vascular resistance

USEFUL CALCULATIONS

1. **Hypotension (systolic blood pressure)**
   a. <1 month: <60 mmHg
   b. 1–12 months (mos): <70 mmHg
   c. 1–10 years (yrs): <70 + [2×age] mmHg
   d. >10 yrs: <90 mmHg
2. **Estimated weight in kg** (APLS 5th ed)
   a. 1–12 mos: [0.5×(age in mos)] + 4
   b. 1–5 yrs: [2×(age in yrs)] + 8
   c. 6–12 yrs: [3×(age in yrs)] + 7
3. **Endotracheal tube (ETT) size**
   a. Uncuffed ETT: [age in yrs/4] + 4
   b. Cuffed ETT: [age in yrs/4] + 3.5
4. **ETT depth**
   a. <1 yr
      i. Oropharyngeal intubation (cm at lip): [(age in yrs)/2] + 8
      ii. Nasopharyngeal intubation (cm at nare): [(age in yrs)/2] + 9
   b. >1 yr
      i. Oropharyngeal intubation (cm at lip): [(age in yrs)/2] + 12 OR [3×ETT diameter]
      ii. Nasopharyngeal intubation (cm at lip): [(age in yrs)/2] + 15

Resuscitation

1

TEAM DYNAMICS

Resuscitation **teamwork**, **communication**, and **leadership** all have a significant impact on patient outcomes.

A. Before a resuscitation
1. **Anticipate needs**
   a. Contact necessary personnel (e.g., respiratory therapy if available, consider anesthesiology) and consider available equipment
   b. Seek help when needed (e.g., contact anesthesiology or otolaryngology if a difficult airway is anticipated)
2. **Assign roles**: clearly define roles and responsibilities of each team member
3. **Know your resources**
   a. Familiarize yourself with the resuscitation equipment of your hospital ward and emergency department
   b. Know your provincial or state resources for coordinating transfer to tertiary care centers, if applicable

B. During a resuscitation
1. A leader should:
   a. Offer **constructive feedback**: "Please perform compressions faster—we're aiming for 100 to 120 per minute."
   b. **Think out loud**: share thoughts and suggestions to create a shared mental model. "I suspect this child has septic shock." Avoid premature fixation on a diagnosis and be ready to shift perspective.
   c. Perform **periodic reviews**: summarize and reevaluate the case. This helps to ensure adherence to algorithms and offers opportunities for new ideas to reduce bias.
   d. **Encourage information sharing** and bidirectional transmission of ideas: "Are there other thoughts about which medications should be used before intubation?"
   e. Remain **"hands off"** (if possible) leaders who focus on coordinating the team rather than participating in the resuscitative efforts perform better. Often this necessitates delegating jobs that can detract from focused leadership (i.e., assigning a specific person to calculate resuscitation medication doses).

✦ PEARL

Closed-loop communication is important in a resuscitation; e.g., when ordering epinephrine during a cardiac arrest:

Provider 1: "The patient's weight is 20 kg; please give 0.2 mg of 1:10,000 epinephrine intravenously, which is 2 mL"
Provider 2: "0.2 mg of 1:10,000 epinephrine, which is 2 mL, now ready to give IV"
Provider 1: "Thank you, please administer that dose"
Provider 2: "Dose administered"

2. All team members should:
   a. Use **closed-loop communication:** improves the safety and efficiency of care provided by removing ambiguity from instructions and allowing for corrections/clarifying questions if needed
   b. Be **respectful!** Evidence suggests rudeness negatively impacts resuscitation teams' performance
   c. **Support family presence** during resuscitation; there is a strong parental preference to be present

C. After a resuscitation
1. Every effort should be made to **conduct a debrief**. Debriefing involves guided reflection of medical issues, emotional impact on care providers, and provides performance feedback to the team.
2. There are many debriefing formats (e.g., standardized forms, "hot" debrief within minutes to hours of the resuscitation, "cold" debrief days to weeks after resuscitation)
3. Ensure your hospital has a culture of safe and nonjudgmental debriefs, which follow a consistent structure to ensure that provider distress is addressed and that constructive feedback is incorporated into future events. If it is clear that team members have experienced distress (e.g., a resuscitation that ends with patient demise), it is important to identify this in the debrief and ensure channels exist to explore and support this further.

CLINICAL ASSESSMENT OF THE ILL CHILD
A. Evaluation of ABCDEs
See Table 1.1

Table 1.1	Assessment of ABCDEs		
	Appearance	**Examination**	**Monitor**
Airway	- Patient position - Respiratory effort - Accessory muscle use - Chest expansion - Drooling - Color	- Stridor - Voice quality - Cough quality - Retractions - Tracheal position	- Respiratory rate - Oxygen saturation (SaO_2)
Breathing	- Respiratory rate, pattern, and effort - Accessory muscle use - Chest expansion - Color	- Breath sounds - Grunting, nasal flaring - Retractions - Crepitus - Tracheal position	- Respiratory rate - Oxygen saturation (SaO_2)
Circulation	- Level of consciousness - Color (pallor, cyanosis) - Mottling	- Pulses (central, peripheral) - Skin temperature - Capillary refill time (perfusion) - Heart sounds	- Heart rate - Blood pressure - Rhythm (ECG monitor)
Disability	Level of consciousness	- Glasgow Coma Score (Table 1.2) - AVPU (Alert, Verbal, Painful stimuli, Unresponsive) - Pupil symmetry/responsiveness - Blood glucose check	Level of consciousness
Exposure	Signs of injury or bleeding	Temperature	

ECG, Electrocardiogram.

© The Hospital for Sick Children, 2019. Adapted from The Hospital for Sick Children Guide to Paediatric Medical Emergencies.

Table 1.2 Pediatric Glasgow Coma Scale

	Child/Adolescent/Adult	Age <2 yrs	Score
Eye opening	Spontaneous	Spontaneous	4
	To voice	To voice	3
	To pain	To pain	2
	None	None	1
Verbal response	Oriented	Appropriate words, smiles, interacts	5
	Confused	Cries, irritable	4
	Inappropriate	Cries to pain	3
	Incomprehensible	Moans to pain	2
	None	None	1
Motor response	Obeys	Spontaneous/obeys	6
	Localizes to pain	Localizes to pain	5
	Withdraws to pain	Withdraws to pain	4
	Abnormal flexion (decorticate)	Abnormal flexion	3
	Abnormal extension (decerebrate)	Abnormal extension	2
	None	None	1

Modified from Teasdale G, Jennett B. Assessment of coma and impaired consciousness. A practical scale. *Lancet.* 1974;2:81; and Holmes JF, Palchak MJ, MacFarlane T, Kuppermann N. Performance of the pediatric Glasgow coma scale in children with blunt head trauma. *Acad Emerg Med.* 2005;12:814.

Resuscitation

B. Pediatric Advanced Life Support (PALS) systematic approach algorithm
Figure 1.1 outlines the approach to caring for a critically ill or injured child. **Note that in the event of an arrest**, the basic approach now recommended by the American Heart Association is **Circulation–Airway–Breathing (C-A-B).**

Figure 1.1 Pediatric Advanced Life Support Systematic Approach Algorithm

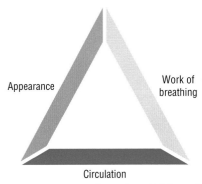

Appearance

Work of breathing

Circulation

(Modified from American Heart Association. *Pediatric Advanced Life Support Provider Manual.* Dallas, TX: American Heart Association; copyright 2016:30.)

RESPIRATORY SUPPORT DURING RESUSCITATION

Most cardiopulmonary arrests in children are caused by respiratory causes. This section covers a number of considerations in providing respiratory support to the acutely ill child.

A. Goals of respiratory support
1. Ventilation: removal of CO_2
2. Oxygenation: adequate oxygenation of the blood

B. Bag-valve-mask (BVM) ventilation
BVM ventilation is an important skill to master because it provides oxygen and also ventilation support to a patient who is making inadequate respiratory efforts
1. **Equipment:** flow-inflating bag (or self-inflating bag with oxygen reservoir) connected to an oxygen source, and appropriately sized mask
2. **Position**
   a. "Sniffing position" (Figure 1.2): slight neck flexion and occipital extension, i.e, lower cervical vertebral flexion and atlantooccipital extension
   b. Consider a shoulder roll in infants or a roll under the occiput in older children (see Figure 1.2)
   c. Additional repositioning techniques: "head tilt-chin lift," "jaw thrust" (Figure 1.3)
3. **Seal**: use E-C placement of hands to create seal, with the E position on the mandible not the neck soft tissues (Figure 1.4)

Figure 1.2 Airway Positioning

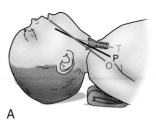 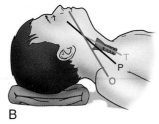

A   B

Preferred airway positioning for (A) infants using shoulder rolls, and (B) children using occipital rolls. (From Urden LD, Stacy KM, Lough ME. *Critical Care Nursing: Diagnosis and Management*. 8th ed. Elsevier; 2018.)

Figure 1.3 Airway Repositioning

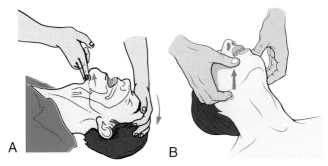

(A) Head tilt chin lift maneuver. (B) Jaw thrust maneuver (A, From Lewis SM, Heitkemper MM, Dirksen SR. *Medical-Surgical Nursing: Assessment and Management of Clinical Problems.* 7th ed. St. Louis: Mosby; 2007. B, From Shimabukuro D, Liu L. Cardiopulmonary resuscitation. In: Stoelting RK, Miller RD, eds. *Basics of Anesthesia.* 5th ed. Elsevier; 2007.)

Figure 1.4 E-C Clamp Technique

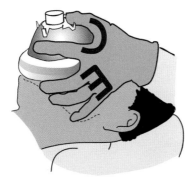

(From Ducanto J, Matioc A. Noninvasive management of the airway. In: Hagberg CA, Artime CA, Aziz MF, eds. *Hagberg and Benumof's Airway Management.* 4th ed. Elsevier; 2018.)

4. **Techniques for improving BVM ventilation:** MRSOPA (Table 1.3)

	Table 1.3	Technique for Improving Positive-Pressure Ventilation by Mask	
	Corrective Steps	**Actions**	
M	Mask readjustment	Be sure there is a good seal of the mask on the face; consider two-hand technique	
R	Reposition airway	Ensure the head is in "sniffing" position	
S	Suction mouth and nose	Suction secretions if present	
O	Open mouth	Ventilate with the patient's mouth slightly open and lift the jaw forward ("jaw thrust")	
P	Pressure increase	Gradually increase the pressure every few breaths until there are bilateral breath sounds and visible chest movement with each breath	
A	Airway alternative	Consider endotracheal intubation or laryngeal mask airway	

Adapted from American Academy of Pediatrics. *Textbook of Neonatal Resuscitation.* 7th ed. 2016.

C. Airway adjuncts

Adjuncts are useful for maintaining a patent airway in cases of obstruction (Figure 1.5)

1. **Oropharyngeal airway**
   a. Sits from mouth to above the vallecula to prevent tongue from touching posterior pharynx
   b. Caution: risk of soft palate injury on insertion, gag reflex limits tolerance in awake patients
2. **Nasopharyngeal airway**
   a. Sits from nare to hypopharynx
   b. Caution: patients with bleeding tendencies, basilar skull fracture, craniofacial trauma/anomalies

Figure 1.5 Oropharyngeal (A) and Nasopharyngeal (B) Airways

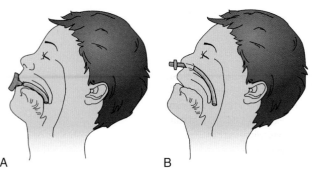

A   B

(From Thompson AE, Salonia R. Airway management. In: Fuhrman BP, Zimmerman JJ, eds. *Pediatric Critical Care.* 5th ed. Elsevier; 2017.)

D. Oxygen delivery systems: see Table 1.4

Table 1.4	Oxygen Delivery Systems		
Mode of O₂ Delivery	Flow Rate (L/min)	FiO₂ Delivered	Comments
Blow-by oxygen	Variable	Variable	Used for well patients that require small amounts of supplemental oxygen
Nasal cannula	<5	~23%–40% [21% + (flow in L/min)×3]	FiO₂ depends on size of child, respiratory rate, tidal volume. With small children, flow is a greater portion of tidal volume, so more FiO₂ is received.
Simple mask	5–10	30%–65%	Open holes allow variable amounts of room air
Venturi mask	5–10	30%–50%	Controls FiO₂ by allowing precise amounts of oxygen and room air
Partial rebreather mask	10–15	Up to 65%	Two open exhalation ports and valveless oxygen reservoir bag. Attached reservoir bag provides higher FiO₂. Needs 10–15 L/min to prevent bag collapse.
Nonrebreather mask	10–15	Up to 95%	Two one-way valve ports: 1 between oxygen reservoir bag and mask, then 1 between mask and exhalation port. May use with oxygen blender to adjust FiO₂ between 50% and 95%.

FiO₂, Fraction of inspired oxygen.

E. Heated humidity high flow therapy
Heated humidity high flow therapy can be delivered through face mask or nasal cannula. Gas is heated and humidified to optimize secretion clearance and tolerance.
1. **Heated high flow face mask** provides oxygenation without the addition of positive pressure ventilation. Adjust FiO_2 as needed.
2. **Heated high flow nasal cannula**
   a. Flow 4 to 60 L/min (maximum depends on machine and mode); typically started at 1 L/kg/min, increase to effect as per manufacturer guidelines

b. Provides potential, variable amounts of positive end-expiratory pressure (higher PEEP achieved with smaller children), reduces breathing effort (assists peak inspiratory flow) and optimizes intended oxygen delivery (limits entrainment of room air)

> **! PITFALL**
>
> A self-inflating bag without a positive-pressure respiratory support valve only delivers oxygen when the bag is squeezed to provide a breath; i.e., it cannot be used to provide continuous positive airway pressure and may not deliver oxygen when the bag is not being depressed.

F. Positive-pressure respiratory support

Positive pressure helps with both ventilation and oxygenation (aerates alveoli, prevents alveolar collapse, increases functional residual capacity). BVM with a flow-inflating bag is an important way to achieve this in emergency situations. Consider insertion of a nasogastric/orogastric tube to minimize gastric distension (which can provoke emesis or reduce FRC caused by intraabdominal pressure).

1. **Continuous Positive Airway Pressure (CPAP)**
   a. Delivered via snug nasal mask or face mask
   b. Useful for low FRC (e.g., atelectasis, pneumonia) and extrathoracic obstruction (e.g., obstructive sleep apnea, postextubation edema, laryngotracheitis)
2. **Bilevel Positive Airway Pressure (BiPAP)**
   a. Provides constant positive pressure during expiration and additional positive pressure support during inspiration
   b. May adjust inspiratory and expiratory pressures separately to change tidal volume
   c. Useful for neuromuscular weakness, spinal injury or ventilation failure

CIRCULATORY SUPPORT DURING RESUSCITATION

> **PEARL**
>
> **Cardiopulmonary Resuscitation Ratios (PALS 2020):**
> Single rescuer:
>   30 compressions: 2 breaths
> Multiple rescuers:
>   15 compressions: 2 breaths
> Advanced airway:
>   Continuous compressions: 1 breath every 2–3 seconds (20–30/min)

A. High-quality CPR
1. **Push hard** ($\geq$1/3 of anteroposterior diameter of chest) and **fast** (100–120/min)
2. Allow complete chest recoil. This is necessary for blood to fill the heart.
3. Minimize interruptions in compressions. Cardiac output increases progressively with consecutive compressions.
4. Avoid excessive ventilation
5. Rotate compressor every 2 minutes or sooner if fatigued
6. End-tidal CO_2 monitoring may be considered to evaluate the quality of chest compressions. PALS 2020 suggests targeting compressions to an $ETCO_2$ value of at least 10 mmHg, and ideally 20 mmHg or greater, may be useful as a marker of CPR quality

B. Vascular access
See Chapter 5 Procedures for all procedure-related details
1. **Peripheral intravenous access** (see Figure 5.1)
   a. General guide: 24 gauge for infants, 22 gauge for children, 20 gauge for adolescents and adults
   b. Trauma/unstable patients: insert the largest gauge possible
2. **Intraosseus access** (see Figure 5.2)
   a. Allows for rapid establishment of access if peripheral intravenous access unsuccessful
   b. Common sites: proximal tibia, distal femur, medial malleolus, proximal humerus, sternum (see Chapter 5 Procedures)
3. **Central venous access** (see Figures 5.3 and 5.4, Table 5.1)
4. **Umbilical catheters:** umbilical vein access usually viable for the first 7 days of life (see Figures 5.5–5.7 and newborn resuscitation in Chapter 27 Neonatology for further details)
5. **Arterial access** (see Figure 5.8)
   a. Provide continuous and accurate blood pressure monitoring
   b. Helpful if frequent arterial gas measurements are needed

C. Inotropic and vasopressor therapy
1. See Table 1.5
2. **Inotropes increase cardiac contractility**, whereas **vasopressors increase systemic vascular resistance** (SVR)

Table 1.5 Vasoactive Agents

Medication	Effects on Myocardium	Effects on Vasculature	Comments/Indications
Dopamine	β_1, β_2 agonist (alpha-adrenergic effects at higher doses)	↑ contractility ↑ HR	Intermediate dose (5–10 mcg/kg/min): β_1, β_2 agonist	↑ contractility, heart rate, cardiac output	Important for cardiogenic shock
		High dose (>10 mcg/kg/min): alpha-adrenergic effects predominate	↑ SVR	Important for distributive shock
Dobutamine	β_1 agonist	↑ contractility ↑ HR	β_1 agonist	Limited effect	Important in heart failure and cardiogenic shock
Epinephrine	β_1, β_2 agonist	↑ contractility ↑ HR	α_1, α_2 agonist At higher doses the alpha-adrenergic receptor effect predominates	↑ SVR (higher dose)	Important in anaphylaxis and cold shock (starting dose typically 0.05 mcg/kg/min)
Norepinephrine	β_1 agonist	Limited effect	α_1, α_2 agonist	↑ SVR	Important in warm septic shock with vasodilation (starting dose typically 0.05 mcg/kg/min)
Vasopressin			Vasopressin receptor 1A (V1AR)	↑ SVR	May be added to norepinephrine to raise mean arterial pressure or decrease norepinephrine dose
Milrinone	PDE III inhibitor	↑ contractility	PDE III Inhibitor	↓ SVR	Potential role in some congenital heart diseases or other conditions in which cardiac afterload should be reduced; use guided by consultation with critical care expertise

HR, Heart rate; *PDE*, phosphodiesterase; *SVR*, systemic vascular resistance.

ADVANCED AIRWAY MANAGEMENT

A. Pediatric airway anatomy and respiratory physiology
1. **Anatomic features of the pediatric airway**: see Box 1.1

> ### Box 1.1 Anatomic Features of the Pediatric Airway
>
> **Anatomic Feature**
> - Occipital prominence (neck flexed in supine position)
> - Narrow nasal passages
> - Large tongue
> - Large tonsils and adenoids
> - Epiglottis large and flaccid with less tensile hyoepiglottic ligament
> - Narrow cricoid
> - Glottis high and superior
> - Short trachea

2. **Pediatric respiratory physiology**
   a. Minute oxygen consumption is higher in children compared with adults (7 mL/kg/min vs. 3 mL/kg/min)
   b. Children have limited ability to adjust tidal volume; alveolar ventilation is primarily controlled by respiratory rate
   c. Children desaturate quickly if apneic because of their higher oxygen consumption and the strong effect of respiratory rate on alveolar ventilation

B. Laryngeal mask airway (LMA)
1. A supraglottic airway device which is not a secure airway (i.e., potential for aspiration of gastric contents) but can be life saving when mask ventilation or intubation is difficult

---

 PEARL

Cuffed ETT Sizing (for 1–10 yrs)
[Age in years/4] + 3.5
(PALS 2020 guidelines now recommend cuffed ETTs for all patients requiring intubation)

ETT Depth (>1 yr):
Length (cm) at lip = [Age/2] +12 OR 3 × diameter of ETT
Length (cm) at nose = [Age/2] +15

C. Endotracheal intubation
1. **Indications**
   a. Inadequate oxygenation or ventilation (despite optimizing noninvasive support)
   b. Inability to maintain and/or protect the airway (e.g., pooling secretions, central nervous system depression with loss of airway reflexes)

c. Potential for loss of airway (e.g., epiglottitis/bacterial tracheitis, severe anaphylaxis, severe burns)

d. Unstable patient requiring transport/prolonged diagnostic studies

> ### ⚡ PEARL
>
> **Intubation Equipment Checklist: SOAP ME**
> **S**uction
> **O**xygen
> **A**irway Equipment: oral/nasal airways, bag-valve-mask, endotracheal tubes, stylets, laryngoscope handles and blades, tape, laryngeal mask airway, video laryngoscope, etc.
> **P**harmacology (Table 1.6)
> **M**onitoring **E**quipment: Electrocardiogram monitor, pulse oximeter, blood pressure (BP) monitor, CO_2 detector/end-tidal CO_2

Table 1.6	Intubation Equipment Sizing by Age and Weight				
Age	Avg Wt (kg)	ETT[a] (mm)	Blade	LMA	Suction (F)
Birth	3.5	2.5–3.5	0 straight	1–1.5	6–8
6 mo	7.5	3.5	1 straight	1.5–2	8
1 yr	10	4.0	1 straight	1.5–2	8
2 yr	12	4.5	2 straight	2	8–10
3 yr	14	4.5–5	2 straight or curved	2	10
4 yr	16	5.0	2 straight or curved	2	10
6 yr	20	5.5	2 straight or curved	2–2.5	10
8 yr	24	5.5 C	2 or 3 curved	2.5	10
9–12 yr	27–40	6.0–6.5 C	3 curved	3–4	10–12

[a]Subtract 0.5 for cuffed ETT size. PALS 2020 guidelines now recommend cuffed ETTs for all patients requiring intubation.

C, Cuffed endotracheal tube; *ETT,* endotracheal tube; *LMA,* laryngeal mask airway; *mo,* month; *yr,* year.

D. Rapid Sequence Intubation (RSI)

RSI refers to a sequential process to facilitate safe emergency tracheal intubation. The steps involved include: **preparation, preoxygenation, premedication (optional), sedation and paralysis, positioning, tube placement and confirmation, postintubation management**.

1. **Preparation**
   a. Focused history and physical to **look for high-risk conditions**
      i. Known difficult airway
      ii. Present/impending upper airway obstruction
      iii. Anatomical challenges (e.g., limited c-spine mobility, macroglossia, micrognathia). Also see Figure 1.6 for Mallampati classification.
      iv. Physiologic risk factors (e.g., hemodynamic instability, severe asthma)

b. **Contingency plan** for failed intubation (back-up approach and additional airway specialists)
c. **Equipment** check ("**SOAP ME**"). Also see Table 1.6 for intubation equipment sizing by age and weight.

Figure 1.6 Mallampati Classification

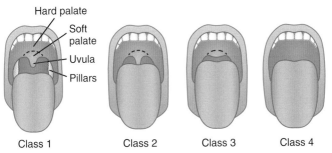

Hard palate
Soft palate
Uvula
Pillars

Class 1   Class 2   Class 3   Class 4

Classes 1 and 2 associated with relatively easy intubation, classes 3 and 4 associated with increased difficulty. (From Johnson BL. Conscious sedation. In: *The University of Cincinnati Residents. The Mont Reid Surgical Handbook: Mobile Medicine Series.* 7th ed. Elsevier; 2018.)

2. **Preoxygenation** (to maximize tolerable apnea time)
   a. Apply 100% O_2 as soon as decision to intubate is made
   b. Non-rebreather mask for spontaneously breathing patients. BVM ventilation for inadequately breathing patients
   c. Apneic oxygenation during intubation process (BVM should be avoided after induction)
3. **Premedication:** these medications are optional for selected patients and *not routinely given*
   a. **Atropine:** no longer routinely recommended for pretreatment before endotracheal intubation (PALS 2015) but may be useful in infants <1 yr of age (predilection for vagal-induced bradycardia) or other patients at risk of progressive unstable bradycardia
   b. Neuroprotective agents (**fentanyl** or **lidocaine**): May attenuate any additional increase in intracranial pressure (ICP) associated with laryngoscopy and intubation in high risk patients. Must be given ~3 minutes before intubation. Clear evidence for effectiveness lacking in children.

 PEARL

There are many strategies available for rapid sequence intubation (RSI) medications. The ideal sedatives and paralytics for RSI will differ depending a variety of clinical factors (hemodynamic instability, status asthmaticus, status epilepticus, increased intracranial pressure, etc.).

Resuscitation

1

4. **Sedation and paralysis** (see Table 1.7 for RSI medications)
   a. Sedation: important to ensure amnesia, analgesia (blunt sympathetic response to laryngoscopy) and to optimize intubating conditions
   b. Sedation should always precede paralysis
   c. Paralytic medications may not be needed if a patient is completely unresponsive

Table 1.7	Medications for Rapid Sequence Intubation	
Premedication		
Atropine	0.02 mg/kg/dose IV/IO (max 0.5 mg single dose, 1 mg cumulative dose)	Not given routinely; consider when there is higher risk for bradycardia
Lidocaine 2%	1–2 mg/kg/dose IV	Not given routinely; consider in cases of increased ICP (evidence inconsistent)
Sedatives		
Etomidate	0.3 mg/kg/dose IV over 30–60 s	Avoid in septic shock (adrenocortical suppression) Maintains hemodynamic stability Decreases ICP (appropriate for head trauma)
Fentanyl	2–5 mcg/kg/dose IV over 30–60 s	If patient is in shock should start at lower dose and titrate to effect
Ketamine	1–2 mg/kg/dose IV	Preferred agent in context of septic shock, and asthma. Appropriate choice for hypotensive patients
Midazolam	0.1–0.2 mg/kg/dose IV	Avoid use in patients with hemodynamic compromise (myocardial depressant) Appropriate choice for status epilepticus
Propofol	1–2 mg/kg/dose IV; dose depends on hemodynamic state of patient. Start low and titrate to effect	Can cause vasodilation/hypotension; avoid use in situations of hemodynamic compromise
Paralytics		
Rocuronium	1–1.2 mg/kg/dose IV for RSI	Fewer side effects than succinylcholine Hypertension or transient hypotension possible Provides longer paralysis
Succinylcholine	1–2 mg/kg/dose IV Give single dose and avoid repeated dosing	Short-acting Side effects: hyperkalemia, hypertension, hypotension, arrhythmia, increased intraocular pressure, increased intragastric pressure DO NOT USE with renal insufficiency, hyperkalemia, burns, crush injuries/polytrauma, extensive denervation of skeletal muscle or upper motor neuron injury, positive personal or family history of malignant hyperthermia CAUTION with unidentified, undiagnosed, or unexplained neurodevelopmental delay or muscular illness

ICP, Intracranial pressure; *IO*, intraosseous; *IV*, intravenous.

Adapted from The Hospital for Sick Children eFormulary, 2020.

5. **Positioning** for direct laryngoscopy
   a. Laryngoscope should be held in operators left hand and inserted into right side of patient's mouth, sweeping the tongue to the left
   b. The laryngoscope blade should be advanced into the vallecula (Macintosh blade, curved) before applying an upward/forward force along the long axis of the laryngoscope, at about 45 degrees, to lift the epiglottis and expose the glottic opening. In infants and younger children, a straight blade (Miller) is used; this is designed for positioning below the epiglottis, to directly lift that structure off the glottic opening (Figures 1.7 and 1.8).
   c. **External laryngeal manipulation** may improve the view in some patients: backward-upward-rightward pressure (BURP) is applied to the larynx by an assistant
   d. In young infants, gentle **cricoid pressure** ("Sellick maneuver") on the anterior neck may improve glottis view (PALS 2020 no longer recommends routine use of cricoid pressure during intubation)

✦ **PEARL**

To Increase Oxygenation
↑ Mean airway pressure (especially PEEP)
↑ FiO₂

To Increase Ventilation
↑ Respiratory rate (RR)
↑ Tidal volume

Figure 1.7 **Direct Laryngoscope Blades**

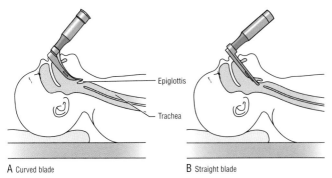

A Curved blade   **B** Straight blade

(A) Curved (Macintosh) blade in vallecula. (B) Straight (Miller) blade underneath epiglottis.
(From Schofield S, Smith H. Endotracheal intubation. In: Cameron P, Browne G, Mitra B, et al., eds. *Textbook of Paediatric Emergency Medicine*. 3rd ed. Elsevier; 2019.)

Figure 1.8 Cormack Lehane Grades

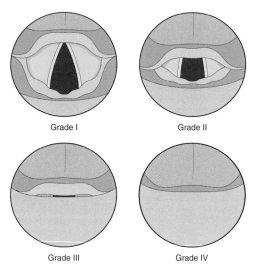

Grade I   Grade II

Grade III   Grade IV

Grade I: full view of glottis; grade II: partial view of glottis; grade III: only epiglottis seen; grade IV: neither glottis nor epiglottis seen. (From Miller RD, Pardo M. *Basics of Anesthesia.* 6th ed. Philadelphia, PA: Saunders; 2012.)

6. **Placement of tube and confirmation**
   a. Confirm tube placement (Box 1.2)
   b. Secure ETT at a corner of the mouth with strong adhesive tape

---

Box 1.2   Verification of Endotracheal Tube Placement[a]

- LOOK: Direct laryngoscopy (gold standard), condensation in ETT, equal chest movement bilaterally
- LISTEN: Bilateral breath sounds (consider right mainstem intubation if breath sounds heard only on right); listen over stomach for gastric insufflation if ETT is esophageal
- MONITOR: Pulse oximetry, end-tidal CO_2 monitoring (capnography or colorimetric CO_2 detectors)
- IMAGE: Chest XR, point-of-care ultrasound

[a]No single method is universally or completely reliable; verification of ETT placement requires a multiple method approach.

ETT, Endotracheal tube; *XR*, x-ray.

---

7. **Postintubation management**
   a. Ongoing sedation, analgesia and paralysis as required
   b. Positive pressure ventilation by hand until transferred to ventilator (seek guidance, as needed, to establish appropriate tidal volumes, pressure and rates on ventilator, Figure 1.9)
   c. For **sudden deterioration** of an intubated patient, address most common causes using the "DOPE" mnemonic

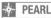
From Pediatric Advanced Life Support. 2010 American Heart Association Guidelines for Cardiopulmonary Resuscitation and Emergency Cardiovascular Care. *Circulation*. 2010;122:S876–S908.

Figure 1.9   General Ventilation Initiation Guidelines

Parameters	Guidelines	
Servo I/U Mode Selection	SIMV PC + PS	PIP is set, Vt is variable
		PIP 15–25 cmH₂O to achieve Vt 6–8 mL/kg
		Common mode for initial ventilation support
	SIMV PRVC + PS	Vt is set, PIP is variable. Vt 6–8 mL/kg
		Potential for barotrauma in patients with decreased lung compliance or significant airway resistance
		An ETT tube leak renders this mode difficult
	CPAP/PS	Patient triggers all breaths
		Continuous PEEP with PS set to obtain Vt 4–8 mL/kg
		Appropriate for spontaneously breathing patients; useful as a weaning mode
RR (set) *use EtCO2/ABG to optimize	• Newborn (term)	25–35
	• 1 mos–1 year	20–30
	• 1 year–6 year	15–25
	• >6 years	15–20
Inspiratory: Expiratory time (sec)	The inspiratory:expiratory (I:E) time ratio is typically 1:2 or 1:3. In obstructive cases such as asthma the expiratory time is set to be proportionally longer (e.g., 1:4, 1:5, 1:6). The absolute inspiratory time will thus depend on the respiratory rate appropriate for age and pathophysiology	
PEEP (cmH₂O)	No pulmonary disease	5	e.g., cardiac, seizures, head trauma
	Pulmonary disease	5–15	e.g., bronchiolitis, pneumonia, ARDS, drowning
	Abdominal distention	5–10	e.g., liver transplant, ascites, fluid overload
FiO₂	• Target SpO₂ range: Generally >92% for those with normal cardiac anatomy	
PS	• General good starting point is 10 cmH₂O (range: 6–20 cmH₂O)	

*This is a general reference only. Optimal settings will vary with patient condition, available equipment and institutional guidelines. *ABG*, Arterial blood gas; *CPAP*, continuous positive airway pressure; *PC*, pressure control; *PIP*, peak inspiratory pressure; *PRVC*, pressure regulated volume control; *PS*, pressure support; *SIMV*, synchronized intermittent mandatory ventilation; *Vt*, tidal volume. (© The Hospital for Sick Children. Adapted from The Hospital for Sick Children Reference for the Ventilation of the Pediatric Patient, 2019.)

Resuscitation

1

E. High-risk intubations
1. **Risk factors on history**
   a. Known history of difficult ventilation or intubation
   b. Present or impending upper airway obstruction (e.g., epiglottitis, airway burns, smoke inhalation, trauma, tumor, abscess, angioedema)

> **! PITFALL**
>
> High-risk intubations should ideally have an airway expert present. This includes specialties, such as otolaryngology, anesthesia, or another provider with airway experience.

2. **Anatomic risk factors**
   a. Atlantoaxial subluxation (e.g., Down syndrome)
   b. Macroglossia (e.g., Down syndrome, Beckwith-Wiedeman)
   c. Retrognathia or micrognathia (e.g., Pierre-Robin, Treacher Collins, and Goldenhar syndrome)
   d. Other abnormalities in craniofacial development (e.g., Apert, Crouzon, and Pfeiffer syndromes)
   e. Limited mouth opening, poor temporomandibular joint function (e.g., juvenile idiopathic arthritis)
   f. Limited cervical spine mobility (e.g., Klippel-Feil, mucopolysaccharidoses) or atlantoaxial instability (e.g., Down syndrome)
   g. Mallampati classification (see Figure 1.6)
      i. May be useful in children >9 yrs; not helpful in small children
      ii. Grades I and II may predict a relatively easy intubation; grades III and IV may predict a difficult intubation
3. **Situational risks**
   a. **Shock**: patients in shock are at high risk of further deterioration and cardiac arrest during intubation. Provision of positive pressure ventilation after intubation can also severely impair venous return and lead to circulatory collapse. Hemodynamic status should be optimized before and after intubation (fluids, vasoactive agents, as needed).
   b. **Asthma**: children with severe acute asthma often have increased intrathoracic pressure from alveolar obstruction and hyperinflation; mechanical ventilation of these patients is challenging and should be avoided unless absolutely necessary
   c. **Bleeding disorders**: children have large tonsils/adenoids that are susceptible to trauma and bleeding, especially with repeated intubation attempts. Children with bleeding disorders should have their coagulation profile optimized before procedures.
   d. **Diabetic ketoacidosis**: children with diabetic ketoacidosis use deep, fast breathing to decrease arterial carbon dioxide levels to compensate for their metabolic acidosis. Intubation is typically

avoided if possible in these patients as it removes the ability of the body to self-regulate its breathing in response to its serum pH. Mechanical ventilation settings must be adjusted accordingly.

e. **Mediastinal mass**: a mass may result in distal tracheal compression, leading to complete airway obstruction, and vascular collapse if thoracic tone is diminished by sedation or paralysis. Sedation and intubation should be avoided and only performed under controlled conditions in consultation with airway experts.

f. **Malignant hyperthermia**: potentially fatal autosomal dominant inherited disorder that leads to a hypermetabolic crisis in susceptible patients exposed to volatile anesthetic or succinylcholine

   i. Signs and symptoms: hypercarbia, tachycardia, tachypnea, muscle rigidity, hyperthermia

   ii. Laboratory findings: mixed respiratory and metabolic acidosis, hyperkalemia, raised creatine kinase, myoglobinuria, renal failure, disseminated intravascular coagulation

   iii. Treatment
  - Cease trigger drug
  - Administer 100% O_2
  - Dantrolene 2.5 mg/kg IV rapidly (further doses of 1 mg/kg IV may be given until clinical improvement, i.e, decreasing temperature, heart rate, muscle rigidity; up to a cumulative dose of 10 mg/kg—although more may be needed under advisement of experienced practitioner)
  - Active cooling: ice bags, cold water lavage, cold IV normal saline
  - Monitor and correct fluid and electrolyte disturbances
  - Treat acidosis, arrhythmias, rhabdomyolysis, and coagulopathy as required
  - Close monitoring (intensive care unit, supportive ventilation)

PALS ALGORITHMS

Resuscitation

1

Figure 1.10 Pediatric Cardiac Arrest Algorithm

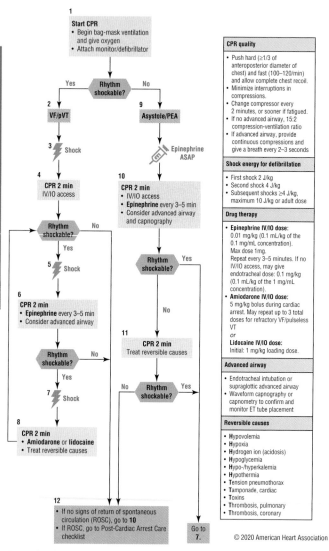

CPR, Cardiopulmonary resuscitation; *IO*, intraosseous; *IV*, intravenous; *PEA*, pulseless electrical activity; *pVT*, pulseless ventricular tachycardia; *VF*, ventricular fibrillation. (From Pediatric Basic and Advanced Life Support. 2020 American Heart Association Guidelines for Cardiopulmonary Resuscitation and Emergency Cardiovascular Care. *Circulation*. 2020;142:S469–S523. Copyright 2020 American Heart Association, Inc.)

Figure 1.11 Pediatric Bradycardia With a Pulse Algorithm

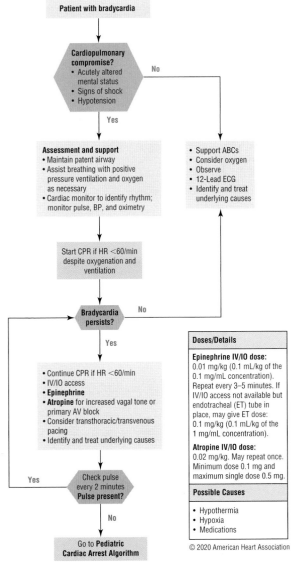

(From Pediatric Basic and Advanced Life Support: 2020 American Heart Association Guidelines for Cardiopulmonary Resuscitation and Emergency Cardiovascular Care. *Circulation*. 2020;142: S469–S523. Copyright 2020 American Heart Association, Inc.)

Figure 1.12 Pediatric Tachycardia With a Pulse Algorithm

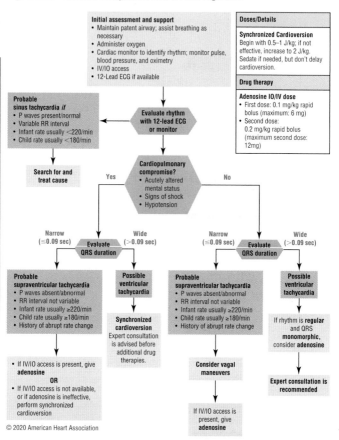

© 2020 American Heart Association

(From Pediatric Basic and Advanced Life Support: 2020 American Heart Association guidelines for cardiopulmonary resuscitation and emergency cardiovascular care. *Circulation*. 2020;142:S469–S523. Copyright 2020 American Heart Association, Inc.)

Figure 1.13 Pediatric Septic Shock Algorithm

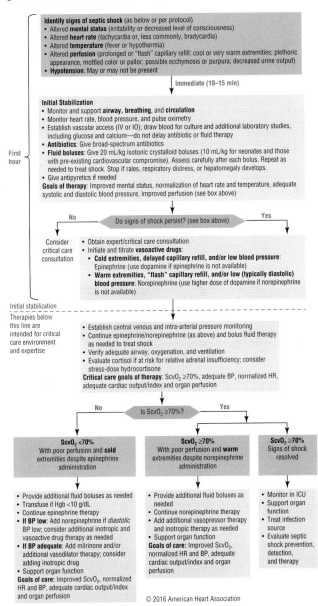

Identify signs of septic shock (as below or per protocol)
- Altered **mental status** (irritability or decreased level of consciousness)
- Altered **heart rate** (tachycardia or, less commonly, bradycardia)
- Altered **temperature** (fever or hypothermia)
- Altered **perfusion** (prolonged or "flash" capillary refill; cool or very warm extremities; plethoric appearance, mottled color or pallor; possible ecchymosis or purpura; decreased urine output)
- **Hypotension**: May or may not be present

Immediate (10–15 min)

Initial Stabilization
- Monitor and support **airway, breathing,** and **circulation**
- Monitor heart rate, blood pressure, and pulse oximetry
- Establish vascular access (IV or IO); draw blood for culture and additional laboratory studies, including glucose and calcium—do not delay antibiotic or fluid therapy
- **Antibiotics**: Give broad-spectrum antibiotics
- **Fluid boluses**: Give 20 mL/kg isotonic crystalloid boluses (10 mL/kg for neonates and those with pre-existing cardiovascular compromise). Assess carefully after each bolus. Repeat as needed to treat shock. Stop if rales, respiratory distress, or hepatomegaly develops.
- Give antipyretics if needed

Goals of therapy: Improved mental status, normalization of heart rate and temperature, adequate systolic and diastolic blood pressure, improved perfusion (see box above)

First hour

Do signs of shock persist? (see box above)

No → Consider critical care consultation

Yes →
- Obtain expert/critical care consultation
- Initiate and titrate **vasoactive drugs**:
  - **Cold extremities, delayed capillary refill, and/or low blood pressure**: Epinephrine (use dopamine if epinephrine is not available)
  - **Warm extremities, "flash" capillary refill, and/or low (typically diastolic) blood pressure**: Norepinephrine (use higher dose of dopamine if norepinephrine is not available)

Initial stabilization

Therapies below this line are intended for critical care environment and expertise

- Establish central venous and intra-arterial pressure monitoring
- Continue epinephrine/norepinephrine (as above) and bolus fluid therapy as needed to treat shock
- Verify adequate airway, oxygenation, and ventilation
- Evaluate cortisol if at risk for relative adrenal insufficiency; consider stress-dose hydrocortisone

Critical care goals of therapy: ScvO₂ ≥70%, adequate BP, normalized HR, adequate cardiac output/index and organ perfusion

Is ScvO₂ ≥70%?

No | Yes

ScvO₂ <70%
With poor perfusion and **cold** extremities despite epinephrine administration

- Provide additional fluid boluses as needed
- Transfuse if Hgb <10 g/dL
- Continue epinephrine therapy
- **If BP low**: Add norepinephrine if *diastolic* BP low; consider additional inotropic and vasoactive drug therapy
- **If BP adequate**: Add milrinone and/or additional vasodilator therapy; consider adding inotropic drug
- Support organ function

Goals of care: Improved ScvO₂, normalized HR and BP, adequate cardiac output/index and organ perfusion

ScvO₂ ≥70%
With poor perfusion and **warm** extremities despite norepinephrine administration

- Provide additional fluid boluses as needed
- Continue norepinephrine therapy
- Add additional vasopressor therapy and inotropic therapy as needed
- Support organ function

Goals of care: Improved ScvO₂, normalized HR and BP, adequate cardiac output/index and organ perfusion

ScvO₂ ≥70%
Signs of shock resolved

- Monitor in ICU
- Support organ function
- Treat infection source
- Evaluate septic shock prevention, detection, and therapy

© 2016 American Heart Association

(Modified from Brierley J, Carcillo JA, Choong K, et al. Clinical practice parameters for hemodynamic support of pediatric and neonatal septic shock: 2007 update from the American College of Critical Care Medicine. *Crit Care Med.* 2009;37:666–688.)

Figure 1.14 Management of shock after return of spontaneous circulation algorithm

Figure 1.14   Post Cardiac-Arrest Care Checklist

Components of Post-Cardiac Arrest Care	Check
Oxygenation and ventilation	
Measure oxygenation and target normoxemia 94%–99% (or child's normal/appropriate oxygen saturation).	☐
Measure and target $Paco_2$ appropriate to the patient's underlying condition and limit exposure to severe hypercapnia or hypocapnia.	☐
Hemodynamic monitoring	
Set specific hemodynamic goals during post-cardiac arrest care and review daily.	☐
Monitor with cardiac telemetry.	☐
Monitor arterial blood pressure.	☐
Monitor serum lactate, urine output, and central venous oxygen saturation to help guide therapies.	☐
Use parenteral fluid bolus with or without inotropes or vasopressors to maintain a systolic blood pressure greater than the fifth percentile for age and sex.	☐
Targeted temperature management (TTM)	
Measure and continuously monitor core temperature.	☐
Prevent and treat fever immediately after arrest and during rewarming	☐
If patient is conatose apply TTM (32°C–34°C) followed by (36°C–37.5°C) or only TTM (36°C–37°C).	☐
Prevent shivering.	☐
Monitor blood pressure and treat hypotension during rewarming.	☐
Neuromonitoring	
If patient has encephalopathy and resources are available, monitor with continuous electroencephalogram.	☐
Treat seizures.	☐
Consider early brain imaging to diagnose treatable causes of cardiac arrest.	☐
Electrolytes and glucose	
Measure blood glucose and avoid hypoglycemia.	☐
Maintain electrolytes within normal ranges to avoid possible life-threatening arrhythmias.	☐
Sedation	
Treat with sedatives and anxiolytcs.	☐
Prognosis	
Always consider multiple modalities (clinical and other) over any single predictive factor.	☐
Remember that assessments may be modified by TTM or induced hypothermia.	☐
Consider electroencephalogram in conjunction with other factors within the first 7 days after cardiac arrest.	☐
Consider neuroimaging such as magnetic resonance imaging during the first 7 days.	☐

(From Pediatric Basic and Advanced Life Support: 2020 American Heart Association Guidelines for Cardiopulmonary Resuscitation and Emergency Cardiovascular Care. *Circulation.* 2020;142:S469–S523. Copyright 2020 American Heart Association, Inc.)

A. Goals of post-resuscitation care

1. **Preserve brain function, prevent secondary hypoxic injury, facilitate transfer** to tertiary care center with appropriate personnel and equipment

   a. Temperature: fever should be aggressively treated after return of spontaneous circulation (ROSC). Continuous temperature monitoring and cooling should be used to maintain normothermia. Therapeutic hypothermia may be indicated in certain cases (discuss with local expert).

   b. Oxygen: providers may wean supplemental oxygen to target saturations of 94% to 99% to avoid both hypoxemia and hyperoxia

   c. Carbon dioxide: limit exposure to severe hypercapnia or hypocapnia

   d. Circulation: use fluids and/or inotropes/vasoactive drugs to maintain systolic blood pressure higher than the percentile for age

   e. Agitation/seizures: treat pain with analgesics (opioids) and keep child sedated (benzodiazepines). Treat clinical seizures and apply electroencephalogram monitoring for patients who remain comatose after resuscitation (potential for subclinical seizures).

FURTHER READING

American Academy of Pediatrics. *Textbook of Neonatal Resuscitation.* 7th ed. Elk Grove Village, IL: American Academy of Pediatrics and American Heart Association; 2016.

American Heart Association. *Pediatric Advanced Life Support Provider Manual.* Dallas, TX: American Heart Association; 2016.

de Caen AR, Berg MD, Chameides L, et al. Part 12: Pediatric Advanced Life Support: 2015 American Heart Association Guidelines Update for Cardiopulmonary Resuscitation and Emergency Cardiovascular Care. *Circulation.* 2015;132:S526.

Kleinman ME, Chameides L, Schexnayder S. et al. Part 14: Pediatric Advanced Life Support: 2010 American Heart Association Guidelines for Cardiopulmonary Resuscitation and Emergency Cardiovascular Care. *Circulation.* 2010; 122:S876–S908.

Topjian A, Raymond T, Atkins D, et al. Part 4: Pediatric Basic and Advanced Life Support: 2020 American Heart Association Guidelines for Cardiopulmonary Resuscitation and Emergency Cardiovascular Care. *Circulation.* 2020;142:S469–S523.

Emergency Medicine

Marie-Pier Lirette • Maya Harel-Sterling • Iwona Baran • Suzanne Beno

COMMON ABBREVIATIONS

Also see page xviii for a list of other abbreviations used throughout this book

0.9% NaCl	0.9% sodium chloride (normal saline)
ABC	airway, breathing, and circulation
ABG	arterial blood gas
ALOC	altered level of consciousness
APLS	advanced pediatric life support
ECMO	extracorporeal membrane oxygenation
ETT	endotracheal tube
GCS	Glasgow Coma Scale
ICP	intracranial pressure
FAST	focused assessment with sonography for trauma
HTN	hypertension
LOC	level of consciousness
PALS	pediatric advanced life support
PRAM	pediatric respiratory assessment measure
PPV	positive pressure ventilation
RSI	rapid sequence intubation
SVR	systemic vascular resistance
tPA	tissue plasminogen activator
VBG	venous blood gas

USEFUL CALCULATIONS AND VALUES

1. **Estimated weight in kilograms (APLS)**
   a. 1–12 months: $[0.5 \times (\text{age in months})] + 4$
   b. 1–5 years: $[2 \times (\text{age in years})] + 8$
   c. 6–12 years: $[3 \times (\text{age in years})] + 7$
2. **Normal ranges for heart rate, respiratory rate, and blood pressure** (BP) for different ages: See figure in back inside cover of book
3. **Hypotension** in children (systolic BP)
   a. Term neonates (<1 month): <60 mmHg
   b. 1–12 months: <70 mmHg
   c. 1–10 years: $<70 + [2 \times (\text{age in years})]$ mmHg
   d. >10 years: <90 mmHg
4. **Fluid bolus** in emergency situations: 20 mL/kg of 0.9% NaCl (normal saline)

CIRCULATORY EMERGENCIES

SHOCK

1. **Definitions**
   a. **Shock:** physiological state in which the cardiovascular system fails to deliver adequate oxygen and nutrients to meet tissue demand
      i. **Compensated shock:** an earlier form of shock characterized by normal BP. Compensatory mechanisms to maintain cardiac output typically include tachycardia (often the most sensitive

marker) and increased systemic vascular resistance (SVR). This is a reversible state but, if unrecognized and untreated, progresses to decompensated shock.

ii. **Decompensated shock:** shock with **hypotension**. This is often a late finding in children because of the ability to compensate as described earlier. If untreated, decompensated shock rapidly leads to organ dysfunction, cardiovascular collapse, and arrest.

2. **Etiology**

a. See Table 2.1 for general classification and common causes of shock

Table 2.1	Types of Shock						
Type	**Common Causes**	**Patho-physiology**	**HR**	**SVR**	**Clinical Features**	**Treatment**
Hypovolemic (most common)	Fluid loss (Gastroenteritis, burns) Hemorrhage	↓ Intravascular volume (decreased preload)	↑	↑	Dry mucous membranes, cool extremities, delayed cap refill, decreased urine output, depressed mental status	Fluids (crystalloid) Hemorrhage control, pRBCs
Cardiogenic	Arrhythmia, Myocarditis, Pericarditis, Cardiomyopathy, Congenital heart disease, Postoperative complications of cardiac surgery, Drug ingestions/metabolic derangements	↓ Cardiac output because of decreased myocardial contractility	↑	↑	Often similar to hypovolemic shock. Features more specific to cardiogenic shock: - Gallop rhythm - Dilated neck veins - Hepatomegaly - CXR: cardiomegaly + pulmonary congestion	Judicious fluid use, Inotropic support, ECMO as needed
Distributive (Derangement in vascular tone)	Anaphylactic shock	IgE-mediated release of histamine (vasodilator)	↑	↓	Signs of anaphylaxis (urticaria, angioedema, wheeze, GI upset)	See Figure 2.4
	Neurogenic shock (Spinal cord trauma)	Loss of sympathetic tone leads to vasodilation	↓	↓	Unopposed vagal activity leads to bradycardia (or absence of reflex tachycardic response to hypotension), flash capillary refill	Fluids, vasoactive agents

Type	Common Causes	Patho-physiology	HR	SVR	Clinical Features	Treatment
Table 2.1	**Types of Shock—cont'd**					
Septic		Severe inflammatory reaction to infection leads to myocardial dysfunction, capillary leak, and vasomotor instability	↑	↑ (cold shock)	"Cold" shock: mottled skin, cool extremities, prolonged capillary refill, weak pulses. Most common in pediatric patients.	Fluids, antibiotics, vasoactive agents. See Figure 2.1
				↓ (warm shock)	"Warm" shock: warm extremities, flash cap refill, bounding pulses, wide pulse pressure. Most common in adults.	
Obstructive	Cardiac tamponade	Mechanical obstruction to left ventricular inflow or outflow	↑	↑	Muffled heart sounds, distended neck veins	Pericardiocentesis
	Tension pneumothorax		↑	↑	Tracheal deviation away from side of pneumothorax, narrow pulse pressure	Needle decompression/ chest tube drainage
Dissociative	Carbon monoxide poisoning, Methemoglobinemia (see Chapter 3 Poisonings and Toxicology)	O_2 not released from hemoglobin	↑	↑↔	Cyanosis, neurological symptoms, coma	Oxygen

CXR, Chest x-ray; ECMO, extracorporeal membrane oxygenation; GI, gastrointestinal; HR, heart rate; IgE, immunoglobulin E; pRBC, packed red blood cell; SVR, systemic vascular resistance.

3. **Clinical manifestations**
   a. All forms of shock involve some degree of absolute or functional hypovolemia (from fluid losses or decreased SVR, respectively) and impaired tissue perfusion
   b. Early clinical manifestations of shock include tachycardia, tachypnea, decreased urine output, and nonspecific symptoms of poor feeding and irritability. Late clinical manifestations of shock include hypotension, altered level of consciousness, and weak pulses.
   c. The various types of shock and aspects of their clinical presentation are shown in Table 2.1

4. **Investigations**
   a. **Laboratory studies**
      i. Signs of infection: CBC + differential, blood culture, ± urine studies
      ii. Signs of organ dysfunction: liver injury (LFTs, coagulation profile), acute kidney injury (urea, creatinine), metabolic disturbance (glucose, calcium), hematological dysfunction (platelets)
      iii. Signs of impaired tissue perfusion: blood gas (pH), lactate
      iv. Sepsis workup as appropriate for age and presentation
   b. **Imaging studies:** CXR for respiratory symptoms ± other additional studies, as guided by history and physical examination ECG, echocardiogram for suspected cardiogenic shock, etc.)

5. **Management**
   a. Successful management relies on rapid recognition, reversal of shock state, and identification and treatment of underlying cause. The clinician should immediately address the ABCs, ensure a secure airway, place supplemental oxygen, and insert two large bore peripheral IV lines for adequate fluid resuscitation. All children should be on continuous cardiac and respiratory monitoring. Urine output should be recorded and patients should be monitored for signs of multiorgan failure. **Resuscitation goals include restoration of normal heart rate, BP, mental status, and perfusion parameters (e.g., cap refill ≤2 s)** (see Table 2.1).

SEPSIS

1. **Definitions**
   a. **Systemic inflammatory response syndrome (SIRS):** inflammatory response with two or more of the following criteria (one of which must be abnormal temperature or leukocyte count)
      i. Core temperature >38.5°C or <36°C
      ii. Tachycardia (or bradycardia if <1 year)
      iii. Tachypnea
      iv. Increased or decreased leukocyte count
   b. **Sepsis:** SIRS with suspected or proven infection
   c. **Severe sepsis (sepsis with associated organ dysfunction):** sepsis associated with *cardiovascular dysfunction* (hypotension, need for vasoactive agent, metabolic acidosis, impaired perfusion) **or** *acute respiratory distress syndrome (ARDS)/need for mechanical ventilation* **or** *dysfunction in ≥2 other systems* (hematological

[thrombocytopenia, disseminated intravascular coagulation], neurological [change in mental status, GCS ≤11], hepatic [elevated bilirubin, AST], renal [increased creatinine])

d. **Septic shock:** sepsis with cardiovascular dysfunction and any signs of impaired tissue perfusion such as altered mental status (irritability, drowsiness, confusion, lethargy), skin, capillary refill, and pulse abnormalities (see Table 2.1), decreased urine output, **or** hypotension

 PEARL

Goals of first hour resuscitation in septic shock are to:
1. Restore/maintain oxygenation and ventilation
2. Restore/maintain circulation
3. Administer broad-spectrum antibiotics (see Chapter 24 Infectious Diseases)

2. **Management**

a. See Figure 2.1 and Chapter 24 Infectious Diseases

b. Clinical targets during resuscitation include improvement of heart rate and BP, mental status, perfusion (cap refill, etc.), lactate, urine output

Figure 2.1   Emergency Room Management of Septic Shock

0 min	Recognize decreased mental status and perfusion. Begin high flow O₂, and establish IO/IV access according to PALS.
5 min	If no hepatomegaly or rales/crackles, then push 20 mL/kg isotonic saline boluses and reassess after each bolus up to 60 mL/kg until improved perfusion. Stop for rales, crackles, or hepatomegaly. Correct hypoglycemia and hypocalcemia. Begin antibiotics.

Fluid refractory shock? (Shock resistant to 40–60 cc/kg IV fluids)

Begin peripheral IV/IO inotrope infusion, preferably Epinephrine 0.05–0.3 μg/kg/min. Use Atropine / Ketamine IV/IO/IM if needed for Central Vein or Airway Access.	**Resuscitation goals include improvement of:** • Heart rate, blood pressure • Mental status • Perfusion (cap refill, etc.) • Urine output • Serum lactate
Titrate Epinephrine 0.05–0.3 μg/kg/min for Cold Shock. (Titrate central Dopamine 5–9 μg/kg/min if Epinephrine not available) Titrate central Norepinephrine from 0.05 μg/kg/min and upward to reverse Warm Shock. (Titrate central Dopamine ≥ 10 μg/kg/min if Norepinephrine not available)	

60 min	**Catecholamine-resistant shock?**
	If at risk for Absolute Adrenal Insufficiency, consider Hydrocortisone. Advanced hemodynamic management in PICU.

IM, Intramuscular; *IO*, intraosseous; *IV*, intravenous; *PALS*, pediatric advanced life support.

(Modified from Davis AL, Carcillo JA, Aneja RK, et al. American College of Critical Care Medicine Clinical Practice Parameters for hemodynamic support of pediatric and neonatal septic shock. *Crit Care Med* 2017;45:1061.)

HYPERTENSIVE CRISIS

1. **Definitions**
   a. See Chapter 28 Nephrology and Urology for age and sex appropriate normal BP values
   b. **Hypertensive urgency:** significantly elevated BP (typically, BP ≥ 95th% + 12 mmHg for age, sex, height, or >140/90 if age ≥13years) *without* severe symptoms or evidence of end-organ injury
   c. **Hypertensive emergency:** significantly elevated BP (typically, BP ≥ 95th% + 12 mmHg for age, sex, height, or >140/90 if age ≥13 years) *with* evidence of severe symptoms or secondary organ injury (most commonly brain, eyes, heart, kidneys)
2. **Etiology**
   a. See Table 2.2 for causes of hypertensive emergencies based on age

Table 2.2	Common Causes of Hypertensive Emergencies Based on Age
Age	**Cause**
Infant/young child	Renovascular causes (thrombosis, stenosis) Coarctation of aorta Renal parenchymal disease Endocrine cause (thyrotoxicosis)
School age/adolescent	Renal parenchymal disease (HUS, HSP, poststrep GN) Renovascular (renal artery stenosis) Endocrine (thyrotoxicosis, pheochromocytoma) Medications/recreational drugs Essential hypertension

HSP, Henoch-Schönlein purpura; *HUS,* hemolytic uremic syndrome; *poststrep GN,* poststreptococcal glomerulonephritis.

3. **Clinical manifestations**
   a. **Neurological dysfunction:** blurred vision, headache, confusion/encephalopathy, seizures, hemiplegia/facial palsy
   b. **Cardiac dysfunction:** congestive heart failure, palpitations, shortness of breath, peripheral edema, weak/absent femoral pulse
   c. **Renal dysfunction:** reduced urine output, edema
   d. **Signs of endocrine disorder:** goiter, abdominal striae, headaches, palpitations, flushing
4. **Investigations**
   a. **Laboratory studies**
      i. **Serum:** CBC, electrolytes, glucose, urea, creatinine. Consider TSH, plasma renin (before initiating therapy) as indicated.
      ii. **Urine:** urinalysis. Toxicology screen, urinary catecholamines as indicated.

b. **Imaging studies:** ECG, CXR, ± echocardiogram if cardiac pathology suspected, CT head for severe neurological dysfunction, renal ultrasound (US) with Doppler for suspected renal artery stenosis

5. **Management**
   a. Adequate IV access should be obtained and cardiorespiratory and BP monitoring initiated
   b. **Exclude increased intracranial pressure (ICP)** before lowering BP (need to have an adequate mean arterial pressure to sustain cerebral perfusion pressure)
   c. **Goal:** initial reduction in BP to stabilize severely symptomatic patients, then gradual decrease: lower BP by maximum 25%, or to 95th percentile for age (whichever is lesser reduction) over first 6 to 8 hours, then gradual decrease to 90th to 95th percentile for age over next 24 to 48 hours
   d. See Table 2.3 for pharmacological management
   e. Children on IV infusions should be monitored in an ICU setting. Consider arterial line or q5–10min noninvasive BP monitoring.
   f. Stop infusions temporarily and ensure fluids (normal saline) are ready for unanticipated large drops in BP

Table 2.3	**Pharmacological Management of Acute Hypertension (See Drug Formulary for Dosing)**			
Medications	**Class**	**Onset of Action**	**Duration of Action**	**Comments**
Intermittent Dosing in Acute Hypertension				
Hydralazine IV	Direct vasodilator	10–30 min	4–12 h	– Adjustment in renal impairment – *Adverse effects:* associated with drug-induced lupus, may cause headaches, tachycardia, increased ICP
Labetolol IV	α_1 and β blocker	5–10 min	2–4 h	– Contraindicated in asthma, pheochromocytoma – *Adverse effects:* Nausea/vomiting, dizziness, scalp tingling, heart block, burning throat sensation
Nifedipine PO	Calcium channel blocker	20–30 min	6 h	– Do not use in neonates – *Adverse effects:* Dizziness, flushing, rebound hypertension

Table 2.3	Pharmacological Management of Acute Hypertension (See Drug Formulary for Dosing)—cont'd			
Medications	**Class**	**Onset of Action**	**Duration of Action**	**Comments**
Continuous Infusion in Hypertensive Emergencies				
Labetalol IV	α_1 and β blocker	5–10 min	2–4 h	– Contraindicated in asthma, pheochromocytoma – *Adverse effects:* Nausea/vomiting, dizziness, scalp tingling, heart block, burning throat sensation
Nitroprusside IV	Direct vasodilator	Within seconds	During infusion only	– Avoid if ↑ ICP or renal failure. – Risk of cyanide toxicity – *Adverse effects:* Nausea/vomiting, diaphoresis, muscle twitching
Esmolol IV	β_1 blocker	Within seconds	10–20 min	– *Adverse effects:* May cause profound bradycardia

Once target BP is reached, options for oral maintenance medications include amlodipine or metoprolol.

BP, Blood pressure; *ICP*, intracranial pressure; *IV*, intravenous; *PO*, orally.

RESPIRATORY EMERGENCIES

ACUTE ASTHMA EXACERBATION

Also see Chapter 35 Respirology for further information on asthma

1. **Definition**
   a. **Status asthmaticus:** severe asthma exacerbation refractory to appropriate medical therapy
2. **Clinical manifestations**
   a. Respiratory failure: ↑ respiratory rate, cough, work of breathing, accessory muscle use, prolonged expiration, wheezing, silent chest (wheezing may be absent in severe exacerbation because of poor air entry from bronchoconstriction)
   b. Cardiovascular: ↑ heart rate
   c. Central nervous system: altered mental status if severe (hypoxia/hypercarbia)
3. **Illness severity**
   a. **PRAM score** (pediatric respiratory assessment measure) can help determine level of severity (Table 2.4)

Table 2.4	Pediatric Respiratory Assessment Measure (PRAM) Score for Asthma Exacerbation Severity			
PRAM Score (Pediatric Respiratory Assessment Measure)				
Signs	**0**	**1**	**2**	**3**
Suprasternal retractions	Absent		Present	
Scalene muscle retractions	Absent		Present	
Air entry	Normal	Decreased at bases	Widespread decrease	Absent/minimal
Wheezing	Absent	Expiratory only	Inspiratory and expiratory	Audible without stethoscope/silent chest with minimal air entry
Oxygen saturation	≥95%	92%–94%	<92%	
Score	**Asthma Severity**			
0–3	Mild			
4–7	Moderate			
8–12	Severe			

From Chalut DS, Ducharme FM, Davis GM. The Preschool Respiratory Assessment Measure (PRAM): a responsive index of acute asthma severity. *J Pediatr*. 2000;137:762–768.

4. **Management**
   a. Assess ABCs and place on monitors (cardiac monitor and O_2 sat monitor)
   b. O_2 to maintain saturation ≥94%
   c. Exclude other causes of wheezing based on history and physical examination (anaphylaxis, foreign body aspiration, pulmonary infection, etc.)
   d. **PRAM score** can help guide management (Figure 2.2)
   e. **Medications**
      i. Initial treatment involves administration of inhaled bronchodilators, such as **short-acting β_2-agonists** (salbutamol), ± **anticholinergics** (ipratropium bromide), as well as **systemic corticosteroids**
      ii. For insufficient response despite maximizing above therapy, **continuous nebulized β_2-agonist**, intravenous **magnesium sulfate**, **intravenous β_2-agonist infusion**, or **heliox** may be needed
   f. **Noninvasive ventilation** (**bilevel positive airway pressure [BiPAP]/continuous positive airway pressure [CPAP]**) may be necessary for tiring patients with impending respiratory failure. Intubation should be avoided if possible and reserved for cases of impending respiratory arrest. Ketamine (bronchodilator) is the preferred agent if sedation is needed.
   g. **CXRs are not routinely indicated** in cases of acute asthma exacerbations

Figure 2.2 Initial Treatment Algorithm for Acute Asthma Exacerbation

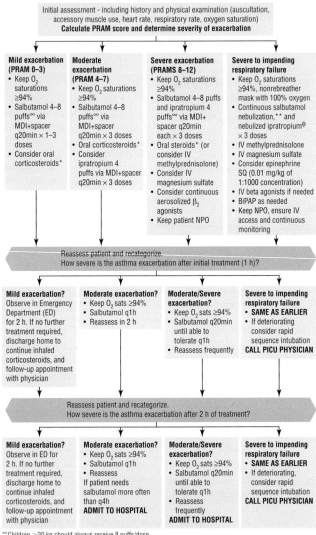

Initial assessment - including history and physical examination (auscultation, accessory muscle use, heart rate, respiratory rate, oxygen saturation)
Calculate PRAM score and determine severity of exacerbation

Mild exacerbation (PRAM 0–3)
- Keep O_2 saturations ≥94%
- Salbutamol 4–8 puffs∞ via MDI+spacer q20min × 1–3 doses
- Consider oral corticosteroids*

Moderate exacerbation (PRAM 4–7)
- Keep O_2 saturations ≥94%
- Salbutamol 4–8 puffs∞ via MDI+spacer q20min × 3 doses
- Oral corticosteroids*
- Consider ipratropium 4 puffs via MDI+spacer q20min × 3 doses

Severe exacerbation (PRAMS 8–12)
- Keep O_2 saturations ≥94%
- Salbutamol 4–8 puffs and ipratropium 4 puffs∞ via MDI+spacer q20min each × 3 doses
- Oral steroids* (or consider IV methylprednisolone)
- Consider IV magnesium sulfate
- Consider continuous aerosolized β_2 agonists
- Keep patient NPO

Severe to impending respiratory failure
- Keep O_2 saturations ≥94%, nonrebreather mask with 100% oxygen
- Continuous salbutamol nebulization,** and nebulized ipratropium$^\phi$ × 3 doses
- IV methylprednisolone
- IV magnesium sulfate
- Consider epinephrine SQ (0.01 mg/kg of 1:1000 concentration)
- IV beta agonists if needed
- BiPAP as needed
- Keep NPO, ensure IV access and continuous monitoring

Reassess patient and recategorize.
How severe is the asthma exacerbation after initial treatment (1 h)?

Mild exacerbation?
Observe in Emergency Department (ED) for 2 h. If no further treatment required, discharge home to continue inhaled corticosteroids, and follow-up appointment with physician

Moderate exacerbation?
- Keep O_2 sats ≥94%
- Salbutamol q1h
- Reassess in 2 h

Moderate/Severe exacerbation?
- Keep O_2 sats ≥94%
- Salbutamol q20min until able to tolerate q1h
- Reassess frequently

Severe to impending respiratory failure
- **SAME AS EARLIER**
- If deteriorating consider rapid sequence intubation
CALL PICU PHYSICIAN

Reassess patient and recategorize.
How severe is the asthma exacerbation after 2 h of treatment?

Mild exacerbation?
Observe in ED for 2 h. If no further treatment required, discharge home to continue inhaled corticosteroids, and follow-up appointment with physician

Moderate exacerbation?
- Keep O_2 sats ≥94%
- Salbutamol q1h
- Reassess
If patient needs salbutamol more often than q4h
ADMIT TO HOSPITAL

Moderate/Severe exacerbation?
- Keep O_2 sats ≥94%
- Salbutamol q20min until able to tolerate q1h
- Reassess frequently
ADMIT TO HOSPITAL

Severe to impending respiratory failure
- **SAME AS EARLIER**
- If deteriorating, consider rapid sequence intubation
CALL PICU PHYSICIAN

∞Children >20 kg should always receive 8 puffs/dose.
*Oral steroids: prednisone 1–2 mg/kg/day ×5 days or dexamethasone 0.6 mg/kg PO daily × 1–2 days.
**Inhalational salbutamol (5 mg/mL): <20 kg: 0.5 mL (2.5 mg) per dose mixed with 3 mL NS; >20 kg: 1 mL (5 mg) per dose mixed with 3 mL NS.
$^\phi$ Inhalational Ipatropium bromide (0.25 mg/mL): 1 mL (0.25 mg) mixed with 3 mL NS.

BiPAP, Bilevel positive airway pressure; *IV*, intravenous; *MDI*, metered-dose inhaler; *NPO*, nothing by mouth; *NS*, normal saline; *PICU*, pediatric intensive care unit; *PRAM*, pediatric respiratory assessment measure. (Modified from Ortiz-Alvarez O, Mikrogianakis A. Canadian Paediatric Society. *Paediatr Child Health*. 2012;17(5):251–255.)

5. **Complications**
   a. Potential complications include pneumothorax, pneumomediastinum, hypoxia, cardiac arrest

---

⭐ **PEARL**

Metered-dose inhaler (MDI) with a mask and spacer is the preferred way to administer bronchodilators. Nebulizer should only be used in cases of impending respiratory failure.

FOREIGN BODY ASPIRATION

See Figure 2.3

Figure 2.3 Management of Suspected Foreign Body Aspiration

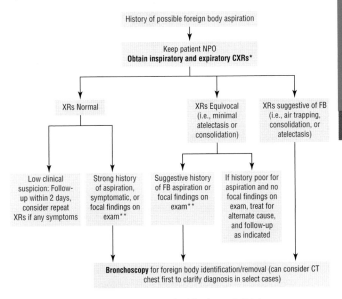

*PA and lateral decubitus chest x-rays (affected side placed down) may substitute in younger or uncooperative patients
**Focal findings include focal wheeze, decreased breath sounds

CT, Computed tomography; *CXR*, chest x-ray; *FB*, foreign body; *FBA*, foreign body aspiration; *NPO*, nothing by mouth. (Adapted from Fleisher GR, Ludwig S, eds. *Textbook of Pediatric Emergency Medicine.* 7th ed. Philadelphia, PA: Lippincott Williams & Wilkins; 2016.)

CROUP, BACTERIAL TRACHEITIS, AND EPIGLOTTITIS

Refer to Table 33.11 in Chapter 33 Otolaryngology

1. **Definition**
   a. **Classic anaphylactic reaction:** life-threatening immunoglobulin IgE-mediated type 1 hypersensitivity reaction, which occurs upon reexposure to an antigen

2. **Etiology**
   a. Most commonly caused by food allergens (peanuts, tree nuts, shellfish, dairy products). Other common triggers include Hymenoptera stings (wasps/bees), drugs (antibiotics), immunotherapy, radiocontrast media, and blood products. The causative agent is unknown in some cases.

3. **Clinical manifestations and diagnosis**
   a. Onset of symptoms can vary from minutes to hours following exposure
   b. **Anaphylaxis should be diagnosed when two or more of the following four systems are affected:**
      i. **Skin/mucous membrane:** urticaria, pruritis, flushing, angioedema, uvula swelling
      ii. **Respiratory** (upper or lower): stridor, voice change/hoarseness, laryngeal edema, throat itching, bronchospasm, wheezing, coughing, chest tightness, shortness of breath
      iii. **Gastrointestinal:** nausea, vomiting, abdominal cramping, diarrhea
      iv. **Circulation:** tachycardia, hypotension, syncope, arrhythmias, cardiac arrest
   c. Other common symptoms include anxiety, dizziness, and sense of impending doom
   d. Up to one-third of patients have biphasic reaction (symptoms recur in 4–72 hours)

4. **Management**
   a. See Figure 2.4 for treatment algorithm
   b. **Discharge planning**
      i. Consider discharge once stable for 4 to 6 hours after IM epinephrine without recurrence of symptoms
      ii. Anaphylaxis education (including MedicAlert bracelet)
      iii. EpiPen teaching and prescription
      iv. Follow-up with an allergist for further testing if not already done

---

 PEARL

Outpatient pediatric EpiPen prescriptions:
EpiPen Jr (0.15 mg) for children 10–25 kg
EpiPen (0.3 mg) for children >25 kg

Figure 2.4   Management Algorithm for Anaphylaxis

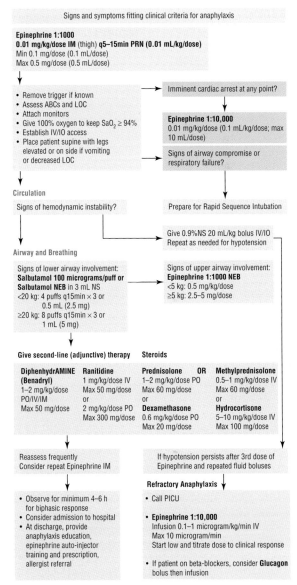

Signs and symptoms fitting clinical criteria for anaphylaxis

Epinephrine 1:1000
0.01 mg/kg/dose IM (thigh) q5–15min PRN (0.01 mL/kg/dose)
Min 0.1 mg/dose (0.1 mL/dose)
Max 0.5 mg/dose (0.5 mL/dose)

- Remove trigger if known
- Assess ABCs and LOC
- Attach monitors
- Give 100% oxygen to keep SaO$_2$ ≥ 94%
- Establish IV/IO access
- Place patient supine with legs elevated or on side if vomiting or decreased LOC

Imminent cardiac arrest at any point?

Epinephrine 1:10,000
0.01 mg/kg/dose (0.1 mL/kg/dose; max 10 mL/dose)

Signs of airway compromise or respiratory failure?

Prepare for Rapid Sequence Intubation

Circulation

Signs of hemodynamic instability?

Give 0.9%NS 20 mL/kg bolus IV/IO
Repeat as needed for hypotension

Airway and Breathing

Signs of lower airway involvement:
Salbutamol 100 micrograms/puff or Salbutamol NEB in 3 mL NS
<20 kg: 4 puffs q15min × 3 or 0.5 mL (2.5 mg)
≥20 kg: 8 puffs q15min × 3 or 1 mL (5 mg)

Signs of upper airway involvement:
Epinephrine 1:1000 NEB
<5 kg: 0.5 mg/kg/dose
≥5 kg: 2.5–5 mg/dose

Give second-line (adjunctive) therapy

DiphenhydrAMINE (Benadryl)	Ranitidine	**Steroids**	
		Prednisolone OR	Methylprednisolone
1–2 mg/kg/dose PO/IV/IM Max 50 mg/dose	1 mg/kg/dose IV Max 50 mg/dose or 2 mg/kg/dose PO Max 300 mg/dose	1–2 mg/kg/dose PO Max 60 mg/dose or Dexamethasone 0.6 mg/kg/dose PO Max 20 mg/dose	0.5–1 mg/kg/dose IV Max 60 mg/dose or Hydrocortisone 5–10 mg/kg/dose IV Max 100 mg/dose

Reassess frequently
Consider repeat Epinephrine IM

- Observe for minimum 4–6 h for biphasic response
- Consider admission to hospital
- At discharge, provide anaphylaxis education, epinephrine auto-injector training and prescription, allergist referral

If hypotension persists after 3rd dose of Epinephrine and repeated fluid boluses

Refractory Anaphylaxis

- Call PICU

- **Epinephrine 1:10,000**
Infusion 0.1–1 microgram/kg/min IV
Max 10 microgram/min
Start low and titrate dose to clinical response

- If patient on beta-blockers, consider **Glucagon** bolus then infusion

IM, Intramuscular; IO, intraosseous; IV, intravenous; LOC, loss of consciousness; PO, orally; PICU, pediatric intensive care unit. (© The Hospital for Sick Children Guide to Mangement of Pediatric Medical Emergencies, 2019.)

Emergency Medicine

2

ACUTE STROKE

1. See Figure 2.5. Also see Chapter 29 Neurology and Neurosurgery.

Figure 2.5 Management of Acute Stroke

Stroke Screening Questions:
Was there abrupt onset of any of:
- **Face** → asymmetrical smile/vision loss/double vision
- **Arms and legs** → unilateral weakness or numbness
- **Speech** → difficulty speaking or understanding/slurred speech
- Dizziness or trouble walking
Did the symptoms have abrupt onset or sudden worsening within the past 24 h?

↓ Yes

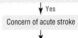

Concern of acute stroke

↓

- Confirm time last seen well (possible candidate for acute intervention* if *≥2 years old __AND__ within 24 h of symptom onset*)
- Confirm accurate body weight
- Apply ECG and BP monitors
- Insert PIV, STAT labs: CBC, INR, PTT, fibrinogen, type and screen, electrolytes, glucose, creatinine, pregnancy test
- Look for stroke risk factors: chronic systemic disease, trauma, infection, congenital heart disease, anemia (iron deficiency, sickle cell disease)
- Contact pediatric stroke center or tertiary care center

↓

Initiate Neuroprotective Measures
- **NPO**, head of bed flat (if tolerated and no signs of increased ICP)
- **Normotension:** Target SBP 50%–95% for age to maintain cerebral perfusion pressure. Treat hypotension (<50% for age): 0.9% NS, inotropes. Treat hypertension (>33% above 95th% for age): labetalol (lower by -25% over 24 h or more rapidly if r-tPA candidate)
- **Normovolemia:** maintenance 0.9% NS, bolus PRN
- **Normothermia:** Treat >37°C with antipyretics +/− cooling
- **Normoglycemia:** No IV glucose unless hypoglycemic, target: 5–10 mmol/L
- **Seizure control:** Treat any suspected seizure activity. Consider EEG.

↓

Obtain Urgent Neuroimaging
- If cooperative, no braces, and access to MRI → obtain STAT MRI/MRA within 1 h
- If MRI not possible and transfer not timely to tertiary care center → obtain CT /CTA within 1 h
- If history of trauma, include vascular imaging of head and neck (MRA or CTA)

*IV r-tPA (if <6 hours since symptom onset) or endovascular therapy in select cases. *BP,* Blood pressure; *CBC,* complete blood count; *CT,* computed tomography; *CTA,* computed tomography angiography; *ECG,* electrocardiogram; *EEG,* electroencephalogram; *ICP,* intracranial pressure; *INR,* international normalized ratio; *IV,* intravenous; *MRA,* magnetic resonance angiography; *MRI,* magnetic resonance imaging; *NS,* normal saline; *PIV,* peripheral intravenous line; *PRN,* as needed; *PTT,* partial thromboplastin time; *NPO,* nothing by mouth; *r-tPA,* recombinant tissue plasminogen activator (thrombolytic), *SBP,* systolic blood pressure. (© The Hospital for Sick Children; Adapted from The Hospital for Sick Children Hyperacute Arterial Ischemic Stroke Pathway, 2020.)

2

2. **Definition**
   a. Acute onset of focal neurological deficit because of either primary ischemic or hemorrhagic insult
3. **Clinical manifestations**
   a. **Hemiparesis, facial paralysis,** and other focal neurological signs, such as vision changes or **aphasia** are common findings in children
   b. **Seizures and altered mental status** may be the presenting sign in infants
4. **Investigations and diagnosis**
   a. **Laboratory tests:** CBC, electrolytes, creatinine, coagulation profile, type, and screen. Consider: hypercoagulability evaluation (protein C and protein S, antithrombin III, etc.), vasculitis evaluation (inflammatory markers, antinuclear antibodies, complement, etc.), and hemoglobin electrophoresis
   b. **Imaging studies**
      i. Urgent diffusion weighted MRI + MR angiography is imaging modality of choice
      ii. When MRI unavailable, cranial CT with CT angiogram can be used to rule out hemorrhage
5. **Management**
   a. **Neuroprotective measures:** see Figure 2.5
   b. **Specific therapy** determined by type of stroke
      i. **Ischemic stroke**
         - Anticoagulation (acetylsalicylic acid, low-molecular-weight heparin, unfractionated heparin)
         - Thrombolysis (tPA) and thrombectomy considered in select cases
      ii. **Hemorrhagic stroke:** catheter-directed embolization for arteriovenous malformations and neurosurgical intervention to control bleeding in select cases
      iii. **Sickle cell disease and ischemic stroke:** transfusion to decrease hemoglobin S to <30%

STATUS EPILEPTICUS

1. **Definition**
   a. Single generalized or focal seizure lasting ≥30 minutes, or a series of seizures during which consciousness is not regained. Urgent treatment should be initiated for seizures lasting longer than 5 minutes.

2. **Etiology**
   a. **Infectious:** fever (prolonged febrile seizure), meningitis, encephalitis, brain abscess
   b. **Metabolic:** hypoglycemia, hyponatremia, hypocalcemia, drug overdose
   c. **Antiepileptic drug noncompliance**, drug withdrawal, overdose, or subtherapeutic levels, refractory/intractable epilepsy
   d. **Trauma:** intracranial hemorrhage/injury
   e. **Other:** intracranial mass lesion, structural brain abnormality, stroke, bleed, idiopathic

3. **Investigations**
   a. **Laboratory studies:** glucose, blood gas, electrolytes, calcium, magnesium, CBC; consider LFTs, ammonia, anticonvulsant levels (if indicated)
   b. **Imaging studies:** consider brain imaging and EEG if appropriate
   c. **Additional tests:** blood, urine, CSF cultures as part of infection workup; toxicology screen

---

PEARL

In the absence of intravenous access in status epilepticus, benzodiazepines can be administered via various routes: intranasal, intramuscular, sublingual (see Figure 2.6).

---

4. **Management**
   a. See Figure 2.6 for management algorithm of status epilepticus

Figure 2.6 Management of Status Epilepticus in Infants (>1 Month), Children, and Adolescents

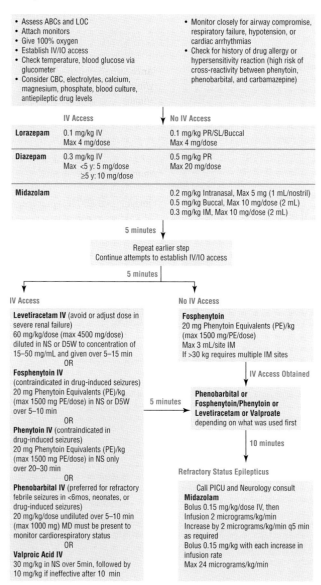

- Assess ABCs and LOC
- Attach monitors
- Give 100% oxygen
- Establish IV/IO access
- Check temperature, blood glucose via glucometer
- Consider CBC, electrolytes, calcium, magnesium, phosphate, blood culture, antiepileptic drug levels

- Monitor closely for airway compromise, respiratory failure, hypotension, or cardiac arrhythmias
- Check for history of drug allergy or hypersensitivity reaction (high risk of cross-reactivity between phenytoin, phenobarbital, and carbamazepine)

	IV Access	No IV Access
Lorazepam	0.1 mg/kg IV Max 4 mg/dose	0.1 mg/kg PR/SL/Buccal Max 4 mg/dose
Diazepam	0.3 mg/kg IV Max <5 y: 5 mg/dose ≥5 y: 10 mg/dose	0.5 mg/kg PR Max 20 mg/dose
Midazolam		0.2 mg/kg Intranasal, Max 5 mg (1 mL/nostril) 0.5 mg/kg Buccal, Max 10 mg/dose (2 mL) 0.3 mg/kg IM, Max 10 mg/dose (2 mL)

5 minutes

Repeat earlier step
Continue attempts to establish IV/IO access

5 minutes

IV Access

Levetiracetam IV (avoid or adjust dose in severe renal failure)
60 mg/kg/dose (max 4500 mg/dose) diluted in NS or D5W to concentration of 15–50 mg/mL and given over 5–15 min
OR
Fosphenytoin IV (contraindicated in drug-induced seizures)
20 mg Phenytoin Equivalents (PE)/kg (max 1500 mg PE/dose) in NS or D5W over 5–10 min
OR
Phenytoin IV (contraindicated in drug-induced seizures)
20 mg Phenytoin Equivalents (PE)/kg (max 1500 mg PE/dose) in NS only over 20–30 min
OR
Phenobarbital IV (preferred for refractory febrile seizures in <6mos, neonates, or drug-induced seizures)
20 mg/kg/dose undiluted over 5–10 min (max 1000 mg) MD must be present to monitor cardiorespiratory status
OR
Valproic Acid IV
30 mg/kg in NS over 5min, followed by 10 mg/kg if ineffective after 10 min

No IV Access

Fosphenytoin
20 mg Phenytoin Equivalents (PE)/kg (max 1500 mg/PE/dose)
Max 3 mL/site IM
If >30 kg requires multiple IM sites

IV Access Obtained

5 minutes

Phenobarbital or Fosphenytoin/Phenytoin or Levetiracetam or Valproate depending on what was used first

10 minutes

Refractory Status Epilepticus

Call PICU and Neurology consult
Midazolam
Bolus 0.15 mg/kg/dose IV, then
Infusion 2 micrograms/kg/min
Increase by 2 micrograms/kg/min q5 min as required
Bolus 0.15 mg/kg with each increase in infusion rate
Max 24 micrograms/kg/min

CBC, Complete blood count; IM, intramuscular; IO, intraosseous; IV, intravenous; LOC, loss of consciousness; NS, normal saline; PICU, pediatric intensive care unit; PR, per rectum; SL, sublingual. (© The Hospital for Sick Children eFormulary: Status epilepticus guidelines for infants and older children, 2020.)

RAISED INTRACRANIAL PRESSURE

1. **Etiology**
   a. Common causes include traumatic brain injury, intracranial hemorrhage, CNS tumors, hydrocephalus, and meningitis

2. **Clinical features**
   a. **Early:** headache (worse in morning, when bending forward, or with valsalva maneuvers), vomiting, ↓LOC, vision changes (double vision, vision loss), gait difficulties, behavioral changes, full fontanelle, or irritability in infants
   b. **Late:** Cushing's triad (↓HR, ↑BP, respiratory depression), unequal or unresponsive pupils, sunsetting eyes, papilledema, cranial nerve VI palsy (can also get CN III and IV deficits), meningismus, head tilt, decorticate (flexed upper limbs + extended lower limbs) or decerebrate posturing (abnormal extension of limbs), coma

3. **Management**
   a. See Figure 2.7

Figure 2.7 Management of Raised Intracranial Pressure

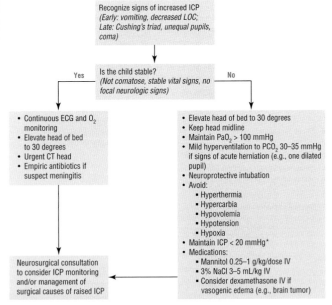

*Cerebral perfusion pressure = (mean arterial pressure) − (intracranial pressure)

CT, Computed tomography; *ECG,* electrocardiogram; *ICP,* intracranial pressure; *IV,* intravenous; *LOC,* loss of consciousness.

COMA AND ALTERED LEVEL OF CONSCIOUSNESS (ALOC)

1. **Definition**
   a. Altered level of consciousness refers to any state other than being awake and aware of oneself and one's surroundings. It includes, but is not limited to, being confused, lethargic, comatose, and delirious.
2. **Etiology**
   a. See Box 2.1 for useful mnemonics.

Box 2.1   Causes of Coma: TIPS and AEIOU

TIPS	AEIOU
T: Trauma	A: Alcohol abuse
I: Insulin/Hypoglycemia, Intussusception, Inborn errors of metabolism	E: Electrolyte abnormalities, Encephalopathy, Endocrinopathy
P: Psychiatric	I: Infection
S: Seizures, Stroke, Shock, Shunt malfunction	O: Overdose/ingestion
	U: Uremia

---

3. **Clinical evaluation**
   a. **History:** presence of fever/infectious symptoms, head trauma, seizure activity, possible ingestions, vomiting, changes in gait or behavior
   b. **Physical examination**
      i. Signs of toxidrome (see Chapter 3 Poisonings and Toxicology)
      ii. Neurological examination (GCS, pupil examination [abnormal size or position may suggest toxic exposure, raised ICP or seizures], nuchal rigidity)
      iii. Signs of head trauma or abuse
4. **Investigations**
   a. Should be guided by clinical assessment and patient condition
   b. Laboratory studies:
      i. Immediate bedside glucose for nontraumatic ALOC
      ii. Electrolytes, BUN, creatinine, calcium, CBC, blood gas, ammonia, lactate
      iii. Toxicological screening for ALOC of unknown origin
      iv. CSF studies if CNS infection suspected (cell count, protein, glucose, gram stain, culture, viral studies). Lumbar puncture is contraindicated if there is evidence of high ICP, hemodynamic instability, low platelets, or coagulopathy.

    c. **Imaging studies**
        i. **CT brain** can reveal many causes of ALOC (cerebral edema, hydrocephalus, malignancy, hematomas, and abscesses). Noncontrast CT head is indicated in cases of trauma. Contrast-enhanced study (CT or MRI) is preferred to detect focal infections and neoplasms.
5. **Management**
    a. **Assess ABCs:** life-threatening hypoxia, hypotension, increased ICP should be addressed first
    b. **Secure airway** if GCS <8, no gag or cough reflexes
    c. **Antidotal therapies:** IV Dextrose for confirmed or suspected hypoglycemia (0.5 g/kg IV); trial of naloxone for suspected opioid overdose
    d. Remainder of management is condition-specific (antibiotics for suspected CNS infection, management of ICP and neurosurgery consult for head trauma, correction of electrolyte disturbances in metabolic disorders, etc.)

> **! PITFALL**
>
> A head computed tomography scan should be performed before lumbar puncture (LP) in a patient with a significantly altered level of consciousness because LP is contraindicated if there is evidence of increased intracranial pressure.

ENVIRONMENTAL EMERGENCIES

DROWNING
1. **Definition**
    a. **Drowning:** the process of experiencing respiratory impairment from submersion/immersion in liquid. It may be fatal or nonfatal.
2. **Pathophysiology**
    a. **Respiratory compromise:** hypoxemia occurs either by means of reflex laryngospasm or aspiration. Aspiration of water disrupts surfactant, leads to pulmonary edema, and decreases lung compliance.
    b. **CNS compromise:** hypoxemia results in altered level of consciousness, which may progress to irreversible CNS damage
    c. **Cardiovascular compromise:** hypoxemia and metabolic acidosis lead to cardiovascular dysfunction and cardiac arrest

3. **Investigations**
   a. **Pulmonary status:** CXR, arterial oxygen saturation, and arterial blood gas
   b. CBC, electrolytes
4. **Management**
   a. **Respiratory** (ventilation is the most important initial treatment)
      i. Alert patients with no respiratory distress, a normal CXR and examination and normal O_2 saturation can be discharged after 6 hours of observation
      ii. Patients with mild respiratory distress should be placed on a cardiorespiratory monitor, provided with supplemental O_2 and chest physiotherapy, and admitted to hospital
      iii. Patients with severe respiratory distress will likely need noninvasive ventilation or intubation with mechanical ventilation and admission to an ICU
   b. **Cardiovascular**
      i. Fluid resuscitation may be needed during initial stages if patient presents in shock
      ii. Once BP is stabilized, fluid restriction and diuretics may improve gas exchange
   c. **Hypothermia should be corrected** to at least 32°C, then allow passive rewarming to 37°C
   d. No benefit to prophylactic antibiotics
   e. Trauma evaluation and C-spine precautions for diving injuries

HYPOTHERMIA

1. **Definition**[a]
   a. **Mild hypothermia:** core temperature 32°C–35°C
   b. **Moderate hypothermia:** core temperature 28°C–32°C
   c. **Severe hypothermia:** core temperature <28°C

---

[a]Special low-reading rectal thermometers are needed for accurate diagnosis

2. **Clinical manifestations**
   a. See Table 2.5

Table 2.5	Clinical Manifestations of Hypothermia		
	Mild Hypothermia (32°C–35°C)	**Moderate Hypothermia (28°C–32°C)**	**Severe Hypothermia (<28°C)**
Cardiac	↑BP (vasoconstriction) and ↑HR	↓BP (vasomotor paralysis at 30°C) ↓HR ECG: prolongation of ECG intervals, pathognomonic J (Osborn) wave	↓HR ECG: sinus bradycardia, asystole, ventricular fibrillation
Respiratory	Initial hyperventilation, then normoventilation	Hypoventilation or apnea	Hypoventilation or apnea
Neurologic	Fatigue, impaired judgment	Decreased LOC, slurred speech, delirium, incoordination	Coma, fixed dilated pupils
Muscular	Shivering and thermogenesis	Extinction of shivering	No shivering, progressive rigidity
Renal	"Cold diuresis," acute tubular necrosis, hypokalemia/hyperkalemia		
Metabolic	Lactic acidosis		

BP, Blood pressure; *ECG,* electrocardiogram; *HR,* heart rate; *LOC,* level of consciousness.

3. **Investigations**
   a. CBC, electrolytes, urea, creatinine, glucose, LFTs, amylase, ABG, drug screen, coagulation screen, CXR, ECG
4. **Management**
   a. **General supportive measures**
      i. Patients with respiratory depression or impaired mental status should be intubated and mechanically ventilated
      ii. Cardiopulmonary resuscitation for any nonperfusing rhythm; defibrillation is often ineffective at <30°C
      iii. Cardiorespiratory monitoring for life-threatening arrhythmias from irritable myocardium
      iv. Fluid replacement with warmed normal saline
      v. Hypoglycemia correction
   b. **Rewarming techniques:** see Table 2.6 for description of passive rewarming and active external and active core rewarming techniques and indications

> **! PITFALL**
>
> Profoundly hypothermic patients may have no signs of life. Resuscitative measures should be continued until patients are rewarmed to >34°C or there is return of spontaneous circulation.

Table 2.6	Rewarming Techniques for Hypothermic Patients		
	Mild Hypothermia (32°C–35°C)	**Moderate Hypothermia (28°C–32°C)**	**Severe Hypothermia (<28°C)**

Rewarming Technique	INITIATE
	- **Passive External Rewarming**
	  - Remove from cold environment, remove wet clothing, cover with warm blankets
		ADD
		- **Active External Rewarming**
		  - Electric blankets/warmers, hot packs (anticipate "afterdrop")
		- **Active Core Rewarming**
		  - Heated humidified oxygen, heated IV normal saline (40°C–43°C)
			ADD
			- **Additional Active Core Rewarming**
			  - Gastric, pleural, peritoneal, bladder lavage with warm IV normal saline
			- ECMO (for absent circulation)

ECMO, Extracorporeal membrane oxygenation; *IV*, intravenous.

HYPERTHERMIA

See Table 2.7 for clinical manifestations and management of hyperthermia

Table 2.7	Clinical Spectrum of Hyperthermia and Management Recommendations	
Type	**Clinical Manifestation**	**Treatment**
Heat cramps	Muscle cramps after exertion; usually because of replacing fluid losses with hypotonic fluids (characterized by ↓Na, ↓Cl)	Cooler environment, rest, oral electrolyte solution or IV fluids, salt replacement
Heat exhaustion	Temperature >39°C, lethargy, thirst, headache, vomiting, tachycardia. Neurological status remains intact **Secondary to water depletion** (characterized by ↑Na, ↑Cl). OR **Secondary to salt depletion** Also characterized by weakness, fatigue, muscle cramps, ↓Na$^+$, ↑urinary Na$^+$	Rest in cool environment and rehydration (see Chapter 15 Fluids and Electrolytes for hypernatremic dehydration correction) Rest in cool environment and high salt intake; IV fluids and salt correction over 12–24 h. Observe in hospital until temperature normalizes
Heat stroke	Life-threatening emergency; rectal temperature >41°C; neurological dysfunction vomiting/diarrhea; hot skin (sweating may stop); ↑HR, ↑RR, ↓BP; circulatory collapse; risk of rhabdomyolysis, acute tubular necrosis, DIC, hepatocellular degeneration; normal or ↑Na$^+$ levels, ↑CPK, Ca^{2+}	Maintain ABCs Elimination of hyperpyrexia: ice packs, active cooling, sedation, and paralysis Cardiovascular support: normal saline ± inotropic support (dobutamine or dopamine) Diuresis for rhabdomyolysis and monitoring for acute renal failure

ABC, Airway, breathing and circulation; *BP*, blood pressure; *HR*, heart rate; *CPK*, creatine phosphokinase; *DIC*, disseminated intravascular coagulation; *IV*, intravenous; *RR*, respiratory rate.

PEARL

Low-risk patients with a brief resolved unexplained event require minimal workup and interventions (see Figure 2.8).

BRIEF RESOLVED UNEXPLAINED EVENT (BRUE)

1. **Definitions:** see Figure 2.8

Figure 2.8 Diagnosis, Risk Classification, and Recommended Management of a Brief Resolved Unexplained Event (BRUE)

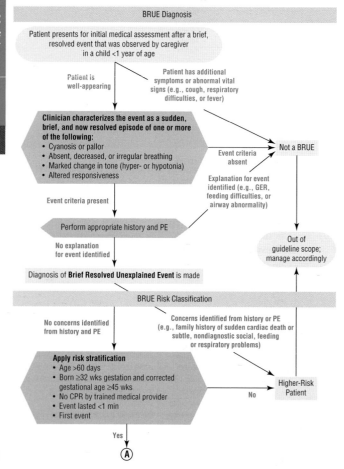

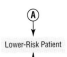

Lower-Risk Patient

Management Recommendations for Lower-Risk Patients	
Should	**Should Not**
• Educate caregivers about BRUEs and engage in shared decision-making to guide evaluation, disposition, and follow-up • Offer resources for CPR training to caregiver	• Obtain WBC count, blood culture, or CSF analysis or culture, serum sodium, potassium, chloride, blood urea nitrogen, creatinine, calcium, ammonia, blood gases, urine organic acids, plasma amino acids or acylcarnitines, chest radiograph, echocardiogram, EEG, studies for GER • Initiate home cardiorespiratory monitoring • Prescribe acid suppression therapy or antiepileptic medications
May	**Need Not**
• Obtain pertussis testing and 12-lead ECG • Briefly monitor patients with continuous pulse oximetry and serial observations	• Obtain viral respiratory test, urinalysis, blood glucose, serum bicarbonate, serum lactic acid, laboratory evaluation for anemia, or neuroimaging • Admit the patient to the hospital *solely* for cardiorespiratory monitoring

CPR, Cardiopulmonary resuscitation; *CSF*, cerebrospinal fluid; *EEG*, electroencephalogram; *GER*, gastro-esophageal reflux; *PE*, physical examination; *WBC*, white blood cell. (Adapted from Tieder JS, Bonkowsky JL, Etzel R, et al. Clinical Practice Source: Guideline: Brief Resolved Unexplained Events (Formerly Apparent Life-Threatening Events) and Evaluation of Lower-Risk Infants: Executive Summary. *Pediatrics*. 2016:137(5):e20160590.)

2. **Risk stratification and management**
   a. **Low-risk patients:** see Figure 2.8 for identification and management
   b. **Higher-Risk patients**
      i. See Box 2.2 for possible concerning findings
      ii. History or examination may suggest a targeted evaluation for specific disorders (respiratory or CNS infection, cardiac arrhythmia, epilepsy or CNS disease, metabolic disease, toxic ingestion, child abuse) and inpatient observation may be warranted

---

Box 2.2 Brief Resolved Unexplained Event: Concerning Findings on History or Physical Examination

Toxic appearance, lethargy, vomiting, respiratory distress at time of evaluation
Significant compromise during the event (need for CPR)
History of recent prior events or recurrent events
Family history of sudden cardiac death, long QT or unexplained drowning or car accident, SIDS or BRUE in sibling
History concerning for seizure
History of paroxysmal cough or exposure to pertussis
Any evidence of trauma or concern for child maltreatment
Unexplained death of sibling or dysmorphic features

BRUE, Brief resolved unexplained event; *CPR,* cardiopulmonary resuscitation; *SIDS,* sudden infant death syndrome.

1. **Definition**
   a. A disturbance in mental state characterized by aberrations in reality testing. Often involves impaired functioning and hallucinations and/or delusions.

2. **Etiology**
   a. See Table 2.8
   b. **Medical causes of psychosis**
      i. **Medical conditions**
         – Metabolic and endocrine disorders: hypoglycemia, hypocalcemia, electrolyte disturbance, thyroid disease, adrenal disease, uremia, diabetes, porphyria
         – CNS lesions: brain tumor, abscess, head trauma, stroke, temporal lobe epilepsy, CNS vasculitis
         – Infection: meningitis, encephalitis, sepsis, malaria
         – Gastrointestinal: hepatic failure
         – Rheumatic/inflammatory diseases: systemic lupus erythematosus
      ii. **Trauma** (acute and chronic)
      iii. **Drug intoxications:** alcohol, cocaine, phencyclidine (PCP), lysergic acid diethylamide (LSD), carbon monoxide poisoning, etc.
      iv. Prescribed medications (misuse, toxicity, side effects)
   c. **Psychiatric causes of psychosis:** schizophrenia, brief psychotic episode, underlying mood/anxiety/trauma disorder

Table 2.8	Differentiating Features of Organic Versus Psychiatric Psychosis	
Evaluation	**Organic Cause**	**Psychiatric Cause**
Onset	Acute	Gradual
Preillness history	May have prior illness/drug use	Prior psychiatric history (self or family)
Pathologic autonomic signs[a]	May be present	Absent
Vital signs	May be abnormal	Normal
Level of consciousness	May be impaired	Normal
Laboratory studies	May be abnormal	Normal
Orientation	Impaired	Intact
Recent memory	Impaired	Intact
Intellectual ability	May be impaired	Intact
Hallucinations	Visual	Auditory
Response to support and medications	Often dramatic	Often limited

[a] ↑ or ↓ in heart rate, respiratory rate, blood pressure, temperature; miosis or mydriasis; skin color changes.

From Fleisher GR, Ludwig S, eds. *Textbook of Pediatric Emergency Medicine.* 7th ed. Philadelphia, PA: Lippincott Williams & Wilkins; 2016: Table 134.23.

3. **Management**
   a. Ensure **patient and staff safety** (may require chemical ± physical restraints)
   b. Investigations to diagnose underlying cause (CBC, extended electrolytes, glucose, TSH, urine toxicology screen and pregnancy test, head imaging as necessary) and hospitalization as needed
   c. Psychiatry consultation
   d. Restraints as needed
      i. **Verbal restraints:** deescalation techniques and reduction of environmental stimulation should always be attempted first
      ii. **Chemical restraints:** drug selection will depend on clinical scenario and drug availability. Commonly used medications include benzodiazepines (e.g., lorazepam IV/IM/SL), atypical antipsychotics (olanzapine or risperdal IM/PO), and typical antipsychotics (haloperidol).
      iii. **Physical restraints:** apply 3-, 4-, or 5-point restraint (recognize risk of skin breakdown and rhabdomyolysis with continuous muscle contractions in restrained individual)
      iv. Involve parent or guardian when present; ensure they understand reasons for use of chemical and/or physical restraints

BURNS

1. See Chapter 34 Plastic Surgery for additional information on burns
2. **Clinical assessment**
   a. Burn mapping and estimation of body surface area (Figure 2.9). Also see Pearl box for rule of palms
   b. Evaluation of burn severity and depth: see Table 34.3
   c. Burn patients should be treated as trauma patients until proven otherwise (see Trauma later)
   d. Electrical burn injuries can be associated with significant internal injuries, which may not be apparent (fractures, rhabdomyolysis, renal failure, compartment syndrome, arrhythmias)
   e. See Chapter 9 Child Maltreatment for concerning burn patterns

 PEARL

Total body surface area (TBSA) can also be estimated using the child's palm. The entire palmar surface of the hand, fingers included, represents ~1% BSA.

Figure 2.9 Estimation of Burn Surface Area in Adults Versus Children

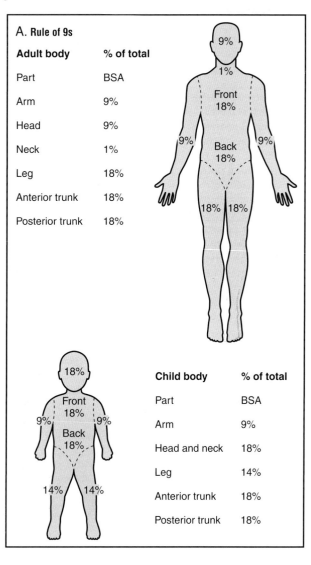

A. Rule of 9s

Adult body Part	% of total BSA
Arm	9%
Head	9%
Neck	1%
Leg	18%
Anterior trunk	18%
Posterior trunk	18%

Child body Part	% of total BSA
Arm	9%
Head and neck	18%
Leg	14%
Anterior trunk	18%
Posterior trunk	18%

B: Lund Browder Chart for Burn Estimates in Infants and Children

Age (in Years)	0–1	2–4	5–9	10–14	15
A: ½ of head	9½%	8½%	6½%	5½%	4½%
B: ½ of one thigh	2¾%	3¼%	4%	4¼%	4½%
C: ½ of one leg	2½%	2½%	2¾%	3%	3¼%

(Modified from Jeschke MG. How should patients with burns be managed in the intensive care unit? In: Deutschman CS, Neligan PJ. *Evidence-Based Practice of Critical Care*. 3rd ed. Elsevier; 2020, Figure 76.1.)

3. **Acute management**
   a. **Evaluate for and treat respiratory compromise**
      i. **Clinical signs of airway involvement:** facial burns, singed nose hairs, intraoral burns, carbonaceous sputum, or any signs of respiratory distress (hoarseness, stridor, cough, hypoxemia)
      ii. **Evaluation:** ABG with cooximetry, carboxyhemoglobin, CXR (as needed)
      iii. **Management**
         – 100% O_2 for all potential smoke inhalation victims; accelerates elimination of carbon monoxide
         – Positive pressure ventilation and early intubation, as needed; anticipate difficult airway (prepare backup equipment and personnel, including potential surgical airway)

- Consider nebulized epinephrine and bronchodilators, as needed, for stridor and wheeze respectively

b. **Fluid resuscitation**
   i. Begin fluid resuscitation using the Parkland formula when TBSA >15% (Box 2.3)
   ii. Maintenance fluids containing dextrose should be added to the aforementioned calculation for children <5 years of age
   iii. Aim for urine output >1 mL/kg/h (2 mL/kg/h if evidence of myoglobinuria)
   iv. Patients with electrical burns and those with inhalational injuries often have increased fluid requirements
   v. Potassium-containing fluids should be avoided in the early stages of therapy

c. **Pain control**
   i. Administer early analgesia (acetaminophen, nonsteroidal antiinflammatory drugs, oral morphine)
   ii. Analgesia ± sedation should be administered before any burn debridement
   iii. For moderate to severe pain, consider IV morphine boluses, IV or intranasal fentanyl boluses, or morphine or hydromorphone infusions, if needed

d. **Wound care**
   i. See Chapter 34 Plastic Surgery for further details on burn debridement and dressings

e. **Infection control**
   i. Tetanus vaccination if immunization status unknown or not up to date (see Chapter 23 Immunoprophylaxis)
   ii. Prophylactic systemic antibiotics are not recommended in the resuscitation period

---

Box 2.3   Parkland Formula for Fluid Resuscitation

- Total amount of fluid in first 24 h (mL) = 3 mL Lactated Ringers × weight (kg) × % TBSA (partial and full thickness burns)
- 50% of total IV fluids should be given over first 8 h (from time of injury)
- Remaining half should be given over next 16 h

IV, Intravenous; *TBSA*, total body surface area.
Data from Recommendations from American College of Surgeons (ACS) Committee on Trauma, Advanced Lifesaving Trauma Support (ATLS) program, 10th edition.

---

4. **Disposition**
   a. See Box 2.4 for burn center referral criteria

> **Box 2.4 Criteria for Referral to a Burn Center**
>
> **Extent:** partial thickness burn >10% TBSA, any full thickness burn
> **Location:** burns on face, neck, hands, feet, perineum, major joints, circumferential burns
> **Type:** chemical, electrical
> **Associated with:** smoke inhalation, head injury, trauma/fractures, preexisting medical conditions
> that could complicate management
> **Social situation:** infants and young children, abuse, self-inflicted, psychological issues

TBSA, Total body surface area.

APPROACH TO TRAUMA

1. **Pediatric injury/trauma**
   a. Leading cause of death and disability in children and youth
   b. Common mechanisms include physical abuse in infants, falls in pre-schoolers, motor vehicle collisions and recreational sports injuries in school-aged children and adolescents
   c. See Box 2.5 for unique pediatric characteristics in trauma

> **Box 2.5 Unique Pediatric Characteristics in Trauma**
>
> **Anatomic**
> - Small body mass with large surface area results in increased heat loss and greater external force per body unit area
> - Proportionally larger and less protected solid organs increase chance of intraabdominal injury (IAI)
> - Pliable ribcage with less musculature and more mobile mediastinum allows for major thoracic injury without obvious external signs of trauma
> - Larger head-to-body ratio results in a higher proportion of head injuries and age-related differences in cervical spine injury patterns
>
> **Physiologic**
> - Higher metabolic rate leads to increased oxygen and glucose demands, increased respiratory rate, and insensible fluid losses
> - Compensated shock is prevalent and often unrecognized as blood pressure remains normal until child displays rapid decompensation and arrest
>
> **Developmental**
> - Normal curiosity in young children and increased risk-taking among adolescents put children and youth at risk of injury
> - Children are often fearful with trauma assessments, and providers have difficulty with communication and examination, especially in young, preverbal children

From Beno S. Bottom Line Recommendation—Mulitsystem Trauma. Translating Emergency Knowledge for Kids TREKK. https://trekk.ca/resources?tag_id=D009104.

PEARL

ATMIST tool for clear communication and handover in trauma:
Age of patient
Time of injury and expected arrival
Mechanism of injury
Injuries suspected
Signs (vitals)
Treatment provided

2. **Prearrival preparation**
   a. **Establish trauma team leader** (TTL), define all roles, and don personal protective equipment
   b. **Multidisciplinary team present:** includes emergency medicine, general surgery, anesthesia, orthopedics ± neurosurgery. Diagnostic imaging, critical care, operating room, and blood bank should also be alerted and available.
   c. **TTL communicates known information** (e.g., ATMIST) and goals for resuscitation
   d. **Prepare** anticipated
      i. **Medications:** consider drawing up medications for analgesia and/or RSI
      ii. **Equipment:** airway support, vascular access/IO, rapid infuser/hotline warmer/pressure bag, chest tube trays, pelvic binder, bair hugger (and other equipment to prevent hypothermia), etc.
      iii. **Fluids:** warmed crystalloid, uncrossmatched pRBCs. If available, activate massive hemorrhage protocol if significant hemorrhage and/or decompensated shock expected.
3. **Trauma assessment and management**
   a. **Primary survey** is C-ABCDE-F (Table 2.9)
      i. Goal: identify and address life-threatening conditions (Table 2.10)
      ii. Assessment and management occur simultaneously
      iii. Change in clinical status should prompt full reassessment of primary survey
   b. **Secondary survey**
      i. **Head-to-toe examination** to define presence, type, and severity of injuries (Table 2.11)
      ii. **SAMPLE** history: **s**ituation, **a**llergies, **m**edications, **p**regnancy and past illnesses, **l**ast meal, **e**vents and environment
      iii. **Imaging** to locate sites of injury and sources of bleeding/shock
         – CXR
         – C-spine XR (Table 2.12)
         – Pelvis XR (Box 2.6)
         – CT head (Figure 2.10 and Box 2.7)
         – CT abdomen/pelvis (Box 2.8)

c. **Disposition:** consider transfer to a pediatric trauma center after stabilization (advanced imaging should not delay transfer, and should preferably be done at a pediatric trauma center)

Table 2.9	Primary Survey of a Trauma Patient
C—Catastrophic bleeding	Apply direct pressure, tourniquet as needed
A—Airway	- Maintain C-spine precautions if indicated - Administer 100% O_2 to all patients initially - Assess patency (clear secretions) and immediate need for intubation - Jaw thrust, suction, oral airway helpful. If BVM necessary, ensure tight fit with good seal. - Protect airway if indicated with RSI
B—Breathing	- Look: Respiratory distress, tension/open pneumothorax, flail chest, penetrating wounds, bruises on chest - Listen: Air entry bilaterally at apex (pneumothorax or hemothorax), - Feel: Tracheal position (take off front of C-collar if necessary) - e-FAST if distress/compromise to assess for pneumothorax, hemothorax, and cardiac tamponade

C—Circulation	- Obtain IV access with two large-bore IVs preferably in upper limbs; obtain IO access if necessary
	- Ensure type and crossmatch sent (other labs as able)
	- Fluid resuscitation if indicated (ensure fluids are warmed)
	  - Compensated shock: 20 mL/kg of IV crystalloid is appropriate initial therapy; give pRBC 10–20 mL/kg if ongoing signs of shock
	  - Decompensated shock (signifies 30%–40% blood loss, hypotension suggests periarrest state): administer blood immediately and activate massive hemorrhage protocol
	- Consider TXA in pediatric patients requiring blood
	- Assess for and control obvious sources of bleeding (internal and external). Bind pelvis if unstable; apply traction to femur fractures; use FAST (positive FAST indicates bleeding, but negative FAST does NOT rule out intraabdominal injury).

D—Disability	- **GCS** or **AVPU** (**A**lert, response to **V**erbal stimulation, response to **P**ainful stimulation, or **U**nresponsive). P or U indicate GCS <9 and merits airway protection - Pupil size and reactivity - Movement/sensation in all four extremities - Blood glucose - Treat pain
E—Exposure	- Fully undress patient to enable complete examination, log roll to examine spine (see secondary survey) - Prevent hypothermia: cover patient with warm blankets, warm room - Rapid MSK examination to identify obvious deformities
F—Family presence	- Requires dedicated personnel to be with family - Can reduce stress and anxiety for both child and family, and allow for a more accurate assessment of child - Enhances communication between medical team and family

BVM, Bag-valve-mask; *FAST,* focused assessment with sonography for trauma; *GCS,* Glasgow Coma Scale; *IO,* intraosseous; *IV,* intravenous; *MSK,* musculoskeletal; *pRBC,* packed red blood cell; *RSI,* rapid sequence intubation; *TXA,* tranexamic acid.

Table 2.10	**Primary Survey Interventions**
Identify	**Intervene**
Airway	
Inadequate airway	Secure and protect
Breathing	
Apnea	Positive pressure ventilation
Hypoxia	Apply supplemental oxygen
Tension pneumothorax	Needle/finger decompression, chest tube
Massive hemothorax	Chest tube
Open pneumothorax	Occlusive dressing, chest tube
Circulation	
Hypovolemic shock	Fluid bolus, blood products
Pericardial tamponade	Fluid bolus, pericardiocentesis, thoracotomy
Cardiac arrest	Chest compressions, thoracotomy if penetrating trauma
Disability	
Spinal cord injury	Immobilization
Cerebral herniation	Hyperventilation, hypertonic saline or mannitol
Exposure	
Hypothermia	Warmed fluid, external warming
Exsanguinating hemorrhage	Direct pressure, tourniquet as needed

Table 2.11	**Secondary Survey of a Trauma Patient**
Head and skull	- Look for: scalp fractures, lacerations, hematomas, hemorrhage or CSF leak (clear fluid) from nose, mouth, ears - Assess pupils, extraocular movements, and gross visual acuity - Assess for midface fracture (contraindication for NG placement) - Assess for dental injuries - Remove contact lenses
Neck	- Assume C-spine fracture until proven otherwise - Examine for C-spine tenderness, subcutaneous emphysema, laryngeal or tracheal injury (abnormal cry, stridor, subcutaneous emphysema, tracheal deviation)
Chest	- Examine for flail segment or penetrating wounds - Crepitus, bruising (note that absence of bruising does not rule out thoracic injury) and rib fractures

Table 2.11	Secondary Survey of a Trauma Patient—cont'd
Abdomen	- Look: Bruises (e.g., seat belt sign), open wounds - Feel: Palpate abdomen for signs of peritonitis (guarding, rebound tenderness, bowel sounds) or liver/spleen/kidney injury - Insert NG or OG tube (use OG if facial injuries or suspected basal skull fractures) - Consider e-FAST examination for free fluid
Perineal	- Examine for vaginal, testicular, and penile injuries - Place urinary catheter to ensure adequate urine output if indicated and no contraindications (pelvic injury, blood visible at urethral meatus)
Musculoskeletal/ pelvis	- Assess for bruising or pelvic instability - Splint unstable pelvic fractures with circumferentially tied cloth or pelvic binder. Apply traction (skin or Thomas splint) for femur fractures. Splint long bone fractures. - Assess for compartment syndrome - Examine spine during log roll (palpate for step defects and assess for point tenderness)
Neurological examination	- Maintain full spinal motion restriction if blunt trauma or concerns for spinal injury with penetrating injury - Reassess GCS or AVPU and pupil size and reactivity - Perform full motor and sensory examination of extremities
Other	- Update family - SAMPLE history - Diagnostic imaging as indicated - Transfer to tertiary trauma center

AVPU, Alert, response to verbal stimulation, response to painful stimulation, or unresponsive; *CSF*, cerebrospinal fluid; *FAST*, focused assessment with sonography for trauma; *GCS*, Glasgow Coma Scale; *NG*, nasogastric; *OG*, orogastric; *SAMPLE*, situation, allergies, medications, pregnancy and past illnesses, last meal, events and environment.

Table 2.12	Management of C-Spine in Trauma
Indication for x-ray	- Altered LOC - Abnormal neurological findings - C-spine, neck or back tenderness - Unexplained hypotension - Predisposing conditions - High-risk injury mechanism If x-ray is abnormal or inconclusive, then do CT C-spine. Patients with altered mental status, neurological deficits, and those who are intubated are at especially high risk and should undergo CT C-spine.
C-spine clearance	**Patients >8 years old:** NEXUS low-risk criteria[a] C-spine imaging indicated unless all of the following criteria met: - No midline cervical spine tenderness, no focal neurological deficit, no intoxication, no painful or distracting injury, normal level of alertness - Able to flex, extend, and rotate neck without pain

Continued

Table 2.12	Management of C-Spine in Trauma—cont'd
	Patients 3–8 years old: PECARN risk factors for CSI[b]
	C-spine imaging indicated for presence of any of following:
	- Altered LOC
	- Focal neurological findings
	- Neck pain
	- Torticollis
	- Substantial coexisting injury (especially torso injury)
	- Predisposing conditions (Down syndrome, Ehlers Danlos)
	- High-risk MVC
	- Diving
	Patients <3 years old: No validated tool. Relies heavily on physical examination

[a]NEXUS C-spine rule: Hoffman JR, Mower WR, Wolfson AB, et al. Validity of a set of clinical criteria to rule out injury to the cervical spine in patients with blunt trauma. National Emergency X-Radiography Utilization Study Group. *N Engl J Med.* 2000;343(2):94–99.

[b]PECARN: Risk Factors for pediatric C-spine injuries: Leonard JC, Kuppermann N, Olsen C, et al. Pediatric Emergency Care Applied Research Network. Factors associated with cervical spine injury in children after blunt trauma. *Ann Emerg Med.* 2011;58(2):145.

CSI, C-spine injury; *CT,* computed tomography; *LOC,* loss of consciousness; *MVC,* motor vehicle collision.

Box 2.6   Low-Risk Rule for Pelvic X-Rays

Pelvic x-rays can be omitted in children at low risk for fracture with a normal GCS and hemodynamic status and **NONE** of the following:
- Signs of abdominal trauma
- Abnormal pelvic examination/pain
- Associated femur fracture
- Hematuria

GCS, Glasgow Coma Scale.

Data from Haasz M, Simone LA, Wales PW, et al. Which pediatric blunt trauma patients do not require pelvic imaging? *J Trauma Acute Care Surg.* 2015;79(5):828–832.

Figure 2.10   PECARN Management Algorithm for Children With Minor Head Trauma (Age <2 Years [A] and ≥2 Years [B])

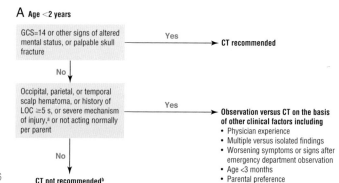

A Age <2 years

GCS=14 or other signs of altered mental status, or palpable skull fracture → **Yes** → CT recommended

No ↓

Occipital, parietal, or temporal scalp hematoma, or history of LOC ≥5 s, or severe mechanism of injury,[a] or not acting normally per parent → **Yes** → Observation versus CT on the basis of other clinical factors including
- Physician experience
- Multiple versus isolated findings
- Worsening symptoms or signs after emergency department observation
- Age <3 months
- Parental preference

No ↓

CT not recommended[b]

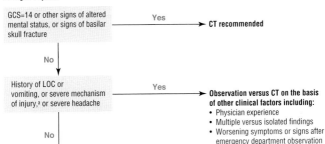

B Age ≥2 years

GCS=14 or other signs of altered mental status, or signs of basilar skull fracture — **Yes** → **CT recommended**

↓ No

History of LOC or vomiting, or severe mechanism of injury,[a] or severe headache — **Yes** → **Observation versus CT on the basis of other clinical factors including:**
- Physician experience
- Multiple versus isolated findings
- Worsening symptoms or signs after emergency department observation
- Parental preference

↓ No

CT not recommended[b]

[a]Severe mechanism of injury is defined as motor vehicle crash with patient ejection, death of another passenger, or rollover; pedestrian or bicyclist without helmet struck by a motorized vehicle; falls of more than 3 feet (A) or more than 5 feet (B); or head struck by a high-impact object. [b]As risk of ciTBI is exceedingly low and may be lower than risk of CT-induced malignancy, CT scans are not recommended for most patients in this group. *ciTBI*, Clinically important traumatic brain injury; *CT*, computed tomography; *GCS*, Glasgow Coma Scale. (A and B, Modified from Kuppermann N, Holmes JF, Dayan PS, et al. Identification of children at very low risk of clinically-important brain injuries after head trauma: a prospective cohort study. *Lancet*. 2009;374:1160.)

Box 2.7 The Canadian Assessment of Tomography for Childhood Head Injury 2 (CATCH2)

CT of the head is required for children with minor head injury[a] and any one of these findings:
- GCS score <15 at 2 h after injury
- Suspected open or depressed skull fracture
- History of worsening headache
- Irritability on examination
- Any sign of basal skull fracture[b]
- Large, boggy hematoma of the scalp
- Dangerous mechanism of injury[c]
- ≥4 episodes of vomiting

[a]Minor head injury is defined as injury within the past 24 h associated with witnessed loss of consciousness, definite amnesia, witnessed disorientation, persistent vomiting (>1 episode) or persistent irritability (in a child <2 years) in a patient with a GCS score of 13–15.
[b]Signs of basal skull fracture include hemotympanum, raccoon eyes, otorrhea or rhinorrhea of the cerebrospinal fluid, and Battle sign.
[c]Dangerous mechanism is a motor vehicle crash. A fall from an elevation ≥3 ft (≥91 cm) or five stairs, or a fall from a bicycle with no helmet.
CT, Computed tomography; *GCS*, Glasgow Coma Scale.
From Osmond MH, Klassen TP, Welss GA, et al. Validation and refinement of a clinical decision rule for the use of computed tomography in children with minor head injury in the emergency department. *CMAJ* 2018;190:816–822.

Box 2.8	Indications for CT Abdomen in Trauma

- Abnormal abdominal examination (peritonitis, distension, seatbelt sign, bruising)
- GCS <14 with blunt abdominal trauma
- Abnormal LFTs, amylase, or unexplained low hemoglobin
- Gross hematuria
- Positive FAST scan (free fluid)
- Pelvic fracture

CT, Computed tomography; *FAST*, focused assessment with sonography for trauma; *GCS*, Glasgow Coma Scale; *LFT*, liver function test.

SPECIFIC INJURIES IN PEDIATRIC TRAUMA

A. Closed head injury

1. **Definitions**
   a. **Minor head trauma:** GCS 14–15 (see Table 1.2 for GCS calculation)
   b. **Moderate head trauma:** GCS 9–13
   c. **Severe head trauma:** GCS ≤8
   d. **Signs of basal skull fracture**
      i. Hemotympanum
      ii. Raccoon eyes (periorbital ecchymosis)
      iii. CSF otorrhea
      iv. CSF rhinorrhea
      v. Battle sign (mastoid ecchymosis)

2. **Investigations**
   a. **Minor head injury:** two validated **clinical decision rules help guide decision for CT head**
      i. **PECARN rule** for findings associated with very low risk of significant traumatic brain injury, in which case CT head can be avoided (see Figure 2.10)
      ii. **CATCH2 rule** (Canadian Assessment of Tomography for Childhood Head Injury) for indications for CT head (see Box 2.7)
   b. **Moderate or severe head trauma:** patients should undergo cranial CT scan

3. **Management**
   a. Low-risk patients and those with a negative CT scan with only mild symptoms may be discharged home with appropriate reasons to return (worsening headache, vomiting, lethargy, neurological signs, etc.)
   b. Patients with negative CT scans, but ongoing severe symptoms, and those with abnormal CT scans should be admitted to hospital
   c. Patients with intracranial injury on CT scan need frequent neurological evaluation and may require treatments for increased ICP (see earlier) ± neurosurgical intervention

B. Concussion

1. **Definition:** characteristic symptoms and signs that individuals may experience after a closed traumatic brain injury. Acute clinical signs (headache, confusion, dizziness, light-headedness, nausea/vomiting, memory impairment, etc.) represent a functional, rather than structural, brain injury and are typically temporary.

2. **Management**
   a. Immediate removal from activity (if applicable)
   b. Rule out coexisting injuries
   c. Routine neuroimaging is not recommended unless there is concern for a structural injury (see above section on closed head injury)
   d. **Restriction of physical activity and neurocognitive rest**. A brief period of physical rest (24–48 hours) should be followed by a gradual and progressive return to regular activities as tolerated (Return to Learn and Return to Play protocols are available at www.parachutecanada.org).
   e. Follow-up with primary care provider

C. Cervical spine injury

1. Also see Chapter 13 Diagnostic Imaging
2. Rare; incidence in pediatric trauma is <2%, but when present, often severe
3. Age-related injury patterns: **upper cervical injuries in infants/ young children, mid-lower cervical injuries in older children/ adolescents**
4. Spinal cord injury without radiological abnormality (SCIWORA): neurological abnormalities without x-ray or CT findings; pathology often seen on MRI
5. No single validated rule exists for pediatric cervical spine clearance. Often considered age-dependent. See Table 2.12 for indications for C-spine x-ray imaging and management of C-spine in trauma.
6. CT imaging is selective rather than standard in pediatric trauma

D. Blunt thoracic injury

1. CXR is an adequate screen in almost all cases (CT not routinely required)
2. Pulmonary contusion is the most common injury
3. Absence of external signs of trauma does not rule out significant thoracic injury

E. Blunt abdominal injury

1. Most common cause of unrecognized hemorrhage in children after trauma
2. **Signs:** bruises in area of handlebar or seatbelt; abdominal tenderness/ distention, polytrauma with hemodynamic instability; up to one-quarter of children have normal examination

3. **Investigations**
   a. **FAST:** specific, but not sensitive; should not be used to rule out intraabdominal injury when there is clinical suspicion
   b. **CT scan:** see Box 2.8 for indications for abdominal CT scan. Note that a CT scan often misses hollow viscous injury. See references for further information on risk stratification (PECARN and PSRC clinical decision rules).
4. **Management:** usually treated conservatively unless hemodynamically unstable (<5% will need surgery)

FURTHER READING AND USEFUL REFERENCES

General

Fleisher GR, Ludwig S, eds. *Textbook of Pediatric Emergency Medicine.* 6th ed. Philadelphia, PA: Lippincott Williams & Wilkins; 2010.
Canadian Pediatric Society Position Statements: www.cps.ca.

Approach to Trauma

Advanced Trauma Life Support: Student Course Manual. 10th ed. Chicago, IL: American College of Surgeons Copyright 2018.

Head Injury

Kuppermann N, Holmes JF, Dayan PS, et al. Identification of children at very low risk of clinically-important brain injuries after head trauma: a prospective cohort study. *Lancet* 2009;374:1160.
Osmond MH, Klassen TP, Welss GA, et al. Validation and refinement of a clinical decision rule for the use of computed tomography in children with minor head injury in the emergency department. *CMAJ* 2018;190:816–822.

C-Spine Clearance

Hoffman JR, Mower WR, Wolfson AB, et al. Validity of a set of clinical criteria to rule out injury to the cervical spine in patients with blunt trauma. National Emergency X-Radiography Utilization Study Group. *N Engl J Med.* 2000;343(2):94–99.
Leonard JC, Kuppermann N, Olsen C, et al. Factors associated with cervical spine injury in children after blunt trauma. *Ann Emerg Med.* 2011;58(2):145.
Trauma Association of Canada Pediatric Subcommittee National Pediatric Cervical Spine Evaluation Pathway: Consensus Guidelines. *J Trauma*, 2011;70:873–884.

Blunt Abdominal Trauma

Haasz M, Simone LA, Wales PW, et al. Which pediatric trauma patients do not require pelvic imaging? *J Trauma Acute Care Surg* 2015;79(5):828.
Holmes JF, Lillith K, Monroe D, et al. Identifying children at very low risk of clinically important blunt abdominal injuries. *Ann Emerg Med.* 2013;62(2):107.
Streck CJ Vogel AM, Zhang J, et al. Identifying children at very low risk for blunt intra-abdominal injury in whom CT of the abdomen can be avoided safely. *J Am Coll Surg.* 2017;224(4):449–458.

Poisonings and Toxicology

Zamin Ladha • Elana Thau • Savithiri Ratnapalan

COMMON ABBREVIATIONS

Also see page xviii for a list of other abbreviations used throughout this book

AC	activated charcoal
ALI	acute lung injury
CO	carbon monoxide
DMPS	2, 3 dimercaptopropane-1-sulfonate
DMSA	dimercaptosuccinic acid
G6PD	glucose-6-phosphate dehydrogenase
GHB	gamma hydroxybutyrate
LOC	level of consciousness
LSD	lysergic acid diethylamide
MAOI	monoamine oxidase inhibitor
MDMA	3,4-methylenedioxymethamphetamine
MetHb	methemoglobin
OSM	osmolality
PaO_2	partial pressure of oxygen
PIC	Poison Information Centre
SSRI	selective serotonin reuptake inhibitor
TCA	tricyclic antidepressants
WBI	whole-bowel irrigation

USEFUL FORMULAS

1. **Anion gap**: $[Na^+] - ([Cl^-] + [HCO_3^-])$. Normal range ~8–12 mEq/L.
2. **Calculated osmolality**
   a. $[2(Na^+) + \text{glucose (mmol/L)}] + [\text{urea (mmol/L)}]$ mOsm/kg H_2O
   b. $[2(Na^+) + \text{glucose (mg/dL)}/18] + [\text{urea (mg/dL)}/2.8]$ mOsm/kg H_2O
3. **Osmolal gap:** Measured Osm – Calculated Osm (>10 mOsmol/kg is considered an elevated osmolal gap)

APPROACH TO THE POISONED CHILD

PEARL

Consider toxic exposure in children presenting with acutely altered mental status, respiratory or cardiac compromise, unexplained acidosis, or seizures.

A. Clinical evaluation

1. **Initial resuscitation and support**
   a. Ensure adequate resuscitation and stabilization of every potentially poisoned patient (see Chapter 1 Resuscitation)
   b. Contact local Poison Information Centre (PIC)

2. **Essential history** (may be provided, but can also be unknown or unwitnessed)
   a. Seven key questions: **who** (age, weight), **what**, **when**, **where**, **why** (intentional or accidental), **how** (route), **how much** (quantity). Some ingestions only cause toxicity at a certain mg/kg dose; however, others can cause substantial toxicity with minimal intake (Box 3.1).
   b. Medication history (past medical history and all substances available in the home)
   c. Thorough review of systems

PEARL

A thorough physical examination may identify a group of signs or symptoms (**toxidrome**) that points to a specific drug or classification of drugs (see Table 3.1).

3. **Physical examination**
   See Table 3.1
   a. **Eyes:** pupil size/reactivity (miosis = constricted pupils, mydriasis = dilated pupils), extra ocular movements
   b. **Mouth:** hydration of mucous membranes, corrosive lesions
   c. **Cardiovascular:** heart rate, blood pressure, rhythm, and perfusion
   d. **Respiratory:** respiratory rate, chest wall movement, air entry, and auscultatory signs
   e. **Gastrointestinal (GI):** motility and presence of bowel sounds, corrosive effects
   f. **Neurologic/Musculoskeletal:** speech, reflexes, muscle tone
   g. **Skin:** colour, burns, diaphoresis, temperature, flushing, and bullae
   h. **Odors:** breath, clothing

Box 3.1 Medications That Can Cause Significant Harm With Only One Dose ("One Pill Can Kill")	
α_2 Adrenergic agonists (e.g., clonidine)	Camphor
Sulfonylureas	Antimalarials (e.g., chloroquine)
Calcium channel blockers	Buprenorphine
β Blockers	Carbamates/organophosphates
Tricyclic antidepressants	Caustics
Opioids	Imidazolines
Toxic alcohols	

Table 3.1   Common Toxic Syndromes (Toxidromes)

Toxic Syndrome	Clinical Signs	Common Causes
Anticholinergic "mad as a hatter, red as a beet, blind as a bat, hot as a hare, dry as a bone"	Tachycardia, hypertension, hyperthermia, dry skin and mucus membranes, mydriasis, urinary retention, ↓ bowel sounds, delirium, hallucinations, mumbling speech, myoclonic jerking, seizures	Antidepressants (tricyclic agents), antihistamines (diphenhydramine), antipsychotic agents, atropine, scopolamine, antiparkinsonism medications (amantadine, benztropine), plants (Jimson weed)
Sympathomimetic	Tachycardia, hypertension, hyperthermia, diaphoresis, mydriasis, hyperreflexia, delusions, agitation, paranoia	Amphetamines, methamphetamines and derivatives (MDMA [ecstasy]), cocaine, decongestants (ephedrine), caffeine, theophylline, withdrawal from sedatives/hypnotics, may be mimicked by ASA toxicity or hypoglycemia
Cholinergic	DUMBELS mnemonic: - **D**iaphoresis, diarrhea - **U**rinary incontinence - **M**iosis - **B**ronchospasm, bronchorrhea, bradycardia - **E**mesis - **L**acrimation - **S**alivation	Organophosphate pesticides, carbamate pesticides, physostigmine, edrophonium, mushrooms (some), nerve gases
Sedative/hypnotic syndrome	Bradycardia, hypotension, variable pupils, hypothermia, ↓ bowel sounds, respiratory and CNS depression, coma, hyporeflexia	Clonidine, methyldopa, barbiturates (phenobarbital), benzodiazepines and other sedatives, hypnotics, ethanol
Hallucinogenic	Tachycardia, hypertension, hyperthermia, tachypnea, nystagmus, mydriasis, hallucinations, perceptual distortions, agitation	LSD, designer amphetamines MDMA (ecstasy), phencyclidine, mescaline
Opioid	Bradycardia, hypotension, hypothermia, bradypnea or apnea, miosis, CNS depression, coma, hyporeflexia	Heroin, morphine, methadone, oxycodone, hydromorphone, diphenoxylate
Serotonin syndrome	- Autonomic dysfunction: Tachycardia, hypertension, hyperthermia, tachypnea, diaphoresis - Altered mental status: confusion, agitation, coma - Neuromuscular excitation: tremors, myoclonus, hyperreflexia, clonus, rigidity	MAOI ± SSRIs, meperidine, dextromethorphan, TCAs, L-tryptophan

ASA, Acetyl salicylic acid; *CNS,* central nervous system; *LSD,* lysergic acid diethylamide; *MAOI,* monoamine oxidase inhibitor, *MDMA,* 3,4-methylenedioxymethamphetamine; *SSRI,* selective serotonin reuptake inhibitor; *TCA,* tricyclic antidepressant.

B. Investigations
1. Most helpful laboratory studies
   a. Bedside glucose
   b. ABG or VBG (acid–base status)
   c. Urea and creatinine (kidney function)
   d. Electrolytes to determine anion gap: $[Na^+] - ([Cl^-] + [HCO_3^-])$. Anion gap >12 mEq/L is considered elevated
   e. Serum osmolality and calculated osmolality to determine osmolar gap (see Useful Formulas above). Increased if >10 mOsm/kg H_2O; only useful if elevated; does not rule out toxic alcohol if within normal range.

See Box 3.2 for differential diagnosis of increased anion gap and osmolal gap

  PEARL

An electrocardiogram should be obtained for all patients for whom poisoning is being considered.

Box 3.2   Differential Diagnosis of Increased Anion Gap and Osmolar Gap

Increased Anion Gap "MUDPILE CATS"
- **M**ethanol
- **U**remia
- **D**iabetic ketoacidosis (also starvation and alcoholic ketoacidosis)
- **P**araldehyde, phenformin (also metformin), paracetamol (acetaminophen)
- **I**ron, isoniazid
- **L**actic acidosis (anything that causes hypotension, seizures)
- **E**thylene glycol
- **C**yanide, carbon monoxide
- **A**cetylsalicylic acid, aminoglycosides
- **T**oluene (gas sniffing)
- **S**olvents, Salicylates

Increased Osmolar Gap
1. **Alcohols**
   - Ethanol
   - Methanol
   - Ethylene glycol
   - Isopropyl alcohol
   - Propylene glycol
   - Acetone (not an alcohol)
2. **Sugars**
   - Mannitol
   - Sorbitol
3. **Lipids**
   - Hypertriglyceridemia
4. **Proteins**
   - Hypergammaglobulinemia

2. Additional laboratory studies to consider (case dependent)
   a. Blood work: CBC, INR, PTT, liver transaminases
   b. Urinalysis to screen for hemoglobin, myoglobin, crystalluria
   c. Urine pregnancy test
3. ECG to evaluate for arrhythmias and prolongation of PR, QT, and QRS intervals

! PITFALL

Do not await results of broad-spectrum toxicology screens to treat suspected poisonings.

4. **Toxicology screening**
   See Table 3.2 for a list of drugs detectable in urine and blood screens
   a. **Broad-spectrum toxicology screening of urine and blood** not **generally recommended**; most poisonings can be managed appropriately without extensive "tox screens"

 PEARL

Acetaminophen and salicylate levels should always be checked in unknown or possible overdose cases as they have few early clinical signs and require prompt intervention.

   b. **Limitations of toxicology screens**
      i. Ability to detect drug or metabolite is dependent on many factors (dose of drug, time and route of ingestion, sample source, analytic method, patient age, fat distribution, liver/kidney function, etc.)
      ii. A number of drugs are not detected by most routine toxicology panels (Box 3.3)
      iii. Cross-reactions occur between drugs with similar metabolites (e.g., dimenhydrinate and diphenhydramine cannot be distinguished)
   c. Toxicology laboratory/PIC can guide clinicians on availability of specific drug tests or levels

Table 3.2	Drugs Commonly Detectable in Blood and Urine Toxicology Screens
Blood	**Urine**[a]
• Volatiles (ethanol, methanol, isopropanol, ethylene glycol must be specifically requested) • Salicylates • Acetaminophen • Barbiturates • Benzodiazepines (qualitative; levels not available) • Antidepressants (tricyclic antidepressants, many false positives and specific levels NOT helpful for acute poisonings; lithium must be specifically requested)	• Opiates (heroin, morphine, codeine) • Barbiturates (specific immunoassay needed) • Benzodiazepines (specific immunoassay needed) • Antidepressants (amitriptyline; many false positives) • Antipsychotics (chlorpromazine) • Stimulants (cocaine, amphetamines) • Hallucinogens (phencyclidine; cannabinoids require specific immunoassay) • Cough/cold remedies • Antihistamines (dimenhydrinate/diphenhydramine) • Some cardiac drugs (verapamil)

[a]Although these substances can be detectable by some assays, few are routinely done and none will affect the care of the acutely poisoned patient.

Box 3.3	Drugs Not Commonly Detected in Routine Blood or Urine Tox Panels

MDMA (ecstasy)	LSD
Methamphetamine	Synthetic cannabanoids
Ketamine	Tryptamines
GHB	Designer amphetamines

GHB, Gamma hydroxybutarate; *LSD*, lysergicacid diethlamide; *MDMA*, 3,4-methylenedioxymethamphetamine.

APPROACH TO DETOXIFICATION

A. Decontamination

1. **Surface decontamination**
   a. **Skin**
      i. Remove contaminated clothing and jewellery
      ii. Flush exposed areas with copious amounts of lukewarm water or 0.9% NaCl for a minimum of 20 minutes starting with area of contamination
   b. **Eyes**
      i. Remove contact lenses
      ii. Flush exposed eye with copious lukewarm water or 0.9% NaCl ($\geq$1 L/eye). Consider use of topical anesthetic drops.
      iii. If exposure to acid or base, continue irrigation until pH of ocular surface is normal (pH 6.5–7.5)
      iv. Refer to ophthalmologist if any abnormalities of cornea/conjunctiva or if exposure to basic (alkaline) substance
   c. **Inhalation**
      i. Remove from source of exposure
      ii. Provide supplemental humidified oxygen
      iii. Watch for worsening cardiorespiratory status (tachypnea, dyspnea, stridor, hoarse voice)

> **✦ PEARL**
>
> Activated charcoal should ideally be used in the first hour following ingestion. It is *not recommended* for **g**lycols, **a**lcohols, **m**etals, **e**lectrolytes (GAME).

2. **GI decontamination** ("get the poison out")
See Table 3.3

Table 3.3	Gastrointestinal Decontamination		
Treatment	**Mechanism of Action**	**Indications/ Contraindications**	**Administration**
Single-dose AC	Highly adsorbent powder that adsorbs toxins	- Within 1 h of potentially toxic ingestion; considered later depending on clinical scenario. - Most drugs - Exceptions: **g**lycols, **a**lcohols, **m**etals (e.g., iron, lead, lithium mercury, arsenic), **e**lectrolytes (Na$^+$, K$^+$), corrosives, hydrocarbons - Contraindications: Risk of aspiration (unprotected airway), GI tract obstruction, perforation. Rarely worth fighting with patient to take	1g/kg PO or by NG tube if unknown amount of toxin; Adult dose: 50 g
WBI	Administration of osmotically balanced polyethylene glycol solution to induce liquid stools and flush toxin out of GI tract	- Consider if large amounts of highly toxic sustained-release/enteric-coated products; toxins poorly adsorbed by charcoal (iron); body packing of illicit drugs - Contraindications: GI obstruction/perforation, unprotected airway, intractable vomiting	Polyethylene glycol (PEG)-electrolyte via NG, until rectal effluent clear - 9 months to 6 years: up to 500 mL/h - 6–12 years: up to 1000 mL/h - Adolescents/adults: up to 1500–2000 mL/h
Gastric lavage	Placement of OG tube to instill/ aspirate small volumes of fluid to aspirate toxin from stomach	- Consider if recent ingestion of ++ toxic substance - Contraindications: Unprotected airway, high aspiration potential, GI hemorrhage/ perforation	*Not* recommended for routine use for any ingestion

AC, Activated charcoal; *GI*, gastrointestinal; *NG*, nasogastric; *OG*, orogastric; *PO*, orally; *WBI*, whole-bowel irrigation.

B. Enhanced elimination

See Table 3.4

Table 3.4	Common Methods for Enhanced Elimination of Poisons		
Treatment	**Indications**	**Contraindications**	**Dose**
Multidose AC	Life-threatening ingestion of: carbamazepine, dapsone, phenobarbital, quinine, theophylline	Unprotected airway, risk of aspiration, GI tract obstruction or perforation	Consult PIC or local drug formulary for dosing; IV antiemetic to prevent vomiting
Urinary alkalization	Salicylates (First-line treatment in moderate–severe salicylate poisoning), severe methotrexate, chlorpropamide poisoning, phenobarbital, selected other poisonings (consult local PIC)	- Renal failure, pulmonary edema, cerebral edema - Caution with fluid overload if preexisting cardiac disease	- 1–2 mEq/kg NaHCO$_3$ bolus followed by continuous infusion: 150 mEq NaHCO$_3$ in 1 L D5W at 1.5–2 × maintenance. - Add 40 mEq KCl/L to maintain K$^+$ ≥4.0. - q2h monitoring of urine pH (goal 7.5–8.5), urine output, serum pH (goal 7.45–7.55), K$^+$, toxin in question. - Insert Foley catheter
Hemodialysis	- Toxic alcohols (ethylene glycol, methanol), lithium, salicylates, valproic acid, theophylline. - Consider in severe poisoning/ poisoning refractory to initial management	Hemodynamic instability, lack of specialized equipment and expertise	

AC, Activated charcoal; *GI,* gastrointestinal; *IV,* intravenous; *PIC,* Poison Information Centre.

 PEARL

Your local poison information center can provide guidance for correct antidote usage and dosing.

C. Antidotes

See Table 3.5

1. Empiric antidotes commonly used during the initial life support phase: **Oxygen** for hypoxia, **glucose** for hypoglycemia, **naloxone** for possible narcotic exposure.

2. Drug-specific antidotes are typically given after patient has been stabilized and a diagnosis has been made.

Table 3.5	Recommended Antidotes in Pediatric Poisoning
Poisoning	**Antidote**
Acetaminophen	NAC
Anticholinergics	Physostigmine
Benzodiazepines	Flumazenil (NOT routinely recommended)[a]
Calcium channel blockers	Calcium gluconate and calcium chloride
Carbon monoxide	100% oxygen; hyperbaric oxygen in severe cases
Cholinergic agents (pesticides)	Atropine Pralidoxime
Cyanide	Hydroxycobalamin (or sodium nitrite + sodium thiosulfate); oxygen
Digoxin	Digoxin immune Fab
Ethylene glycol	Fomepizole (or ethanol)
Hypoglycemics (insulin oral hypoglycemics)	Dextrose (0.5–1.0 g/kg/dose)
Iron	Deferoxamine
Mercury	DMSA DMPS
Methanol	Fomepizole (or ethanol)
Methemoglobin	Methylene blue (contraindicated in G6PD deficiency)
Opiates	Naloxone
Oral hypoglycemic (sulfonylurea)	Octreotide
Tricyclic antidepressants	Sodium bicarbonate
Salicylates	Sodium bicarbonate
Warfarin	Vitamin K

Consult your local poison information center or clinical pharmacist for dosing.
[a]Can precipitate seizures or arrhythmias.

DMPS, 2,3 Dimercaptopropane-1-sulfonate; *DMSA*, dimercaptosuccinic acid; *G6PD*, glucose-6-phosphate dehydrogenase; *NAC*, n-Acetyl cysteine.

SELECTED POISONINGS

See Table 3.6 for clinical presentation and management of selected poisonings
See Figure 3.1 for acetaminophen nomogram

(Text continued on page 86)

Figure 3.1 Semilogarithmic Plot of Plasma Acetaminophen Versus Time

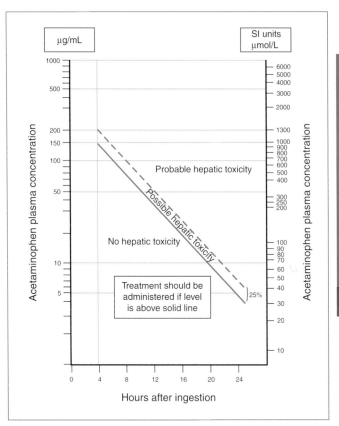

The solid blue line represents the treatment line, the level at which N-acetylcysteine therapy is indicated. (Data from Rumack BH, Matthew H. Acetaminophen poisoning and toxicity. *Pediatrics.* 1975;55:871–876.)

Table 3.6	**Selected Poisonings, Clinical Presentation, Workup, and Management**		
Toxin/Exposure	**Clinical Presentation**	**Key Investigations**	**Management**

Acetaminophen
Toxic dose: >200 mg/kg in children, >7.5 g in large children and adults
	Stage I: 0.5–24 h
	- Asymptomatic, nausea, vomiting, lethargy, pallor, diaphoresis, malaise; rarely change in LOC
	Stage II: 24–72 h
	- Initial symptoms resolve: RUQ pain, liver enlargement/tenderness; ↑AST/ALT, bilirubin, INR; oliguria, renal function abnormalities
	Stage III: 72–96 h
	- Stage I symptoms reappear; jaundice, encephalopathy; peak elevation of AST/ALT, coagulation defects, lactic acidosis, hypoglycemia; acute renal failure; death
	Stage IV: 4 days to 2 weeks
	- Symptoms resolve, liver/renal function normalize
		- Obtain 4 h postingestion acetaminophen level, plot on Rumack-Matthew nomogram (see Figure 3.1)
		- Baseline electrolytes, glucose, urea, creatinine, liver transaminases, INR
		- Repeat acetaminophen level, liver transaminases, INR at regular intervals per PIC recommendations
			1. Administer AC
			2. NAC:
			  a. Indications:
			    i. A 4 h or greater level above the possible hepatotoxic line on nomogram (see Figure 3.1)
			    ii. History of ingestion of >200 mg/kg and no level available ever
			    iii. History of ingestion of >200 mg/kg and presentation >8–10 h; start empirically and stop if level below the line once available
			    iv. Presentation >24 h postingestion with detectable acetaminophen level and evidence of hepatotoxicity
			  b. *Ontario IV protocol* for acute ingestion[a]
			    i. Standard protocol: 60 mg/kg/h × 4 h followed by 6 mg/kg/h until advised to stop by poison center
			    ii. High risk protocol: 60 mg/kg/h × 4 h followed by 12 mg/kg/h until advised to stop by poison center
			  c. Consult PIC for dosing in delayed overdose presentations
			  d. Outcome excellent if NAC started within 8–10 h of ingestion; treatment initiated >8 h postingestion beneficial, but effectiveness diminishes with time

Barbiturates and Anticonvulsants	- CNS depression: lethargy, ataxia, slurred speech, nystagmus - Respiratory depression (apnea, hypoxia), hypotension - Other: delirium, bullous skin lesions, hypothermia	Stat and serial anticonvulsant levels if available (peak often delayed by 24–48 h)	1. Support ventilation, circulation; watch for seizures, arrhythmias 2. Consider AC 3. Consider multidose AC for phenobarbital, carbamazepine (see Table 3.4) 4. Consider urinary alkalinization (see Table 3.4) for phenobarbital 5. Consider dialysis for carbamazepine, valproic acid, phenobarbital

Calcium Channel Blockers	- Hypotension, bradycardia, dysrhythmias, noncardiogenic pulmonary edema, coma, seizures (severe)
	- Hyperglycemia, metabolic acidosis
		- ECG: PR prolongation, bradyarrhythmia
		- Continuous cardiorespiratory monitoring
		- Electrolytes (especially K^+, Ca^{2+}), glucose, urea, creatinine, ABG
		- CXR if signs of pulmonary edema
			1. GI decontamination
			  a. AC is preferred method
			  b. Consider WBI for large ingestions of sustained-release preparations (see Table 3.3)
			2. IV fluid resuscitation
			3. Specific drugs and antidotes
			  a. 10% $CaCl_2$ 20 mg/kg IV OR 10% calcium gluconate 60 mg/kg IV slow push for symptomatic hypotension/bradycardia
			  b. If response to Ca^{2+}, repeat bolus or continuous infusion
			  c. High-dose regular insulin (0.5–1.0 units/kg IV bolus followed by 0.5–1.0 units/kg/h infusion, titrating as necessary) if inadequate response to aforementioned measures (frequent glucose checks, may require glucose infusion)
			  d. Vasopressors and inotropes for hypotension unresponsive to aforementioned treatments
			  e. Consider intralipids (consult PIC)

Insecticides (Organophosphates)	- Cholinergic signs muscarinic: DUMBELS, see Table 3.1; nicotinic: weakness, muscle fasciculations, - CNS signs (coma, convulsions), respiratory insufficiency		1. Airway management/suctioning 2. AC once airway secured 3. Surface decontamination 4. Atropine 0.05 mg/kg IV (1–5 mg/dose); double dose q5min until bronchial secretions dry, wheezing stops (if no IV access, give IM, then start an infusion (10%–20% of total dose needed/h) 5. Pralidoxime 20–50 mg/kg/dose (max 2g) IV slowly; repeat dose and/or continuous infusions may be necessary 6. Benzodiazepines for seizures

Continued

Poisonings and Toxicology

3

Table 3.6　Selected Poisonings, Clinical Presentation, Workup, and Management—cont'd

Toxin/Exposure	Clinical Presentation	Key Investigations	Management

Iron
- Elemental iron: 33% in ferrous fumarate; 20% in ferrous sulfate; 12% in ferrous gluconate
- Potentially toxic dose: 20–60 mg/kg elemental iron
- Highly toxic dose: >60 mg/kg
- Lethal dose: 60–300 mg/kg
	- *Gastrointestinal phase* (30 min–6 h): direct injury to GI mucosa; vomiting, bloody diarrhea, abdominal pain, hypotension, shock, metabolic acidosis
	- *Quiescent phase* (6–24 h): resolution of GI symptoms; may not be seen in severe poisoning
	- *Delayed phase* (4 h to 4 days): abrupt relapse with multiple organ failure: shock, profound metabolic acidosis, coagulopathy, hepatic dysfunction, renal failure, pulmonary failure, CNS dysfunction
	- *Hepatotoxicity* (within 4 days): coma, coagulopathy, jaundice
	- *Bowel obstruction* (2–8 weeks): GI scarring ± obstruction, classically at gastric outlet
		- Serum iron concentration at 4–6 h
		- CBC, electrolytes, urea, creatinine, blood gas, liver enzymes, glucose, INR, PTT type and crossmatch
		- Abdominal x-ray (looking for radiopaque pills)
			1. Supportive care for nausea, vomiting, diarrhea, fluid loss
			2. GI decontamination: WBI if tablets seen on x-ray (see Table 3.3)
			3. If asymptomatic, normal laboratory values, and ingested <20 mg/kg, may discharge home; otherwise, observe for at least 8 h
			4. Deferoxamine indicated if any of the following (call PIC for dosing):
			  a. Severe symptoms: altered mental status, hemodynamic instability, persistent vomiting and/or diarrhea
			  b. Serum iron level >90 μmol/L (>500 mcg/dL); brief chelation may be necessary if level 63–90 μmol/L (300–500 mcg/dL) and symptomatic
			  c. Iron level not available and >60 mg/kg elemental iron ingested and symptomatic
			  d. Anion gap metabolic acidosis

Opiates and Opioids (Narcotics) (e.g., morphine, heroin, codeine, hydrocodone, fentanyl, meperidine, methadone, dextromethorphan)	- Mild to moderate: sedation, miosis, hypotension, bradycardia, flushing, nausea - Severe: respiratory depression, apnea, coma, ALI - Seizures: rare, but may occur with meperidine and dextromethorphan ingestions	- Positive response to naloxone (consider qualitative urine screen for verification and identification of coingestions)	1. Airway/ventilatory support 2. AC 3. Naloxone 0.1 kg/kg/dose IV/ETT (max 2 mg/dose); repeat prn to maintain reversal; contact PIC for continuous naloxone infusion 4. Infants/young children requiring naloxone, patients symptomatic from long-acting opioids (e.g., methadone), and those with any recurrence of symptoms at 2–3 h should be admitted to hospital

Salicylates - Sources include ASA, salicylic acid, bismuth salicylate, methyl salicylate (oil of wintergreen) - Toxic dose of ASA: >150 mg/kg - Lethal dose: >500 mg/kg - Oil of wintergreen: 1 mL = 1.4 g ASA - Most patients show signs intoxication when plasma concentration >2.9–3.6 mmol/L	- Common symptoms: tachypnea, nausea, vomiting, diaphoresis, tinnitus - Severe cases: tachycardia, hyperthermia, hyperventilation, lethargy, confusion - May progress to convulsions, coma, ALI, and death	- Blood glucose (usually low) - INR (elevated); lactate (elevated) - VBG/ABG: initially can see mixed picture of respiratory alkalosis and metabolic acidosis; as condition progresses metabolic acidosis becomes primary abnormality - CBC, electrolytes, urea, creatinine, Ca^{2+}, acetaminophen level - Serum salicylate level on presentation and q2h until peak and declining × 2 - Urine pH and ketones - VBG/ABG and electrolytes q1h while alkalinization therapy in progress	1. AC, consider multiple doses 2. Supplemental glucose as needed 3. Volume resuscitation; add KCl once voided/catheterize if needed 4. Airway intervention (if required) followed by hyperventilation (iatrogenic respiratory alkalosis) → decreases brain salicylate levels, cerebral edema 5. Urinary alkalinization: $NaHCO_3$ 1–2 mEq/kg IV bolus, then start infusion (150 mEq $NaHCO_3$ in 1L D5W) at 1.5–2 times maintenance IV fluid rate. Add 40 mEq/L KCl to maintain K ≥ 4.0. Titrate to normal urine output and urine pH 7.5–8.5. Indicated if any of the following: a. Symptomatic ingestion (other than tinnitus) if level not available b. Acute ingestion and a salicylate level of >3.5 mmol/L c. Metabolic acidosis 6. Hemodialysis indicated for sick patients unable to undergo alkalinization (cerebral edema, renal failure), failure of alkalinization after 2 h of therapy, clinical deterioration/refractory acidosis despite appropriate supportive care or critical salicylate levels (>7.2 mmol/L acute; >5.0 mmol/L chronic)

Continued

Table 3.6 Selected Poisonings, Clinical Presentation, Workup, and Management—cont'd

Toxin/Exposure	Clinical Presentation	Key Investigations	Management

Toxic Alcohols	- *Methanol:* retinal injury, visual disturbances (blurring, central scotomata), blindness, abdominal pain and vomiting, metabolic acidosis
	- *Ethylene glycol:* flank pain, hematuria, oliguria, renal failure, metabolic acidosis
	- *Both:* inebriation, hyperventilation (Kussmaul), seizures, coma, death
		- Stat serum ethylene glycol, methanol, ethanol levels
		- Electrolytes, blood gas, glucose, urea, creatinine, amylase, serum osmolality, Ca^{2+}, urinalysis
		- Anion gap (latent period up to 40 h for methanol, 4–24 h for ethylene glycol)
		- Osmolal gap (increased early, disappears as toxic alcohol is metabolized)
			1. Consider gastric lavage if early
			2. Fomepizole (preferred antidote): 15 mg/kg loading dose. Repeat dosing per PIC guidelines.
			3. Ethanol infusion (second-line antidote); consult local PIC for dosing
			4. Cofactor therapy (adjunctive to antidotal therapy):
			  a. Methanol ingestion: Folic acid
			  b. Ethylene glycol ingestion: Pyridoxine and thiamine
			5. Hemodialysis indicated if:
			  a. Evidence of end-organ damage (any degree of visual impairment, renal failure, or high anion gap metabolic acidosis)
			  b. Other indications for hemodialysis should be reviewed with PIC and nephrology

| Tricyclic Antidepressants (e.g., amitriptyline, imipramine) | Three major toxic syndromes:
- Anticholinergic (see Table 3.1)
- CNS: confusion, delirium, hallucinations, hyperreflexia: late—seizures, obtundation, coma
- Cardiovascular: tachycardia, hypotension, QRS prolongation (>100 ms), ventricular arrhythmias; hallmark ECG pattern: deep S wave in I, aVR and tall R wave in aVL | Cardiac monitor × 24 h, and hourly ECGs until 6 h after ingestion | 1. Administer AC if stable
2. Fluid resuscitation for hypotension
3. Sodium bicarbonate for hypotension, prolonged QRS, arrhythmias: $NaHCO_3$ 1–2 mEq/kg IV bolus (repeat as necessary), then titrate infusion (150 mEq $NaHCO_3$ in 1 L D5W) to QRS duration and serum pH 7.45–7.55
4. Vasopressors for refractory hypotension: norepinephrine first line
5. Consider lidocaine for refractory arrhythmias
6. Treat seizures with benzodiazepines (phenobarbital as second line)
7. Consider intralipids; contact local PIC for dosing |

[a]NAC dosing regimens, starting criteria in situations different from the acute one time overdose, the stopping criteria, and the duration of treatment vary across the US and Canada. Clinicians should always consult their local PIC before starting a NAC protocol.

ABG, Arterial blood gas; *AC*, activated charcoal; *ALI*, acute lung injury; *ALT*, alanine transaminase; *ASA*, acetyl salicylic acid; *AST*, aspartate transaminase; *CBC*, complete blood count; *CNS*, central nervous system; *CXR*, chest x-ray; *ECG*, electrocardiogram; *ETT*, endotracheal tube; *GI*, gastrointestinal; *IM*, intramuscular; *INR*, international normalized ratio; *IV*, intravenous; *LOC*, level of consciousness; *NAC*, n-Acetyl cysteine; *PIC*, Poison Information Centre; *PR*, *prn*, as needed; *PTT*, partial thromboplastin time; *RUQ*, right upper quadrant; *VBG*, venous blood gas; *WBI*, whole-bowel irrigation.

See Table 3.7

Table 3.7	Common Environmental Contaminants, Presentation, and Management	
Substance	**Clinical Presentation**	**Management**
Carbon monoxide (smoke inhalation, combustion, appliances, car exhaust)	- PaO_2 and SaO_2 likely normal - Young age: fussiness, feeding difficulty - 20% COHb: headache, dyspnea, confusion - 20%–40% COHb: Drowsiness, nausea, vomiting - 40%–60% COHb: weakness, incoordination, imminent neuro and cardiovascular collapse - >60% COHb: coma, convulsions, death	- Remove from contaminated environment - ECG in all patients - Carboxyhemoglobin (COHb) level - Provide 100% supplemental O_2 - Consider hyperbaric oxygen for COHb >25%, loss of consciousness, pH < 7.1, or end-organ damage

Lead (paint, gasoline, folk remedies, cosmetics)	- Headache, abdominal pain, constipation, poor appetite
	- *Severe:* loss of milestones, poor coordination, hearing loss, renal insufficiency; lead encephalopathy: ataxia, persistent vomiting, lethargy, stupor, coma, seizures
		- Venous lead level, CBC (microcytic anemia), reticulocyte, serum iron, TIBC, ferritin, abdominal XR ("lead flecks")
		- Based on lead level[a]:
		  - <0.24 μmol/L (<5 mcg/dL): no treatment
		  - 0.24–2.12 μmol/L (5–44 mcg/dL): remove environmental lead sources, follow levels
		  - >2.17 μmol/L (≥45 mcg/dL) Acute lead poisoning toxic level in pediatric population: immediate medical evaluation, consider treatment with chelation therapy, especially if symptomatic (discuss with PIC)
		  - >19 years: >3.38 μmol/L (>70 mcg/dL) is critical value requiring consideration of chelation
		- Chelating agents: dimercaprol (BAL), calcium disodium edetate, succimer (DMSA). Consult PIC/refer local drug dosing guidelines.

BAL, British antilewisite; *CBC*, complete blood count; *DMSA*, dimercaptosuccinic acid; *ECG*, electrocardiogram; *PaO₂*, partial pressure of oxygen; *PIC*, Poison Information Centre; *SaO₂*, oxygen saturation; *TIBC*, total iron binding capacity; *XR*, x-ray.
[a]https://www.cps.ca/en/documents/position/lead-toxicity#ref16

SUBSTANCES OF ABUSE (RECREATIONAL DRUGS)

See Table 3.8

Table 3.8	Common Substances of Abuse, Presentation and Management	
Substance	**Clinical Presentation**	**Management**

Amphetamines ("speed," "crystal meth," Ritalin, ephedrine) and synthetic cathiones ("bath salts")	- Sympathomimetic toxidrome (see Table 3.1)
	- Other:
	  - Hallucinations, seizures, coma, myoclonus
	  - Rhabdomyolysis,
	  - Electrolyte abnormalities, renal injury
		- AC benzodiazepines for agitation, seizures, hypertension
		- Aggressive cooling
		- Short-acting IV antihypertensives for refractory hypertension
		- Avoid β-blockers
		- Monitoring of sodium and glucose

Cocaine	- Sympathomimetic toxidrome (see Table 3.1)
	- Other:
	  - Cardiac ischemia, arrhythmias
	  - Seizures, focal neurological deficits, coma, stroke
	  - Respiratory distress, airway disease, pulmonary infarctions
	  - Perforated intestinal ulcers
	  - Rhabdomyolysis
		- Judicious use of benzodiazepines for seizures, hypertension, and/or agitation
		- Aggressive cooling
		- Short-acting IV antihypertensives for refractory hypertension
		- Serial ECGs and cardiac enzymes, if chest pain
		- Avoid β-blockers and succinylcholine

MDMA ("ecstasy," "M," "E," "love drug," "rave drug")	- Sympathomimetic and hallucinogenic toxidromes (see Table 3.1)
	- Other:
	  - Euphoria, increased alertness, hyperactivity, anxiety, hallucinations, delirium, seizures, cerebrovascular accident
	  - Hyponatremia
	  - Rhabdomyolysis
	  - Hepatotoxicity
	  - Serotonin syndrome: autonomic dysfunction, neuromuscular hyperactivity, altered mental status
		- Single-dose AC if recent ingestion
		- Benzodiazepines for hyperthermia, agitation, hypertension, and/or seizures
		- Cautious fluid resuscitation (check serum Na); tachycardia cannot be used as a sign of dehydration
		- Aggressive cooling
		- 3% NaCl for severe, symptomatic hyponatremia
		- Avoid β-blockers

Ethanol (a child not used to exposure may get serious toxic effects with as little as 10–15 mL/kg beer, 4–6 mL/kg wine, 1–2 mL/kg 80-proof liquor)	- *Mild:* sedation, impaired judgment, slurred speech, ataxia - *Moderate:* hypotension, hypothermia, respiratory distress, coma hypoglycemia, hypokalemia - *Severe:* death in 50% hypoglycemia, metabolic acidosis, increased osmolar gap	- Consider AC only if suspect drug coingestion - Treat hypoglycemia, hypokalemia - Consider hemodialysis if ethanol level >110 mmol/L (>500 mg/dL)

Continued

Table 3.8	Common Substances of Abuse, Presentation and Management—cont'd	
Substance	**Clinical Presentation**	**Management**
GHB	- Bradycardia, hypotension, hypothermia, bradypnea - Dose-dependent CNS depression, ataxia, agitation, amnesia, seizures, coma, and death - Miosis, nystagmus	- Supportive care - Benzodiazepines for seizures
Heroin	See Table 3.1	
Ketamine ("special K")	- Low dose: tachycardia, hypertension - High dose (>5 mg/kg): tachycardia and hypertension; OR bradycardia and hypotension if severely catecholamine depleted - Respiratory depression, apnea, laryngospasm, salivation - Dissociative anesthetic, analgesia, amnesia, nystagmus, hallucinations, myoclonic jerks, rhabdomyolysis	- Respiratory support - Atropine for bradycardia - Frequent suctioning - Benzodiazepines for tachycardia, psychomotor agitation

LSD ("acid") and other Hallucinogens	- Hallucinogenic toxidrome (Table 3.1)
	- Other:
	  - Psychosis, seizures
	  - Rhabdomyolysis
		- Benzodiazepines for seizures and/or anxiety
		- Otherwise treat as per sympathomimetic

Cannabis (Marijuana)	- Sleepiness, euphoria, irritability - Tachycardia, hypertension, - Nausea, vomiting, conjunctival injection, nystagmus, ataxia, slurred speech, dry mouth, ↑ appetite - Coma	- Benzodiazepines for psychotic reactions/acute delirium - Observation: general improvement in 4–6 h - For coma, consider naloxone to exclude opioid ingestion; duration 1–2 days with full recovery expected

AC, Activated charcoal; *CNS*, central nervous system; *ECG*; electrocardiogram; *GHB*, gamma hydroxybutyrate; *IV*, intravenous; *LSD*, lysergic acid diethylamide; *MDMA*, 3,4-methylenedioxymethamphetamine.

METHEMOGLOBINEMIA

1. **Pathophysiology**
   a. Increased amounts of methemoglobin (MetHb): a form of hemoglobin in which iron is oxidized to the ferric (Fe^{3+}) state, rendering it unable to reversibly bind oxygen
   b. Oxygen affinity of remaining ferrous (Fe^{2+}) hemoglobin is increased; hemoglobin-dissociation curve is left shifted, and oxygen delivery to tissues is impaired

2. **Etiology**
   a. Congenital
   b. Acquired: Ingestion or topical exposure to oxidizing drugs or chemicals (benzocaine, lidocaine, dapsone, sulphonamides, chloroquine, nitrates)
3. **Clinical presentation**
   a. Should be suspected when **cyanosis is present in setting of normal arterial PaO$_2$**; or when cyanosis occurs in the absence of obvious pulmonary or cardiac disease and **does not respond to oxygen therapy**
   b. Symptoms depend on the amount of MetHb and % of total haemoglobin in the blood:
      i. <20% MetHb: generally asymptomatic, unless preexisting condition (anemia)
      ii. 20%–50% MetHb: cyanosis, headache, fatigue, dyspnea, lethargy
      iii. >50% MetHb: respiratory depression, altered consciousness, shock, seizures, death
4. **Investigations**
   a. ABG: PaO$_2$ normal despite presence of cyanosis or decreased O$_2$ saturation measured via pulse oximetry (SpO$_2$)
   b. **MetHb detection by co-oximetry**; confirm with Evelyn-Malloy method
5. **Treatment:** Major goals are to removal of causative agent, optimize end organ oxygenation and promote reduction of MetHb back to Hb
   a. Asymptomatic: no active treatment other than removal of causative agent
   b. Symptomatic patients, or those with MetHb >20% should be treated:
      i. Symptomatic and no history glucose-6-phosphate dehydrogenase (G6PD) deficiency: intravenous methylene blue (1–2 mg/kg IV over 5 minutes; may repeat q30–60 min if necessary)
      ii. Symptomatic and known/suspected G6PD deficiency: ascorbic acid
   c. Consider blood transfusion or exchange transfusion if patient in shock

> **! PITFALL**
>
> Methylene blue should not be used in glucose-6-phosphate dehydrogenase deficiency because it may be ineffective and can induce hemolysis.

FURTHER READING

Nelson LS, Hoffman RS, Howland MA, et al, eds. *Goldfrank's Toxicologic Emergencies*. 11th ed. New York, NY: McGraw-Hill; 2019.

Klaasen CD, ed. *Casarett and Doull's Toxicology: The Basic Science of Poisons*. 8th ed. New York, NY: McGraw-Hill; 2013.

Olson KR, ed. *Poisoning & Drug Overdose*. 7th ed. New York, NY: Lange Medical Books/McGraw-Hill; 2018.

USEFUL WEBSITES

Agency for Toxic Substances and Disease Registry. Available at: http://www.atsdr.cdc.gov.

American Academy of Clinical Toxicology. Available at: http://www.clintox.org.

TOXNET Toxicology Data Network from US National Library of Medicine. Available at: https://www.nlm.nih.gov/toxnet/.

Toxic Plant Index. Available at: http://chppm-www.apgea.army.mil/ento/plntndx.htm.

The Vaults of Erowid (information about psychoactive plants and chemicals). Available at: http://www.erowid.org.

Pain and Sedation

Tahira Daya • Lisa Isaac

COMMON ABBREVIATIONS

Also see page xviii for a list of other abbreviations used throughout this book

PCA   patient-controlled analgesia
NSAID   nonsteroidal antiinflammatory drug

PAIN ASSESSMENT

See Figure 4.1

Figure 4.1 Pain Assessment and Management of the Child

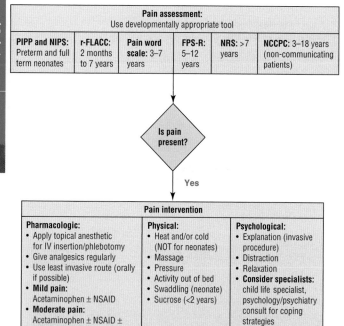

FPS-R, Faces Pain Scale—Revised; *IV*, intravenous; *NCCPC*, noncommunicating children's pain checklist; *NIPS*, Neonatal Infant Pain Scale; *NRS*, Numeric Rating Scale; *NSAID*, nonsteroidal antiinflammatory drug; *PIPP*, premature infant pain profile; *r-FLACC*, revised—Faces Legs Activity Cry Consolability. (Adapted from The Hospital for Sick Children eFormulary: Sedation and Analgesia Guidelines, 2019.)

A. General principles of assessment
1. Obtain pain history from child and/or parents
2. Assess children based on developmental level, situation, and context (e.g., a child may be crying because a toy was taken away, not necessarily because of pain)
3. Assess pain routinely and regularly to tailor therapy; tools and results must be charted

B. Vital signs
1. Physiologic measures (e.g., heart rate, respiratory rate, blood pressure) can be used as adjuncts to self-reported and behavioral observations but are NOT sensitive or specific indicators of chronic pain
2. Vital signs should be interpreted in context of the situation (e.g., if the patient has a fever, they may also have tachycardia)

 PEARL

Developmentally typical children ≥4 years can self-report pain and those ≥7 to 8 years can use numeric scale reporting.

C. Pain assessment tools
1. Self-report tools should be used whenever possible
2. Behavioral observation tools (e.g., vocalization, facial expression, motor response, activity, appearance) can be used with preverbal/nonverbal children and as adjuncts to older children's self-report

D. Pain scales
Many different scales are available based on age and developmental level (see Figure 4.1)
1. **PIPP** (premature infant pain profile) and **NIPS** (Neonatal Infant Pain Scale) are used for neonates and use mainly objective markers, including changes in vital signs, to assess pain
2. **r-FLACC** (revised—Face, Legs, Activity, Cry, Consolability) is commonly used between ages 2 months and 7 years
3. **Verbal Rating Scale** uses words (from no pain at all to extremely intense pain) instead of numbers to describe pain levels and is typically used between ages 3 and 7 years
4. **FPS-R, Faces** pain scale, revised (https://www.iasp-pain.org/resources/faces-pain-scale-revised/?ItemNumber=1519) is frequently used between ages 5 and 12 years

5. **NRS** (Numerical Rating Scale) involves selecting a number between 0 (no pain) and 10 (worst pain) to reflect the intensity of the pain and is commonly used above the age of 7 years

6. **NCCPC** (Noncommunicating Children's Pain Checklist) is designed for pain assessment in cognitively impaired children and adolescents and is typically used between ages 3 and 18 years

GENERAL PRINCIPLES OF PAIN MANAGEMENT

A multifaceted approach should include pharmacological, physical, and psychological therapies.

 PEARL

Analgesics should be given early and regularly using the least invasive route.

A. Principles of pharmacological therapy

1. **Pain prevention is the primary goal**: sufficient analgesia should be given intraoperatively or before painful procedures to minimize stress response and decrease postprocedure analgesia requirements

2. **Give analgesics early and regularly**: when pain is expected to be constant (e.g., postsurgical), analgesics should be provided as scheduled medications ("around the clock"); PRN dosing should be used for breakthrough pain (i.e., perambulation, preprocedures)

3. **Use the least invasive route** to provide analgesics: oral route is preferred (if possible); intramuscular is least acceptable

4. **Follow the analgesic ladder** (Figure 4.2) to match severity of pain to appropriate analgesics, and use more than one class of analgesic (e.g., acetaminophen and nonsteroidal antiinflammatory drugs [NSAIDs]) to improve pain relief

5. **Use equianalgesic doses when changing routes or switching** from one opioid to another (Table 4.1)

Figure 4.2 Analgesic Ladder

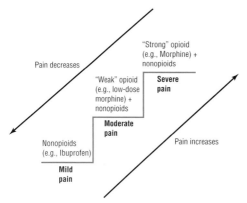

(Adapted from The Hospital for Sick Children eFormulary: Sedation and Analgesia Guidelines, 2019.)

Table 4.1	Opioid Equianalgesic Conversion Chart[a]		
Opioid	**Equipotent IV/IM Dose**	**Equipotent PO Dose**	**Parenteral to Oral Ratio**
Morphine	10	30	1/3
Hydromorphone	1.5	10	1/5
Oxycodone	NA	15	NA
Fentanyl	0.1	NA	NA

[a]Based on a single dose. When changing from one opioid to another, consider decreasing the dose of the converted opioid by 25%–50% for incomplete cross tolerance.

IM, Intramuscular; *IV,* intravenous; *PO,* orally.

Adapted from The Hospital for Sick Children eFormulary: Sedation and Analgesia Guidelines, 2019.

B. Physical interventions

1. Deep breathing, use of heat and/or cold, massage, pressure or vibration, repositioning, and activity out of bed as tolerated

C. Psychological interventions

1. Distraction, relaxation, and child life specialists.
2. For complex or chronic pain, consider consultation with anesthesiologists, psychologists, psychiatrists

> ❗ **PITFALL**
>
> Codeine should not be used before the age of 12 years because of variability in metabolism, which can lead to overdose and respiratory depression.

A. First-line agents

1. See Figure 4.1 and Table 4.2 for recommended type and dosing of analgesics for mild, moderate, and severe pain. Also see Section IV Chapter 40 Pediatric Drug Dosing Guidelines.
2. See Tables 4.3 and 4.4 for opioid side effects and dosing of neonatal opioid infusions, respectively

Table 4.2	Oral Analgesia Dosage Guidelines for Infants and Children[a]			
Medication	**Dosage**	**Route**	**Frequency**	**Maximum Dose**
Acetaminophen	- 10–15 mg/kg/dose - 10–20 mg/kg/dose	PO PR	q4–6h	75 mg/kg/day or 4 g/day, whichever is less
NSAIDs[b]				
Ibuprofen (>6 months of age)	5–10 mg/kg/dose	PO	q6–8h	40 mg/kg/day or 2400 mg/day
Naproxen	- 5–10 mg/kg/dose - 25–49 kg: 250 mg/dose - >50 kg: 500 mg/dose	PO PR PR	q12h	1 g/day
Ketorolac	0.5 mg/kg/dose	IV	q6–8h for only 48h	<16 years: 15 mg/dose ≥16 years: 30 mg/dose
Opioids[c]				
Morphine[d,e]	- 0.2–0.5 mg/kg/dose - 0.05–0.1 mg/kg/dose - 0.01–0.04 mg/kg/h	PO/PR IV IV infusion	q4–6h q2–4h Continuous infusion	15 mg/dose 5 mg/dose

Table 4.2	Oral Analgesia Dosage Guidelines for Infants and Children[a]—cont'd			
Medication	**Dosage**	**Route**	**Frequency**	**Maximum Dose**
Hydromorphone[e]	- 0.04–0.08 mg/kg/ dose	PO	q3–4h	4 mg/dose
	- 0.01–0.02 mg/kg/ dose	IV	q2–4h	1 mg/dose

[a]Refer to Section IV: Drug Dosing Guidelines for neonatal dosing.

[b]Use of NSAIDs may decrease opioid usage by 30%–50%; ensure adequate hydration and renal function with NSAID use.

[c]For nonintubated infants <3 months, initial opioid dose should be reduced to one-third to one-fourth of recommended dose.

[d]Dosages recommended are initial doses: IV dose may be repeated q10min, until child is comfortable, then administer q2–4h; when around the clock or continuous morphine is ordered, 0.01–0.04 mg/kg IV q2–4h prn may be prescribed for breakthrough pain.

Institutions should develop standardized dosing regimens for infusion.

[e]Oral dosing based on children <50 kg. Maximum doses for patients with prior opioid exposure can be higher.

IV, Intravenous; *NSAID*, nonsteroidal antiinflammatory drug; *PO*, orally; *PR*, rectally; *prn*, as needed.

Adapted from The Hospital for Sick Children eFormulary, 2020

Pain and Sedation

4

Table 4.3	Adverse Effects of Opioid Analgesics
Adverse Effect	**Management**
Nausea/vomiting	• Antihistamine (e.g., dimenhydrinate)[a] • Serotonin receptor antagonist (e.g., ondansetron) prn IV/PO
Constipation	• Laxatives (e.g., Polyethylene Glycol 3350)
Pruritus	• Antihistamine (e.g., diphenhydramine)[a]
Somnolence	• Reduce dose of opioid • Consider naloxone (start low to avoid reversal of analgesia; see Opioid Reversal in text)
Respiratory depression	• Stop opioid • Mild: stimulation and oxygen • Severe: respiratory support • Naloxone: see Section IV Chapter 40 Drug Dosing Guidelines
Chest wall rigidity	• Short-acting neuromuscular blockade • Naloxone: see Section IV Chapter 40 Drug Dosing Guidelines

[a]When dimenhydrinate and diphenhydramine are used in combination, reduce the dose of each to 0.5 mg/kg/dose to avoid sedation.

IV, Intravenous; *PO*, orally; *prn*, as needed.

From Zeltzer LK, Krane EJ, Palermo TM. Pediatric pain management. In: *Nelson's Textbook of Pediatrics*. 20th ed. Philadelphia, PA: Elsevier; 2016:430–447, chap 62.

Table 4.4	Neonatal Opioid Infusion Guidelines		
Population	**Pain Severity**	**Morphine (mcg/kg/h)**	**Fentanyl (mcg/kg/h)**
Preterm neonate	Mild	0–2	0.5
	Moderate	2–5	0.5
	Severe	5–10	1
Term neonate	Mild	0–5	0–0.5
	Moderate	5–10	0.5–1
	Severe	10–40	1–2

Adapted from The Hospital for Sick Children eFormulary, 2020

B. Adjuvant therapy

1. Other medications can be used for certain types of pain, in addition to first-line agents:
   a. Certain anticonvulsants (gabapentin), tricyclic antidepressants (amitriptyline), ketamine, and clonidine may be important in treatment of neuropathic pain
   b. Benzodiazepines may be helpful for treatment of painful muscle spasms
   c. Oral sucrose/glucose reduces procedural pain in neonates and young infants

MANAGEMENT OF PATIENTS TAKING OPIOIDS

A. Monitoring

1. All patients taking medications with potential cardiorespiratory compromising effects should be monitored according to institution-specific guidelines

PEARL

When naloxone is used to reverse adverse opioid effects other than respiratory depression, use lowest dose possible to avoid rebound hypertension, arrhythmias, and pulmonary edema.

B. Opioid reversal

1. **Naloxone** (opioid antagonist) should be available for reversal of adverse opioid effects (Table 4.5)

Table 4.5	Naloxone Administration
Step	**Comment**
1. Discontinue opioids and other sedation	
2. Evaluate ABCs	See Chapter 1 Resuscitation

Table 4.5	Naloxone Administration—cont'd
Step	**Comment**
3. Administer naloxone IV over 30–60 s	• Respiratory arrest: • 0.1 mg/kg to a maximum of 2 mg; repeat PRN • Respiratory depression: • 0.001–0.01 mg/kg; repeat PRN • In the absence of respiratory compromise, use lowest effective dose to reverse respiratory effects and not analgesia
4. Observe for response and titrate naloxone	• Patient should open eyes and respond within 2 min • If no effect after 0.01 mg/kg has been given, consider nonopioid causes of unresponsiveness
5. Discontinue naloxone	• When patient responds
6. Observation	• Monitor for at least 2 h • Naloxone duration is less than that of most opioids (30–90 min), and repeated doses may be necessary
7. Replacement analgesia	• Consider use of naloxone infusion • Use nonopioids during observation

IV, Intravenous; *PRN*, as needed.

Modified from McCaffery M, Pasero C. *Pain: Clinical Manual.* St. Louis: Mosby; 1999; and from Yaster M, Krane EJ, Kaplan RF, Coté CJ, Lappe DG. *Pediatric Pain Management and Sedation Handbook.* St. Louis: Mosby; 1997:48–49.

C. Opioid tapering

1. Consider tapering for any patient who has received opioids >5 days
2. Switch to per mouth (PO) if possible (see Table 4.1)
3. Weaning: for PO or intermittent intravenous (IV), **decrease daily dose by 10% to 20% of *initial daily dose* every day**
4. Consider IV morphine boluses for breakthrough pain

D. Outpatient opioid management

1. Healthcare providers should prescribe the lowest effective dose and minimum quantity of prescription opioid medications and parents should be instructed on how to safely dispose of leftover opioids (return to the pharmacy or, if unable, flush down the toilet)
2. Close follow-up with a healthcare provider should be scheduled
3. Long-acting or extended release preparations should only be used for long-term pain management in special cases (e.g., cancer treatment)
4. Adjuvant therapy should be used to reduce or eliminate the requirement of opioids, especially in neuropathic and chronic pain

PATIENT/NURSE-CONTROLLED ANALGESIA (PCA/NCA)

1. **Definition:** device that primarily provides patient or nurse administered boluses for breakthrough pain with an optional additional basal opioid infusion
2. **Common indications:** postoperative pain, sickle cell pain crises, burns, cancer pain, before dressing changes
3. **General guideline:** in the absence of contraindications, initiate PCA using morphine; hydromorphone or fentanyl may be used in cases of morphine intolerance (nausea, vomiting) or renal impairment (Table 4.6)

Table 4.6	Patient-Controlled Analgesia Initiation in Opioid-Naïve Patients			
Drug	**Basal Rate (mcg/kg/h)**	**Bolus Dose (mcg/kg)**	**Lockout Period (min)**	**Maximum Dose**
Morphine	4–30	10–30	6–14	Lockout period of 6–14 min when 80% of potential dose reached (basal + boluses) in 2 h period
Hydromorphone	3–5	3–5	6–14	
Fentanyl	0.15–1	0.2–0.5	6–14	

Adapted from The Hospital for Sick Children eFormulary: Pain Service Dosing Guidelines, 2020.

LOCAL ANESTHETICS

See Table 4.7 for list of commonly used subcutaneous and topical anesthetic medications.

Table 4.7	Local Anesthetic Dosage Guidelines		
Medication	**Maximum Dose**	**Duration After Infiltration**	**Route**
Lidocaine plain 1% or 2%	5 mg/kg	1–2 h	SC
Lidocaine with epinephrine 1:200,000	7 mg/kg	2–6 h	SC
Bupivacaine 0.25% or 0.5% (± epinephrine 1:200,000)	2–3 mg/kg	4–8 h	SC
Topical Anesthesia			
EMLA (intact skin): 1 g patch contains lidocaine 25 mg, prilocaine 25 mg	See Section IV Chapter 40 Pediatric Drug Dosing Guidelines	1–2 h	Under occlusive dressing for 60 min; not for abraded skin, mucous membranes; risk of methemoglobinemia in infants and neonates

	Table 4.7 Local Anesthetic Dosage Guidelines—cont'd			

Medication	Maximum Dose	Duration After Infiltration	Route
LET (lacerated skin): 1 mL contains lidocaine 40 mg, epinephrine HCl 0.5 mg, tetracaine 5 mg	3 mL	20–30 min	Not for mucous membranes or infants; avoid over areas of end-arterial perfusion[a]— risk of ischemia
Tetracaine HCl (Ametop) 4% gel (intact skin)	>1 month: 1 g (1 tube) per 30 m² skin	4–6 h	Not for abraded skin; not for mucous membranes or infants; under occlusive dressing for 30–40 min
Maxilene: 4% Liposomal Lidocaine (intact skin)	2.5 g (1 g/ day for infants 0–3 months)	1–2 h	Not for mucous membranes or abraded skin

[a]Areas of end-arterial perfusion: pinna, tip of nose, fingers, toes, penis. Not for use in premature or infant <1 month of age.

EMLA, Lidocaine and prilocaine topical; *LET*, lidocaine, epinephrine, tetracaine; *SC*, subcutaneous; *TAC*, tetracaine, adrenaline and cocaine.

Adapted from The Hospital for Sick Children eFormulary: Sedation and Analgesia Guidelines, 2019.

SEDATION

A. Definitions
1. **Minimal sedation**: anxiolysis with maintenance of consciousness; often obtained from a single drug, given once, at a low dose
2. **Moderate sedation**: medically controlled depressed consciousness in which the patient maintains protective reflexes (swallowing, coughing, gagging), an independently patent airway, and the ability to respond appropriately to stimulation or command. Usually achieved with a combination of sedative and analgesic drugs.
3. **Deep sedation**: medically controlled depressed consciousness in which the patient *may not* maintain protective reflexes, an independent airway, or the ability to respond
4. **General anesthesia**: medically controlled depressed consciousness in which the patient is unarousable even with painful stimulation, and frequently cannot maintain spontaneous ventilation or protective reflexes. Cardiovascular function may be impaired.

Note: Sedation is a continuum in which patients can easily progress into deeper levels of sedation and fluctuate between levels of sedation.

 PEARL

Only patients who are American Society of Anesthesiologists (ASA) classification I (normal healthy) or II (mild systemic disease) should undergo *elective* sedation in the emergency department.

Pain and Sedation

4

B. Preparation

1. **History/Physical Exam**: allergies, medications, medical history, conditions associated with difficult airway (see Advanced airway management in Chapter 1 Resuscitation), previous adverse reactions to sedatives, time of last oral intake
2. **Airway examination**: see Chapter 1 Resuscitation
3. **NPO guidelines**:
   a. For elective sedation: see Table 4.8
   b. For emergent and urgent sedations commonly performed in the emergency room (ER), there are no absolute guidelines regarding the duration of preprocedural fasting. Generally speaking, procedural sedation in the ER should not be delayed based on fasting time.
4. **Monitoring**: continuous saturation and cardiac monitoring, pulse oximetry, and capnography
5. **Equipment** for airway management and resuscitation: bag valve mask, endotracheal tube, O_2, suction, laryngoscope, intubation medications (see Tables 1.6 and 1.7)
6. **Personnel**: at least two qualified individuals trained in the sedation, procedure, and monitoring

Table 4.8 Fasting Guidelines for Sedation	
Ingested Material	**Minimum Fasting Period**
Clear liquids	2 h
Breast milk	4 h
Infant formula/nonhuman milk	6 h
Light meal[a]	6 h
Fried foods, fatty foods, or meat	8+ h

[a]Light meal: typically consists of toast and clear liquids

From American Society of Anesthesiologists. Practice guidelines for preoperative fasting and the use of pharmacologic agents to reduce the risk of pulmonary aspiration: application to healthy patients undergoing elective procedures. *Anesthesiology.* 2017;126:376–393.

C. Sedation drugs

1. See Table 4.9 for common medications

D. Discharge criteria post-sedation

1. Independent patent airway and stable cardiovascular function
2. Intact protective reflexes (swallowing, coughing, gagging) and easy arousability
3. Able to talk and sit unaided, if developmentally appropriate
4. Adequate hydration

Table 4.9	Drugs for Sedation of Infants and Children Outside the Operating Room[a]			
Drug	**Characteristics**	**Route**	**Dosage**	**Comments**
Benzodiazepines				
Midazolam	• Sedative, amnestic, anxiolytic with NO analgesic effects (useful for procedures that do not require full immobility)	IV	• Pediatric/infant/neonate: 0.05 mg/kg IV; may be repeated × 1 prn (max total dose 0.15 mg/kg dose IV)	• Adverse effects: Respiratory depression, apnea, laryngospasm, hypotension, paradoxical reactions (agitation, inconsolable crying)
		IN	• Pediatric/infant: 0.2–0.5 mg/kg IN; may be repeated q5–15min to maximum 0.5 mg/kg total (Dose limit: 5 mg per nostril or 10 mg total)	
		PO	• Pediatric/infant: <20 kg: 0.5–0.75 mg/kg PO (max dose 20 mg) >20 kg: 0.3–0.5 mg/kg PO (max dose 20 mg) • Administer 15–30 min before procedure	
Diazepam	• Sedative, anxiolytic with NO analgesic effects.	IV	• Pediatric/infant: 0.1 mg/kg IV; may be repeated × 1 prn (max total dose 20 mg IV)	• Adverse effects: Ataxia, respiratory depression, laryngospasm, hypotension, blurred vision, diplopia, paradoxical excitement
		PO	• Pediatric/infant: 0.2 mg/kg (PO max dose 20 mg) • Administer 45–60 min before procedure	
Lorazepam	• Sedative, anxiolytic, amnesic but NO analgesic effects	IV	• Pediatric/infant: 0.03–0.05 mg/kg IV (max dose 4 mg)	• Same as diazepam
		SL	• Pediatric/infant: 0.05 mg/kg SL 30–60 min before procedure (max dose 4 mg)	

Continued

Table 4.9	Drugs for Sedation of Infants and Children Outside the Operating Room[a]—cont'd			
Drug	**Characteristics**	**Route**	**Dosage**	**Comments**
Opioids				
Fentanyl	• Potent analgesic with sedative effects	IV	• Pediatric/infant: 0.5–1 mcg/kg/dose IV; may repeat q10min PRN (max dose 3 mcg/kg) Administer slowly over at least 60 s	• Adverse effects: Respiratory depression, apnea, chest wall rigidity
		IN	• 1.5 mcg/kg/dose IN; may repeat q5min prn for total of 3 doses; max volume 0.5 mL/nostril in infants and 1 mL/nostril in children	
Dissociative Agents				
Ketamine	• Sedative, amnestic, analgesic, dissociative agent	IV	• Pediatric/infant >3 months: 0.5–1.5 mg/kg IV slowly over 1–2 min; incremental doses of 0.5 mg/kg may be given (max dose 100 mg/dose)	• Adverse effects: Nausea/vomiting, respiratory depression, laryngospasm, apnea • Absolute contraindications: Age <3 months, psychosis
Sedative Hypnotics				
Propofol	• Ultra short-acting sedative hypnotic with NO analgesic effects	IV	• Pediatric/infant: 1 mg/kg IV • Administer over 1–2 min followed by 0.5 mg/kg supplemental doses as needed	• Adverse effects: Hypotension, bradycardia, apnea, airway obstruction, anaphylaxis in patients with soybean oil or egg phosphatide allergy • Narrow therapeutic range
Etomidate	• Sedative hypnotic	IV	• Pediatric/infant: 0.1–0.2 mg/kg IV • Administer slow over 1 min, repeat doses of 0.05 mg/kg may be needed	• Reduces ICP • Possible adrenal suppression
Chloral hydrate[b]	• Sedative with NO analgesic effects	PO/PR	• Pediatric/infants: 80–100 mg/kg PO/PR; administer 20–45 min before procedure; may repeat with 40 mg/kg in 1 h (max 2 g/dose)	• Adverse effects: Respiratory depression, hypotension, GI discomfort, residual sedation, paradoxical excitement

Table 4.9	Drugs for Sedation of Infants and Children Outside the Operating Room[a]—cont'd			
Drug	**Characteristics**	**Route**	**Dosage**	**Comments**
Other				
Nitrous oxide	• Sedative, anxiolytic, amnestic (mild analgesic effects)	INH	• 50-50 mixture of N_2O-oxygen (via face mask or nose mask); 100% oxygen must be administered for at least 5 min following discontinuation of nitrous oxide	• Adverse effects: vomiting and dysphoria • Contraindications: conditions with trapped gas in body cavity (pneumothorax, otitis media)

[a]See Section IV Drug Dosing Guidelines for neonatal dosing.

[b]Should not be used in patients with hepatic, renal, or pulmonary disease.

GI, Gastrointestinal; *ICP*, intracranial pressure; *IN*, intranasal; *INH*, inhalational; *IV*, intravenous; *PO*, orally; *PR*, rectally; *prn*, as needed; *SL*, sublingual.

Adapted from The Hospital for Sick Children eFormulary: Sedation and Analgesia Guidelines 2019.

Pain and Sedation

4

FURTHER READING

Committee on Fetus and Newborn and Section on Anesthesiology and Pain Medicine. Prevention and management of procedural pain in the neonate: an update. *Pediatrics*. 2016;137(2):e20154271. doi:10.1542/peds.2015-4271.

Coté CJ, Wilson S, American Academy of Pediatrics, American Academy of Pediatric Dentistry. Guidelines for monitoring and management of pediatric patients before, during, and after sedation for diagnostic and therapeutic procedures. *Pediatrics*, 2019;143(6), e20191000. http://doi.org/10.1542/peds.2019-1000.

Cravero JP, Agarwal R, Berde C, et al. The Society for Pediatric Anesthesia recommendations for the use of opioids in children during the perioperative period. *Paediatr Anaesth*, 2019;29(6):547–571. https://doi.org/10.1111/pan.13639.

Friedrichsdorf SJ, Goubert L. Pediatric pain treatment and prevention for hospitalized children. *Pain Rep*. 2019;5(1):e804. https://doi.org/10.1097/PR9.0000000000000804.

Hammill JK, Lyndon M, Liley A, Hill AG. Where it hurts: a systematic review of pain-location tools for children. *Pain*. 2014;155(5):851–858.

Verghese ST, Hannallah RS. Acute pain management in children. *J Pain Res*. 2010;3:105–123.

Procedures

Zachary Pancer • Meghan Gilley • Jonathan Pirie

COMMON ABBREVIATIONS

Also see page xviii for a list of other abbreviations used throughout this book

0.9% NaCl	isotonic sodium chloride (normal saline)
ASIS	anterior superior iliac spine
Fr	French
IJ	internal jugular
IO	intraosseous
IVC	inferior vena cava
LET	lidocaine, epinephrine, tetracaine
NG	nasogastric
SCM	sternocleidomastoid muscle
SVC	superior vena cava
UAC	umbilical artery catheter
UVC	umbilical venous catheter

PREPARATION BEFORE PROCEDURE

1. **Consent:** Consent must be obtained before any procedure is undertaken. Valid consent must be voluntary, and the medical decision maker must be properly informed and have the capacity to give consent. In emergency situations, physicians may have to perform procedures before consent is obtained if deemed medically necessary.
2. **Pain control and anxiolysis:** Many procedures may be painful or anxiety provoking in pediatric patients. Clinicians should consider analgesic and anxiolytic medications, and distraction techniques by parents or multidisciplinary team, before performing any invasive procedures. Also see Chapter 4 Pain and Sedation.
3. **Restraint:** Restraints should be appropriate for age, cognitive ability, and behavior of the child. Physical and chemical restraints are variable in their application and dependent on nurse and physician experience, age of the patient, urgency of the procedure, and type of treatment performed (refer to your organizational policies for restraints).
4. **Monitoring:** Monitoring is dependent on the nature of the procedure, as well as the patient's preprocedural status. Procedures requiring sedative or anxiolytic medication should only be completed in the presence of individuals skilled in airway management and cardiopulmonary resuscitation and may require cardiac and respiratory monitoring, depending on the depth of sedation and medications used.
5. **Aseptic techniques:** Unless otherwise mentioned, all procedures should be performed using aseptic technique

VASCULAR PROCEDURES

PERIPHERAL INTRAVENOUS CATHETERIZATION

1. **Indications:** Intravenous (IV) administration of medications, fluids, or blood products

Procedures

5

2. **Equipment**
   a. Tourniquet, tape
   b. 16- to 24-gauge IV over-the-needle catheter
   c. Syringe with 0.9% NaCl, IV fluid setup
3. **Method**
   a. Choose the vein to be accessed; in a resuscitation scenario, this is ideally the largest vein that does not interfere with resuscitation. Scalp veins may be used in cases of difficult IV access in infants <3 months (but can often be used up to 9 months). Figure 5.1 outlines common sites for IV access.
   b. Immobilize the extremity and prepare the site with antiseptic solution
   c. Apply tourniquet and squeeze limb above the site to distend veins (Trendelenburg position may be used when attempting to distend/access *external* jugular vein)
   d. Puncture skin 0.5 to 1 cm distal to desired site of entry to vein at an angle of 15 to 45 degrees
   e. When blood returns, decrease angle of IV catheter so that it is almost parallel to the skin and advance further by 1 to 2 mm; then feed the plastic cannula over the needle while keeping needle steady so only the catheter advances into the vein
   f. Release tourniquet, remove needle, tape cannula into place, flush cannula with 0.9% NaCl to ensure position, attach line tubing
4. **Complications:** Bleeding, infection, extravasation (see Chapter 34 Plastic Surgery)

Figure 5.1 Sites for Peripheral Intravenous Access

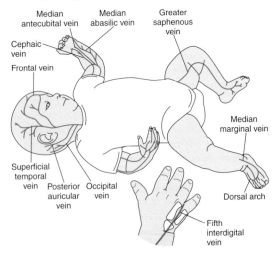

(From Baldwin GA. *Handbook of Pediatric Emergencies.* 3rd ed. Philadelphia, PA: Lippincott Williams & Wilkins; 2001:19.)

INTRAOSSEOUS ACCESS

1. **Indications:** Parenteral administration of medications, fluids, or blood products. Used as second-line procedure when peripheral IV insertion is unsuccessful, or when access is urgent.

2. **Equipment**
   a. EZ-intraosseous (IO) battery-powered drill, or if unavailable can use 14- to 20-gauge IO infusion needle (various models available), or bone marrow aspiration needle, or 20-gauge spinal needle
   b. Syringe with sterile 0.9% NaCl

3. **Insertion sites**
   a. **Proximal tibia:** Anteromedial surface of proximal tibia, 1 to 2 cm distal to tibial tuberosity (Figure 5.2A)
   b. **Distal tibia:** Medial surface of distal tibia, 1 to 2 cm proximal to the medial malleolus
   c. **Distal femur:** In the midline, 1 to 2 cm proximal to the superior border of the patella (Figure 5.2B)
   d. **Proximal humerus:** Into the greater tubercle, 2 cm below the acromion process (with arm held in adduction and internal rotation)

Figure 5.2 Intraosseous Infusion Sites: Proximal tibia (A) and distal femur (B)

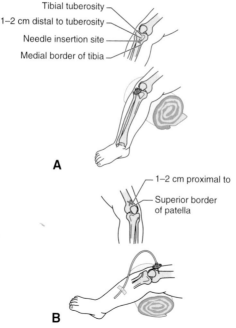

(From King C, Henretig FM, eds. *Textbook of Pediatric Emergency Procedures*. 2nd ed. Baltimore, MD: Lippincott Williams & Wilkins; 2008:284, 285 (Figure 21.3, Figure 21.4, Figure 21.5).)

4. **Method**
   a. Prepare site using antiseptic solution and provide local anesthesia with 1% lidocaine if patient is awake and time permits
   b. Choose drill-powered IO or manual IO
      i. If using EZ-IO, ensure device charged and attach appropriate needle to drill. Hold needle perpendicular to bony cortex and manually insert needle through skin until needle tip touches bone. Ensure that at least 5 mm of the catheter (look for a black line on the catheter) is visible outside the skin. If line is not visualized or hub is flush with skin, choose larger needle. Squeeze drill trigger and apply gentle pressure into bone until you feel "give". STOP once this sudden decrease in resistance is felt.
      ii. If using manual needle, hold needle and stylet securely. Insert needle at 90-degree angle to bony surface or angled slightly away from joint space. Use steady back-and-forth "screwing" motion until there is a decrease in resistance, indicating entry into the marrow.
   c. Remove stylet while leaving needle in place
   d. Aspirate marrow to confirm needle placement or infuse small amount of saline and ensure flushes easily. Once placement confirmed, can provide analgesia by slow administration of 0.5 mg/kg of lidocaine (max 40 mg).
   e. Secure the line and attach to IV infusion set up
   f. Remove the IO as soon as other IV access is established or within 24 hours of insertion
5. **Complications:** Bleeding, infection, extravasation, osteomyelitis, subcutaneous abscess, epiphyseal damage, fracture, fat embolism, compartment syndrome

INTERNAL JUGULAR CATHETERIZATION

1. **Indication:** Administration of large volumes of IV fluids, vasoactive medications or hypertonic fluids (TPN, chemotherapy), long-term vascular access or frequent use, monitoring of central venous pressure
2. **Equipment**
   a. Central line kit (3–5 Fr Cook catheter, metal needle, blade, guidewire, infusion catheter). See Table 5.1 for catheter sizes.

Table 5.1	Central Catheter Diameters for Pediatric Patients	
Age	Internal Jugular (Fr)	Femoral (Fr)
0–6 months	3	3
6 months–2 years	3	3–4
3–6 years	4	4
7–12 years	4–5	4–5

From King C, Henretig FM, eds. *Textbook of Pediatric Emergency Procedures.* 2nd ed. Baltimore, MD: Lippincott Williams & Wilkins; 2008.

b. 5 mL syringe, IV line, and fluid

c. 2-0 suture, sterile dressing

d. Ultrasound machine

3. **Method (Seldinger technique)**

a. Right internal jugular (IJ) cannulation is preferred because the right IJ assumes a relatively straight course into the right atrium, the left dome of the lung is higher, and the thoracic duct is on the left. Position patient in 15 to 20 degrees Trendelenburg; place a roll under the shoulders and turn head away from site of line placement.

b. Use sterile technique to prepare and drape site

c. Identify insertion site

   i. **Ultrasound-guided** central line insertion is now standard practice and should always be used if available. Use a linear probe with sterile cover to identify the IJ vein, which will usually be a larger, compressible structure lateral and anterior to the pulsating carotid artery. Use the probe to visualize the vessel throughout the insertion process.

   ii. **Landmark-guided** approach (Figure 5.3): Enter at the apex of the triangle formed by the middle third of the clavicle and the two bellies of sternocleidomastoid muscle, and direct needle toward the ipsilateral nipple at an angle of 30 degrees; alternatively, the needle can be inserted along the anterior margin of the sternocleidomastoid muscle, halfway between the mastoid process and suprasternal notch, and directed toward the ipsilateral nipple

d. Attach the entry needle to 5 mL syringe and insert needle at 30-degree angle toward ipsilateral nipple. Slowly advance needle while gently applying negative pressure to syringe.

e. When blood return is seen, advance the needle only 1 to 2 mm farther. Then carefully remove the syringe and steady needle with the other hand. Expect venous flow; cover hub with a finger to prevent blood loss.

f. Insert guidewire through needle several centimeters past needle tip; if it does not advance easily, remove wire, reconfirm needle position within the vessel, then replace wire. The proximal end of the guidewire must always be visible.

g. Remove the needle, firmly holding the guidewire; keep pressure on vein to limit blood loss

h. Use a scalpel blade to enlarge the skin puncture, then thread dilator over the wire until beneath skin, then remove dilator

i. Thread the *preflushed* (primed) intravascular catheter over the wire. Once the wire emerges from the proximal end of the catheter, gently thread the catheter into the vessel in a twisting motion. Once in place, remove the guidewire.

j. Check for adequate retrograde blood flow through the catheter lumen; attach infusion setup

Figure 5.3 Internal Jugular Vein Cannulation

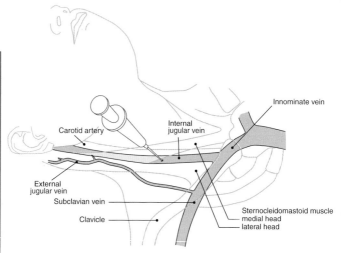

(From Kohl BA, Lanken PN, Hanson CW, Manaker S. *The Intensive Care Unit Manual.* 2nd ed. Philadelphia, PA: Elsevier; 2013.)

k. Secure the cannula with sutures; apply sterile dressing
l. Ensure proper placement with chest x-ray

4. **Complications:** Venous laceration, arterial line placement, pneumothorax, hemothorax, air embolism, right atrial irritation, arrhythmias

FEMORAL VEIN CATHETERIZATION

1. **Indications:** See IJ catheterization earlier
2. **Equipment:** See IJ catheterization earlier
3. **Method**
   a. Position the patient: With patient lying supine, flex and externally rotate hip. Ultrasound should be used to identify the femoral vein, which lies medial to the femoral artery. One can also identify landmarks by palpating the femoral pulse 2 cm below the inguinal ligament, halfway between symphysis pubis and anterior superior iliac spine (ASIS) (Figure 5.4).
   b. Insert needle into femoral vein, which is typically 0.5 to 1 cm *medial to femoral pulse,* at 30-degree angle directed toward the umbilicus
   c. Setup and Seldinger technique as per IJ cannulation section earlier
4. **Complications:** Vascular laceration, arterial line placement, air embolism, bowel perforation, infection (including osteomyelitis), avascular necrosis of hip

Figure 5.4   Femoral Vein Cannulation

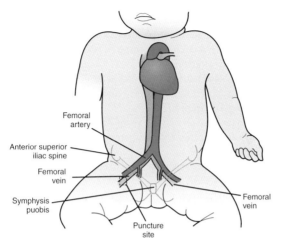

Anterior superior
iliac spine

Femoral
artery

Femoral
vein

Symphysis
puobis

Femoral
vein

Puncture
site

(From Beno S, Nadel F. Central venous access. In: Chiang VW, Zaoutis LB, eds. *Comprehensive Pediatric Hospital Medicine.* Philadelphia, PA: Elsevier Inc.; 2007.)

UMBILICAL VEIN AND UMBILICAL ARTERY CATHETERIZATION (UVC, UAC)

1. **Indications:** UVC: emergent delivery of resuscitative medications, volume expanders or blood products in neonates; UAC: arterial blood gas sampling in neonates requiring respiratory support, IV access for fluids, medications
2. **Equipment**
   a. 5 Fr umbilical UVC or 3.5 Fr UAC insertion kit (smaller-size catheters may be required for premature infants)
   b. Three-way stopcock
   c. 0.9% NaCl
3. **Method**
   a. Prepare site using sterile technique
   b. Prepare equipment: Attach UA and UV catheters to tubing lines, prime and flush setup with 0.9% NaCl; ensure the system is closed to avoid loss of priming
   c. Estimate catheter insertion length using the "shoulder-umbilical" graph (Figures 5.5 and 5.6), or formula of Shukla:
      i. High UAC insertion length $(3 \times \text{birthweight in kg}) + 9$
      ii. UVC insertion length: $[(3 \times \text{birthweight in kg} + 9) / 2] + 1$
   d. Tie a loose knot with an umbilical tie at base of stump; cut stump with a clean stroke of the scalpel 1 to 2 cm from stump base (Figure 5.7A)
   e. Evert edges of stump with mosquito forceps (Figure 5.7B)

115

f. Identify two arteries and one thin-walled larger vein. Gently use dilator to open vessels if needed, especially arteries.

g. Grasp catheter 1 cm from its tip with toothless forceps, and gently insert catheter into vessel to desired distance (Figure 5.7C and D). If catheter does not insert easily, suspect a false tract and check for blood flow by aspirating.

h. Once easy blood return is confirmed at the desired insertion depth, secure the catheter with a suture to cord, and secure with "bridge-tape" support (Figure 5.7E)

i. Confirm the position with two view CXR/AXR (ultrasound confirmation can also be performed by experienced providers). Also see Figures 5.5 and 5.6.

   i. High UAC placement (preferred): catheter tip between T6 and T9 (above the diaphragm)

   ii. Low UAC placement: catheter tip between L3 and L5 (above aortic bifurcation)

   iii. UVC placement: catheter tip at junction of inferior vena cava (IVC) and right atrium, projecting just above diaphragm on AP CXR

   iv. To differentiate UAC from UVC on x-ray: UAC turns down and then upward (as it enters internal iliac artery); UVC takes only a cephalad (upward) direction, toward the liver.

j. Remove line as soon as it is no longer needed. Ensure pressure at umbilical site for 3 to 5 minutes to prevent bleeding.

Figure 5.5 Umbilical Vein Catheter Insertion Length

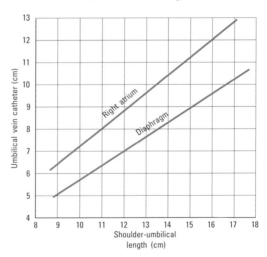

(Data from Dunn PM. Localization of the umbilical catheter by post-mortem measurement. *Arch Dis Child.* 1966;41:70–71.)

Figure 5.6   Umbilical Artery Catheter Insertion Length

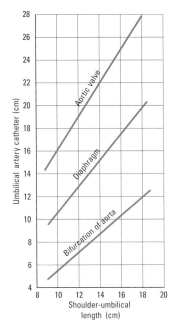

(Data from Dunn PM. Localization of the umbilical catheter by post-mortem measurement. *Arch Dis Child*. 1966;41:70–71.)

Figure 5.7 (A–E)   Insertion of Umbilical Vein and Artery Catheters

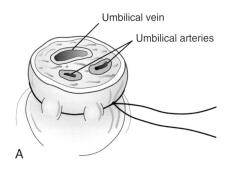

Continued

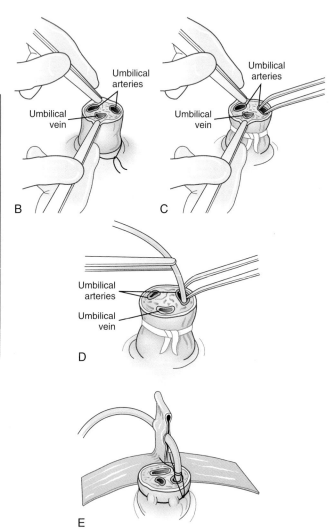

(A) Tie a loose knot at the base of the stump; use scalpel to cut cleanly 1 to 2 cm from the base of the stump; identify two arteries and one thin-walled larger vein. (B) Use two hemostats to grasp opposite sides of the umbilicus to stabilize vessels. (C) Gently dilate vessel lumen using smooth curved forceps. (D) Insert primed catheter into vessel lumen. (E) Secure the catheter in place with a suture and bridge-tape support. (From Cameron P, et al. *Textbook of Paediatric Emergency Medicine*. 3rd ed. Elsevier; 2019.)

4. **Complications:** Bleeding, infection, vessel perforation, thrombus formation, ischemia of lower limbs with arterial spasm or stenosis, necrotizing enterocolitis, air embolus

PERIPHERAL ARTERIAL ACCESS

1. **Indications:** Continuous blood pressure monitoring, frequent blood sampling, arterial blood gas sampling
2. **Equipment**
   a. 23- to 25-gauge butterfly needle with 1 to 3 mL syringe for single sampling
   b. 20- to 24-gauge angiocatheters for artery catheterization (or full arterial line kit, including guidewire)
   c. Heparinized infusion setup for indwelling catheter
3. **Method**
   a. Identify the artery: Feel for pulse at radial, femoral, dorsalis pedis, or posterior tibial arteries
   b. Position and assess the site
      i. Radial artery: Place wrist in 30 degree extension and immobilize the wrist (Figure 5.8). Ensure collateral flow in the hand with Allen test: Elevate fisted hand for 30 seconds, and then apply pressure, to occlude both radial and ulnar arteries. Open hand, release ulnar pressure, and color should return within 5 seconds (if pallor persists beyond 5 seconds do not access radial artery at this site).
      ii. Femoral artery: The femoral triangle contains the femoral nerve, artery, and vein (lateral to medial). The borders consist of the inguinal ligament (superior), adductor longus (medial), and sartorius (lateral). The common femoral artery can be palpated inferior to the mid-inguinal point, half way between the ASIS and the symphysis pubis (see Figure 5.4).
      iii. Posterior tibialis: Identify the artery running posterior to the medial malleolus while holding a foot in dorsiflexion
   c. Clean area, and insert needle at 30-degree angle, bevel up
   d. For sampling only, use butterfly needle, and aspirating syringe to assist with blood return
   e. For artery cannulation, insert catheter and advance 1 to 2 mm once blood return is seen. If blood return ceases or slows, distal wall of the artery may have been punctured. If this occurs, pull back very slowly until flashback is seen again.
   f. Advance plastic catheter with twisting motion; remove needle and ensure arterial flow. Alternatively, one can use the Seldinger technique (see IJ catheterization earlier). Once flashback is seen, the needle is removed, and a guidewire inserted. The plastic catheter is then advanced over the guidewire into the vessel lumen.
   g. Attach heparinized infusion; secure with tape or operation-site dressing
   h. Apply firm constant pressure to vessel for 5 minutes after removal of any butterfly or catheter
4. **Complications:** Infection, bleeding, arterial spasm, distal ischemia

Figure 5.8 Insertion of a Radial Arterial Catheter

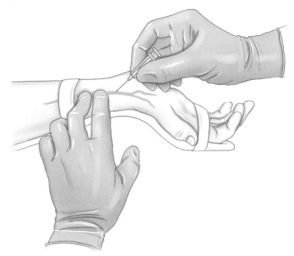

(Modified from Sills JR. *The Comprehensive Respiratory Therapist Exam Review*, 6th ed. Elsevier Inc. 2016.)

CARDIORESPIRATORY PROCEDURES

NEEDLE ASPIRATION OF PNEUMOTHORAX

1. **Indications:** Tension pneumothorax, spontaneous pneumothorax in neonates
2. **Equipment**
   a. 16- to 24-gauge angiocatheter (based on patient size)
   b. 5 mL syringe filled with sterile 0.9% NaCl
   c. Optional: three-way stopcock with tubing
3. **Method**
   a. Locate insertion site: second intercostal space in the midclavicular line (Figure 5.9) on the affected side
   b. With the syringe attached to the angiocath device, insert needle just superior to the third rib to avoid the neurovascular bundle on the inferior aspect of second rib
   c. Remove air by drawing back on syringe, visualizing air bubbles (if catheter device is used without syringe attached, listen for "rush of air")
   d. When the pleural space is entered, the needle can be withdrawn and a three-way stopcock attached to the catheter and a syringe. Closing the stopcock to the environment ensures that air is not unintentionally pulled from the outside into the pleural space (risk of pneumothorax). Air can be aspirated out of pleural cavity into syringe (stopcock closed to environment), and then disposed of (stopcock closed to pleural space).

e. If significant pneumothorax is found, a catheter or tube thoracostomy
      should be placed for definitive management

Figure 5.9   Needle Aspiration of Tension Pneumothorax

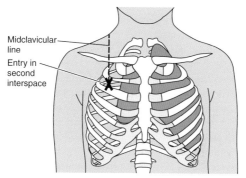

Midclavicular line
Entry in second interspace

(Adapted from Henretig FM, King C, eds. *Textbook of Pediatric Emergency Procedures.*
Baltimore, MD: Williams & Wilkins; 1997:395.)

4. **Complications:** Pneumomediastinum, bleeding, hematoma, lung laceration

CHEST TUBE INSERTION

1. **Indications**: Pneumothorax, hemothorax, pleural effusion
2. **Equipment**
   a. Chest tube (Table 5.2)
   b. Chest tube insertion kit (scalpel, hemostat, Kelly forceps, 2-0 silk
      suture), sterile drainage/suction system
   c. Local anesthetic

Table 5.2 Chest Tube Sizes by Age	
Age	Size (F)
Newborn	10–12
6 months	10–12
1 year	16–20
4 years	20–28
10 years	28–32
>14 years	28–32

From Fleisher GR, Ludwig S, eds. *Textbook of Pediatric Emergency Medicine.* 7th ed. Philadelphia, PA:
Lippincott Williams & Wilkins; 2015.

Procedures

5

3. **Method**
   a. Locate insertion site: With patient supine and ipsilateral arm behind the head, locate the fifth intercostal space between the anterior and midaxillary lines
   b. Anesthetize the skin, periosteum, and pleura below the interspace of intended tube placement
   c. Make 1- to 2-cm incision over rib below interspace of intended tube placement (Figure 5.10A)
   d. Use Kelly forceps to bluntly dissect subcutaneously and superiorly over the superior aspect of rib until pleura is penetrated (Figure 5.10B and C). One may then insert finger to confirm entry and feel for adhesions.
   e. Use Kelly forceps to grip proximal tip of chest tube and guide tube through pleural opening, aiming the cephalad to avoid viscus injury (see Figure 5.10D)
   f. Advance the tube 4 to 10 cm, depending on size of child or until fluid/condensation appears in tube (also ensure all side holes on the chest tube lie completely within chest cavity), then attach to drainage device
   g. Alternately, if a smaller diameter catheter is needed (to drain air or simple fluid), one can use the wire-guided Seldinger technique (outlined in the Internal Jugular Catheterization section). Attach syringe with saline to needle and insert needle above superior edge of rib until air of fluid is aspirated (Figure 5.11A); remove syringe, and thread guidewire through the needle lumen (Figure 5.11B); remove needle and use dilator over guidewire to widen opening (Figure 5.11C and D); remove dilator, then thread thoracostomy catheter over guidewire into chest (Figure 5.11E); remove guidewire wire and secure catheter in place.
   h. Distal end of tube should be clamped until attached to drainage system (e.g., Pleur-evac) to prevent inspiration of air into pleural cavity
   i. Fix chest tube with suture and cover with sterile occlusive dressing
   j. CXR postprocedure to assess size of pneumothorax, intrapleural fluid volume

Figure 5.10 Insertion of a Chest Tube

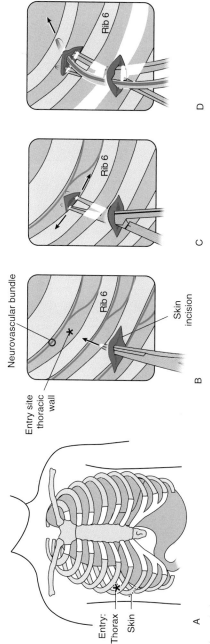

A

Entry: Thorax
Skin

B

Entry site thoracic wall
Neurovascular bundle
Skin incision
Rib 6

C

Rib 6

D

Rib 6

(From Fleisher GR, Ludwig S, eds. *Textbook of Pediatric Emergency Medicine*. 7th ed. Philadelphia, PA: Lippincott Williams & Wilkins; 2015.Section VIII, Chapter 141, Figure 141.23.)

Figure 5.11 Insertion of a Chest Tube With Seldinger Technique

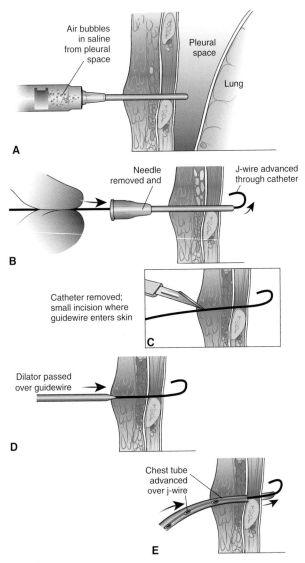

A — Air bubbles in saline from pleural space; Pleural space; Lung

B — Needle removed and; J-wire advanced through catheter

C — Catheter removed; small incision where guidewire enters skin

D — Dilator passed over guidewire

E — Chest tube advanced over j-wire

(From King C, Henretig FM, eds. *Textbook of Pediatric Emergency Procedures.* 2nd ed. Baltimore, MD: Lippincott Williams & Wilkins; 2008:370, Figure 29.7.)

4. **Complications:** Injury to lungs, heart, mediastinal vessels, diaphragm, liver, spleen, pneumothorax, hemothorax, infection

NASOGASTRIC TUBE INSERTION

1. **Indications**: Passage to GI tract for enteral nutrition or medications if unable to swallow, drain gastric contents, decompress stomach
2. **Equipment**
   a. 8 to 12 Fr NG tube
   b. Lubricant
3. **Method**
   a. Estimate length of insertion by measuring distance from nose to earlobe to below left costal margin, and mark on tube
   b. Lubricate tip of tube and insert through either nostril; use oral route if suspicion of facial injury, skull fracture, or dysmorphic facies
   c. Watch for coiling in pharynx; if older, ask patient to swallow during insertion
   d. Confirm placement
      i. Aspirate gastric fluid and check pH (<4) to confirm gastric placement
      ii. While listening with stethoscope over stomach, rapidly instill 5 mL of air through tube; listen for a "pop" when appropriately positioned in the stomach
      iii. X-ray to ensure placement if uncertain
4. **Complications:** Intracranial, esophageal, or bronchial insertion, perforation, bleeding

REPLACEMENT OF A GASTROSTOMY TUBE WITH FOLEY CATHETER

1. **Indications:** *Temporizing measure* to maintain tract patency of recently dislodged or blocked tube and allow for feeding/meds while awaiting replacement gastrostomy feeding device.
   Note: replacement should not be attempted if tube has recently been placed in last 6–8 weeks (risk of formation of false tract) or if tube has been out of place for an extended period of time (tract may have narrowed).
2. **Equipment**
   a. Foley catheter matched to size of child's gastrostomy tube (or 1 Fr size smaller)
   b. 0.9% NaCl or sterile water, syringe
   c. Lubricant, absorbent dressing, tape
3. **Method**
   a. Gently insert a cotton-tipped swab with lubricant to assess tract patency
   b. Grasp the distal end of the tube between the index finger and thumb of one hand and stabilize it by placing the heel of this hand against the abdominal wall to prevent slippage.
   c. Position lubricated tip of Foley catheter perpendicular to the abdominal wall
   d. Insert catheter, applying gentle steady pressure, directing along previously assessed tract
   e. A decrease in resistance will be felt once catheter enters stomach

Procedures

5

f. Insert catheter far enough to allow inflation of balloon with 0.9% NaCl (Figure 5.12)
g. Ensure appropriate position by aspirating stomach contents through catheter, with option of instilling 30 mL of 0.9% NaCl before aspirating. pH of gastric contents should be <6. If in doubt or with difficult placements, consider a contrast study to assess location of the tube tip.

Figure 5.12 Replacement of a Gastrostomy Tube with a Foley Catheter

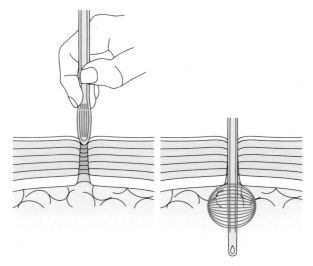

(Adapted from Fleisher GR, Ludwig S, eds. *Textbook of Pediatric Emergency Medicine.* Philadelphia, PA: Lippincott Williams & Wilkins; 2000:1852.)

4. **Complications:** Bleeding, insertion of tube between stomach and anterior abdominal wall, obstruction of stomach outlet with balloon of newly replaced tube

GENITOURINARY PROCEDURES

BLADDER CATHETERIZATION

1. **Indications:** Collect sterile urine sample, relieve bladder distension, track urine output, postsurgical or critically ill
2. **Equipment**
    a. Sterile Foley catheter set (Table 5.3)
    b. Lubricant, sterile water

Table 5.3 Urinary Catheter Sizes	
Infant and Child Size (kg)	**Catheter Size (F)**
Term neonate (3–5 kg)	5[a]–6
Small infant (6–7 kg)	6–8
Infant (8–9 kg)	6–8
Toddler (10–11 kg)	8–10
Small child (12–14 kg)	10
Child (15–23 kg)	10–12
Large child (24–29 kg)	12
Adult (30–36 kg)	12

[a] 5 Fr feeding tube can be used.

© Hospital for Sick Children; adapted from *Patient Care Guideline for Urinary Catheterization*, 2017.

3. **Method**
   a. Apply gentle traction to penis to straighten the urethra in males (Figure 5.13A); or separate labia to visualize urethra under clitoral hood in females (Figure 5.13B)
   b. Swab area with antiseptic; drape sterile towel above and below
   c. Lubricate catheter, apply traction to surrounding skin, and introduce catheter into urethral meatus
   d. Advance until urine returns
   e. For in-and-out catheterization, remove tube after urine obtained
   f. To instill indwelling Foley catheter, inflate balloon with 3 to 5 mL of sterile water, pull back gently to ensure that inflated balloon stays in bladder (Figure 5.13C), and attach outlet to sterile closed collecting system

Figure 5.13   Catheterization of the Bladder

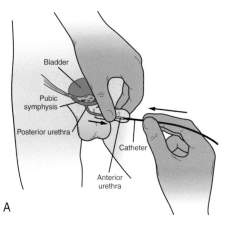

Bladder

Pubic
symphysis

Posterior urethra

Catheter

Anterior
urethra

A

Continued 127

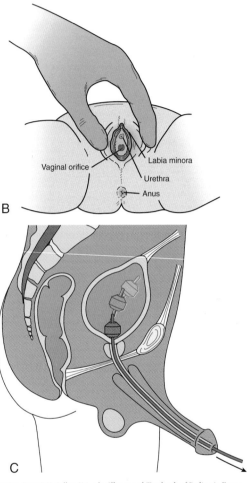

B

Vaginal orifice · · · · · · · · · · Labia minora

· · · · · · Urethra

· · · · · · Anus

C

(A, From Dieckmann RA, Fiser DH, Selbst SM, eds. *Illustrated Textbook of Pediatric Emergency and Critical Care Procedures*. St Louis: Mosby; 1997. B, From Dieckmann RA, Fiser DH, Selbst SM, eds. *Illustrated Textbook of Pediatric Emergency and Critical Care Procedures*. St Louis: Mosby; 1997. C, Modified from Fleisher GR, Ludwig S, eds. *Textbook of Pediatric Emergency Medicine*. Philadelphia, PA: Lippincott Williams & Wilkins; 2000:1856. Reprinted by permission of Lippincot Williams and Wilkins.)

4. **Complications:** Trauma, bleeding, perforation, infection, urethral stenosis

LUMBAR PUNCTURE

1. **Indications:** To obtain cerebrospinal fluid (CSF) for diagnostic purposes (infectious, bleeding, oncologic, metabolic), measure intracranial pressure, instill therapeutic medications, introduction of anesthesia
   Note: Ensure no evidence of raised intracranial pressure or infection over site of lumbar puncture before procedure

2. **Equipment**
   a. Appropriate spinal needle with stylet (infants: 22-gauge 1.5 inch; children: 22 gauge 2.5 inch; larger children and adolescents: 20- to 22-gauge 3.5 inch), CSF specimen tubes
   b. Manometer, three-way stopcock (only needed for measuring opening pressure)

3. **Method**
   a. Positioning
      i. **Lateral decubitus position:** Place child on their side with hips, knees, and neck flexed; have assistant holding feet and head while curving the spine to achieve maximum flexion; ensure shoulders/hips are perpendicular to bed to avoid rotating the spine (Figure 5.14A)
      ii. **Sitting position:** (Figure 5.14B)
   b. Locate insertion site: Locate superior edges of both iliac crests and draw an imaginary line between them to intersect spine at L4–L5; palpate this or the next intervertebral space upward (L3–L4); insertion of needle in L3–L4 or L4–L5 disk space ensures that needle entry is below level of spinal cord
   c. With sterile technique, cleanse skin with antiseptic solution; use sterile drapes
   d. Anesthetize area appropriately with topical anesthetic patch (placed before sterilization) or injection of local anesthetic
   e. Confirm landmarks and insert needle and stylet slowly with bevel up and angled slightly cephalad toward the umbilicus; resistance will increase as needle passes through fascia
   f. Advance the needle slowly and remove stylet frequently to check for CSF flow. Alternatively, needle may be advanced without stylet once skin is completely punctured. If bony resistance is felt, withdraw needle carefully to just below skin surface and redirect angle slightly. Often a slight "pop" and a "give" is felt when needle passes through dura (not always felt in small infants).
   g. If indicated, attach three-way stopcock and manometer to measure opening pressure. Note: Measurements are only accurate when patient is in *quiet, non-flexed, lateral decubitus* position.
   h. Let CSF drain into sterile tubes and send for relevant investigations (e.g., Gram stain/culture, protein/glucose, cell count [usually last tube], virology [as needed])
   i. Reinsert stylet, and then remove needle. Apply pressure to site for 1 to 2 minutes.

Figure 5.14 Lumbar Puncture Positioning

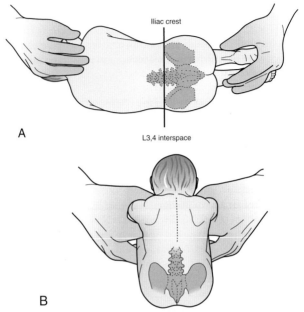

(Modified from Cameron P, Browne G, Biswadev M, Dalziel S, Craig S. *Textbook of Pediatric Emergency Medicine*. 3rd ed. Elsevier; 2019.)

4. **Complications:** Headache, epidermal cyst, CSF leakage, bleeding, infection, brainstem herniation

MUSCULOSKELETAL PROCEDURES

ARTHROCENTESIS

1. **Indications:** Diagnostic evaluation of synovial fluid (e.g., suspected septic arthritis, autoimmune arthropathy, hemarthrosis), introduction of medications
2. **Equipment**
   a. 18- to 20-gauge needle with 10-mL syringe
   b. Specimen collection tubes (ideally EDTA or heparinized tubes for cell count)
3. **Method**
   a. Clean area and anesthetize with topical anesthetic and injection of local anesthetic
   b. Restrain child if necessary, and have an assistant hold joint stable

c. Positioning/insertion sites
   i. Knee (superolateral approach): Extend the knee. Insert needle slightly lateral to superolateral border of patella. Needle should be directed at a 10- to 20-degree downward angle (to pass underneath the patella) (Figure 5.15A).
   ii. Elbow: Flex elbow to 90-degree angle. Insert needle into the center of the triangle formed by head of radius, lateral epicondyle of humerus, and olecranon (Figure 5.15B).
   iii. Ankle (medial approach): Place patient supine with ankle in plantar flexion. Insert needle between anterior tibialis tendon and medial malleolus. Direct needle posterolaterally (Figure 5.15C).
   iv. Shoulder: Patient should be seated upright with arm in external rotation. Insert needle inferior and lateral to coracoid process (Figure 5.15D).
d. Advance needle with syringe suction until synovial fluid is obtained. Send fluid for desired studies.
4. **Complications:** Infection, bleeding, epiphyseal damage

Figure 5.15 Arthrocentesis of the Knee (A), Elbow (B), Ankle (C), and Shoulder (D)

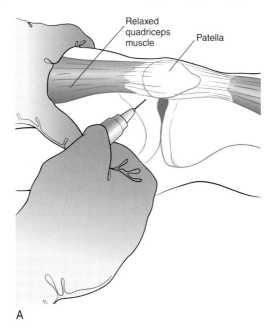

A

Continued

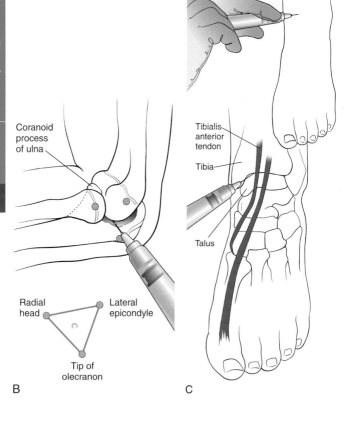

Coranoid process of ulna

Radial head

Lateral epicondyle

Tip of olecranon

B

Tibialis anterior tendon

Tibia

Talus

C

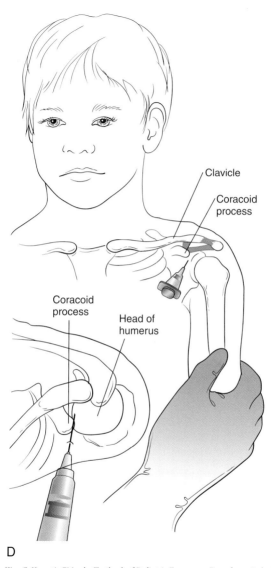

Clavicle

Coracoid process

Coracoid process

Head of humerus

D

(From King C, Henretig FM, eds. *Textbook of Pediatric Emergency Procedures*. 2nd ed. Baltimore, MD: Lippincott Williams & Wilkins; 2008:956 (Figure 104.1), 958 (Figure 104.6), 957 (Figure 104.3), 958 (Figure 104.5).)

REDUCTION OF RADIAL HEAD SUBLUXATION ("PULLED ELBOW")

1. **Indications:** Radial head subluxation (often presenting as toddler refusing to move arm after sudden longitudinal traction on forearm or minor fall)
2. **Equipment:** None
3. **Method**
   a. **Hyperpronation technique**
      i. Place thumb over the radial head of the affected elbow, applying gentle pressure with one hand. Hold the child's hand/wrist with your other hand.
      ii. Fully pronate the forearm at the wrist while applying gentle pressure at the radial head
      iii. A "click" may be felt over the radial head. Flex the elbow.
      iv. Review for full range of motion after 10 minutes
   b. **Supination technique**
      i. Place hands as with the hyperpronation technique
      ii. Fully supinate the forearm and flex the elbow
      iii. A "click" may be felt over the radial head
      iv. Review for full range of motion after 10 minutes
4. **Complications:** Failed reduction

SPLINTING

1. **Indications:** Immobilization of injured extremity
2. **Equipment**
   a. Splinting material (stockinette, cotton padding, elastic [ACE] bandage, plaster, or fiberglass)
   b. Bucket of water at room temperature
3. **Method**
   a. Determine type of splint
      i. Upper extremity examples: Long-arm posterior splint for proximal forearm and elbow injuries, short arm splint or distal sugar tong for wrist injuries, thumb spica for scaphoid fractures, radial or ulnar guttar splints for metacarpal and/or proximal phalangeal injuries (Figure 5.16A)
      ii. Lower extremity examples: Posterior ankle splint for distal fibula, ankle, foot (Figure 5.16B)
   b. Measure and cut stockinette and plaster to appropriate length
   c. Use stockinette that will extend slightly farther than splint so that it can fold back over the ends of plaster
   d. Wrap circumferentially with cotton padding; overlap each turn by 50%, adding extra padding at bony prominences
   e. Keep joints in neutral positions (e.g., elbow at a 90-degree angle, wrist in slight dorsiflexion)
   f. Immerse plaster in cool or tepid water, squeeze out extra water, and mold slab into place (perform initial splint shaping at large joints)

g. Wrap the cling or elastic wrap around the splint while continuing to mold

h. Splint must be kept in position until the plaster or fiberglass has hardened

4. **Complications:** Pressure sores, dermatitis, neurovascular compromise

Figure 5.16 Long-Arm Posterior Splint (A) and Posterior Ankle Splint (B)

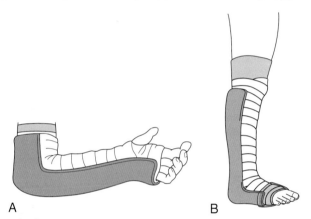

A   B

(From The Johns Hopkins Hospital, Hughes HK, Kahl LK. *The Harriet Lane Handbook: A Manual for Pediatric House Officers*; 1969.)

LACERATION REPAIR

GLUING

1. **Indications**
   a. For repair of *clean*, *well-approximated*, *superficial* lacerations <4 cm length and <0.5 cm width
   b. Should not be used in wounds in which dehiscence is likely to occur (over/near a joint), where there is increased risk of infection, or areas with dense hair or crossing mucocutaneous borders

2. **Equipment**
   a. Tissue adhesive (e.g., 2-octylcyanoacrylate [Dermabond])
   b. Topical anesthetic (e.g., LET, lidcaine epinephrine tetracaine) if desired

3. **Method**
   a. LET topical anesthetic may be used for pain control; will also aid in vascular constriction and hemostasis; apply 20 to 30 minutes before procedure
   b. Preparation of wound should include irrigation (~50–100 mL of irrigation fluid for each 1 cm of laceration) and cleansing area with antiseptic solution

c. After cleaning, wound should be dried and hemostasis attained

d. Appose wound edges with slight eversion, using forceps or fingers

e. Apply thin layer of tissue adhesive over wound edges, holding wound in apposition for 30 to 60 seconds to allow polymerization

f. Repeat this maneuver 2 to 3 times to allow optimal wound closure, holding wound in apposition for 2 to 3 minutes after final application

4. **Complications:** Wound infection, wound dehiscence, accidental adhesion of procedural materials (e.g., gauze) to glued wound

SUTURING

1. **Indications:** Closure of simple lacerations in the absence of wound contamination, injury to deeper structures, or impaired blood supply

   Note: Consultation with a specialist should be considered for wounds involving tendons, nerves, or blood vessels; wounds involving an open fracture, and complicated lacerations to face, lips, or genitalia. Also see Chapter 34 Plastic Surgery for further discussion of bite wounds.

2. **Equipment**

   a. Suture material: In general, nonabsorbable sutures for superficial laceration repair (although absorbable may be suitable for infants and young children for whom removal is difficult) and absorbable synthetic sutures for deeper (layered) repair. See Table 5.4 for suture size recommendations and Table 5.5 for common suture types.

   b. Needle holder, tissue forceps, tissue scissors

   c. Sterile gauze dressing

   d. Irrigation equipment (0.9% NaCl or sterile water, syringe attached to a 18- to 20-gauge angiocatheter (without needle)

   e. Antibiotic ointment

Table 5.4	Suture Size by Region
Wound Location	**Suture Size**
Intraoral mucosa	4-0–5-0
Scalp, torso, extremities	
- Superficial sutures	4-0–5-0
- Deep sutures	3-0–4-0
Face (eyelid, lip)	
- Superficial sutures	6-0
- Deep sutures	5-0–6-0
Face (forehead, chin)	5-0–6-0
Digits	5-0
Trunk/extremity wounds under tension	
- Superficial	3-0–4-0
- Deep	3-0–4-0

Table 5.5	Common Suture Types

Nonabsorbable

Synthetic monofilament
   Polypropylene (Prolene)
   Nylon (Dermalon, Ethilon)
Nonsynthetic
   Silk

Absorbable

Synthetic
   Polyglactin (Vicryl)
   Polyglactin 910 (Vicryl Rapide)
   Polyglycolic Acid (Dexon)
   Poliglecaprone (Monocryl)
Nonsynthetic
   Catgut (Fast absorbing, Plain, and Chromic)

Modified from Hollander JE, Singer AJ. Laceration management. *Ann Emerg Med.* 1999;34(3):356–367.

3. **Method**
   a. Preparation of wound should include cleansing area with antiseptic solution, irrigation of wound (~50–100 mL of irrigation fluid for each 1 cm of laceration)
   b. Ensure edges of wound can be approximated with good alignment; edges should be everted to avoid depressed scar once healed
   c. Basic suture techniques include simple interrupted (may be used to repair superficial skin wounds, with knots placed to side to avoid irritation and inflammation of wound), horizontal mattress, vertical mattress, and deep dermal
   d. Simple skin lacerations should be dressed with sterile gauze and antibacterial ointment
   e. Tetanus prophylaxis should be administered if appropriate (see Chapter 23 Immunoprophylaxis)
   f. Removal of nonabsorbable sutures is dependent on location of wound (Table 5.6)
4. **Complications:** Wound infection, wound dehiscence

Table 5.6	Timely Suture Removal
Wound Location	**Time of Removal (Days)**
Neck	3–4
Face	5
Scalp	7–10
Upper extremities, trunk	7–10
Lower extremities	8–10
Joint surface	10–14

From Fleisher GR, Ludwig S, eds. *Textbook of Pediatric Emergency Medicine*. 6th ed. Philadelphia, PA: Lippincott Williams & Wilkins; 2010.

ABSCESS INCISION AND DRAINAGE

1. **Indications:** Treatment of superficial cutaneous abscess. Surgical consultation should be sought for very large abscesses, deep abscesses in sensitive areas (e.g., perirectal), or abscesses in nasolabial folds or palmar or deep plantar spaces.
2. **Equipment**
   a. Scalpel (No. 11 or 15 blade), hemostat, syringe with 18-gauge needle
   b. 0.9% NaCl
   c. Packing/gauze if needed
3. **Method**
   a. Anesthetize area with application of topical anesthetic and injection of local anesthetic
   b. Define area of maximum fluctuation; can try aspirating with 18-gauge needle
   c. Make incision over the abscess with scalpel, cutting parallel to natural crease of skin
   d. Spread abscess cavity open with hemostat and dissect loculations
   e. Irrigate with 0.9% NaCl to help remove purulent material
   f. Pack with sterile packing strip if indicated (this is *not* necessary for most abscesses <5 cm)
4. **Complications:** Bleeding, scarring, nerve or vessel damage

FURTHER READING

Bachur RG, Shaw KN. *Fleisher & Ludwig's Textbook of Pediatric Emergency Medicine.* 7th ed. Philadelphia, PA: Lippincott Williams & Wilkins; 2015.
King C, Henretig FM. *Textbook of Pediatric Emergency Procedures.* Philadelphia, PA: Lippincott Williams & Wilkins; 2008.

Procedures

5

Section II

Subspecialty Pediatrics

Adolescent Medicine

Valene Singh • Samantha Martin • Alene Toulany

COMMON ABBREVIATIONS

Also see page xviii for a list of other abbreviations used throughout this book

AN	anorexia nervosa
AN-R	anorexia nervosa restricting subtype
ARFID	avoidant/restrictive food intake disorder
BED	binge eating disorder
BMI	body mass index
BN	bulimia nervosa
CBT	cognitive behavioral therapy
COC	combined oral contraceptives
DBT	dialectical behavior therapy
DSM-5	*Diagnostic and Statistical Manual of Mental Disorders*, 5th Edition
FBT	family based therapy
FSH	follicle-stimulating hormone
FTT	failure to thrive
LFT	liver function test
LH	luteinizing hormone
NAAT	nucleic acid amplification test

INTERVIEWING THE ADOLESCENT

1. **HEADSSS** and **THRxEADSS** framework for all adolescents and those with chronic illness or disability (Table 6.1)

Table 6.1	Approach to the Adolescent Interview: HEADSSS and THRxEADSS Framework	
		HEADSSS	THRxEADSS
T	Transition		What is your health condition? Can you explain the important things about your condition in three or four sentences? How much of your health care is your responsibility? What do you think you need to get ready for adult healthcare?
H	Home	Who lives with you? Where do you live? What are your relationships like at home? What are your responsibilities at home? Does home ever feel stressful or unsafe?	Are there any issues with housing and your health (accessibility/allergens/others)? Do you have concerns about how your condition affects your family's function? Who knows about your condition (family members/friends)?
Rx	Medication, Treatment	What medications do you take? What are the dosages? Who is in charge of your medications? What is your role? How do your medications/treatments fit in your routine during the week/weekend? What happens when you miss a dose? What do you like and dislike about your medications?	

Continued

		HEADSSS	**THRxEADSS**
Table 6.1		**Approach to the Adolescent Interview: HEADSSS and THRxEADSS Framework—cont'd**	
E	Education/ Employment	Tell me about school. How are your grades? What do you like to learn? What are your future education/employment plans? Do you feel you belong at school? Any issues with bullying? Do you feel safe at school? Are you working/have a job?	Does your condition make things different or difficult for you at school? Is there someone you can talk to or go see for help/support at school? How often do you have to miss school because of your condition?
	Eating	How do you feel about your body? Does your weight or body shape concern you? Have you had recent changes to your weight? Have you done anything to try to change your weight? Tell me about your exercise routine.	How does your condition or medications affect your diet and appetite? Does your condition affect how your body looks? In what way?
A	Activities	What do you do for fun? What are your hobbies/interests? Do you spend time with friends outside of school? Tell me what you like to do online.	Does your condition get in the way of participating in activities that your friends do? Do you have friends or talk to people who have similar health/disability issues? Do you use the internet to connect with other teens with health conditions or learn about your condition? Does your condition have an effect on your sleep?
D	Drugs	Some teenagers your age drink alcohol, use tobacco/e-cigarettes/vape, smoke marijuana, or other drugs—what has your experience been? Do any of your family members use tobacco/alcohol/other drugs? Do you take over-the-counter/herbal medications? Have you ever taken medications not prescribed to you? Consider CRAFFT screen (see Table 6.7).	What do you know about the effect of alcohol/cigarettes/street drugs on your condition or treatments? Do you ever use alcohol/cigarettes/street drugs to treat your condition, symptoms, or medication side effects?

Table 6.1		**Approach to the Adolescent Interview: HEADSSS and THRxEADSS Framework—cont'd**	
		HEADSSS	**THRxEADSS**
S	Sexuality	Have you ever been in a romantic relationship? Tell me about the people you have dated. Are you interested in boys/girls/both/unsure? Have any of your relationships ever been sexual relationships (such as involving kissing or touching)? What does "safe sex" mean to you? How are you protecting yourself from getting pregnant? Have you ever been tested for an STI?	What do you know about the effect of your condition on your sexual health? Are there any limits on contraception you can use because of your condition Have you talked about the genetics of your condition (i.e., can it be passed on to your children)?
	Suicide/ depression	How is your mood (scale of 1–10)? Do you feel sad/down more than usual? Do you feel stressed or worried more than usual? How is your sleep? Appetite? Have you ever felt so low that you have thoughts about hurting or killing yourself?	Does your condition make you sad, angry, or anxious? Have you ever had suicidal thoughts or tried to hurt yourself because of your condition?
	Safety	Do you feel safe at home? School? Have you ever been bullied or experienced violence at school or at home? Do you text and drive? Have you ever driven a car while high or been a passenger in a car of a driver who was high? Do you wear a seatbelt?	
	Strengths	What do you think are your strengths? What skills/unique attributes do you have?	

STI, Sexually transmitted infection.

2. Interview adolescent alone, also ensure time to hear from family/caregivers
3. **Confidentiality:** ensure confidentiality and state limits up front (e.g., at risk of serious and imminent harm to self or others, any child <16 years living in the patient's home at risk of harm)
4. **Motivational interviewing:** can be used as a way to encourage "change talk" (Table 6.2). Goal is to highlight a discrepancy between the patient's current behavior and their treatment goal.

Table 6.2	Motivational Interviewing
Technique	**Examples**
Open-ended questions	How does drinking on the weekends affect getting your homework done?
Reflective listening	It sounds like you are very upset about the conflict at home with your parents. Do you think you are more likely to use when you are upset?
Affirmations	Deciding to smoke less because of how it makes you feel sounds like a good choice.
Summary statements	Hanging out with your friends is important. What other activities do you like to do together?
Eliciting change talk	What are some things you would like to change?

AGE OF CONSENT

1. No legal age of consent for medical treatment in Canada (exception Quebec, age of consent is 14 years old)
2. Consent is based on whether the patient can fully appreciate the nature and consequences of the proposed treatment or lack of treatment
3. Parent/caregiver involvement is strongly recommended when the treatment involves serious risks or there is potential to have serious/permanent effects on the patient
4. Age of consent for sexual activity in Canada is 16 years (includes all forms—kissing to intercourse)
   a. Anyone <18 years cannot consent for sexual activity that is exploitative (e.g., trading goods for sex, pornography)
   b. A 16- or 17-year-old cannot consent to sexual activity if there is a relationship of trust/authority/dependency/exploitation with the partner
   c. A 14- or 15-year-old can consent to sexual activity as long as their partner is less than 5 years older and there is no relationship of trust/authority/dependency/exploitation
   d. A 12- or 13-year-old can consent to sexual activity with a partner as long as the partner is less than 2 years older and there is no relationship of trust/authority/dependency/exploitation

EATING DISORDERS

1. See Table 6.3 for comparison of common eating disorders
2. **History**
   a. **Weight loss:** intentional? Is it a result of decreased intake versus increased output?
   b. **Weight history:** acuity of weight loss, highest and lowest weights, social environment just before and at start of weight loss, attitudes about size and shape
   c. **Growth chart:** get historical growth charts

Table 6.3

Table 6.3 Comparison of Common Pediatric and Adolescent Eating Disorders

	Anorexia Nervosa	Bulimia Nervosa	Binge Eating Disorder	Avoidant/ Restrictive Food Intake Disorder
Diagnostic criteria	1. Restriction of energy intake relative to requirement, leading to a significantly low body weight 2. Intense fear of gaining weight or of becoming fat, or *persistent behavior* that interferes with weight gain, even though at a significantly low body weight 3. Disturbance in the way in which one's body weight or shape is experienced, or persistent lack of recognition of the seriousness of the current low body weight Classifications: Restrictive subtype and binge/purge subtype	1. Recurrent episodes of binge eating: consuming large amount in a discrete period of time; feeling out of control during episodes 2. Recurrent inappropriate compensatory behavior to prevent weight gain (e.g., self-induced vomiting; misuse of laxatives, diuretics, enemas, or other medications; fasting; excessive exercise) 3. Occurs regularly: at least once per week for 3 months 4. Self-evaluation is unduly influenced by body shape and weight	1. Recurrent episodes of binge eating without compensatory behaviors 2. Episodes occur regularly: at least *once per week* for 3 months	1. Eating or feeding disturbance (e.g., apparent lack of interest in eating or food; avoidance based on the sensory characteristics of food; concern about aversive consequences of eating) as manifested by *persistent* failure to meet appropriate nutritional and/or energy needs associated with at least one of: a. Significant weight loss (or failure to achieve expected weight gain or faltering growth in children) b. Significant nutritional deficiency c. Dependence on enteral feeding or oral nutritional supplements d. Marked interference with psychosocial functioning 2. The disturbance is not better explained by lack of available food or by an associated culturally sanctioned practice 3. There is no evidence of a disturbance in the way in which one's body weight or shape is experienced
Management	1. FBT 2. SSRI, atypical antipsychotics for comorbidities	1. FBT 2. CBT 3. Fluoxetine	1. CBT, DBT and interdisciplinary weight loss management 2. Imipramine, topiramate, SSRIs to reduce binge eating	1. FBT

CBT, Cognitive behavioral therapy; *DBT,* dialectical behavior therapy; *FBT,* family-based therapy; *SSRI,* selective serotonin reuptake inhibitor.

Data from *Diagnostic and Statistical Manual of Mental Disorders,* 5th Edition.

Adolescent Medicine

6

d. **Dietary history:** food choices and portion size; history of uncontrolled eating, purging, exercise (types and frequency); diet aids, laxative use, smoking/drug use

e. **Menstrual history:** age at menarche, regularity of menstruation, weight at time of last normal menstrual period

f. **Review of systems:** fever, night sweats, blurry vision, headache, dizziness, syncope, chest pain, dyspnea, palpitations, abdominal pain, hematemesis, constipation, bloody stool, heat/cold intolerance, hair loss, arthralgia, rashes, alopecia

g. **Psychiatric and social/family history:** family history of eating disorders, mental health conditions

3. **Clinical manifestations**

   a. See Table 6.4 for clinical features of anorexia nervosa (AN), avoidant/restrictive food intake disorder (ARFID) and bulimia nervosa (BN)

   b. Features of AN, ARFID, and BN often overlap

Table 6.4	Clinical Features of Anorexia Nervosa, Avoidant/Restrictive Food Intake Disorder and Bulimia Nervosa	
Features	**Anorexia Nervosa and Avoidant/Restrictive Food Intake Disorder**	**Bulimia Nervosa**
General examination	Hypothermia and cold extremities, dry skin, lanugo, carotenemia, alopecia	Eroded tooth enamel (posterior aspect upper teeth), Russell's sign (callus on knuckles), subconjunctival hemorrhages, parotid enlargement
Gastrointestinal	Delayed gastric emptying, constipation	Esophagitis, gastric dilatation, Mallory-Weiss tear, esophageal rupture (rare), vocal cord dysfunction
Cardiovascular system	Sinus bradycardia, arrhythmias, hypotension, pericardial effusion, poor peripheral perfusion, edema, cardiac muscle atrophy, murmur (mitral valve prolapse)	Cardiomyopathy (suspect ipecac poisoning), edema
Endocrine	Amenorrhea, growth delay/failure, delayed puberty	Irregular menses
Neurological	Structural brain changes, atrophy in severe cases, seizure, syncope, poor concentration	

4. **Physical examination**

   a. **Growth parameters:** weight, height, body mass index (BMI)

   b. **Physical examination**

      i. **Vital signs:** resting heart rate (HR), orthostatic changes in HR and blood pressure (BP) (taken after lying down for approximately 3 minutes followed by standing for 2 minutes), temperature

      ii. Assess for features in Table 6.4

PEARL

Plot weight, height, and body mass index at every visit: children should NOT maintain or lose weight. Rapid weight loss, crossing percentiles, persistent failure to gain weight, and any parental eating or weight concerns should be taken seriously.

5. **Differential diagnosis:** see Table 6.5 for differential diagnosis of eating disorders

Table 6.5	Differential Diagnosis for Eating Disorders
System	**Differential Diagnosis**
Endocrine	- Thyroid disease (hypo- or hyper-) - Diabetes mellitus - Adrenal insufficiency - Hypercortisolism
Gastrointestinal disorders	- Inflammatory bowel disease - Celiac disease - Infectious diarrhea - Immunodeficiency or chronic infections (tuberculosis, human immunodeficiency virus)
Psychiatric	- Depression - Anxiety - Obsessive compulsive disorder - Substance abuse
Other	- Malignancy (prolactinoma) - Rheumatological disease (systemic lupus erythematosus) - Pregnancy - Chronic renal disease - Wilson disease - Porphyria

6. **Initial workup**
   a. Complete blood count (CBC) and differential, electrolytes, bicarbonate, calcium, magnesium, phosphate, glucose, urea, creatinine, amylase, albumin, liver enzymes, bilirubin, erythrocyte sedimentation rate (ESR), vitamin D
   b. Thyroid-stimulating hormone (TSH), follicle-stimulating hormone (FSH), luteinizing hormone (LH), estradiol, prolactin, pregnancy test
   c. Consider cortisol (am) and celiac screen
   d. 12-Lead electrocardiogram (ECG)
   e. Urinalysis (particularly for specific gravity, hematuria, proteinuria)
   f. Other investigations based on history and physical examination
   g. See Table 6.6 for laboratory features of eating disorders

Table 6.6	Laboratory Features of Anorexia Nervosa, Bulimia Nervosa, and Avoidant/Restrictive Food Intake Disorder	
Features	**Anorexia Nervosa and Avoidant/ Restrictive Food Intake Disorder**	**Bulimia Nervosa**
Gastrointestinal	Hypercholesterolemia, ↑liver enzymes	
Cardiovascular system	Sinus bradycardia, arrhythmias, hypotension, low-voltage ECG with flattened or inverted T waves, prolonged QTc interval	Prolonged QTc interval
Endocrine	Hypercortisolemia, sick euthyroid syndrome (↓TSH, normal T_4, T_3), partial DI	
Metabolic	↑Na secondary to dehydration, ↓Na from ↑H_2O intake, ↓ renal function, hypophosphatemia, ↓K, hypoglycemia, ↓Ca, ↓Mg	Hypochloremic hypokalemic metabolic alkalosis if vomiting; hyperchloremic metabolic acidosis if laxative abuse; ↑ amylase; ↑Na secondary to dehydration
Hematological	B12 and folate deficiency, vitamin K deficiency, coagulopathy, pancytopenia, ↓ESR	

DI, Diabetes insipidus; *ECG*, electrocardiogram; *ESR*, erythrocyte sedimentation rate; T_3, triiodothyronine; T_4, thyroxine; *TSH*, thyroid-stimulating hormone.

7. **Indications for hospitalization**
   a. Bradycardia (daytime HR <50 beats/min; night time HR <45 beats/min) or hypotension
   b. Orthostatic changes (↓ in systolic BP >20 mmHg, ↑ in HR >35 beats/min)
   c. Arrhythmias, including prolonged QTc interval
   d. Moderate to severe dehydration
   e. Electrolyte or acid–base abnormalities
   f. Absolute weight <75% (or <80%) target weight
   g. Arrested growth and development
   h. Acute food refusal
   i. Suicidal ideation

✦ PEARL

To determine target weight, prior growth (weight, height, body mass index [BMI]) curve most predictive. Can also use weight for 50th percentile BMI, weight at same percentile as height percentile, or weight at which patient became amenorrheic +2 kg. Reassess regularly as treatment progresses.

8. **Initial inpatient management**
   a. **Bed rest:** advance activity as soon as possible based on vital signs and symptoms
   b. **Monitoring:** continuous cardiac monitoring until stable, orthostatic vital signs
   c. **Judicious use of fluids:** avoid boluses of IV fluids unless patient is severely dehydrated or in shock; avoid dextrose containing solution because it may contribute to refeeding syndrome
   d. **Nutrition:** start on the approximate caloric intake before hospitalization divided into three meals and three snacks. Slowly increase by 250 kcal/day increments, if no evidence of refeeding syndrome. Determine total fluid intake based on weight, determine fluid content of meals and give difference as additional water throughout the day. Eventual goal of ~1 to 2 kg weight gain per week.
   e. **Supplements:** calcium, vitamin D, multivitamin, consider thiamine if very low BMI
   f. **Refeeding bloodwork** (see Section 9 below)
   g. **Multidisciplinary team approach**
9. **Refeeding syndrome**
   a. Potentially fatal shifts in fluids and electrolytes that can occur upon initiating feeds in a malnourished patient (orally, enterally or parenterally)
   b. **Highest risk:** admission at <70% target weight
   c. **Refeeding bloodwork:** Na, K, Cl, glucose, Ca, Mg, PO_4 daily for 5 days after initiation of feeding (oral or nasogastric); as necessary, supplement PO_4, Ca, Mg, K
      i. ↓ Phosphate: nadir typically on day 4 of refeeding
   d. **Cardiovascular**
      i. ↓ Potassium, ↓ magnesium: can lead to cardiac arrhythmias
      ii. Increased metabolic demand can lead to heart failure
   e. **Neurological:** delirium can occur during or after second week of refeeding, even after electrolytes have normalized
10. **Outpatient management**
    a. Family-based therapy (FBT) (first-line treatment): pediatrician's role is to be a consultant to parents and therapist. Goal weight gain as an outpatient is 0.2 to 0.5 kg/week. Cognitive behavior therapy (CBT) and dialectical behavior therapy (DBT) can be considered for patients that do not qualify for FBT (e.g., BN).
11. **Pharmacological therapy**
    a. Medication is used as second-line or adjunct treatment
    b. Depressive or obsessive compulsive disorder (OCD) symptoms may improve or resolve with weight restoration

c. Atypical antipsychotics (i.e., olanzapine, risperidone)—used for treatment of comorbid psychiatric conditions or excessive rigidity/anxiety impeding recovery

d. Selective serotonin reuptake inhibitors (SSRIs, i.e., fluoxetine) treatment of comorbid depression/anxiety/OCD in AN-R (ideally when weight restored for improved efficacy), BN, binge eating disorder (BED)

SUBSTANCE USE

1. **Screening tools**
   a. **CRAFFT:** behavioral health screening tool (CRAFFT) to identify problematic substance use in adolescents (Table 6.7). Two or more positive answers suggests problematic use and need for further assessment.
   b. **Global Appraisal of Individual Needs—Short Screener (GAIN-SS):** self-reported questionnaire to identify youth at risk of having a substance abuse or dependence disorder and screen for mental health disorders

Table 6.7	CRAFFT Screen for Problematic Substance Use
C	Have you ever driven a *CAR* or driven with someone else while high or drunk?
R	Do you ever drink or use drugs to *RELAX*, feel better, or fit in?
A	Do you ever drink or get high *ALONE*?
F	Do you ever *FORGET* things while drinking or using drugs?
F	Do your *FAMILY* or *FRIENDS* ever tell you to cut down on drinking or drug use?
T	Has your alcohol or drug use ever gotten you in *TROUBLE*?

Adapted from Knight JR et al. A new brief screen for adolescent substance abuse. *Arch Pediatr Adolesc Med.* 1999;153(6):591–596.

2. **Risk factors**
   a. **Social:** academic failure, family/friends who use, history of abuse
   b. **Protective factors:** sense of connectedness to school, family or community
   c. **Biological:** concurrent mental health disorder, incentive/reward neuronal pathways are very active and immature prefrontal cortex
   d. **Genetic predisposition**

3. **Diagnosis**
   a. DSM-5 combines previous substance abuse and substance dependence disorders into a single disorder
   b. Behaviors contributing to diagnosis include: impaired control, social impairment, risky use, and pharmacological indicators, such as tolerance and withdrawal

4. **Management**
   a. See Chapter 3 Poisonings and Toxicology for acute overdose management
   b. **Harm reduction:** accepts that a continuing level of drug use is inevitable, thus the goal is to reduce adverse consequences if abstinence is not possible. Emphasis is on the measurement of health, social, and economic outcomes, as opposed to drug consumption.

CONTRACEPTION

1. Types of contraception (Table 6.8)
2. Regardless of the contraceptive method, encourage condom use to reduce risk for sexually transmitted infections

Table 6.8	**Types of Contraception**		
Types	**Examples**	**Failure Rate (Typical use)**	**Side Effects**
No method		94%	
Barrier	1. Female Condom 2. Male Condom 3. Diaphragm 4. Sponge	1. 21% 2. 18% 3. 12% 4. 12%–28%	- Recurrent UTI, vaginal DC, irritation from spermicide (diaphragm) - May damage vaginal mucosa; more prone to yeast infections and BV (sponge)
Hormonal	1. Combined oral contraceptive/progestin only pill 2. NuvaRing 3. Patch 4. Depo-Provera	1. 9% 2. 9% 3. 9% 4. 6%	- Irregular bleeding/spotting, breast tenderness, bloating, nausea, headaches - Local skin irritation (patch) - Weight gain, irregular bleeding, decreased bone density (Depo)
Intrauterine device	1. IUD (Copper) 2. Hormonal IUS (e.g., Mirena)	1. 0.8% 2. 0.2%	- Risk for perforation, expulsion, PID, ectopic pregnancy - Irregular bleeding, pain/dysmenorrhea
Emergency	1. Levonorgestrel (Plan B) 2. Ulipristal Acetate (e.g., Ella) 3. Yuzpe (estrogen and progestin) 4. Copper IUD	Failure rate increases with length of time between intercourse and first dose	- Nausea/vomiting - Cramping (copper IUD)

BV, Bacterial vaginosis; *DC*, discharge; *IUD*, intrauterine device; *IUS*, intrauterine system; *PID*, pelvic inflammatory disease; *UTI*, urinary tract infection.

Data from Di Meglio et al. Contraceptive care for Canadian youth. *Paediatr Child Health*. 2018: 23(4):271–277.

3. Long-acting reversible contraceptives, such as intrauterine devices (IUDs), are the recommended first choice for contraception in adolescents, even if nulliparous

4. Absolute contraindication to estrogen-containing contraception (COCs, transdermal patch, or vaginal ring) is migraine with aura. Progestin only pill can be used. See Box 6.1 for absolute contraindications to COCs.

> **Box 6.1   Absolute Contraindications to Combined Oral Contraceptives in the Pediatric Population**
>
> 1. Migraine headache with focal neurological symptoms (i.e., aura)
> 2. Hypertension (systolic >160 mmHg or diastolic >100 mmHg)
> 3. Current or previous history of thromboembolism
> 4. Systemic lupus erythematosus, positive or unknown antiphospholipid antibodies
> 5. History of cerebrovascular accident
> 6. Current or history of ischemic heart disease
> 7. Complicated valvular heart disease (pulmonary hypertension, atrial fibrillation, history of subacute bacterial endocarditis)
> 8. Liver disease or hepatoma
> 9. Known or suspected pregnancy
> 10. Major surgery with prolonged immobilization
> 11. <21 days postpartum if breastfeeding
> 12. Undiagnosed abnormal uterine bleeding
> 13. Known/suspected breast cancer
> 14. Diabetes with retinopathy/nephropathy/neuropathy

Data from https://www.cdc.gov/reproductivehealth/contraception/pdf/summary-chart-us-medical-eligibility-criteria_508tagged.pdf

5. Ulipristal acetate (Ella) is the most effective *emergency contraceptive pill*, whereas the copper IUD is the most effective mode of emergency contraception. BMI may affect the efficacy of emergency contraception. Offer ulipristal acetate and the copper IUD to women with higher BMI.

6. Consider providing the following websites for patient education and resources: "Sex & U" www.sexualityandu.ca and "Go Ask Alice" www.goaskalice.columbia.edu

SEXUALLY TRANSMITTED INFECTIONS

See Genital Infections in Chapter 20 Gynecology

Allergy

Stephanie Erdle • Melanie Conway • Adelle Atkinson

COMMON ABBREVIATIONS

Also see page xviii for a list of other abbreviations used throughout this book

AAE	acquired angioedema
ACE	angiotensin converting enzyme
AD	atopic dermatitis
DRESS	drug rash with eosinophilia and systemic symptoms
EBV	Epstein-Barr virus
FPE	food protein enteropathy
FPIAP	food protein-induced allergic proctocolitis
FPIES	food protein-induced enterocolitis syndrome
FTT	failure to thrive
HAE	hereditary angioedema
HIV	human immunodeficiency virus
IDT	intradermal test
IgE	immunoglobulin E
IgG	immunoglobulin G
IgM	immunoglobulin M
JIA	juvenile idiopathic arthritis
SCIT	subcutaneous immunotherapy
SJS	Stevens-Johnson syndrome
SLE	systemic lupus erythematosus
SPT	skin prick test
SSLR	serum sickness-like reaction
TEN	toxic epidermal necrolysis
VIT	venom immunotherapy

ALLERGY INVESTIGATIONS

See Box 7.1 for common investigations for evaluation of allergies

---

Box 7.1   Common Investigations for Evaluation of Allergy

Skin Prick Testing
1. Most sensitive screening method to detect IgE antibodies if history of reaction to allergen
2. Positive reaction: wheal ≥3 mm larger than the saline control, read 15 min after application of reagents, positive histamine control ensures reliable testing
3. Antihistamines should be held for 1 week before skin testing
4. False positives may occur with skin conditions such as atopic dermatitis, dermatographism

Allergen-Specific Immunoglobulin E Tests
1. Quantifies in vitro specific IgE to a particular allergen (e.g., to follow food-specific IgE antibody concentrations)
2. Useful when SPT not possible, not as sensitive or specific as standardized SPT
3. Useful with the SPT when making decisions about provocation testing

Provocation Testing
1. Administering the allergen in question (e.g., food, drug, or vaccine) in graded steps
2. Gold standard in the diagnosis of IgE-mediated hypersensitivity
3. Should be conducted in a controlled setting equipped to deal with anaphylaxis

---

Ig, Immunoglobulin; *SPT,* skin prick testing.

HYPERSENSITIVITY IMMUNE RESPONSES

See Table 7.1 for classification of hypersensitivity immune responses

Table 7.1	Classification of Hypersensitivity Immune Responses			
Type of Hypersensitivity	Pathologic Immune Mechanisms	Timing After Exposure	Culprit Agents	Examples
I: Anaphylactic or immediate hypersensitivity reactions	IgE antibody	Minutes to several hours	Food, drugs, vaccines, insect stings, pollens	Anaphylaxis, allergic rhinitis, allergic asthma, acute urticaria
II: Cytotoxic reactions	IgM, IgG antibodies against antigens bound to cell membrane structures	Varies depending on specific entity	ABO blood group antigens, Rh D antigen, drugs (e.g., penicillin, cephalosporins)	Immune hemolytic anemia, Rh hemolytic disease in newborn, autoimmune hyperthyroidism, myasthenia gravis, Goodpasture syndrome, penicillin-induced hemolytic anemia
III: Immune-complex mediated	Complexes of circulating antigens and IgM or IgG antibodies (pathogenesis unknown for SSLR)	5–21 days	Serum sickness: Equine or rabbit ATG SSLR: drugs (e.g., antibiotics, antiepileptics), vaccines, viral infections	Serum sickness and SSLR, post-streptococcal glomerulonephritis
IV: Delayed Hypersensitivity	T lymphocytes	2 days to 8 weeks	Drugs (e.g., antibiotics, antiepileptics), viral infections (EBV, HIV), nickel	Tuberculin skin test reactions, contact dermatitis, exanthematous drug eruption, DRESS

ATG, Antithyroglobulin; *DRESS*, drug rash with eosinophilia and systemic symptoms; *EBV*, Epstein-Barr virus; *HIV*, human immunodeficiency virus; *Ig*, immunoglobulin; *SSLR*, serum sickness-like reaction.

ANAPHYLAXIS

See Chapter 2 Emergency Medicine for emergent management of anaphylaxis

FOOD ALLERGIC REACTIONS

IgE-MEDIATED FOOD REACTIONS

1. **Epidemiology**
   a. Most common food allergens (in descending order): cow's milk, eggs, peanuts, wheat, soy, tree nuts, fish, shellfish, sesame

155

    b. Early childhood allergies to cow's milk, egg, wheat, and soy typically resolve (resolution ranges from toddlerhood to adolescence)
    c. Peanut, tree nut, sesame, fish, and shellfish allergies tend to be persistent; ~20% of peanut allergy may resolve, usually by age 8 years
2. **Clinical manifestations**
    a. Rapid in onset, typically within minutes to 2 hours from time of ingestion
    b. Signs and symptoms can affect many systems (Table 7.2)
3. **Evaluation for suspected food allergy**
    a. **Detailed history:** timing, foods ingested, characterization of reaction, similar past reactions, treatments given/required
    b. **Investigations:** skin prick test (SPT), allergen-specific IgE (sIgE) tests, provocation tests

Table 7.2	Signs and Symptoms of IgE-Mediated Reactions
System	**Signs and Symptoms**
General/central nervous system	Fussiness, irritability, drowsiness, lethargy, reduced level of consciousness, somnolence
Skin	Urticaria, pruritus, angioedema, flushing
Upper airway	Stridor, hoarseness, oropharyngeal or laryngeal edema, uvular edema, swollen lips/tongue, sneezing, rhinorrhea, upper airway obstruction
Lower airway	Coughing, dyspnea, bronchospasm, tachypnea, respiratory arrest
Cardiovascular	Tachycardia, hypotension, dizziness, syncope, arrhythmias, diaphoresis, pallor, cyanosis, cardiac arrest
Gastrointestinal	Nausea, vomiting, diarrhea, abdominal pain

4. **Management**
    a. Treat anaphylaxis with IM epinephrine (see Chapter 2 Emergency Medicine)
    b. **Elimination:** strict elimination of the food identified as the allergen (including "may contain")
    c. **Epinephrine:** prescribe autoinjectable epinephrine (e.g., EpiPen®) to be carried at all times
        i. EpiPen® Jr (0.15 mg) for 10 to 25 kg (and <10 kg if needed)
        ii. EpiPen® (0.3 mg) for ≥25 kg
    d. Medical alert bracelet
    e. Referral to an allergist
    f. **"Allergy-aware" or "allergy-safe" classroom:** do not trade/share foods, hand washing before and after eating, no food allowed in activities, scrutinize ingredient labels
5. **Food allergy prevention guidelines in high risk infants**
    a. **High risk infants:** infants with a personal history of atopy or one first-degree relative with atopy
    b. No restrictions in the maternal diet during pregnancy or lactation

c. Exclusive breastfeeding for the first 4 to 6 months of life, if possible

d. If formula is required, may consider hydrolyzed cow's milk formula

e. No delay in the introduction of any solids

f. Based on developmental readiness, consider introducing common allergenic solids between 4 and 6 months of age

   i. Evidence supports significant prevention of peanut allergy with early introduction

   ii. Evidence supports possible prevention of egg allergy with early introduction

   iii. Lack of evidence for other allergenic foods

g. If the infant tolerates a common allergenic food, advise parents to offer it a few times per week to maintain tolerance

6. **Pollen-food allergy syndrome (oral allergy syndrome, pollen fruit syndrome)**

a. **Description:** localized IgE mediated allergy associated with ingestion of uncooked fruits/vegetables and certain nuts in patients with allergies to certain pollens (food proteins cross react with pollen proteins)

b. **Symptoms:** typically limited to the oropharynx with immediate onset pruritus, tingling, irritation, and mild swelling of the lips, tongue, palate, and oropharynx; rarely systemic symptoms

c. **Investigations:** SPT to fresh food and inhalant aeroallergens

d. **Management**

   i. If fruits or vegetables, heated forms generally tolerated

   ii. If nuts, avoidance

> **! PITFALL**
>
> Adverse immune response to food proteins: must distinguish between immunoglobin (Ig)E-mediated (allergic) and non–IgE-mediated (intolerance or toxic reactions).

NON-IgE-MEDIATED FOOD REACTIONS

1. **Clinical presentation:** subacute and/or chronic symptoms, typically isolated to the gastrointestinal tract and/or skin

a. Examples: food protein-induced enterocolitis syndrome (FPIES—entire gastrointestinal tract), food protein-induced allergic proctocolitis (FPIAP—rectum and colon) and food protein enteropathy (FPE—small bowel) (Table 7.3)

2. **Investigations:** food-specific IgE antibody levels and SPT typically negative

a. Cow's milk and soy proteins most commonly implicated

3. **Complications:** some patients with FPIES can go on to develop Type 1-mediated allergy

Table 7.3	Non–IgE-Mediated Reactions		
	FPIES	**FPIAP**	**FPE**
Symptoms	Profuse, repetitive vomiting 1–3 h after ingestion, ± diarrhea; dehydration and lethargy (acute), weight loss/ FTT (chronic)	Blood-tinged stools and mucus in otherwise healthy and thriving infant	Protracted diarrhea, malabsorption, intermittent vomiting, FTT; rarely bloody stools
Most common triggers	Early: cow's milk formula (uncommon in exclusively breastfed infants), soy formula Late: milk, soy, grains	Cow's milk (cow's milk in mother's diet if breast fed), soy formula	Cow's milk formula (uncommon in exclusively breastfed infants), soy formula
Age of onset	Most within first 3 months of life; later for solid food FPIES	Days–6 months; most 2–8 weeks	Most 1–2 months
Diagnosis	Based on history, with clinical improvement with withdrawal of suspected causal protein	Based on history, with clinical improvement with withdrawal of suspected causal protein	Based on history, confirmed with endoscopy and biopsy
Management	Food elimination, change to hydrolyzed formula	Food elimination from the maternal diet if breast-fed, hydrolyzed formula	Food elimination; change to hydrolyzed formula
Natural history	Most resolve by age 3–5 years	Majority resolve by 1 year	Majority resolve by 2–3 years

FPE, Food protein enteropathy; *FPIAP,* food protein-induced allergic proctocolitis; *FPIES,* food protein-induced enterocolitis syndrome; *FTT,* failure to thrive.

DRUG ALLERGIC REACTIONS

A. Types of immunologic drug reactions

1. **Type I**
   a. **Description:** presence of a drug-specific IgE, causing mast cell degranulation of histamine when drug is encountered
   b. **Clinical presentation**: see Table 7.1
   c. **Timing**: minutes to hours following drug exposure
   d. **Common culprit drugs:** beta-lactams, quinolones, chemotherapeutics, neuromuscular blocking agents
   e. **Management:** intramuscular (IM) epinephrine for anaphylaxis, withdrawal of offending drug, avoid drug in the future

2. **Serum sickness-like reaction (Type III)**
   a. **Description:** clinically resembles serum sickness, but pathogenesis unknown
   b. **Clinical presentation:** urticarial rash that lasts >24 hours and may leave bruising, arthralgias, fever, edematous hands and feet
   c. **Timing:** 5 to 21 days after drug exposure
   d. **Common culprit drugs:** cefaclor, penicillins, septra

e. **Management:** withdrawal of offending drug, supportive care with antihistamines and nonsteroidal antiinflammatory drugs (NSAIDs), steroids for severe arthritis, avoid drug in the future

3. **Exanthematous (morbilliform) drug eruption (Type IV)**
   a. **Clinical presentation:** morbilliform rash without mucosal involvement
   b. **Timing:** 5 to 14 days after drug exposure, but may occur sooner in previously sensitized patients
   c. **Common culprit drugs:** large variety of drugs, viral infections may contribute (e.g., Epstein-Barr virus [EBV])
   d. **Management:** discontinue drug, symptomatic treatment, not a contraindication for graded challenge at a later date

4. **Drug rash with eosinophilia and systemic symptoms (Type IV)**
   a. **Clinical presentation:** fever, malaise, lymphadenopathy, morbilliform rash; in severe cases, can affect liver, kidneys and lungs. Can be life-threatening a small percentage of the time.
   b. **Timing:** within 2 to 8 weeks after drug exposure
   c. **Common culprit drugs:** antiepileptic agents, sulfonamides
   d. **Laboratory features:** high eosinophils, atypical lymphocytes, elevated alanine transaminase (ALT)
   e. **Management:** withdrawal of offending drug, high potency topical corticosteroids, avoid medication in the future

5. **Steven-Johnson syndrome/toxic epidermal necrolysis (Type IV)**
   a. See Chapter 11 Dermatology

B. Specific drug allergies

1. **Penicillin allergy**
   a. Majority of persons deemed penicillin allergic from history are not truly allergic—confirm with intradermal test (IDT) and oral challenge
   b. If negative IDT to major and minor determinants of penicillin, rare chance of having allergic reaction

2. **Cephalosporin allergy**
   a. ~2% of patients with penicillin allergy AND positive SPT/IDT will react to cephalosporins
   b. If required in penicillin-sensitive patient, consider graded challenge as majority will tolerate cephalosporins

C. Evaluation for suspected drug allergy

1. **History:** timing; all prescription, nonprescription, biological (e.g., monoclonal antibodies, intravenous immunoglobulin [IVIG]) drugs; characterization of reaction, similar past reactions

2. **Investigations:** skin testing to evaluate IgE-mediated reactions (if available for particular drug) may be indicated; negative SPT confirmed with IDT, then provocative drug challenge

3. **Management**
   a. Discontinue suspected medication immediately
   b. Treat with IM epinephrine (if anaphylaxis), antihistamines, and/or corticosteroids
   c. Educate to avoid future exposure—consider cross reactivity with other drugs
   d. If mild reaction and not felt to be IgE-mediated, suppressive therapy (antihistamines ± corticosteroids) with continuation of offending drug may be appropriate (consult allergist)
   e. Consult allergist for consideration of desensitization of IgE-mediated drug allergy if medication required in the future with no acceptable alternatives. Perform in controlled hospital setting.
   f. Most non–IgE-mediated adverse drug reactions are contraindicated for in vivo challenge or desensitization (consult allergist)
   g. Medical alert bracelet

LATEX ALLERGIC REACTIONS

1. **Risk factors:** contact with mostly stretchable latex articles, multiple surgical procedures (e.g., spina bifida, genitourinary anomalies, repeated catheterizations, contact with healthcare workers), atopy
2. **Investigations:** SPT, specific IgE
3. **Management:** avoidance (especially stretchable latex [e.g., balloons, gloves]), latex-free surgery, prescribe autoinjectable epinephrine if risk of anaphylaxis

INSECT STING ALLERGIC REACTIONS

1. **Epidemiology:** most common Hymenoptera allergies: honeybee, yellow jacket, yellow hornet, white-faced hornet, paper wasp
2. **Clinical manifestations:** see Table 7.4
3. **Investigations:** for patients that are candidates for venom immunotherapy (VIT), perform IDT with Hymenoptera venom to identify specific causative insect. Consider baseline serum tryptase for those with severe anaphylaxis.
4. **Management of acute local reactions**
   a. **Local reactions:** resolve spontaneously; symptomatic treatment with cold compresses, oral analgesics, antihistamines
   b. **Large local reactions:** cold compresses, elevation of affected limb, analgesia, antihistamines; if extensive and disabling, consider oral steroids (2–4 days)
   c. **Systemic reactions:** treat anaphylaxis with IM epinephrine (see Chapter 2 Emergency Medicine)
   d. If stinger is visible, remove carefully to avoid further venom injection

Table 7.4	**Types of Reactions to Insect Stings**			
	IMMEDIATE			
Type	**Local Reactions**	**Large Local Reactions**	**Cutaneous Systemic Reaction or Anaphylaxis**	**Delayed**
Timing	Within minutes up to about 4 h after sting			Develop days after the sting
Clinical	Swelling, erythema, burning sensation at site	Cover two large joints or involve an entire limb	"Cutaneous systemic reactions" are limited to skin manifestations, such as: urticaria, pruritus, and angioedema. Anaphylaxis may also involve vomiting, dyspnea, wheezing, hypotension.	Rare; serum sickness, vasculitis, glomerulonephritis, Guillain-Barré syndrome, encephalitis, or myocarditis
Course	Resolve within hours or few days	Swelling may increase over 24–48 h, resolves in 5–10 days	IgE mediated; mild symptoms to life-threatening	Variable course
Risk with subsequent sting	Not predictive of systemic reactions to subsequent stings	<5% risk of anaphylaxis to subsequent stings	30%–60% recurrence of anaphylaxis with subsequent sting, unless symptoms are purely cutaneous	Variable, depending on initial reaction

5. **Prophylactic management**
   a. Avoidance measures (e.g., avoid drinking from straws, cans, or bottles when outdoors, avoid flowering plants, cover trashcans, avoid bare feet outdoors)
   b. Prescribe epinephrine autoinjector to patients with a history of an anaphylactic reaction
   c. Refer to a pediatric allergist for consideration of VIT
      i. VIT recommended in all patients with a history of an anaphylactic reaction and who have specific IgE to venom allergens
      ii. Patients with a history of cutaneous systemic reactions generally do not require VIT, but this may be considered when high-risk factors are present

VACCINE ALLERGIC REACTIONS

See Table 23.4 in Chapter 23 Immunoprophylaxis.

ALLERGIC RHINITIS AND CONJUNCTIVITIS

1. **Clinical description**
   a. **Allergic rhinitis symptoms:** sneezing, rhinorrhea, congestion, nasal itch, postnasal drip, cough, itchy palate, itchy ears
   b. **Allergic conjunctivitis symptoms:** itching, tearing, burning, conjunctival injection

c. **Characteristic signs:** horizontal nasal crease ("allergic salute"); allergic shiners (dark circles beneath eyes); Dennie-Morgan folds (creases on lower eyelid parallel to lower lid margin); pale, bluish, edematous nasal turbinates; cobblestoning of posterior pharynx and eyelids

d. **Comorbidities:** asthma, sinusitis, otitis media, atopic dermatitis, lymphoid hypertrophy/obstructive sleep apnea, nasal polyps, oral allergy syndrome

e. **Perennial allergic rhinoconjunctivitis:** year-round symptoms
   i. Includes: dust mites, indoor moulds, pets, cockroaches
   ii. Age of onset: ≥1 year

f. **Seasonal allergic rhinoconjunctivitis:** symptoms occur during particular seasons of allergen exposure (generally spring, summer, and/or fall)
   i. Includes: tree pollen, grass pollen, ragweed pollen, outdoor moulds
   ii. Age of onset: ≥2 years

2. **Investigations:** SPT to inhalant aeroallergens

3. **Management**
   a. Allergen avoidance measures (e.g., dust mite covers for mattress and pillows, closing windows during pollen seasons, removing pets from the home)
   b. Address comorbidities
   c. Pharmacologic management (Table 7.5) for children ≥2 years old. Medications can be used throughout the patient's allergy season(s) or year-round for patients with perennial allergic rhinoconjunctivitis.
   d. Immunotherapy if appropriate: subcutaneous immunotherapy or sublingual immunotherapy

Table 7.5	**Pharmacologic Management of Allergic Rhinoconjunctivitis**
Type of Medication	**Comments**
First-Generation Oral Antihistamines *Diphenhydramine* *Hydroxyzine*	Effective but generally avoided because of adverse side effects, such as somnolence and central nervous system depression
Second-Generation Oral Antihistamines (Examples) *Cetirizine* *Loratadine*	Fewer side effects (non-sedating), preferred as first-line therapy; may be given once daily
Intranasal Corticosteroids (examples) *Budesonide* *Fluticasone propionate*	Effective in relieving symptoms of allergic and non-allergic rhinitis, especially congestion. May also be effective for symptoms of allergic conjunctivitis
Combined Intranasal Corticosteroid and Intranasal Antihistamine	Effective in relieving symptoms of allergic rhinitis and conjunctivitis
Eye Drops (Antihistamines and Mast Cell Stabilizers)	Topical medications effective in relieving symptoms of allergic conjunctivitis

A. Acute urticaria

1. **Definition:** urticaria lasting for <6 weeks, may be associated with angioedema (face, lips, extremities, genitals)
2. **Etiologies:** infection (especially viral, but also bacterial and parasitic), idiopathic, type I hypersensitivity reaction (e.g., food, drug or insect sting allergy), direct mast cell activation (e.g., NSAIDs, vancomycin, opioids), physical urticaria (e.g., dermatographism, cold urticaria, cholinergic urticaria, solar urticaria, aquagenic urticaria, exercise-induced urticaria)
3. **Investigations:** allergy testing may be indicated if concerns of type I hypersensitivity reaction
4. **Management:** eliminate trigger if identified, second-generation oral antihistamines are first-line therapy (see Table 7.5), referral to allergist if becomes chronic

B. Chronic urticaria

1. **Definition:** urticaria occurring on most days of the week for >6 weeks (may be associated with angioedema)
2. **Etiology:** idiopathic (spontaneous) most common etiology
   a. Other etiologies include infection (hepatitis B/C, EBV, herpes simplex virus [HSV], *Helicobacter pylori*, helminthic parasitic infections), autoimmunity (SLE, JIA, hypo/hyperthyroidism, Sjögren, celiac), autoinflammatory, physical urticarias, malignancy
3. **Evaluation:** history and physical examination to rule out signs and symptoms of an identifiable etiology
4. **Investigations:** often not indicated, unless specific etiology suspected; may order complete blood count (CBC), erythrocyte sedimentation rate (ESR), and C-reactive protein (CRP) to screen for autoimmune/autoinflammatory diseases; allergy testing via SPT or specific IgE is not indicated
5. **Management**
   a. Second generation oral antihistamines (prescribe daily rather than as needed). Often dose needs to be increased up to 2 to 4 times the standard dose; consult an allergist.
   b. Omalizumab for refractory cases

C. Angioedema without urticaria

1. **Definition:** isolated angioedema without urticaria/pruritus is generally bradykinin-mediated (not mast cell/histamine-mediated)
2. **Etiology**
   a. Most common: idiopathic angioedema, angioedema associated with angiotensin-converting enzyme (ACE) inhibitors

Allergy

7

   b. Less common: hereditary angioedema (HAE), acquired angioedema (AAE)
3. **Symptoms:** recurrent episodes of angioedema without urticaria/pruritus; most often skin or mucosal tissues of the gastrointestinal and upper respiratory tracts; laryngeal involvement can lead to fatal asphyxiation if untreated
4. **Investigations:** diagnosis of HAE and AAE should include C4 level (the natural substrate for C1), C1 esterase inhibitor level $\pm$ C1 esterase inhibitor functional level
5. **Treatment**
   a. Discontinue ACE inhibitors
   b. Idiopathic angioedema may respond in the acute setting to second-generation oral antihistamines or glucocorticoids
   c. HAE/AAE do not respond to epinephrine, antihistamine, or glucocorticoids. Treat with C1 esterase inhibitor concentrate or drugs that act on the bradykinin pathway.

FURTHER READING

Abrams EM, Hildebrand K, Blair B, Chan ES. Timing of introduction of allergenic solids for infants at high risk. *Paediatr Child Health*. 2019;24(1):56–57.

Chan ES, Cummings C. Dietary exposures and allergy prevention in high-risk infants. *Paediatr Child Health*. 2013;18(10):545–549.

Cheng A. Emergency treatment of anaphylaxis in infants and children. *Paediatr Child Health*. 2011;16(1):35–40.

Dykewicz MS, Wallace DV, Baroody F, et al. Treatment of seasonal allergic rhinitis: an evidence-based focused 2017 guideline update. *Ann Allergy Asthma Immunol*. 2017:1–23.

Golden DB, Demain J, Freeman T, et al. Stinging insect hypersensitivity: a practice parameter update 2016. *Ann Allergy Asthma Immunol*. 2017;118:28–54.

Nowak-Wegrzyn A, Katz Y, Mehr SS, Koletzko S. Non-IgE-mediated gastrointestinal food allergy. *J Allergy Clin Immunol*. 2015;135(5):1114–1124.

Togias A, Cooper SF, Acebal ML, et al. Addendum guidelines for the prevention of peanut allergy in the United States: report of the National Institute of Allergy and Infectious Diseases—sponsored expert panel. *World Allergy Organ J*. 2017;10(1):1.

Zuberbier T, Aberer W, Asero R, et al. The EAACI/GA^{2}LEN/EDF/WAO guideline for the definition, classification, diagnosis and management of urticaria. *Allergy*. 2018;73(7):1393–1414.

Cardiology

Michael D. Fridman • Jonathan Wong • Koyelle Papneja • Jennifer L. Russell

COMMON ABBREVIATIONS

Also see page xviii for a list of other abbreviations used throughout this book

A-fib	atrial fibrillation
A-flutter	atrial flutter
ABC	airway, breathing, circulation
AoV	aortic valve
AS	aortic stenosis
ASD	atrial septal defect
AVSD	atrioventricular septal defect
BTT	Blalock-Taussig-Thomas
CHD	congenital heart disease
CHF	congestive heart failure
CoA	coarctation of the aorta
DCM	dilated cardiomyopathy
GXT	graded exercise test
HCM	hypertrophic cardiomyopathy
HLH	hypoplastic left heart
IE	infective endocarditis
IVC	inferior vena cava
JVP	jugular venous pressure
LA	left atrium
LAD	left axis deviation
LAE	left atrial enlargement
LBBB	left bundle branch block
LLSB	left lower sternal border
LPA	left pulmonary artery
LQTS	long QT syndrome
LUSB	left upper sternal border
LV	left ventricle
LVH	left ventricular hypertrophy
LVOTO	left ventricular outflow tract obstruction
MAPCA	major aortopulmonary collateral arteries
MV	mitral valve
PA	pulmonary artery
PAC	premature atrial contraction
PDA	patent ductus arteriosus
PGE_1	prostaglandin E_1
PPHN	persistent pulmonary hypertension of the newborn
PPS	peripheral pulmonary stenosis
PS	pulmonary stenosis
PVC	premature ventricular contraction
PVR	pulmonary vascular resistance
RA	right atrium

RAD	right axis deviation
RAE	right atrial enlargement
RBBB	right bundle branch block
RCM	restrictive cardiomyopathy
RPA	right pulmonary artery
RUSB	right upper sternal border
RV	right ventricle
RVH	right ventricular hypertrophy
RVOTO	right ventricular outflow tract obstruction
SBE	subacute bacterial endocarditis
SEM	systolic ejection murmur
SVC	superior vena cava
SVR	systemic vascular resistance
SVT	supraventricular tachycardia
TAPVD	total anomalous pulmonary venous drainage
TGA	transposition of the great arteries
TOF	tetralogy of Fallot
TR	tricuspid regurgitation
TV	tricuspid valve
V-fib	ventricular fibrillation
VSD	ventricular septal defect
VT	ventricular tachycardia
WPW	Wolff-Parkinson-White

FOCUSED CARDIOLOGY ASSESSMENT

1. **History**
   a. **Presenting illness:** difficulty feeding, failure to thrive, lethargy, exercise intolerance, tachypnea, dyspnea, orthopnea, cyanosis, palpitations, syncope, chest pain
   b. **Family history:** congenital heart disease (CHD), sudden death, unexplained deaths (possible familial arrhythmia), pacemakers, implantable cardioverter defibrillators, premature myocardial infarction/stroke (age <55 years in males, age <60 years in females), decreased ventricular function, cardiomyopathy
2. **Physical examination**
   a. **General examination:** dysmorphic features, growth parameters, color, clubbing
   b. **Vital signs:** respiratory rate (RR), heart rate (HR), four-limb blood pressure (BP; abnormal if right arm systolic >20 mmHg above lower limbs), oxygen saturation (abnormal if <95% and if >3% difference between preductal and postductal saturations if PDA is open)
   c. **Head/neck:** jugular venous pressure, central cyanosis, bruits (carotid, cranial)

d. **Cardiac:** perfusion, peripheral pulses, left ventricle (LV) apex location, right ventricle (RV) heave, thrills, S_1, S_2 (normal splitting), S_3, S_4, murmurs (Table 8.1 and Box 8.1)—timing, location, radiation, pitch, intensity, additional heart sounds (e.g., click, gallop), thrill, peripheral edema

e. **Respiratory:** respiratory distress or increased work of breathing, crackles, wheezes (can be cardiac)

f. **Abdominal:** hepatomegaly, splenomegaly, bruits

3. **Investigations**

a. Electrocardiogram

b. Chest x-ray (CXR): cardiac size/shape/location, pulmonary vascularity, position of aortic arch

c. Echocardiography: real-time two-dimensional and Doppler images of cardiac anatomy, function, pericardial effusions

d. Holter: correlate symptoms with rhythm disturbance, assess for asymptomatic arrhythmia in at-risk populations, response to antiarrhythmic medication; assess pacemaker function

e. Graded exercise test (GXT): response to exercise (i.e., HR, BP, arrhythmia, ischemic changes), quantitative functional assessment

f. Computed tomography (CT) scan: cardiac, vascular, and airway anatomy, pericardial abnormalities, lung parenchyma

g. Cardiac magnetic resonance imaging (CMR): cardiac anatomy and function, vascular and airway anatomy, quantitative measures of blood flow

Table 8.1	Characteristics of Innocent and Pathological Murmurs	
Characteristics	**Innocent (Box 8.2)**	**Pathological**
Timing	Systolic	Systolic or diastolic
Intensity (systolic)	Grade 1–2	Grade 3–6
Associated sounds	None	Click, gallop rhythm
Response to inspiration	Louder after inspiration	No change
Response to change in position	Quieter when upright compared with supine	No change

Box 8.1	Systolic Murmur Intensity Grading
Grade 1	Soft, barely audible
Grade 2	Same intensity as heart sounds
Grade 3	Greater intensity than heart sounds
Grade 4	Grade 3 + thrill
Grade 5	Heard with diaphragm of stethoscope at 45 degrees to chest wall + thrill
Grade 6	Heard with diaphragm of stethoscope completely off chest wall

Still's: musical vibratory systolic murmur along left sternal border (young children)
Pulmonary flow: soft blowing murmur at upper left sternal border (older children)
Peripheral pulmonary stenosis: same as pulmonary flow but radiates to back (infancy, resolves by 3–6 months)
Carotid bruit: 2/6 intensity systolic murmur above clavicles, along carotids (all ages)
Venous hum: continuous murmur above or below clavicles; intensity changes with rotation of head and compression of jugular vein; disappears when supine (young children)

CARDIAC APPROACH TO CHEST X-RAY

See Table 8.2

Table 8.2	Cardiac Characteristics on Chest X-Ray
Characteristics	**Chest X-Ray Findings**
Situs	Normal left-sided structures: heart, stomach bubble
	Normal right-sided structures: liver, minor fissure of right middle lobe of lung
Cardiac position	Levocardia: apex of heart directed to left
	Dextrocardia: apex of heart directed to right
Cardiothoracic ratio	Ratio of diameter of cardiac silhouette to diameter of thoracic cage
	Newborn <0.6; outside newborn period <0.5
Aortic arch sidedness	Left- or right-sided aortic arch (relative to trachea)
Pulmonary markings	Normal, ↑ or ↓

ELECTROCARDIOGRAM

ELECTROCARDIOGRAM INTERPRETATION

1. See Table 8.3 for summary of electrocardiogram (ECG) normal values

170

Table 8.3	Normal Electrocardiogram Values for Age									
Age	Heart Rate Minimum–Maximum[a] (beats/min)	Mean Frontal Plane QRS Axis[a] (degrees)	PR Interval[a] (seconds)	QRS Duration[a] (seconds)	Lead V₁ R Wave Amplitude[a] (mm)	Lead V₁ S Wave Amplitude[a] (mm)	R/S Ratio[a]	Lead V₆ R Wave Amplitude[a] (mm)	Lead V₆ S Wave Amplitude[a] (mm)	R/S Ratio[a]
0–1 months	100–180 (120)	+75 to +180 (+120)	0.08–0.12 (0.10)	0.04–0.08 (0.06)	4–25 (15)	1–20 (10)	0.5–∞ (1.5)	1–21 (6)	0–12 (4)	0.1–∞ (2)
2–3 months	110–180 (120)	+35 to +135 (+100)	0.08–0.12 (0.10)	0.04–0.08 (0.06)	2–20 (11)	1–18 (7)	0.3–10.0 (1.5)	3–20 (10)	0–6 (2)	1.5–∞ (4)
4–12 months	100–180 (150)	+30 to +135 (+160)	0.09–0.13 (0.12)	0.04–0.08 (0.06)	3–20 (10)	1–16 (8)	0.3–4.0 (1.2)	6–20 (13)	0–4 (2)	2.0–∞ (6)
1–3 years	100–180 (130)	0 to +110 (+60)	0.10–0.14 (0.12)	0.04–0.08 (0.06)	1–18 (9)	1–27 (13)	0.5–1.5 (0.8)	3–24 (12)	0–4 (2)	3.0–∞ (20)
4–5 years	60–150 (100)	0 to +110 (+60)	0.11–0.15 (0.13)	0.05–0.09 (0.07)	1–18 (7)	1–30 (14)	0.1–1.5 (0.7)	4–24 (13)	0–4 (1)	2.0–∞ (20)
6–8 years	60–130 (100)	−15 to +110 (+60)	0.12–0.16 (0.14)	0.05–0.09 (0.07)	1–18 (7)	1–30 (14)	0.1–1.5 (0.7)	4–24 (13)	0–4 (1)	2.0–∞ (20)
9–11 years	50–110 (80)	−15 to +110 (+60)	0.12–0.17 (0.14)	0.05–0.09 (0.07)	1–16 (6)	1–26 (16)	0.1–1.0 (0.5)	4–24 (14)	0–4 (1)	4.0–∞ (20)
12–16 years	50–100 (75)	−15 to +110 (+60)	0.12–0.17 (0.15)	0.05–0.09 (0.07)	1–16 (5)	1–23 (14)	0.0–1.0 (0.3)	4–22 (14)	0–5 (1)	2.0–∞ (9)
>16 years	50–90 (70)	−15 to +110 (+60)	0.12–0.20 (0.15)	0.05–1.0 (0.08)	1–14 (3)	1–23 (10)	0.0–1.0 (0.3)	4–21 (10)	0–6 (1)	2.0–∞ (9)

[a]Mean values are noted in brackets.

From the Texas Children's Hospital. In: Carson A, Gilette PC, McNamara DB, eds. *A Guide to Cardiac Dysrhythmias in Children*. New York, NY: Grune and Stratton; 1980.

2. **Heart rate**
   a. 300 divided by number of "large" squares on the ECG (assuming regular rhythm and paper speed is 25 mm/s) (Figure 8.1)
   b. If rhythm irregular, count total number of QRS complexes on the 10-second rhythm strip and multiply by 6

Figure 8.1   How to Count Heart Rate Based on Electrocardiogram

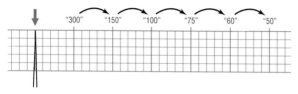

(Modified from Dubin D. *Rapid Interpretation of EKGs*. St Louis, MO: Mosby; 1991. Revised and updated 4th ed. Tampa, FL: Cover Publishing Company; 1991:60.)

3. **Rhythm**
   a. Regular versus irregular, narrow complex versus wide complex QRS, sinus rhythm versus other
   b. Criteria for sinus rhythm: P wave for every QRS complex, QRS complex for every P wave; normal P wave axis (upright P wave in II and usually I and aV_F)

4. **Axis**
   a. Use limb leads (I, II, III, aV_R, aV_L, aV_F) to determine cardiac axis (Figure 8.2)
   b. See Table 8.3 for normative values for different ages

5. **P wave**
   a. Represents atrial activation
   b. Tall P wave (>3 mV in height): RAE
   c. Wide (>0.12 ms in width) or bifid P wave: LAE

Figure 8.2 Determining Cardiac Axis

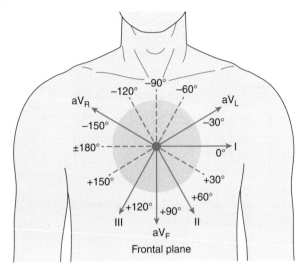

Frontal plane

6. PR interval

a. Represents physiological delay in atrioventricular (AV) node

b. First-degree AV block: see Figure 8.3, PR interval greater than normal value for age (Table 8.3)

c. Second-degree AV block

   i. Mobitz type I (Wenckebach): progressive prolongation of PR interval with eventual nonconducted P wave followed by a conducted sinus beat with shorter PR interval (Figure 8.4)

   ii. Mobitz type II: nonconducted P waves that occur outside the ventricular refractory period, without progressive prolongation of the PR interval (Figure 8.5)

d. Third-degree AV block (complete heart block): no relationship between P waves and QRS complexes (Figure 8.6)

Figure 8.3 First-Degree Atrioventricular Block

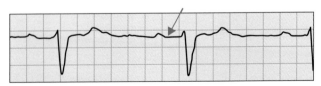

Figure 8.4 Mobitz Type I Atrioventricular Block (Wenckebach)

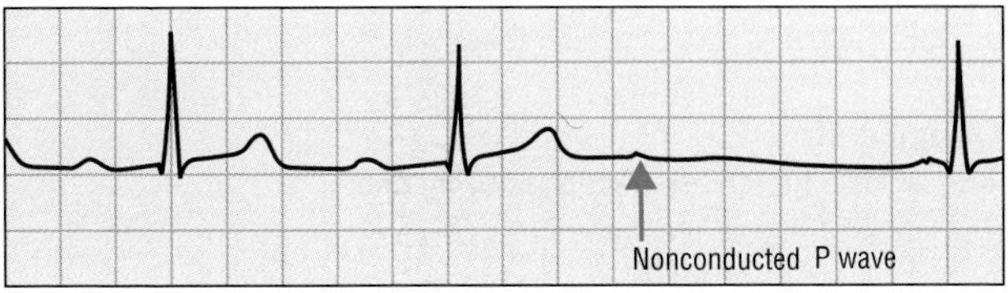

Nonconducted P wave

Figure 8.5 Mobitz Type II Atrioventricular Block

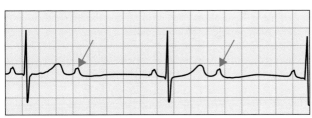

Figure 8.6 Complete Heart Block

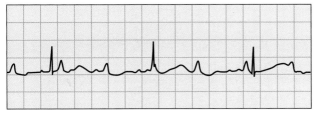

7. **QRS complex**
   a. Q waves in leads II, III, aV_F, V_5–V_6: usually narrow, low voltage
   b. QRS complex duration should be <60 ms in infants and <80 ms in children. Post-pubertal adolescents should have durations <120 ms (similar to adults).

   c. RBBB: right axis, rSR' in leads V_4R, V_1, V_2; wide slurred S in I, V_5, V_6

   d. LBBB: left axis, wide slurred R in leads I, aV_L, V_5, V_6; wide S in V_1, V_2

8. **QT interval**

   a. Corrected for HR using the Bazett equation:

$$QTc = \frac{QT}{\sqrt{RR\ interval}}$$

   b. QTc $\leq$ 440 ms in children (>6 months) and adults, no consensus for expected QTc in infants <6 months

   c. Causes of QTc prolongation: congenital, hypothermia, $\downarrow K^+$, $\downarrow Ca^{2+}$, medications, brain injury

9. **ST segments**

   a. Normal ST segments may be ↑ up to 1 mm in the limb leads

   b. Diffuse ST segment elevation: pericarditis, myocarditis, or pericardial effusion

   c. Local ST segment elevation: coronary ischemia

10. **T waves**

   a. From birth to 7 days, T wave may be upright in V_1

   b. From 7 days to approximately 7 years, T wave in V_1 should be inverted

   c. In adolescents, T wave should be upright in V_1

11. **Ventricular hypertrophy:** see Table 8.4

8

Table 8.4	Electrocardiogram Findings Suggestive of Hypertrophy
RVH	**LVH**
RAD	S wave in V_1 >95th percentile for age
rSR' pattern with R' >R in V_1, V_3R, V_4R	R wave in V_6 >95th percentile for age
Q waves in V_3R, V_4R	Deep Q waves in V_5–V_7
Monophasic R wave in V_1, V_3R, V_4R	ST depression or T wave inversion in V_5–V_7
Abnormal T wave orientation in V_1	
R wave in V_1 >95th percentile for age	
S wave in V_6 >95th percentile for age	

LVH, Left ventricular hypertrophy; *RAD*, right axis deviation; *RVH*, right ventricular hypertrophy.

ELECTROCARDIOGRAM CHANGES IN SELECTED DISORDERS

See Table 8.5

Table 8.5	Electrocardiogram Changes in Selected Disorders
Abnormality	**Electrocardiogram Findings**
AVSD	Left or northwest axis deviation
ASD	RBBB pattern in V_1 and inferior leads
HLH	Low-amplitude QRS voltages in lateral leads
Anomalous left coronary artery from the pulmonary artery (ALCAPA)	Deep Q waves in I, aV_L, V_6; ST segment and T wave abnormalities in inferolateral leads
Hyperkalemia	Peaked T waves
Hypokalemia	Flat T waves or U waves
Hypercalcemia	Shortened QTc, lengthened QRS, bradycardia
Hypocalcemia	Lengthened QTc

ASD, Atrial septal defect; *AVSD*, atrioventricular septal defect; *HLH*, hypoplastic left heart; *RBBB*, right bundle branch block.

ARRHYTHMIAS

TACHYCARDIAS

1. See Figure 8.7 for approach to tachycardias
2. **Supraventricular tachycardia (SVT)**
   a. See Figure 8.8 and Table 8.6

176

Figure 8.7 Approach to Tachycardias

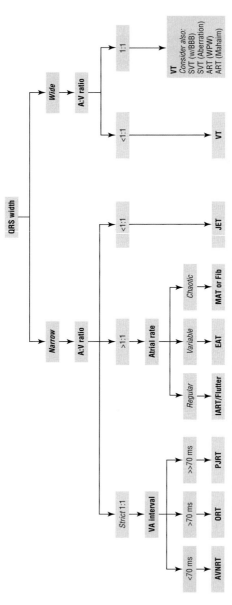

ART, Antidromic re-entrant tachycardia; *AVNRT*, AV node re-entrant tachycardia; *EAT*, ectopic atrial tachycardia; *IART*, intra-atrial re-entrant tachycardia; *JET*, junctional ectopic tachycardia; *MAT*, multifocal atrial tachycardia; *ORT*, orthodromic re-entrant tachycardia; *PJRT*, paroxysmal junctional re-entrant tachycardia; *SVT*, supra-ventricular tachycardia; *VT*, ventricular tachycardia; *WPW*, Wolff-Parkinson-White; *VA*, ventriculoatrial.

Figure 8.8 Supraventricular Tachycardia

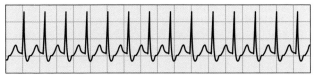

Table 8.6	Different Types of Supraventricular Tachycardia and Their Differentiating Characteristics				
Characteristics	**AVNRT**	**AVRT**	**AET**	**A-Flutter**	**A-Fib**
Frequency	15% of SVT	70% of SVT	Uncommon	Rare	Rare
Population at risk	Older children	Younger children		Postoperative CHD	Postoperative CHD, WPW
Onset	Sudden	Sudden	Warm up (slow increase)	Sudden	Sudden
Offset	Sudden	Sudden	Cool down (slow decrease)	Incessant	Incessant
Heart rate (HR) variability	Fixed HR	Fixed HR	Variable HR	Fixed atrial rate with variable QRS	Irregularly irregular
P wave morphology	May have retrograde P wave close to QRS complex	May have retrograde P wave close to QRS complex	P waves different compared with normal sinus rhythm	Saw-tooth pattern (best seen in II, V$_2$)	No discernible P waves
Response to adenosine or vagal maneuvers	Terminates	Terminates	Blocks temporarily but resumes quickly	Blocks at AV node; flutter waves persist	Blocks at AV node, but A-fib continues

AET, Atrial ectopic tachycardia; *A-fib*, atrial fibrillation; *AV*, atrioventricular; *AVNRT*, atrioventricular node reentrant tachycardia; *AVRT*, atrioventricular reentrant tachycardia; *CHD*, congenital heart disease; *SVT*, supraventricular tachycardia; *WPW*, Wolff-Parkinson-White.

b. **Management of SVT**
   i. **Unstable:** see Chapter 1 Resuscitation
   ii. **Acute, stable:** attempt vagal maneuvers, adenosine
   iii. **Long-term:** beta blockade; electrophysiological study and abla-
        tion for definitive diagnosis and management for recurrent and
        symptomatic SVT or if nonresponsive to medical management
3. **Ventricular tachycardia (VT)**
   a. **Definition:** >3 sequential ventricular beats at rate above upper
      limit of normal for age
   b. **Causes:** electrolyte abnormalities (e.g., $\uparrow K^+$, $\downarrow Mg^{2+}$), CHD, long QT
      syndrome, idiopathic ventricular tachycardia (VT), arrhythmogenic
      RV cardiomyopathy
   c. **ECG characteristics:** wide complex tachycardia, AV dissociation,
      ventricular rate faster than atrial rate (Figure 8.9)
   d. Management of VT
      i. **Unstable:** see Chapter 1 Resuscitation
      ii. **Acute, stable:** amiodarone loading dose then continuous infusion
      iii. **Long term:** amiodarone, automated implantable cardiac defibrilla-
           tor, electrophysiological study for intracardiac mapping for possible
           ablation

Figure 8.9   Ventricular Tachycardia

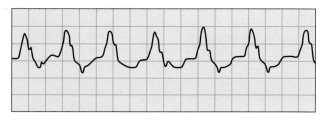

BRADYCARDIAS
1. **Sinus arrhythmia**
   a. Normal finding, requires no treatment
   b. **ECG characteristics:** normal variation of HR with respiration,
      slower during expiration (Figure 8.10)
2. **Sinus bradycardia**
   a. **Definition:** HR less than lower limit of normal for age
   b. **Causes:** hypothermia, hypothyroidism, anorexia nervosa, malnutrition,
      hypokalemia, hypoxia, central nervous system (CNS) injury, atrial
      cardiac surgery

c. **Management:** treat reversible cause if present; consider atropine or pacing if symptomatic

Figure 8.10   Sinus Arrhythmia

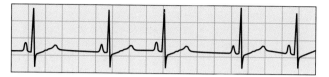

3. **AV block**
   a. **Causes:** maternal lupus (congenital heart block), rheumatic fever, infective endocarditis, myocarditis, Lyme disease, cardiomyopathies, atrial septal defect (ASD), Ebstein anomaly, atrioventricular septal defect (AVSD), congenitally corrected transposition of the great arteries (TGA), cardiac surgery, digoxin toxicity
   b. **Types:** first degree, second degree, third degree
   c. **Pathophysiology:** no conduction of electrical signal from atria to ventricles; resultant ventricular escape rate may be too slow to maintain adequate cardiac output
   d. **Acute management:** airway, breathing, circulation (ABCs), isoproterenol infusion, or transcutaneous pacing to ↑HR and cardiac output
   e. **Long-term management**
      i. No treatment for first-degree or Mobitz I second-degree heart block (Wenckebach)
      ii. Permanent pacemaker for high-grade, Mobitz II second-degree, or complete heart block

ECTOPIC BEATS

1. See Table 8.7
2. Benign versus worrisome premature ventricular contractions (PVCs)
   a. **Benign:** monomorphic (i.e., QRS morphology same for each one), disappear or become less frequent with exercise
   b. **Worrisome:** underlying CHD, polymorphic PVCs, personal or family history of sudden death or syncope, incessant or very frequent PVCs

Table 8.7	Premature Ectopic Beats	
Characteristics	PACs	PVCs
Epidemiology	Common in children with normal hearts	50%–70% of children with normal hearts (with Holter)
Causes	Stimulants, caffeine, hypoxia, hyperthyroidism, digoxin, amphetamines	Hypoxia, inflammation, cardiomyopathy, electrolyte abnormalities, cardiac tumors
ECG characteristics	P wave with different morphology than normal sinus rhythm P wave, followed by narrow QRS complex; P wave may not be conducted if ventricle is refractory	Wide QRS complex with no preceding P wave; appears earlier than anticipated with change in T wave morphology
Management	No treatment required; treat reversible underlying causes	No treatment required; treat reversible underlying causes

ECG, Electrocardiogram; *PACs*, premature atrial contractions; *PVCs*, premature ventricular contractions.

ARRHYTHMIA SYNDROMES
See Table 8.8

Table 8.8	Characteristics of Selected Arrythmia Syndromes	
Characteristics	WPW	LQTS
Associated abnormalities	Ebstein anomaly	Deafness (Jervell and Lange-Nielson syndrome)
Inheritance pattern	Not usually inherited	AD or AR (6 subtypes)
Baseline ECG findings	Short PR interval, delta wave	QTc >upper limit of normal
Risk of sudden death	1/1000 patient-years	⅔ higher risk of death than general population
Commonly associated arrhythmias	SVT (atrioventricular re-entrant tachycardia); rarely can present with pre-excited A-fib (wide complex, irregularly irregular rhythm); pre-excited A-fib can degenerate into V-fib, especially with drugs that block the AV node	Torsades de pointes
Management	Beta blockade, catheter ablation	Beta blockade, implantable defibrillator
Additional information	Risk factors for sudden death: family history of sudden death, A-fib, delta wave at high HRs	30% can have normal baseline QTc with LQTS apparent with provocation testing; only 75% are gene positive

AD, Autosomal dominant; *A-fib*, atrial fibrillation; *AR*, autosomal recessive; *AV*, atrioventricular; *ECG*, electrocardiogram; *HR*, heart rate; *LQTS*, long QT syndrome; *SVT*, supraventricular tachycardia; *V-fib*, ventricular fibrillation; *WPW*, Wolff-Parkinson-White.

CONGENITAL HEART DISEASE

NEWBORN PRESENTING WITH CYANOSIS

1. **History, physical examination, ECG, CXR, hyperoxia test**
   a. **Hyperoxia test:** place infant in 100% FiO_2 (via oxyhood, continuous positive airway pressure, endotracheal tube) for 10 minutes and measure preductal PaO_2 (arterial blood gas) before and after application of oxygen. Preductal $PaO_2 < 150$ mmHg after oxygen suggests cyanotic CHD.
2. **Approach:** see Figure 8.11

Figure 8.11   Approach to the Cyanotic Newborn

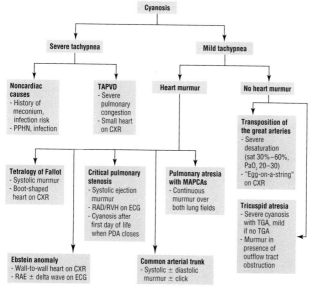

CXR, Chest x-ray; ECG, electrocardiogram; MAPCAs, major aortopulmonary collateral arteries; PDA, patent ductus arteriosus; PPHN, persistent pulmonary hypertension of the newborn; RAD, right axis deviation; RVH, right ventricular hypertrophy; TAPVD, total anomalous pulmonary venous drainage; TGA, transposition of the great arteries.

3. **Noncardiac causes of cyanosis:** PPHN, sepsis, lung disease, hypoglycemia
4. **Common cyanotic heart lesions:** see Table 8.9
5. **Acute management**
   a. Prostaglandin E_1 (PGE_1) for any suspected cyanotic heart lesion
   b. Accept saturations of >70% acutely; if intubated, aim for CO_2 ~45 mmHg
   c. Transfer emergently to pediatric cardiologist for evaluation and management

✦ PEARL

Start PGE_1 at 0.01 mcg/kg/min. Side effects include apnea, fever, hypotension (secondary to vasodilation).

Table 8.9 Congenital Cyanotic Heart Lesions

Characteristics	TGA (Figure 8.12)	TOF (Figure 8.13)	Common Arterial Trunk (Figure 8.15)	Tricuspid Atresia (Figure 8.16)	TAPVD (Figure 8.17)
Epidemiology	1. Most common cyanotic lesion in neonates	1. Most common cyanotic lesion in children			1. Supracardiac (50%) 2. Cardiac (20%) 3. Infracardiac (20%) 4. Mixed types (10%)
Structural abnormalities	1. Aorta arises from RV and out aorta 2. Pulmonary venous blood returns to LV and out PA	1. Large unrestrictive VSD 2. RVOTO 3. RVH 4. Overriding aorta	1. Systemic and pulmonary vessels from single great vessel 2. Large VSD	1. No connection between RA and RV	1. Pulmonary veins drain to site other than LA
Pathophysiology	1. Systemic venous blood returns to RV and out aorta 2. Pulmonary venous blood returns to LV and out PA 3. Mixing occurs at PFO/ASD	1. RVOTO limits pulmonary blood flow 2. R→L shunting across VSD 3. "Pink Tets" have mild RVOTO and CHF rather than cyanosis	1. Ratio of SVR:PVR determines symptoms 2. Lower PVR results in more pulmonary blood flow, higher saturations, heart failure ± coronary ischemia	1. Mixing between desaturated blood from RA and fully saturated blood from pulmonary veins in LA	1. Pulmonary blood drains to other venous structure 2. ASD with R→L shunt causing cyanosis 3. Infracardiac TAPVD always obstructed
Associated lesions	1. ASD 2. VSD 3. PS 4. PDA	1. Right aortic arch in 25%	1. Truncal valve stenosis or insufficiency 2. Arch interruption 3. Coronary abnormalities	1. Pulmonary atresia 2. PS/AS 3. CoA 4. TGA	1. ASD 2. Right atrial isomerism 3. Complex heart disease with AVSD or DORV

Clinical features	1. Single loud S_2 ± soft SEM 2. Degree of cyanosis depends on mixing of blood across ASD	1. Single loud S_2, 2–3/6 SEM (because of RVOTO) 2. Degree of cyanosis depends on RVOTO 3. See Figure 8.14 for management of hypercyanotic spells ("Tet spells")	1. Cyanosis, CHF 2. 3/6 SEM, ±click, diastolic murmur (truncal valve insufficiency)	1. Cyanosis, normal S_1, single S_2 2. 2–3/6 systolic murmur at LLSB	1. Severe obstruction: severe tachypnea, cyanosis 2. Mild obstruction: CHF, cyanosis
CXR findings	1. "Egg on a string"	1. "Boot-shaped" heart	1. Cardiomegaly 2. ↑ pulmonary flow 3. Right aortic arch (25%)	1. Normal cardiac silhouette 2. Enlarged RA, ↑ pulmonary vascularity	1. ↑ pulmonary markings 2. Bilateral white-out if obstructed 3. "Snowman sign" in supracardiac TAPVD
ECG findings	1. Most commonly normal but can have RAD and RVH	1. RAD 2. RVH	1. RAD 2. RVH 3. LVH 4. ST depression	1. LAD 2. RAE 3. LVH 4. ↓ voltages in V_1–V_3	1. RVH 2. RAE
Treatment	1. PGE_1, ± balloon septostomy 2. Arterial switch operation in newborn period	1. Repair at 4–6 months	1. Definitive surgical treatment within 2–4 weeks	1. PGE_1 and surgery	1. If obstructed, emergent surgery 2. If unobstructed, repair in first 4–6 weeks

Continued

184

Table 8.9 Congenital Cyanotic Heart Lesions—cont'd

Characteristics	TGA (Figure 8.12)	TOF (Figure 8.13)	Common Arterial Trunk (Figure 8.15)	Tricuspid Atresia (Figure 8.16)	TAPVD (Figure 8.17)
Long-term complications	1. Aortic/PA dilation 2. Pulmonary artery stenosis 3. AI 4. Rarely coronary artery stenosis	1. Residual RVOTO 2. PI 3. RV dilation 4. Poor RV function 5. Ventricular arrhythmias	1. Truncal valve insufficiency 2. RVOTO 3. Ventricular arrhythmias	1. Arrythmias 2. Decreased cardiac function 3. Protein-losing enteropathy 4. Thromboembolic complications	1. Residual or recurrent pulmonary vein stenosis 2. Atrial arrhythmia

AI, Aortic insufficiency; *ASD*, atrial septal defect; *AS*, aortic stenosis; *CCTGA*, congenitally corrected transposition of the great arteries; *CHF*, congestive heart failure; *CoA*, coarctation of the aorta; *CXR*, chest x-ray; *DORV*, double outlet right ventricle; *ECG*, electrocardiogram; *LA*, left atrium; *LAD*, left axis deviation; *LLSB*, left lower sternal border; *LV*, left ventricle; *MVP*, mitral valve prolapse; *PA*, pulmonary artery; *PDA*, patent ductus arteriosus; *PFO*, patent foramen ovale; *PGE₁*, prostaglandin E₁; *PI*, pulmonary insufficiency; *PS*, pulmonary stenosis; *PVR*, pulmonary vascular resistance; *RA*, right atrium; *RAD*, right axis deviation; *RAE*, right atrial enlargement; *RBBB*, right bundle branch block; *RV*, right ventricle; *RVH*, right ventricular hypertrophy; *RVOTO*, right ventricular outflow tract obstruction; *SEM*, systolic ejection murmur; *SVR*, systemic vascular resistance; *TAPVD*, total anomalous pulmonary venous drainage; *TGA*, transposition of the great arteries; *TOF*, tetralogy of Fallot; *TR*, tricuspid regurgitation; *TV*, tricuspid valve; *VSD*, ventricular septal defect.

Figure 8.12   Transposition of the Great Arteries

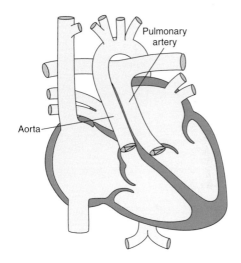

Figure 8.13   Tetralogy of Fallot

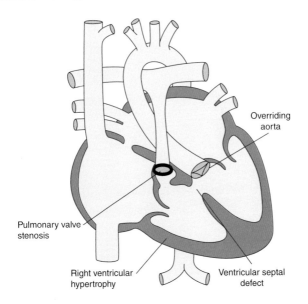

Figure 8.14 Management of Hypercyanotic Spells ("Tet" Spells)[a]

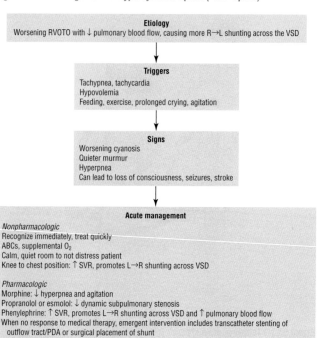

Etiology
Worsening RVOTO with ↓ pulmonary blood flow, causing more R→L shunting across the VSD

Triggers
Tachypnea, tachycardia
Hypovolemia
Feeding, exercise, prolonged crying, agitation

Signs
Worsening cyanosis
Quieter murmur
Hyperpnea
Can lead to loss of consciousness, seizures, stroke

Acute management
Nonpharmacologic
Recognize immediately, treat quickly
ABCs, supplemental O₂
Calm, quiet room to not distress patient
Knee to chest position: ↑ SVR, promotes L→R shunting across VSD

Pharmacologic
Morphine: ↓ hyperpnea and agitation
Propranolol or esmolol: ↓ dynamic subpulmonary stenosis
Phenylephrine: ↑ SVR, promotes L→R shunting across VSD and ↑ pulmonary blood flow
When no response to medical therapy, emergent intervention includes transcatheter stenting of
   outflow tract/PDA or surgical placement of shunt

[a]Occurs in tetralogy of Fallot and other cardiac defects with pulmonary/subpulmonary stenosis and a ventricular septal defect. *ABC*, Airway, breathing, circulation; *RVOTO*, right ventricular outflow tract obstruction; *SVR*, systemic vascular resistance; *VSD*, ventricular septal defect.

Figure 8.15   Common Arterial Trunk

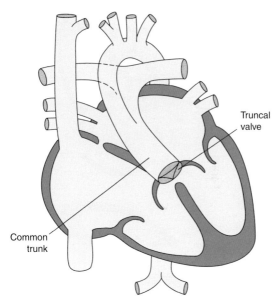

Truncal valve

Common trunk

Figure 8.16   Tricuspid Atresia

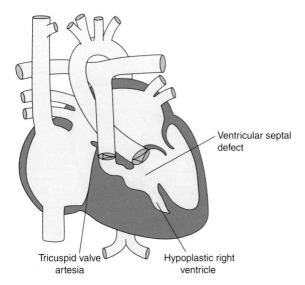

Ventricular septal defect

Tricuspid valve artesia

Hypoplastic right ventricle

Figure 8.17 Types of Total Anomalous Pulmonary Venous Return

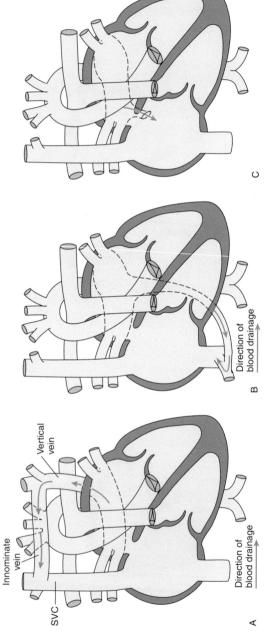

(A) Supracardiac TAPVR with vertical vein to the innominate vein. (B) Infracardiac TAPVR with vertical vein draining below the diaphragm into the hepatic vein. (C) Cardiac TAPVR with vertical vein to the coronary sinus. *SVC,* Superior vena cava.

NEWBORN OR CHILD PRESENTING WITH CARDIOGENIC SHOCK

Cardiogenic shock is typically caused by congenital left heart obstructive lesions (see Table 8.10)

Table 8.10	Congenital Left Heart Obstructive Lesions		
Characteristics	**CoA**	**Aortic Stenosis**	**HLH (Figure 8.18)**
Structural abnormalities	1. Discrete narrowing of aortic arch at level of PDA	1. Valvular AS (70%): thickened, dysplastic AoV 2. Subvalvular AS (25%): muscle or membrane 3. Supravalvular (5%)	1. MV, LV, AoV are small; function like single ventricle physiology 2. AoV or MV can be stenotic or atretic 3. Aortic arch is hypoplastic
Pathophysiology	1. Pressure load on LV, if severe, can lead to LV dysfunction 2. Descending aorta may be supplied via PDA, as PDA closes→cardiogenic shock	1. Pressure load on LV, if severe can lead to LV dysfunction 2. In neonatal critical AS, systemic blood flow supplied via PDA, as PDA closes→cardiogenic shock	1. Fully saturated blood from LA mixes with venous blood from RA, is ejected out RV to PA, and through PDA to body, as PDA closes, ↓ systemic perfusion
Associated lesions	1. Hypoplasia of transverse arch 2. VSD 3. Bicuspid AoV (85%)		
Clinical features	1. Gradient >20 mmHg systolic BP ± gradient >3% oxygen saturation between right arm and lower extremities 2. Systolic murmur at LUSB border radiating to back 3. Weak/absent femoral pulses 4. Gallop rhythm if CHF	1. Can be asymptomatic (only newborns with critical AS present in shock) 2. Exercise intolerance 3. Normal S1, narrow S2 4. 2/6–4/6 SEM at RUSB ± thrill that radiates to carotids 5. CHF if severe and ↓ heart function	1. Normal S1, single loud S2 2. Usually no murmur 3. Poor perfusion, weak pulses
CXR findings	1. Cardiomegaly 2. Rib notching (in older children) 3. "3 sign" (indentation in aorta)	1. Dilated aorta 2. Cardiomegaly 3. Pulmonary edema if severe CHF	1. Moderate cardiomegaly 2. ↑ pulmonary vascular markings

Cardiology

8

Continued

Characteristics	CoA	Aortic Stenosis	HLH (Figure 8.18)
Table 8.10 — Congenital Left Heart Obstructive Lesions—cont'd			
ECG findings	1. Neonates: RVH (can be normal) 2. Older children: may have LVH	1. LVH ± strain, coronary ischemia, if obstruction severe and function poor	1. RAD 2. RVH 3. Poor left-sided forces (i.e., no Q wave in V_6, small QRS voltages in lateral precordial leads)
Treatment	1. If in shock, resuscitation 2. Neonates: use PGE_1 to keep PDA open 3. Surgery in neonates or balloon dilation ± stents in older children	1. If cardiogenic shock, resuscitation 2. Neonates: PGE_1 3. AoV balloon dilation or surgical repair/replacement	1. Resuscitation 2. PGE_1 infusion 3. Single ventricle palliation (Norwood/Hybrid → Glenn → Fontan)
Long-term complications	1. Recurrent/residual CoA 2. Hypertension 3. Aortic aneurysms	1. Recurrent stenosis 2. Aortic insufficiency related to treatment	1. Arrythmias 2. Decreased cardiac function 3. Protein-losing enteropathy 4. Thromboembolic complications

AoV, Aortic valve; *AS,* aortic stenosis; *BP,* blood pressure; *CHF,* congestive heart failure; *CoA,* coarctation of the aorta; *CXR,* chest x-ray; *ECG,* electrocardiogram; *HLH,* hypoplastic left heart; *LA,* left atrium; *LUSB,* left upper sternal border; *LV,* left ventricle; *LVH,* left ventricular hypertrophy; *LVOTO,* left ventricular outflow tract obstruction; *MV,* mitral valve; *PA,* pulmonary artery; *PDA,* patent ductus arteriosus; *PGE₁,* prostaglandin E₁; *RA,* right atrium; *RAD,* right axis deviation; *RUSB,* right upper sternal border; *RV,* right ventricle; *RVH,* right ventricular hypertrophy; *SEM,* systolic ejection murmur; *VSD,* ventricular septal defect.

Figure 8.18 Hypoplastic Left Heart

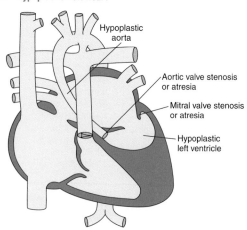

Hypoplastic aorta

Aortic valve stenosis or atresia

Mitral valve stenosis or atresia

Hypoplastic left ventricle

NEWBORN OR CHILD PRESENTING WITH CONGESTIVE HEART FAILURE

See Table 8.11

Table 8.11 Congenital Lesions Causing Congestive Heart Failure

Characteristics	VSD (Figure 8.19)	AVSD (Figure 8.20)	PDA (Figure 8.21)
Structural abnormalities	1. Perimembranous (70%) 2. Outlet (5%) 3. Inlet (5%) 4. Muscular (5%–20%)	1. Complete: single "common" AV valve 2. Partial: two separate orifices	1. Arterial duct between descending aorta and LPA (most common)
Pathophysiology	1. L→R shunting between ventricles 2. Degree of shunt depends on size of VSD 3. Volume overload to left-sided structures and pulmonary vasculature	1. L→R shunting between atria or ventricles 2. Often large ASD and VSD 3. Primum ASD along spectrum of AVSD 4. Causes volume overload, leads to pulmonary hypertension	1. L→R shunting 2. Degree of shunting depends on size of PDA and pressure difference between aorta and PA
Associated lesions		1. TOF 2. DORV 3. Right or left isomerism	
Clinical features	1. Depends on size 2. Small: pansystolic murmur ± thrill 3. Moderate/large: CHF, pulmonary hypertension	1. Signs of CHF 2. Pansystolic murmur (because of VSD or valvular regurgitation)	1. Bounding pulses 2. Wide pulse pressure 3. Normal S_1, loud S_2 4. Neonates: systolic murmur 5. Older children: continuous murmur (if small–moderate)
CXR findings	1. Cardiomegaly 2. Increased pulmonary blood flow	1. Cardiomegaly 2. Increased pulmonary blood flow	1. Mild cardiomegaly 2. Increased pulmonary blood flow

Continued

Continued

Cardiology

8

191

Table 8.11 Congenital Lesions Causing Congestive Heart Failure—cont'd

Characteristics	VSD (Figure 8.19)	AVSD (Figure 8.20)	PDA (Figure 8.21)
ECG findings	1. Can be normal 2. LAE 3. LVH	1. Superior QRS axis 2. Long PR interval 3. RVH/LVH	1. Normal 2. With larger PDA: can have LAE, LVH, RVH
Treatment	1. 40% perimembranous and 80% muscular VSDs close by 2 years 2. Treat CHF 3. Surgical/device closure at 4–6 months, earlier if refractory CHF	1. Treat CHF 2. Should be repaired by 6 months	1. Treat CHF 2. Follow for closure 3. If small/moderate: transcatheter device closure 4. If large or symptomatic in neonates: surgical ligation
Long-term complications	1. Subaortic stenosis 2. Aortic insufficiency 3. Pulmonary hypertension (if treated/diagnosed late) 4. Postoperative heart block	1. Pulmonary hypertension 2. Valvular regurgitation or stenosis	1. Pulmonary hypertension if very large

ASD, Atrial septal defect; AV, atrioventricular; AVSD, atrioventricular septal defect; CHF, congestive heart failure; CXR, chest x-ray; DORV, double outlet right ventricle; ECG, electrocardiogram; LAE, left atrial enlargement; LPA, left pulmonary artery; LVH, left ventricular hypertrophy; PA, pulmonary artery; PDA, patent ductus arteriosus; PFO, patent foramen ovale; RA, right atrium; RAD, right axis deviation; RBBB, right bundle branch block; RV, right ventricle; RVH, right ventricular hypertrophy; SEM, systolic ejection murmur; TOF, tetralogy of Fallot; VSD, ventricular septal defect.

Figure 8.19   Ventricular Septal Defect

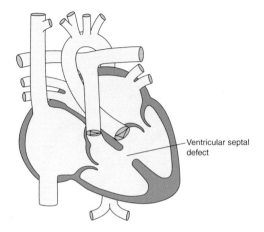

Ventricular septal defect

Figure 8.20   Atrioventricular Septal Defect

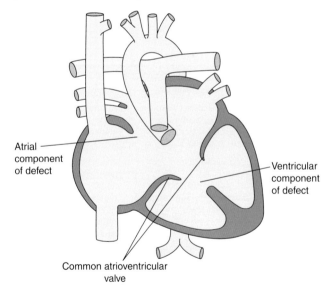

Atrial component of defect

Ventricular component of defect

Common atrioventricular valve

Figure 8.21 Patent Ductus Arteriosus

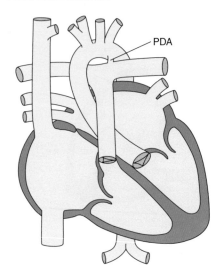

PDA

OTHER CARDIAC LESIONS
See Table 8.12

Table 8.12 Other Cardiac Lesions

Characteristics	Ebstein Anomaly (Figure 8.22)	ASD (Figure 8.23A and B)
Structural abnormalities	1. TV displaced downward into RV with septal leaflet adherent to interventricular septum and portion of RV being "atrialized"	1. Secundum (50%–70%) 2. Primum (15%) 3. Sinus venosus (10%)
Pathophysiology	1. TV has variable degree of regurgitation 2. Clinical course dependent on TV apparatus, RV function, RV size, and presence of ASD	1. Secundum: defect near PFO 2. Primum: defect in inferior atrial septum 3. Sinus venosus: defect in upper atrial septum 4. L→R shunt causing RV volume overload
Associated lesions	1. ASD 2. Bicuspid or atretic aortic valve 3. PS/PA/hypoplastic pulmonary artery 4. Subaortic stenosis 5. CoA 6. MVP 7. VSD 8. CCTGA	1. Sinus venosus ASD associated with anomalous pulmonary veins 2. VSD

Table 8.12	Other Cardiac Lesions—cont'd	
Characteristics	Ebstein Anomaly (Figure 8.22)	ASD (Figure 8.23A and B)
Clinical features	1. Cyanosis at birth/plethora 2. Digital clubbing 3. Displaced apical impulse 4. Holosystolic murmur from TR at LLSB 5. Quadruple rhythm (split S_1 and split S_2) 6. CHF	1. Asymptomatic 2. Soft SEM at upper left sternal border 3. Widely fixed split S_2
CXR findings	1. Range from normal to severe cardiomegaly 2. Diminished vascular markings 3. "Wall to wall heart"	1. Can be normal 2. Mild cardiomegaly 3. Enlarged RA and RV 4. Increased pulmonary blood flow
ECG findings	1. Tall, wide P waves 2. RBBB 3. First-degree AV block 4. Preexcitation 5. Absence of RBBB suspicious for preexcitation	1. Incomplete RBBB in V_1, II, III, aV_F, RVH, RAD
Treatment	1. If cyanotic newborn, may require O_2, PGE_1 2. No intervention for mild cases, surgical intervention on TV is challenging 3. Preexcitation patients should undergo ablation	1. If no CHF, follow for closure 2. If no RV enlargement, no indication to intervene 3. Small–moderate: closure in cath lab 4. Large, primum, or sinus venosus ASDs: surgery
Long-term complications	1. Atrial arrhythmias 2. Permanent pacemaker 3. Ventricular dysfunction 4. TV regurgitation (residual or worsening)	1. Atrial arrhythmia 2. Pulmonary hypertension (occurring at age 20–30)

ASD, Atrial septal defect; *AV,* atrioventricular; *CCGTA,* congenitally corrected transposition of the great arteries; *CoA,* coarctation of the aorta; CHF, congestive heart failure; *LLSB,* left lower sternal border; *MVP,* mitral valve prolapse; PGE_1, prostaglandin E_1; *PA,* pulmonary atresia; *PFO,* patent foramen ovale; *PS,* pulmonary stenosis; *RBBB,* right bundle branch block; *RA,* right atrium; *RV,* right ventricle; *SEM,* systolic ejection murmur; *TR,* tricuspid regurgitation; *TV,* tricuspid valve; *VSD,* ventricular septal defect.

Cardiology

8

Figure 8.22 Ebstein Anomaly

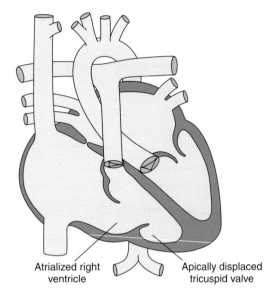

Atrialized right ventricle

Apically displaced tricuspid valve

Figure 8.23 A. Atrial Septal Defect B. Sinus Venosus Atrial Septal Defect

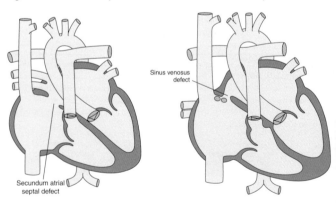

Sinus venosus defect

Secundum atrial septal defect

1. **Staged surgical palliation for single ventricle physiology (e.g., hypoplastic left heart [HLH])**
   a. **Stage 1 (first week of life)**
      i. **Norwood:** aortopulmonary connection, aortic arch reconstruction, atrial septectomy, and shunt to the disconnected pulmonary arteries (PAs) (Figure 8.24)
      ii. **Hybrid (alternative):** bilateral pulmonary artery bands and ductal stenting
      iii. Saturations: 75% to 85%
   b. **Stage 2 (4–6 months)—Bidirectional cavopulmonary connection (bidirectional Glenn):** superior vena cava (SVC) to PA connection (Figure 8.25)
      i. Saturations: 80% to 85%
      ii. If bilateral SVCs, left SVC anastomosed to left pulmonary artery (LPA)—increased risk of thrombus formation in pulmonary artery segment between the two SVCs
   c. **Stage 3 (2–4 years)—Fontan:** IVC-to-PA connection (extracardiac conduit or lateral tunnel) $\pm$ fenestration (Figure 8.26)
      i. Saturations: >90%
      ii. Long-term complications: rhythm disturbances, thromboembolic complications, ↓ cardiac function, valve regurgitation, protein-losing enteropathy

Cardiology

8

8

Figure 8.24 Norwood Procedure

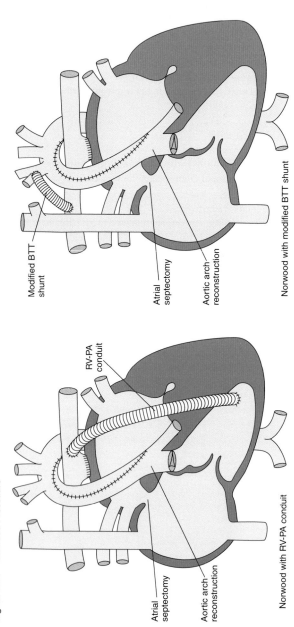

Modified BTT shunt

Atrial septectomy

Aortic arch reconstruction

Norwood with modified BTT shunt

RV-PA conduit

Atrial septectomy

Aortic arch reconstruction

Norwood with RV-PA conduit

Figure 8.25 Bidirectional Cavopulmonary Connection

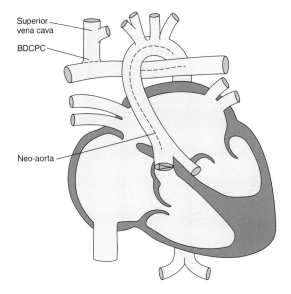

Superior vena cava

BDCPC

Neo-aorta

Figure 8.26 Fontan Procedure

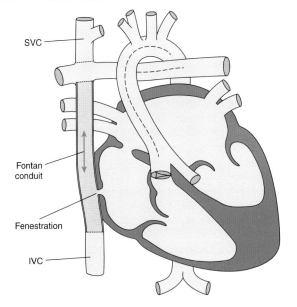

SVC

Fontan conduit

Fenestration

IVC

2. **Blalock-Taussig-Thomas shunt (modified):** polyethylene terephthalate (Dacron) shunt from innominate artery to PA to increase pulmonary blood flow (e.g., as part of Norwood stage I)
3. **Arterial switch operation (formerly Jatene procedure):** correction of complete TGA
4. **Ross:** aortic valve (AoV) replacement with pulmonary autograft, then pulmonary valve replacement with tissue valve (homograft or bovine jugular vein graft)
5. **Konno:** aortic root enlargement
6. **Balloon atrial septosomy:** transcatheter balloon to create/enlarge ASD
7. **Rastelli operation:** placement of valved conduit-graft between RV and PA and intraventricular tunnel to direct LV blood to the aorta via VSD (for TGA with VSD and PS)

INFECTIVE ENDOCARDITIS

1. **Etiology**
   a. Usually associated with structural heart disease
   b. **Risk factors:** artificial valves (tissue or mechanical), indwelling lines, intravenous (IV) drug use, immunocompromised patients
   c. **Organisms:** *Viridans streptococci* (most common), *Staphylococcus*, the HACEK group of organisms (*Haemophilus* species, *Aggregatibacter actinomycetemcomitans* [formerly *Actinobacillus*], *Cardiobacterium hominis, Eikenella corrodens, Kingella* species), which are commensal oropharyngeal flora known to cause infective endocarditis; gram-negative organisms and fungi uncommon unless neonate, immunocompromised, or IV drug user
2. **Clinical features**
   a. **Symptoms:** fever, myalgia, arthralgia, malaise
   b. **Signs:** new heart murmur or change in murmur, congestive heart failure (CHF), embolic phenomena (petechiae, hepatosplenomegaly, splinter hemorrhages, Janeway lesions, Osler nodes, pulmonary emboli)
3. **Investigations**
   a. **Blood tests:** three successive separate blood cultures, complete blood count (CBC), C-reactive protein (CRP), creatinine
   b. **Echocardiogram:** underlying structural disease, vegetations, cardiac function
      i. Transthoracic echocardiogram adequate and often do not need transesophageal echocardiogram
      ii. Negative findings on echocardiogram does not rule out endocarditis
4. **Diagnosis:** Modified Duke Criteria (see Figure 8.27)

Figure 8.27 Modified Duke Criteria for the Diagnosis of Infective Endocarditis

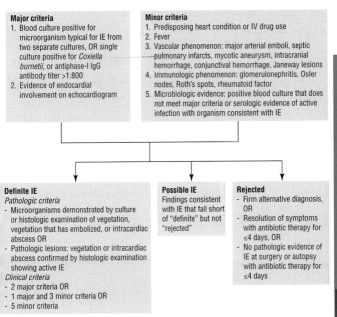

Major criteria
1. Blood culture positive for microorganism typical for IE from two separate cultures, OR single culture positive for *Coxiella burnetii*, or antiphase-I IgG antibody titer >1:800
2. Evidence of endocardial involvement on echocardiogram

Minor criteria
1. Predisposing heart condition or IV drug use
2. Fever
3. Vascular phenomenon: major arterial emboli, septic pulmonary infarcts, mycotic aneurysm, intracranial hemorrhage, conjunctival hemorrhage, Janeway lesions
4. Immunologic phenomenon: glomerulonephritis, Osler nodes, Roth's spots, rheumatoid factor
5. Microbiologic evidence: positive blood culture that does not meet major criteria or serologic evidence of active infection with organism consistent with IE

Definite IE
Pathologic criteria
- Microorganisms demonstrated by culture or histologic examination of vegetation, vegetation that has embolized, or intracardiac abscess OR
- Pathologic lesions: vegetation or intracardiac abscess confirmed by histologic examination showing active IE
Clinical criteria
- 2 major criteria OR
- 1 major and 3 minor criteria OR
- 5 minor criteria

Possible IE
Findings consistent with IE that fall short of "definite" but not "rejected"

Rejected
- Firm alternative diagnosis, OR
- Resolution of symptoms with antibiotic therapy for ≤4 days, OR
- No pathologic evidence of IE at surgery or autopsy with antibiotic therapy for ≤4 days

IE, Infective endocarditis; *IV,* intravenous. (Data from Li JS, Sexton DJ, Mick N, et al. Proposed modifications to the Duke criteria for the diagnosis of infective endocarditis. *Clinical Infectious Diseases.* 2000;30:633–638.)

5. **Management**
   a. **Acute**
      i. Antibiotics
      ii. Treatment of CHF
      iii. Surgery if severe valvular regurgitation, aortic root abscess, large vegetation, embolic phenomena, or persistent bacteremia
   b. **Long-term:** management of residual lesions or sequelae
   c. **Antibiotic prophylaxis:** see Endocarditis Prophylaxis in Chapter 40 Drug Dosing Guidelines

ACUTE RHEUMATIC FEVER

1. **Background**
   a. Autoimmune sequelae of group A streptococcal (GAS) pharyngitis
   b. Diagnosis based on Jones criteria (Table 8.13)

Table 8.13	2015 Jones Criteria	
For all patients with evidence of preceding GAS infection		
Initial ARF diagnosis: 2 major OR 1 major plus 2 minor manifestations **Recurrent ARF diagnosis:** 2 major OR 1 major plus 2 minor OR 3 minor manifestations		
Major criteria	**Low-Risk Population[a]**	**Moderate and High-Risk Population**
Carditis	Clinical and/or subclinical	Clinical and/or subclinical
Arthritis	Polyarthritis	Monoarthritis, polyarthritis, and/or polyarthraglia
Movements	Chorea	Chorea
Skin findings	Erythema marginatum Subcutaneous nodules	Erythema marginatum Subcutaneous nodules
Minor criteria		
Cardiac	Prolonged PR interval (if no carditis)	Prolonged PR interval (if no carditis)
Arthralgia	Polyarthralgia	Monoarthralgia
Fever	$\geq 38.5°C$	$\geq 38°C$
Markers of inflammation	Peak ESR ≥ 60 mm/h and/or CRP ≥ 30 mg/L	Peak ESR ≥ 30 mm/h and/or CRP ≥ 30 mg/L

[a]ARF incidence ≤ 2 per 100,000 school-aged children or all-age RHD prevalence of ≤ 1 per 1000 population per year.
ARF, Acute rheumatic fever; *CRP*, C-reactive protein; *ESR*, erythrocyte sedimentation rate; *GAS*, group A streptococcal; *RHD*, rheumatic heart disease.

Data from Gewitz MH, Baltimore RS, Tani LY, Sable CA, Shulman ST, Carapetis J, Remenyi B, Taubert KA, Bolger AF, Beerman L, Mayosi BM, Beaton A, Pandian NG, Kaplan EL; and on behalf of the American Heart Association Committee on Rheumatic Fever, Endocarditis, and Kawasaki Disease of the Council on Cardiovascular Disease in the Young. Revision of the Jones criteria for the diagnosis of acute rheumatic fever in the era of Doppler echocardiography: a scientific statement from the American Heart Association. *Circulation*. 2015;131:1806–1818.

2. **Investigations**
   a. CBC, CRP, ESR, antistreptolysin O titer (ASOT) throat culture
   b. ECG: prolonged PR interval
   c. Echocardiogram: function, pericardial effusion, valvular regurgitation
3. **Management**
   a. Acute: see Table 8.14
   b. Long term: see Table 8.15

Table 8.14	Management of Acute Rheumatic Fever
Immediate treatment of pharyngitis	- Penicillin VK OR amoxicillin for 10 days - If non-type 1 hypersensitivity to betalactams: cephalexin - If life-threatening or type I hypersensitivity to betalactams: macrolide (azithromycin for 5 days OR clarithromycin for 10 days)
Continued antibiotic prophylaxis	- Benzathine Penicillin G intramuscularly every 4 weeks - Penicillin VK or erythromycin (if penicillin allergy)
Antiinflammatory therapy	- ASA - Prednisone (if carditis present)
Heart failure therapy	- Diuretics and/or ACE inhibitors in patients with severe symptoms - May need valve repair or replacement if severe/chronic rheumatic valve disease
Chorea	- Consider neuroleptics, benzodiazepines, antiepileptics if severe - Usually considered self-limiting and benign

ACE, Angiotensin-converting enzyme; *ASA*, acetyl salicylic acid.

Table 8.15	Duration of Prophylaxis for People Who Have Had Acute Rheumatic Fever
Category	**Duration**
Rheumatic fever without carditis	5 years or until 21 years of age, whichever is longer
Rheumatic fever with carditis but without residual heart disease	10 years or until 21 years of age, whichever is longer
Rheumatic fever with carditis and residual heart disease	10 years or until 40 years of age, sometimes lifelong

From Dajani A, Taubert K, Ferrieri P, et al, and Committee on Rheumatic Fever, Endocarditis and Kawasaki Disease of the Council on Cardiovascular Disease in the Young, and American Heart Association. Treatment of acute streptococcal pharyngitis and prevention of rheumatic fever: a statement for health professionals. *Pediatrics*. 1995;96:758–764.

MYOCARDITIS

1. **Background:** characterized by inflammatory changes in myocardium and necrosis of adjacent myocytes
2. **Etiology**
   a. **Infectious:** viral infection (coxsackievirus, adenovirus, echovirus, cytomegalovirus [CMV], Epstein-Barr virus [EBV], measles, human immunodeficiency virus [HIV]); bacterial, fungal, protozoal
   b. **Autoimmune/inflammatory:** lupus, Kawasaki disease, rheumatic fever
   c. **Drugs/toxins:** lead, allergic drug hypersensitivity reaction

3. **Clinical features:** fever, tachycardia, signs of CHF, exercise intolerance, palpitations, chest pain, cardiogenic shock
4. **Investigations**
   a. Blood tests: CBC, ESR, blood culture, troponins, viral studies
   b. ECG: tachycardia, low QRS voltage, ST-T wave changes, heart block, arrhythmias
   c. CXR: cardiomegaly, ↑ pulmonary vascular markings
   d. Echocardiogram: decreased function, chamber enlargement, AV valve regurgitation, thrombus, pericardial effusion
   e. Endomyocardial biopsy
5. **Management**
   a. Acute: ABCs, inotropes, mechanical support
   b. Intermediate: diuretics, angiotensin-converting enzyme (ACE) inhibitors, β-blockers
   c. Controversial therapies: steroids, intravenous immune globulin (IVIG), immunotherapy
6. **Prognosis**
   a. Outcomes for neonates poor
   b. Patients with mild inflammation generally recover completely
   c. 25% to 30% will progress to dilated cardiomyopathy (DCM) requiring transplantation

CARDIOMYOPATHY

1. **Investigations**
   a. Echocardiogram: functional or structural abnormalities, hemodynamic parameters
   b. ECG: ischemia, hypertrophy, chamber enlargement
   c. Holter: arrhythmias, ischemia
   d. GXT: arrhythmias, ischemia, decreased aerobic capacity
   e. Investigations (as indicated): CBC, troponins, B-type natriuretic peptide (BNP), blood gas, calcium/vitamin D levels, thyroid stimulating hormone (TSH), acylcarnitines, carnitine (total and free), amino acids, CK, ALT, AST, lactate, trace metals, urine organic acids
   f. Endomyocardial biopsy/skeletal muscle biopsy may be considered
   g. Genetic testing may be considered
2. See Tables 8.16 and 8.17 for types of cardiomyopathies, clinical features and management

Table 8.16	Cardiomyopathies		
Characteristics	**HCM**	**DCM**	**RCM**
Epidemiology	AD (30%–60%); mutations in muscle proteins; can be caused by metabolic diseases or infant of diabetic mother	60% idiopathic, 30% familial; see Table 8.17 for other causes	Rare in children; can be idiopathic or secondary to systemic disease (e.g., scleroderma, sarcoidosis, metabolic diseases, radiation)
Structural abnormalities	Hypertrophied ventricular septum leading to LVOTO	Dilated, poorly contractile ventricle	Dilated atria
Pathophysiology	Stiff hypertrophied ventricle that does not fill well; LVOTO caused by sub-AS; subendocardial ischemia caused by severe hypertrophy	Dilated, poorly contractile ventricle leads to congestion and poor systemic perfusion	Noncompliant ventricle results in poor filling
Associated lesions	LVOTO, mitral insufficiency		
Clinical features	Sudden death can be initial presentation; exercise intolerance, syncope, chest pain, or dyspnea on exertion; SEM at left sternal border	Dyspnea, orthopnea, poor exercise tolerance, 90% present with CHF, gallop, hepatomegaly	Dyspnea, orthopnea, poor exercise tolerance, CHF, gallop, sudden death, arrhythmia
CXR findings	LVE	Cardiomegaly, ↑ pulmonary blood flow	Dilated atria, ↑ pulmonary vascular markings
ECG findings	LVH, ST-T wave changes, abnormal Q waves	Sinus tachycardia, nonspecific ST changes, low voltage, LVH	RAE/LAE, arrhythmia
Treatment	Activity restriction; β-blockers; myectomy for severe LVOTO, implantable defibrillator	Management of CHF (diuretics, β-blockers, ACE inhibitors), transplantation if end stage	Manage CHF, arrhythmia; transplantation if end-stage
Long-term complications	Sudden death, worsening LVOTO	Arrhythmia, sudden death	Arrhythmia, sudden death

ACE, Angiotensin-converting enzyme; *AD,* autosomal dominant; *CHF,* congestive heart failure; *CXR,* chest x-ray; *DCM,* dilated cardiomyopathy; *ECG,* electrocardiogram; *HCM,* hypertrophic cardiomyopathy; *LAE,* left atrial enlargement; *LVOTO,* left ventricular outflow tract obstruction; *LVE,* left ventricular enlargement; *LVH,* left ventricular hypertrophy; *RAE,* right atrial enlargement; *RCM,* restrictive cardiomyopathy; *SEM,* systolic ejection murmur; *sub-AS,* sub-aortic stenosis.

Cardiology

8

Table 8.17	Causes of Dilated Cardiomyopathy
Infectious	Viral: coxsackievirus, adenovirus, echovirus, EBV, CMV, HIV
	Bacterial: diphtheria, *Mycoplasma*, meningococcus
	Fungal: histoplasmosis, coccidioidomycosis
	Parasites: Chagas disease, toxoplasmosis
Metabolic	Lysosomal storage disease, mitochondrial disease
Endocrine	Hyperthyroidism, pheochromocytoma, vitamin D deficiency
Autoimmune	Lupus, scleroderma, rheumatic fever
Neuromuscular/myopathic	Muscular/myotonic dystrophy, Friedreich ataxia
Hematological	Anemia, sickle cell anemia, beta thalassemia
Toxin induced	Anthracyclines, radiation, cyclophosphamide, chloroquine, hemosiderosis
Other	Chronic tachyarrhythmia, coronary artery abnormality/chronic ischemia

CMV, Cytomegalovirus; *EBV*, Epstein-Barr virus; *HIV*, human immunodeficiency virus.

Data from Allen HD, Adams FH, Moss AJ. *Moss and Adams' Heart Disease in Infants, Children and Adolescents: Including the Fetus and Young Adults.* 6th ed. Philadelphia, PA: Lippincott Williams and Wilkins; 2001, and from Behrman RE, Kliegman RM, Jenson HB. *Nelson Textbook of Pediatrics.* 17th ed. Philadelphia, PA: Saunders; 2004:1572–1576.

PULMONARY HYPERTENSION

1. **Definition**
   a. **Pulmonary hypertension:** elevated pulmonary arterial (PA) pressure (mean $\geq$25 mmHg at sea level)
   b. **Measurement**
      i. Cardiac catheterization: normal PA systolic pressure $\leq$30 mmHg and mean $\leq$25 mmHg
      ii. Echocardiography using tricuspid regurgitation jet velocity and Bernoulli equation (often overestimates PA pressure): normal PA systolic pressure $\leq$37 mmHg
2. **Classification:** see Table 8.18 for clinical classification
3. **Clinical features**
   a. **Symptoms:** exertional dyspnea, fatigue, headache, presyncope, syncope, chest pain, cough
   b. **Physical examination**
      i. General: cyanosis with exertion or rest, failure to thrive, digital clubbing
      ii. Cardiac examination: parasternal heave, loud single or narrowly split S_2, systolic murmur (tricuspid regurgitation) or diastolic murmur (pulmonary regurgitation)
      iii. Signs of heart failure: jugular venous distension, hepatomegaly, peripheral edema

Table 8.18	Classification of Pulmonary Hypertension
Category	**Etiology**
Pulmonary arterial hypertension (intrinsic vessel abnormalities)	- Idiopathic - Heritable - Induced by drugs or toxins - Associated with connective tissue disease, congenital heart disease, portal hypertension - Pulmonary venoocclusive disease and/or pulmonary capillary hemangiomatosis - Persistent pulmonary hypertension of the newborn
Pulmonary hypertension caused by left heart disease	- Systolic left ventricular failure - Left ventricular diastolic dysfunction - Valvular diseases - Congenital/acquired left heart inflow/outflow tract obstruction and congenital cardiomyopathies
Pulmonary hypertension caused by lung diseases and/or hypoxia	- Chronic obstructive pulmonary disease - Interstitial lung disease - Sleep apnea - Developmental lung diseases
Chronic thromboembolic pulmonary hypertension	
Pulmonary hypertension with unclear multifactorial mechanisms	- Hematological disorders: chronic hemolytic anemia, myeloproliferative disorders, splenectomy - Systemic disorders: sarcoidosis, pulmonary histiocytosis, lymphangioleiomyomatosis - Metabolic disorders: glycogen storage disease, Gaucher disease, thyroid disorders - Others: tumoral obstruction, fibrosing mediastinitis, chronic renal failure, segmental pulmonary hypertension

4. **Investigations**
   a. Electrocardiogram: right axis deviation, right ventricular hypertrophy, right atrial hypertrophy, arrhythmias (late)
   b. Chest radiograph: normal or slightly enlarged heart, dilated PA branches, pulmonary edema if heart failure
   c. Echocardiogram: RA/RV enlargement, IV septal flattening, estimates of RV and/or PA pressure
   d. Cardiac catheterization for confirmation

5. **Management**
   a. Treat underlying causes
      i. Adenoidectomy and tonsillectomy for sleep-disordered breathing
      ii. Surgical repair of CHD if still a surgical candidate
   b. Timely expert consultation for management
      i. Medications: nifedipine, prostacyclines, endothelin receptor antagonists, phosphodiesterase inhibitors, nitric oxide
      ii. Surgery

SYNCOPE

1. Common in childhood, usually benign
2. Etiologies
   a. Neurally mediated: vasovagal, orthostatic
   b. Cardiovascular
   c. Noncardiovascular: seizure, hypoglycemia, electrolyte abnormality, psychogenic (e.g., hyperventilation)
3. See Table 8.19 for approach

Table 8.19	Approach to Syncope		
	Vasovagal	**Orthostatic**	**Cardiac**
Etiology	Neurally mediated	Neurally mediated	Arrhythmia (LQTS, extreme tachycardia/bradycardia), obstructive (severe AS, PS, HOCM, pulmonary HTN), myocardial dysfunction (infarction, Kawasaki disease, coronary anomalies)
History	1. Associated with fright, pain, heat, prolonged standing, crowding 2. Prodrome of dizziness, pallor, diaphoresis, hyperventilation 3. Loss of consciousness usually <1 min, with gradual awakening	1. Usually occurs on changing position 2. May have history of prolonged bed rest, dehydration, medications (e.g., antihypertensives, vasodilators)	1. Exercise induced 2. Syncope when supine 3. Associated chest pain 4. Family history of sudden death 5. History of structural heart disease
Physical findings	Normal	1. Orthostatic BP and HR (record BP and HR when supine, and again after standing for 5–10 min) 2. 10–15 mmHg drop in BP is abnormal, especially if HR does not increase	Focused cardiac examination
Investigations to consider	No investigations necessary	1. Electrolytes, fasting blood glucose 2. Orthostatic BP and HR 3. EEG if suspect seizure	ECG, GXT, 24-h Holter monitor, cardiac event recorder, echocardiogram

Table 8.19	Approach to Syncope—cont'd		
	Vasovagal	**Orthostatic**	**Cardiac**
Management	1. Reassurance 2. Cross legs if prodromal signs 3. Encourage fluids 4. Frequent severe episodes despite nonpharmacological interventions, consider medication (β-blocker, fludrocortisone)	1. Stand up slowly 2. Encourage fluids, ↑ salt in diet	Etiology specific

AS, Aortic stenosis; *BP*, blood pressure; *ECG*, electrocardiogram; *EEG*, electroencephalogram; *GXT*, graded exercise test; *HOCM*, hypertrophic obstructive cardiomyopathy; *HR*, heart rate; *HTN*, hypertension; *LQTS*, long QT syndrome; *PS*, pulmonary stenosis.

SYNDROMES ASSOCIATED WITH CARDIAC DISEASE

See Table 8.20

Table 8.20	Syndromes Associated With Congenital Heart Disease	
Syndrome	**% Risk of Heart Disease**	**Associated Lesions**
45 XO (Turner syndrome)	15	CoA
47 XXY (Klinefelter syndrome)	50	VSD, PDA, MVP, TOF
Alagille	>90	Peripheral PS, PA, TOF
Apert	10	VSD, TOF
Asplenia/polysplenia	Almost 100	AVSD, TGA, TAPVR
CFC	75	PS, ASD, HCM
Charge syndrome (CHD7)	75–85	TOF, PDA, AVSD, DORV, VSD
Crouzon syndrome		PDA, CoA
Cutis laxa		PS, pulmonary hypertension
Deletion 4p	50	ASD, VSD, PDA
Deletion 5p (Cri du Chat syndrome)	30	VSD, ASD, PDA
Deletion 22q (DiGeorge)	85	Conotruncal anomalies (TOF, common arterial trunk)
Ehlers-Danlos (some types)	50	MVP, dilated aortic root
Ellis-van Creveld	50–60	Common atrium, ASD
Fragile X	50–75	MVP (in older patients)
Goldenhar	32	VSD, PDA, TOF, COA, conotruncal defects

Continued 209

Table 8.20	Syndromes Associated With Congenital Heart Disease—cont'd	
Syndrome	**% Risk of Heart Disease**	**Associated Lesions**
Holt-Oram	50–100	ASD, VSD, AV block
Hurler/Hunter/other MPS		Valvular insufficiency
LEOPARD	50	PS
Marfan	60–80	MVP, AI, dilated aortic root
Noonan	75	Dysplastic PS, ASD, TOF, AVSD, HCM, VSD, PDA
Osteogenesis imperfecta	5–10	Aortic incompetence
Rubinstein-Taybi	33	PDA, VSD, ASD, HLH, BAV
Smith-Lemli-Opitz	50	AVSD, HLH, ASD, PDA, VSD
TAR	20	TOF, ASD
Trisomy 13	90	VSD, ASD, PDA
Trisomy 18	95	VSD, DORV, PDA
Trisomy 21	40	AVSD (15%), VSD, ASD, TOF
Tetrasomy 22 (cat eye syndrome)	40	TAPVR, TOF, VSD
Tuberous sclerosis	30	Cardiac rhabdomyoma
VATER/VACTERL	>50	VSD, TOF, ASD, PDA
Williams (deletion 7q)	80	AS (supravalvular), PS, VSD, ASD

AI, Aortic insufficiency; *AS,* aortic stenosis; *ASD,* atrial septal defect; *AV,* atrioventricular; *AVSD,* atrioventricular septal defect; *BAV,* bicuspid aortic value; *CFC,* cardiofaciocutaneous; *CHARGE,* Coloboma, Heart defects, Atresia choanae, Retarded growth, Genital abnormalities, and Ear abnormalities; *CoA,* coarctation of the aorta; *DORV,* double outlet right ventricle; *HCM,* hypertrophic cardiomyopathy; *HLH,* hypoplastic left heart; LEOPARD Syndrome (Lentigines, Electrocardiographic conduction defects, Ocular hypertelorism, Pulmonary stenosis, Abnormalities of the genitals, Retarded growth, and Deafness/hearing loss; also known as Noonan syndrome with multiple lentigines); *MPS,* mucopolysaccharidosis; *MVP,* mitral valve prolapse; *PA,* pulmonary atresia; *PDA,* patent ductus arteriosus; *PS,* pulmonary stenosis; *TAPVR,* total anomalous pulmonary venous return; *TAR,* thrombocytopenia with absent radius; *TGA,* transposition of the great arteries; *TOF,* tetralogy of Fallot; *VACTERL,* Vertebral defects, Anal atresia, Cardiac defects, Tracheo-Esophageal fistula, Renal anomalies, and Limb abnormalities; *VATER,* Verterbral defects, Anal atresia, Tracheo-Esophageal fistula, Limb abnormalities; *VSD,* ventricular septal defect.

Data from Freedom RM, Benson LN, Smallhorn JF, eds. *Neonatal Heart Disease.* New York, NY: Springer-Verlag; 1992:8, and Pierpont ME, Brueckner M, Chung WK, et al. Genetic basis for congenital heart disease: revisited: a scientific statement from the American Heart Association. *Circulation.* 2018;138(21):e563–e711.

NEWBORN PULSE OXIMETRY SCREENING

1. Screening guidelines for the detection of critical CHD in the newborn
   a. The optimal screening should include prenatal ultrasound, physical examination and pulse oximetry screening
   b. See Figure 8.28 for screening protocol
   c. Referral to a pediatric cardiologist if a cardiac diagnosis cannot be confidently excluded

Figure 8.28   Critical Congenital Heart Disease Screening Protocol

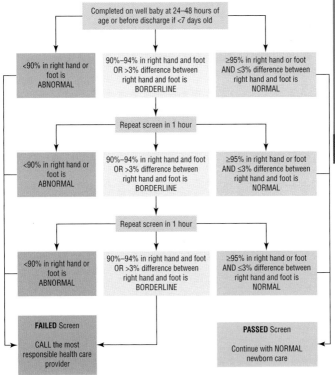

(Data from Kemper AR, Mahle WT, Martin GR, et al. Strategies for implementing screening for critical congenital heart disease. *Pediatrics*. 2011; 128(5):e1259.)

CARDIAC SCREENING BEFORE USE OF STIMULANT MEDICATIONS

1. Little evidence that stimulant medications increase the risk of sudden death in pediatric patients with attention-deficit hyperactivity disorder (ADHD)

2. Children and adolescents with ADHD should undergo a careful history and physical examination by their primary care physician to identify those at increased risk of sudden death
3. Routine ECG assessment not recommended
4. For patients with known cardiac disease followed by a cardiologist, the physician with expertise in ADHD is the appropriate person to recommend medication
5. Discussion of treatment options with the cardiologist to form a consensus decision is appropriate
6. For patients with ADHD and suspected cardiac disease or risk factors for sudden cardiac death, assessment by a cardiologist is recommended (as with any non-ADHD patient)

LIPID SCREENING

1. See Table 8.21 for screening recommendations
2. See Table 8.22 for interpretation of results. If abnormal, refer to lipid specialist and dietitian.

Table 8.21	Lipid Screening Recommendations
Birth–2 years	No lipid screening
2–9 years	Targeted lipid screening (Box 8.3)
9–11 years	Universal lipid screening (Box 8.4)
12–16 years	Targeted lipid screening (see Box 8.3)
17–21 years	Universal lipid screening (see Box 8.4)

Data from Expert Panel on Integrated Guidelines for Cardiovascular Health and Risk Reduction in Children and Adolescents: Summary Report. *Pediatrics*. 2011; 128(s5):s213.

Table 8.22	Laboratory Parameters for Lipid Screening Results		
Laboratory Parameter	**Acceptable (mmol/L)**	**Borderline (mmol/L)**	**Abnormal (mmol/L)**
Total cholesterol	<4.4	4.40–5.19	≥5.20
LDL-C	<2.85	2.85–3.34	≥3.35
HDL-C	>1.15	1–1.15	<1
Triglycerides (<10 years of age)	<0.85	0.85–1.14	≥1.15
Triglycerides (10–19 years of age)	<1	1–1.44	≥1.45
Non-HDL-C	<3.1	3.10–3.74	≥3.75

HDL, High-density lipoprotein; *LDL*, low-density lipoprotein.

Data from Expert Panel on Integrated Guidelines for Cardiovascular Health and Risk Reduction in Children and Adolescents: Summary Report. *Pediatrics*. 2011; 128(s5):s213.

Box 8.3 Targeted Lipid Screening

Measure fasting lipid profile twice (2–12 weeks apart) and average the results, if
1. Parent, grandparent, aunt/uncle, or sibling with MI, angina, stroke, CABG/stent/angioplasty at <55 years in males and <65 years in females
2. Parent with total cholesterol ≥6.2 mmol/L or known dyslipidemia
3. Child has diabetes, hypertension, BMI ≥95th percentile (2–9 years)/85th percentile (12–16 years) or smokes tobacco products
4. Child has a moderate- or high-risk condition (see Table 8.23)

BMI, Body mass index; *CABG*, coronary artery bypass graft; *MI*, myocardial infarction.
Data from Expert Panel on Integrated Guidelines for Cardiovascular Health and Risk Reduction in Children and Adolescents: Summary Report. *Pediatrics*. 2011; 128(s5):s213.

Box 8.4 Universal Lipid Screening (Nonfasting or Fasting)

Nonfasting lipid screen: calculate non-HDL cholesterol
1. Non-HDL cholesterol = Total cholesterol – HDL
2. If non-HDL ≥3.75 or HDL <1.05 mmol/L, then obtain fasting lipid profile twice (2–12 weeks apart) and average the results
Fasting lipid screen
1. Repeat fasting lipid profile in 2–12 weeks, and average the results if any of
   a. LDL ≥3.35 mmol/L
   b. Non-HDL ≥3.75 mmol/L
   c. HDL <1.05 mmol/L
   d. Triglycerides ≥1.15 mmol/L (≤9 years) or ≥1.45 mmol/L (≥10 years)

HDL, High-density lipoprotein; *LDL*, low-density lipoprotein.
Data from Expert Panel on Integrated Guidelines for Cardiovascular Health and Risk Reduction in Children and Adolescents: Summary Report. *Pediatrics*. 2011; 128(s5):s213.

Table 8.23 Moderate or High-Risk Conditions for Lipid Screening

Moderate-Risk Conditions	High-Risk Conditions
Kawasaki disease with regressed coronary aneurysms	Chronic kidney disease/end-stage renal disease/postrenal transplant
Chronic inflammatory disease (SLE, JRA)	T1DM and T2DM
HIV infection	Postorthotopic heart transplant
Nephrotic syndrome	Kawasaki disease with current aneurysms

HIV, Human immunodeficiency syndrome; *JRA*, juvenile rheumatoid arthritis; *SLE*, systemic lupus erythematosus; *T1DM*, type 1 diabetes mellitus; *T2DM*, type 2 diabetes mellitus.

Data from Expert Panel on Integrated Guidelines for Cardiovascular Health and Risk Reduction in Children and Adolescents: Summary Report. *Pediatrics*. 2011; 128(s5):s213.

PREPARTICIPATION SCREENING IN ATHLETES

1. American Heart Association (AHA)
   a. Screening for high school and college athletes preparticipation and at 2 to 4 year intervals
   b. Cardiac-focused history and physical examination
2. European Society of Cardiology (ESC)
   a. Routine preparticipation screening of athletes
   b. Cardiac-focused history, physical examination and resting 12-lead ECG

ANTIARRYTHMIC MEDICATIONS

See Table 8.24 for common antiarrythmic agents

Table 8.24	Cardiac Antiarrythmic Agents	
Medication Class	**Examples**	**Side Effects**
Class I—Na Channel Blockade		
Ia	- Quinidine - Procainamide	Blood dyscrasias, cinchonism (quinidine), depressed myocardial contractility, drug-induced lupus (procainamide), nausea and vomiting, prolonged QRS complex, ventricular arrhythmias
Ib	- Lidocaine - Phenytoin - Mexiletine	Anxiety, drowsiness, hypotension, respiratory depression, seizure, shock
Ic	- Flecainide	Bradycardia, AV block, dizziness, blurred vision, dyspnea, nausea, headache, increased PR and QRS duration
Class II—Beta Blockade		
	- Nadolol - Propranolol - Esmolol - Atenolol	Bronchospasm, CHF, hypotension, nausea and vomiting, fatigue, depression in adolescents
Class III—K Channel Blockade		
	- Amiodarone - Sotalol	Amiodarone: ataxia, corneal microdeposits, heart block, hepatotoxicity, hypotension, nausea, and vomiting, photosensitivity, pulmonary fibrosis, thyroid dysfunction Sotalol: bradycardia, bronchospasm, chest pain, depression, dizziness, heart block, hypoglycemia, hypotension, QT prolongation, torsades de pointes

Table 8.24	Cardiac Antiarrhythmic Agents—cont'd	
Medication Class	**Examples**	**Side Effects**
Class IV—Ca Channel Blockade		
	- Verapamil - Diltiazem	Arrhythmias, dizziness, edema, headache, nausea and vomiting
		Contraindicated in second- and third-degree heart block, sinus node dysfunction
Class V—Other Mechanism		
	- Adenosine - Digoxin - Magnesium sulfate	

AV, Atrioventricular; *CHF*, congestive heart failure.

HEART TRANSPLANTATION

See Chapter 38 Transplantation

Child Maltreatment

Tanvi Agarwal • Rebecca Wang • Elodie April • Romy Cho • Jennifer Smith

| NAAT | nucleic-acid amplification test |
| STI | sexually transmitted infection |

REPORTING AND DOCUMENTATION

A. Reporting

1. If you suspect child abuse or neglect is occurring, you have met the legal threshold to report to the appropriate child welfare agency
2. Reports should be directly made by the concerned healthcare provider; in most cases, families should be informed about the report being made to child welfare agency
3. Child welfare agencies will determine the need for police involvement
4. Healthcare professionals have an ongoing duty to report any new concerns

B. Documentation

1. Medical records can be used for legal purposes: document history and physical examination carefully and objectively, write legibly, include times and dates
2. Include relevant statements in quotes, drawings, measurements, body diagrams (Figure 9.1), photographs (consent required)

Figure 9.1 Body Diagram

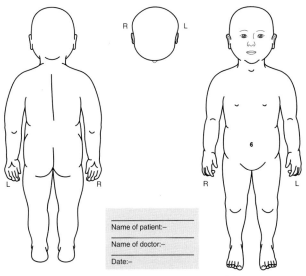

Name of patient:–

Name of doctor:–

Date:–

(From The Faculty of Forensic & Legal Medicine of the Royal College of Physicians. Source: https://fflm.ac.uk/publications/pro-forma-body-diagrams/.)

RED FLAGS

1. Injury not consistent with history provided and/or age/developmental stage of child
2. Inconsistent/changing history for a significant injury
3. Delay in seeking medical attention
4. Multiple injuries or injuries of different ages
5. Evidence of neglect or failure to thrive
6. Absence of a history of trauma in a child with obvious injury

PHYSICAL ABUSE

Any act that causes injury or trauma to a child through bodily contact

A. History

1. **Sentinel injuries:** relatively minor, suspicious injuries (e.g., frenulum tears or bruises in precruising infants) that may identify those who are at risk for suffering more serious abusive injuries
2. **Injury:** detailed history of sequence of events leading up to injury (nonleading, open-ended questions), event details (timing, location, response of child/caregiver, witnessed/unwitnessed), symptom progression, when the child last fed/acted normally
3. **Past medical history:** previous trauma/injury, chronic illnesses, birth history, administration of vitamin K at birth, bleeding history, and/or predisposition to fractures
4. **Development:** ambulation, level of functioning, ability to express pain
5. **Family history:** family members with easy bleeding, bruising, fractures, bleeding disorder, collagen vascular diseases, bone disorders, metabolic or genetic disorders; consanguinity
6. **Social:** caregivers, discipline practices, substance or alcohol abuse, mental illness, domestic violence, stressors, prior criminal or child protection agency involvement, other children in the home who may need to be assessed for maltreatment

B. Physical examination

A thorough examination is necessary to respond to life-threatening injuries, consider the differential diagnoses, assess for other injuries (including sentinel injuries). Consider conducting the examination following consultation with a clinician who has expertise in the evaluation of suspected child maltreatment.

1. **Anthropometrics:** growth parameters (weight, height, head circumference) and percentiles
2. **Skin:** undress and examine entire body, including pinnae, behind ears, soles and palms, genitals and buttocks. Describe location, distribution, color, shape, size of each skin finding.
3. **ENT:** frenula (between lips and gums, under tongue), oral injuries, dentition

4. **Neurologic:** level of consciousness, fontanelle, fundi
5. **MSK:** skull fractures, scalp swelling, bony tenderness, limb swelling

C. Injury patterns
1. **Bruising**
   a. Cannot be dated
   b. **Features concerning for inflicted injury:** preambulatory infant, located on areas that are padded by soft tissue or less exposed (e.g., buttocks, neck, genitalia, ears, chest, back, abdomen), clustered or patterned (e.g., looped or parallel linear bruises), large or numerous, causal mechanism does not correlate
   c. **Differential:** birthmarks (congenital dermal melanocytosis, café-au-lait macules), cultural practices (coining or cupping), bleeding disorders
2. **Bites**
   a. Characteristic pattern involves two opposing convex arcs of bruising or change in pigmentation, may or may not have a central bruise
   b. **Concerning features:** multiple bites, no explanation for bites, bites on inaccessible areas (self-inflicted are often on the hands)
3. **Burns**
   a. Injury can be affected by multiple factors, such as temperature, mechanism, duration of exposure, presence of clothing, first aid applied (see Burn Management in Chapter 34 Plastic Surgery)
   b. **Concerning features:** burns in nonmobile infants, clear delineation between burned and healthy skin (e.g., immersion), patterned burns (e.g., clothing irons, radiators), burns on buttocks/perineum, glove/stocking distribution. Absence of splash marks does not provide additional information about mechanism of scald burns.
   c. **Differential:** skin infections (e.g., staphylococcus scalded skin syndrome, dermatitis herpetiformis, varicella, impetigo), drug eruptions, insect bites, photosensitive dermatitis, allergic/irritant contact burn, chilblains or sunburn, cultural practices (e.g., moxibustion, chemical burns from home remedies), senna (typically in diapered children)
4. **Fractures**
   a. **Concerning features:** fractures in nonambulatory children, multiple fractures, different stages of healing, delay in seeking treatment, fracture does not fit with described mechanism, specific locations—ribs (especially posterior), metaphyseal, vertebral spinous process, scapula, sternum
      i. **Rib fractures:** typical mechanism is anterior–posterior compression of rib cage with forceful squeezing or shaking; can also include direct impact to chest (Figure 9.2)

Figure 9.2   Mechanism of Rib Fractures in Child Maltreatment

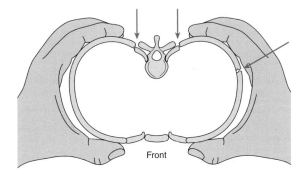

Front

ii. **Metaphyseal fractures** (classic metaphyseal lesion, corner fracture, bucket-handle fracture): caused by shearing of new bone formation from ends of long bones; typical mechanism is tractional/torsional force (e.g., yank, pull, twist) applied to the limb (Figure 9.3)

b. **Differential**: osteopenia, osteogenesis imperfecta, metabolic and nutritional disorders (e.g., vitamin D deficiency rickets), Menkes disease, copper deficiency, osteomyelitis, neoplasia

Figure 9.3   Mechanism of Metaphyseal Fractures

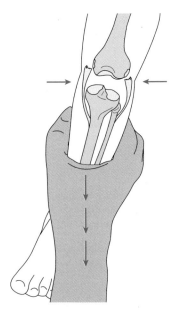

9

5. **Traumatic head injury**
   a. **Description:** subdural hemorrhages may be caused by direct impact to head and/or head acceleration-deceleration (e.g., forceful shaking). Symptoms range from nonspecific fussiness/crying to persistent vomiting to life-threatening symptoms (e.g., coma, seizures, respiratory arrest).
   b. **Other findings**: retinal hemorrhages (especially extensive and multilayered), complex skull fractures, other cutaneous/skeletal/ visceral injuries
   c. **Differential**: bleeding disorder, birth trauma, infection, metabolic conditions (glutaric aciduria type 1), tumor, arteriovenous malformations
6. **Abdominal injury**
   a. **Features:** solid organ (such as liver, pancreas, and spleen), hollow organs (duodenal perforation, transection, hematoma)

D. Investigations

Determine investigations based on patient age, history, physical examination, differential diagnoses. Exclude the presence of other traumatic injuries, which may be occult.

1. **Laboratory**
   a. **Bleeding/bruising:** complete blood count (CBC), international normalized ratio (INR)/partial thromboplastin time (PTT), peripheral blood smear, fibrinogen, Von Willebrand antigen and activity, blood group, factor VIII, factor IX, liver enzymes, and renal function tests
   b. **Fractures:** bone health (calcium, magnesium, phosphate, alkaline phosphatase [ALP], parathyroid hormone [PTH], vitamin D)
   c. **Subdural hemorrhages/retinal hemorrhages:** coagulation workup (see bleeding/bruising workup), Factor XIII, metabolic workup (urine organic acids, plasma amino acids, plasma acylcarnitines)
   d. **Abdominal trauma:** liver enzymes (alanine transaminase [ALT] and/or aspartate transaminase [AST] >80 U/L concerning for occult injury), pancreatic enzymes (lipase and amylase)
   e. **Altered mental status:** urine toxicology for overdose, if relevant
2. **Radiologic**
   a. **Skeletal survey** (see Chapter 13 Diagnostic Imaging): children <2 years old (index case and siblings) and in children >2 years old, based on clinical suspicion and developmental level. Repeat skeletal survey after 14 days to assess for healing fractures.
   b. **Neuroimaging:** head CT and/or MRI for facial injuries or concern of head injury. Screening head CT and/or MRI for all children <1 year of age (head ultrasound is not sufficient to assess for traumatic brain injury).

     c. **Abdominal imaging:** CT if abnormally elevated AST/ALT/ pancreatic enzymes or abdominal bruising (abdominal ultrasound not sufficient)

3. **Ophthalmologic**: dilated fundoscopic examination for retinal hemorrhages if subdural hemorrhages on neuroimaging (should be completed by ophthalmologist)

E. Management

1. Stabilize patient, manage acute injuries, and consult experts (e.g., child maltreatment clinician, hematology, neurosurgery, orthopedics)
2. Objectively document clinical information and report case to local child welfare agency
3. Consider hospitalization for additional medical testing, subspecialty consultation, treatment of known injuries, at request from local child welfare agency

SEXUAL ABUSE

A. Approach

1. Sexual abuse is any sexual behavior or action that is unwanted or exploitative
2. Sexual abuse does not have to involve direct touching or contact. Showing pornography to a child, photographing/filming a child in sexually explicit poses, or encouraging a child to perform sex acts also constitutes as sexual abuse.
3. See Age of Consent in Chapter 6 Adolescent Medicine
4. Sexualized behaviors that raise concern for possible sexual abuse:
   a. Developmentally inappropriate knowledge of sexual activities
   b. Developmentally inappropriate play/sexual acts
   c. Sexual behavior that results in emotional distress or physical pain
   d. Sexual behaviors associated with other physically aggressive behavior
   e. Sexual behaviors that involve coercion

B. History

Do not ask leading questions, avoid asking the child directly, and avoid repeated questioning.

1. **Injury:** what happened, when did it happen
2. **Genitourinary (GU) symptoms:** vaginal or anal symptoms (bleeding, pain, discharge)
3. **Past medical history:** medical (infection, eczema), gynecologic (vulvovaginitis, STI, foreign body)
4. **Psychological:** current level of distress, suicidality
5. **Social:** living situation, prior child welfare agency involvement

6. **Special consideration:** forensic interview should be completed by police and child welfare agency

C. Physical examination
1. **Acute assault or pain/bleeding/discharge**: urgent evaluation by a sexual assault specialist examiner
2. **Nonacute, asymptomatic cases**: in consultation with sexual assault specialist examiner, can likely defer examination until interview has been completed by child welfare agency
3. Limit unnecessary or multiple examinations. Most genital examination findings are normal or nonspecific; this does not confirm or rule out the possibility of sexual abuse/assault.
4. **General:** other injuries (e.g., skin injuries), sexual maturity rating
5. **GU:** perform in the most comfortable manner. Supine frog leg, prone knee-chest, or lithotomy positions to assess external genital, hymen (configuration, rim, edges, injuries), anal examination. No role for speculum examination.
   a. Redness in the anogenital region is not diagnostic for sexual abuse. Other causes of anogenital redness include vulvovaginitis, streptococcus infections, yeast infections.
   b. If anogenital warts present, obtain detailed history including family members or caregivers with warts, maternal Pap smear results, maternal history of genital warts. Absence of maternal genital warts on history does not exclude the possibility of perinatal transmission. Consider vertical transmission if child is <5 years of age.
   c. Consult sexual assault specialist examiner for interpretation of genital findings

D. Investigations
Laboratory tests and STI screening are based on the sexual abuse/assault disclosed, pubertal development of the child, perpetrator risk factors, and parent/patient concern or request for testing. Consult sexual assault specialist examiner to assist with these recommendations.
1. **Sexual assault evidence kit**: requires patient consent and police involvement, should be done in consultation with a sexual assault specialist examiner
2. **Laboratory:** serologies (human immunodeficiency virus [HIV], hepatitis B, hepatitis C, syphilis), pregnancy testing
3. **STI:** consider swabs for STIs (gonorrhea, chlamydia, trichomonas); vaginal swabs (technically difficult) in symptomatic prepubertal females
   a. Gonorrhea/chlamydia: urine nucleic acid amplification test (NAAT), vaginal/vestibule/discharge (girls) and meatus (boys) swabs for NAAT and/or culture, pharynx/rectum swabs for NAAT and/or culture

    b. Trichomonas vaginalis: vaginal/vestibule/discharge (girls) or meatus (boys) culture
    c. Herpes simplex virus (HSV) viral lesion swab if ulcers present

E. Management
1. **Report to child welfare agency:** if the child is under the age of 16 years and any of the following applies:
    a. Suspected sexual abuse by a person in position of authority (e.g., teacher, employer) OR
    b. If assault is by a stranger and parents are not believing, or are unsupportive of disclosure
    c. Ongoing concerns of child safety
2. **Pharmacological agents:** consider STI prophylaxis (risk of exposure based on history and ability to follow-up, particularly in adolescents), emergency contraception, hepatitis B immunization and immunoglobulin, HIV prophylaxis for high-risk cases (requires expert consultation with sexual assault specialist examiner and/or infectious disease specialist)

NEGLECT AND CAREGIVER FABRICATED ILLNESS

A. Neglect
1. **Definition**: omission in care that results in actual or potential harm
    a. **Physical:** failure to provide necessities (e.g., shelter, food), abandonment or inadequate supervision, repeated accidents/toxicities
    b. **Emotional:** lack of nurturing or affection
    c. **Educational:** child not involved in any educational programs
    d. **Medical:** failure to seek timely care of illness/injury, failure to comply with medical recommendations
2. **History**: evidence of harm (e.g., injury, ingestion), indications that basic needs have not been adequately met (e.g., poor hygiene, poor growth), nature and pattern of neglect, risk factors for neglect (e.g., parental depression, substance abuse, violence)
3. **Assessment**: complete physical examination (including growth, mental status)
4. **Management**: target interventions at apparent medical concerns (may need hospitalization), address risk factors, report to local child welfare agency

B. Caregiver-fabricated illness
1. **Definition:** when a parent or adult simulates or causes disease in a child and falsely presents a child for medical attention (sometimes called *medical child abuse*, *Munchausen syndrome by proxy*, *factitious disorder by proxy*)

2. **Clinical manifestations**: presentation varies in nature and severity. Examples include bleeding (adding dyes to samples), seizures (fabricated history, toxin induced), apnea (partial suffocation, toxin induced), gastrointestinal symptoms (forced ingestion of substances, laxative use), recurrent sepsis (contaminating intravenous lines, blood, urine samples).

3. **Possible features**: suspect if signs/symptoms occur only in the presence of a single caregiver, failure of illness to respond to normal treatments, caregiver not relieved if child improves, and/or caregiver insists on invasive/painful procedures and hospitalizations

4. **Approach:** review all the child's medical records, look for discrepancies between objective and described findings. Close observation and detailed clinical documentation of events is essential.

5. **Management:** work collaboratively with providers with expertise in child maltreatment for treatment plan

10

Dentistry

Rodd Morgan • Jane Ho • Shonna Masse

CHILDHOOD DENTAL CARE AND CARIES

A. Recommendations for dental care

1. Children should have dental home and first dental visit by age one
2. Encourage parents to lift the lip to check for tooth decay
3. Wipe gums with damp washcloth until first tooth erupts
4. Children <3 years should have their teeth brushed twice daily, starting at first tooth eruption. Fluoride toothpaste smear, no larger than a grain of rice, should be used if child is at risk of caries.
5. Children aged 3 to 6 years should have adult assistance and use adult fluoridated toothpaste
6. Non-nutritive sucking habits should be discouraged as young as possible

B. Early childhood caries

1. **Diagnosis:** may appear as chalky white spots through to brown/black holes in enamel. Parents may not be aware of cavities until teeth discolor or enamel "chips."
2. **Risk factors:** bottle feeding with any liquid other than water while being put to sleep; using bottle as pacifier; not brushing after feeding; breastfeeding on demand and special healthcare needs. Children on long-term medications containing sucrose or high calorific dietary supplements are at elevated risk. Sugar-free formulations should be used when possible.
3. **Prevention:** dental care outlined earlier. Cessation of a bottle and use of a cup should be encouraged by age one.

 PEARL

A child's first dental check-up should occur by 1 year of age

TEETHING, NATAL/NEONATAL TEETH, AND EARLY TOOTH LOSS

A. Teething

1. **Clinical features**
   a. Children have two sets of teeth (primary and permanent)
   b. Teeth tend to follow a pattern of eruption although variance in timing is common. The earliest eruption is typically around 6 months (Figure 10.1 and Table 10.1).
   c. Some children may present with drooling, irritability, and discomfort in the area of an erupting primary tooth

2. **Management**
   a. Chilled teething rings and oral analgesics may help alleviate discomfort
   b. Avoid teething gels and topical anaesthetics because of risk of methemoglobinemia, aspiration, and overdose

Figure 10.1   Identification System for Primary and Permanent Teeth

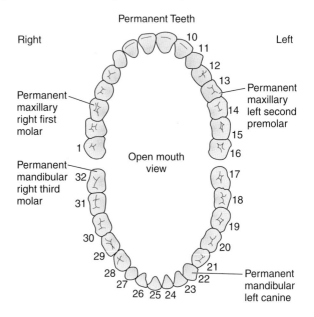

Permanent Teeth

Right

Left

Permanent maxillary right first molar

Permanent maxillary left second premolar

Open mouth view

Permanent mandibular right third molar

Permanent mandibular left canine

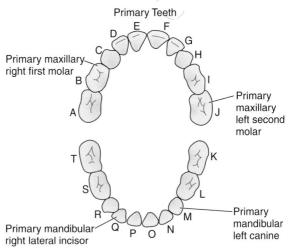

Primary Teeth

Primary maxillary right first molar

Primary maxillary left second molar

Primary mandibular right lateral incisor

Primary mandibular left canine

(Modified from Benko, Kip R. Emergency dental procedures. In: *Roberts and Hedges' Clinical Procedures in Emergency Medicine and Acute Care*. 7th ed. Philadelphia, PA: Elsevier; 2017.)

Table 10.1	Chronology of Human Dentition	
Teeth	**Eruption (Exfoliation)**	
Primary Teeth	**Maxillary**	**Mandibular**
Central incisors	6–10 months (*7–8 years*)	5–8 months (*6–7 years*)
Lateral incisors	8–12 months (*8–9 years*)	7–10 months (*7–8 years*)
Canines	16–20 months (*11–12 years*)	16–20 months (*9–11 years*)
First molars	11–18 months (*9–11 years*)	11–18 months (*10–12 years*)
Second molars	20–30 months (*9–12 years*)	20–30 months (*11–13 years*)
Permanent Teeth	**Maxillary**	**Mandibular**
Central incisors	7–8 years	6–7 years
Lateral incisors	8–9 years	7–8 years
Canines	11–12 years	9–11 years
First premolars	10–11 years	10–12 years
Second premolars	10–12 years	11–13 years
First molars	5.5–7 years	5.5–7 years
Second molars	12–14 years	12–14 years
Third molars	17–30 years	17–30 years

Modified from AAPD Dental Growth and Development Resource 2018.

B. Natal/neonatal teeth

1. **Clinical features**

    a. May be present at birth (natal) or within 30 days postpartum (neonatal) and are most commonly in the region of mandibular incisors. Most are prematurely erupted primary incisors. The exact etiology is unknown.

    b. Riga-Fede disease is a lesion on the ventral tongue caused by abrasion from neonatal teeth. May be associated with dehydration and insufficient nutrient intake.

2. **Management:** natal teeth may warrant extraction if they interfere with feeding, present an aspiration risk, or cause Riga-Fede disease. A dental consult is recommended.

C. Early tooth loss

1. Primary teeth may be lost (exfoliate) early because of advanced dental development of underlying permanent successors or, less commonly because of underlying systemic causes, such as immunological defects. A dental consult is recommended.

DENTAL TRAUMA

1. **Clinical features**

    a. See Table 10.2 for description of common injuries

b. Multiple teeth and oral structures (mucosa, gingiva, bone) may be injured concurrently

2. **Management**

a. Please see Table 10.2 for indications for dental referral. Trauma management may include tooth replantation, splinting, extractions, suturing, root canal therapy, and restorations.

b. Children may require advanced behavioral management, including sedation and support of other services, such as child life specialists

Table 10.2	Description and Management of Dental Trauma	
Type of Injury	**Description**	**Management of Dental Trauma**
Crown fractures	No pulpal exposure (enamel and dentine only)	Permanent and primary teeth: referral to dentist within 24 h
	With pulpal exposure (enamel, dentine, pulp)	Permanent and primary teeth: immediate referral to dentist
Nondisplacement injuries	Concussion: injury to tooth/ supporting structures, NO abnormal loosening/displacement	Permanent and primary teeth: referral to dentist within 24 h
	Subluxation injury to tooth/ supporting structures, abnormal loosening, but NO displacement	Permanent teeth: immediate referral to dentist
		Primary teeth: in significantly loose immediate referral, if minimally loose referral within 24 h
Displacement injuries	Extrusion: partial displacement of tooth from socket	Permanent and primary teeth: immediate referral to dentist
	Luxation: displacement of tooth in direction other than axially	Permanent and primary teeth: immediate referral to dentist
	Intrusion: displacement of tooth apically into alveolar bone	Permanent and primary teeth: immediate referral to dentist
Avulsion	Complete displacement of tooth from socket	Permanent teeth: immediate replantation within 5 min; if not, store and transport in chilled milk, immediate referral to dentist
		Primary teeth: immediate referral if caregivers cannot find tooth (rule out intrusion); avulsed tooth should not be replanted (infection and ankylosis risk)

> **! PITFALL**
>
> Failure to reflect the lips to assess the soft tissue surrounding teeth and the sulcus may result in missed oral soft tissue injuries (these may be more extensive than they appear!)

ODONTOGENIC INFECTIONS/DENTAL ABSCESS

1. **Etiology:** infection in the teeth and supporting structures may originate from a chronic or acute source, typically from a tooth with either decay, a dental anomaly, trauma, or failed dental treatment.
2. **Clinical features:** pain, swelling, erythema, and suppuration localized to tooth
3. **Management**
   a. Antibiotics
      i. Oral antibiotics for localized swelling: amoxicillin/clavulanate is typically the antibiotic of choice. Clindamycin is an alternative for children with penicillin allergy.
      ii. IV antibiotics (Clindamycin) in cases of failed oral antibiotics, rapid progression, or signs of complications (see later)
   b. Urgent referral to dentist: most cases will require extraction, pulp therapy (root canal), and/or incision and drainage
4. **Complications:** untreated dental abscesses can spread to local soft tissues (facial cellulitis, Ludwig's angina), bone (jaw osteomyelitis), or spread hematogenously (sepsis, meningitis). Early management (IV antibiotics and dental evaluation) is essential because of potential for rapid systemic involvement.

 PEARL

A spreading odontogenic infection can lead to facial cellulitis which is a dental emergency

COMMON DENTAL PROBLEMS

A. Soft tissue lesions of the oral cavity

1. **Eruption cyst/hematoma:** soft tissue cyst often found in the posterior mandible or where a tooth is about to erupt. Color varies from coral pink to blue-black depending on extent of blood within cyst. Self-resolving lesion requires no treatment unless infected.
2. **Mucocele:** small bluish/translucent (white if longstanding) swelling caused by extravasation of mucous from a severed minor salivary gland. Usually midline of the lower lip. Sometimes on inner cheek surface, ventral tongue, and floor of mouth. May spontaneously resolve. Excision of nonresolving lesions and associated gland.
3. **Ranula:** painless swelling that occurs as a result of extravasation of mucous from a severed sublingual gland. Larger bluish/translucent swelling on the floor of the mouth lateral to the tongue. Consult for excision or marsupialization.

B. Ulcers

1. **Minor recurrent aphthous ulcers (i.e., canker sores):** cause not clear; may be genetic or related to stress, trauma, hematinic deficiency

(B12, folate, iron). Small ulcers with a red halo and yellow/grey floor. Self-limiting lesions that do not scar. Management is symptomatic, topical anesthetic mouthwash (e.g., lidocaine) may reduce discomfort.

2. **Acute herpetic gingivostomatitis (HSV-1):** self-limited manifestation of primary herpes simplex virus (HSV) infection lasting 7 to 14 days. Characterized by gingivitis (inflamed, friable gums) and stomatitis (oral and lip ulcers). Vesicles rupture leaving painful pseudomembranous lesion with adjacent erythema. Patients typically demonstrate malaise, cervical lymphadenopathy, headache, and fever during prodromal phase. Management is symptomatic: soft diet, good oral hygiene, ensure adequate hydration, and analgesia (acetaminophen, ibuprofen; morphine in severe cases). Antibiotics contraindicated. Consider antivirals in immunocompromised patients.

CONDITIONS ASSOCIATED WITH DENTAL ANOMALIES AND PERIODONTAL DISEASE

Numerous syndromes have associated dental and or craniofacial anomalies. Inherited dental anomalies may be expressed in an excess or reduced number of teeth, size or shape of teeth, or qualitative defects of the formation of tooth structure. Several systemic conditions are also associated with periodontal disease (Table 10.3).

Table 10.3	Systemic Conditions With Manifestation of Periodontal Disease
Systemic Condition	**Dental/Periodontal Features**
Hypophosphatasia	Premature loss of primary teeth
Ehler-Danlos syndrome	Premature loss of primary teeth, gingival recession, periodontal disease
Neutropenia	Fiery red gingiva, periodontal disease, increased susceptibility to oral ulcerations and infections
Leukemia	Acute oral infections, spontaneous gingival bleeding, oral mucosal petechiae, periodontal disease
Leukocyte adhesion deficiency syndrome	Premature loss of primary teeth, periodontal disease, linear gingival erythema, recurrent oral infections, oral ulcerations
Chediak-Higashi syndrome	Severe gingival inflammation, periodontal disease, oral ulceration, increased tooth mobility
Papillon-Lefèvre syndrome	Premature loss of primary teeth, periodontal disease

DENTAL CARE OF MEDICALLY COMPROMISED PATIENTS

A risk/benefit analysis should be performed before performing elective

dental care on patients who are medically compromised

A. Immunocompromised patients

1. Ideally, dental assessment and management should be performed before initiation of oncology care, immunosuppression, or organ transplantation to eliminate potentially life-threatening infection sources
2. Excellent oral hygiene is required, as is regular dental follow-up. Oral hygiene should be maintained and monitored by parents.
3. Because of expediency of oncology management, nonemergent dental care may need to be delayed until cell counts are adequate for it to be performed
4. For patients with mucositis, when use of a soft toothbrush is not possible because of bleeding, a sodium bicarbonate rinse may be used as a rinse or on damp, clean washcloth
5. Foam swabs are inferior to toothbrushes, and should only be used when toothbrush is contraindicated
6. Lines of communication should be kept open between dentistry and the physician managing the child regarding precautions and health changes

B. Cardiac patients

1. Consultation and definitive dental management (caries and periodontal) should be performed before elective cardiac surgery
2. Considerations when planning care include hemodynamic stability, anticoagulants, and specific anesthesia requirements, including the availability of the extracorporeal membrane oxygenation (ECMO) team
3. Cardiac dental patients may or may not require antibiotic prophylaxis before dental procedures, and need is dependent on cardiology guidance and endocarditis guidelines (see Chapter 8 Cardiology)

USEFUL WEBSITES

American Academy of Pediatric Dentistry: http://www.aapd.org/policies/
Canadian Dental Association: http://www.cdc-adc.ca

Dermatology

Laura Morrissey • Kimberly Tantuco • Rebecca Levy

COMMON ABBREVIATIONS

Also see page xviii for a list of other abbreviations used throughout this book

AD	atopic dermatitis
BSA	body surface area
CM	capillary malformation
CNI	calcineurin inhibitors
CS	corticosteroids
GAS	group A *streptococcus*
HSV	herpes simplex virus
KOH	potassium hydroxide
PCR	polymerase chain reaction
SJS/TEN	Stevens Johnson syndrome/toxic epidermal necrolysis
SSSS	staphylococcal scalded skin syndrome
ung	ointment
VZV	varicella zoster virus

MORPHOLOGY

1. **Macule (<1 cm in diameter) and patch (>1 cm):** A flat, nonpalpable change in the normal color of the skin
2. **Papule (<1 cm) and plaque (>1 cm):** An elevated, well-circumscribed, palpable change above the skin surface
3. **Vesicle (<1 cm) and bulla (>1 cm):** A raised, well-demarcated, fluid filled change in the skin; fluid can be clear, yellow and/or hemorrhagic
4. **Pustule:** A <1 cm in diameter lesion, raised above the skin surface filled with seropurulent fluid
5. **Nodule:** A >1 cm in diameter lesion, with deeper involvement than a plaque, extending into the deep dermis and subcutaneous tissue
6. **Purpura:** Nonblanchable erythematous to violaceous discoloration of the skin; represents extravasated blood

NEONATAL/INFANTILE ERUPTIONS

VESICULOPUSTULAR ERUPTIONS

See Table 11.1

Table 11.1	Differential Diagnosis of Infantile Vesicopustular Eruptions
Diagnosis	**Clinical Presentation**
Acropustulosis of infancy	Pustules/vesicles on palms and soles; presents/recurs birth to 3 years
Erythema toxicum neonatorum	Discrete vesicles, papules, pustules on erythematous base; spares palms and soles; new lesions up to 10 days
Infantile acne	Presents at 3–6 months; erythematous papules and pustules (primarily on face/upper chest)

Dermatology

11

Continued 235

Table 11.1	Differential Diagnosis of Infantile Vesicopustular Eruptions—cont'd
Diagnosis	**Clinical Presentation**
Infections: Bacterial Impetigo neonatorum	Flaccid, well-demarcated bullae; leaves erosions, crust, collarette of scale
Fungal Congenital candida	Usually systemically unwell; generalized erythematous papules, vesicles, pustules, erythroderma; presents on first day of life
Viral Neonatal HSV	Grouped vesicles on erythematous base
Neonatal varicella	Macules and papules evolving to vesicles that crust over; presents within 5 days of birth
Miliaria	Blockage of eccrine ducts, associated with excess heat/humidity Miliaria crystillina: 1–2 mm superficial vesicles without skin erythema Miliaria rubra ("heat rash"): small erythematous papules and pustules
Neonatal cephalic pustulosis	Formerly known as "neonatal acne"; Presents in first 4 weeks of life Generally resolves spontaneously; severe cases may require topical ketoconazole to treat Malasezzia furfur
Scabies	Papules, vesicles, pustules, burrows in axillae, neck, web spaces, palms, and soles
Sucking blister	Solitary ovoid blister or erosion on noninflamed skin
Transient neonatal pustular melanosis	Pustules that rupture and leave a collarette of scale, pigmented macules; more common in black infants; presents at birth

HSV, Herpes simplex virus.

SUBCUTANEOUS FAT NECROSIS OF THE NEWBORN (SCFN)

1. **Etiology:** Panniculitis of unknown etiology; thought to be related to hypoxia/hypothermia/trauma at birth
2. **Clinical presentation**: Onset in first few weeks of life, benign, self-limited. Erythematous plaques/nodules over cheeks, arms, trunk, buttocks, and/or legs. May be tender to palpation.
3. **Management**: Resolves spontaneously without scarring within weeks. Monitor serum calcium for up to 6 months

PEARL

Hypercalcemia is common in infants with subcutaneous fat necrosis of the newborn and may be severe and life-threatening. Serum calcium levels should be monitored for up to 6 months.

DIAPER DERMATITIS

See Table 11.2

Table 11.2 — Etiology and Management of Diaper Dermatitis

	Etiology	Clinical Presentation	Investigations	Management
Irritant contact dermatitis	Prolonged contact with urine and feces, friction	- Bright red erythema ± scale, erosions - Convex surfaces, often spares the folds	None necessary	- Decrease contact time between skin and wet diaper - Zinc oxide - Topical corticosteroids
Candidiasis	Candida albicans	- Intense erythema with desquamation/ superficial erosions; satellite pustules - Favors folds, genitalia	If diagnosis uncertain: KOH preparation, Fungal culture	Topical antifungal (e.g., clotrimazole)
Seborrheic dermatitis	- Malassezia furfur - Sebum over-production	- Well-defined pink to erythematous patches; thin plaques with flaky or greasy yellowish scales - Intertriginous areas, scalp	None necessary	- Good skin hygiene - Ketoconazole cream or - Combination of topical antifungal + corticosteroids
Bullous impetigo	Staphylococcus aureus	- Flaccid bullae, vesiculopustules, superficial erythematous erosions with collarette of scale	Gram stain and bacterial culture	Antibiotics
Acrodermatitis enteropathica	Autosomal recessive inherited disorder	- Triad of acral and periorificial skin lesions (erythematous, scaling, crusted, psoriasiform, eczematous, or vesiculobullous eruption) diarrhea and alopecia - Localized around body orifices, buttocks and extensor surface of major joints	Zinc levels (50 mcg/dL or lower)	Zinc supplementation
Langerhans cells histiocytosis	Clonal proliferative disorder	- Pink to skin colored papules, pustules, vesicles, erosions, and/or ulcers - Petechiae/purpura - Fissures in perineal area	- Skin biopsy - Check hematologic (bone marrow), pulmonary, hepatosplenic, renal, skeletal, CNS systems	For single-system skin disease: - Topical corticosteroids - Topical antimicrobials - Narrowband UVB, PUVA

CNS, Central nervous system; KOH, potassium hydroxide; PUVA, psoralen and ultraviolet A; UVB, ultraviolet B.

Dermatology

11

SEBORRHEIC DERMATITIS

1. **Clinical manifestations**
   a. Lesions: erythematous plaques with yellow greasy scales
   b. Sites: scalp, axilla, trunk, and/or flexural areas
2. **Management**
   a. Education and reassurance because it resolves spontaneously in most infants
   b. Application of gentle emollient or baby shampoo followed by careful removal of scales using a soft toothbrush or comb
   c. If extensive or resistant may try limited course of low potency topical steroid (1% hydrocortisone) or topical antifungal azole (Ketoconazole 2%)

NEONATAL/INFANTILE VASCULAR LESIONS

INFANTILE HEMANGIOMA

1. **Definition**: Benign tumor of endothelial cells
2. **Clinical manifestations**
   a. Superficial (bright red, papular), deep (bluish, nodular), and mixed
   b. Presents at birth or in weeks thereafter as macular lesion
   c. Rapid proliferation phase continues until average 6 months, then growth plateaus
   d. Subsequent slow involution over several years (complete involution in 30% by 3 years; 50% by 5 years, and 90% by 9 years)
3. **Complications:** Ulceration, functional impairment depending on location, airway involvement, aesthetic complications, and complex associations (see below)
4. **Management**
   a. **No intervention** for majority
   b. **Pharmacological treatment** indicated for functional impairment, potential poor cosmetic outcome, ulceration
      i. Topical timolol maleate 0.5% gel twice daily for superficial lesions not requiring systemic therapy
      ii. Oral beta blockers (nadolol or propranolol) for all other lesions requiring treatment
         - Contraindications include extreme prematurity, significant reactive airway disease, infants <2 kg, bradycardia/heart block, pheochromocytoma
         - Monitor vitals regularly. Discuss signs hypoglycemia.
         - Average course of treatment 1 year; continued until complete resolution or lack of effect, and then tapered slowly to prevent rebound growth
      iii. Plastic surgery or laser as needed for cutaneous residua after involution is complete
5. **Prognosis**: Majority completely resolve without complication or residua

6. **Associations**
    a. **PHACE(S) syndrome:** *P*osterior fossa brain malformations, large, segmental facial *h*emangioma, *a*rteriopathy, *c*ardiac anomalies, *e*ye abnormalities, *s*ternal defects (requires MRI/MRA of the head and neck, ophthalmology evaluation, and echocardiogram)
    b. **PELVIS syndrome:** *P*erineal hemangioma (large, segmental), *e*xternal genitalia malformations, *l*ipomyelomeningocele, *v*esicorenal abnormalities, *i*mperforate anus, *s*kin tag
    c. **Neonatal hemangiomatosis:** multiple cutaneous hemangiomas (often small; >5) associated with visceral hemangiomas (liver most common; GI tract, brain rarely). Screen all infants with >5 hemangiomas with abdominal ultrasound to look for liver hemangiomas; others (endoscopy, echo) only if symptoms; monitor thyroid function when liver lesions present (associated with hypothyroidism).

CAPILLARY MALFORMATIONS (CM)

A. Nevus simplex (salmon patch/stork bite)
1. **Epidemiology**: 40% of all newborns
2. **Clinical manifestations**: Pink/red patches with poorly defined borders; common sites include nape of neck, glabella and eyelids
3. **Investigations:** Lumbosacral lesions accompanied by other stigmata of spinal dysraphism should undergo spinal imaging (US <6 months, MRI >6 months)
4. **Prognosis**: Frequently fade or disappear by 1 to 2 years of age

B. Nevus flammeus (port-wine stain)
1. **Epidemiology:** 0.2% of newborns
2. **Clinical presentation:** Blanchable red to pink patch, often segmental/ unilateral and respecting midline. Present at birth, grows proportionately with child.
3. **Associations**
    a. Sturge-Weber syndrome in 10% of facial V1/V2 distribution (facial CM + leptomeningeal angiomatosis + eye involvement)
    b. Klippel-Trénaunay syndrome (CM + venous and lymphatic malformations + soft tissue overgrowth/ asymmetry)
    c. Macrocephaly-CM syndrome
4. **Management:** Laser improves redness and prevents nodularity/ thickening from occurring in adulthood

DERMATITIC ERUPTIONS

ATOPIC DERMATITIS (AD)
1. **Risk factors:** Family or personal history of atopy, gene mutations

2. **Clinical manifestations**
    a. **Cutaneous features:** Pruritis and dry skin are major features. Appearance and distribution otherwise dependent on age and chronicity.
        i. ≤2 years: scaly erythematous, crusted plaques to extensor surfaces, cheeks, and/or scalp. Vesicles and significant exudate may be presents. Diaper area is typically spared.
        ii. Childhood: more chronic, lichenified plaques to flexural surfaces
    b. **Aggravating factors**: Cold weather, concurrent illness, sweating, contact sensitivity and/or secondary infection
    c. **Course of disease:** Chronic illness that waxes and wanes. Many remit by adulthood, but family history of AD, persistence in childhood, more severe disease are risk factors for persistence in adulthood.
3. **Management**
    a. **Skin care**
        i. Moisturizers: minimum 2 to 3 times daily during flares and as maintenance; ointments and creams preferred to lotions and oils.
        ii. Regular bathing (5–10 minutes, lukewarm water, 1–3 × daily), with immediate application of emollient (prescribed topical medicines to active areas and moisturizers to other areas)
        iii. Cotton clothing, keep room cool, humidifier
        iv. Avoid irritants: use mild soaps, detergents; double rinse; avoid bleaches, fabric softeners, wool and/or synthetic fibers
        v. Petroleum jelly around mouth to avoid irritation from contact when eating
        vi. Lack of evidence for food triggers; avoid elimination diets because of risk of malnutrition

 PEARL

Select your vehicle for topical steroids thoughtfully. Ointment provides optimal absorption of medication. Creams and lotions may sting when applied on open skin. Lotions or oils may be useful for hairy surfaces (scalp).

    b. **Topical medicines**
        i. Topical corticosteroids (CS). See Table 11.10. Potency and vehicle dependent on age, severity and location; cover all affected areas with thin layer and treat to complete resolution; first-line option for infants and/or mild to moderate disease in childhood:
            • Face and folds: 1% hydrocortisone ointment to affected areas twice daily until clear
            • Body: 0.05% betamethasone valerate ointment to affected areas twice daily until clear

ii. Topical calcineurin inhibitors (CNI): alternative to topical steroids as steroid-sparing agents; may sting on application
- Pimecrolimus 1% cream (off-label use in <2 years) twice daily until clear (mild to moderate AD)
- Tacrolimus 0.03% (off-label use in <2 years) or 0.1% (off-label use in <17 years) ointment twice daily until clear (moderate to severe AD)

iii. Maintenance therapy: topical CS or CNI 1 to 2 times/week to areas that commonly flare during periods of remission increases duration between flares compared with moisturizing alone

c. **Adjunctive measures**
   i. Bleach baths: in patients with recurrent skin infections
   ii. Wet wraps: over petroleum jelly or mild topical CS for severe, lichenified areas
   iii. Oral antihistamines (hydroxyzine or diphenhydramine) for severe pruritis resulting in loss of sleep
   iv. Phototherapy: option for older patients with moderate to severe disease

4. **Complications**
   a. **Bacterial superinfection** (most often *Staphylococcus aureus*)
      i. Clinical presentation: weeping, oozing, honey-crusting, pustules
      ii. Treatment: topical mupirocin 2% cream twice daily for localized disease, empiric oral cephalexin for more extensive infection
   b. **Eczema herpeticum** (superinfection with HSV-1 or -2)
      i. Clinical presentation: punched-out erosions, hemorrhagic crusts, vesicles; often unwell with fever and lymphadenopathy
      ii. Investigations: swab for viral PCR and/or culture

! PITFALL

Eczema herpeticum involving the nasal tip can lead to ocular complications (i.e., herpes kerato-conjunctivitis) because of innervation by V1 branch of trigeminal nerve.

---

iii. Treatment: IV acyclovir for extensive involvement, periorbital involvement, younger patients; PO acyclovir for milder mucocutaneous involvement. Avoid topical steroids to affected areas until all lesions are crusted over.

c. **Other complications**: extensive molluscum, mental health issues, anemia of chronic disease

ALLERGIC CONTACT DERMATITIS

1. **Etiology**
   a. Delayed type hypersensitivity reaction. Allergen specific and requires prior exposure.
   b. Common allergens: urshiol (in poison ivy/oak), latex, nickel
2. **Clinical manifestations:** Erythematous, pruritic plaques ± vesicles and bullae in areas of allergen contact but may spread more diffusely
3. **Management:** Avoid contact allergen. Antihistamines for itch. Topical CS or CNI. Two-week course of systemic steroids with slow taper for more extensive cases with blistering involvement (often required for poison ivy/oak).

PAPULOSQUAMOUS ERUPTIONS

PSORIASIS

1. **Clinical presentation**
   a. Lesions: well-demarcated erythematous plaques with adherent silvery scale ± itch + Koebner phenomenon (the appearance of skin lesions in areas of trauma)
   b. Distribution: extensor surfaces, scalp, umbilicus, flexures/folds (inverse psoriasis); nail involvement (variants include palmar-plantar, pustular, guttate [may follow GAS infection])

> **! PITFALL**
>
> Psoriasis can be confused with other papulosquamous skin conditions, including eczematous dermatitis, seborrheic dermatitis, tinea corporis, and pityriasis rosea.

2. **Management**
   a. **Comorbidity screening:** Per American Academy of Pediatrics guidelines, for associated obesity, diabetes, dyslipidemia, hypertension, nonalcoholic fatty liver, polycystic ovary syndrome, inflammatory bowel disease (IBD), arthritis, mood disorders
   b. **Topical CS**
      i. low potency (i.e., desonide ung twice daily) for face and folds; mid- to high-potency (i.e., betamethasone valerate 0.1% ung twice daily) for body
      ii. Incorporate topical vitamin D analog (calcipotriene twice daily or mixed with potent CS [Dovobet])
      iii. May add keratolytics (CS compounded with 6% salicylic acid)
      iv. For scalp: tar shampoo and fluocinolone acetonide oil daily

c. **Topical CNI**: useful as steroid-sparing agent, for face/folds (tacrolimus 0.1% ung twice daily to affected areas)

d. **Phototherapy**

e. **Systemic agents**
   i. No systemic CS (cause erythroderma on withdrawal)
   ii. Methotrexate, cyclosporine, retinoids (acitretin), biologics (ustekinumab)
   iii. Guttate psoriasis: throat/perianal swab for *Streptococcus*, treat appropriately

ACNE VULGARIS

1. **Pathogenesis**: Follicular hyperkeratinization, increased sebum production, inflammation, *Cutibacterium acnes (*formerly *Propionibacterium acnes)* growth

2. **Clinical manifestations**
   a. Noninflammatory: open and closed comedones
   b. Inflammatory: papules, pustules, nodules
   c. Postinflammatory erythema and hyperpigmentation
   d. Scarring with nodulocystic lesions
   e. Location: predominantly located on the face may involve the upper chest and back

3. **Investigations**
   a. Usually not indicated unless clinical signs of hyperandrogenism
   b. All acne presenting between 1 and 6 years of age requires bloodwork (total and free testosterone, DHEAS, 17-hydroxyprogesterone), bone age, endocrinology referral

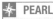 **PEARL**

Female patients with acne and oligomenorrhea should undergo work-up for polycystic ovary syndrome.

4. **Management:** Depends on primary morphology, severity, clinician experience and patient preference. Combination therapy often preferred (Table 11.3).
   a. **Topical retinoids**: tretinoin, adapalene, tazarotene
   b. **Topical antimicrobials**: erythromycin/clindamycin (not recommended as monotherapy), dapsone, benzoyl peroxide
   c. **Oral antibiotics**: tetracycline/doxycycline/minocycline (not recommend for use under the age of 8 years old), alternatives are azithromycin, trimethoprim-sulfamethoxazole

d. **Oral isotretinoin**: 0.5 mg/kg/day × 1 month, then 1 mg/kg/day. Continue until cumulative dose between 120 and 150 mg/kg
   i. Tests needed before initiation and monthly: LFTs, urinalysis, CBC, cholesterol, triglycerides, β-HCG
   ii. Highly teratogenic, avoid conception during and 1 month posttreatment; need two forms of contraception during active treatment
   iii. Side effects: cheilitis, xerostomia, xerophthalmia, conjunctivitis, myalgia, headache, teratogenicity, hepatitis, hypercholesterolemia, hypertriglyceridemia, pseudotumor cerebri, exacerbation of IBD flares, premature epiphyseal closure, depression
e. **Hormonal therapy**: oral contraceptive pill, spironolactone
5. **Complications:** Permanent scarring, mental health issues

Table 11.3	First-Line Treatment for Acne	
Mild Comedonal or Inflammatory	**Moderate**	**Severe (Scarring/Nodulocystic)**
Topical retinoid[a] **OR** Benzoyl peroxide (BP)[b] **OR** Topical combination[c]	Topical combination[c] with or without systemic antibiotics[d] **OR** Oral contraceptive (females)	Oral isotretinoin

[a]Example: adapalene 0.1% gel QHS.
[b]Example: benzoyl peroxide 5% gel daily.
[c]Options include topical retinoid + BP, topical clindamycin + BP, or topical retinoid + clindamycin + BP.
[d]Example: doxycycline 100 mg PO daily-BID × 3–4 months.

CUTANEOUS BACTERIAL INFECTIONS

See Table 11.4. Also see Chapter 24 Infectious Disease

> **PEARL**
>
> Impetigo presents with yellow-gold or "honey" crusts.

Table 11.4	Cutaneous Bacterial Infections		
Diagnosis	**Clinical Features**	**Investigations**	**Management**
Cellulitis	- Infection of dermis and subcutaneous tissue - Poorly demarcated erythema, warmth, induration ± tenderness, fever - *Streptococcus pyogenes* and S*taphylococcus aureus* most common		Oral cephalexin or IV cefazolin depending on severity
Impetigo	- Superficial infection - Erythematous papules, vesicles, pustules with thick honey-crusting - Bullous variant involves progression to large, flaccid bullae that may rupture - *S. aureus* or *S. pyogenes* are most common	Swab for C&S if diagnosis uncertain	- Topical antibiotics if mild/focal (e.g., mupirocin ointment) - If more severe or extensive, then PO antistaphylococcal coverage (e.g., cephalexin, cloxacillin) - IV antibiotics if systemically unwell
Staphylococcal scalded skin syndrome	- *S. aureus* exfoliative toxin causes skin exfoliation at granular layer - Tender erythematous eruption of central face, neck, axillae, groin, torso, followed by flaccid bullae, generalized desquamation; typically, spares conjunctivae and mucous membranes	Swab potential foci of infection (nares, conjunctivae, umbilicus (neonates), throat and perianal), collect blood culture. Swabs of bullae are sterile!	- Usually benign self-limited course - Minimize handling. - Petroleum jelly to affected skin ± nonstick gauze - IV cefazolin OR cloxacillin. Complete 7–10 days course with PO cephalexin after clinical improvement and no new lesions
Toxic shock syndrome	- Acute, toxin-mediated illness caused by *S. aureus* or *S. pyogenes* - Extensive macular erythema/ erythroderma involving mucous membranes, fever, hypotension, multiorgan involvement; late desquamation (particularly palms and soles) ± hair loss and nail shedding	Laboratory testing reflective of shock and organ dysfunction. Skin swabs positive in majority of cases, rarely positive blood culture	- 3%–5% mortality - Supportive care, including hemodynamic support. - Empiric IV ceftriaxone PLUS vancomycin PLUS Clindamycin (anti-toxin effect) - Consider IVIG

C&S, Culture and susceptibility; *IV*, intravenous; *IVIG*, intravenous immunoglobulin; *PO*, by mouth.

Also see Table 11.5 for childhood exanthems

HSV MUCOCUTANEOUS INFECTIONS

Also see Chapter 10 Dentistry (herpetic gingivostomatitis) and Chapter 24 Infectious Diseases

1. **Etiology:** HSV-1 and -2
2. **Clinical manifestations:** Primary eruption (most severe) followed by recurrences at same site
   a. **Herpes labialis**
      i. Pain, burning, tingling or itchiness, may precede eruption
      ii. Grouped vesicles on an erythematous base → pustules → erosions and crusts with scalloped border involving mouth and lips
      iii. Heals within 2 to 6 weeks
   b. **Herpetic whitlow**: grouped vesicles, pustules, erosions, crusts and paronychia involving the digits
3. **Investigations:** Tzanck smear from early lesion (multinucleated giant cells); swab for viral culture and PCR; bacterial culture to rule out alternative diagnoses/secondary bacterial infection
4. **Management:** Antivirals initiated within 24 to 48 hours of eruption onset reduce viral shedding and shortens duration
   a. Topical acyclovir 5% 4 times daily × 7 days may hasten resolution
   b. Oral acyclovir or valacyclovir
   c. Chronic suppressive therapy may be considered for frequent recurrences

MOLLUSCUM CONTAGIOSUM

1. **Etiology:** Poxvirus
2. **Clinical manifestations**: Flesh-colored, dome-shaped umbilicated papules
3. **Management:** Spontaneous regression after 2 years; majority require no treatment. Options for extensive disease or significant distress: cantharidin, podophyllin, cryotherapy, and/or curettage

VERRUCAE (WARTS)

1. **Etiology**: HPV (human papilloma virus)
2. **Epidemiology**: Vertical transmission (i.e., contracted from mother with genital warts) possible up to 5 years of age. Infection via direct skin contact (during diapering)
3. **Clinical manifestations:** Vulgaris (anywhere on body), plantar (palms and soles), accuminata (genitals), and flat (sites of trauma, face, or extremities)

4. **Management**
    1. Vulgaris and plantar: 60% salicylic acid under duct tape for 1 week, debride and continue with weaker over-the-counter preparations. Cryotherapy in older children/adolescents.
    2. Accuminata: topical Veregen twice daily or imiquimod 5 times per week until resolution. Consider child abuse if >5 years, lack of household contact with warts, or risk factors present.

HAND, FOOT, AND MOUTH (HFM) DISEASE

1. **Etiology**: Coxsackievirus. Fecal-oral route of transmission
2. **Clinical manifestations**
    a. Classic HFM: Fever, diarrhea, oral vesicles/ulcers and erythematous macular or papulovesicular rash to palms, soles and groin/buttocks
    b. Atypical HFM: Coxsackievirus A6. More severe skin involvement than classical HFM (papular, vesiculobullous and/or erosive lesions that extend beyond the palms and soles; can be accompanied by petechial and purpuric eruption; may favor sites of skin trauma, i.e., eczema).

 PEARL

Onychomadesis (shedding of the nails) may occur 1–2 months after infection with coxsackievirus infection. Nails regrow normally thereafter.

---

3. **Investigations**: Rule out HSV as needed, swab for C&S if suspicion for secondary bacterial infection, can do stool enterovirus PCR if diarrhea (but not necessary in most cases)
4. **Management:** Supportive

CHILDHOOD EXANTHEMS

See Table 11.5

 PITFALL

Varicella is highly contagious and is transmitted via direct contact or aerosolized droplets of nasopharyngeal secretions. Airborne precautions are indicated when infection is suspected.

Dermatology

11

Table 11.5	Classic Childhood Exanthems					
Diagnosis	**Infectious Agent**	**Incubation Period**	**Rash Appearance**	**Other Features**	**Investigations**	**Management**	**Complications**
Measles	Measles virus	10–14 days	Erythematous macules and papules that first appear on head/face and spreads cephalocaudally and fade after 5 days in order of appearance	- Prodrome: Fever, cough, coryza, conjunctivitis - Koplik spots (gray-white papules on the buccal mucosa) during prodrome	Serology (IgM, IgG), PCR for virus isolation (throat or nasopharyngeal swabs, blood, urine)	WHO recommends Vitamin A (once daily for 2 days) to decrease morbidity and mortality	Measles-associated immunosuppression, diarrhea, pneumonia, acute disseminating encephalomyelitis, subacute sclerosing panencephalitis (7–10 years later)
Rubella	Rubella virus	16–18 days	Erythematous macules and papules that begin on the face, spreading cephalocaudally and fade after 2–3 days in order of appearance	- Prodrome: fever, headache, upper respiratory symptoms - Forchheimer spots: petechial macules on the soft palate	Serology (IgG, IgM) and PCR (throat or nasopharyngeal swabs preferred; blood and urine also possible)	Supportive	- Arthralgia and arthritis - Rarely: hepatitis, myocarditis, pericarditis, hemolytic anemia and thrombocytopenia, encephalitis

| Erythema infectiosum (Fifth Disease) | Human parvovirus B19 | 4–14 days | - Erythematous macules on the cheeks, spares the nasal bridge and perioral area ("slapped cheek")
- Second stage occurs 1–4 days later: erythematous macules and papules in lacy reticular pattern on the trunk and limbs for 1–3 weeks, may wax and wane
- Papular purpuric gloves and socks syndrome: petechial and purpuric eruption on acral sites and flexures | Prodrome occurs 7–10 days before exanthem appears: low-grade fever, myalgia, headache | PCR testing for parvovirus B19 (preferred test); Serum serology (IgM, IgG) | Supportive | Transient aplastic crises, thrombocytopenia, neutropenia, and pancytopenia; fetal hydrops |
| Roseola infantum | HHV6, HHV7 | 9–10 days | Exanthem appears after fever resolution: rose-pink macules and papules on the neck, trunk, proximal extremities and occasionally the face | - Prodrome: High fever occurs for 3–5 days
- Nagayama spots: red papules on the soft palate and uvula
- Characteristic finding: uvular and palatoglossal junctional ulcers | HHV-6 PCR (*NOT* routinely needed) | Supportive care | Febrile seizures common |

Continued

250

Table 11.5 Classic Childhood Exanthems—cont'd

Diagnosis	Infectious Agent	Incubation Period	Rash Appearance	Other Features	Investigations	Management	Complications
Scarlet fever	GAS	1–7 days	- Red, finely textured sandpaper rash. Spreads from face to rest of body. - Perioral pallor, strawberry tongue - Pastia's lines in antecubital and axillary folds	- Fever - Sore throat - Headache - Nausea - Vomiting	Throat swab for GAS	- Antibiotic treatment of GAS if throat swab positive - Supportive care	- Rheumatic fever (very rare) - Arthritis - Poststreptococcal glomerulonephritis
Varicella (chickenpox)	Varicella zoster virus	10–21 days	Crops of pruritic macules, papules, and vesicles that leave crusts and erosions after rupture. Lesions present at various stages concurrently	Prodrome of fever, malaise	Viral PCR for VZV from vesicles and/or blood	- Supportive for healthy patients. IV antivirals for immunocompromised. - Prevention with vaccine and/or VZIG for exposed at-risk patients (See Chapter 23 Immunoprophylaxis)	Increased risk of invasive group A streptococcal infections, encephalitis, Reye syndrome, pneumonia, hepatitis

GAS, Group A streptococcus; HHV, human herpesvirus; Ig, immunoglobulin; PCR, polymerase chain reaction; VZV, varicella zoster virus; VZIG, varicella zoster immune globulin; WHO, World Health Organization.

FUNGAL ERUPTIONS

See Table 11.6

Table 11.6	Tinea Capitis Versus Corporis	
	Tinea Capitis (Head)	**Tinea Corporis (Body)**
Etiology	- *Trichophyton tonsurans* or *Microsporum canis*	- *M. canis, T. mentagrophytes, T. tonsurans, T. rubrum*
Clinical features	- 5 Clinical patterns: diffuse scaling, circumscribed alopecia with scale, black dot (broken hairs), kerion (boggy mass), pustular	- Pruritic annular scaly plaques with active border and central clearing
Management	- Scraping for KOH and fungal culture - Systemic treatment only! Terbinafine PO for 4–6 weeks (<20 kg, 62.5 mg daily; 20–40 kg, 125 mg daily; >40 kg, 250 mg daily)	- Scraping for KOH and fungal culture - Systemic treatment rarely needed - Topical terbinafine, ciclopirox, clotrimazole, ketoconazole all efficacious applied BID - Resolution may take up to 4 weeks

BID, Twice daily; *KOH*, potassium hydroxide.

INFESTATIONS

See Table 11.7

Table 11.7	Cutaneous Infestations	
Diagnosis	**Clinical Features**	**Treatment**
Scabies	- *Sarcoptes scabiei* var. *hominis* mite - Intensely pruritic papules/burrows, nodules, dermatitis - Favors abdomen, dorsa of hands, web spaces, genitalia, skin folds	- Treat all household contacts - 5% permethrin cream/lotion, from neck down (include head in infants) for 8–14 h then wash off; repeat after 7 days - Wash bedding/clothing in hot water - Treat pruritus with antihistamines, topical mid-potency corticosteroid if needed
Pediculosis (lice)	- Pediculosis louse 3–4 mm long and mobile; eggs 1 mm long and firmly adherent to hair shaft - Can be capitis (*Pediculus capitis*), or pubis (*Pthrius pubis*; crab louse)	- Wash and towel-dry hair; apply permethrin 1% for 10 min and rinse; repeat in 7 days - Vinegar-and-water (1:1) soaks and fine-tooth comb - If eyelash involvement, apply petroleum jelly BID to TID for 10 days - Soak combs, hair accessories in permethrin shampoo or boil for 10 min; wash clothing/bedding in hot water

> **! PITFALL**
>
> Persistent pruritis after treatment does not necessarily indicate treatment failure; postscabetic pruritis may persist for up to 4 weeks and can be managed with topical corticosteroids.

ALOPECIA

See Figure 11.1 for general approach to hair loss

Figure 11.1 Approach to Nonscarring Hair Loss

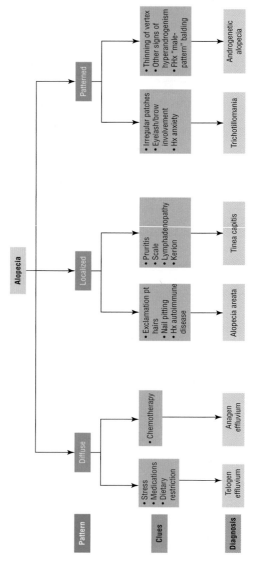

Pattern					

Alopecia

Diffuse → Localized → Patterned

Clues

- Stress
- Medications
- Dietary restriction

- Chemotherapy

- Exclamation pt hairs
- Nail pitting
- Hx autoimmune disease

- Pruritis
- Scale
- Lymphadenopathy
- Kerion

- Irregular patches
- Eyelash/brow involvement
- Hx anxiety

- Thinning of vertex
- Other signs of hyperandrogenism
- FHx "male-pattern" balding

Diagnosis

- Telogen effluvium
- Anagen effluvium
- Alopecia areata
- Tinea capitis
- Trichotillomania
- Androgenetic alopecia

ACUTE BLISTERING REACTIONS

See Box 11.1 and Table 11.8

> ### Box 11.1 Differential Diagnosis of Most Common Acute Bullous Eruptions
>
> - Stevens Johnson syndrome/toxic epidermal necrolysis
> - Mycoplasma-induced rash and mucositis
> - Erythema multiforme
> - Bullous impetigo/staphylococcal scalded skin syndrome
> - Autoimmune blistering diseases (linear immunoglobulin A/chronic bullous dermatosis of childhood; pemphigus; pemphigoid; bullous cutaneous lupus)
> - Dermatitis herpetiformis
> - Bullous fixed drug eruption
> - Friction blisters
> - Burns

Table 11.8	Comparison of Erythema Multiforme, Mycoplasma-Induced Rash and Mucositis, Stevens-Johnson Syndrome, and Toxic Epidermal Necrolysis		
	Erythema Multiforme (EM)	**Mycoplasma-Induced Rash and Mucositis (MIRM)**	**Stevens-Johnson Syndrome (SJS) and Toxic Epidermal Necrolysis (TEN)**
Etiology	HSV, *Mycoplasma pneumoniae*, drugs	*Mycoplasma pneumoniae*	Drugs: NSAIDs, antibiotics, anticonvulsants
Prodrome	May have preceding herpes labialis	Fever, cough precede mucosal and skin eruption	Fever, skin tenderness precedes the skin eruption by 1–3 days

Clinical features	- Typical target lesion: three distinct concentric zones with dusky erythematous center
	- Typically develops over the extremities (upper > lower), face, and/or trunk.
	- *EM minor:* mild to no mucosal symptoms, limited systemic symptoms
	- *EM major:* severe mucosal involvement, fever, malaise, arthralgias
		- Prominent mucositis (≥2 mucosal sites involved), most often eyes and mouth
		- Variable cutaneous involvement; vesiculobullous, targetoid or morbiliform
			- Tender erythematous, dusky, purpuric patches → flaccid bullae → erosions → desquamated plaques
			- Extent of skin detachment:
			  - SJS: 10% BSA
			  - SJS-TEN overlap: 10%–30% BSA
			  - TEN: >30% BSA
			- ≥2 mucosal surfaces (oral, ocular, genital)
			- Systemic manifestations: fever, lymphadenopathy, hepatitis, cytopenia and cholestasis

Clinical course	Appears within 24–72 h and usually clears within 1–2 weeks. Recurrences possible	Skin lesions heal without sequelae, complete resolution within 2 weeks	Rapid progression of disease; higher mortality

Continued

	Table 11.8	Comparison of Erythema Multiforme, Mycoplasma-Induced Rash and Mucositis, Stevens-Johnson Syndrome, and Toxic Epidermal Necrolysis—cont'd	
	Erythema Multiforme (EM)	**Mycoplasma-Induced Rash and Mucositis (MIRM)**	**Stevens-Johnson Syndrome (SJS) and Toxic Epidermal Necrolysis (TEN)**
Management	- Antiseptic/local anesthetic solutions for oral lesions - Antihistamines or topical CS for itch - Antivirals if confirmed HSV infection - Consider oral steroids for severe/extensive disease - Ophthalmology if ocular involvement	- Antiseptic/local anesthetic solutions for oral lesions - Antihistamines for itch - Treat underlying mycoplasma infection to prevent other complications but does not alter course of cutaneous disease - Ophthalmology if ocular involvement	- ICU or burn unit admission for supportive care (infection, fluid and electrolyte instability, respiratory distress, multiorgan failure) - Early identification and withdrawal of offending drug - Early involvement of dermatology, ophthalmology and urology/gynecology - Potential systemic agents: IVIG, cyclosporine, systemic steroids, TNF-α inhibitors

BSA, Body surface area; *CS,* corticosteroids; *HSV,* Herpes simplex virus; *ICU,* intensive care unit; *IVIG,* intravenous immunoglobulin; *NSAID,* nonsteroidal antiinflammatory drug; *TNF,* tumor necrosis factor.

GENODERMATOSES (GENETIC SKIN CONDITIONS)

See Table 11.9

Table 11.9	Most Common Neurocutaneous Syndromes		
	Neurofibromatosis (NF1 and NF2)	**Tuberous Sclerosis**	**Sturge-Weber Syndrome**
Inheritance	Autosomal dominant (high rate of de novo mutations)	Autosomal dominant (high rate of de novo mutations)	Sporadic
Cutaneous findings	NF1: - Cafe au lait macules (>5 mm before puberty, >15 mm after puberty) - Freckling (axilla and groin) - Neurofibromas (cutaneous, subcutaneous, plexiform) NF2: - Cutaneous and subcutaneous tumors, skin plaques	- Hypomelanotic macules (≥5 mm, "ash-leaf spots") - Angiofibromas - Periungual fibromas - Fibrous plaque of forehead - Shagreen patch - "Confetti" skin lesions - Dental enamel pits	Segmental facial capillary malformation/ port wine stain
Other findings	NF1: - Lisch nodules (iris hamartomas), macrocephaly, learning disabilities, seizures, sphenoid sysplasia, pseudoarthrosis and bone dysplasia, scoliosis, congenital heart disease, hypertension NF2: - Cataracts, retinal hamartomas	Seizures/infantile spasms, developmental delay, cortical dysplasia, retinal hamartomas	Ipsilateral lepto-meningeal angioma, seizures, glaucoma, hemiparesis and hemihypertrophy, intracranial AVM, developmental delay
Tumors	NF1: - Peripheral neurofibromas (cutaneous, plexiform, nodular), optic gliomas, malignant peripheral nerve sheath tumors, astrocytomas, pheochromocytoma, leukemia, gastrointestinal stromal tumor, rhabdomyosarcoma NF2: - Schwannomas (vestibular, other cranial, peripheral nerve), neurofibromas, cranial/spinal meningiomas, gliomas, spinal cord ependymomas	SEGA, glioneuronal hamartomas (cortical tubers), subependymal nodules, cardiac rhabdomyomas, renal angiomyolipomas, lymphangioleiomyomatosis	

AVM, Arteriovenous malformation; *NF*, neurofibromatosis; *SEGA*, subependymal giant astrocytoma.

EPIDERMOLYSIS BULLOSA (EB)

⭐ PEARL

Always consider epidermolysis bullosa on the differential of congenital blistering. Note that severity of disease in the newborn is not reflective of overall subtype or long-term prognosis.

1. **Definition:** Group of heterogeneous mechanobullous diseases characterized by extreme skin fragility; usually present at birth or in infancy

2. **Severity:** Ranges from more benign, nonscarring (EB simplex), to more severe scarring with multisystem involvement, which is often fatal (junctional ED, dystrophic EB)

3. **Management:** Multidisciplinary support, including education, symptomatic management, support; special attention to temperature control, airway involvement, nutrition, fluid balance, secondary infections, functional impairments

TOPICAL STEROIDS

1. **Potency**
   a. See Table 11.10 for topical CS potencies

Table 11.10	Classes of Topical Corticosteroids
Class/Group	**Representative Examples**
Super-high potency/group 1	clobetasol propionate 0.05% ung
High potency/group 2	fluocinonide 0.05% ung
High potency/group 3	betamethasone valerate 0.1% ung mometasone furoate 0.1% ung
Medium potency/group 4	hydrocortisone valerate 0.2% ung mometasone furoate 0.1% cream
Lower-mid potency/group 5	betamethasone valerate 0.05% ung hydrocortisone valerate 0.2% cream
Low potency/group 6	desonide cream
Least potent/group 7	hydrocortisone 1% ung

ung, Ointment.

2. **Side effects:** Increase with potency and duration; atrophy, striae, hypertrichosis, perioral dermatitis, delayed wound healing, exacerbation of skin infections

3. **Vehicle**
   a. Ointment most potent, greasy, and hydrating; use on thick dry skin, avoid on hairy areas or face
   b. Creams less potent than ointment, can be used on face, may sting on open skin
   c. Lotions, oils and gels more drying, much less potent, good for scalp

4. **Quantity**
   a. Fingertip unit (FTU) used to estimate quantity required
   b. One FTU = amount of cream squeezed out of tube onto tip of index finger (from DIP to distal aspect) = ~0.5 g
   c. One FTU treats the size of 1 palm (i.e., for isolated bilateral hand involvement = 2 FTU × BID = 4 FTU/day × 30 days = 120 FTU/month = 60 g for 1 month)

FURTHER READING

Darrow DH, Greene AK, Mancini AJ, Nopper AJ. Diagnosis and management of infantile hemangioma. *Pediatrics*. 2015;136(4):e1060–e1104.

Eichenfield LF, Krakowski AC, Piggott C, et al. Evidence-based recommendations for the diagnosis and treatment of pediatric acne. *Pediatrics*. 2013;131(suppl 3):S163–S186.

Eichenfield LF, Boguniewicz M, Simpson EL, et al. Translating atopic dermatitis management guidelines into practice for primary care providers. *Pediatrics*. 2015;136(3):554–565.

Paller AS, Mancini AJ. *Hurwitz Clinical Pediatric Dermatology*. 5th ed. Philadelphia, PA: Elsevier; 2016.

USEFUL WEBSITES

Dermnet New Zealand, dermnetnz.org
Eczema Society of Canada, eczemahelp.ca

Dermatology

11

Development

Audrey Tilly-Gratton • Claire Nguyen • Jenna Doig • Amber Makino

COMMON ABBREVIATIONS

Also see page xviii for a list of other abbreviations used throughout this book

ABA	applied behavior analysis
ADHD	attention deficit/hyperactivity disorder
ADOS	autism diagnostic observation schedule
ASD	autism spectrum disorder
CO-OP	cognitive orientation to daily occupational performance
CP	cerebral palsy
DSM-V	*Diagnostic and Statistical Manual of Mental Disorders,* 5th Edition
EDI	early developmental impairment
GMFCS	gross motor function classification system
ID	intellectual disability
IEM	inborn error of metabolism
IEP	individual education plan
PECS	picture exchange communication system
REM	rapid eye movement

NORMAL PATTERNS OF DEVELOPMENT

1. **Developmental domains**
   a. **Gross motor:** movements using the large muscles
   b. **Fine motor:** movements using the hands and smaller muscles, often involving self-help skills
   c. **Communication:** receptive and expressive language, speech, nonverbal communication
   d. **Cognitive:** reasoning, memory, problem-solving skills
   e. **Social-emotional and behavioral:** attachment, self-regulation, interaction with others
2. **Developmental milestones:** see Table 12.1 for average developmental milestones from birth to 5 years

Development

12

Table 12.1 Emerging Developmental Milestones From Birth to 5 Years

Age	Gross Motor	Fine Motor	Social	Language and Communication	Self-Help
Birth	Kicks legs and thrashes arms; Moro, stepping, placing and grasp reflexes present	Looks at objects or faces	Responds positively to feeding and comforting	Cries; startled by loud sudden sounds	Alert: interested in sights and sounds
1 month	Raises head and chest when lying on stomach	Follows moving objects with eyes	Social smile; becomes active when sees human face	Cries in distinct way when hungry	Sucks well; responds to voices: turns head toward voice
2 months	Ventral suspension: head sustained in plane of body; pull to sitting: head lags; holds head steady when held sitting	Holds objects put in hand; hand regard; follows moving object 180 degrees	Recognizes mother/primary caregiver; listens to voice and coos	Makes sounds: "ah," "eh," "ugh"; laughs	Reacts to sight of bottle or breast
3 months	Ventral suspension: lifts head and chest, arms extended; tonic neck posture predominant; pull to sitting: head lag partially compensated; early head control with bobbing motion; back rounded	Shakes rattle; reaches toward and misses objects; waves at toy	Recognizes most familiar adults	Says "ahh," "ngah"	Increases activity when shown toy
4 months	Turns around when lying on stomach; in prone position, lifts head and chest—head in approximate vertical axis, legs extended; pull to sitting: no head lag; head steady, held forward; sitting with full truncal support; when held in standing/erect position, pushes with feet	Puts toys or other objects in mouth	Interested in own image in mirror—smiles, playful; laughs out loud; may show displeasure if social contact is broken; excited at sight of food	Squeals, "ah-goo" sounds	Reaches for larger objects; sees small objects but makes no move to them
5 months	Rolls from stomach to back	Picks up objects with one hand	Reacts differently to strangers (stranger anxiety)	Makes razzing sounds—gives "raspberries"	

6 months	Rolls from back to stomach	Transfers objects from one hand to another	Reaches for familiar persons	Babbles; turns to own name	Looks for object after it disappears from sight
7 months	Sits without support; may support most of weight when standing; bounces actively	Holds two objects (one in each hand) at same time; grasps using radial palm; rakes at small object	Gets upset and afraid if left alone	Makes sounds, such as "da," "ba," "ga," "ka," "ma"	Anticipates being lifted by raising arms
8 months	Crawls on hands and knees	Uses forefinger to poke, push, or roll small objects	Plays "peek-a-boo"	Makes sounds like "ma-ma," "da-da," "ba-ba" (two-syllable babbling)	Feeds self cracker or cookie
9 months	Pulls self to standing position	Picks up small objects using only finger and thumb (pincer grasp)	Resists having toy taken away	Imitates speech sounds	
10 months	Sidesteps/walks around furniture while holding on	Picks up two small objects in one hand	Plays "pat-a-cake"		
11 months	Stands alone well	Puts small objects in cup or other container	Shows or offers toy to adult	Uses "Mama" or "Dada" specifically for parent	Picks up spoon by handle
12 months	Climbs up on chairs or other furniture; walks with one hand held; "cruises"	Turns pages of books a few at a time	Imitates simple acts, such as hugging or loving doll; plays simple ball game; makes postural adjustment to dressing	Says one word clearly; points in response to word	Removes socks
13 months	Walks without help	Builds tower of two or more blocks	Plays with other children	Shakes head to express "no"; hands object to you when asked	Lifts cup to mouth and drinks

Continued

Development

12

Table 12.1 Emerging Developmental Milestones From Birth to 5 Years—cont'd

Age	Gross Motor	Fine Motor	Social	Language and Communication	Self-Help
14 months	Stoops and recovers	Marks with pencil or crayon	Gives kisses	Asks for food or drink with sounds or words	Insists on feeding self
15 months	Runs	Scribbles with pencil or crayon	Greets people with "hi" or similar; hugs parents	Says two words besides "Mama" or "Dada"; makes sounds in sequences that sound like sentences	Feeds self with spoon
18 months	Sits on small chair; walks upstairs with one hand held; kicks a ball—good balance and coordination; moves toys into and out of container	Builds tower of four or more cubes; imitates vertical strokes; dumps small object from bottle	Sometimes says "no" when interfered with; kisses parent with puckering of lips; exhibits shared attention (points to share interesting observation with another)	Uses five or more words as names of things (i.e., water, cookie, clock); follows a few simple instructions; understands phrases such as "Give me that" when gestures are used; recognizes names of common objects; identifies one or more parts of body	Feeds self; eats with a fork; seeks help when in trouble; may complain when wet or soiled; knows use of toothbrush and comb
24 months	Runs well; walks up and down stairs, one step at a time; opens doors; climbs on furniture; throws and kicks ball	Builds tower of six cubes; performs circular scribbling; imitates horizontal stroke; folds paper once imitatively	Tells immediate experiences; listens to stories with pictures	Puts two to three words together; knows "I"; points to appropriate picture when someone says "Show me the dog"; has expressive vocabulary of 50–250 words	Handles spoon well; helps to undress

30 months	Jumps	Builds tower of eight cubes; makes horizontal and vertical strokes but generally will not join them to make a cross; imitates circular stroke, forming closed figure	Pretends in play	Refers to self by pronoun "I"; knows full name	Helps put things away
36 months	Goes up stairs alternating feet; rides tricycle; stands momentarily on one foot	Builds tower of nine cubes; imitates construction of "bridge" of three cubes; copies circle; imitates cross	Plays simple games (in "parallel" with other children)	Knows age and sex; counts three objects correctly; repeats three numbers or sentence of six syllables; expressive vocabulary of over 1000 words; remembers some recent past events	Toilet trained; helps in dressing (unbuttons clothing, puts on shoes); washes hands
48 months	Hops on one foot; throws ball overhand; uses scissors to cut out pictures; climbs well	Imitates construction of "gate" of five cubes; copies cross and square; draws person with two or four parts besides head; can name longer of two lines	Plays with several children—beginning of social interaction and role-playing	Counts four pennies accurately; tells story; asks many questions; uses four- to five-word sentences; uses plurals; can repeat three or four numbers; knows four colors	Uses toilet alone
60 months	Skips	Copies triangle; can name heavier of two weights	Asks questions about meaning of words; participates in domestic role-playing	Repeats sentence of 10 syllables; counts 10 pennies correctly; follows three-part instructions; can name penny, nickel, and dime; uses pronouns properly	Dresses and undresses

Modified from Parker S, Zuckerman B, eds. *Behavioural and Developmental Pediatrics: A Handbook for Primary Care*. Boston, MA: Little, Brown; 1995:420–421.

DEVELOPMENTAL RED FLAGS

See Table 12.2

Table 12.2	Developmental Red Flags		
Time Period	**Language/ Cognitive**	**Gross Motor, Fine Motor, and Self Care**	**Social-Emotional**
Neonatal period	Infant does not respond to loud sounds	Muscle tone too low to feed	Caregiver shows indifference or disinterest in infant
6 months	Not starting to coo, does not turn towards voices	Not holding head and shoulders up with good control when lying on tummy, not holding head with control in supported sitting, does not bring hands together at midline	Does not smile, laugh or interact with people
9 months	Lack of babbling with consonants	Not rolling, not sitting independently/without support, does not pass object from one hand to another	Not sharing enjoyment with others using eye contact or facial expression
12 months	No babbled phrases that sound like talking, no response to familiar words (e.g., bottle, daddy)	No form of independent mobility (e.g., crawling, commando crawling, bottom shuffle), not pulling to stand independently and holding on for support, does not feed self finger foods or hold own bottle/cup, unable to pick up small items using index finger and thumb	Does not notice someone new, does not play early turn-taking games
18 months	No clear words, not able to understand short requests (e.g., "Where is the ball?")	Not standing independently, not attempting to walk without support	Lacks interest in playing and interacting with others, absence of pointing to show interest or showing gestures
2 years	Lack of words and not putting words together, inability to follow simple commands.	Not able to walk well, does not attempt to feed self using a spoon and/or help with dressing	Does not imitate actions or words of caregivers, tends to bang, throw or drop toys rather than use toys for their purpose
3 years	Speech difficult for familiar people to understand, not using simple sentences (e.g., "Big car go")	Not able to walk up and down stairs independently, not able to run or jump, does not attempt everyday self-care skills (such as feeding or dressing)	No interest in pretend play or interacting with other children, difficulty noticing and understanding feelings in themselves and others
4 years	Speech difficult to understand, does not answer simple questions, not able to follow directions with two steps	Not toilet trained by day, not able to draw lines and circles, not able to walk, run, climb, jump and use stairs confidently, not able to catch, throw or kick a ball	Unwilling or unable to play cooperatively

Table 12.2   Developmental Red Flags—cont'd

Time Period	Language/ Cognitive	Gross Motor, Fine Motor, and Self Care	Social-Emotional
5 years	Not able to answer questions in a simple conversation, inability to recognize shapes, letters, colors	Poor balance, concerns from teacher about school readiness	Play is different than their friends, unusually fearful, sad, shy, angry
Any age	Loss of previously acquired skill Low tone or high tone impacting on development and functional motor skills Lack of response to sound or visual stimuli Differences between right and left sides of body in strength, movement or tone Lack of or limited eye contact Poor interactions with adults or other children Parental concerns		

Data from www.childrens.health.qld.gov.au/wp-content/uploads/PDF/red-flags-a3.pdf.

DEVELOPMENTAL ASSESSMENT

1. **History**
   a. Presenting issue, parental concerns
   b. **Pregnancy and birth history**
      i. Antenatal investigations (bloodwork, ultrasounds)
      ii. Maternal illness, including pregnancy related (e.g., hypertension, gestational diabetes), exposure to teratogens (e.g., alcohol, nicotine, other drugs, TORCH infections)
      iii. Delivery (gestational age, type of delivery, birthweight, resuscitation, complications)
      iv. Neonatal history (e.g., neonatal intensive care unit stay, establishment of feeding, issues encountered and treatment needed, e.g., jaundice, hypoglycemia, seizures, infection)
   c. **Medical history:** previous interactions with healthcare (hospitalizations including surgeries, emergency room, primary care attendance, subspeciality consultations, and investigations), medications, vaccinations
   d. **Developmental history:** see Box 12.1
   e. **Day care/school history:** grades, individual education plan (IEP), special supports (e.g., educational assistant), extracurricular activities
   f. **Supports and services:** rehabilitation services (e.g., physiotherapy, occupational therapy, speech and language therapy), funding, equipment
   g. **Family history:** three-generation pedigree, consanguinity, miscarriages/stillbirths, presence of developmental disability, neurological and psychiatric conditions
   h. **Social history:** home environment, parental education and employment, involvement of child protection services
   i. Review of systems including vision, hearing, sleep, diet, dental, diapering/toileting, feeding, activities of daily living

---

⚡ **PEARL**

Collateral information from teachers, therapists, and other practitioners is valuable.

Box 12.1 Developmental History

1. For each domain outlined in Table 12.1 determine: when milestones were achieved, current level of function, presence of any regression
2. Assessment of
   a. Gross motor (e.g., head control, sitting, walking, running, stairs, sports)
   b. Fine motor (e.g., handedness, pincer grasp, utensil use, zippers/buttons, printing skills)
   c. Communication: languages to which the child is exposed, expressive language (e.g., babbling, age of first words, number of words, grammar, conversational abilities), receptive language (e.g., response to name, following simple and multistep commands), speech (articulation, fluency), and nonverbal (e.g., eye contact, gestures, pointing)
   d. Social and play (e.g., joint attention, interest in peers, pretend play, favourite toys and activities)
   e. Adaptive/self-help (e.g., feeding, dressing, toileting, hygiene)
   f. Behavior (e.g., aggression, self-injury, hyperactivity, impulsivity, repetitive behaviors or mannerisms, temper tantrums, discipline strategies, sensory interests or aversions)
   g. Cognitive (e.g., cause-and-effect, puzzles, body parts, colors, shapes, letters, numbers, academic performance, attention)

---

2. **Physical examination**
   a. Informal observation: parental and professional interaction with child, observe skills in each developmental domain. Toys, crayons, and books can be helpful.
   b. Growth parameters
   c. Dysmorphology examination: see Chapter 18 Genetics and Teratology
   d. Neurological examination: cranial nerves, tone, strength, reflexes, sensory, coordination, gait
   e. Head to toe: head and neck (e.g., cleft palate, strabismus), cardiorespiratory (e.g., murmur), abdominal (e.g., organomegaly), genitourinary (e.g., inguinal hernia, undescended testes), musculoskeletal (e.g., scoliosis, contractures), skin (e.g., café-au-lait macules, hypomelanotic macules, fibromas)
3. **Investigations:** depends on specific clinical context
4. **Management**
   a. Multidisciplinary team-based care, including input from physiotherapists, occupational therapists, psychologists, behavioral therapists, registered dietitians, paediatricians, psychiatrists, and social workers, is a mainstay of care
   b. Diagnosis-specific early intervention to optimize infant motor and cognitive plasticity, prevent secondary complications, and enhance caregiver well-being

c. Consider educational needs, including an IEP
d. Family support, including counselling about diagnosis and progress, system navigation, access to necessary supports (e.g., allowances, respite)
e. Consideration of comorbid conditions (e.g., seizure disorder, sleep, constipation, mental health)
f. Clear communication with primary care providers is an important aspect of continuing care

BEHAVIOR ISSUES

A. Night terrors
1. **Description:** non-REM sleep disorder; presents as an abrupt awakening from sleep, typically within 1 to 3 hours of falling asleep; often associated with screaming and agitation; child may be flushed, sweating, and tachycardic; child does not respond to attempts at comforting by the caregiver and does not remember the episode in the morning
2. **Epidemiology:** common in preschoolers; family history common
3. **Management:** supportive (parental reassurance and education, sleep hygiene); avoid waking the child during an episode; if occurring on a nightly basis, may consider scheduled awakenings

B. Behavioral insomnia of childhood
1. **Definition**
   a. **Sleep-onset association type:** difficulty initiating sleep independently; child associates falling asleep with certain conditions or circumstances (e.g., caregiver presence, feeding from a bottle)
   b. **Limit-setting type:** child delays bedtime; caregiver has difficulty setting limits
   c. **Combined type:** both of the aforementioned
2. **Management:** parent education, sleep hygiene (see Chapter 25 Mental Health), consistent routines, gradual extinction

C. Temper tantrums
1. **Definition:** extreme episodes of frustration or anger. Examples of manifestations can include shouting, screaming, crying, and falling to the floor.
2. **Epidemiology:** frequency peaks around 3 years of age; typically a transient developmental stage
3. **Assessment**
   a. Distinguish developmentally normative behaviors from atypical behaviors; explore frequency, intensity, and duration
   b. Features which indicate problematic, disruptive behaviors include: atypical behavior for the child's developmental age that persists for

at least 6 months, occurs across situations and impairs functioning, causes significant distress for the child and family

4. **Management**
    a. Anticipatory guidance for positive parenting and effective discipline strategies: regular praise for good behavior, reducing triggers, distraction/redirection, ignoring the tantrum as long as the child is safe
    b. First-line management are parent behavior training programs

EARLY DEVELOPMENTAL IMPAIRMENT AND INTELLECTUAL DISABILITY

1. **Description**
    a. **Early developmental impairment (EDI):** failure to meet expected developmental milestones in at least two areas of functioning (e.g., motor, speech/language, cognition, social, adaptive functioning) in an individual under 5 years of age. Requires reassessment after a period of time. Also referred to as *global developmental delay* (GDD).
    b. **Intellectual disability** (all three criteria must be met, adapted from DSM-V)
        i. Deficits in intellectual functions, such as reasoning, problem solving, planning, abstract thinking, judgment, academic learning, and learning from experience; confirmed by both clinical assessment and individualized, standardized intelligence testing
        ii. Deficits in adaptive functioning that result in failure to meet developmental and socio-cultural standards for personal independence and social responsibility. Without ongoing support, the adaptive deficits limit functioning in one or more activities of daily life, such as communication, social participation, and independent living, across multiple environments, such as home, school, work, and community.
        iii. Onset of intellectual and adaptive deficits occur during the developmental period

2. **Approach to investigations** (see Figure 12.1)
    a. When a more specific diagnosis is suspected following clinical evaluation, investigations to confirm that etiology should be ordered first
    b. For unexplained EDI, chromosomal microarray and Fragile X testing are first-line investigations
    c. When no etiological diagnosis has been identified following history, physical examination and initial genetic tests (Fragile X, chromosomal microarray), consider metabolic testing for diagnosis of treatable inborn errors of metabolism (IEM) even in the absence of red flags for a metabolic condition (Table 12.3) ± brain imaging (see also www.treatable-id.org)

Figure 12.1 An Approach to Investigation of Early Developmental Impairment and Intellectual Disability

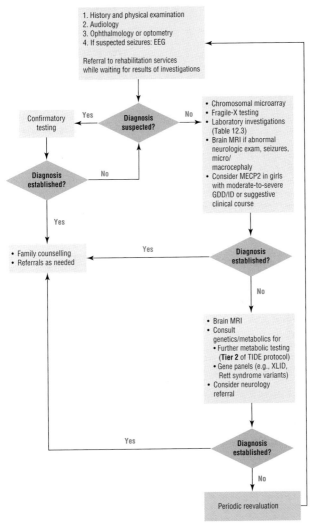

EEG, Electroencephalogram, *GDD/ID*, global developmental delay/intellectual disability; *MECP2*, methyl CpG binding protein 2; *MRI*, magnetic resonance imaging; *TIDE*, Treatable Intellectual Disability Endeavor (https://www.tidebc.org/resources/Early-Ident-Paediatr-Child-Health-2014.pdf); *XLID*, X-linked intellectual disability. (Modified from Bélanger SA, Caron J. Evaluation of the child with global developmental delay and intellectual disability. *Paediatr Child Health.* 2018;23(6):403–410.)

Table 12.3	Laboratory Investigations for Unexplained Early Developmental Impairment/Intellectual Disability	
Blood[a]		**Urine[a]**
- Complete blood count - Glucose - Blood gas - Urea, creatinine - Electrolytes (to calculate anion gap) - AST, ALT - TSH - Creatine kinase - Ammonia - Lactate - Amino acids - Acylcarnitine profile, carnitine (free and total) - Homocysteine - Copper, ceruloplasmin[b] - Biotinidase[c] - Ferritin, vitamin B12 when dietary restriction or pica are present - Lead level when risk factors for exposure are present		- Organic acids - Creatine metabolites - Purines, pyrimidines - Glycosaminoglycans

[a]Perform testing after 4–8 h of fasting.

[b]Recommended tier-1 test in the Treatable Intellectual Disability Endeavor (TIDE) protocol, but not by the American Academy of Pediatrics (AAP), the American Academy of Neurology (AAN). Consider as a first-line investigation when hepatomegaly, dystonia, abnormal liver function findings are present.

[c]Clinical expert recommendation only. Consider biotinidase testing when severe hypotonia, seizures are present.

ALT, Alanine aminotransferase; *AST,* aspartate aminotransferase; *TSH,* thyroid-stimulating hormone.

From Bélanger SA, Caron J. Evaluation of the child with global developmental delay and intellectual disability. *Paediatr Child Health.* 2018;23(6):403–410.

3. **Management:** early intervention programs with family education and support, routine health evaluations, anticipate and plan for future level of independent functioning

> ✦ **PEARL**
>
> Preschool developmental scales are not always predictive of future intelligence quotient (IQ). IQ cannot be accurately determined before 5 years of age.

AUTISM SPECTRUM DISORDER

1. **Description:** persistent deficits in social communication and social interaction across multiple contexts, and restricted, repetitive patterns of behavior, interests, or activities (see Box 12.2 for diagnostic criteria)

A. Persistent deficits in social communication and social interaction across multiple contexts, as manifested by the following, currently or by history. Examples include:
1. Deficits in social-emotional reciprocity, e.g., abnormal social approach, and failure of normal back-and-forth conversation
2. Deficits in nonverbal communicative behaviors used for social interaction, e.g., poorly integrated verbal and nonverbal communication, abnormalities in eye contact
3. Deficits in developing, maintaining, and understanding relationships, e.g., difficulties adjusting behavior to suit various social contexts: severity is based on social communication impairments and restricted, repetitive patterns of behavior
B. Restricted, repetitive patterns of behavior, interests, or activities, as manifested by at least two of the following, currently or by history. Examples include:
1. Stereotyped or repetitive motor movements, use of objects, or speech (e.g., simple motor stereotypies, lining up toys or flipping objects, echolalia, idiosyncratic phrases)
2. Insistence on sameness, inflexible adherence to routines, or ritualized patterns of verbal or nonverbal behavior (e.g., extreme distress at small changes, difficulties with transitions, rigid thinking patterns, greeting rituals, need to take same route or eat same food every day)
3. Highly restricted, fixated interests that are abnormal in intensity or focus (e.g., strong attachment to or preoccupation with unusual objects)
4. Hyper- or hyporeactivity to sensory input or unusual interest in sensory aspects of the environment (e.g., apparent indifference to pain/temperature, adverse response to specific sounds or textures, excessive smelling or touching of objects, visual fascination with lights or movement)
C. Symptoms must be present in the early developmental period (but may not become fully manifest until social demands exceed limited capacities or may be masked by learned strategies in later life)
D. Symptoms cause clinically significant impairment in social, occupational, or other important areas of current functioning
E. These disturbances are not better explained by ID or EDI. ID and ASD frequently cooccur; to make comorbid diagnoses of ASD and ID, social communication should be below that expected for general developmental level.

ASD, Autism spectrum disorder, *EDI*, early developmental impairment, *ID*, intellectual disability.

Data from *Diagnostic and Statistical Manual of Mental Disorders*, 5th Edition.

2. **Autism spectrum disorder (ASD) red flags**
   a. Reduced/atypical eye gaze, sharing of emotion, social interest/connectedness, response to name, babbling, language comprehension and production, gestures, and imitation
   b. Excessive/unusual manipulation or visual exploration of objects, repetitive actions, under/overreaction to sensory stimuli, or delayed fine/gross motor skills
3. **Approach to diagnosis**
   a. Full development assessment (see the Developmental Assessment section)
   b. Diagnosis can include standardized assessments (e.g., autism diagnostic observation schedule)

4. **Management**
   a. Consider investigations for underlying etiology, especially if co-occurring EDI or regression (see Figure 12.1 and Table 12.3)
   b. Multidisciplinary team-based care
      i. Early intervention is important and can include particular methodologies, such as parent coaching of social communication skills and behavior therapy (i.e., applied behavioral analysis)
      ii. Occupational therapy: to improve fine motor deficits, and improve academic and self-care skills. Addresses issues with the integration of sensory of information.
      iii. Speech and language pathology: to improve verbal and nonverbal communication. May include sign language and augmentative communication techniques, such as picture exchange communication system (PECS).
   c. At higher risk for comorbid conditions including
      i. Sleep disorders, constipation, nutritional deficiencies (from restricted diet)
      ii. Mental health: anxiety, attention deficit/hyperactivity disorder (ADHD), obsessive-compulsive behaviors, disruptive behaviors

CEREBRAL PALSY

1. **Definition**
   a. A group of permanent disorders of the development of movement and posture, causing activity limitations
   b. Attributed to nonprogressive disturbances that occurred in the developing fetal or infant brain
   c. Often accompanied by disturbances of sensation, perception, cognition, communication, and behavior, by epilepsy, and by secondary musculoskeletal problems

2. **Diagnosis**
   a. Full developmental assessment (see the Developmental Assessment section)
   b. Standardized tools helpful in identifying infants at risk for cerebral palsy (e.g., Hammersmith infant neurological evaluation, Prechtl's general movements assessment)

3. **Classification systems**
   a. See Figure 12.2 for classification of subtypes
   b. See Table 12.4 for different CP classification tools
      i. Gross motor functional classification system (GMFCS): gross motor grading system describing self-initiated movement, emphasis on sitting, transfers and mobility. Relatively stable after 2 years of age, can be used for prognosticating and goal setting.

Figure 12.2 Classification for Subtypes of Cerebral Palsy

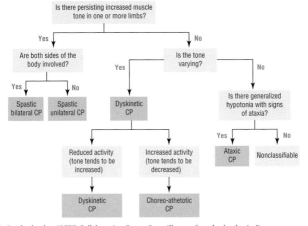

CP, Cerebral palsy. (SCPE Collaborative Group. Surveillance of cerebral palsy in Europe: a collaboration of cerebral palsy surveys and registers. *Developmental Medicine and Child Neurology.* 2000;42:816–824.)

Table 12.4	**Functional Classification Systems Used in Cerebral Palsy**			
	GMFCS	**MACS**	**CFCS**	**EDACS**
I	Walks without limitation	Handles objects easily and successfully	Effective sender and receiver	Eats and drinks safely and efficiently
II	Walks with limitations (no mobility aid by 4 years)	Handles most objects with reduced speed/quality	Effective but slow paced sender and receiver	Eats and drinks safely but with some limitations to efficiency
III	Walks with handheld mobility device	Handles objects with difficulty, help to prepare or modify activity	Effective sender and receiver with familiar partners	Eats and drinks with some limitations to safely; there may also be limitations to efficiency
IV	Self-mobility with limitations, may use power	Handles limited number of objects in adapted setting	Inconsistent sender and receiver with familiar partners	Eats and drinks with significant limitations to safety
V	Transported in manual wheelchair	Does not handle objects	Seldom effective sender and receiver with familiar partners	Unable to eat or drink safely, consider feeding tube

CFCS, Communication, Function Classification System; *EDACS*, Eating and Drinking Ability Classification System; *GMFCS*, Gross Motor Functional Classification System; *MACS*, Manual Ability Classification System.

From Paulson A, Vargus-Adams, J. Overview of four functional classification systems commonly used in cerebral palsy. *Children* (Basel). 2017;4(4):30.

ii. Manual ability classification system (MACS): used to classify a child's typical use of both hands and upper limbs for children >4 years of age

iii. Communication, function classification system (CFCS): assesses everyday communication, allowing all methods of communication (e.g., vocalizations, manual signs, eye gaze, pictures, communication boards, speech generating devices) to be included during classification

iv. Eating and drinking ability classification system (EDACS): assesses eating and drinking safety (aspiration and choking), as well as efficiency (amount of food lost and time taken to eat) in children >3 years of age. Addresses the amount of assistance a person needs: independent, requires assistance, or dependent for eating and drinking.

4. **Management**
   a. Early multidisciplinary team input
   b. Compensatory and environmental adaptation approaches including environmental modifications or specialized equipment (e.g., orthotics, walkers, specialized seating)
   c. Surveillance and management of common musculoskeletal complications including pain, contractures, hip subluxation (www.aacpdm.org/publications/care-pathways/hip-surveillance-in-cerebral-palsy), scoliosis, and osteoporosis (www.aacpdm.org/publications/care-pathways/osteoporosis-in-cerebral-palsy)
   d. Tone management: may require oral medications (e.g., baclofen) or botulinum toxin A injections to manage hypertonia if it is causing pain, limiting function or participation, or impacting caregiving (pathways.nice.org.uk/pathways/spasticity-in-children-and-young-people for care pathway for spasticity and www.aacpdm.org/publications/care-pathways/dystonia-in-cerebral-palsy for care pathway for dystonia)
   e. Siallorhea care pathway (www.aacpdm.org/publications/care-pathways/sialorrhea-in-cerebral-palsy)

ATTENTION DEFICIT/HYPERACTIVITY DISORDER

1. **Description:** a persistent pattern of inattention and/or hyperactivity-impulsivity that interferes with functioning or development, and negatively impacts directly on social and academic/occupational activities

2. **Approach to diagnosis:** see Table 12.5

12

Table 12.5	Clinical Process and Diagnosis of Attention Deficit/Hyperactivity Disorder	
Step	**Considerations**	
Schedule multiple office visits to complete the diagnostic evaluation		
Obtain detailed information on prenatal/perinatal events, medical and mental health history		
Obtain developmental/behavioral history (motor, language, social milestones, and behavior, including temperament/emotional regulation and attachment)	In preschool children, impaired attention and hyperactivity may also be features of a neurodevelopmental disorder	
Perform thorough physical, neurological, and dysmorphology assessments		
Evaluate family medical and mental health, family functioning and coping styles of primary caregivers	Do comorbid symptoms meet criteria for a separate disorder that is the main diagnosis, OR exist in tandem with ADHD as the main diagnosis, OR are they secondary symptoms (stemming from the ADHD)?	
Evaluate for comorbid disorder(s) (psychiatric, neurodevelopmental and physical)		
Review academic progress (e.g., report cards, sample assignments), look for symptoms of a learning disorder	Clinical impressions and use of standardized scales are the most effective tools for diagnosis	
Obtain standardized behavior rating scale(s) that evaluate DSM-V criteria from primary caregivers, teachers, and the adolescent being assessed Find screening tools and rating scales at https://www.cps.ca/en/tools-outils/condition-specific-screening-tools-and-rating-scales	Rating scales are not diagnostic of ADHD but help quantify the degree to which a behavior may deviate from the norm and can be used to evaluate the effects of interventions in home or school	
Unless indicated by history and physical examination, do NOT: - Order laboratory tests, genetic testing, EEG, or neuroimaging - Order psychological, neuropsychological, or speech-language assessments - Use psychological tests or measures of executive function to diagnose ADHD and/or as a means to evaluate the effects of interventions		

Development

12

Continued

Table 12.5	Clinical Process and Diagnosis of Attention Deficit/Hyperactivity Disorder—cont'd	
Step		**Considerations**
Refer to DSM-V criteria for core symptoms and characteristics: 1. Symptoms are severe, persistent (i.e., present before 12 years of age and continuing >6 months), and inappropriate for the patient's age and developmental level 2. Symptoms are associated with impairment in academic achievement, peer and family relations, and adaptive skills 3. If there is a discrepancy of symptoms across settings, it is important to identify why the discrepancy exists		Consider the demands and expectations being placed on the child and what the child's innate capabilities are to meet these expectations. What will this child look like over time?

4. Specify the type of ADHD presentation as per the DSM-V:
   i. Combined presentation (criteria are met for inattention, hyperactivity-impulsivity)
   ii. Predominantly inattentive presentation (criteria are met for inattention)
   iii. Predominantly hyperactive-impulsive presentation (criteria are met for hyperactivity-impulsivity)
5. Specify current severity (mild, moderate, or severe) based on the symptoms and degree of functional impairment
		The abilities to self-control attention, activity and impulses emerge in a developmental process. The DSM-V does not provide for developmental level differences, which may lead to overdiagnosis of ADHD in preschool-aged children.
		
		Impairment implies greater severity and frequency of symptoms that interfere with the ability to function across major life domains

ADHD, Attention deficit/hyperactivity disorder; *DSM-V, Diagnostic and Statistical Manual of Mental Disorders,* 5th Edition; *EEG,* electroencephalogram.

Modified from Belanger SA, Andrews D, et al. ADHD in children and youth: part 1—etiology, diagnosis, and comorbidity. *Paediatr Child Health.* 2018;23(7):447–453.

3. **Management**
   a. **Children <6 years of age**
      i. Parent behavior training
      ii. Poor evidence for psychostimulants in this age group
   b. **Children >6 years of age**
      i. *Nonpharmacological interventions:* psychoeducation, parent behavior training, classroom management, daily report card, behavioral peer interactions, organizational skills training, cognitive training, exercise
      ii. *Pharmacological interventions:* see Table 12.6

- Reserve medications for those diagnosed with ADHD whose learning or academic performance are impaired by attention difficulties or whose behaviors and social interactions are impaired by lack of impulse control and hyperactivity
- In addition to nonpharmacological interventions, extended release stimulants are recommended as first-line therapy
- See Chapter 8 Cardiology for cardiac screening before stimulant use
- When initiating pharmacological therapy, use standardized checklists to monitor treatment response

 PEARL

ADHD medications are controlled substances. In Ontario, prescriptions for controlled substances must be prescribed as the total quantity to be dispensed. Refills are permitted if the refill quantity and refill date or interval between refills is included in the prescription. Consider having the interval as just less than the quantity to be dispensed to give families time to pick up the medication.

Example:
Ritalin 20 mg
Take one tablet (20 mg) by mouth once daily
Total quantity: 90 tablets
Dispense as 30 tablets every 25 days

Development

12

Table 12.6 Psychostimulant and Non-Psychostimulant Pharmacological Treatment for ADHD

Medication	Formulations	Delivery	Duration of Action[a]	Starting Dose[b]	Dose Titration[c]
Amphetamine-Based Psychostimulants (First Line Options)					
Adderall XR	Capsules 5, 10, 15, 20, 25, 30 mg	Granules can be sprinkled	~12 h	0.25 mg/kg or 5–10 mg qam	↑5–10 mg at weekly intervals *Usual dose range:* 0.4–0.7 mg/kg *Maximum dose/day:* Children = 1 mg/kg or 30 mg Adolescents and adults = 20–30 mg
Vyvanse	Capsules 10, 20, 30, 40, 50, 60 mg Chewable Tablets 10, 20, 30, 40, 50, 60 mg	Capsule content can be diluted in liquid or sprinkled Chewable tablets should be chewed thoroughly	~13–14 h	0.5 mg/kg or 20–30 mg qam	↑10–20 mg by clinical discretion at weekly intervals *Usual dose range:* 0.8–1.5 mg/kg *Maximum dose/day:* 2 mg/kg or 60 mg
Methylphenidate-Based Psychostimulants (First Line Options)					
Biphentin	Capsules 10, 15, 20, 30, 40, 50, 60, 80 mg	Granules can be sprinkled	~10–12 h	0.5 mg/kg or 10–20 qam	↑5–10 mg at weekly intervals *Usual dose range:* 0.8–1.5 mg/kg *Maximum dose/day:* Children and adolescents = 2 mg/kg or 60 mg Adults = 80 mg
Concerta	Extended Release Tablets 18, 27, 36, 54 mg	Osmotic-Controlled Release Oral Delivery System (OROS)	~12 h	0.5 mg/kg or 18 mg qam	↑9–18 mg at weekly intervals *Usual dose range:* 0.8–1.5 mg/kg *Maximum dose/day:* Children and adolescents = 2 mg/kg or 54 mg Adults = 72 mg

Foquest	Capsules 25, 35, 45, 55, 70, 85, 100 mg	Granules can be sprinkled	~16 h	25 mg qam	↑10–15 mg in intervals of no less than 5 days *Maximum dose/day:* Children and adolescents = 70 mg Adults = 100 mg

Non-Psychostimulant–Selective Norepinephrine Reuptake Inhibitor

Strattera (Atomoxetine)	Capsules 10, 18, 25, 40, 60, 80, 100 mg	Capsule needs to be swallowed whole to reduce GI side effects	Up to 24 h	6–17 years and <70 kg = 0.5 mg/kg Adults or >70 kg = 40 mg daily	Maintain dose for a minimum of 7–14 days before adjusting Children and adolescents: ↑ by 0.3 mg/kg intervals Adults or >70 kg: ↑ by 20 mg intervals *Usual dose range:* 0.5–1.2 mg/kg *Maximum dose/day:* 1.2 mg/kg or 80 mg

Non-Psychostimulant–Selective Alpha-2A Adrenergic Receptor Agonist

Intuniv XR (Guanfacine XR)	Extended Release Tablets 1, 2, 3, 4 mg	Pills need to be swallowed whole to keep delivery mechanism intact	Up to 24 h	1 mg/day (morning or evening)	Maintain dose for a minimum of 7 days before adjusting by no more than 1 mg increment weekly *Usual dose range:* 0.05–0.12 mg/kg *Maximum dose/day for monotherapy:* 6–12 years = 4 mg 13–17 years = 7 mg *Maximum dose/day as adjunctive therapy with stimulants:* 6–17 years = 4 mg *To discontinue:* Taper dose in decrements of 1 mg every 3–7 days

[a] Pharmacokinetic and pharmacodynamic responses vary from individual to individual.
[b] CADDRA recommends starting with the lowest dose available.
[c] Dose titration per product monograph. For specific details on how to start, adjust and switch ADHD medications, clinicians should refer to the Canadian ADHD Practice Guidelines (www.caddra.ca). Children refers to 6–12 years of age. Adolescents refers to 13–17 years of age.

Data from https://www.caddra.ca/wp-content/uploads/Final-Laminate-Card-2019_9-1.pdf and Feldman et al. ADHD in children and youth: Part 2 - treatment. *Paediatr Child Health* 2018, 23(7):462–472.

Development

12

279

SPECIFIC LEARNING DISORDERS

1. **Description:** see Box 12.3
2. **Assessment:** diagnosis requires psychoeducational assessment (Box 12.4)
3. **Management:** IEP with child-specific accommodations and modifications

---

Box 12.3 Types and Diagnosis of Specific Learning Disorders

1. Difficulty in at least one of the following areas, despite targeted help:
   a. Inaccurate or slow and effortful word reading (e.g., reads single words aloud incorrectly or slowly and hesitantly)
   b. Difficulty understanding the meaning of what is read (e.g., may read text accurately but not understand the deeper meanings of what is read)
   c. Difficulties with spelling (e.g., may add, omit, or substitute vowels or consonants)
   d. Difficulties with written expression (e.g., makes multiple grammatical or punctuation errors within sentences)
   e. Difficulties mastering number sense, number facts, or calculation (e.g., has poor understanding of numbers)
   f. Difficulties with mathematical reasoning (e.g., has severe difficulty applying mathematical concepts)
2. Academic skills are substantially below what is expected for the child's age and impair everyday function
3. Learning difficulties begin during school-age years (may not fully manifest until later when demands are greater)
4. Learning difficulties are caused by other conditions such as intellectual disabilities, uncorrected visual or auditory acuity, other mental or neurological disorders, psychosocial adversity, lack of proficiency in the language of academic instruction, or inadequate educational instruction.

Modified from the *Diagnostic and Statistical Manual of Mental Disorders*, 5th Edition.

Box 12.4 Components of a Psychoeducational Assessment

1. **Cognitive Assessment** (e.g., Weschler Intelligence Scales for Children, Stanford-Binet, Leiter)
2. **Academic Assessment** (e.g., Woodcock Johnson, Wide Range Achievement Test)
3. **Emotional/Behavioral Assessment** (Conners, Child Behavior Checklist)
4. **Adaptive Assessment** (e.g., Vineland Adaptive Behaviour Scale, Adaptive Behaviour Assessment System)

SPEECH AND LANGUAGE DISORDERS

1. **Description**
   a. **Language disorder:** persistent difficulties acquiring/using language (limited vocabulary, sentence structure, discourse) with linguistic abilities below what is expected for age
   b. **Speech sound disorder:** early onset, persistent difficulty with speech sound production affecting intelligibility of communication and interfering with social, academic, or personal accomplishment

c. **Child-onset fluency disorder (stuttering):** sustained disturbance speech fluency and time pattern (repetitions, prolongations, or broken words) out of keeping with age and language skills causing significant distress

d. **Social (pragmatic) communication disorder:** persistent difficulties in use of verbal/nonverbal communication for social interaction including using language in the appropriate context, responding to verbal/nonverbal signals, or understanding metaphors/multiple meanings

2. **Epidemiology:** children with speech/language disorders are at increased risk for later learning difficulties

3. **Assessment and management**
   a. Early introduction of reading and provision of a language rich environment
   b. Involve a speech language pathologist and/or psychologist to help with diagnosis and ruling out alternative diagnoses (e.g., EDI, ASD) while providing therapy
   c. Alternative or augmentative communication may be used (sign language, PECS, or computerized devices)

DEVELOPMENTAL COORDINATION DISORDER

1. **Description:** acquisition and execution of coordinated motor skills is substantially below that expected for the patient's age and opportunities for learning. Motor skills deficit significantly and persistently interferes with activities of daily living appropriate to chronological age. The onset of symptoms is in the early developmental period.

2. **Assessment**
   a. Developmental coordination disorder questionnaire
   b. Referral to trained occupational therapist and/or physiotherapist for standardized assessment of motor abilities (e.g., Movement Assessment Battery for Children)

3. **Management:** individualized and task-oriented approach focusing on direct teaching of functional skills (such as CO-OP technique); typically delivered by occupational or physiotherapist

Diagnostic Imaging

Alisha Jamal • Jeffrey Traubici

COMMON ABBREVIATIONS

Also see page xviii for a list of other abbreviations used throughout this book

AP	anterior to posterior
AXR	abdominal x-ray
C+ CT	contrast-enhanced computed tomography
C− CT	non-enhanced computed tomography
C+MR	contrast-enhanced magnetic resonance imaging
CTA	computed tomography angiography
CXR	chest x-ray
ETT	endotracheal tube
GA	general anesthesia
MRA	magnetic resonance angiography
MRCP	magnetic resonance cholangiopancreatography
NEC	necrotizing enterocolitis
NG	nasogastric
NJ	nasojejunal
PA	posterior to anterior
PICC	peripherally inserted central catheter
RLQ	right lower quadrant
RUQ	right upper quadrant
UGI	upper gastrointestinal (series)
US	ultrasonography
VCUG	voiding cystourethrogram

GENERAL PRINCIPLES

1. **Imaging modalities**
   a. See Table 13.1

2. **Contrast agents**
   a. Definition: agents used to increase the contrast of soft tissue structures and of fluids, to aid in differentiating adjacent structures, as well as characterize abnormal lesions in the body during medical imaging
   b. See Table 13.2 for description of various contrast agents and their modes of administration

Table 13.1	**Imaging Modalities**		
Modality	**Advantages**	**Disadvantages**	**Contraindications**
Plain film x-ray	- Inexpensive, noninvasive - Readily available	- Radiation exposure - Poor at distinguishing soft tissues	Pregnancy
CT	- Excellent delineation of bones and soft tissue - Spiral CT: fast data acquisition - May allow 3D reconstruction - CT angiography less invasive than conventional catheter angiography	- High radiation exposure - Sedation/GA may be needed - Relatively expensive - Caution with contrast in renal failure/allergy - Metal causes artifact	- Pregnancy - Contraindication to contrast agents
MRI	- Excellent soft tissue resolution and discrimination - No ionizing radiation involved - MR angiography provides noninvasive assessment of vessels and flow	- Claustrophobia - Sedation/GA may be needed - Metal causes artifact - May be less readily available	- Ferromagnetic metal - Foreign bodies - Cardiac pace-maker
US	- Inexpensive, noninvasive - No ionizing radiation involved - Determines cystic vs. solid - Real-time imaging useful for interventions	- Highly operator dependent - Air in bowel may prevent imaging of midline abdominal structures	
Nuclear medicine	Functional imaging data	- Radioactive substance injected/ingested/inhaled - Frequently needs IV ± sedation urine - Body fluids radioactive	Pregnancy
PET-CT	Excellent tumor detection	High radiation dose ± IV sedation/GA	Pregnancy
Fluoroscopy (GI/GU)	- Real time - Rarely requires sedation	- Radiation involved - Bladder catheterization for VCUG	Pregnancy

3D, Three-dimensional; *CT*, computed tomography; *GA*, general anesthesia; *GI*, gastrointestinal; *GU*, genitourinary; *MRI*, magnetic resonance imaging; *PET*, positron emission tomography; *US*, ultrasound; *VCUG*, voiding cystourethrogram.

Modality	Agent	Routes and Study Type	Contraindications
X-ray	Barium	PO/PR—routine GI studies	Perforation, toxic megacolon
	Iodinated contrast	PO/PR—suspected perforation in GI/GU studies, suspected bowel obstruction, delineate fistula/sinus tract Via urinary catheter—GU studies, VCUG, retrograde urethrogram	- Allergy (consult radiology regarding alternative options; consider premedication in select cases) - Anaphylactoid-like reactions have been reported in GI/GU imaging
CT	Iodinated contrast	IV—highlights vessels, enhances solid and hollow viscera, inflammation	- Renal failure - Allergy (discussion with radiologist regarding potential alternative modality or pretreatment)
MRI	Gadolinium	IV—specific angiographic sequences, enhances solid and hollow viscera, inflammation	Renal failure (risk of nephrogenic systemic fibrosis—NSF)

Table 13.2 Types and Uses of Contrast in Imaging

CT, Computed tomography; *GI*, gastrointestinal; *GU*, genitourinary; *MRI*, magnetic resonance imaging; *VCUG*, voiding cystourethrogram.

APPROACH TO IMAGING

HEAD

1. **X-ray skull:** most common indications include assessing trauma, workup of syndromes, metabolic disorders and dysplasias, abnormal skull shape, craniosynostosis, or focal craniofacial lesion (including occasionally metastatic disease)

2. **Ultrasound**
   a. Preterm babies and term neonates: used to evaluate intraventricular hemorrhage (IVH), ventricular enlargement/macrocephaly, white matter abnormalities (i.e., periventricular leukomalacia), and as an initial screening test for pathologies of the central nervous system
   b. Transcranial Doppler: used to measure cerebral blood flow noninvasively (i.e., sickle cell disease)

3. **Computed tomography**
   a. C– CT: typically the initial imaging modality for acute trauma and emergent situations to assess for skull fractures, traumatic brain injuries, hemorrhages, or masses

    b. C+ CT: typically used for the evaluation of head and neck masses, intracranial infection, inflammatory diseases

    c. Computed tomography angiography (CTA): used to evaluate blood vessel patency (i.e., for pediatric stroke, vasculitis, or vascular malformations)

4. **Magnetic resonance imaging**

    a. Most sensitive and specific noninvasive test to provide detailed imaging of the brain; often used as the imaging modality of choice for CNS pathologies, bypassing CT

    b. MRA: used to evaluate blood vessel patency (similar to CTA)

CERVICAL SPINE

1. Also see Chapter 2 Emergency Medicine for C-spine trauma

2. **Plain radiographs (anterior to posterior [AP], cross table lateral, and,** when obtainable, **open mouth odontoid view)** are typically the initial imaging modality of choice to detect fractures or dislocations

    a. **Injury location:** axial (occiput to C2) cervical spine injuries are most common in children <8 years. Older children tend to sustain subaxial (C3–C7) injuries.

    b. **Approach to C-spine x-ray interpretation:** see Figure 13.1 and Table 13.3

    c. **Pseudosubluxation** of C2 on C3 can be differentiated from true subluxation by evaluating Swischuk's line: line drawn from the spino-laminar point of C1 to spinolaminar point C3. True subluxation should be suspected if this line misses the spinolaminar point of C2 by >2 mm. See Figure 13.2.

    d. **Odontoid views:** Examine dens for fractures and ensure lateral aspects of C1 are symmetric (have equal amounts of space on both sides of the dens [lateral atlantodental interval]) and that lateral masses align

    e. **Flexion/extension x-rays** are very useful to detect ligamentous injury

3. **CT C-spine** is the most sensitive modality to detect bony injuries

    a. Used to confirm suspicious or abnormal C-spine x-rays (or when high suspicion for injury despite normal x-rays), or instead of x-rays in cases of severe head trauma or acute neurological deficits

    b. C+ CT useful when associated vascular injury suspected

4. **MRI spine** is the most sensitive modality to detect injuries to soft tissues of spinal column and spinal cord. Indicated for patients with neurological deficit or ongoing symptoms despite negative x-rays/CT (can have significant spinal cord injury WITHOUT radiological abnormalities).

Figure 13.1   Normal Lateral X-Ray of C-Spine

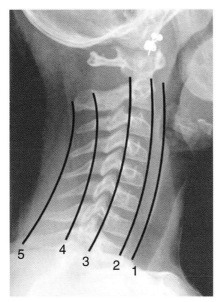

Line 1, Prevertebral soft tissue line: runs along the posterior border of airway through the first few vertebral bodies, then widens around laryngeal cartilage, and parallels the remaining cervical vertebrae. *Line 2*, Anterior spinal line: demarcates anterior border of cervical vertebral bodies. *Line 3*, Posterior spinal line: demarcates posterior border of cervical vertebral bodies. *Line 4*, Spinolaminar line: connects junction of lamina and spinous process. *Line 5*, Spinous process line: joins the tips of spinous processes. These lines should run smooth and parallel, with no abrupt step-offs.

Table 13.3	ABCDS for Reading C-Spine X-Rays
Alignment	Look for continuous lines with smooth contour and no step-offs - Anterior vertebral body (spinal) line - Posterior vertebral body (spinal) line - Facet line - Spinolaminar line - Spinous process line
Bones	Chips or fractures
Count	Must visualize all seven cervical vertebral bodies in entirety
Disk spaces	Look for consistent distance between each vertebral body
Soft tissue	Look for swelling, especially prevertebral

Figure 13.2   Lateral Cervical Spine X-Ray with Swischuk's Line

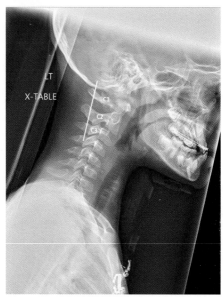

Demonstration of pseudosubluxation (physiological displacement of C2 on C3). A true subluxation should be considered if spinolaminar point of C2 is deviated >2 mm from this line (see text above).

CHEST

1. **Plain x-rays** are initial imaging study for nearly all suspected thoracic disease
   a. **Standard x-ray views:** upright PA and left lateral (supplemental views may be obtained as needed: oblique, lordotic, left or right lateral decubitus)
   b. **Basic CXR interpretation:** see Table 13.4
   c. **X-ray finding of common pulmonary pathologies:** see Table 13.5
2. **US** is the most sensitive modality for pleural effusions (i.e., detecting pleural fluid, extent, loculations, septations, and pleural thickening)
3. **CT chest:** used for assessment of complex pleural disease, vascular disease, congenital malformations, complex chest infections, trauma, inflammatory diseases, interstitial lung diseases, and for oncological staging
4. **MRI chest:** used for detailed assessment of the mediastinum, cardio-vascular system, chest wall, and pleura. Less useful for evaluation of the lung parenchyma.

Table 13.4 Basic Approach to Chest X-Ray

Identification	Date, patient name, indications, technique of examination
Exposure	Thoracic disk spaces should be just visible through heart
Rotation	- Medial ends of clavicles should be equidistant from spinous process - Anterior and posterior aspects of the ribs should appear symmetric
Inspiration	- Poor inspiration: poor aeration, vascular crowding, compressed and widened central shadow - Older children: six anterior and eight posterior ribs normally seen (general rule) - Hyperinflation: lucent lungs, flattened diaphragm, small heart
Soft tissues	- Look for air in the soft tissues - Swelling, calcification, foreign bodies
Abdomen	- Look for free air under diaphragm in upright CXR - Displacement of the gastric air bubble medially suggests splenomegaly
Bones	Check cervical and thoracic spine, shoulder girdle, ribs, sternum
Mediastinum	- Trachea, heart, great vessels, thymus - Look for mediastinal or tracheal shift, widened mediastinum
Hila	Pulmonary vessels, mainstem and segmental bronchi, lymphadenopathy
Lungs	Lung parenchyma, pleura, diaphragm
Lines/tubes	Presence + positioning of ETT, CVLs, UAC/UVC, feeding tubes

CVLs, Central venous lines; *CXR*, chest x-ray; *ETT*, endotracheal tube; *UAC*, umbilical artery catheter; *UVC*, umbilical vein catheter.

Table 13.5 Pathologic Findings on Chest X-Ray

Finding	Pathology
Pulmonary opacity	Cells or fluid in the bronchoalveolar airspace results in a confluent density (i.e., pneumonia, mass, pulmonary edema, hemorrhage, atelectasis)
Silhouette sign	Opacity, by virtue of its presence, obscures a normal anatomic landmark
- Loss of right heart border	Right middle lobe
- Loss of right hemidiaphragm	Right lower lobe
- Loss of left heart border	Lingula
- Loss of left hemidiaphragm	Left lower lobe
Air bronchograms	Radiolucent branching bronchi visible through opacified airspace disease (i.e., pneumonia, edema, infarct, hemorrhage)
Peribronchial cuffing	Interstitial infiltrate, edema, and/or bronchial inflammation (i.e., bronchiolitis, asthma)
Volume loss/atelectasis	- Indicates collapse of a portion of the lung - May see rib crowding - Indirect signs: hilar/mediastinal shift toward collapse, ± hemidiaphragm elevation - Often difficult to differentiate volume loss from other pulmonary opacity in children

Continued 289

Table 13.5	Pathologic Findings on Chest X-Ray—cont'd
Finding	**Pathology**
Pleural effusion	Blunting of costophrenic angle, fluid in horizontal or oblique fissures. Can see meniscus in uncomplicated effusions.
Pneumothorax	- Air enters pleural space (ie. the space between visceral and parietal pleura), separating partially collapsed lung from the chest wall - Mediastinal shift away from the pneumothorax and diaphragmatic inversion indicate tension pneumothorax

ABDOMEN

1. **Plain x-rays** are initial imaging modality of choice for many abdominal conditions, especially NEC, bowel obstruction, bowel perforation, radio-opaque renal tract/biliary tract calculi and foreign bodies
   a. **Standard x-ray views:** AP supine, PA erect (others include: lateral decubitus, dorsal decubitus, PA prone)
   b. **Basic AXR interpretation:** see Table 13.6 and Figure 13.3

Table 13.6	Basic Approach to Abdominal X-Ray
Identification	Date, patient name, indications, technique of examination
Exposure	Whole abdomen should be visible from diaphragm to pelvis

Stomach, small and large bowel	- Stomach seen left of the midline, below hemidiaphragm with variable amount of air
	- Small bowel
	  - Usually more central with the large bowel creating a "frame" around the periphery
	  - Mucosal folds are seen across the full width of the small bowel (valvulae conniventes)
	- Large bowel
	  - The ascending and descending colon will be in fixed positions laterally (and posteriorly in the retroperitoneum); transverse and sigmoid positions can vary (each with a "mesocolon")
	  - Look for haustra (folds that protrude only part way through the lumen) and the spaces between the haustra
	  - Look for the presence of gas to the level of the rectum and for signs of obstruction (i.e., air/fluid levels, dilated loops of bowel, transition zone), as well as intramural gas and intraperitoneal gas

Other organs	- Lungs–check lung bases for pathology (i.e., consolidation) as a source of abdominal pain - Liver: seen in RUQ - Gallbladder: often not seen, but can see calcified gallstones - Kidneys: often visible (if sufficient perirenal fat), the right will be lower than left because of liver - Spleen: seen in LUQ

Table 13.6	Basic Approach to Abdominal X-Ray—cont'd
Bones	Check ribs, lumbar vertebrae, sacrum, coccyx, pelvis, proximal femurs
Calcifications/artifacts	Look for renal, ureteric, bladder stones/calcifications, gallstones (RUQ)
Lines/tubes	Presence and positioning of NG tubes, NJ tubes, G-tubes, GJ tubes, femoral lines, etc.

AXR, Abdominal x-ray; *GI*, gastrointestinal; *GJ*, gastro-jejunal; *LUQ*, left upper quadrant; *NG*, nasogastric; *NJ*, nasojejunal; *RUQ*, right upper quadrant.

Figure 13.3   Posteroanterior Abdominal X-Ray

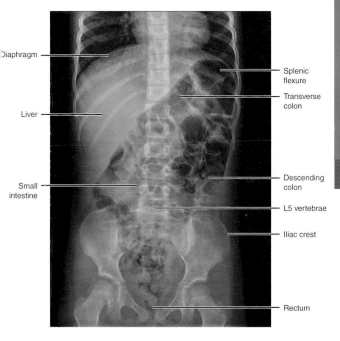

2. **US:** generally used as a first-line screening test for evaluation of liver, spleen, bowel (intussusception, appendicitis, etc.), biliary tract and gallbladder, and renal pathologies
3. **CT abdomen:** used sparingly because of radiation risk but valuable for oncologic workup, abdominal trauma, and surgical planning
4. **MRI abdomen:** useful for detailed evaluation of solid organ pathology, intra- and extraluminal bowel pathology, oncologic workup
5. **Magnetic resonance cholangiopancreatography:** used as a noninvasive technique to assess the biliary tree and pancreatic duct system

(i.e., choledocholithiasis, congenital anomalies of the bile and pancreatic ducts, choledochal cysts, primary sclerosing cholangitis)

6. **Meckel scan** (Tc-pertechnetate scintigraphy): generally used as a first-line screening test for a Meckel diverticulum. The radiopharmaceutical has an affinity for gastric mucosa and can be used to identify ectopic gastric mucosa.

7. **Upper GI (UGI) ± small bowel follow-through:** oral contrast administered under fluoroscopic visualization. Various indications, including workup of abdominal pain, vomiting, bleeding, failure to thrive. In neonates, often used in the workup of congenital obstruction/malrotation/midgut volvulus.

8. **Barium enema:** contrast administered per rectum via a rectal catheter under fluoroscopic visualization. Various indications include workup of chronic constipation, Hirschsprung disease, or bleeding. In neonates, often used in the workup of congenital obstruction (i.e., distal bowel atresia, Hirschsprung disease, meconium ileus).

MUSCULOSKELETAL SYSTEM

1. Also see Chapter 32 Orthopedics for further description of fractures, hip disorders, and bone and joint infections

2. **Plain x-rays** are initial imaging modality of choice for most musculoskeletal complaints (trauma, infection, congenital abnormalities, and malignancy)
   a. **Standard x-ray views** for fractures: AP and lateral x-ray (oblique views may be helpful in select cases)
   b. **Bone age:** obtain single **AP x-ray of left hand and wrist** (radiologist then compares x-ray with images in standard atlas of bone development)
   c. **Skeletal survey:** ≥12 x-ray views (skull, spine, chest, abdomen, extremities). Mainly performed in skeletal dysplasias, metabolic disorders, histiocytosis, and child abuse (see Chapter 9 Child Maltreatment).

3. **CT scan**
   a. Useful to evaluate certain fractures (e.g., pelvic and select ankle fractures) for treatment planning
   b. Useful for detailed evaluation of congenital bone malformations, tumors, foreign bodies, and osteochondral lesions
   c. Often used when MRI is unavailable

4. **MRI**
   a. Most sensitive and specific noninvasive test for evaluation of bone, cartilage, soft tissue, and ligamentous changes
   b. Most useful modality to evaluate extent of bony tumors and metastases
   c. Best modality to diagnose osteoarticular infections such as osteomyelitis, septic arthritis (x-ray relatively insensitive in the early stages of osteomyelitis)

d. Best modality to assess for muscle pathologies and inflammatory conditions (i.e., dermatomyositis)

e. Best modality to assess marrow disorders

GENITOURINARY TRACT

See Chapter 28 Nephrology and Urology

RADIOGRAPHIC APPEARANCE OF LINES AND TUBES

See Table 13.7

Table 13.7	Appropriate Positioning of Lines and Tubes on X-Ray	
Line/Tube	**Imaging Study**	**Appropriate Position**
ETT	CXR AP and lateral	Midway between thoracic inlet and carina
Chest tube	CXR AP and lateral	- Pneumothorax: anterior and apical - Pleural Effusion: posterior and inferior to the fluid to enable drainage
PICC	CXR AP ± lateral	- Arm PICC: end should be in the SVC (T4–T6), avoid right atrium. SVC/RA junction at T6 (or interspace above/below) in 93% of patients - Leg PICC: in IVC, (T9–T11) above renal veins (L1, L2), avoid right atrium
UAC	Chest/abdominal AP ± lateral	- High: T6–T9 (preferred), Low: L3–L4 - Avoid major branches of abdominal aorta (celiac axis to inferior mesenteric artery)
UVC	Chest/abdominal lateral ± AP	- Should be between the level of the diaphragm and the IVC/RA junction, lateral radiograph very useful for localizing tip
NG	Chest/abdominal AP ± lateral	- Should overlay the gastric bubble

AP, Anteroposterior; *CXR,* chest x-ray; *ETT,* endotracheal tube; *IVC,* inferior vena cava; *NG,* nasogastric; *PICC,* peripherally inserted central catheter; *RA,* right atrium; *SVC,* superior vena cava; *UAC,* umbilical artery catheter; *UVC,* umbilical vein catheter.

13

FURTHER READING

Coley B. *Caffey's Pediatric Diagnostic Imaging.* 13th ed. Canada: Elsevier Canada; 2018.

USEFUL WEBSITE

Resource for additional information and radiographic examples: https://radiopaedia.org.

Endocrinology

Joju Sowemimo • Julia Sorbara • Jonathan D. Wasserman

COMMON ABBREVIATIONS

Also see page xviii for a list of other abbreviations used throughout this book

17-OHP	17-hydroxyprogesterone
ACTH	adrenocorticotropic hormone
ADH	antidiuretic hormone
AI	adrenal insufficiency
ATD	antithyroid drugs
BG	blood glucose
CAH	congenital adrenal hyperplasia
CHO	carbohydrate
DDAVP	desmopressin (*1-deamino-8-D-arginine vasopressin*)
DHEAS	dehydroepiandrosterone sulfate
DI	diabetes insipidus
DKA	diabetic ketoacidosis
DSD	disorders of sex development
ED	emergency department
FSH	follicle-stimulating hormone
GAD	glutamic acid decarboxylase
GFR	glomerular filtration rate
GH	growth hormone
GnRH	gonadotropin-releasing hormone
HbA1c	hemoglobin A1c
hCG	human chorionic gonadotropin
IAI	intermediate-acting insulin
iCa	ionized calcium
IUGR	intrauterine growth restriction
LAI	long-acting insulin
LH	luteinizing hormone
MEN	multiple endocrine neoplasia
OGTT	oral glucose tolerance test
PCOS	polycystic ovarian syndrome
RAI	rapid-acting insulin
T1DM	type 1 diabetes mellitus
T2DM	type 2 diabetes mellitus
TDD	total daily dose (of insulin)
TPO	thyroid peroxidase
TSH	thyroid-stimulating hormone
TSI	thyroid-stimulating immunoglobulin (TSH receptor-stimulating antibodies)

1. **Diagnosis:** see Box 14.1

Box 14.1   Diagnostic Criteria for Diabetes

Fasting BG ≥7.0 mmol/L (i.e., no caloric intake for ≥8 h) **OR**
BG ≥11.1 mmol/L 2 h following OGTT (75 g oral carbohydrate) **OR**
Random BG ≥11.1 mmol/L

BG, Blood glucose; *OGTT*, oral glucose tolerance test.

TYPE 1 DIABETES MELLITUS

1. **Definition:** hyperglycemia resulting from absolute or relative insulin deficiency
2. **Presentation**
   a. Polyuria, polydipsia, polyphagia, weight loss
   b. Abdominal pain, nausea, vomiting
   c. Asymptomatic, incidental finding
   d. May present in diabetic ketoacidosis (DKA)
3. **Onset:** peaks in early childhood (4–6 years) and around puberty (10–14 years)
4. **Diagnosis**
   a. Symptomatic random hyperglycemia ≥11.1 mmol/L: diagnostic, no confirmatory testing required
   b. Asymptomatic: perform second confirmatory test on a different day
   c. If high suspicion, confirmatory testing should not delay treatment
   d. HbA1c not useful for diagnosis—may be normal in early Type 1 diabetes mellitus (T1DM)
5. **Investigations**
   a. **Blood:** hyperglycemia (see Box 14.1) ± ketonemia
   b. **Urine:** glucosuria ± ketonuria
   c. **Electrolyte abnormalities:** may have hyponatremia, hypokalemia
   d. **Additional tests:** not required to establish diagnosis but may be helpful if etiology unclear
      i. Low/undetectable fasting insulin and C-peptide
      ii. Positive pancreatic β-cell autoantibodies: anti-GAD, anti-insulin, islet cell antibodies

A. Management of Type 1 diabetes mellitus without DKA

1. **Monitor blood glucose (BG):** before meals and before bed
   a. Additional checks if symptoms of hypoglycemia (see later)
   b. Check overnight if concern for nocturnal hypoglycemia

   c. May use continuous or flash glucose monitors to augment capillary BG monitoring

   d. **Target BG**

      i. 6 to 10 mmol/L in initial education period and/or younger patients

      ii. 4 to 8 mmol/L for established patients

2. **Insulin initiation**

   a. Initial total daily dose (TDD): 0.3 to 0.6 units/kg/day

   b. Anticipate decreasing requirements during first year after diagnosis because of "honeymoon period"

   c. **Insulin preparations:** see Table 14.1

Table 14.1	Characteristics of Insulin Preparations		
Insulin (Trade Name in Parentheses)	**Onset**	**Peak**	**Duration**
Ultra-Rapid-Acting			
Aspart (Fiasp)	4 min	30–90 min	3–5 h
Rapid-Acting (RAI)			
Lispro (Humalog)	10–15 min	1–2 h	3–5 h
Aspart (Novolog, Novorapid)	10–15 min	1–2 h	3–5 h
Glulisine (Apidra)	10–15 min	1–2 h	3–5 h
Insulin regular (Humulin R)	30 min	2–3 h	6.5 h
Intermediate-Acting (IAI)			
Isophane (Humulin N, Novolin)	1–3 h	5–8 h	Up to 18 h
Long-Acting (LAI)			
Glargine (Lantus, Basaglar, Toujeo)	90 min	No peak	Up to 24 h
Detemir (Levemir)	90 min	No peak	16–24 h
Degludec (Tresiba)	90 min	No peak	42 h

3. **Multiple daily injection (basal-bolus) regimen**

   a. Give half TDD as LAI (basal insulin) administered once daily, and half as RAI (bolus insulin) divided equally among three meals

      E.g., 60 kg child: TDD 0.5 units/kg/day = 30 units

         Half as basal insulin = 15 units, given as LAI q24h

         Half as bolus insulin = 15 units, divided by 3 daily meals = 5 units given as RAI before each meal (may distribute differently, relative to sizes of meals, e.g., 4 units at breakfast, 5 at lunch, 6 at dinner)

4. **BID or TID regimens**

   a. Used if a child cannot administer their own insulin and no caregiver is available to administer pre-lunch insulin at school

   b. Give two-thirds TDD in morning, one-third in evening

c. Divide each dose: two-thirds IAI, one-third RAI

E.g., 30 kg child: TDD 0.5 units/kg/day = 15 units

Morning dose: ⅔ of 15 = 10 units

⅔ (7 units) as IAI before breakfast

⅓ (3 units) as RAI before breakfast

Evening dose: ⅓ of 15 = 5 units

⅔ (3.5 units) as IAI before dinner (toddler) or before bed (school-age child)

⅓ (1.5 units) as RAI before dinner

5. **Continuous subcutaneous insulin infusion (insulin pump)**

   a. Delivers RAI as continuous infusion (basal insulin), with boluses before each meal

   b. Bolus calculated using carbohydrate (CHO) ratio and insulin sensitivity factor

   c. DKA evolves quickly if insulin delivery interrupted

6. **Long-term management:** education and multidisciplinary team involvement essential

   a. Treatment can begin as outpatient, provided patient is medically stable and there are no barriers prohibiting follow-up

B. Hypoglycemia in Type 1 diabetes mellitus

1. Families should receive hypoglycemia education and keep glucagon kits at home

2. **Presentation**

   a. Mild: sweating, weakness, tachycardia, tremors, feelings of nervousness/hunger

   b. Severe: irritability, confusion, lethargy, abnormal behavior, seizure, obtundation

   c. May be asymptomatic (hypoglycemia unawareness)

3. **Management of mild hypoglycemia**

   a. Treat BG <4 mmol/L, even if asymptomatic

   b. Oral treatment preferred in an alert child who is otherwise well: 10 to 15 g CHO (e.g., 125 mL juice, 2–3 dextrose tablets, 250 mL milk or 2 teaspoons of sugar)

   c. Recheck BG in 10 to 15 min, if <4 mmol/L: repeat 10 to 15 g CHO

   d. May require mini-dose glucagon if unable to tolerate fluids (see later)

4. **Management of severe hypoglycemia**

   a. Give glucagon immediately (subcutaneous [SC] or intramuscular [IM])

   b. Avoid oral CHO until the child is awake and alert

   c. Continue monitoring BG for several hours afterward (glucagon half-life: 8–18 minutes)

5. **ED management:** (Figure 14.1); refer if
   a. Persistent hypoglycemia despite treatment
   b. Suspected prolonged hypoglycemia (LAI overdose)
   c. Ongoing hypoglycemia and not tolerating oral therapy

Figure 14.1 Emergency Department Management of Hypoglycemia in Type 1 Diabetes Mellitus

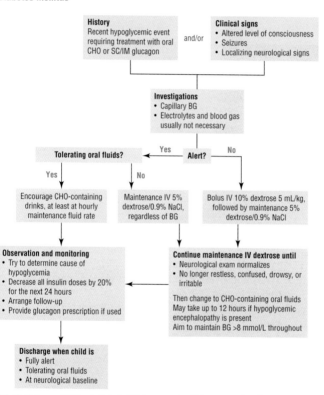

BG, Blood glucose; *CHO,* carbohydrate; *IM,* intramuscular; *IV,* intravenous; *NaCl,* sodium chloride; *SC,* subcutaneous.

6. Remind families to carry glucagon *en route* to ED
7. Recurring hypoglycemia may warrant insulin dose adjustment by diabetes team

C. Management of intercurrent illness in T1DM

1. BG may be high or low in the setting of illness
2. Check BG and urine ketones q4h, including overnight
3. Ensure fluid and calorie intake, ideally 10 g CHO per hour (can be provided as fluid)
4. Insulin doses may require adjustment (Table 14.2), but should *not* be omitted

Table 14.2	Insulin Adjustment for Illness			
BG (mmol/L) Check q4 Hourly	<6	6–14	>14	>14
Urine ketones	Negative or positive	Negative or positive	Negative or small (+)	Moderate or large (+ +)
Action	Decrease TDD by 20% until BG 6–11	Continue to monitor, give insulin as usual	Give insulin as usual plus 10% TDD as RAI	Give insulin as usual plus 20% TDD as RAI

BG, Blood glucose; *RAI*, rapid-acting insulin; *TDD*, total daily dose.

5. Consider mini-dose glucagon for mild or recurrent hypoglycemia (BG <4 mmol/L)
   a. <2 years old: 2 units (20 mcg)
   b. ≥2 years: 1 unit/year of age (e.g., 6-years-old = 6 units) to maximum 15 units (150 mcg)
   c. Double dose if initial administration does not result in BG >4 mmol/L
6. **ED management:** Figure 14.2; refer if
   a. ≥2 vomits within 6 to 8 hours
   b. Refusing oral intake
   c. Multiple doses of glucagon required

Figure 14.2   Emergency Department Management of Intercurrent Illness in Type 1 Diabetes Mellitus

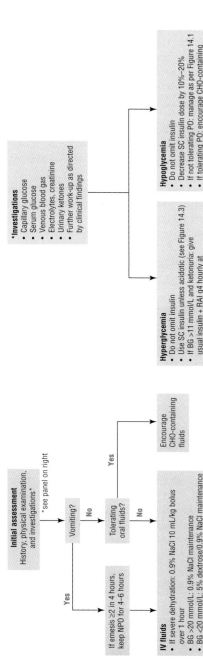

BG, blood glucose; *CHO*, carbohydrate; *KCl*, potassium chloride; *NaCl*, sodium chloride; *NPO*, nil per os (nil by mouth); *PO*, per os (by mouth); *RAI*, rapid-acting insulin; *SC*, subcutaneous; *TDD*, total daily dose.

301

D. Managing hyperglycemia on insulin pump therapy

1. **Administer insulin bolus via pump:** recheck after 2 hours; lack of response suggests insulin pump malfunction
2. **Check pump:** empty reservoir, expired insulin, error messages, dead battery; contact manufacturer for replacement if necessary
3. **Check tubing:** leaks, cracked tubing, air bubbles; change infusion set, reprime
4. **Check pump site:** leakage, dislodged catheter, cellulitis; change site
5. **Convert to insulin injections:** until pump is functioning reliably
   - a. If family has IAI: give ⅔–¾ total daily basal insulin as single IAI dose at bedtime
   - b. If family has LAI: give total daily basal insulin as single LAI dose
   - c. Total daily basal insulin = average basal pump rate × 24 hours (determine by interrogating pump settings)
   - d. Give RAI with meals and to correct hyperglycemia, according to ratios set in pump
6. Once pump issue resolved, restart basal rate 18 to 24 hours after LAI

 PEARL

Assume hyperglycemia with ketonuria reflects pump failure until proven otherwise

E. Perioperative management of Type 1 diabetes mellitus

1. Schedule as first case of the day to minimize duration of fasting
2. Monitor BG closely before and during procedure
   - a. **Hyperglycemia:** correct with insulin, especially if associated ketosis
   - b. **Hypoglycemia:** correct with oral fluids during window for clear fluids
3. **IV fluid selection**
   - a. 5% dextrose/0.9% NaCl if BG in target range of 5 to 10 mmol/L
   - b. 10% dextrose/0.9% NaCl if concerns about hypoglycemia
   - c. 0.9% NaCl if BG >14 mmol/L
   - d. Choice of IV fluid may require adjustment intraoperatively based on BG
4. Insulin adjustments for surgery are based on the patient's insulin regimen; specific recommendations should be provided by the patient's primary diabetes team for elective surgeries

DIABETIC KETOACIDOSIS

1. **Definition:** hyperglycemia (BG >11 mmol/L), detectable ketones (urine/blood), acidosis
2. **Classification**
   - a. **Mild:** pH <7.3 or HCO_3 <15 mmol/L
   - b. **Moderate:** pH <7.2 or HCO_3 <10 mmol/L
   - c. **Severe:** pH <7.1 or HCO_3 <5 mmol/L

3. **Presentation and management:** see Figure 14.3

Figure 14.3 Management of Pediatric Diabetic Ketoacidosis (DKA)

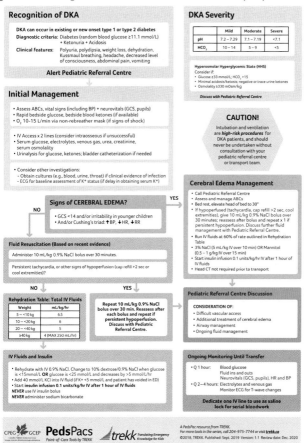

ABCs, airway breathing, circulation; *BP,* blood pressure; *CT,* computerized tomography;
ECG, electrocardiogram; *ED,* emergency department; *GCS,* Glasgow coma scale; *HR,* heart rate;
IV, intravenous; *KCl,* potassium chloride; *NaCl,* sodium chloride; *RR,* respiratory rate.
(Modified with permission from Translating Emergency Knowledge for Kids.)

4. **Useful calculations**

   a. Effective osmolarity = $2 \times$ [Na (mmol/L)] + glucose (mmol/L)

   b. Corrected sodium = measured Na + $2 \times$ [(glucose − 5.6)/5.6]

TYPE 2 DIABETES MELLITUS

1. **Definition:** hyperglycemia (see Box 14.1) associated with insulin resistance and relative impairment in insulin secretion

2. **Presentation**
   a. Polyuria, polydipsia
   b. Incidental finding: asymptomatic hyperglycemia
   c. Occasional clinical overlap with T1DM: distinguished by presence of obesity, signs/symptoms of insulin resistance (Box 14.2), and strong family history
   d. May present with DKA (less likely than T1DM) or hyperosmolar hyperglycemic state (HHS)

> **Box 14.2   Risk Factors for Type 2 Diabetes Mellitus**
>
> Obesity (BMI ≥95th percentile for age and gender)
> High-risk ethnic group (Aboriginal, African, Asian, Hispanic, Pacific Islander, or South Asian descent)
> Family history of Type 2 diabetes mellitus and/or *in utero* exposure to hyperglycemia
> Clinical evidence of insulin resistance:
> - Acanthosis nigricans
> - Hypertension
> - Dyslipidemia
> - Non-alcoholic fatty liver disease (ALT >3× upper limit of normal, or fatty liver on ultrasound)
> - Polycystic ovarian syndrome

ALT, Alanine aminotransferase; *BMI,* body mass index.

3. **Investigations:** as in T1DM
   a. Additional investigations useful to differentiate from T1DM: high fasting insulin, high C-peptide levels, absence of pancreatic autoantibodies
4. **T2DM screening:** Diabetes Canada recommends screening q2 yearly using fasting BG in children with any of
   a. ≥3 risk factors in pre-pubertal children, or ≥2 in pubertal children (see Box 14.2)
   b. Impaired fasting glucose (BG 6.1–6.9 mmol/L) or impaired glucose tolerance (BG 7.8–11 mmol/L 2 hours post-oral glucose tolerance test [OGTT])
   c. Use of atypical antipsychotic medications
5. **Management**
   a. **Non-pharmacological:** weight reduction, dietary intervention, increased physical activity to improve insulin sensitivity
   b. **Metformin:** decreases hepatic glucose production, increases insulin sensitivity
      i. Alternative oral antihyperglycemic agents not yet approved for use in children
   c. **SC insulin:** as in T1DM, particularly if HbA1c >9%
   d. **Multidisciplinary approach:** as in T1DM

A. Hyperosmolar hyperglycemic state

1. **Definition:** substantially elevated BG (>33.3 mmol/L) and hyperosmolarity (>320 mOsm/kg), often without significant ketosis or acidosis
   a. Metabolic emergency in the context of severe insulin resistance, often requires ICU-level care

2. **Presentation**
   a. Polyuria, polydipsia, severe dehydration
   b. Altered level of consciousness, seizures
   c. Clinical overlap with DKA, usually without hyperventilation, vomiting, or abdominal pain

3. **Management**
   a. Aggressive fluid resuscitation
   b. Correct electrolyte abnormalities, frequent electrolyte monitoring
   c. Insulin administration, once BG no longer improving with fluids alone

4. **Complications:** rhabdomyolysis, renal failure, deteriorating mental status, ventricular arrhythmias, thrombosis, malignant hyperthermia-like picture (rising CK and fever), death

OTHER FORMS OF DIABETES

A. Monogenic diabetes

1. Previously known as maturity-onset diabetes of the young (MODY)
2. Rare, autosomal dominant defect in pancreatic beta-cell genes
3. **Classic characteristics:** <25 years of age at diagnosis, average weight, absence of features of insulin resistance, absent β-cell autoantibodies, often multi-generational family history
4. **Treatment:** depends on specific gene affected
   a. Some forms require no treatment, others require lifestyle and diet modifications, as well as sulfonylureas or insulin

B. Medication-induced hyperglycemia

1. Many medications impair glucose tolerance by
   a. Decreasing insulin secretion
   b. Increasing hepatic glucose production
   c. Promoting insulin resistance
   d. Exerting cytotoxic effects on pancreatic β-cells
   e. Enhancing counter-regulatory responses
2. **Common causes:** corticosteroids, immunosuppressants, atypical antipsychotics
3. **Treatment:** monitoring alone versus SC or IV insulin, depending on degree of hyperglycemia and anticipated duration of medication use
   a. Adjust insulin dose as doses of hyperglycemia-inducing medication(s) are altered

HYPOGLYCEMIA

1. **Neonatal hypoglycemia:** see Chapter 27 Neonatology
2. **Non-neonatal hypoglycemia:** see Chapter 26 Metabolic Disease

> **PEARL**
>
> Determining the presence or absence of ketones is central to determining the etiology of hypoglycemia. Urine ketones may remain detectable several hours after hypoglycemia, thus a urine sample is valuable, even if a serum sample cannot be obtained (see details of critical samples required for BG <2.7; Hypoglycemia section, Chapter 26 Metabolic Disease).

THYROID DISORDERS

CONGENITAL HYPOTHYROIDISM

1. May be permanent or transient, depending on etiology
2. Asymptomatic at birth because of transplacental passage of maternal T4
3. **If untreated:** may lead to
   a. Neurodevelopmental delay
   b. Prolonged neonatal jaundice
   c. Feeding difficulties, constipation, abdominal distension, umbilical hernia
   d. Macroglossia, wide anterior fontanelle
   e. Hypotonia, hypothermia, lethargy, apneic episodes
4. **Newborn screening (NBS):** allows identification before symptoms develop
   a. All abnormal results require confirmatory serum thyroid function tests (TSH, free T4)
   b. **NBS TSH >40 mIU/L:** require prompt physician assessment, initiate treatment without delay if confirmatory testing remains abnormal
   c. **NBS TSH 15–40 mIU/L:** perform confirmatory labs, subsequent management determined by results
5. NBS programs using TSH alone may miss congenital central hypothyroidism
   a. Send TSH, free T4 if clinical suspicion for hypothyroidism despite normal NBS
6. **Further investigations:** TSH, free T4 ± thyroid radionuclide scan, ideally before or within 1 week of starting treatment
7. **Treatment:** commence thyroxine replacement promptly once diagnosis confirmed—do not delay to accommodate imaging
   a. **Levothyroxine:** once daily as tablet (Table 14.3)
   b. **Dose adjustment:** if TSH >5 mIU/L or <0.5 mIU/L
   c. Cognitive function unlikely to be impacted if treatment initiated by 10 days of age

Table 14.3	Levothyroxine Starting Dose Recommendations
Age	**Dose (mcg/kg/day)**
0–6 months	10–15
6–12 months	6–10
1–5 years	5–7
6–12 years	3–5
>12 years	2–3
Adult	1.7

8. **Monitoring:** free T4, TSH, and growth
   a. Two weeks after starting treatment
   b. At 2, 3, 6, 9, 12 months of age
   c. Every 6 months from 1 to 3 years of age
   d. Yearly after 3 years
   e. Check TSH 4 to 6 weeks after any dose adjustment

 PEARL

Stable suspensions of levothyroxine do not exist. Do not prescribe liquid—crush tablets and mix with breastmilk/formula instead.

ACQUIRED HYPOTHYROIDISM

1. **Primary hypothyroidism**
   a. Hashimoto (lymphocytic) thyroiditis: most common cause in North American youth
      i. Female:male ratio 4:1
      ii. High risk with trisomy 21, Turner, DiGeorge, and Williams syndromes, other autoimmune diseases, e.g., T1DM, celiac disease, first-degree relatives with autoimmune thyroiditis
   b. Iodine deficiency: most common cause worldwide
   c. Iodine excess
   d. Medications, e.g., lithium, amiodarone, antiepileptic drugs, tyrosine kinase inhibitors
   e. Thyroid injury, e.g., following therapeutic radiation
2. **Central hypothyroidism**
   a. Hypothalamic/pituitary tumors
   b. Congenital variant, e.g., septo-optic dysplasia
   c. Infiltrative processes, e.g., Langerhans cell histiocytosis
   d. Central nervous system (CNS) trauma/surgery
   e. Sequelae of craniospinal radiation

3. **Presentation:** see Box 14.3

Box 14.3	Clinical Manifestations of Hypothyroidism
Lethargy, somnolence	Diffuse goiter
Constipation	Sinus bradycardia
Linear growth failure	Proximal muscle weakness
Delayed or precocious puberty	Delayed relaxation of deep tendon reflexes
Cold intolerance; cool, dry extremities	Dry skin, hair, myxedema

4. **Investigations**
   a. **TSH:** sole recommended screening test for primary hypothyroidism
   b. **Free T4:** request if TSH outside reference range, congenital hypothyroidism or suspicion for central hypothyroidism
   c. **Anti-TPO antibodies:** if suspecting autoimmune thyroid disease
   d. **MRI brain:** if new central hypothyroidism in child without known risk factors
   e. **Thyroid US:** not routine; consider only if thyroid asymmetry on exam, cervical lymphadenopathy or palpable nodule
5. **Diagnosis**
   a. **Primary hypothyroidism:** ↑ TSH with ↓ free T4
   b. **Subclinical hypothyroidism:** ↑ TSH with normal free T4
      i. Repeat mildly ↑ TSH values (5–10 mIU/L) after at least 4 weeks, as spontaneous normalization is common
      ii. Typically does not merit treatment unless clearly attributable symptoms
   c. **Central hypothyroidism:** ↓ or inappropriately normal TSH, ↓ free T4 or progressively declining free T4 following CNS insult
6. **Treatment:** levothyroxine (see Table 14.3)
   a. Initiate when TSH >10 mIU/L and low free T4; consider earlier based on free T4 level and presence of attributable symptoms
7. **Goals of treatment**
   a. **Primary hypothyroidism:** normalize TSH
   b. **Central hypothyroidism:** free T4 within upper half of reference range; not useful to follow TSH

THYROTOXICOSIS

1. **Etiology**
   a. Graves' disease: most common cause
   b. Hashitoxicosis: Hashimoto thyroiditis with early thyrotoxic phase
   c. Subacute thyroiditis: usually viral
   d. Suppurative thyroiditis: bacterial or viral
   e. Toxic adenoma: autonomously functioning solitary nodule
   f. Amiodarone-induced
   g. Toxic multinodular goiter: rare in children

2. **Presentation:** see Box 14.4

Box 14.4	Clinical Manifestations of Hyperthyroidism

Anxiety
Palpitations
Hypertension
Fatigue, weakness
Sweating, heat intolerance
Tremor

Insomnia
Increased appetite
Frequent stools
Weight loss
Exophthalmos
Goiter

3. **Investigations**
   a. ↓ TSH, ↑ free T4
   b. T3: not part of initial workup; consider if free T4 normal in the setting of ↓ TSH
   c. Thyrotropin receptor antibody (TRAb) or thyroid stimulating antibody (TSI) titers
   d. Radioactive iodine uptake and scan: consider if TRAb/TSI not elevated, or palpable nodule present
      i. High diffuse uptake: Graves'
      ii. Localized uptake: toxic nodule
      iii. Low/absent uptake: Hashitoxicosis or other forms of thyroiditis

4. **Medical management**
   a. **Methimazole:** first-line anti-thyroid drug (ATD); adjust initial dose based on free T4 or T3 levels
   b. **Propylthiouracil:** may be useful in thyroid storm; black box warning in children because of risk of fulminant hepatic failure
   c. **Propranolol:** if significant symptoms, particularly at onset of ATD therapy
   d. **Remission rate:** up to 30% after 2 years with medical management (lower than adults)

5. **Monitoring**
   a. Before starting ATDs: CBC, ALT
   b. Side effects of both ATDs: idiosyncratic; include agranulocytosis, lupus-like syndrome, jaundice, rashes
   c. Check CBC if patient is febrile or develops pharyngitis/stomatitis while on ATDs

GRAVES' DISEASE

1. **Autoimmune pathogenesis:** TSIs bind to TSH-receptors, leading to autonomous production of thyroid hormone; associated with other forms of autoimmunity

2. **Presentation:** see Box 14.4
   a. Associated ophthalmopathy in ⅓ children: usually less severe than in adults, without vision loss; improves when remission achieved

3. **Highest incidence:** adolescent females

4. **Medical management:** as earlier
   a. If low-dose methimazole is effectively controlling thyroid function without side effects, prolonged ATD therapy may be considered
5. **Definitive management**
   a. **¹³¹I (radioactive iodine) therapy:** remission may take weeks/months, ongoing ATD often required until hypothyroidism achieved
      i. Avoid <10 years of age or in pregnancy
   b. **Thyroidectomy:** immediate control of hyperthyroidism
      i. Surgical risks: hypocalcemia because of hypoparathyroidism, recurrent laryngeal nerve palsy

CALCIUM DISORDERS

HYPOCALCEMIA

1. **Normal calcium range:** see Chapter 39 Laboratory Reference Values
2. **Relevant history:** see Table 14.4

Table 14.4	Relevant History in Hypocalcemia
Features from History	**Diagnosis to Consider**
Congenital anomalies Developmental delay	DiGeorge (22q11.2 deletion) syndrome
Neck surgery/trauma	Surgical/traumatic hypoparathyroidism
Dietary limitations, decreased sunlight exposure	Vitamin D deficiency
Gastrointestinal, hepatobiliary, or pancreatic disease	Decreased calcium or vitamin D absorption
Renal disease	Increased calcium excretion
Positive family history	Hypocalcemic genetic disorders

3. **Presentation**
   a. Tetany, muscle cramps, carpopedal spasm (Trousseau sign), facial twitch (Chvostek sign), acral paresthesias, numbness, seizures, papilledema
   b. Laryngeal stridor
   c. ECG abnormalities, e.g., prolonged QT, widened T-waves, bradycardia
   d. Psychiatric manifestations
4. **Differential diagnosis:** see Hypocalcemia in Chapter 27 Neonatology (neonates), and Box 14.5 (infants and children)

Box 14.5 Differential Diagnosis of Hypocalcemia in Infants and Children

Hypoparathyroidism
- Genetic, e.g., late presentation of DiGeorge syndrome
- Autoimmune polyglandular syndrome type 1
- Injury to parathyroid glands because of surgery, iron deposition, radiation
- Idiopathic

Defect in calcium-sensing receptor (autosomal dominant)
Pseudo-hypoparathyroidism, i.e., end-organ resistance to parathyroid hormone
Vitamin D deficiency, resistance or impaired synthesis
Hyperphosphatemia, e.g., tumor lysis syndrome
Hypomagnesemia
Drugs, e.g., bisphosphonates, some chemotherapeutic drugs, calcimimetics
Pancreatitis

Modified from Sperling M. *Pediatric Endocrinology*. 4th ed. Philadelphia, PA: WB Saunders; 2014.

5. **Investigations**
   a. Ca, albumin, iCa, PO_4, Mg, ALP, PTH, 25-(OH)-vitamin D, spot urine calcium:creatinine ratio, renal function
   b. 1,25-$(OH)_2$-vitamin D should not be performed during initial workup
6. **Diagnosis:** see Table 14.5

Table 14.5 Laboratory Findings in Hypocalcemia

Diagnosis	Ca	PO$_4$	25-(OH)-D$_3$	1,25-(OH)$_2$-D$_3$	PTH	ALP
Vitamin D deficiency	↓	N or ↓	↓	N or ↑	↑	↑↑↑
Hypoparathyroidism	↓	↑	N	↓	↓[a]	N or ↑
Pseudo-hypoparathyroidism	↓	↑	N	↓	↑	↑

[a]Or inappropriately normal in the setting of hypocalcemia

ALP, Alkaline phosphatase; *Ca*, calcium; *N*, normal; *PO$_4$*, phosphate; *PTH*, parathyroid hormone.
Data from Alario A. *Practical Guide to the Care of the Pediatric Patient*. St. Louis, MO: Mosby; 1997.

7. **Management**
   a. **Oral calcium supplementation:** calcium carbonate
      i. Effective monotherapy in mild hypocalcemia
      ii. May require doses exceeding recommended daily intake
   b. **Cholecalciferol:** 25-(OH)-vitamin D
      i. Treat vitamin D deficiency, even if not thought to be the cause of hypocalcemia
      ii. May require IM formulation if concern for fat malabsorption

c. **Alfacalcidol** (1α-(OH)-vitamin D) or **Calcitriol** (1,25-(OH)$_2$-vitamin D): active form of vitamin D
   i. Required in conditions associated with defects in vitamin D activation, e.g., renal disease, hypoparathyroidism
   ii. Often used in settings of severe hypocalcemia, even if defective vitamin D activation not suspected
d. **Calcium infusion:** for severe and/or symptomatic hypocalcemia (e.g., seizures, arrhythmia) or inability to use oral treatment
   i. Central venous access preferred due to risk of severe extravasation injuries, e.g., tissue necrosis, burns, venous thrombosis; lower risk with calcium gluconate than calcium chloride
   ii. Never give IV calcium bolus, because of risk of rebound hypocalcemia
   iii. Monitor levels q4h until stable: aim for total Ca >2 mmol/L, and/or iCa >1 mmol/L; wean as tolerated; repeat bloodwork 4 to 6 hours after any change in rate
   iv. During infusion: monitor cardiac rhythm, IV site
   v. Incompatible solutions: sodium bicarbonate and ceftriaxone; never infuse ceftriaxone with calcium, even in different IV lines, because of risk of potentially fatal calcium-ceftriaxone precipitates in lungs and kidneys

14

> ⭐ **PEARL**
>
> Plasma calcium concentration falls by 0.2 mmol/L for every 10 g/L fall in plasma albumin—measure iCa if serum protein or pH is abnormal.

HYPERCALCEMIA

1. **Definition:** total calcium above upper limit of reference range for age, once corrected for albumin, i.e., Ca >2.64 (<1 year), >2.54 (1–18 years), or iCa >1.37 mmol/L
2. **Presentation**
   a. Nonspecific weakness, hypotonia, mental status changes
   b. Abdominal pain, bone pain
   c. Hematuria (nephrolithiasis), polyuria
   d. Neonates: poor feeding, jittery, increased urine output; assess for subcutaneous fat necrosis, especially if history of instrument-assisted delivery
3. **Differential diagnosis:** see Table 14.6
4. **Investigations**
   a. Serum total Ca, albumin, iCa, PO$_4$
   b. PTH, 25-(OH)-vitamin D, renal function

c. Spot urine calcium:creatinine ratio
d. Consider 1,25-$(OH)_2$-vitamin D level if PTH suppressed/low-normal, or if suspicion for systemic inflammatory process (e.g., sarcoidosis) or malignancy

Table 14.6	Differential Diagnosis of Hypercalcemia	
↑ Intestinal Ca Absorption	↑ Bone Resorption	Other

Increased Ca intake
Hypervitaminosis D
Granulomatous disease
- Sarcoidosis
- Subcutaneous fat
  necrosis (neonates)
	Maternal hypoparathyroidism
	  (neonates)
	Hyperparathyroidism
	- Parathyroid adenoma/
	  hyperplasia
	- Genetic, e.g., MEN,
	  McCune-Albright syndrome
	Hyperthyroidism
	Hypervitaminosis A
	Malignancy
	- Paraneoplastic PTH-related
	  peptide production
	- Bony metastases
		Drugs
		- Thiazide diuretics
		- Lithium
		Phosphate depletion
		Idiopathic infantile
		  hypercalcemia
		Familial hypocalciuric
		  hypercalcemia
		Primary adrenal
		  insufficiency
		Renal failure
		Rhabdomyolysis
		Immobilization
		Total parenteral nutrition

MEN, Multiple endocrine neoplasia; *PTH,* parathyroid hormone.

5. **Management**
   a. Hold vitamin D, calcium supplements
   b. **Formula-fed infants:** switch to low-calcium formula
   c. **Hyperhydration:** IV fluids at 2 to 3 times maintenance, if normal renal function
   d. **If no improvement in 12 to 24 hours:** consider bisphosphonate ± subcutaneous calcitonin (use limited to 2–3 days, because of tachyphylaxis)
   e. **Steroids:** inhibit hydroxylation of 25-(OH)-vitamin D; may be useful in circumstances of increased 1,25-$(OH)_2$-vitamin D production, e.g., subcutaneous fat necrosis, sarcoidosis

PUBERTY

NORMAL PUBERTAL DEVELOPMENT

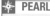 **PEARL**

Puberty is defined by the appearance of a palpable breast bud in females and enlargement of testes ≥4 mL (2.5 cm long axis) in males.

1. **Definition:** see Tables 14.7 and 14.8

Table 14.7		**Normal Pubertal Development**	
		Female	**Male**
Age of onset (years)	Average	10.5	11.5
	Range	8–13	9–14
Stage	1	Thelarche: development of breast tissue	Increased testicular volume: >4 mL
	2	Pubarche: appearance of pubic hair	Pubarche: appearance of pubic hair
	3	Growth spurt: 8–14 cm/year	Elongation of penis
	4	Menarche: first menstrual bleed, approximately 2 years after thelarche	Growth spurt: 8–14 cm/year

Table 14.8	**Tanner Staging**		
	Male	**Female**	**Both Sexes**
Stage	**Genital Development**	**Breast Development**	**Pubic Hair**
I	Prepubertal: testes, scrotum, and penis as in early childhood	Prepubertal: papillary elevation only	Prepubertal: no pubic hair
II	Enlargement of scrotum and testes	Breast bud stage: elevation of breast and papilla	Sparse growth of downy hair at base of penis/along labia
III	Penile lengthening, further growth of testes and scrotum	Further enlargement and elevation of breast and areola	Darker, coarser, more curled; spreads over junction of pubes
IV	Increased breadth of penis, development of glans; scrotal skin darkened	Projection of areola and papilla to form a secondary mound	Adult-type hair, no spreading to medial surface of thighs
V	Adult genitalia	Adult breast: projection of papilla only, areola within general contour of breast	Adult quantity and type; spreading to medial surface of thighs

PRECOCIOUS PUBERTY

1. **Definition:** onset of puberty 2 to 2.5 standard deviations before population average, i.e., thelarche before age 8 years in females, testicular enlargement before age 9 years in males
   a. **Ethnic variation common:** earlier onset of puberty may be typical
2. **History**
   a. **Secondary sexual characteristics:** breast development, pubic hair, facial hair, testicular enlargement, penile enlargement
   b. **Growth velocity:** measured as cm/year
   c. **Family history:** pubertal timing of parents and siblings

d. **Red flags:** changes in behavior or vision, headaches, seizures, history of CNS disease/radiation, head trauma, abdominal pain, exposure to exogenous sex steroids (e.g., oral contraceptives, testosterone gel)

3. **Physical:** height, weight, Tanner stage, acne, facial/axillary hair, body odor

4. **Differential diagnosis:** see Table 14.9
   a. Precocious puberty less common in males, more likely to be associated with underlying pathology
   b. Isosexual pubertal changes occurring in sequence: most likely central in origin
   c. Out of sequence isosexual or contrasexual pubertal changes: more likely peripheral

Table 14.9	Differential Diagnosis of Precocious Puberty	
Normal Variants	**Central (Gonadotropin-Dependent)**	**Peripheral (Gonadotropin-Independent)**
Premature thelarche Premature adrenarche	Idiopathic (most common in females) CNS malformation, trauma or tumor CNS infection CNS radiation Genetic/familial Previous sex steroid exposure	CAH Exogenous sex-steroid exposure Ovarian cyst/tumor Testosterone-producing tumor (e.g., Leydig cell tumor, adrenal adenoma or carcinoma) hCG-producing tumor (e.g., germinoma, teratoma, hepatoblastoma) Familial male-limited precocious puberty Severe hypothyroidism McCune-Albright syndrome

CAH, Congenital adrenal hyperplasia; *CNS*, central nervous system; *hCG*, human chorionic gonadotropin.

Modified from Sperling M. *Pediatric Endocrinology*. 4th ed. Philadelphia, PA: WB Saunders; 2014.

5. **Investigations**
   a. **LH:** ≥0.3 IU/L predicts progression of central puberty within 6 months; <0.3 IU/L suggests peripheral etiology (or benign variant)
   b. **FSH:** may be helpful, but elevated levels not specific for central puberty
   c. **Testosterone** or **estradiol**
   d. **17-OHP, androstenedione, DHEAS:** if male patient or female with evidence of androgenization
   e. **TSH**
   f. **Bone age**
   g. **Pelvic and abdominal US (in females):** if low FSH, LH or estrogen elevated for age

h. **MRI sella turcica:** if diagnosis of central precocious puberty suspected or established; particularly if <6 years at pubertal onset or where pubertal timing is out of keeping with ethnicity and family history

6. **Management**
   a. Treat underlying cause, if identified
   b. **Central precocious puberty:** consider GnRH analogues, e.g., leuprolide
   c. **Peripheral precocious puberty:** treatment varies with cause, consider aromatase inhibitors

7. **Goals of treatment**
   a. Optimize final adult height: limited/no benefit if treatment started after age 8 years
   b. Psychosocial: ensure age-appropriate sexual/behavioural maturation

DELAYED PUBERTY

1. **Females:** lack of breast development by age 13 years, primary amenorrhea by age 16 years or 2 years post-thelarche
2. **Males:** lack of testicular enlargement by age 14 years
3. **Clinical evaluation:** as for precocious puberty, plus
   a. Diet, exercise intensity, weight changes, chronic medical illness
   b. Midline defects, cryptorchidism, skeletal abnormalities, anosmia
   c. History of alkylating chemotherapy or cranial/craniospinal radiation
   d. Features of Turner or Klinefelter syndromes (see Selected Genetic Conditions in Chapter 18 Genetics and Teratology)
4. **Differential diagnosis**
   a. Constitutional delay of growth and puberty: more common in males
   b. Functional hypogonadotropic hypogonadism: may be related to chronic illness, nutritional state, hypothyroidism, vigorous exercise
   c. Syndromic hypogonadotropic hypogonadism: e.g., Kallmann syndrome (anosmia), Prader-Willi, CHARGE, Noonan syndrome
   d. Damage to hypothalamic-pituitary-gonadal axis: CNS tumor or radiation
   e. Hyperprolactinemia
   f. Idiopathic hypogonadotropic hypogonadism
   g. Hypergonadotropic hypogonadism (primary gonadal failure): Klinefelter syndrome, Turner syndrome, autoimmune ovarian failure, gonadal dysgenesis, alkylating chemotherapy, gonadal radiation
   h. Delayed puberty less common in females, more likely to be pathological
5. **Investigations**
   a. **LH, FSH:** ↑in primary gonadal failure; ↓in central hypogonadism
   b. **Testosterone** or **estradiol**
   c. **Bone age**
   d. **Prolactin, TSH**

e. **Karyotype**

f. **Pelvic US (in females):** if ↑LH, FSH; to determine presence/absence of internal/Mullerian structures

g. **Brain MRI:** if ↓LH, FSH; to assess for hypothalamic or pituitary disease

6. **Management**

a. Treat underlying cause, if identified

b. **Watchful waiting:** for constitutional delay

c. **Induction of puberty:** sex steroid replacement; may be required transiently or life-long, depending on underlying etiology

   i. Males: IM testosterone q2 or 4 weekly

   ii. Females: PO or transdermal estradiol, with addition of progesterone (as Provera) after 1 to 2 years or if menstruation begins

DISORDERS OF SEX DEVELOPMENT

1. **Definition:** congenital conditions in which the development of chromosomal, gonadal, or anatomic sex is atypical

2. **Classification:** see Table 14.10

Table 14.10	Classification of Disorders of Sex Development	
	Sex Chromosome DSD	**46 XY DSD**	**46 XX DSD**
Causes	45 X: Turner syndrome 47 XXY: Klinefelter syndrome 45 X/46 XY: mixed gonadal dysgenesis, ovotesticular DSD 46 XX/46 XY: chimeric, ovotesticular DSD	Disorders of gonadal (testicular) development Disorders of androgen synthesis/action - Enzyme defect in adrenal steroid synthesis - Leydig cell dysgenesis/agenesis 5α-reductase deficiency Complete/partial androgen insensitivity	Disorders of gonadal (ovarian) development Androgen excess - Congenital adrenal hyperplasia - Maternal androgen exposure - Maternal virilizing tumors
Details	Often have mix of streak gonad, ovarian or testicular tissue	Testes present, location may vary	Account for up to 70% DSD

DSD, Disorders of sex development.

Adapted from Hughes IA et al. Consensus statement on management of intersex disorders. *Arch Dis Child.* 2006;91:554–562.

3. **Clinical evaluation**

a. **Antenatal:** prenatal androgen exposure, maternal virilization and medication use, antenatal US including details about infant sex

b. **Neonatal:** feeding difficulty, poor weight gain, vomiting, lethargy

c. **Family:** unexplained infant death, spontaneous abortions, consanguinity, family history of atypical genitalia, parental ethnicity

d. **Physical:** appearance of genitalia, presence of palpable gonads (including inguinal canal), other anomalies or dysmorphic features

e. **Features suggestive of disorders of sex development (DSD)**

   i. Apparent female genitalia with clitoral enlargement (>1 cm in term newborn), posterior labial fusion, inguinal/labial mass

   ii. Apparent male genitalia with bilateral undescended testes, micropenis, isolated perineal hypospadias or mild hypospadias with undescended testis

4. **Investigations**

   a. **Newborn screening results:** review

   b. **Karyotype and fluorescent in situ hybridization (FISH) for SRY:** expedite

   c. **Abdominal and pelvic US:** presence of uterus, vagina, gonads, anomalies of urinary tract, adrenal glands (pathognomonic "cerebriform" appearance in CAH)

   d. **Within first 3 days of life:** 17-OHP, androstenedione, testosterone, dihydrotestosterone, estradiol, FSH, LH, serum electrolytes (normal electrolytes do not exclude salt-wasting CAH)

5. **Management principles**

   a. **Psychosocial emergency:** expedite investigations and consult tertiary care center with multidisciplinary team (pediatrician/pediatric endocrinologist, urologist, gynecologist, geneticist, social worker)

   b. **Delay gender assignment:** (including name selection) until investigations and expert evaluation completed; encourage terms such as "the baby" rather than "he/she"

CONGENITAL ADRENAL HYPERPLASIA

1. Most common DSD in females

2. **Etiology:** autosomal recessive defects in enzymes involved in adrenal steroidogenesis

   a. All forms associated with cortisol deficiency

   b. Depending on enzyme involved, may have mineralocorticoid (aldosterone) and/or adrenal androgen deficiency/excess

   c. ↑ ACTH secretion may cause hyperpigmentation and adrenal hyperplasia

3. **21-hydroxylase deficiency:** most common defect

   a. Impaired glucocorticoid and mineralocorticoid synthesis with accumulation of biosynthetic precursors (17-OHP), which are instead shunted into androgen synthesis pathways, leading to virilization

   b. Three subtypes

      i. **Severe (salt-wasting) congenital adrenal hyperplasia (CAH):** impaired cortisol and mineralocorticoid production; hyponatremia, hyperkalemia, hypoglycemia, dehydration, acidosis, vascular collapse

ii. **Simple virilizing CAH:** inadequate cortisol production, adequate mineralocorticoid activity without salt-wasting

iii. **Non-classic CAH:** later onset, milder form; present with virilization only (overlap with PCOS in adolescents) or infertility

4. **Investigations**

a. **17-OHP, androstenedione, testosterone:** all increased in 21-hydroxylase deficiency

i. Different precursors elevated in other forms of CAH

b. **Serum 17-OHP:** unreliable <36 hours of age

i. **False positive:** preterm, low birthweight infants, perinatal stress

ii. **False negative:** possible if mother received antenatal steroids

c. **Serum electrolytes:** typically normal before day 5 to 7 of life in salt-wasting CAH

d. **Karyotype:** consider for phenotypic males if suspicion for severe CAH (may be virilized female)

5. **Management**

a. Glucocorticoid $\pm$ mineralocorticoid replacement

b. Salt (NaCl) supplementation often required in neonatal period

c. Management of intercurrent illness: see next section on Adrenal Insufficiency

ADRENAL DISORDERS

ADRENAL INSUFFICIENCY

1. **Etiology:** see Box 14.6

Box 14.6   Etiology of Adrenal Insufficiency

Primary Adrenal Insufficiency
Congenital: congenital adrenal hyperplasia, adrenal hypoplasia congenita
Autoimmune: Addison disease, autoimmune polyglandular syndromes
ACTH resistance syndromes: triple A syndrome, familial glucocorticoid deficiencies
Infection: sepsis, tuberculosis, viral, fungal
X-linked adrenoleukodystrophy
Disorders of cholesterol metabolism: Smith-Lemli-Opitz syndrome
Mitochondrial: Kearns-Sayre syndrome
Amyloidosis
Adrenal hemorrhage: Waterhouse-Friderichsen syndrome
Drugs inhibiting steroid biosynthesis, e.g., mitotane, ketoconazole

Secondary Adrenal Insufficiency
Prolonged glucocorticoid therapy
Hypothalamic/pituitary tumors, surgery, radiation
Congenital hypopituitarism
Isolated ACTH deficiency

ACTH, Adrenocorticotropic hormone.
Modified from Sperling M. *Pediatric Endocrinology.* 4th ed. Philadelphia, PA: WB Saunders; 2014.

2. **Presentation:** insidious onset, may have symptoms for months before diagnosis
   a. Anorexia, weight loss
   b. Nausea, vomiting, abdominal pain
   c. Hypoglycemia
   d. Slowing of linear growth
   e. Muscle weakness, fatigue
   f. Hypotension (orthostatic), dizziness
   g. Skin and mucous membrane hyperpigmentation
   h. **Adrenal crisis:** acute onset or exacerbation of insufficiency with electrolyte abnormalities, metabolic acidosis and hypotensive shock
3. **Investigations:** see Table 14.11
   a. Electrolytes, urea, creatinine
   b. Morning cortisol (8 a.m.), ACTH
   c. Confirmation: ACTH stimulation test

Table 14.11	Laboratory Findings in Adrenal Insufficiency	
	Primary AI	**Secondary AI**
Etiology	Adrenal failure	Decreased ACTH release because of impaired synthesis or exogenous suppression
Cortisol	↓	↓
ACTH	↑	↓
Mineralocorticoid deficiency	May be present	Never present

ACTH, Adrenocorticotropic hormone; *AI,* adrenal insufficiency.

4. **Long-term management**
   a. **Hydrocortisone:** divided BID or TID
   b. **Fludrocortisone:** if mineralocorticoid-deficient
   c. **Sodium supplements:** for salt-wasting phenotypes in infancy
5. **Management of adrenal crisis**
   a. **Fluid resuscitation**
   b. **IV hydrocortisone:** 100 mg/m^2 (max. dose 100 mg), followed by 25 mg/m^2 (max. 25 mg) q6h × 24 hours or until patient is stable
   c. **Monitor BG:** treat as needed
   d. Fludrocortisone "stress-dose" not required
   e. Treat underlying illness

6. **Management of intercurrent illnesses**
   a. Additional "stress-dose" hydrocortisone required for
      i. Febrile illness
      ii. Vomiting or diarrhea
      iii. Drowsiness or decreased energy
   b. **Hydrocortisone stress-dosing:** 40 mg/m^2/day divided q8h until symptoms resolve
   c. No change to fludrocortisone dose
   d. Significant vomiting, diarrhea or inability to tolerate oral meds requires admission for IV hydrocortisone
   e. **IM hydrocortisone:** may be required in emergency situations, home supply can be given by family or emergency services
7. **Management during anesthesia**
   a. **Minor procedures:** 40 mg/m^2 IV hydrocortisone once at induction of anesthesia
   b. **Major procedures:** 100 mg/m^2 (max. 100 mg) IV hydrocortisone at induction, then 25 mg/m^2 q6h $\times$ 24 to 48 hours

CUSHING SYNDROME

1. **Definition:** clinical syndrome associated with glucocorticoid excess
2. **Etiology**
   a. Iatrogenic (most common): because of prolonged supraphysiological glucocorticoid exposure, including topical/inhaled steroids
   b. ACTH-producing pituitary tumor: Cushing disease
   c. Tumors producing ectopic ACTH or corticotropin-releasing hormone
   d. Adrenocortical adenomas, carcinomas (very rare)
3. **Presentation**
   a. Hypertension
   b. Hyperglycemia, glucose intolerance, weight gain
   c. Slowing of linear growth, delayed sexual development
   d. Increased facial and abdominal fat stores, supraclavicular fat pad
   e. Osteoporosis
   f. Wasting of extremities, proximal muscle weakness
   g. Menstrual irregularities
   h. Signs of adrenal androgen excess: hirsutism, oily skin, acne to face, neck, shoulders $\pm$ hyperpigmentation
   i. Skin: violaceous striae, bruising, skin thinning, acanthosis nigricans, facial plethora

4. **Screening investigations**
   a. 24-hour urinary free cortisol
   b. Midnight salivary cortisol
   c. Perform at least twice, as hypercortisolism can be variable
5. **Diagnosis:** dexamethasone suppression test
   a. Give 1 mg dexamethasone between 10 p.m. and midnight, measure next day early-morning cortisol
   b. Normal response: serum cortisol <50 nmol/L
   c. If abnormal: refer to endocrinologist to confirm diagnosis and etiology
6. **Management**
   a. Treat underlying cause
   b. If caused by exogenous steroids: wean gradually; stress-dosing may be required during intercurrent illness

SHORT STATURE

1. **Definition:** height ≥2 standard deviations below mean (<2.5 percentile)
   a. Normal growth parameters: see Assessment of Growth in Chapter 19 Growth and Nutrition
2. **Differential diagnosis:** may be normal variant or pathological (Table 14.12)

Table 14.12	Differential Diagnosis of Short Stature		
Onset	**Differential**		
Prenatal	IUGR: placental disease, congenital infection, teratogens, e.g., ethanol, medications		
	Chromosomal disorders, e.g., Turner syndrome, trisomy 21		
	Syndromic, e.g., Russell-Silver syndrome		
Postnatal	Disproportionate growth	Skeletal dysplasia, e.g., achondroplasia	
		Rickets	
	Proportionate growth	Normal growth velocity	Constitutional growth delay (bone age < chronological age)
			Familial short stature (bone age = chronological age)
			Idiopathic short stature (diagnosis of exclusion)
		Abnormal growth velocity	Chronic disease, e.g., GI, renal, cardiac, malignancy
			Malnutrition/malabsorption
			Endocrinopathies: hypothyroidism, GH deficiency, glucocorticoid excess
			Psychosocial short stature
			Drugs, e.g., steroids
			Genetic, e.g., Prader-Willi, Noonan syndrome

GH, Growth hormone; *GI*, gastrointestinal; *IUGR*, intrauterine growth restriction.

14

3. **Clinical evaluation**
   a. **History:** prenatal insults, birth weight, features of underlying systemic, genetic or endocrine disease, nutritional intake, symptoms of malabsorption or GI inflammation, pubertal changes
   b. **Growth velocity:** review longitudinal growth charts
   c. **Family history:** parental heights, pubertal timing
   d. **Mid-parental height (cm):** ½ [mother's height + father's height + 13 (males) **OR** − 13 (females)]
   e. **Physical examination:** height, weight, pubertal stage, dysmorphic features
   f. Psychosocial burden of short stature
4. **Investigations:** based on history and physical; see Table 14.13

Table 14.13	Investigation of Short Stature
Investigation	**Possible Etiology**
CBC, ESR	Chronic disease, e.g., IBD
IGF-1	GH deficiency
TSH	Hypothyroidism
Creatinine	Renal disease
Anti-TTG, IgA	Celiac disease
Karyotype in females	Turner syndrome
LH/FSH if signs of sexual precocity	Precocious puberty
Bone age x-ray	May differentiate between constitutional delay, familial short statue, precocious puberty

CBC, Complete blood count; *ESR,* erythrocyte sedimentation rate; *FSH,* follicle stimulating hormone; *GH,* growth hormone; *IBD,* inflammatory bowel disease; *IgA,* immunoglobulin A; *IGF-1,* insulin-like growth factor 1; *LH,* luteinizing hormone; *TSH,* thyroid stimulating hormone; *TTG,* tissue transglutaminase.

GROWTH HORMONE DEFICIENCY

1. **Congenital growth hormone (GH) deficiency**
   a. Birth length normal or slightly reduced: insulin, not GH, is the primary antenatal growth factor
   b. Growth failure may not be obvious until 3 years or later
   c. May have history of hypoglycemia, micropenis, prolonged neonatal jaundice
   d. Assess for midline defects (hypopituitarism); hypoglycemia more pronounced if concomitant ACTH deficiency

2. **Acquired GH deficiency**
   a. Growth failure
   b. Delayed bone age
   c. Slow growth velocity for age
   d. Increased weight/height ratio
   e. Immature "cherubic" face, infantile voice
   f. Most common pituitary deficiency following cranial radiation
3. **Investigations:** as in Table 14.13
   a. Exclude other causes of growth failure (see Table 14.12)
   b. Evaluate for other pituitary hormone deficiencies: TSH, free T4, cortisol, prolactin, sodium, urine specific gravity if GH deficiency suspected/demonstrated
   c. May require referral for dynamic GH testing
4. **Indications for GH treatment**
   a. GH deficiency
   b. Small for gestational age with failure to catch-up by age 3 years
   c. Chronic renal failure
   d. Turner, Noonan, Prader-Willi syndromes
   e. Idiopathic short stature (controversial)
   f. No benefit in trisomy 21, most skeletal dysplasias
5. **Risks of GH treatment**
   a. Benign intracranial hypertension
   b. Slipped capital femoral epiphyses
   c. Progression of scoliosis
   d. Transaminitis
   e. Glucose intolerance, may progress to medication-induced diabetes
   f. Increase in growth and pigmentation of nevi
   g. No evidence for increasing risk of malignancy: avoid during active treatment for malignancy and for ≥1 year following treatment

DISORDERS OF WATER BALANCE

DIABETES INSIPIDUS
1. **Central:** defect in vasopressin synthesis and/or secretion; 90% of pediatric DI
2. **Nephrogenic:** see Tubular Disorders in Chapter 28 Nephrology and Urology
3. **Etiology:** see Table 14.14

Table 14.14	Etiology of Diabetes Insipidus	
Central	**Nephrogenic**
Genetic	Genetic
Infiltrative disease, e.g., LCH	Drug-induced, e.g., lithium, amphotericin
Neoplasm, e.g., germinoma	Renal failure
CNS trauma/surgery	Obstructive uropathy
CNS infection	Fanconi syndrome
Midline brain defects	Sickle cell disease/trait
	Sarcoidosis

CNS, Central nervous system; *LCH*, Langerhans cell histiocytosis.

4. **Presentation**
   a. **Polyuria:** >2 L/m^2/day, dilute urine
   b. **Dehydration, hypernatremia:** if no access to water or impaired thirst, e.g., hypothalamic injury
   c. $\pm$ failure to thrive
5. **Investigations**
   a. **Serum:** osmolality, glucose, Na, K, Ca
   b. **Urine:** osmolality $\pm$ specific gravity, glucose
6. **Consider differential diagnosis for polyuria**
   a. Primary polydipsia: keep fluid intake diary
   b. Hyperglycemia, hypercalcemia
   c. Diuresis post-renal injury or urinary tract obstruction
   d. Increased GFR, e.g., hyperthyroidism, febrile illness
   e. Medications, e.g., diuretics
   f. Fanconi syndrome
7. **Diagnosis**
   a. Serum osmolality >300 with urine <300 mOsm/kg = highly suspicious for DI
   b. Serum osmolality <270 or urine >600 mOsm/kg = DI highly unlikely
   c. Confirm with water deprivation test (only in experienced centers)
   d. Brain MRI, renal US or genetic testing as indicated
8. **Management of central DI**
   a. Desmopressin (DDAVP); via PO, SL, SC, or intranasal route
   b. Thiazide diuretics, low-solute formula often used in neonates
   c. Treat underlying disorder
9. **Management of nephrogenic DI**
   a. Access to free water, low-solute diet
   b. Thiazide diuretics
   c. Indomethacin

SYNDROME OF INAPPROPRIATE ANTIDIURETIC HORMONE SECRETION

1. See Euvolemic Hyponatremia in Chapter 15 Fluids, Electrolytes, and Acid-Base

FURTHER READING

Daneman D, Barret S, Harrington J. *When a Child Has Diabetes.* Toronto, ON: Robert Rose; 2018.

USEFUL WEBSITES

Diabetes Canada. www.diabetes.ca
International Society for Pediatric and Adolescent Diabetes. www.ispad.org

Fluids, Electrolytes, and Acid–Base

Laura Betcherman • Emma Ulrich • Katie Sullivan • Damien Noone

COMMON ABBREVIATIONS

Also see page xviii for a list of other abbreviations used throughout this book

ADH	antidiuretic hormone
ATN	acute tubular necrosis
BSA	body surface area
CK	creatine kinase
DI	diabetes insipidus
DKA	diabetic ketoacidosis
ECF	extracellular fluid
ECF_{Osm}	ECF osmolality
FE	fractional excretion
GFR	glomerular filtration rate
HCO_3^-	bicarbonate ion
ICF	intracellular fluid
ICF_{Osm}	ICF osmolality
ISF	interstitial fluid
NG	nasogastric
ORT	oral rehydration therapy
PCO_2	partial pressure of carbon dioxide
PO_4^-	phosphate
P_{K^+}	plasma potassium
P_{Na^+}	plasma sodium
P_{Osm}	plasma osmolality
PTH	parathyroid hormone
RDI	recommended daily intake
RTA	renal tubular acidosis
SAG	serum anion gap
SIADH	syndrome of inappropriate antidiuretic hormone
TBW	total body water
TRP	tubular reabsorption of phosphate
TTKG	transtubular potassium gradient
U_{Cl^-}	urinary chloride
U_{K^+}	urinary potassium
U_{Na^+}	urinary sodium
UAG	urinary anion gap
UNC	urinary net charge
U_{Osm}	urinary osmolality

Fluids, Electrolytes, and Acid–Base

15

COMPONENTS OF FLUID THERAPY

1. **Water:** homeostasis depends on ADH, renal function, and intake
   a. Losses come from insensible losses, diarrhea, emesis, gastric aspiration, surgical drains
2. **Electrolytes:** Na^+, K^+, Cl^-
   a. Losses mainly through urinary and gastrointestinal (GI) tract, very little through insensible losses
3. **Dextrose:** added in intravenous (IV) solutions, may not be necessary in patients with hyperglycemia, older teenagers or on ketogenic diet
4. Fluids can be administered parenterally (Table 15.1) or enterally

Table 15.1	Commonly Used Intravenous Fluid Solutions					
Fluid	**[Na⁺]**	**[K⁺]**	**[Cl⁻]**	**Other**	**Glucose**	**Tonicity Versus Plasma**
D5W	0	0	0	0	5 g/100 mL	Hypotonic
D10W	0	0	0	0	10 g/100 mL	Hypotonic
0.9% NaCl	154	0	154	0	0	Isotonic
0.45% NaCl	77	0	77	0	0	Hypotonic
0.2% NaCl	33	0	33	0	0	Hypotonic
Ringer's	130	4	109	Lactate 28 Ca 3	0	Isotonic

Note: Electrolyte concentration and relative tonicity of available IV fluids. All concentrations in mmol/L; any dextrose solution may be mixed with any of the NaCl or Ringer's solutions; KCl may be added at 10, 20, or 40 mmol/L.

APPROACH TO FLUID MANAGEMENT

1. Maintenance fluids (fluid balance at homeostasis)
2. Replacing fluid losses
   a. Ongoing losses (urine, GI—diarrhea, nasogastric [NG]/enterostomy tube output, surgical drains, other body cavities)
   b. Insensible (physiological) losses from sweat, evaporation, breathing
3. Deficit replacement

A. Maintenance requirements

1. **Definition:** fluid and electrolyte requirements with normal hydration status. Volume of "maintenance fluid" is an estimate of normal insensible losses and urine output in a healthy euvolemic child.
2. Based on estimated daily fluid and electrolyte requirements (Table 15.2)
3. Insensible fluid losses are ↑ in fever or overhead warmer, ↓ with humidified ventilation

Table 15.2	Recommended Daily Intake[a] of Na+, K+, and Water		
Parameter	**Weight Range**	**RDI**	**Example for a 47-kg Child**
Na+	Any weight	2–3 mmol/kg/day	94–141 mmol/day
K+	Any weight	1–3 mmol/kg/day	47–141 mmol/day
H_2O	1–10 kg	100 mL/kg/day	1000 mL/day
	11–20 kg	50 mL/kg/day	500 mL/day
	Each kg >20 kg	20 mL/kg/day	540 mL/day
	The values above are additive		Total = 2040 mL/day

[a]Recommended daily intake for healthy children beyond the neonatal period.

RDI, Recommended daily intake.

PEARL

Use the "4-2-1" rule for calculation of hourly maintenance rate (mL/h)

4 mL/kg/h for the first 10 kg

2 mL/kg/h for the next 10 kg

1 mL/kg/h each additional kg

For weight >20 kg, hourly maintenance rate is weight (kg) + 40

B. Principles of intravenous maintenance fluids

1. No single solution will precisely give the required water and electrolytes in all situations

2. Reevaluate frequently based on clinical picture, weight, plasma and urine electrolytes

3. Include oral fluids in fluid balance

4. Infants and young children have limited glycogen stores, so saline solutions with added dextrose are required to prevent hypoglycemia and ketosis (dextrose may be contraindicated in specific situations, for example, patients on a ketogenic diet)

5. Hospitalized children are at high risk of SIADH. Although hypotonic fluids have enough sodium to meet daily requirements, administration can lead to hyponatremia.

   a. Groups particularly at risk include children undergoing surgery, in intensive care units (ICU) and those with acute illnesses including meningitis, encephalitis, bronchiolitis, and pneumonia

6. See Figure 15.1 for prescribing recommendations

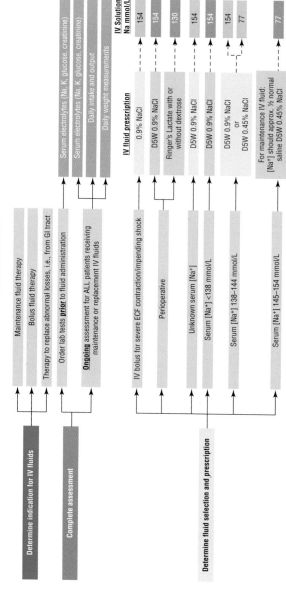

	IV Solution Na mmol/L

Determine indication for IV fluids
- Maintenance fluid therapy
- Bolus fluid therapy
- Therapy to replace abnormal losses, i.e., from GI tract

Complete assessment
- Order lab tests **prior** to fluid administration
- **Ongoing** assessment for ALL patients receiving maintenance or replacement IV fluids
  - Serum electrolytes (Na, K, glucose, creatinine)
  - Serum electrolytes (Na, K, glucose, creatinine)
  - Daily intake and output
  - Daily weight measurements

Determine fluid selection and prescription

IV fluid prescription

IV fluid	Na mmol/L
IV bolus for severe ECF contraction/impending shock → 0.9% NaCl	154
Perioperative → D5W 0.9% NaCl	154
Perioperative → Ringer's Lactate with or without dextrose	130
Unknown serum [Na⁺] → D5W 0.9% NaCl	154
Serum [Na⁺] <138 mmol/L → D5W 0.9% NaCl	154
Serum [Na⁺] 138–144 mmol/L → D5W 0.9% NaCl	154
Serum [Na⁺] 138–144 mmol/L → or D5W 0.45% NaCl	77
Serum [Na⁺] 145–154 mmol/L → For maintenance IV fluid: [Na⁺] should approx. ½ normal saline D5W 0.45% NaCl. If dehydration: D5W 0.9% NaCl	77

Potassium (KCl) may need to be added to IV fluid prescription; maintenance requirement is approximately 20 mEq/L, but exact amount will depend on individual factors including serum K, serum Cr, and urine output.

ECF, Extracellular fluid. (Adapted from The Hospital for Sick Children Fluid and Electrolyte Administration in Children, Clinical Practice Guideline, 2019.)

Fluids, Electrolytes, and Acid-Base

15

C. Fluid losses

1. Identify type of physiological fluid lost (Table 15.3)

Table 15.3	Approximate Electrolyte Composition of Gastrointestinal Fluids[a]			
Fluid	**[Na⁺]**	**[K⁺]**	**[Cl⁻]**	**[HCO₃⁻]**
Normal stool	20–30	55–75	15–25	0
Vomitus/stomach drainage	20–100	10–15	120–160	0
Inflammatory diarrhea	50–100	15–20	50–100	10
Secretory diarrhea	40–140	15–40	25–105	20–75
Ileostomy drainage				
New	115–140	5–15	95–125	30
Existing	40–90	5	20	15–30

[a]in mmol/L

Data from Gennari FJ and Wiese WJ. Acid-base disturbances in gastrointestinal disease. *Clin J Am Soc Nephrol.* 2008;3(6):1861–1868.

2. Choose IV fluid (see Table 15.1) that approximates expected losses
3. Replace ongoing losses (GI, diarrhea, other body cavities)
   a. If volume unknown, can estimate 10 mL/kg for each diarrhea and 2 mL/kg for each emesis

⚡ PEARL

Use 0.45% saline with potassium to replace gastric or diarrheal losses. It should not be used to replace ileostomy losses, as it will be hypotonic to the ostomy output, putting the patient at risk of hyponatremia. Instead, aim to replace ileostomy losses with 0.9% normal saline + 20 mEq/L KCl.

D. Insensible losses

1. Includes sweat, evaporation, breathing
2. Approximated by BSA (m²)

$$BSA = \sqrt{\frac{weight \times height}{3600}}$$

weight (kg); height (cm)

3. Estimates (mL/day)
   a. Neonates = 500–600 mL/m² × BSA (↑ with overhead warmer)
   b. Ventilated (non-neonates) = 300 mL/m² × BSA
   c. Nonventilated (non-neonates) = 400 mL/m² × BSA

E. Deficit replacement

1. Determine deficit (degree of dehydration) based on
   a. Weight loss
      i. Water deficit (L) = pre-illness weight (kg) – illness weight (kg)
      ii. % dehydration = 100 × water deficit (L) / preillness weight (kg)

b. Clinical assessment: see Table 15.4. Each 1% dehydration corresponds to 10 mL/kg of fluid deficit.

2. After initial stabilization, replace remaining deficit slowly over next 24 to 48 hours

Table 15.4	Clinical Assessment of Degree of Dehydration[a]	
Mild (<5%)	**Moderate (5%–10%)**	**Severe (>10%)**
- Slightly decreased urine output - Slightly increased thirst - Slightly dry mucous membranes - Slightly elevated heart rate	- Decreased urine output - Moderately increased thirst - Dry mucous membranes - Elevated heart rate - Decreased skin turgor - Sunken eyes - Sunken anterior fontanelle	- Markedly decreased or absent urine output - Greatly increased thirst - Very dry mucous membranes - Greatly elevated heart rate - Decreased skin turgor - Very sunken eyes - Very sunken anterior fontanelle - Lethargy - Cold extremities - Hypotension - Coma

[a]These findings are for patients with a serum sodium in the normal range. Clinical manifestations may differ with hypernatremia or hyponatremia. Not all signs may be present.

Data from Leung A, Prince T. Oral rehydration therapy and early refeeding in the management of childhood gastroenteritis. *Paediatr Child Health.* 2006;11(8):527–531.

DEHYDRATION

1. Oral rehydration therapy is as effective as IV therapy for mild to moderate dehydration from acute gastroenteritis and is first line
2. Oral rehydration solutions (ORS) contains glucose, which enhances Na^+ and H_2O transport across intestinal mucosa
3. See Table 15.5 for components of different ORS and commonly consumed fluids

Table 15.5	Composition of Oral Rehydration Solutions and Clear Liquids				
Solution	**Carbohydrate (mmol/L)**	**Na+ (mmol/L)**	**K+ (mmol/L)**	**Base (mmol/L)**	**Osmolality (mOsm/L)**
Pedialyte (ORS)	140	45	20	30	250
WHO/UNICEF (ORS)	111	90	20	30	310
Cola	700	2	0	13	750
Apple juice	690	3	32	0	730
Chicken broth	0	250	8	0	500
Sports beverage	255	20	3	3	330
Ginger ale	500	3	1	4	540

ORS, Oral rehydration solution, *UNICEF,* United Nations International Children's Fund; *WHO,* World Health Organization.

4. See Figure 15.2 for algorithm for managing acute dehydration based on degree of dehydration
5. Considerations
    a. Early refeeding
        i. Commence 4 hours into therapy; breastfeeding should continue despite diarrhea
        ii. Extra ORS may be given: 5 to 10 mL/kg for each diarrhea and 2 mL/kg for each emesis
        iii. Appropriate foods: complex carbohydrates, lean meat, yogurt, fruits, vegetables
        iv. Avoid foods high in simple sugars
    b. Vomiting
        i. Administer small volume of ORS frequently (5 mL every 1–2 minutes)
        ii. Consider oral ondansetron therapy if vomiting persists
        iii. If vomiting continues, IV hydration is indicated
    c. Refusal to take ORS
        i. Give solution in small amounts to get used to salty taste
        ii. Add 30 mL of juice to 120 mL of ORS to improve compliance
        iii. NG tube may be used to administer ORS

Figure 15.2   Algorithm for Managing Acute Dehydration

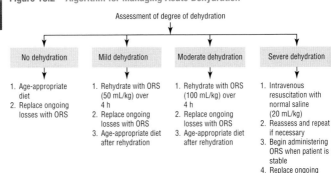

ORS, Oral rehydration solution. (Adapted from Leung A, Prince T. Oral rehydration therapy and early refeeding in the management of childhood gastroenteritis. *Paediatr Child Health.* 2006;11(8): 527–531.)

SALT AND WATER

1. **Osmolality**
    a. Measure of the concentration of a solute in a given weight of water
    b. Units: mOsm/kg

   c. Main constituents: Na^+, accompanying anions, urea (blood urea nitrogen [BUN]), glucose

   d. Most important plasma osmole is P_{Na^+}

   e. P_{Osm} either measured in the laboratory or calculated *("Two salts and a sticky BUN")*

      i. $P_{Osm} = (2 \times P_{Na^+}) + glucose + BUN$ (all in mmol/L)

2. **Water**

   a. As percentage of body weight, total body water (TBW) varies inversely with age (Table 15.6)

   b. Composition of TBW (see Figure 15.3)

Table 15.6	Total Body Water by Age	
Age	**% of Body Weight**	**L/kg**
In utero	85%	0.85
Term infants	70%	0.7
Toddlers/children	65%	0.65
Adolescents/adults	60%	0.6

Figure 15.3 **Composition of Total Body Water**

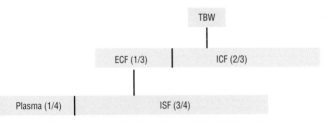

ECF, Extra-cellular fluid; *ICF,* intracellular fluid; *ISF,* interstitial fluid; *TBW,* total body water.

3. Dynamics of fluid shifts between compartments

   a. At equilibrium, $ECF_{Osm} = ICF_{Osm}$

   b. Change in P_{Osm} in either compartment causes rapid H_2O shifts until $ECF_{Osm} = ICF_{Osm}$

   c. Acute changes (minutes) in P_{Osm} occur only in the ECF. ICF_{Osm} changes occur slowly (hours to days) and are generally not the primary problem.

   d. Changes in P_{Na^+} always result in proportional alterations in ICF_{volume} because Na remains largely outside the cell membrane (and is therefore a very effective osmolyte)

      i. Hypernatremia results in ICF_{volume} contraction (water shifts from $ICF \rightarrow ECF$)

      ii. Hyponatremia results in ICF_{volume} expansion (water shifts from $ECF \rightarrow ICF$)

HYPONATREMIA

1. **Definition:** $P_{Na^+} < 135$ mEq/L
   a. Acute (<48 h) or chronic (>48 h)
   b. Most common electrolyte abnormality in hospitalized patients
2. **Pathophysiology:** typically a result of free water retention. Rarely, because of excess loss of urinary sodium.
3. **Clinical manifestations**
   a. See Figure 15.4
   b. Mostly asymptomatic with mild (>125 mEq/L) or chronic hyponatremia
   c. Symptoms imply acute onset and/or cerebral edema, and occur because a rapid $\downarrow ECF_{Osm}$ has caused H_2O to shift to the ICF
   d. Hyponatremia may exaggerate signs of hypovolemia because fluid shifts from $ECF \rightarrow ICF$ (circulatory compromise occurs earlier than expected)

Figure 15.4 Clinical Manifestations of Hyponatremia

Sodium level	Symptoms
>125 mEq/L	-----
	Headache
	Nausea or vomiting
	Lethargy/altered LOC
	Ataxia
	Psychosis
<120 mEq/L	Seizure
	Coma

LOC, Level of consciousness.

4. **Approach to diagnosis**
   a. See Figure 15.5 for diagnostic algorithm and etiology of hyponatremia
   b. Physical examination: volume status (weight, blood pressure, general appearance, mucous membranes, capillary refill)
   c. Investigations: blood Na^+, K^+, creatinine, urea, osmolality, glucose; urinary Na^+, creatinine, osmolality; urinalysis
   d. Accurate measurements of all inputs and outputs
5. **General management**
   a. Based on etiology, severity of symptoms (symptomatic—seizures, altered level of consciousness), and timing (acute or chronic)

Figure 15.5 Hyponatremia Diagnostic Algorithm

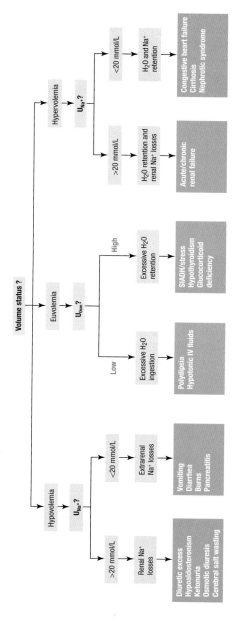

Volume status?

Hypovolemia

U_{Na^+}?

- >20 mmol/L → Renal Na⁺ losses → **Diuretic excess, Hypoaldosteronism, Ketonuria, Osmotic diuresis, Cerebral salt wasting**
- <20 mmol/L → Extrarenal Na⁺ losses → **Vomiting, Diarrhea, Burns, Pancreatitis**

Euvolemia

U_{Osm}?

- Low → Excessive H₂O ingestion → **Polydipsia, Hypotonic IV fluids**
- High → Excessive H₂O retention → **SIADH/stress, Hypothyroidism, Glucocorticoid deficiency**

Hypervolemia

U_{Na^+}?

- >20 mmol/L → H₂O retention and renal Na⁺ losses → **Acute/chronic renal failure**
- <20 mmol/L → H₂O and Na⁺ retention → **Congestive heart failure, Cirrhosis, Nephrotic syndrome**

Fluids, Electrolytes, and Acid–Base

15

A. Acute symptomatic hypovolemic hyponatremia

1. Immediate goal: prevent cerebral edema by acutely increasing P_{Na^+} by 6 to 8 mmol/L or until resolution of symptoms
2. See Table 15.7 for management steps

Table 15.7	Management of Acute Symptomatic Hypovolemic Hyponatremia
STEP 1	Keep NPO
STEP 2	1. Give hypertonic saline (3% NaCl) 2–4 mL/kg over 10 min 2. Repeat 1–2 times, as needed, until symptoms improve 3. Stop other IV fluids
STEP 3	1. Monitor urine output, serum and urine Na$^+$ q2–4h 2. Intermediate goal: ↑P_{Na^+} by a maximum of 0.5 mmol/L/h (to a max of 8–10 mmol/L/day) Note: Increased urinary output may herald an overly rapid correction of hyponatremia as ADH is suppressed when intravascular volume is restored, resulting in an increase in free water clearance
Other treatment options	1. Fluid restriction 2. Oral salt supplementation 3. Coadministration of furosemide (to increase free water loss)

ADH, Antidiuretic hormone; *NPO*, nil per os (nothing by mouth).

B. Asymptomatic hypovolemic hyponatremia

1. Management: Saline infusion for salt loss or hypovolemic hyponatremia using the formula:

$$\text{Change in serum Na}^+ \text{ from 1 L solution} = [\text{infusate Na}^+ - \text{serum Na}^+] \div [\text{TBW (L)} + 1]$$

2. Do not exceed increase in P_{Na^+} of 8 to 10 mmol/L/day
   a. Too rapid P_{Na^+} correction may result in osmotic demyelination syndrome
   b. Monitor electrolytes to avoid over correction
3. See Box 15.1 for sample calculation

Box 15.1 Hyponatremia Sample Calculation

You are seeing a 10 kg child with a serum sodium of 117 mmol/L
1. Weight = 10 kg
2. Total body water (L) = 0.65 L/kg (see Table 15.6) × 10 kg = 6.5 L
3. Change in [Na$^+$] with 1 L of 0.9% saline = [154 mmol/L – 117 mmol/L] ÷ [6.5 L + 1] = 5 mmol/L
4. 1 L 0.9% saline over next 24 h would raise the serum sodium by 5 mmol/L or 1.5 L 0.9% saline over next 24 h by 7.5 mmol/L

---

4. Other treatment options
   a. Enteral salt tabs or liquid: starting dose depends on the degree of hyponatremia, usually starts at 2 to 8 mmol/kg/day PO/IV divided q6–8h (for premature neonates), 2 to 5 mmol/kg/day PO/IV divided q6–8h (for term neonates) and 3 to 4 mmol/kg/day PO/IV divided q12–24h (for infants and older children)

C. Euvolemic hyponatremia (urine Na >20)

1. Indicates inappropriate activity of ADH (SIADH): will have low measured serum osmolality (usually <280 mOsm/kg) and high urine osmolality (usually >300 mOsm/kg)
2. See Table 15.8 for management steps

Table 15.8	Management of Euvolemic Hyponatremia
STEP 1	Stop all other intravenous fluids
STEP 2	Treat underlying cause
STEP 3	Fluid restriction to less than the urine output for the previous 24 h, or if that is unknown, then to twice calculated insensible losses

HYPERNATREMIA

1. **Definition:** P_{Na^+} >150 mmol/L
   a. Acute (<48 hours) or chronic (>48 hours)
2. **Pathophysiology:** failure to replace water loss (GI or renal) where water loss exceeds the loss of Na^+ ions, OR excess Na^+ intake (rare)
3. **Clinical manifestations**
   a. Most patients are asymptomatic if Na^+ <160 mmol/L
   b. May have symptoms of fluid loss and hypovolemia (i.e., hypernatremic dehydration)
   c. Acute hypernatremia with Na^+ >160 mmol/L may present with central nervous system (CNS) symptoms, including high-pitched cry, lethargy, confusion, seizures, coma
   d. Severity of symptoms depends on magnitude and rate of rise: a rapid ↑ in ECF_{Osm} causes H_2O to shift out of the ICF, brain shrinkage, and risk of vascular rupture with demyelination or subarachnoid hemorrhage
   e. More severe hypernatremia may minimize signs of hypovolemia because of fluid shifts from ICF → ECF (circulatory compromise occurs later than expected)
4. **Approach to diagnosis**
   a. See Figure 15.6 for diagnostic algorithm of hypernatremia
   b. Physical examination: weight, hydration status, neurologic impairment
   c. Investigations: blood Na^+, K^+, creatinine, urea, osmolality, glucose; urinary Na^+, creatinine, osmolality; urinalysis
   d. Accurate measurements of all inputs and outputs

Figure 15.6 Hypernatremia Diagnostic Algorithm

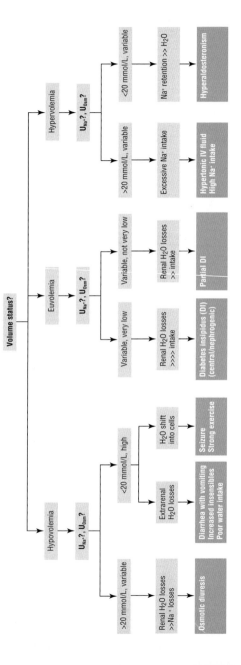

5. Management

a. Based on etiology, severity of symptoms, and timing (acute or chronic)

i. Hypervolemic hypernatremia: reduce Na^+ intake

ii. See Table 15.9 for management steps of hypo- or euvolemic hypernatremia

iii. No evidence-based guidelines for therapy for severe (>160 mmol/L) or extreme (>175 mmol/L) hypernatremia. Consider nephrology consultation.

Table 15.9	Management of Hypo- or Euvolemic Hypernatremia
STEP 1	For patients with hemodynamic compromise, restore intravascular volume with fluid resuscitation
STEP 2	Calculate free water deficit (provides the amount of electrolyte-free fluid needed to restore normal [Na^+])
	Free water deficit (L) = TBW (L) × ([measured P_{Na^+} – ideal P_{Na^+}] ÷ [ideal P_{Na^+}])
STEP 3	Replace the deficit slowly, aim to correct over 48 h
	Note: Do not ↓ P_{Na^+} by >0.5 mmol/h (12 mmol/L/day) because of risk of cerebral edema. This is especially true in chronic hypernatremia, where osmotic equilibrium between ECF and ICF has already occurred. Rapid correction causes cells to swell, raising intracranial pressure, and increasing the risk of brain herniation.

STEP 4	Choose an intravenous solution (see Table 15.1) and determine the volume needed to correct the free water deficit
	     1 L D5W = 100% free water
	     1 L 0.2%NS = 80% free water
	     1 L 0.45%NS = 50% free water
	     1 L 0.9%NS = 5% free water

	Example: If the free water deficit is 250 mL and you want to use 0.45%NS Free water deficit ÷ (% free water in 1 L of the chosen solution ÷ 100) 250 mL ÷ (50 ÷ 100) = 500 mL 500 mL of 0.45%NS is needed to correct the deficit
STEP 5	1. Replace the volume to correct free water deficit over 48 h 2. Choose an IV fluid for maintenance and insensible losses. Add dextrose and potassium as per needs. 3. Add in replacement for ongoing losses (emesis, diarrhea) with 1:1 ratio, choose a fluid similar to the composition of the fluid lost (see Table 15.3)
STEP 6	Recheck electrolytes q2–4h
Other treatment options	1. DDAVP for central diabetes insipidus 2. Dialysis for refractory cases

DDVAP, Desmopressin; *ECF*, extracellular fluid; *ICF*, intracellular fluid; *TBW*, total body water.

POTASSIUM

1. Major intracellular cation; crucial for many cellular functions
   a. Maintains cellular membrane potential and regulating electrical excitability (muscles, heart, neurons)
2. Input mainly from diet (60–100 mmol/day, 90% absorbed), output mainly via kidneys
3. Potassium is in part regulated by aldosterone (high aldosterone = more potassium excretion)
4. Use transtubular potassium gradient (TTKG) (Box 15.2) to estimate the degree of aldosterone activity, renal excretory mechanisms

---

Box 15.2   Calculation of Transtubular Potassium Gradient

$$TTKG = \frac{[Urine\ K^+] \times P_{Osm}}{[Plasma\ K^+] \times U_{Osm}}$$

Requirements for accuracy: $U_{Osm}/P_{Osm} >1$, $U_{Na^+} >25$ mmol/L
Interpretation:
  TTKG = 6 is normal
  TTKG > 6 suggests presence of aldosterone
  TTKG < 5 suggests low aldosterone levels

HYPOKALEMIA

1. **Definition:** $P_{K^+} <3.5$ mmol/L
2. **Etiology**
   a. K^+ loss (urine or GI)
   b. ↑ shifts of K^+ to the intracellular compartment
3. **Clinical manifestations**
   a. Symptoms usually occur when $P_{K^+} <3$ mmol/L
   b. Physical symptoms: weakness, muscle cramping, constipation, respiratory failure, cardiac arrhythmias
   c. Electrocardiogram (ECG): ↓ST segments, ↓T waves, U wave elevation, ↑QT intervals, VF
4. **Approach to diagnosis**
   a. See Figure 15.7
   b. Characteristic ECG changes mandate rapid treatment
   c. Investigations
      i. Plasma Na^+, K^+, Cl^-, Ca^{2+}, PO_4^-, Mg^{2+}, creatinine, urea, osmolality, pH, HCO_3^-
      ii. Urinary K^+, osmolality, pH
      iii. ECG

Figure 15.7 Hypokalemia Diagnostic Algorithm

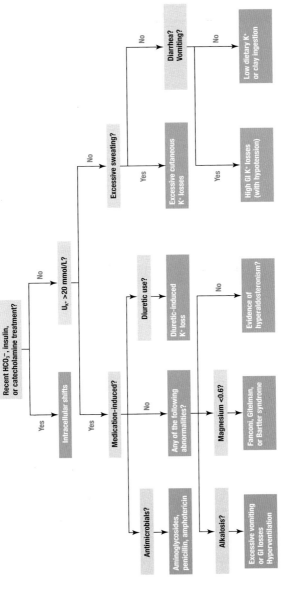

GI, Gastrointestinal.

5. **Management:** see Table 15.10 for management steps

Fluids, Electrolytes, and Acid-Base

Table 15.10	Management of Hypokalemia
STEP 1	Cardiac monitoring
STEP 2	Potassium replacement 1. If symptomatic or K^+ <2.9 mmol/L: consider parenteral treatment, including adding 20–60 mEq/L of K^+ to intravenous (IV) fluid. Avoid IV boluses of potassium to protect the heart. 2. If asymptomatic and K^+ >3.0 mmol/L: enteral or slow IV K^+ supplementation 3. If chronic and/or stable: may consider enteral treatment
STEP 3	Frequently measure serum K^+
STEP 4	Treat underlying cause
STEP 5	Check magnesium, calcium, phosphate, and treat accordingly Untreated hypomagnesemia may aggravate the adverse effects of hypokalemia Treatment of concomitant acidosis with bicarbonate will worsen hypokalemia secondary to transcellular shifts

HYPERKALEMIA

1. **Definition:** P_{K^+} >5.5 mmol/L (in neonates > 6 mmol/L)
2. **Etiology**
   a. ↓ Urinary K^+ excretion (e.g., renal failure)
   b. ↑ GI absorption of K^+ or ↑ intake
   c. Cellular shift (hyperglycemia, acidosis)
   d. Pseudohyperkalemia: hemolysis, severe leucocytosis/thrombocytosis
3. **Clinical manifestations**
   a. Symptoms usually occur in the context of severe hyperkalemia
   b. Physical symptoms: muscle weakness, paralysis, palpitations, syncope
   c. ECG changes include
      i. P_{K^+} > 5.5 mEq/L: peaked T waves
      ii. P_{K^+} > 6.5 mEq/L: P wave widens and flattens, PR lengthens, P waves eventually disappear
      iii. P_{K^+} > 7.0 mEq/L: QRS prolongation, any conduction abnormality, sinus bradycardia, ventricular fibrillation, ventricular tachycardia
4. **Approach to diagnosis**
   a. See Figure 15.8 diagnostic algorithm
   b. Characteristic ECG changes mandate rapid treatment

15

c. Investigations
  i. Plasma Na^+, K^+, Cl^-, Ca^{2+}, PO_4^-, Mg^{2+}, glucose, creatinine, urea, osmolality, pH, HCO_3^-, CK, CBC
  ii. Urinary K^+, osmolality, pH
  iii. ECG
5. **Management:** see Figure 15.9 for management algorithm

Figure 15.8 Hyperkalemia Diagnostic Algorithm

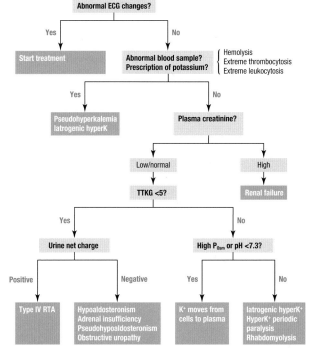

ECG, Electrocardiogram; *RTA*, renal tubular acidosis; *TTKG*, transtubular potassium gradient. See Box 15.6 for urine net charge calculation.

Figure 15.9 Management of Hyperkalemia

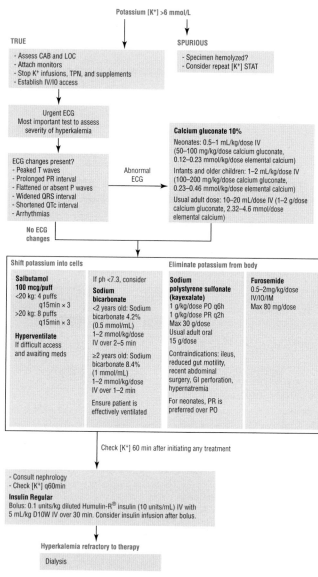

Potassium [K⁺] >6 mmol/L

TRUE
- Assess CAB and LOC
- Attach monitors
- Stop K⁺ infusions, TPN, and supplements
- Establish IV/IO access

SPURIOUS
- Specimen hemolyzed?
- Consider repeat [K⁺] STAT

Urgent ECG
Most important test to assess severity of hyperkalemia

ECG changes present?
- Peaked T waves
- Prolonged PR interval
- Flattened or absent P waves
- Widened QRS interval
- Shortened QTc interval
- Arrhythmias

Abnormal ECG →

No ECG changes

Calcium gluconate 10%

Neonates: 0.5–1 mL/kg/dose IV (50–100 mg/kg/dose calcium gluconate, 0.12–0.23 mmol/kg/dose elemental calcium)

Infants and older children: 1–2 mL/kg/dose IV (100–200 mg/kg/dose calcium gluconate, 0.23–0.46 mmol/kg/dose elemental calcium)

Usual adult dose: 10–20 mL/dose IV (1–2 g/dose calcium gluconate, 2.32–4.6 mmol/dose elemental calcium)

Shift potassium into cells

Salbutamol
100 mcg/puff
<20 kg: 4 puffs
q15min × 3
>20 kg: 8 puffs
q15min × 3

Hyperventilate
If difficult access and awaiting meds

If ph <7.3, consider
Sodium bicarbonate
<2 years old: Sodium bicarbonate 4.2% (0.5 mmol/mL)
1–2 mmol/kg/dose IV over 2–5 min

≥2 years old: Sodium bicarbonate 8.4% (1 mmol/mL)
1–2 mmol/kg/dose IV over 1–2 min

Ensure patient is effectively ventilated

Eliminate potassium from body

Sodium polystyrene sulfonate (kayexalate)
1 g/kg/dose PO q6h
1 g/kg/dose PR q2h
Max 30 g/dose
Usual adult oral 15 g/dose

Contraindications: ileus, reduced gut motility, recent abdominal surgery, GI perforation, hypernatremia

For neonates, PR is preferred over PO

Furosemide
0.5–2mg/kg/dose IV/IO/IM
Max 80 mg/dose

Check [K⁺] 60 min after initiating any treatment

- Consult nephrology
- Check [K⁺] q60min

Insulin Regular
Bolus: 0.1 units/kg diluted Humulin-R® insulin (10 units/mL) IV with 5 mL/kg D10W IV over 30 min. Consider insulin infusion after bolus.

Hyperkalemia refractory to therapy

Dialysis

CAB, Circulation, airway and breathing; *ECG,* electrocardiogram; *GI,* gastrointestinal; *LOC,* level of consciousness; *TPN,* total parenteral nutrition. (Adapted from The Hospital for Sick Children Guide to Management of Paediatric Medical Emergencies, 2019.)

MAGNESIUM

1. Input mainly from diet (20–40 mmol/day, of which 30% is absorbed), output mainly via kidneys
2. Magnesium depletion is often because of gastric losses
3. Important for calcium and potassium homeostasis
   a. Hypomagnesemia can cause hypocalcemia because of impaired PTH release
4. To change concentration of Mg^{2+} from mmol/L to mg/dL, multiply by 2.4
5. See Box 15.3 for calculating the fractional excretion of magnesium

---

Box 15.3   Calculation of Fractional Excretion of Magnesium

$$FE\text{-}Mg^{2+} = \frac{Urine\ Mg^{2+} \times P_{Cr}}{Plasma\ Mg^{2+} \times U_{Cr}} \times 100$$

$FE\text{-}Mg^{2+}$
Low <5%
High >5%

FE, Fractional excretion.

HYPOMAGNESEMIA

1. **Definition:** Mg <0.7 mmol/L (<1.7 mg/dL)
2. **Etiology**
   a. GI causes: ↓ GI absorption of Mg^{2+}, ↓ intake (starvation), acute pancreatitis, excess GI losses (vomiting/diarrhea)
   b. Renal losses: ↑ urinary Mg^{2+} loss (diuretics, nephrotoxic medications), Gitelman/Bartter syndrome, metabolic acidosis, hypercalcemia, familial hypomagnesemia with hypercalciuria
3. **Clinical manifestations**
   a. Usually asymptomatic
   b. If associated with hypokalemia or hypocalcemia, presents with their associated symptoms
   c. ECG: prolonged QTc interval
   d. Severe risks include: seizures, cardiac arrhythmias (torsades de pointes)
4. **Approach to diagnosis**
   a. Investigations
      i. Plasma Mg^{2+}, Na^+, K^+, Ca^{2+}, PO_4^-, creatinine, urea
      ii. Urinary Mg^{2+} (usually timed collection), Ca^{2+} (spot or timed), creatinine
      iii. Renal ultrasound for nephrocalcinosis if there is also hypercalcemia
   b. Calculate the $FE\text{-}Mg^{2+}$ (see Box 15.3) to determine if GI or renal loss
      i. If $FE\text{-}Mg^{2+}$ >5% in a patient with normal renal function, renal magnesium wasting most likely
   c. See Figure 15.10 for diagnostic algorithm

Figure 15.10 Hypomagnesemia Diagnostic Algorithm Based on Fractional Excretion of Magnesium

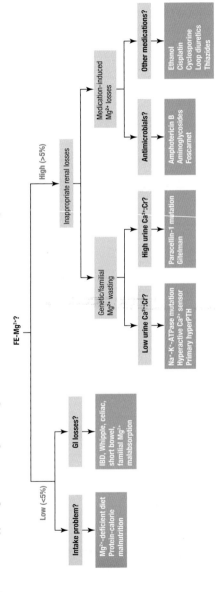

FE, Fractional excretion; GI, gastrointestinal; IBD, inflammatory bowel disease; PTH, parathyroid hormone.

5. **Management**
   a. Asymptomatic: enteral Mg^{2+} supplements
   b. Symptomatic: parenteral treatment, measure Mg^{2+} every 6 to 12 hours after each dose of IV Mg^{2+}
   c. Treat underlying cause, discontinue diuretics
   d. Correct coexisting electrolyte abnormalities
   e. Monitor for hypermagnesemia, especially in patients with abnormal renal function
   f. Chronic hypomagnesemia implies a decrease in both intracellular and extracellular Mg^{2+} and requires long-term supplementation

HYPERMAGNESEMIA

1. **Definition:** Mg^{2+} >0.85 mmol/L (>2.1 mg/dL)
2. **Etiology**
   a. ↓ urinary Mg^{2+} loss
   b. ↑ intake (including IV administration of $MgSO_4$, Mg^{2+} containing antacids)
3. **Clinical manifestations**
   a. Mild hypermagnesemia: asymptomatic, cutaneous flushing, mild hypotension
   b. Severe hypermagnesemia (>2.5 mmol/L): muscle weakness, hyporeflexia, ↓ BP, nausea, vomiting, paralytic ileus, hypocalcemia
   c. Extreme hypermagnesemia (>6 mmol/L) associated with complete heart block and respiratory muscle paralysis
   d. ECG abnormalities: bradycardia, prolonged PR and QTc, increased QRS duration (typically seen at levels >2.5 mmol/L)
4. **Approach to diagnosis**
   a. Investigations
      i. Plasma Mg^{2+}, Na^+, K^+, Ca^{2+}, PO_4^-, creatinine, urea
      ii. Urinary Mg^{2+} (usually timed collection), Ca^{2+} (spot or timed), creatinine
      iii. Renal ultrasound for nephrocalcinosis
   b. See Figure 15.11 for diagnostic algorithm
   c. FE-Mg^{2+} (see Box 15.3) <5% implies suboptimal renal Mg^{2+} excretion
5. **Management**
   a. Stop Mg^{2+} infusions or supplementation
   b. For rapid correction or if severe, consider dialysis

Figure 15.11 Hypermagnesemia Diagnostic Algorithm

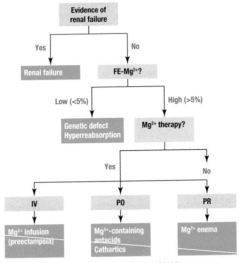

FE, Fractional excretion; *IV*, intravenous; *PO*, per os (by mouth); *PR*, per rectum.

PHOSPHATE

1. Central role in adenosine triphosphate (ATP), deoxyribonucleic acid (DNA), and ribonucleic acid (RNA) biology; major constituent of bone
2. Vitamin D and PTH are main hormones involved in PO_4^- homeostasis (Table 15.11)

Table 15.11	Ca^{2+} and PO_4^- Regulation			
Hormones	**Origin (Trigger)**	**Effect**	**Target(s)**	**End Result**
↑ PTH	Parathyroid gland (↓ Ca^{2+} and to a lesser extent ↑ PO_4^-, ↓ 1, 25-Vitamin D and ↓ Mg^{2+})	↑ Ca^{2+}	Kidney Bone Vitamin D	↑ Reabsorption ↑ Mobilization ↑ Production
		↓ PO_4^-	Kidney	↑ Excretion
↑ Vitamin D	Liver/kidney (↑ PTH, ↓ PO_4^-)	↑ Ca^{2+}	GI tract	↑ Reabsorption
		↑ PO_4^-	GI tract Kidney	↑ Absorption ↑ Reabsorption
Calcitonin	Thyroid C cells (↑ Ca^{2+})	↓ Ca^{2+}	GI tract Kidney Bone	↓ Reabsorption ↓ Reabsorption ↓ Osteoclasts
		↑ PO_4^-	Kidney	↑ Reabsorption

GI, Gastrointestinal; *PTH*, parathyroid hormone.

3. To change concentration of PO_4^- from mmol/L to mg/dL, multiply by 3.1
4. See Box 15.4 for calculating the tubular reabsorption of phosphate (TRP)

Box 15.4 Calculation of Tubular Reabsorption of Phosphate

$$FE\text{-}PO_4^- = \frac{U_{PO_4^-} \times P_{Cr}}{P_{PO_4^-} \times U_{Cr}}$$

$$TRP\% = 100 \times (1 - FE\text{-}PO_4^-)$$

TRP
High >95%
Low <95%

FE, Fractional excretion; *TRP,* tubular reabsorption of phosphate.

HYPOPHOSPHATEMIA

1. **Definition:** PO_4^- <0.85 mmol/L (<2.6 mg/dL)
2. Most commonly seen in patients with diabetes (DKA or DKA recovery) or anorexia (refeeding syndrome)
3. **Etiology**
   a. Inadequate intake: starvation, ↓ GI absorption of PO_4^- (70% of dietary PO_4^- is absorbed), antacid use
   b. Renal losses: ↑ urinary PO_4^- loss, hyperparathyroidism, diuretics, Fanconi syndrome
   c. Shift into ICF: recovery from metabolic acidosis, respiratory alkalosis, refeeding syndrome (insulin stimulated)
4. **Clinical manifestations**
   a. Most asymptomatic
   b. Chronic severe hypophosphatemia (PO_4^- < 0.35 mmol/L): muscle weakness, myalgia. Can lead to rhabdomyolysis, skeletal deformities with rickets.
5. **Approach to diagnosis**
   a. Laboratory
      i. Plasma Na^+, K^+, Ca^{2+}, PO_4^-, Mg^{2+}, alkaline phosphatase, PTH, vitamin D, albumin, creatinine, urea, blood gas, CK
      ii. Urinary Ca^{2+}, PO_4^-, glucose, creatinine, pH
   b. See Figure 15.12 for diagnostic algorithm
6. **Management**
   a. Based on etiology and severity of symptoms
      i. Mild, asymptomatic: enteral (preferred)
      ii. Severe, symptomatic: parenteral PO_4^-
   b. Stop PO_4^- binders (calcium carbonate, sevelamer hydrochloride)
   c. Correction of coexisting electrolyte abnormalities

Fluids, Electrolytes, and Acid–Base

Figure 15.12 Hypophosphatemia Diagnostic Algorithm

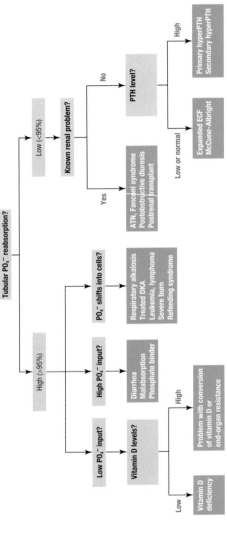

ATN, Acute tubular necrosis; *DKA,* diabetic ketoacidosis; *ECF,* extracellular fluid; *PTH,* parathyroid hormone.

HYPERPHOSPHATEMIA

1. **Definition:** PO_4^- >1.45 mmol/L (>4.5 mg/dL)
2. Most commonly seen in patients with renal failure or cellular lysis
3. **Etiology**
   a. Increased PO_4^- load: ↑GI absorption of PO_4^- (laxatives), IV phosphate/iatrogenic, cell lysis (tumor lysis syndrome, rhabdomyolysis, hemolysis)
   b. ↓ Renal clearance: acute/chronic renal failure, ↓ urinary PO_4^- loss (bisphosphonates, vitamin D toxicity), hypoparathyroidism
   c. Pseudohyperphosphatemia: hyperglobulinemia, hyperlipidemia, hyperbilirubinemia
4. **Clinical manifestations**
   a. No obvious symptoms
   b. Phosphate retention begins early as GFR declines in renal failure
   c. Often associated with hypocalcemia and hyperparathyroidism
   d. Chronic ↑ PO_4^- is associated with $CaHPO_4$ precipitation (metastatic calcifications)
5. **Approach to diagnosis**
   a. Laboratory
      i. Plasma Na^+, K^+, Ca^{2+}, PO_4^-, Mg^{2+}, alkaline phosphatase, PTH, vitamin D, albumin, creatinine, urea, CBC, CK, LDH, blood gas
      ii. Urinary Ca^{2+}, PO_4^-, glucose, creatinine, urinalysis (for hemoglobinuria/myoglobinuria)
   b. See Figure 15.13 for diagnostic algorithm
6. **Management**
   a. Treat underlying cause
      i. ↓ GI absorption by ↓ dietary PO_4^- intake or using PO_4^- binders (calcium carbonate, aluminum-based salts, sevelamer hydrochloride)
      ii. Treat concomitant hypocalcemia
      iii. Use dialysis if severe ↑PO_4^-, especially in context of end-stage renal failure

Figure 15.13 Hyperphosphatemia Diagnostic Algorithm

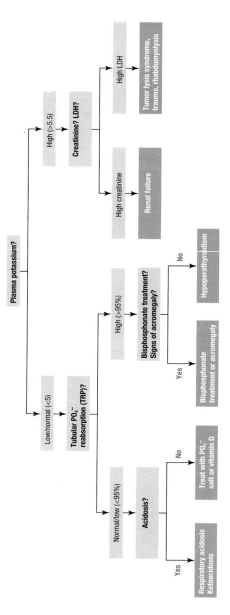

CALCIUM

See Chapter 14 Endocrinology

ACID–BASE DISTURBANCES

1. Main acid–base disturbances
   a. Acidemia: ↓ serum pH <7.35 (i.e., a gain or excess of H^+ ions)
   b. Alkalemia: ↑ serum pH >7.45 (i.e., a loss or deficit of H^+ ions)
2. pH changes are prevented by buffering systems
   a. CO_2: regulated by pulmonary system ("respiratory" component)
      i. Respiratory acidosis: PCO_2 >45 mm Hg
      ii. Respiratory alkalosis: PCO_2 <35 mm Hg
   b. HCO_3: regulated by the renal system ("metabolic" component)
      i. Metabolic acidosis: measured bicarbonate <22 mmol/L
      ii. Metabolic alkalosis: measured bicarbonate >26 mmol/L
3. Acid–base disturbances may be respiratory/metabolic/mixed, acute/
   compensated
   a. Respiratory compensation for a metabolic disorder can occur quickly,
      metabolic compensation for a respiratory disorder can take at least a
      few days
4. Base excess: calculated amount of acid required to return the blood pH
   to 7.4 (normal range: −2 to 2 mmol/L)

BLOOD GAS INTERPRETATION

1. Determine the primary disturbance (Figure 15.14): acidosis/alkalosis,
   metabolic/respiratory

Figure 15.14 Algorithm to Distinguish Primary Acid-Base Disturbances

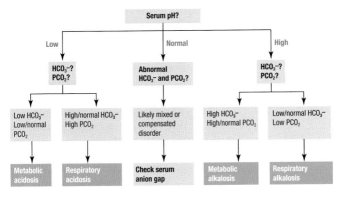

2. Evaluate compensation (Table 15.12)
    a. Compensation is always in same direction as primary disturbance
    b. Compensation rarely overshoots (correcting for acidosis does not cause alkalosis). Consider mixed disturbance or other pathologies if compensation seems inappropriate.

Table 15.12	Predicted Compensation in Primary Acid-Base Disturbances	
Respiratory	**Change in HCO_3^-**	**Change in PCO_2**
Acute respiratory acidosis	↑ 1 mmol/L	↑ 10 mmHg
Acute respiratory alkalosis	↓ 2 mmol/L	↓ 10 mmHg
Chronic respiratory acidosis	↑ 3 mmol/L	↑ 10 mmHg
Chronic respiratory alkalosis	↓ 5 mmol/L	↓ 10 mmHg
Metabolic	**Change in HCO_3^-**	**Change in PCO_2**
Metabolic acidosis	↓ 1 mmol/L	↓ 1 mmHg
Metabolic alkalosis	↑ 10 mmol/L	↑ 5–7 mmHg

METABOLIC ACIDOSIS

1. **Definition:** low blood pH (<7.4) and low plasma HCO_3^-
    a. Compensatory hyperventilation should occur, resulting in ↓PCO_2
2. **Etiology:** processes that generate either a gain of H^+ or a loss of HCO_3^- from plasma
3. **Approach:** see Figure 15.15 for diagnostic algorithm
    a. **Causes of anion gap metabolic acidosis (MUDPILES):** methanol, uremia, diabetic or starvation ketoacidosis, paraldehyde, isopropyl alcohol/iron, lactic acidosis, ethylene glycol, salicylates
    b. **Causes of non-anion gap metabolic acidosis (HARDUP):** hyperalimentation, hyperchloremia, acetazolamide, RTA, diarrhea, ureteroenteric fistula, pancreaticoduodenal fistula
4. **Management**
    a. Treat underlying cause of acidosis and associated electrolyte disorders (correct K^+ and Ca^{2+}, if applicable). Always correct electrolyte disturbances prior to bicarbonate therapy.
    b. If plasma pH <7.0, HCO_3^- <12, and cardiovascular compromise (does not apply to DKA) or to replace significant ongoing renal HCO_3^- losses, consider treatment with bicarbonate
    c. Calculate HCO_3^- deficit = 0.4 × body weight (kg) × (24 – serum HCO_3^-)
        i. Rate of correction depends on target HCO_3^- and clinical scenario: can start with 1 to 2 mmol/kg of $NaHCO_3$, followed by half of calculated HCO_3^- deficit over the next 24 hours
        ii. Risks include hypokalemia and hypocalcemia

Figure 15.15   Metabolic Acidosis Diagnostic Algorithm

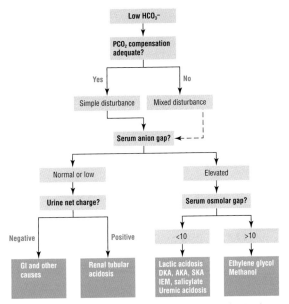

AKA, Alcoholic ketoacidosis; *DKA*, diabetic ketoacidosis; *GI*, gastrointestinal; *IEM*, inborn error of metabolism; *SKA*, starvation ketoacidosis. See Box 15.5 for serum anion gap calculation, Box 15.6 for urine net charge calculation and Box 15.7 for serum osmolar gap calculation. (Adapted from Halperin ML, Goldstein MB. *Fluid, Electrolyte, and Acid-Base Physiology: A Problem-Based Approach.* 3rd ed. Philadelphia, PA: WB Saunders; 1999.)

Box 15.5   Serum Anion Gap and Delta Ratio Calculations

$$SAG = Na^+ - Cl^- - HCO_3^-$$

Normal range: 12 ± 2 mmol/L
Correct for serum albumin: $\downarrow$ 2.5–3 mmol/L SAG for every $\downarrow$ 10 g/L albumin

If SAG is elevated, calculate the delta ratio to help determine if there is a coexistent normal anion gap metabolic acidosis or metabolic alkalosis

$$\text{Delta ratio} = \frac{\text{Actual SAG} - \text{Expected SAG (12)}}{\text{Expected HCO}_3^- \text{ (24)} - \text{Actual HCO}_3^-}$$

Delta ratio <1: consider combined acidosis (wide anion gap + normal anion gap acidosis)
Delta ratio 1–2: uncomplicated wide anion gap metabolic acidosis
Delta ratio >2: consider combined metabolic acidosis and alkalosis

Box 15.6 Urine Net Charge Calculation

$$UNC = U_{Na^+} + U_{K^+} - U_{Cl^-}$$

Indirect measure of urine ammonium concentration. Useful in clarifying whether the renal response to acidosis is appropriate. In patients with normal anion gap metabolic acidosis, negative UNC suggests increased ammonium secretion (i.e., diarrhea); positive UNC indicates impaired ammonium secretion (i.e., distal RTA)

Box 15.7 Serum Osmolar Gap Calculation

Serum osmolar gap = Measured osmolality − Calculated osmolality
Calculated osmolality = $2 \times Na^+$ + glucose + urea
Normal range: <10 mOsm/kg H_2O

RENAL TUBULAR ACIDOSIS

1. Metabolic acidosis secondary to impaired urinary acidification
2. Suspect in child with failure to thrive and/or normal anion gap metabolic acidosis
3. See Table 15.13 for types of RTA

Table 15.13 Types of Renal Tubular Acidosis

Renal Tubular Acidosis Type	Problem	Etiologies	Diagnostics	Treatment
Type 1: distal	↓ H^+ secretion by the distal tubule, leading to ↓ NH_4^+ excretion and ↑ HCO_3^- urine losses	Genetic, medications, infection, autoimmune diseases	Urine pH >5.8 ↓ serum K^+ ↓↓ serum HCO_3^- ↑ urine Ca^{2+}	Alkali therapy with Na^+ or K^+ salts Monitor for nephrocalcinosis
Type 2: proximal	Proximal HCO_3^- reabsorption defect causing bicarbonaturia	Fanconi syndrome, genetic disorders	Urine pH <5.8 ↓ serum K^+ ↓ serum HCO_3^-	As with distal RTA, but tend to have higher alkali requirements
Type 4: hyperkalemic	↓ production or response to aldosterone	Obstructive uropathy, Sickle Cell nephropathy, adrenal insufficiency, medications	Urine pH <5.5 High serum K^+	Treat hyperkalemia K^+ restriction Fludrocortisone

METABOLIC ALKALOSIS

1. **Definition:** high blood pH (>7.4) and high plasma HCO_3^-
   a. Compensatory hypoventilation may occur (resulting in increased PCO_2) but is limited by a strong competing interest (oxygenation)
2. **Etiology:** loss of H^+ or gain of HCO_3^-
   a. See Figure 15.16 for approach

Figure 15.16 Metabolic Alkalosis Diagnostic Algorithm

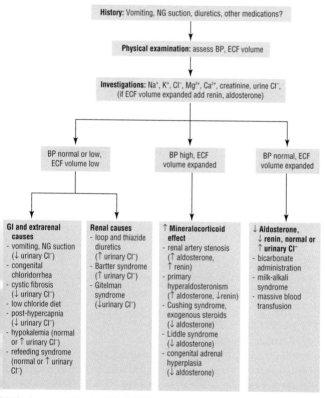

History: Vomiting, NG suction, diuretics, other medications?

↓

Physical examination: assess BP, ECF volume

↓

Investigations: Na^+, K^+, Cl^-, Mg^{2+}, Ca^{2+}, creatinine, urine Cl^-, (if ECF volume expanded add renin, aldosterone)

BP normal or low, ECF volume low

GI and extrarenal causes
- vomiting, NG suction (↓ urinary Cl^-)
- congenital chloridorrhea (↓ urinary Cl^-)
- cystic fibrosis (↓ urinary Cl^-)
- low chloride diet
- post-hypercapnia (↓ urinary Cl^-)
- hypokalemia (normal or ↑ urinary Cl^-)
- refeeding syndrome (normal or ↑ urinary Cl^-)

Renal causes
- loop and thiazide diuretics (↑ urinary Cl^-)
- Bartter syndrome (↑ urinary Cl^-)
- Gitelman syndrome (↓urinary Cl^-)

BP high, ECF volume expanded

↑ Mineralocorticoid effect
- renal artery stenosis (↑ aldosterone, ↑ renin)
- primary hyperaldosteronism (↑ aldosterone, ↓renin)
- Cushing syndrome, exogenous steroids (↓ aldosterone)
- Liddle syndrome (↓ aldosterone)
- congenital adrenal hyperplasia (↓ aldosterone)

BP normal, ECF volume expanded

↓ Aldosterone, ↓ renin, normal or ↑ urinary Cl^-
- bicarbonate administration
- milk-alkali syndrome
- massive blood transfusion

BP, Blood pressure; *ECF*, extracellular fluid; *NG*, nasogastric.

RESPIRATORY ACIDOSIS

1. **Definition:** ↓ pH and ↑PCO_2
2. **Etiology:** caused by ↓ in minute ventilation and CO_2 retention
   a. Chronic respiratory acidosis leads to ↑ renal reabsorption of HCO_3^-
   b. See Table 15.14 for approach to diagnosis

3. **Clinical manifestations**
   a. CNS: drowsiness, somnolence (because of hypercarbia), restlessness, irritability, confusion, headache, fatigue, sweating
   b. Respiratory: compensatory tachypnea (if able), irregular breathing, cyanosis
   c. Cardiac: tachycardia
   d. Long-term complications include respiratory failure, pulmonary hypertension
4. **Management**
   a. Support ventilation: may require positive pressure ventilation or intubation. Heated-high flow nasal cannula has not been shown to reduce PCO_2.
   b. Identify and treat the underlying cause

Table 15.14	Approach to Diagnosis for Respiratory Acidosis	
Problem	**Anatomical Correlate**	**Differential Diagnosis**
Breathing problem	Central control of breathing	Anesthetics, sedatives, opioids, brain injury, central hypoventilation, ventilator dysfunction
	Respiratory muscles	Spinal cord injury, Guillain-Barré syndrome, myasthenia gravis, botulism, tetanus, poliomyelitis, spinal cord tumor, organophosphate poisoning
	Chest wall weakness	Muscular dystrophy, spinal muscular atrophy
	Chest well restriction	Kyphoscoliosis, extreme obesity, thoracic cage injury
Lung failure	Lung restriction	Pulmonary fibrosis, sarcoidosis, pneumothorax, hemothorax, massive pleural effusion, pulmonary hypertension
	Parenchyma	Pneumonia, pulmonary edema, chronic lung disease
	Airway	Severe acute asthma, upper airway obstruction

Adapted from Rose BD, Post TW. *Clinical Physiology of Acid-base and Electrolyte Disorders.* 5th ed. New York: McGraw-Hill; 2001.

RESPIRATORY ALKALOSIS

1. **Definition:** $\uparrow$pH and $\downarrow PCO_2$
2. **Etiology:** caused by $\uparrow$ minute ventilation and "blowing off" CO_2
   a. Hypoxemia: pulmonary disease (pneumonia, pulmonary edema, pulmonary embolism), severe anemia, heart failure, altitude, mechanical ventilation
   b. Stimulation of respiratory center: sepsis, CNS disorders, drugs (salicylates, catecholamines, psychotropics), anxiety/pain
3. **Clinical manifestations**
   a. Depends on underlying etiology
   b. Risk of respiratory muscle fatigue with prolonged increased work of breathing
4. **Management:** treat underlying cause

Gastroenterology and Hepatology

Ameilia Kellar • Eileen Crowley • Thomas Walters

COMMON ABBREVIATIONS

Also see page xviii for a list of other abbreviations used throughout this book

5-ASA	5-aminosalicylate
AFP	alpha fetoprotein
ALP	alkaline phosphatase
α1-AT	alpha-1 antitrypsin
AXR	abdominal x-ray
CD	Crohn's disease
C. difficile	*Clostridium difficile*
CF	cystic fibrosis
CMPA	cow's milk protein allergy
CMV	cytomegalovirus
CRP	C-reactive protein
EM	electron microscopy
ERCP	endoscopic retrograde cholangiopancreatography
EoE	eosinophilic esophagitis
FAPDs	functional abdominal pain disorders
FTT	failure to thrive
G tube	gastrostomy tube
GER	gastroesophageal reflux
GERD	gastroesophageal reflux disease
GI	gastrointestinal
GGT	gamma-glutamyl transpeptidase
HCC	hepatocellular carcinoma
IBD	inflammatory bowel disease
Ig	immunoglobulin
LGI	lower gastrointestinal
MCT	medium chain triglycerides
MRCP	magnetic resonance cholangiopancreatography
MRE	magnetic resonance enterography
NAFLD	nonalcoholic fatty liver disease
NEC	necrotizing enterocolitis
NG	nasogastric
O&P	ova and parasites
PEG	polyethylene glycol
PLE	protein-losing enteropathy
PPI	proton-pump inhibitor
PUD	peptic ulcer disease
SBFT	small bowel follow-through
SBP	spontaneous bacterial peritonitis
SLE	systemic lupus erythematosus
UC	ulcerative colitis
UGI	upper gastrointestinal

GASTROINTESTINAL TRACT INVESTIGATIONS

1. **Abdominal x-ray:** first line to assess for obstruction, free air (perforation), nephrocalcinosis, foreign body or mass
2. **Transabdominal ultrasound (US):** visualization of solid organs, vessels, inflammation/abscesses, bowel wall thickening, pyloric stenosis, intussusception, necrotizing enterocolitis (NEC), biliary system and kidneys for stones, dilatation. Images can be obstructed by gas and adipose tissue.
3. **Upper gastrointestinal (GI) series:** radiocontrast agent (barium sulfate) is ingested or instilled into the GI tract. Fluoroscopy is used to examine the structure (e.g., malrotation, web, strictures, esophageal atresia, tracheoesophageal fistula, hiatal hernia) and function of aspects of the GI tract (e.g., swallowing, peristalsis, sphincter closure). Small bowel follow-through (SBFT) to image the small intestine.
4. **Gastric emptying studies:** nuclear medicine study to assess stomach emptying, can be performed to assess suspected complications postoperatively, gastroesophageal reflux disease (GERD), gastroparesis
5. **Motility studies:** esophageal manometry assesses intraluminal esophageal pressures, ideal for evaluation of dysphagia, GERD, and noncardiac chest pain. Anorectal manometry assesses anal sphincter, rectal pressure and function for fecal incontinence, constipation, and biofeedback therapy.
6. **Computed tomography (CT):** useful for visualizing small bowel, colon, solid organs, vessels, inflammation (appendix, peritoneum), abscesses, stones
7. **Magnetic resonance imaging (MRI):** useful for assessing fatty tissue, masses, abscesses, characterizing focal liver lesions, detecting edema and inflammation, fistulas (for inflammatory bowel disease [IBD])
8. **Magnetic resonance enterography (MRE):** uses gadolinium-based intravenous (IV) contrast to perform dynamic imaging. Provides localization of structural bowel lesions and mucosal detail, especially in the small bowel to assess for IBD.
9. **Endoscopy:** esophagogastroduodenoscopy to examine to the level of the duodenum or colonoscopy (requires bowel preparation) to examine distal rectum to intubation of the terminal ileum. Performed under general anesthetic. Risks: bleeding, infection, perforation, or infection postoperatively.
   a. Esophagogastroduodenoscopy (EGD) indications: foreign body retrieval, control of GI bleeding, dilatation of esophageal strictures, biopsies (e.g., for celiac disease, eosinophilic esophagitis, IBD)

b. Colonoscopy indications: control of lower GI bleeding, polypectomy, biopsies (e.g., for IBD)

c. Video capsule endoscopy: to diagnose obscure bleeding, polyps, and ulcers in the small bowel

10. **Endoscopic retrograde cholangiopancreatography (ERCP):** uses endoscopy and fluoroscopy to visualize the stomach, duodenum, bile ducts and pancreas. For diagnosis and therapeutic management of suspected gallstones, strictures, postoperative complications, trauma, and malignancy.

11. **Magnetic resonance cholangiopancreatography (MRCP):** noninvasive use of MRI to visualize the biliary ducts and pancreas, primary use is to determine if gallstones are obstructing the ducts surrounding the gallbladder

12. **Liver biopsy:** percutaneous liver biopsy performed for diagnosis or staging of liver disease, identifying nonalcoholic fatty liver disease (NAFLD), chronic hepatitis B or C, autoimmune hepatitis, primary biliary cirrhosis, primary sclerosing cholangitis, hemochromatosis, Wilson disease

13. **Cholangiogram:** x-ray imaging of the bile ducts through insertion of a needle into the liver, carrying contrast medium to identify blockage in the liver and bile ducts. Diagnostic for biliary atresia.

GASTROINTESTINAL EMERGENCIES

ACUTE GASTROINTESTINAL BLEEDING

1. **Locations**
   a. Upper gastrointestinal (UGI) bleeding: proximal to ligament of Treitz
   b. Lower gastrointestinal (LGI) bleeding: distal to ligament of Treitz

2. **Terminology**
   a. Hematemesis: emesis of blood
   b. Melena: black, tarry, foul-smelling stool caused by degradation of blood in LGI tract
   c. Hematochezia: passage of fresh blood through the rectum with or without passing stool, typically seen with LGI bleeding or vigorous UGI bleeding

3. **Differential diagnosis:** see Table 16.1

4. **Approach:** see Figure 16.1

Table 16.1	Differential Diagnosis of Gastrointestinal Bleeding		
Age	Infant	Child	Adolescent
Common causes	- Infectious enterocolitis (bacterial >viral) - Allergic gastroenteritis (CMPA most common) - Intussusception - Swallowed maternal blood - Anal fissure - Lymphoid hyperplasia	- Infectious enterocolitis (bacterial >viral) - Anal fissure - Colonic polyps - Intussusception - PUD/gastritis - Epistaxis - Mallory-Weiss syndrome	- Infectious enterocolitis (bacterial >viral) - IBD - PUD/gastritis - Mallory-Weiss syndrome - Colonic polyps

Table 16.1   Differential Diagnosis of Gastrointestinal Bleeding—cont'd

Age	Infant	Child	Adolescent
Less common causes	- Volvulus - NEC - Meckel diverticulum - Coagulopathy (hemorrhagic disease of the newborn)	- Esophageal varices - Esophagitis - Meckel diverticulum - Lymphoid hyperplasia - HSP - Foreign body - Vascular malformation - Hemangioma - Trauma/abuse - HUS - IBD - Coagulopathy	- Hemorrhoids - Esophageal varices - Esophagitis - Telangiectasia-angiodysplasia - Graft-versus-host disease

CMPA, Cow's milk protein allergy; *HSP,* Henoch-Schönlein purpura; *HUS,* hemolytic uremic syndrome; *IBD,* inflammatory bowel disease; *NEC,* necrotizing enterocolitis; *PUD,* peptic ulcer disease.

From Berhman RE, Kliegman RM, Jenson HB. *Nelson's Textbook of Pediatrics.* 17th ed. Philadelphia, PA: Elsevier Science; 2004.

Figure 16.1   Approach to Gastrointestinal Bleeding

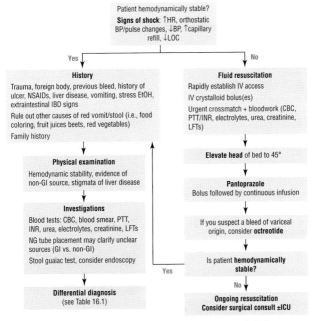

BP, Blood pressure; *CBC,* complete blood count; *eTOH,* alcohol; *GI,* gastrointestinal; *HR,* heart rate; *IBD,* inflammatory bowel disease; *ICU,* intensive care unit; *INR,* international normalized ratio; *LFT,* liver function test; *LOC,* level of consciousness; *NG,* nasogastric; *NSAID,* nonsteroidal antiinflammatory drug; *PTT,* partial thromboplastin time.

ACUTE ABDOMINAL PAIN

See Figure 16.2

Figure 16.2 Approach to Acute Abdominal Pain

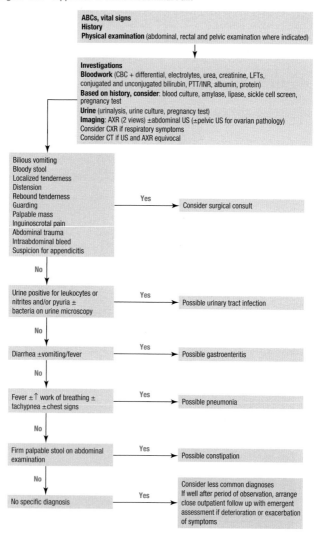

ABC, Airway, breathing and circulation; *AXR*, abdominal x-ray; *CBC*, complete blood count; *CT*, computed tomography; *CXR*, chest x-ray; *INR*, international normalized ratio; *LFT*, liver function test; *PTT*, partial thromboplastin time. (Adapted from Policy Directive: *Children and Infants With Acute Abdominal Pain—Acute Management*. North Sydney, Australia: New South Wales Government, Department of Health; 2013.)

BILIOUS VOMITING

1. Green emesis indicating larger amounts of bile within the stomach, suggestive of intestinal obstruction
2. See Table 16.2 for differential diagnosis and initial management

Table 16.2	Differential Diagnosis of Bilious Vomiting		
Etiology	**Description**	**Diagnosis**	**Management**
Intestinal atresia	Congenital defect of hollow viscus resulting in obstruction of the intestinal lumen	AXR, UGI series	NPO, NG, surgical approach dependent on site/extent of atresia
Hirschsprung disease	Failure of neural crest cells to migrate	Contrast enema and rectal biopsy	Surgical resection of aganglionic segment and preservation of internal anal sphincter
Malrotation (with or without volvulus)	Cecum abnormally positioned facilitating volvulus: twisting of intestine on the mesentery	AXR, UGI series	Ladd procedure
Intussusception	Invagination of part of intestine into itself	US	Ileocolic: hydrostatic or pneumatic pressure enema, surgical intervention only if nonoperative reduction fails Ileoileal: can be found incidentally, may spontaneously reduce. May require surgical intervention.
Pancreatitis	Inflammation of the pancreas	Amylase/lipase, US, CT	See Pancreatitis section
Obstruction	Causes include: incarcerated hernia, peritoneal adhesions, ileus	AXR, CT	Depending on underlying cause (see Chapter 17 General Surgery)

AXR, Abdominal x-ray; *CT*, computed tomography; *NG*, nasogastric; *NPO*, nil per os (nothing by mouth); *UGI*, upper gastrointestinal; *US*, ultrasound.

GASTROINTESTINAL TRACT PRESENTATIONS

CHRONIC ABDOMINAL PAIN

See Figure 16.3 for approach to chronic abdominal pain

Figure 16.3 Approach to Chronic Abdominal Pain

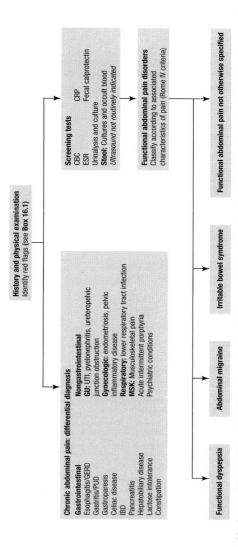

History and physical examination
Identify red flags (see **Box 16.1**)

Chronic abdominal pain: differential diagnosis

Gastrointestinal
Esophagitis/GERD
Gastritis/PUD
Gastroparesis
Celiac disease
IBD
Pancreatitis
Hepatobiliary disease
Lactose intolerance
Constipation

Nongastrointestinal
GU: UTI, pyelonephritis, ureteropelvic
junction obstruction
Gynecologic: endometriosis, pelvic
inflammatory disease
Respiratory: lower respiratory tract infection
MSK: Musculoskeletal pain
Acute intermittent porphyria
Psychiatric conditions

Screening tests
CBC   CRP
ESR   Fecal calprotectin
Urinalysis and culture
Stool: Cultures and occult blood
Ultrasound not routinely indicated

Functional abdominal pain disorders
Classify according to associated
characteristics of pain (Rome IV criteria)

Functional dyspepsia

Abdominal migraine

Irritable bowel syndrome

Functional abdominal pain not otherwise specified

CBC, Complete blood count; *CRP,* c-reactive protein; *ESR,* erythrocyte sedimentation rate; *GU,* genitourinary; *IBD,* inflammatory bowel disease; *GERD,* gastroesophageal reflux disease; *PUD,* peptic ulcer disease; *UTI,* urinary tract infection.

| Box 16.1 | Red Flags in Evaluating Abdominal Pain |

1. Well-localized pain away from umbilicus
2. Pain awakening from sleep
3. Radiation of pain to back, shoulder, scapula, lower extremities
4. Altered bowel pattern (diarrhea, constipation) or vomiting
5. Involuntary weight loss or growth deceleration
6. Gastrointestinal bleeding, constitutional symptoms (e.g., fever, arthralgias, rash) or specific physical findings (e.g., distention, hepatomegaly, positive rectal examination results, perianal disease, joint swelling, clubbing)
7. Consistent sleepiness after pain attacks
8. Positive family history of peptic ulcer, inflammatory bowel disease, celiac disease

Data from Miranda A. Chapter 10: Abdominal pain. In: Kliegman RM, Lye PS, Bordini BJ, Toth H, Basel D, eds. *Nelson Pediatric Symptom-Based Diagnosis.* Elsevier; 2018:161–181.e2.

FUNCTIONAL ABDOMINAL PAIN DISORDERS

1. Classified according to Rome IV criteria, can generally be clinically diagnosed if normal physical examination and no red flags (see Box 16.1)
2. May be caused by abnormal reactivity of enteric nervous system to physiological and stressful stimuli (visceral hyperalgesia)
3. See Table 16.3 for subtypes. Essential criteria for ALL subtypes: after appropriate medical evaluation, symptoms cannot be attributed to another medical condition.
4. No agreement on universally proven management that will help everyone; strategies include
   a. Nonpharmacological: dietary interventions, probiotics, biopsychosocial modifying therapies, multidisciplinary team approach
   b. Pharmacological: no convincing evidence to support the use of drugs to treat RAPDs in children

Table 16.3	Functional Abdominal Pain Disorders Subtypes
Subtype	**Criteria**
Functional dyspepsia	One or more of the following symptoms at least 4 days per month, for at least 2 months 1. Postprandial fullness 2. Early satiety 3. Epigastric pain or burning not associated with defecation
Irritable bowel syndrome	All of the following for at least 2 months 1. Abdominal pain at least 4 days per month associated with one or more of the following: related to defecation, change in frequency of stool, change in appearance of stool 2. In children with constipation, pain does not resolve with relief of constipation (functional constipation rather than IBS)
Abdominal migraine	All of the following occurring at least twice in the 6 months before diagnosis 1. Paroxysmal episodes of intense, acute periumbilical, midline, or diffuse abdominal pain lasting 1 h or more which is incapacitating and interferes with normal activities 2. Episodes separated by weeks to months and stereotypical in the individual patient 3. Pain is associated with two or more of the following: anorexia, nausea, vomiting, headache, photophobia, pallor
Functional abdominal pain not otherwise specified	All of the following at least 4 times per month for at least 2 months 1. Episodic or continuous abdominal pain that does not occur solely during physiological events 2. Insufficient criteria for one of the other three FAPDs

FAPD, Functional abdominal pain disorder; *IBS,* irritable bowel syndrome.

Modified from Hyams JS, Di Lorenzo C, Saps M, et al. Childhood functional gastrointestinal disorders: child/adolescent. *Gastroenterology.* 2016;150:1456–1468.

VOMITING

1. **Differential diagnosis:** see Figure 16.4
2. **History:** presence of other GI and systemic symptoms, quality, timing, presence of bile/blood in vomitus
3. Investigations guided by history and physical exam
   a. Blood tests: complete blood count (CBC), electrolytes, blood gas, creatinine, glucose, liver function tests (LFTs), lipase, metabolic workup depending on history
   b. Urine: urinalysis, culture, toxicology screen
   c. Stool: virology (EM), occult blood, eosinophils
   d. Radiology: abdominal x-ray (AXR) (2 views), UGI series ±SBFT, gastric emptying time, abdominal US, neuroimaging
   e. Consider pH probe, upper endoscopy
4. See Figure 16.5 and Table 16.4 for approach and management of cyclic vomiting syndrome

Figure 16.4   Differential Diagnosis of Vomiting

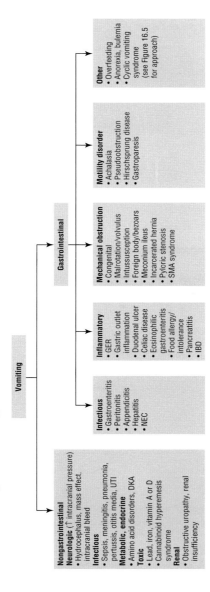

Vomiting

Nongastrointestinal

Neurologic (↑ intracranial pressure)
• Hydrocephalus, mass effect, intracranial bleed

Infectious
• Sepsis, meningitis, pneumonia, pertussis, otitis media, UTI

Metabolic, endocrine
• Amino acid disorders, DKA

Toxic
• Lead, iron, vitamin A or D
• Cannabinoid hyperemesis syndrome

Renal
• Obstructive uropathy, renal insufficiency

Gastrointestinal

Infectious
• Gastroenteritis
• Peritonitis
• Appendicitis
• Hepatitis
• NEC

Inflammatory
• GER
• Gastric outlet inflammation
• Duodenal ulcer
• Celiac disease
• Eosinophilic gastroenteritis
• Food allergy/intolerance
• Pancreatitis
• IBD

Mechanical obstruction
• Congenital
• Malrotation/volvulus
• Intussusception
• Foreign body/bezoars
• Meconium ileus
• Incarcerated hernia
• Pyloric stenosis
• SMA syndrome

Motility disorder
• Achalasia
• Pseudoobstruction
• Hirschsprung disease
• Gastroparesis

Other
• Overfeeding
• Anorexia, bulimia
• Cyclic vomiting syndrome
(see Figure 16.5 for approach)

DKA, Diabetic ketoacidosis; *GER,* gastroesophageal reflux; *IBD,* inflammatory bowel disease; *NEC,* necrotizing enterocolitis; *SMA,* superior mesenteric artery; *UTI,* urinary tract infection.

Gastroenterology and Hepatology

16

371

Figure 16.5 Approach to Cyclic Vomiting Syndrome in Patients Over 2 Years Old

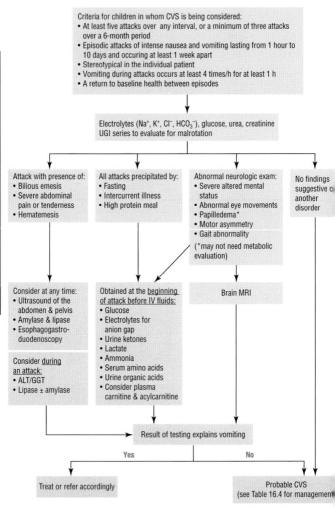

Criteria for children in whom CVS is being considered:
- At least five attacks over any interval, or a minimum of three attacks over a 6-month period
- Episodic attacks of intense nausea and vomiting lasting from 1 hour to 10 days and occuring at least 1 week apart
- Stereotypical in the individual patient
- Vomiting during attacks occurs at least 4 times/h for at least 1 h
- A return to baseline health between episodes

Electrolytes (Na⁺, K⁺, Cl⁻, HCO₃⁻), glucose, urea, creatinine UGI series to evaluate for malrotation

Attack with presence of:
- Bilious emesis
- Severe abdominal pain or tenderness
- Hematemesis

All attacks precipitated by:
- Fasting
- Intercurrent illness
- High protein meal

Abnormal neurologic exam:
- Severe altered mental status
- Abnormal eye movements
- Papilledema*
- Motor asymmetry
- Gait abnormality

(*may not need metabolic evaluation)

No findings suggestive of another disorder

Consider at any time:
- Ultrasound of the abdomen & pelvis
- Amylase & lipase
- Esophagogastro-duodenoscopy

Consider during an attack:
- ALT/GGT
- Lipase ± amylase

Obtained at the beginning of attack before IV fluids:
- Glucose
- Electrolytes for anion gap
- Urine ketones
- Lactate
- Ammonia
- Serum amino acids
- Urine organic acids
- Consider plasma carnitine & acylcarnitine

Brain MRI

Result of testing explains vomiting

Yes

No

Treat or refer accordingly

Probable CVS (see Table 16.4 for management)

ALT, Alanine aminotransferase; *CVS,* cyclic vomiting syndrome; *GGT,* gamma-glutamyl transpeptidase; *IV,* intravenous; *MRI,* magnetic resonance imaging; *UGI,* upper gastrointestinal. (From Li BUK, Lefevre F, Chelimsky, GG, et al. North American Society for Pediatric Gastroenterology, Hepatology, and Nutrition Consensus Statement on the diagnosis and management of cyclic vomiting syndrome. *J Pediatr Gastroenterol Nutr.* 2008;47(3).)

Table 16.4	Management of Cyclic Vomiting Syndrome	
	Therapy: Mild Disease[a]	**Therapy: Moderate-Severe Disease**[b]
Lifestyle measures	1. Trigger avoidance 2. >Maintenance fluids 3. Exercise 4. Sleep hygiene 5. Stress reduction	Same as for mild disease plus Hospital Abortive Plan
Abortive	1. Sumatriptan nasal/subcutaneous 2. Ondansetron	In emergency department or hospital settings, an example abortive plan would include: 1. Darkened, quiet room 2. Initial fluid bolus 10 mL/kg normal saline if dehydrated and repeat as clinically necessary 3. IV fluids at 1.5 times maintenance rates 4. Intravenous ondansetron 5. Intravenous lorazepam 6. If moderate to severe abdominal pain, intravenous ketorolac Admit if >5% dehydrated, no urine output >12 h, Na^+ <130 mEq/L, anion gap >18 mEq/L, or inability to stop emesis Allow fluid oral intake
Prophylactic	Optional (if poor response to abortive therapy) - Coenzyme Q10	**<5 years** 1. Antihistamines: cyproheptadine (first choice) - Side effects: increased appetite, weight gain, sedation. Alternatives: pizotifen (available in UK, Canada). 2. β-Blockers: propranolol (second choice) - Monitor: resting heart rate maintains ≥60 beats/min - Side effects: lethargy, reduced exercise intolerance. Contraindications: asthma, diabetes, heart disease, depression. - Discontinuation: tapered for 1–2 weeks **≥5 years** 1. Tricyclic antidepressants: amitriptyline (first choice) - Monitor: QT_c interval before starting and 10 days after peak dose - Side effects: constipation, sedation, arrhythmia, behavioral changes (especially in young children) - Alternatives: nortriptyline (available in liquid) 2. β-Blocker: propranolol (second choice)

Continued

Table 16.4	Management of Cyclic Vomiting Syndrome—cont'd
Therapy: Mild Disease[a]	**Therapy: Moderate-Severe Disease[b]**
	3. Other agents: - Anticonvulsants: phenobarbital (side effects: sedation, cognitive impairment. Alternatives: topiramate, valproic acid, gabapentin, levetiracetam (consult neurologist). - Supplements: L carnitine (side effects diarrhea, fishy body odor), Coenzyme Q10

[a]Mild disease: no emergency visits or hospital admits; <6 episodes/year and <24 h duration.
[b]Moderate-severe disease: occasional-frequent emergency visits and/or hospital admits; ≥6 episodes/year and ≥24 h.

Modified from Li BUK. Managing cyclic vomiting syndrome in children: beyond the guidelines. *Eur J Pediatr*. 2018;177(10):1435–1442 and from Li BUK, Lefevre F, Chelimsky GG, et al. North American Society for Pediatric Gastroenterology, Hepatology, and Nutrition consensus statement on the diagnosis and management of cyclic vomiting syndrome. *J Pediatr Gastroenterol Nutr*. 2008;47(3):379–393.

GASTROESOPHAGEAL REFLUX

1. **Gastroesophageal reflux (GER):** effortless nonbilious emesis after some or every feeding ("happy spitter")
   a. History and physical examination sufficient for diagnosis in majority of cases
   b. No investigations
   c. Reassurance and education for developmental of warning signs
   d. Positioning therapy (upright after feeds)
   e. Can consider thickened formula
2. **Gastroesophageal reflux disease (GERD):** when reflux leads to troublesome symptoms and/or complications (Table 16.5)
   a. Differential diagnosis: assess for "red flag" symptoms and signs (Table 16.6) suggestive of disorders other than GERD
   b. Investigations: consider UGI series and abdominal US to rule out anatomic causes (malrotation, annular pancreas, hiatal hernia, esophageal stricture), not to diagnose GERD
   c. Management
      i. Symptomatic infants: avoid overfeeding and thicken feeds if not breastfeeding. If no improvement, consider 2–4 week trial hydrolyzed or amino acid based formula or cow's milk elimination from mother's diet. If no improvement, consider trial of acid suppression and refer to gastroenterology.
      ii. Older children: Provide lifestyle and dietary education. If no improvement, trial of acid suppression for 4–8 weeks. If no improvement, refer to gastroenterology for endoscopy.

d. Pharmacological therapy
   i. Acid suppression: proton-pump inhibitor (PPI) (omeprazole, lansoprazole, pantoprazole, esomeprazole, rabeprazole) superior to H$_2$-receptor antagonist (ranitidine, famotidine). Choice based on availability, cost, palatability (lansoprazole preferred oral medication), feeding tube use (omeprazole preferred feeding tube medication).
   ii. Prokinetic medications: include domperidone, metoclopramide, cisapride. Not recommended as first-line treatment. Concerns for serious cardiac arrhythmias, many drug interactions.
e. Surgical treatment: transpyloric/jejunal feedings, fundoplication

Table 16.5	Signs and Symptoms Associated With Gastroesophageal Reflux Disease	
Symptoms	**Signs**	
General	**General**	
Discomfort/irritability[a]	Dental erosion	
Failure to thrive	Anemia	
Feeding refusal		
Dystonic neck posturing (Sandifer syndrome)		
Gastrointestinal	**Gastrointestinal**	
Recurrent regurgitation with/without vomiting in older children	Esophagitis	
Heartburn/chest pain[b]	Esophageal stricture	
Epigastric pain[b]	Barrett esophagus	
Hematemesis		
Dysphagia/odynophagia		
Airway	**Airway**	
Wheezing	Apnea spells	
Stridor	Asthma	
Cough	Recurrent pneumonia associated with aspiration	
Hoarseness	Recurrent otitis media	

[a]If excessive irritability and pain is the only symptom, it is unlikely to be related to GERD.
[b]Typical symptoms of GERD in older children.

GERD, Gastroesophageal reflux disease.

From Rosen R, Vandelplas Y, Singendonk M, et al. Pediatric gastroesophageal reflux clinical practice guidelines: Joint Recommendations of the North American Society for Pediatric Gastroenterology, Hepatology, and Nutrition and the European Society for Pediatric Gastroenterology, Hepatology, and Nutrition. Pediatric Gastroenterology, Hepatology, and Nutrition. *J Pediatr Gastroenterol Nutr.* 2018;66(3):516–554.

Table 16.6	"Red Flag" Symptoms and Signs That Suggest Disorders Other Than Gastroesophageal Reflux Disease
Symptoms and Signs	**Remarks**
General	
Weight loss	Suggesting a variety of conditions, including systemic infections
Lethargy	
Fever	
Excessive irritability/pain	
Dysuria	May suggest urinary tract infection, especially in infants and young children
Onset of regurgitation/vomiting >6 months or increasing/persisting >12–18 months of age	Late onset, as well as symptoms increasing or persisting after infancy, based on the natural course of the disease, may indicate a diagnosis other than GERD
Neurological	
Bulging fontanel/rapidly increasing head circumference	May suggest raised intracranial pressure, for example, because of meningitis, brain tumor, or hydrocephalus
Seizures	
Macro/microcephaly	
Gastrointestinal	
Persistent forceful vomiting	Indicative of hypertrophic pyloric stenosis (infants up to 2 months old)
Nocturnal vomiting	May suggest increased intracranial pressure
Bilious vomiting	Regarded as symptom of intestinal obstruction. See Table 16.2 for differential diagnosis.
Hematemesis	Suggests a potentially serious bleed from the esophagus, stomach, or upper gut, possibly GERD-associated, occurring from peptic ulcer disease,[a] Mallory-Weiss tear,[b] or reflux-esophagitis
Chronic diarrhea	May suggest food protein-induced gastroenteropathy[c]
Rectal bleeding	Indicative of multiple conditions, including bacterial gastroenteritis, inflammatory bowel disease, as well as acute surgical conditions and food protein-induced gastroenteropathy rectal bleeding (bleeding caused by proctocolitis)
Abdominal distension	Indicative of obstruction, dysmotility, or anatomic abnormalities

[a]Especially with NSAID use.

[b]Associated with vomiting.

[c]More likely in infants with eczema and/or a strong family history of atopic disease.

GERD, Gastroesophageal reflux disease; *NSAID*, nonsteroidal antiinflammatory drug.

Modified from Rosen R, Vandelplas Y, Singendonk M, et al. Pediatric gastroesophageal reflux clinical practice guidelines: Joint Recommendations of the North American Society for Pediatric Gastroenterology, Hepatology, and Nutrition and the European Society for Pediatric Gastroenterology, Hepatology, and Nutrition. *J Pediatr Gastroenterol Nutr.* 2018;66(3):516–554.

DYSPHAGIA

1. **Description:** difficulty swallowing secondary to
   a. Oropharyngeal causes: structural, neuromuscular, infectious/inflammatory
   b. Esophageal causes
      i. Abnormal esophageal motility: both liquids and solids affected
      ii. Mechanical obstruction: usually solids, relieved by vomiting
   c. Odynophagia: pain with swallowing, indicates esophageal mucosal disease
2. **Differential diagnosis:** see Table 16.7

Table 16.7	Differential Diagnosis of Dysphagia Resulting From Esophageal Causes	
Mechanism	**Etiology**	**Description**
Mechanical	Achalasia	Functional obstruction of esophagogastric junction
	External compression	Foreign body, mediastinal mass, pulmonary sling, vascular ring
	Esophageal stricture or stenosis	Often past history of GERD or caustic ingestion
	Lower esophageal (Schatzki) ring	Intermittent dysphagia; can be acute with large food bolus
Motor dysfunction	Infectious esophagitis (*Candida*, HSV)	Severe odynophagia, often unable to swallow
	GERD	See Gastroesophageal Reflux section
	Caustic ingestion	May lead to erosive esophagitis and stricture
	Eosinophilic esophagitis	Often associated with atopic/asthma history
	Collagen vascular disease	Classically associated with scleroderma
	Aperistalsis	History of tracheoesophageal fistula, esophageal atresia
Other	Globus pharyngeus	Painless sensation of a lump in the throat, or a tightening or choking feeling

GERD, Gastroesophageal reflux disease; *HSV*, herpes simplex virus.

3. Investigations guided by history and physical exam. Clinical feeding assessment and videofluoroscopic swallow study for children with oropharyngeal dysphagia to assess feeding safety.
4. Management depends on underlying cause

EOSINOPHILIC ESOPHAGITIS

1. **Description:** chronic, local immune-mediated disease of the esophagus
   a. Present with symptoms of esophageal dysfunction
   b. Histological evidence of eosinophil-predominant inflammation ($\geq$15 Eosinophils in 1 high-power field)
   c. Exclude other systemic and local causes of esophageal eosinophilia
   d. Eosinophilic esophagitis (EoE) may coexist with GERD
2. Leading cause of dysphagia and food impaction in children and adolescents—if untreated may result in stricture formation and functional abnormalities
3. **Investigations**
   a. Endoscopy: mucosal friability, edema, white exudates, longitudinal shearing, furrowing and circular rings (presence of $\geq$1 features is highly suggestive of EoE)
   b. Histology: total of at least six biopsies should be obtained from at least two different locations in the esophagus
   c. No available, reliable noninvasive markers, and clinical symptoms unreliable measure of disease activity
   d. Upper endoscopy and biopsy are required to assess for disease relapse or response
4. **Management**
   a. High dose PPI therapy may induce and maintain remission in some patients
   b. Empiric elimination diets or amino acid-based formula induces and maintains remission in the majority of patients
   c. Topical steroids typically resolve pathological features of EoE. When discontinued, disease generally recurs.
   d. Esophageal dilatation for esophageal narrowing and fixed strictures

INFLAMMATORY BOWEL DISEASE

1. **Description:** characterized by relapsing and remitting episodes of GI inflammation
   a. Crohn's disease (CD) is characterized by transmural inflammation that can affect any part of the GI tract from mouth to anus
   b. Ulcerative colitis (UC) affects the superficial mucosa, starting with the rectum, in a continuous pattern, limited to the colon
   c. See Table 16.8 for comparison of CD and UC
2. **Evaluation:** see Figure 16.7
3. **Management:** individualized based on disease location, severity, and comorbidities (e.g., growth delay, medication allergies)

Table 16.8	Crohn's Disease Versus Ulcerative Colitis	
Investigations	**Crohn's Disease**	**Ulcerative Colitis**
Clinical history, physical examination	1. GI symptoms: abdominal pain, weight loss, vomiting, diarrhea (may be bloody) 2. Growth failure, pubertal delay, anemia, weight loss, fever 3. Extraintestinal manifestations (see Figure 16.6) 4. Perianal lesions common (skin tags, fissures, abscesses, fistulae)	1. GI symptoms: bloody diarrhea ± predefecatory abdominal pain 2. Extraintestinal manifestations (see Figure 16.6)
Laboratory	1. ↑ ESR, CRP, platelets 2. ↓ serum protein, albumin 3. Iron deficiency anemia 4. Stool culture negative 5. Fecal calprotectin elevated	1. ↑ ESR, CRP, platelets 2. Serum protein, albumin results normal unless severe 3. Iron deficiency anemia 4. Stool culture negative 5. Fecal calprotectin elevated
Radiology (AUS, MRI, MRE)	1. Mucosal inflammation of any part of small bowel, most commonly terminal ileum	1. Normal
Endoscopy	1. Affects any part of GI tract 2. Classically segmental GI disease with skip lesions, relative rectal sparing	1. No small-bowel disease 2. Begins in rectum and extends proximally for variable distance
Histopathology	1. Focal transmural inflammation 2. Fissures, fistulae 3. Noncaseating granulomas	1. Diffuse mucosal inflammation
Complications	1. Abscess, fistula, stricture, obstruction 2. Toxic megacolon 3. Increased colon cancer risk	1. Toxic megacolon 2. Severe abdominal pain, tenderness, vomiting, fever 3. Increased colon cancer risk
Management[a]	1. Goals: reduce symptoms, achieve mucosal healing, optimize nutrition, bone health, and growth 2. Induction agents: exclusive enteral nutrition, oral/IV steroid (prednisone, budesonide) 3. Maintenance of remission: immunomodulator (methotrexate, azathioprine), biologic agent (i.e., Infliximab/Remicade; Adalimumab/Humira; Vedolizumab/Entyvio; Ustekinumab/Stelara) 4. Surgery (not curative) reserved for complications (e.g., obstruction, abscesses)	1. Avoid opioid-derived analgesia in fulminant colitis 2. Induction agents: oral/IV steroid (prednisone), oral 5-ASA ± rectal therapy 3. Maintenance of remission: oral 5-ASA ± rectal therapy (i.e., Sulfasalazine, Mesalazine), immunomodulator (Azathioprine, 6-mercaptopurine), biologic agent (i.e., Infliximab/Remicade; Adalimumab/Humira; Vedolizumab/Entyvio; Ustekinumab/Stelara; Golimumab/Simponi) 4. Colectomy indicated for fulminant and medically refractory disease or complications associated with colitis ("curative")

[a]Not all medications approved for pediatric use.

AUS, Abdominal ultrasound; CRP, C-reactive protein; ESR, erythrocyte sedimentation rate; GI, gastrointestinal; MRE, magnetic resonance enterography; MRI, magnetic resonance imaging. Modified from Zachos M, Critch J, Jackson R. Gastroenterology and hepatology. In: Laxer RM, ed. *The Hospital for Sick Children Atlas of Pediatrics*. Philadelphia, PA: Current Medicine LLC; 2005:401.

Figure 16.6 Extraintestinal Manifestations of Inflammatory Bowel Disease

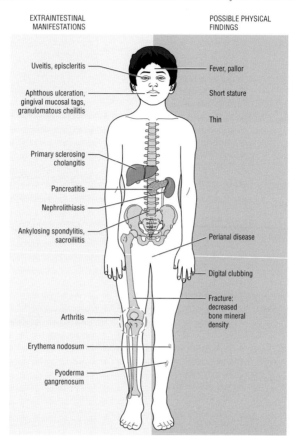

EXTRAINTESTINAL MANIFESTATIONS

Uveitis, episcleritis

Aphthous ulceration, gingival mucosal tags, granulomatous cheilitis

Primary sclerosing cholangitis

Pancreatitis

Nephrolithiasis

Ankylosing spondylitis, sacroiliitis

Arthritis

Erythema nodosum

Pyoderma gangrenosum

POSSIBLE PHYSICAL FINDINGS

Fever, pallor

Short stature

Thin

Perianal disease

Digital clubbing

Fracture: decreased bone mineral density

Figure 16.7 Evaluation of a Patient Suspected of Having Inflammatory Bowel Disease

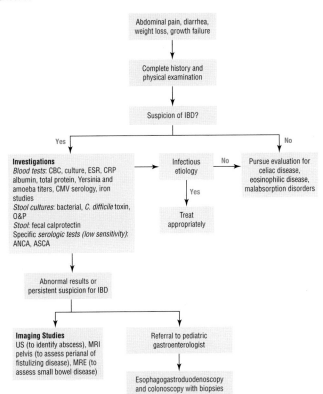

ANCA, Antinuclear cytoplasmic antibody; *ASCA*, antisaccharomyces cerevisiae antibody; *CBC*, complete blood count; *CMV*, cytomegalovirus; *ESR*, erythrocyte sedimentation rate; *IBD*, inflammatory bowel disease; *MRI*, magnetic resonance imaging; *MRE*, magnetic resonance enterography. (Data from Glick SR, Carvalho RS. Inflammatory bowel disease. *Pediatr Rev.* 2011;32(1):14–25.)

CELIAC DISEASE

1. **Description:** chronic immune-mediated disorder that develops in genetically susceptible persons when gluten (major protein found in wheat, barley, and rye) is ingested
2. **Clinical manifestations:** see Table 16.9 for common clinical manifestations of gluten-related disorders (celiac disease, non-celiac gluten sensitivity, and wheat allergy)

Table 16.9	Common Clinical Manifestations of Gluten-Related Disorders		
Time From Exposure to Symptoms	**Celiac** Hours-Months	**NCGS** Hours-Days	**WA** Minutes-Hours
Gastrointestinal	X	X	X
Diarrhea	X	X	X
Abdominal pain	X	X	X
Constipation	X	X	X
Gas/bloat/distention	X	X	X
Poor weight gain	X	X	X
Malodorous fatty stools	X		
Vomiting	X	X	X
Extraintestinal			
Pubertal delay	X		
Unexplained weight loss	X	X	X
Poor height gain	X		
Bone/joint pain	X	X	X
Rash of dermatitis herpetiformis	X		
Eczema		X	X
Hives/atopic dermatitis			X
Fatigue	X	X	X
Headache/migraine	X	X	X
Foggy mind	X	X	
Angioedema			X
Anaphylaxis			X
Respiratory			
Asthma			X
Cough			X
Postnasal drip, throat clearing, rhinitis			X

NCGS, Non-celiac gluten sensitivity; *WA*, wheat allergy.

From Hill ID, Fasano A, Guandalini S, et al. NASPGHAN clinical report on the diagnosis and treatment of gluten-related disorders. *J Pediatr Gastroenterol Nutr.* 2016;63(1):156–165.

3. **Diagnosis**
   a. History and physical examination
   b. Serological testing
      i. Tissue transglutaminase (tTG) IgA: sensitivity 90% to 98%, specificity 94% to 97%
      ii. False-negative serological testing in patients with selective IgA deficiency → check IgA

iii. Endomysial antibody (EMA): sensitivity 89% to 98%, specificity 97% to 100%

iv. Antigliadin antibody and deamidated gliadin antibody not recommended (poor sensitivity and specificity)

c. Consider HLA testing if a diagnostic dilemma

   i. Discrepancy between serological and histological findings

   ii. If a gluten-free diet has been started before any testing

   iii. Screening asymptomatic people at increased risk for celiac disease (family members of an index case)

d. Small intestinal biopsy (gold standard) to confirm diagnosis when tTG or EMA elevated

   i. Blunting/atrophy of small intestinal villi; crypt elongation, intraepithelial lymphocytes

   ii. Must be on gluten-containing diet at time of biopsy

4. **Treatment**

a. Lifelong gluten-free diet

b. Check celiac disease serology 3 to 6 months after starting the gluten-free diet and every 6 months thereafter until celiac disease serology has normalized. Then check annually after symptom resolution and normalization of celiac disease serology.

SMALL BOWEL BACTERIAL OVERGROWTH

1. **Description:** small bowel is colonized by an increased number of aerobic and anaerobic bacteria normally found in the colon (streptococci, bacteroides, escherichia, lactobacillus)

2. **Clinical manifestations**: bloating, abdominal pain, flatulence, chronic watery diarrhea

3. **Etiology**

a. Motility disorders (secondary to irritable bowel syndrome, diabetes, narcotics, intestinal pseudoobstruction)

b. Anatomic disorders (adhesions, strictures)

c. Immune disorders (combined variable immunodeficiency, immunoglobin [Ig]A deficiency, human immunodeficiency virus [HIV])

d. Gastric hypochlorhydia (secondary to long-term PPI use or autoimmune etiology)

e. Metabolic and systemic disorders (pancreatic insufficiency, cirrhosis)

4. **Investigations**

a. Carbohydrate breath test

b. Jejunal aspirate culture containing $>10^5$ colony forming units/mL

5. **Treatment:** antibiotic therapy based on pattern of bacterial overgrowth

a. Hydrogen predominant: rifaximin

b. Methane predominant: neomycin and rifaximin

c. Other antibiotics: metronidazole, amoxicillin with clavulanic acid, clindamycin, ciprofloxacin, trimethoprim with sulfamethoxazole

d. Probiotics: no pediatric studies to date have proven efficacy

MALABSORPTON

1. **Description:** may be caused directly by impaired nutritional uptake from intestine or indirectly as a result of incomplete enzymatic digestion of macronutrients
   a. May have failure to thrive (FTT), chronic diarrhea/steatorrhea, abdominal pain, edema, ascites
   b. Suspect in FTT even in absence of chronic diarrhea, especially if adequate intake
2. **Differential diagnosis:** classified according to the phase of digestion and absorption (Table 16.10)

Table 16.10	Differential Diagnosis for Nutrient Malabsorption	
Phase	**Mechanism**	**Etiology**
Luminal phase	Impaired nutrient hydrolysis—impaired fat and protein absorption	1. Pancreatic insufficiency (chronic pancreatitis, CF, Shwachman-Diamond syndrome, pancreatic resection) 2. Decreased luminal transit time (intestinal resection, short-bowel syndrome) 3. Decreased enzyme activation (rare: trypsinogen and/or enterokinase deficiencies)
	Impaired micelle formation—impaired fat absorption	1. Decreased bile acid production (parenchymal liver disease, fatty liver disease, liver cirrhosis) 2. Decreased bile acid secretion (TPN cholestatic liver disease, biliary atresia, primary biliary cirrhosis, primary sclerosing cholangitis) 3. Impaired enterohepatic bile circulation (intestinal resection) 4. Increased bile acid deconjugation (bacterial overgrowth)
	Decreased luminal substrate availability	1. Bacterial overgrowth
Mucosal phase	Impaired brush border enzyme activity	1. Disaccharidase deficiency (primary or postinfectious), IgA deficiency
	Impaired nutrient absorption	1. Congenital (e.g., galactosemia, fructosemia, immunodeficiency syndromes, abetalipoproteinemia, cystinuria) 2. Acquired (e.g., short-bowel syndrome, celiac disease, IBD, AIDS enteropathy, lymphoma)
Postabsorptive phase	Lymphatic obstruction	1. Congenital (intestinal lymphangiectasia) 2. Acquired (e.g., lymphoma, TB, Whipple disease)

AIDS, Acquired immunodeficiency syndrome; *CF,* cystic fibrosis; *IBD,* inflammatory bowel disease; *IgA,* immunoglobulin A; *TB,* tuberculosis; *TPN,* total parenteral nutrition.

3. **Investigations**
   a. Assess caloric intake and requirements (calorimetry)
   b. Blood: complete blood count (CBC), blood film, electrolytes and extended electrolytes, total protein, albumin, immunoglobulins, fat-soluble vitamins, INR, zinc, iron, ferritin, folate

c. Stool: consistency (pink color may indicate phenolphthalein, present in some laxatives), pH, reducing substances, microscopy for fecal leukocytes, fat globules and red blood cells, O&P (minimum 3 samples), culture, *Clostridium difficile* toxin, 3 day fecal fat collection, α1-AT clearance, electrolytes

d. Urinalysis, urine culture

e. If indicated: celiac testing, LFTs, lipid panel, trypsinogen, thyroid stimulating hormone (TSH), urine vanillylmandelic acid (VMA) and homovanillic acid (HVA), HIV, lead

f. Specialized tests: upper endoscopy with small-bowel biopsy, exocrine pancreatic testing

PROTEIN-LOSING ENTEROPATHY

1. **Description:** hypoproteinemia secondary to GI protein loss or decreased uptake of protein by intestinal lymphatics (implies loss of intestinal mucosal integrity)

2. **Clinical manifestations**
   a. Diarrhea, FTT, abdominal distension, ascites, abdominal pain
   b. Edema, hypoproteinemia, but no proteinuria (exclude renal causes)

3. **Etiology**
   a. Common causes: cow's milk/soy protein intolerance, celiac disease, IBD
   b. Less common: Hirschsprung disease, Ménétrier disease, Henoch-Schönlein purpura (HSP), lymphangiectasia, congestive heart failure, restrictive pericarditis, eosinophilic gastroenteritis

4. **Investigations**
   a. Blood tests: CBC, blood film, erythrocyte sedimentation rate (ESR), albumin, immunoglobulins, ferritin, serum α1-AT, celiac serology
   b. Urinalysis: exclude proteinuria
   c. Fecal α1-AT clearance: endogenous protein not normally excreted in stool—detection in stool is abnormal (measure serum α1-AT during stool collection)
   d. Stool for occult blood

COW'S MILK PROTEIN ALLERGY

1. **Description**
   a. Precipitated by cow, soy, or goat milk protein
   b. Not lactose intolerance (result of mucosal lactase deficiency)

2. **Clinical features**
   a. Younger infants most often present with proctocolitis
   b. Immediate reactions may be indicative of IgE-mediated process
   c. May have hypoalbuminemia ±iron deficiency anemia

3. **Workup and management:** see Figure 16.8 (formula fed infants) and Figure 16.9 (breastfed infants)

4. **Prognosis:** most tolerate cow's milk by 2 years, rarely persists after 3 years

Figure 16.8 Algorithm for Formula Fed Infants Under 1 Year With Suspected Mild-Moderate Cow's Milk Protein Allergy

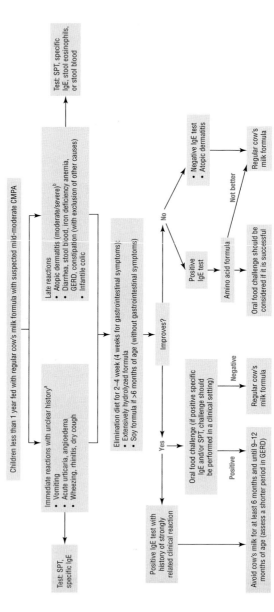

CMPA, Cow's milk protein allergy; GERD, gastroesophageal reflux disease; IgE, immunoglobulin E; SPT, skin prick test.

[a]If history is clear, initiate elimination diet. Oral food challenge is not necessary.

[b]For mild atopic dermatitis: restricted diet is not required if there is no history of reactions to cow's milk.

Figure 16.9 Algorithm for Breastfed Infants Under 1 Year With Suspected Non–IgE Mediated Reactions to Cow's Milk Protein

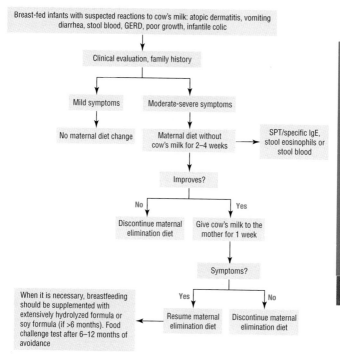

GERD, Gastrointestinal reflux disease. (Adapted from Caffarelli C, Baldi F, Bendandi B, et al. Cow's milk protein allergy in children: a practical guide. *Ital J Pediatr.* 2010;36:5.)

> ⁙ **PEARL**
>
> In older infants and children, hypoalbuminemia in the setting of severe iron deficiency anemia can be from excessive cow's milk intake. Iron supplementation and decreasing milk intake should improve anemia and albumin without the need for an amino acid-based formula.

DIARRHEA (ACUTE AND CHRONIC)

1. **Etiology:** infectious or malabsorptive, osmotic or secretory
   a. Osmotic: stool volume depends on diet, decreases with fasting
   b. Secretory: increased stool volume, does not vary with diet
2. See Figure 16.10 for differential diagnosis

Figure 16.10 Differential Diagnosis for Acute and Chronic Diarrhea

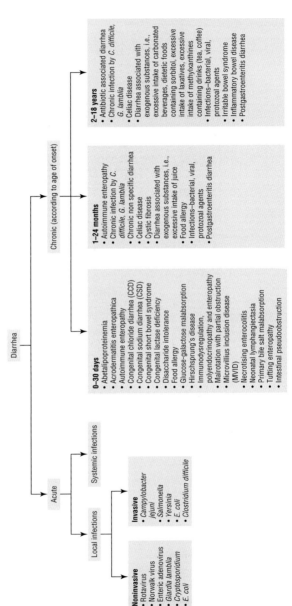

Diarrhea

Acute

Systemic infections

Local infections

Noninvasive
- Rotavirus
- Norwalk virus
- Enteric adenovirus
- *Giardia lamblia*
- *Cryptosporidium*
- *E. coli*

Invasive
- *Campylobacter jejuni*
- *Salmonella*
- *Yersinia*
- *E. coli*
- *Clostridium difficile*

Chronic (according to age of onset)

0–30 days
- Abetalipoproteinemia
- Acrodermatitis enteropathica
- Autoimmune enteropathy
- Congenital chloride diarrhea (CCD)
- Congenital sodium diarrhea (CSD)
- Congenital short bowel syndrome
- Congenital lactase deficiency
- Disaccharide intolerance
- Food allergy
- Glucose-galactose malabsorption
- Hirschsprung's disease
- Immunodysregulation, polyendocrinopathy and enteropathy
- Malrotation with partial obstruction
- Microvillus inclusion disease (MVID)
- Necrotising enterocolitis
- Neonatal lymphangiectasia
- Primary bile salt malabsorption
- Tufting enteropathy
- Intestinal pseudoobstruction

1–24 months
- Autoimmune enteropathy
- Chronic infection by *C. difficile, G. lamblia*
- Chronic non specific diarrhea
- Celiac disease
- Cystic fibrosis
- Diarrhea associated with exogenous substances, i.e., excessive intake of juice
- Food allergy
- Infections–bacterial, viral, protozoal agents
- Postgastroenteritis diarrhea

2–18 years
- Antibiotic associated diarrhea
- Chronic infection by *C. difficile, G. lamblia*
- Celiac disease
- Diarrhea associated with exogenous substances, i.e., excessive intake of carbonated beverages, dietetic foods containing sorbitol, excessive intake of laxatives, excessive intake of methylxanthines containing drinks (tea, coffee)
- Infections–bacterial, viral, protozoal agents
- Irritable bowel syndrome
- Inflammatory bowel disease
- Postgastroenteritis diarrhea

(Data from Thiagarajah J, Kamin D, Acra S et al. Advances in evaluation of chronic diarrhea in infants. *Gastroenterology.* 2018;154(8):2045–2059.)

3. **Acute diarrhea**
   a. Intestinal infections most common
   b. **Approach**
      i. History (include travel, recent antibiotic use) and physical examination, assess degree of dehydration
      ii. Stool: examination for consistency, fecal leukocytes (microscopy), virology (EM and cultures), bacterial culture, O&P, *C. difficile* toxin
      iii. Blood (if severe): CBC, blood film, electrolytes, blood gas, urea, creatinine, blood culture
      iv. Urine: microscopy, culture
   c. **Management**
      i. Prevention and treatment of dehydration (see Chapter 15 Fluids, Electrolytes, and Acid-Base)
      ii. Transient lactose intolerance possible, secondary to villus damage; avoidance of lactose-containing formulas and foods may be required for 48 to 72 hours
      iii. Antidiarrheal medications not indicated
      iv. Antibiotic therapy for specific organisms (see Chapter 24 Infectious Diseases)

4. **Chronic diarrhea**
   a. **Definition:** diarrhea lasting >14 days
   b. **Investigations**
      i. Serial height, weight, growth percentiles
      ii. Stool examination
      iii. Investigations guided by differential diagnosis
   c. **Management**
      i. Diarrhea of infancy/toddler: no specific therapy, restrict high sorbitol–containing fruit juices, stools usually form by 3 years and/or when toilet trained
      ii. Management depends on underlying cause. Pathological chronic diarrhea may require electrolyte, water, nutrient replacement.

CONSTIPATION

1. **Description:** difficult and infrequent passage of hard stool
2. **Differential diagnosis:** see Table 16.11
3. **History and physical examination**
   a. Precipitating factors (functional constipation): coinciding with the start of symptoms: fissure, change of diet, infections, changing house, starting school, fears and phobias, major change in family, new medicines, travel
   b. Weight and height, abdominal examination, position and appearance of anus and surrounding area, appearance of skin and anatomic structures of lumbosacral/gluteal regions, gait, tone, strength and reflexes in lower limbs

c. Digital rectal examination: anal tone and sensation, rectal size. Tight empty rectum in presence of abdominal fecal mass and/or explosive stool on withdrawal suggests Hirschsprung disease (see Chapter 17 General Surgery)

4. **Investigations:** consider further investigations and gastroenterology or general surgery referral if alarm signs or no response to conventional treatment

   a. **Alarm signs:** constipation starting extremely early in life, passage of meconium >48 hours, ribbon stools, bilious vomiting, blood in the stool in the absence of anal fissures, abnormal thyroid gland, FTT, abnormal position of the anus, perianal fistula, decreased lower extremity tone/strength/reflexes, sacral dimple/tuft of hair on spine/gluteal cleft deviation

5. **Management algorithm:** see Figure 16.11

Table 16.11	Differential Diagnosis of Constipation	
Neonate (<1 Month)	**Infant**	**Child/Adolescent**
1. Hypothyroidism 2. Meconium ileus/plug (rule out cystic fibrosis) 3. Intestinal atresia or stricture/stenosis 4. Hirschsprung disease 5. Cow's milk protein intolerance 6. Vitamin D intoxication, hypercalcemia 7. Anal stenosis 8. Imperforate anus 9. Spinal cord anomalies (e.g., tethered cord) 10. Visceral myopathies/neuropathies	1. Cow's milk protein intolerance 2. Hirschsprung disease 3. Botulism 4. Drugs (e.g., opiates, phenobarbital, anticholinergics) 5. Spinal cord pathology 6. Visceral myopathies/neuropathies 7. Heavy metal toxicity	1. Functional 2. Situational (phobia, abuse) 3. Depression 4. Constitutional (colonic inertia, genetic predisposition) 5. Celiac disease, hypothyroidism, hypercalcemia, hypokalemia 6. Drugs (e.g., opiates, phenobarbital, anticholinergics, antidepressants, sympathomimetics)

 PEARL

Onset of symptoms in infants <1 month old raises the suspicion for the presence of an organic condition, such as Hirschsprung disease.

Figure 16.11 Algorithm for Management of Constipation

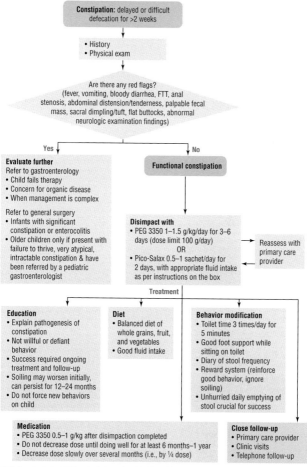

Constipation: delayed or difficult defecation
In the absence of organic pathology, at least two of the following must occur:

For a child with a developmental age <4 years
1. ≤ 2 defecations per week
2. At least 1 episode of fecal incontinence per week after the acquisition of toileting skills
3. History of excessive stool retention
4. History of painful or hard bowel movements
5. Presence of a large fecal mass in the rectum
6. History of large-diameter stools that may obstruct the toilet

Accompanying symptoms may include irritability, decreased appetite, and/or early satiety which may disappear immediately following passage of a large stool

For a child with a developmental age ≥4 years
1. ≤ 2 defecations in the toilet per week
2. At least 1 episode of fecal incontinence per week
3. History of retentive posturing or excessive volitional stool retention
4. History of painful or hard bowel movements
5. Presence of a large fecal mass in the rectum
6. History of large-diameter stools that may obstruct the toilet

Constipation: delayed or difficult defecation for >2 weeks

- History
- Physical exam

Are there any red flags?
(fever, vomiting, bloody diarrhea, FTT, anal stenosis, abdominal distension/tenderness, palpable fecal mass, sacral dimpling/tuft, flat buttocks, abnormal neurologic examination findings)

Yes

Evaluate further
Refer to gastroenterology
- Child fails therapy
- Concern for organic disease
- When management is complex

Refer to general surgery
- Infants with significant constipation or enterocolitis
- Older children only if present with failure to thrive, very atypical, intractable constipation & have been referred by a pediatric gastroenterologist

No

Functional constipation

Disimpact with
- PEG 3350 1–1.5 g/kg/day for 3–6 days (dose limit 100 g/day)
  OR
- Pico-Salax 0.5–1 sachet/day for 2 days, with appropriate fluid intake as per instructions on the box

Reassess with primary care provider

Treatment

Education
- Explain pathogenesis of constipation
- Not willful or defiant behavior
- Success required ongoing treatment and follow-up
- Soiling may worsen initially, can persist for 12–24 months
- Do not force new behaviors on child

Diet
- Balanced diet of whole grains, fruit, and vegetables
- Good fluid intake

Behavior modification
- Toilet time 3 times/day for 5 minutes
- Good foot support while sitting on toilet
- Diary of stool frequency
- Reward system (reinforce good behavior, ignore soiling)
- Unhurried daily emptying of stool crucial for success

Medication
- PEG 3350 0.5–1 g/kg after disimpaction completed
- Do not decrease dose until doing well for at least 6 months–1 year
- Decrease dose slowly over several months (i.e., by ¼ dose)

Close follow-up
- Primary care provider
- Clinic visits
- Telephone follow-up

FTT, Failure to thrive; *PEG*, polyethylene glycol. (Adapted from The Hospital for Sick Children Management of Functional Constipation Clinical Practice Guideline, 2015. With permission.)

Gastroenterology and Hepatology

16

PANCREATITIS

1. **Clinical presentation:** abdominal pain that may radiate to back or shoulder, vomiting
2. **Etiology:** see Box 16.2
3. **Investigations**
   a. Amylase/lipase ($\geq$3 times upper limits of normal)
      i. Elevated amylase also found in pancreatic pseudocyst, parotitis, biliary tract disease, duodenal ulcer, peritonitis, renal failure, burns, stress
   b. Trypsinogen, liver enzymes, conjugated/unconjugated bilirubin, gamma-glutamyl transferase (GGT), glucose, electrolytes/extended electrolytes, creatinine, triglycerides, blood gas, CBC, blood culture
   c. US for detecting obstruction (stones) or bile duct dilatation
4. **Management**
   a. Analgesia, IV fluids, antiemetics
   b. Control of metabolic complications (hyperglycemia, hypocalcemia)
   c. Nasogastric suction, consider early reintroduction of clear fluids to solids as tolerated

---

Box 16.2   Etiology of Acute Pancreatitis

Trauma
Infection
- Virus (e.g., mumps, coxsackievirus B, EBV, hepatitis A, influenza A)
- Bacteria
- Parasites (e.g., malaria)

Drugs
- Furosemide, steroids, azathioprine

Obstruction
- Gallstones
- Choledochal cyst
- Pancreas divisum
- Sclerosing cholangitis

Systemic diseases
- CF (pancreatic sufficient)
- IBD
- Vasculitis (HSP, SLE)
- Hyperparathyroidism, hypercalcemia
- Hyperlipoproteinemia I, IV

Idiopathic

CF, Cystic fibrosis; *EBV,* Epstein-Barr virus; *HSP,* Henoch-Schönlein purpura; *IBD,* inflammatory bowel disease; *SLE,* systemic lupus erythematosus.

1. Laboratory evaluation: see Table 16.12
   a. Liver cell injury: aspartate aminotransferase (AST), alanine aminotransferase (ALT), lactate dehydrogenase (LDH)
   b. Cholestasis: bilirubin (total, conjugated/direct), GGT, alkaline phosphatase (ALP)
   c. Synthetic function
      i. ↓: albumin, clotting factors (I, II, V, VII, IX, X), cholesterol, glucose
      ii. ↑: INR, partial thromboplastin time (PTT), ammonia

Table 16.12	Laboratory Evaluation of the Liver		
Lab	Source	Increased in	Comments
ALT AST	Predominantly liver but also heart, skeletal muscle, kidney, pancreas, lung, brain, leukocytes, erythrocytes	1. Hepatocellular inflammation 2. Muscle disease 3. Rhabdomyolysis 4. Hemolysis 5. Anorexia nervosa 6. Celiac disease (mild)	1. ALT more sensitive than AST for detecting liver damage 2. Concurrent increase in CK or LDH suggests primary muscle source 3. AST > ALT in hemolysis, muscle disorders
ALP	Liver, bone, intestine, kidney, leukocytes	1. Cholestasis 2. Infiltrative liver disease 3. Bone growth or disease 4. Trauma 5. Pregnancy	1. Must differentiate from bone source (i.e., history/ examination suggestive of bone disease, no elevation in GGT) 2. Subnormal levels in Wilson disease
GGT	Liver, kidney, pancreas, seminal vesicles, spleen, heart, brain	1. Cholestasis 2. Newborn period 3. Drug induced (e.g., phenytoin, phenobarbital, erythromycin, nitrofurantoin, alcohol)	1. Most sensitive indicator of biliary tract disease 2. Not present in bone
INR (PT)		1. Liver disease 2. Vitamin K deficiency 3. Factor II, V, VII, X, or fibrinogen deficiency 4. Dysfibrinogenemia	1. Factor VII earliest to be depleted in liver disease; INR prolonged before PTT

ALP, Alkaline phosphatase; *ALT*, alanine aminotransferase; *AST*, asparate aminotransferase; *GGT*, gamma-glutamyl transferase; *CK*, creatine kinase; *INR*, international normalized ratio; *LDH*, lactate dehydrogenase; *PT*, prothrombin time; *PTT*, partial thromboplastin time.

Gastroenterology and Hepatology

16

VIRAL HEPATITIS

See Table 16.13 for a comparison of hepatotropic viruses

Table 16.13	Comparison of Major Hepatotropic Viruses		
	Hepatitis A	**Hepatitis B**	**Hepatitis C**
Transmission	Fecal-oral	Parenteral, vertical, sexual	Parenteral, vertical, sexual
Incubation	15–50 days	60–180 days	14–180 days
Risk factors	1. Contaminated water or food 2. Travel to endemic countries	1. Infant born to infected mother 2. Child/parents from country where HBV endemic 3. Sex partners of infected persons 4. Injection drug use 5. Tattoos	1. Injection drug use 2. Infant born to infected mother 3. Needle-stick injury in health care settings
Diagnostic tests	See Figure 16.12	See Figure 16.13	See Figure 16.14
Presentation	1. Acute, self-limited illness 2. Fulminant hepatic failure (<1%)	1. Mostly asymptomatic 2. Fulminant hepatitis rare	1. Asymptomatic to clinical hepatitis 2. Fulminant hepatic failure rare
Signs and symptoms of acute infection	Fever, malaise, jaundice, anorexia, nausea, abdominal discomfort	Fatigue, jaundice, arthralgia, arthritis, rashes	Nonspecific, onset usually mild, <20% jaundiced
Characteristics of infection by age	1. Children <6 years: 30% symptomatic (2–3 weeks), few jaundiced 2. Older children/adults: most symptomatic (lasting 1 week to 6 months), >70% jaundiced	1. Higher rates of chronic infection in younger individuals	1. Chronic infection in 50%–60% children, 60%–70% adults (usually asymptomatic) 2. 5% risk of vertical transmission
Chronic infection	No	HBsAg/HBeAg/HBV DNA +ve for >6 months or HBsAg/HBeAg/HBV DNA +ve and anti-HBc IgM negative	HCV RNA positive for >6 months

Table 16.13	Comparison of Major Hepatotropic Viruses—cont'd		
	Hepatitis A	**Hepatitis B**	**Hepatitis C**
Monitoring		1. AST/ALT every 6–12 months 2. HBeAg, anti-HBe, HBV DNA every 6–12 months 3. AFP every 6–12 months (at risk for HCC) 4. Liver US periodically 5. Increased frequency of US surveillance for HCC, if cirrhosis 6. Screen before starting immunosuppressive medications 7. Transient elastography every 6–12 months	1. AST/ALT every 6–12 months 2. Quantitative HCV RNA assay periodically 3. AFP yearly (at risk for HCC) 4. Liver US every 2 years 5. Increased frequency of US surveillance for HCC, if cirrhosis 6. Transient elastography every 6–12 months
Vaccine, pre- and postexposure prophylaxis	See Chapter 23 Immunoprophylaxis	1. See Chapter 23 Immunoprophylaxis 2. Vaccinate against HAV	1. No HCV vaccine available 2. Vaccinate against HAV and HBV
Management	Supportive	1. Counseling 2. Surveillance for disease progression and complications 3. Treatment depending on age, availability	1. Counseling 2. Surveillance for disease progression and complications 3. Treatment depending on age, availability
Long-term complications		1. Cirrhosis, HCC 2. Rare skin manifestations (Gianotti-Crosti), kidney disease	1. Cirrhosis, HCC 2. Rare extrahepatic manifestations (e.g., thyroid dysfunction, kidney disease)

AFP, Alpha fetoprotein; *ALT*, alanine aminotransferase; *anti-HBc IgM*, hepatitis B core antibody immunoglobulin M; *anti-HBe*, hepatitis B e-antibody; *AST*, aspartate aminotransferase; *DNA*, deoxyribonucleic acid; *HAV*, hepatitis A virus; *HBeAg*, hepatitis B e-antigen; *HBsAg*, hepatitis B surface antigen; *HBV*, hepatitis B virus; *HCC*, hepatocellular carcinoma; *HCV*, hepatitis C virus; *RNA*, ribonucleic acid; *US*, ultrasound.

Figure 16.12 Hepatitis A Serological Markers

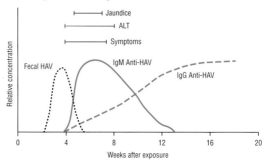

ALT, Alanine aminotransferase; *HAV,* hepatitis A virus; *Ig,* immunoglobulin. (From depts.washington. edu/labweb/Divisions/Viro/images/page33a.jpg.)

Figure 16.13 Hepatitis B Virus Serological Markers

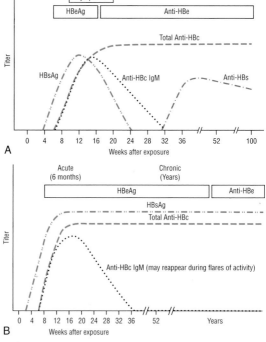

(A) Acute hepatitis B virus (HBV) with recovery. (B) Chronic HBV. *anti-HBc,* Hepatitis B core antibody; *anti-HBe,* hepatitis B e-antibody; *anti-HBs,* hepatitis B surface antibody; *HBeAg,* hepatitis B e-antigen; *HBsAg,* hepatitis B surface antigen; *HBV,* hepatitis B virus; *IgM,* immunoglobulin M. (From Andonov A, Butler, G, Ling R, et al. *Primary Care Management of Hepatitis B—Quick Reference (HBV-QR).* Government of Canada; February 2014.)

Figure 16.14 Hepatitis C Virus Laboratory Markers

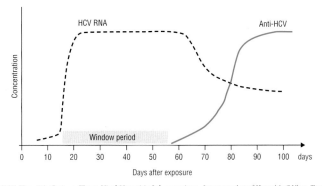

HCV, Hepatitis C virus. (From Viral Hepatitis Subcommittee. *Interpretation of Hepatitis C Virus Test Results: Guidance for Laboratories.* Association of Public Health Laboratories; January 2019.)

NONALCOHOLIC FATTY LIVER DISEASE

1. **Description:** characterized by fat accumulation (steatosis), absence of alcohol consumption, occurring with or without inflammation and fibrosis
2. **Screening**
   a. Screen with ALT, if normal, rescreen every 2 to 3 years
   b. Begin screening at age 9 years for all obese children (BMI >95th percentile) and for overweight children (BMI 85th–94th percentile) with additional risk factors (central adiposity, insulin resistance, prediabetes or diabetes, dyslipidemia, sleep apnea, or family history of NAFLD/nonalcoholic steatohepatitis [NASH])
   c. Consider earlier screening in younger patients with risk factors (severe obesity, family history of NAFLD/NASH, or hypopituitarism)
3. **Investigations** (see Figure 16.15 for screening algorithm)
   a. Bloodwork: ALT, AST, total bilirubin, lipid profile, CBC, GGT, ALP, INR, albumin, total protein, hemoglobin (Hb)A1c
   b. Imaging: abdominal US
   c. Liver biopsy: differentiates between simple steatosis and NASH, determines severity of hepatic fibrosis, and provides prognostic information for disease progression
4. **Management:** dietary modification, exercise, weight loss, diabetes management

Figure 16.15 Nonalcoholic Fatty Liver Disease Screening Algorithm

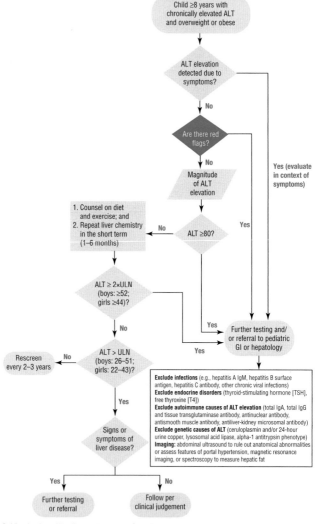

Red flags for advanced liver disease—chronic fatigue, GI bleeding, jaundice, splenomegaly, firm liver on examination, enlarged left lobe of the liver, low platelets, low white blood cell count, elevated direct bilirubin, elevated INR, long history of elevated liver enzymes (>2 years).

ALT, Alanine aminotransferase; *GI*, gastrointestinal; *Ig*, immunoglobulin ; *ULN*, upper limit of normal. (From Vos MB, Abrams SH, Barlow SE, et al. NASPGHAN clinical practice guideline for the diagnosis and treatment of nonalcoholic fatty liver disease in children: recommendations from the expert committee on NAFLD (ECON) and the North American Society of Pediatric Gastroenterology, Hepatology and Nutrition (NASPGHAN). *J Pediatr Gastroenterol Nutr.* 2017;64(2):319–334.)

ACUTE LIVER FAILURE

1. **Definition**
   a. Children: biochemical evidence of acute liver injury and hepatic-based coagulopathy not responsive to vitamin K (INR ≥1.5 with clinical hepatic encephalopathy or INR ≥2.0, regardless of clinical hepatic encephalopathy) and no evidence of known liver disease
   b. Neonates: severe hepatic dysfunction with coagulopathy, metabolic instability, and signs of liver damage in the first 60 days of life
2. **Clinical presentation:** see Box 16.3
3. **Investigations:** see Figure 16.16
4. **Management:** see Figure 16.17

Box 16.3   Suggestive Signs and Symptoms of Acute Liver Failure

- Anorexia, nausea, vomiting
- Fatigue, malaise, lethargy, irritability
- Fever, flulike symptoms
- Jaundice (± dark urine, pale stools, pruritus)
- Hepatic encephalopathy; alterations in sleep and/or behavior
- Asterixis
- Fetor hepaticus (sweetish, slightly fecal smell of exhaled breath)
- Bleeding (varices, gastrointestinal tract, cutaneous, mucous membranes)
- Ascites, hepatomegaly, splenomegaly

Figure 16.16   Acute Liver Failure Investigations

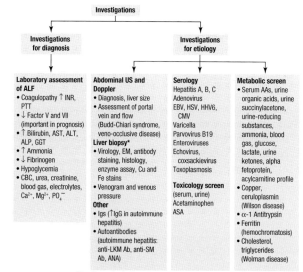

*Consider transjugular biopsy if percutaneous biopsy contraindicated because of coagulopathy.

AA, Amino acid; *ALF*, acute liver failure; *ALP*, alkaline phosphatase; *ALT*, alanine aminotransferase; *ANA*, anti-nuclear antibody; *ASA*, acetylsalicylic acid; *AST*, aspartate aminotransferase; *CBC*, complete blood count; *CMV*, cytomegalovirus; *EBV*, Epstein-Barr virus; *EM*, electron microscopy; *GGT*, gamma-glutamyl transferase; *HHV6*, human herpes virus 6; *HSV*, herpes simplex virus; *IgG*, immunoglobulin G; *INR*, international normalized ratio; *LKM*, liver kidney microsome; *PTT*, partial thromboplastin time; *SM*, smooth muscle.

Figure 16.17 Acute Liver Failure Management

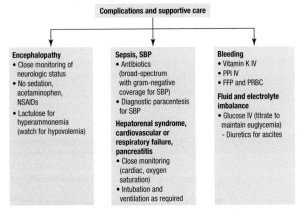

FFP, Fresh frozen plasma; *IV*, intravenous; *NSAID*, nonsteriodal antiinflammatory drug; *PPI*, proton-pump inhibitor; *PRBC*, packed red blood cells; *SBP*, spontaneous bacterial peritonitis.

CHRONIC LIVER FAILURE

1. **Clinical manifestations:** see Figure 16.18
2. **Management**
   a. Slow or reverse progression of liver disease, prevent additional liver insults
   b. Immunizations: scheduled vaccines, hepatitis A and B vaccines
   c. Avoid hepatotoxic medications (e.g., acetaminophen, nonsteroidal antiinflammatory drugs [NSAIDs], methotrexate, valproic acid)
   d. Prevent and treat complications (Table 16.14)
   e. Early assessment with transplant team

Figure 16.18 Stigmata of Chronic Liver Failure

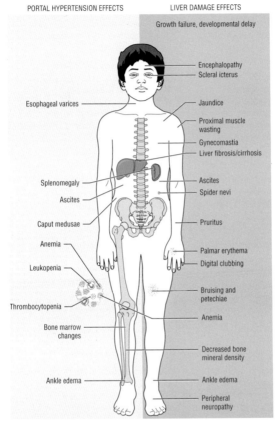

PORTAL HYPERTENSION EFFECTS

LIVER DAMAGE EFFECTS

Growth failure, developmental delay

Encephalopathy
Scleral icterus

Esophageal varices

Jaundice
Proximal muscle wasting
Gynecomastia
Liver fibrosis/cirrhosis

Splenomegaly
Ascites
Caput medusae

Ascites
Spider nevi

Pruritus

Anemia
Leukopenia

Palmar erythema
Digital clubbing

Thrombocytopenia

Bruising and petechiae
Anemia

Bone marrow changes

Decreased bone mineral density

Ankle edema

Ankle edema
Peripheral neuropathy

(Modified from Zachos M, Critch J, Jackson R. Gastroenterology and hepatology. In: Laxer RM, ed. *The Hospital for Sick Children Atlas of Pediatrics*. Philadelphia, PA: Current Medicine LLC; 2005:390–413.)

Table 16.14	Complications and Management of Chronic/End-Stage Liver Disease
Problem	**Approach**
Malnutrition and growth failure	1. Adequate caloric intake (MCT and branch chain AA supplementation) 2. May require supplemental NG feedings or TPN to prevent catabolic state, rickets, coagulopathy, xerophthalmia
Fat soluble vitamin deficiency	1. Vitamin A, D, E, K supplementation

Continued

Table 16.14	Complications and Management of Chronic/ End-Stage Liver Failure—cont'd
Problem	**Approach**
Cholestasis (jaundice, pruritus, xanthomas, xanthelasma)	1. Choleretic agents (ursodiol, cholestyramine) 2. Antihistamines, rifampin
Bleeding - Thrombocytopenia (hypersplenism) - Prolonged INR±PTT - Vitamin K deficiency - Esophageal varices (portal hypertension)	1. Avoid antiplatelet drugs (ASA, NSAIDs) 2. Platelet transfusion 3. FFP and activated factor VIIa for active bleeding 4. Vitamin K 5. PPIs/octreotide (UGI bleeding) 6. Endoscopic sclerotherapy/banding, portosystemic shunting for varices
Ascites (±edema/pleural effusions) - Fluid is transudative (↑ serum/ascitic albumin gradient ≥11 g/L)	1. Sodium restriction 2. Diuretics 3. Water restriction (insensible losses + output) if dilutional hyponatremia prominent 4. Albumin and furosemide in cases of azotemia and intravascular volume depletion 5. Paracentesis for respiratory distress
Increased susceptibility to infections	1. Prevention (inactivated vaccines and live vaccines before transplant) 2. Appropriate antibiotic treatment
SBP (presentation: ±fever, abdominal pain, ↓ bowel sounds, altered mental status)	1. Early recognition and treatment
Renal insufficiency	1. Prerenal failure: volume expansion 2. ATN: ±dialysis 3. At risk for hepatorenal syndrome
Impaired drug clearance (hepatic and renal failure, portal–systemic shunting, hypoalbuminemia)	1. Reduce dosage, monitor toxicity, choose alternative agents
Hepatic encephalopathy (precipitating factors: GI hemorrhage, hypokalemia [especially with alkalosis], sepsis, high-protein diet, constipation, sedative-hypnotic medications, azotemia, pancreatitis, surgery)	1. Identify, remove/correct, and avoid precipitants 2. Tight fluid and electrolyte control 3. Dietary: protein restriction 4. Lactulose (PO/PR): ↓ ammonia resorption 5. Antibiotics (neomycin, metronidazole): ↓ available bacterial urease

AA, Amino acid; *ASA,* acetylsalicylic acid; *ATN,* acute tubular necrosis; *FFP,* fresh frozen plasma; *GI,* gastrointestinal; *INR,* international normalized ratio; *MCT,* medium chain triglycerides; *NG,* nasogastric; *NSAID,* nonsteroidal antiinflammatory drug; *PO,* per os (by mouth); *PR,* per rectum; *PPI,* proton-pump inhibitor; *PTT,* partial thromboplastin time; *TPN,* total parenteral nutrition; *SBP,* spontaneous bacterial peritonitis; *UGI,* upper gastrointestinal.

HYPERBILIRUBINEMIA/CHOLESTASIS IN INFANCY

1. Measure total, conjugated/direct bilirubin in all jaundiced infants
   a. If breastfed, at 3 weeks of life
   b. If formula fed, at 2 weeks of life
   c. At any age, if pale stools or dark urine
2. Conjugated/direct bilirubin abnormal if
   a. >18 mmol/L if the total bilirubin is <85 mmol/L
   b. >20% total bilirubin if total bilirubin is >85 mmol/L
3. See Figure 16.19 for approach
4. Treatment depends on etiology. For biliary atresia, timely diagnosis important for prognosis.

Figure 16.19   Approach to Cholestasis in Infancy

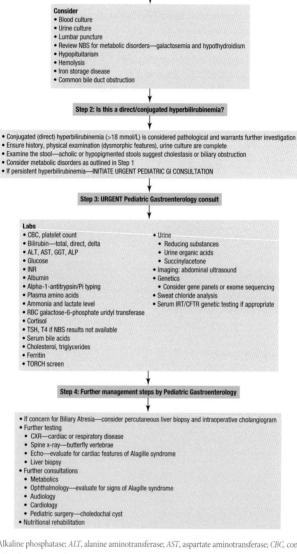

Step 1: Rule out acute illness

Consider
- Blood culture
- Urine culture
- Lumbar puncture
- Review NBS for metabolic disorders—galactosemia and hypothyroidism
- Hypopituitarism
- Hemolysis
- Iron storage disease
- Common bile duct obstruction

Step 2: Is this a direct/conjugated hyperbilirubinemia?

- Conjugated (direct) hyperbilirubinemia (>18 mmol/L) is considered pathological and warrants further investigation
- Ensure history, physical examination (dysmorphic features), urine culture are complete
- Examine the stool—acholic or hypopigmented stools suggest cholestasis or biliary obstruction
- Consider metabolic disorders as outlined in Step 1
- If persistent hyperbilirubinemia—INITIATE URGENT PEDIATRIC GI CONSULTATION

Step 3: URGENT Pediatric Gastroenterology consult

Labs
- CBC, platelet count
- Bilirubin—total, direct, delta
- ALT, AST, GGT, ALP
- Glucose
- INR
- Albumin
- Alpha-1-antitrypsin/Pi typing
- Plasma amino acids
- Ammonia and lactate level
- RBC galactose-6-phosphate uridyl transferase
- Cortisol
- TSH, T4 if NBS results not available
- Serum bile acids
- Cholesterol, triglycerides
- Ferritin
- TORCH screen

- Urine
  - Reducing substances
  - Urine organic acids
  - Succinylacetone
- Imaging: abdominal ultrasound
- Genetics
  - Consider gene panels or exome sequencing
- Sweat chloride analysis
- Serum IRT/CFTR genetic testing if appropriate

Step 4: Further management steps by Pediatric Gastroenterology

- If concern for Biliary Atresia—consider percutaneous liver biopsy and intraoperative cholangiogram
- Further testing
  - CXR—cardiac or respiratory disease
  - Spine x-ray—butterfly vertebrae
  - Echo—evaluate for cardiac features of Alagille syndrome
  - Liver biopsy
- Further consultations
  - Metabolics
  - Ophthalmology—evaluate for signs of Alagille syndrome
  - Audiology
  - Cardiology
  - Pediatric surgery—choledochal cyst
- Nutritional rehabilitation

LP, Alkaline phosphatase; *ALT*, alanine aminotransferase; *AST*, aspartate aminotransferase; *CBC*, complete blood count; *CXR*, chest x-ray; *GGT*, gamma-glutamyl transferase; *GI*, gastroenterology; *INR*, international normalized ratio; *IRT*, immunoreactive trypsin; *NBS*, newborn screen; *RBC*, red blood cell; *TSH*, thyroid-stimulating hormone; *TORCH* screen, Toxoplasma gondii, other viruses, rubella, cytomegalovirus, herpes simplex virus.

HYPERBILIRUBINEMIA OUTSIDE OF INFANCY

1. Investigate new onset jaundice to delineate conjugated hyperbilirubinemia (obstructive or hepatocellular causes) versus unconjugated hyperbilirubinemia (hemolysis or inadequate bilirubin conjugation)
   a. **Obstructive:** stones, choledochal cyst, primary sclerosing cholangitis, tumors, parasitic infections
   b. **Hepatocellular:** viral, medication induced, Wilson disease, autoimmune hepatitis
2. See Table 16.15 for differential diagnoses and approach
3. Treatment depends on underlying etiology

Table 16.15	Differential Diagnosis of Conjugated Hyperbilirubinemia Outside of Infancy
Disease	**Major Diagnostic Strategy**
Obstructive Cholestasis	
Choledochal cyst or other congenital bile duct anomaly	US, cholangiogram
Gallstones or biliary sludge	US
Tumor	US or CT abdomen
Hepatocellular Cholestasis	
Autoimmune	
Autoimmune hepatitis	Increased ANA, ASMA, LKM-1, serum protein electrophoresis, quantitative immunoglobulins
Primary sclerosing cholangitis (PSC)	Increased ALP, GGT, immunoglobulins, ERCP/MRCP
Primary biliary cholangitis (PBC)	Increased AMA, ANA, liver enzymes, liver biopsy
Disorders of Intrahepatic Bile Ducts	
Alagille syndrome (paucity of intrahepatic bile ducts)	Echocardiogram (peripheral pulmonic stenosis), eye examination (posterior embryotoxon), CXR (butterfly vertebrae), liver biopsy (paucity of small ducts), typical facial appearance (broad forehead, pointed chin, elongated nose with bulbous tip), genetic testing
Nonsyndromic paucity of the intrahepatic bile ducts	US, cholangiogram
Congenital hepatic fibrosis/Caroli disease	US, cholangiogram, liver biopsy, renal US (associated abnormalities)
Genetic and Metabolic Disorders	
Wilson disease	CBC, liver enzymes, decreased serum ceruloplasmin, increased copper level, ocular slit lamp examination, 24 h urinary copper excretion
Dubin-Johnson syndrome	Urinary coproporphyrin excretion, CT (liver is densely black, shows higher attenuation), liver biopsy

Table 16.15	Differential Diagnosis of Conjugated Hyperbilirubinemia Outside of Infancy—cont'd
Disease	**Major Diagnostic Strategy**
Rotor syndrome	Urinary coproporphyrin excretion, oral cholecystography
Mitochondrial disorders	CBC, elevated CK, liver enzymes, albumin, lactate, pyruvate, serum amino acids, serum acylcarnitine, urine organic acids
α1-AT deficiency	↓α1-AT level, Pi genotyping (ZZ, Znul, nul deficient)
Hemochromatosis	↑Ferritin, ↓ total iron binding
Cystic fibrosis	Sweat chloride test
Progressive familial intrahepatic cholestasis	Liver biopsy, GGT (↓/normal in types 1 and 2, ↑ in type 3), genetic testing
Endocrine	
Hypothyroidism	↑TSH, ↓ T$_4$
Panhypopituitarism	↓ cortisol, ↓TSH, ↓T$_4$
Toxic/Secondary	
Parenteral nutrition–associated cholestasis	
Drugs (e.g., acetaminophen, anticonvulsants) and toxins (e.g., alcohol, organophosphates)	Urine and serum toxicology testing
Infectious	
Hepatitis A, B, C, D, E, nontypeable hepatitis	HAV-IgM, HBsAg, anti-HBs, HBeAg, Anti-HBe, Anti-HBc, HBV-DNA, anti-HBc-IgM, anti-HCV, HDV-IgM, HEV-IgM, HEV-IgG
HIV	HIV DNA PCR, serology, CD4 count
Sepsis	Blood cultures
Other	
Vascular anomalies	Doppler US
Budd-Chiari syndrome	Doppler US, prothrombotic work-up
Hemangioma	Doppler US
Cardiac insufficiency and hypoperfusion	Echocardiogram

α1-AT, Alpha-1 antitrypsin; *ALP,* alkaline phosphatase; *AMA,* antimitochondrial antibody; *ANA,* antinuclear antibody; *ASMA,* antismooth muscle antibody; *CBC,* complete blood count; *CK,* creatine kinase; *CT,* computed tomography; *CXR,* chest x-ray; *DNA,* deoxyribonucleic acid; *ERCP,* endoscopic retrograde cholangiopancreatography; *GGT,* gamma-glutamyl transpeptidase; *HIV,* human immunodeficiency virus; *LKM-1,* liver kidney microsome type 1; *MRCP,* magnetic resonance cholangiopancreatography; *PCR,* polymerase chain reaction; *TSH,* thyroid stimulating hormone; *US,* ultrasound.

ACUTE ASCENDING CHOLANGITIS

1. **Description:** characterized by fever, jaundice and right upper quadrant abdominal pain secondary to stasis/obstruction and infection in the biliary tract
2. **Associations:** biliary atresia, calculi, benign stricture, sclerosing cholangitis, postliver transplant
3. **Diagnosis:** ↑ white blood cell (WBC) count, cholestatic pattern of LFTs, blood culture, US
4. **Treatment:** broad-spectrum antibiotics to cover gram-negative bacteria and enterococci ± anaerobes (e.g., ampicillin, gentamicin, and metronidazole), biliary drainage in select cases (e.g., cholangitis secondary to biliary calculi)

GALLSTONES (CHOLELITHIASIS)

1. **Etiology:** hemolytic disease, TPN, Wilson disease, epilepsy medications, malabsorption, NEC, hepatobiliary diseases, obesity, abdominal surgery, acute leukemia, cystic fibrosis (CF)
   a. Stone features: cholesterol (risk factors: hyperlipidemia, obesity, CF, pregnancy, octreotide use), black pigment (risk factors: hemolytic anemia, TPN, ceftriaxone use), or brown pigment (bacterial infections, parasitic infections, bile duct anomaly, use of birth control)
2. **Clinical manifestations**
   a. Children predominantly asymptomatic, found incidentally on US
   b. If symptomatic, likely secondary to cholecystitis, cholangitis, or cholestasis causing abdominal pain, nausea, vomiting, icterus, and positive Murphy's sign
3. **Investigations:** abdominal US
4. **Treatment:** based on location of the stone, severity of symptoms, cause of stone formation, comorbidities, evidence of inflammatory change and age. See Table 16.16 for therapeutic options.

Table 16.16	Therapeutic Approaches for Cholelithiasis
Approach	Description
Surgical	
Cholecystectomy	Method of choice if symptomatic
Cholecystostomy	For acute gallbladder drainage (i.e., acalculous cholecystitis)
ERCP	
Basket removal	Bile duct stone removal
Mechanical basket lithotripsy	Stone crushing within the bile ducts
Electrohydraulic or laser lithotripsy	Stone destruction within the bile ducts

Table 16.16	Therapeutic Approaches for Cholelithiasis—cont'd
Approach	Description
Dissolution	
Oral medication	Ursodeoxycholic acid and chenodeoxycholic acid
Contact	Methyl tert-butyl-ether (cholesterol stones) or bile acid-EDTA solution (pigment stones)
Preventative Measures	
Enteral feeding	Trophic feeds can decrease stone formation while on TPN
Weight loss	In obese patients

EDTA, Ethylenediaminetetraacetic acid; *ERCP,* endoscopic retrograde cholangiopancreatography; *TPN,* total parenteral nutrition.

Data from Karami H, Kianifar H, Karami S. Cholelithasis in children: a diagnostic and therapeutic approach. *J Pediatr Rev.* 2017;5(1):e9114.

LIVER TRANSPLANT

1. Most common indication: biliary atresia
2. See Chapter 38 Transplantation

General Surgery

Jonathon Hagel • Justyna M. Wolinska • Georges Azzie

Also see page xviii for a list of other abbreviations used throughout this book

CDH	congenital diaphragmatic hernia
EA	esophageal atresia
NG	nasogastric
OR	operating room
RLQ	right lower quadrant
RUQ	right upper quadrant
SMA	superior mesenteric artery
SMV	superior mesenteric vein
TEF	tracheoesophageal fistula
UGI	upper gastrointestinal (series)
VACTERL	*v*ertebral defects, *a*norectal malformation, *c*ardiac anomalies, *t*racheoesophageal fistula with *e*sophageal atresia, *r*enal anomalies, *l*imb anomalies

OBSTRUCTION—NEONATAL

TRACHEOESOPHAGEAL FISTULA (TEF) AND ESOPHAGEAL ATRESIA (EA)

1. **Definition and etiology**
   a. Congenital anomalies caused by a defect in septation of the foregut into the esophagus and trachea
   b. Classified according to the anatomic configuration (Figure 17.1)
   c. Associated anomalies in 55% of cases (often as part of vertebral defects, anorectal malformation, cardiac anomalies, tracheoesophageal fistula with esophageal atresia, renal anomalies, limb anomalies [VACTERL])

2. **Presentation**
   a. Cases of EA (~95%) present in the newborn period:
      i. History of maternal polyhydramnios
      ii. **Excessive oral secretions** and **choking/cyanosis with feeding**
   b. **H type TEF may be a delayed diagnosis:** rare subtype that uniquely presents with recurrent aspiration pneumonia

3. **Investigations**
   a. **Inability to pass nasogastric (NG) tube into stomach** (except H type) **often diagnostic**
   b. **CXR**
      i. Upper esophageal pouch dilated with air (for two most common types)
      ii. Curled OG/NG in upper esophagus
   c. **AXR:** air in the GI tract confirms the presence of a TEF versus pure EA
   d. Contrast studies are rarely ever required (if necessary, use water soluble contrast because of risk of aspiration)

Figure 17.1 Most Common Forms of Esophageal Atresia and Tracheoesophageal Fistula

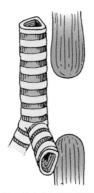

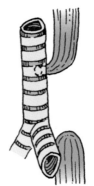

Type A: isolated EA (9%)

Type B: proximal fistula with distal atresia (1%)

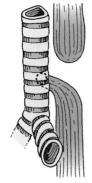

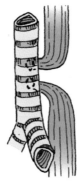

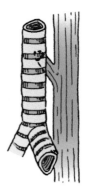

Type C: proximal atresia with distal fistula (82%)

Type D: double fistula with intervening atresia (2%)

Type E: isolated fistula (H-type) (6%)

(From Liacouras CA, Wendel D, Jump C, et al. Gastroenterology. In: Polin RA, Ditmar MF, eds. *Pediatric Secrets.* 6th ed. Philadelphia, PA: Elsevier; 2016.)

4. **Management**
   a. NPO on maintenance fluids
   b. Replogle tube set to low suction
   c. Consider antibiotics if concern for aspiration
   d. **VACTERL screen** (abdominal US, cardiac ECHO, spine x-ray and US, examination for limb anomalies)
   e. Operative repair

5. **Complications**
   a. Anastomotic leak, esophageal stricture, recurrent TEF
   b. Long-term surveillance for feeding intolerance, growth, gastroesophageal reflux disease (GERD), and tracheomalacia

INTESTINAL ATRESIA

1. **Definition**
   a. Congenital defect resulting in obstruction in a hollow viscous lumen: duodenal atresia (most common), jejunoileal atresia, colonic atresia
   b. Duodenal atresia associated with trisomy 21 and other cardiac, renal, GI anomalies; jejunoileal atresia associated with cystic fibrosis

2. **Presentation**
   a. Bilious vomiting (most common), abdominal distension, failure to pass meconium in first 24 hours

3. **Investigations**
   a. Duodenal atresia: AXR shows "double bubble" sign (distension of stomach and proximal duodenum); often visible on prenatal US. Upper gastrointestinal series can confirm diagnosis.
   b. Jejunoileal/colonic atresia: AXR shows diffuse air fluid levels in multiple loops of dilated intestine. Contrast enema rules out both isolated and associated colonic atresias.

4. **Management**
   a. Decompression of proximal GI tract with NG tube, IV fluids
   b. Surgical repair

HIRSCHSPRUNG DISEASE

1. **Definition and etiology**
   a. Absence of ganglion cells beginning at anorectal junction (and extending proximally for variable distance), leading to functional obstruction
   b. Location of aganglionic segment: rectosigmoid (75%), colonic extension (15%–20%), total colon (5%)
   c. Associated with trisomy 21, Waardenburg syndrome, congenital central hypoventilation syndrome, cardiovascular anomalies

2. **Presentation**
   a. Majority present in neonatal period with signs of distal intestinal obstruction: **failure to pass meconium** in first 24 hours, **abdominal distension**, **vomiting**

   b. **Hirschsprung enterocolitis:** potentially life-threatening complication presenting with diarrhea, anorexia, abdominal distension, and fever with lethargy or shock

   c. Explosive release of stool and gas on rectal examination ("blast sign") which may temporarily relieve obstruction

   d. Late presentation with chronic refractory constipation

3. **Investigations**

   a. **AXR:** may show nonspecific findings of distal bowel obstruction (diffusely dilated bowel with air; air fluid levels)

   b. **Contrast enema** can suggest diagnosis and location of transition zone

     i. Small-caliber rectum (rectum should always be more dilated than sigmoid)

     ii. Dilation of colon proximal to narrowed (aganglionic) segment (diameter of colon > diameter of rectum) with **transition zone** (present in 80% of cases)

   c. **Gold standard: rectal biopsy** (absence of ganglion cells)

   d. **Anorectal manometry:** absence of anorectal inhibitory reflex may aid in diagnosis in older patients able to cooperate

4. **Management**

   a. Anal stimulation or rectal irrigations for obstructive symptoms (enemas should NOT be used because these infants cannot spontaneously pass stool)

   b. Definitive management is surgical: most common surgical treatment is **one-stage pull-through** procedure

   c. If **enterocolitis** present: IV fluid resuscitation, broad spectrum antibiotics, rectal irrigations to decompress (30 cc/kg normal saline q6h); may require urgent diverting ostomy if no response

MECONIUM ILEUS

1. **Definition and etiology**

   a. Obstruction of the small intestine at the level of the terminal ileum with inspissated meconium

   b. More than 80% of patients with meconium ileus have cystic fibrosis (CF) but it is the presenting feature in only 10% to 20% of patients with CF

> ✴ **PEARL**
>
> All cases of meconium ileus should prompt a sweat chloride test to rule out cystic fibrosis.

2. **Presentation**

   a. In general, presents within first 3 days of life: **failure to pass meconium** in the setting of a patent anus, **abdominal distension**, ± **bilious emesis**

3. **Investigations**
    a. **AXR**
        i. Dilated loops of small bowel **without air–fluid levels**
        ii. **"Soap-bubble" appearance** of intestinal contents proximal to the obstruction (air mixed with meconium)
    b. **Contrast enema**
        i. Microcolon (unused colon)
        ii. Small pellets of meconium outlined by contrast material in terminal ileum
4. **Management**
    a. Nonoperative: water-soluble enemas to break up meconium and relieve obstruction
    b. Operative: if nonoperative management fails or "complicated" cases (perforation with meconium peritonitis, volvulus, intestinal atresia)

ANORECTAL MALFORMATION (ARM)

1. **Definition and etiology**
    a. Abnormalities in anorectal development, including imperforate anus, perineal fistula, and persistent cloaca (a single orifice in females; often associated with a hydrocolpos)
    b. Anal atresia (rare) also associated with VACTERL
2. **Investigations**
    a. Look for meconium excreted from urethra, vestibule of vagina, or on perineal skin, including the scrotum (via fistula)

> **PEARL**
>
> 80% to 90% of anorectal malformation cases can be determined by good clinical evaluation. All cases must, however, have thorough investigations for VACTERL associations. In males, eventual distal contrast study via the mucus fistula is required to define the precise anatomy.

3. **Management**
    a. At presentation: npo, decompress the GI tract, urine assessment for stool, and VACTERL screen (see TEF section for details). Antibiotics if urethral fistula suspected.
    b. **Usually three-stage surgical treatment** involving colostomy, anorectoplasty, and colostomy closure. Select cases may be amenable to single-stage procedure.

OBSTRUCTION—EARLY INFANCY

HYPERTROPHIC PYLORIC STENOSIS

1. **Definition and etiology**
    a. Hypertrophy of pylorus leading to gastric outlet obstruction
    b. Risk factors: males > females (4:1), firstborn, familial tendency

Presentation

a. 2 weeks to 2 months of life

b. Classic presentation: postprandial **nonbilious projectile vomiting** followed by desire to feed ("hungry vomiter")

c. Acute weight loss and dehydration can be seen with prolonged symptoms

d. Laboratory evaluation: **hypochloremic hypokalemic metabolic alkalosis**

e. Other findings: "olive-like" like mass in epigastrium and upper abdominal peristaltic waves (late finding)

Physical examination

a. Epigastric "olive" (i.e., the hypertrophied pylorus) may be palpable under the costal margin in the midline when infant is calm and abdominal muscles relaxed

Investigations

a. **Abdominal ultrasound** (first line)
   i. Pylorus measurements: thickness >3 mm, length >15 mm
   ii. Failure to see gastric emptying through the pyloric channel

b. Upper GI contrast study only if US not available (looking for elongated pyloric channel: "string sign")

Management

a. NPO ± NG tube for decompression

b. Fluid resuscitation: fluid bolus (as needed), 1.5 × maintenance fluids (may require 48–72 hours to correct electrolyte abnormalities and fluid deficit)

c. Surgery should be delayed in the setting of dehydration and/or electrolyte derangements (risk of hypotension at induction or apnea)

d. Operative repair: pyloromyotomy

OBSTRUCTION—CHILDHOOD

INTUSSUSCEPTION

Definition and etiology

a. Telescoping or invagination of proximal portion of intestine into more distal portion

b. Most commonly **ileocolic** (85%). Ileoileal or jejunoileal intussusceptions usually not significant (usually incidental abdominal US finding) and generally no treatment necessary.

c. ~75% of cases considered to be idiopathic (GI lymphoid hyperplasia from viral infection may serve as lead point)

d. Pathologic lead points: Meckel diverticulum, appendix, polyps, duplications, submucosal hemorrhage (e.g., Henoch-Schönlein purpura), lymphomas, tumors, hamartoma (Peutz Jaeger)

e. If the intussusception is secondary to a gastrostomy-jejunostomy (GJ) tube lead point, interventional radiology should be asked to manipulate the tube

2. **Presentation**
   a. Typically presents **3 months to 3 years** of age
   b. Cyclic **episodes of sudden, crampy, severe abdominal pain** q5–30min (often accompanied by crying and drawing legs up to abdomen). Patient may appear calm, pain free, or lethargic between episodes
   c. **Vomiting:** may become bilious as obstruction progresses
   d. **Bloody stools:** grossly bloody or occult blood positive ("red currant jelly" stools are a late sign because of intestinal mucosal congestion, ischemia, or mucosal sloughing)
   e. Palpable right sided abdominal mass
3. **Investigations**
   a. **Ultrasound** is diagnostic ("target sign"): 97% sensitivity, 95% specificity when intussuscepted
4. **Management**
   a. **Ileocolic** (most common) and **colocolic** (very rare) **intussusceptions should be treated**. Small bowel-small bowel intussusceptions do not generally require treatment.
   b. NPO, fluid resuscitation as needed; then proceed to air enema. Consider broad spectrum antibiotics only if unstable or suspected perforation.
   c. **Nonoperative enema reduction**
      i. Pneumatic (air) enema reduction under ultrasound or fluoroscopic guidance is procedure of choice
      ii. Contrast (barium enema) can be used (slightly lower success rates and complications if intestinal perforation occurs)
      iii. Delayed repeat enema for partly reduced intussusceptions in stable patients often successful and avoids surgery (performed at discretion of treating physicians)
      iv. Postprocedure: advance to clear fluids when awake; discharge home after 2 to 4 hours, if asymptomatic
      v. Absolute contraindications to air enema: hemodynamic instability, pneumoperitoneum, peritonitis
   d. **Operative management** indicated for patients who are acutely ill/unstable, those with signs of bowel perforation, or for failed non-operative management

e. **Recurrence risk:** 5% to 10% after successful nonoperative reduction, 1% to 4% after surgical reduction

BOWEL OBSTRUCTION

1. **Definition and etiology**
   a. **Mechanical obstruction:** partial or complete blockage of the bowel resulting in failure of intestinal contents to pass through lumen
   b. **Paralytic ileus** (nonmechanical bowel obstruction): functional blockage of the bowel because of paralysis of intestinal muscles
2. **Causes**
   a. Mechanical obstruction
      i. Extrinsic causes: adhesions, hernias, inflammatory mass (5% lifetime risk of adhesive small bowel obstruction for postsurgical patients; most common in first 2 years after abdominal surgery)
      ii. Intrinsic causes: intestinal atresia, meconium ileus, Hirschsprung disease, foreign body, mass, duplication
   b. Paralytic ileus: may occur postoperatively, as a side effect of drugs, or reaction to various injuries, illnesses, infections
3. **Presentation**
   a. **Small bowel obstruction:** large-volume frequent emesis (bilious emesis when distal to ampulla of Vater), crampy abdominal pain relieved by vomiting, minimal distension if proximal, more distended if distal. Fundoplication patients may be unable to vomit.
   b. **Large bowel obstruction:** abdominal distension, emesis that is **progressively feculent**, crampy abdominal pain
   c. **Complete obstruction:** obstipation (unable to pass gas/stool) versus **incomplete obstruction:** loose stools
   d. **Peritonitis** (surgical emergency) should be suspected if patient develops fever, tachycardia, hypotension, hematemesis, bleeding from rectum, or clinical peritoneal signs (rebound, guarding)

> **! PITFALL**
>
> Failure to consider obstruction in a patient with vomiting and abdominal distension but who is still passing stools can lead to missed diagnosis.

4. **Investigations**
   a. **AXR** (at least two views: flat and upright views or flat and left lateral decubitus)
      i. dilated loops of bowel
      ii. air–fluid levels
      iii. paucity of gas in colon

    b. **Computed tomography (CT) abdomen may be required** in cases of mechanical obstruction to fully determine the level/cause of an obstruction and assess for compromised bowel

5. **Management**
    a. **NPO** and IV fluids as needed, bloodwork (CBC, electrolytes)
    b. **NG tube** for decompression of the stomach
    c. Antibiotics for any signs of bowel perforation
    d. **Surgical consultation:** indications for urgent surgical consultation (and possible operative intervention) include: peritonitis, free air on AXR, radiologic evidence of non-evolving gas pattern (sign of high grade obstruction), obstruction in patients with virgin abdomen (i.e., no prior abdominal surgeries)

ACUTE ABDOMEN

NEONATAL NECROTIZING ENTEROCOLITIS

See necrotizing enterocolitis in Chapter 27 Neonatology for further details

MALROTATION AND MIDGUT VOLVULUS

1. **Definition and etiology**
    a. **Intestinal malrotation:** congenital anomaly of rotation of the embryonic gut, which results in abnormal positioning of small and large intestine with a narrow-based mesentery (Figure 17.2)
    b. **Midgut volvulus** (a true surgical emergency): narrow mesenteric base permits twisting of the small intestine, which obstructs mesenteric blood vessels and causes gut ischemia and infarction

2. **Presentation**
    a. **Volvulus**
        i. Bilious vomiting, sudden onset of abdominal pain, scaphoid abdomen which eventually progresses to abdominal distension as a **late sign**
        ii. Signs of progression from ischemia to infarction and necrosis: fever, peritonitis, abdominal distension, dehydration, hemodynamic instability, metabolic acidosis, septic appearance
        iii. Some 30% of patients with symptomatic malrotation present in first week of life, >65% in first month, but may present at any age
    b. **Malrotation:** older children with uncorrected malrotation can present with chronic, vague symptoms, such as recurrent intermittent vomiting, crampy abdominal pain, failure to thrive, or constipation
    c. Malrotation can also be asymptomatic!

Figure 17.2 Intestinal Malrotation

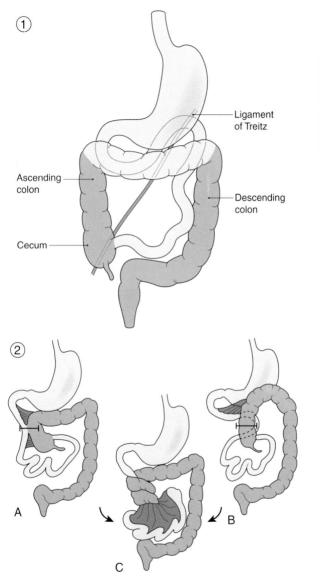

1: Normal intestinal anatomy and mesenteric fixation. 2: Abnormal mesenteric fixation in nonrotation (A) and incomplete rotation (B), leading to intestinal volvulus (C). (From Evans S. *Surgical Pitfalls*. Saunders; 2009; and Wyllie R, Hyams J. *Pediatric Gastrointestinal and Liver Disease*. 4th ed. Philadelphia, PA: Saunders; 2004.)

3. **Investigations**
   a. **AXR:** should be used to rule out perforation if there is clinical suspicion
   b. **Upper GI series is the gold standard** in stable patients
      i. Findings in malrotation: duodenojejunal flexure is to the right of the midline and lower than level of pylorus
      ii. Findings in malrotation with volvulus: duodenum stays to right of spine and has a "corkscrew" appearance. Contrast fails to fill jejunum as a result of obstruction.
   c. **Imaging adjuncts**
      i. Ultrasound: inversion of the superior mesenteric vein to superior mesenteric artery relationship may suggest malrotation; "whirlpool sign" suggests volvulus
      ii. Contrast enema: can be used to identify abnormal position of cecum (however high false positive and false negative rate)
      iii. AXR: may be normal or show nonspecific findings (intestinal dilatation, gasless abdomen) or rarely, diagnostic findings, such as "double bubble" sign, signifying duodenal obstruction

> **! PITFALL**
> Normal abdominal x-ray findings do not rule out a malrotation or volvulus.

4. **Management**
   a. NPO with fluid resuscitation as needed
   b. NG tube
   c. Broad-spectrum IV antibiotics
   d. Stable patients should undergo immediate radiologic assessment
   e. Critically ill or unstable patients, with high suspicion for volvulus, should be rapidly resuscitated and taken directly to the operating room (OR) for exploration and repair
   f. OR repair: laparotomy and Ladd's procedure

APPENDICITIS
1. **Definition and etiology**
   a. Inflammation of the appendix most commonly caused by nonspecific obstruction of the appendiceal lumen
   b. Peak incidence 10 to 12 years of age
2. **Presentation**
   a. Periumbilical dull constant pain, followed by anorexia and vomiting
   b. Pain moves to the RLQ as inflammation progresses (however 15% have atypically located appendix)
   c. May be accompanied by watery diarrhea, low-grade fever

d. RLQ tenderness with localized peritonitis is most valuable finding on examination
e. Generalized peritonitis may occur with noncontained perforation
f. Perforation correlates with duration of symptoms (may occur 36–48 hours after onset of symptoms); infants and children <5 years of age have highest rates of perforation

3. **Investigations**
   a. **Laboratory tests**
      i. WBC and absolute neutrophil count (ANC) frequently elevated but not specific nor sensitive enough to rule diagnosis in nor out
      ii. β-hCG to rule out ectopic pregnancy in adolescent females
      iii. Urinalysis: can help rule out UTI; however sterile pyuria is commonly seen in appendicitis
   b. **Imaging**
      i. **Ultrasound** should be used as first-line diagnostic study in stable patients: noncompressible tubular structure, diameter >7 mm, hyperemia, ± calcified appendicolith, surrounding echogenic fat, free fluid, fluid collections if perforation
      ii. **CT scan or MRI** for cases with inconclusive US findings and high clinical suspicion

4. **Management**
   a. **NPO** with IV fluids
   b. **IV antibiotics**
      i. Cefoxitin if not perforated
      ii. Broad spectrum antibiotics if perforated (e.g., ceftriaxone and metronidazole)
   c. **Nonperforated appendicitis** or advanced appendicitis without appendiceal abscess: urgent appendectomy
   d. **Delayed presentation associated with perforation and phlegmon or abscess**
      i. Broad spectrum IV antibiotics until afebrile and clinically improved
      ii. If no clinical improvement: obtain additional imaging to rule out abscess formation, consider drainage and additional antibiotics
      iii. Interval appendectomy can be considered after minimum of 6 to 8 weeks

General Surgery

17

BOCHDALEK HERNIA

1. **Definition and etiology**
   a. Herniation through posterolateral foramen of Bochdalek (most common)
   b. Left-sided defects most common (70%–85%); occasionally bilateral (<5%)
   c. Associated anomalies (15%–25%): CNS lesions, esophageal atresia, omphalocele, cardiac lesions, trisomy 21, lethal syndromes

2. **Presentation**
   a. **Prenatal diagnosis:** most commonly diagnosed on routine US
   b. **Postnatal presentation:** severe respiratory distress in first hours of life, secondary to pulmonary hypoplasia and resultant pulmonary hypertension (causes R→L shunt and persistent fetal circulation)
   c. **Physical findings**
      i. Absent breath sounds on affected side with barrel-shaped chest
      ii. Scaphoid abdomen secondary to abdominal contents in the chest
      iii. Shifted heart sounds (mediastinal shift)

3. **Investigations**
   a. **CXR/AXR**
      i. Loops of air-filled intestine within thoracic cavity
      ii. Absence of intestine in abdominal cavity
      iii. Shifted mediastinum
      iv. NG tube in chest (if stomach above diaphragm)
   b. **Measurement of pre- and postductal saturations**
   c. **ECHO** to assess pulmonary hypertension (associated cardiac anomaly increases mortality)

4. **Management**
   a. Avoid bag and mask ventilation (leads to gastric distension, lung compression)
   b. Rapid endotracheal intubation if breathing compromised
      i. Ventilate with low peak inspiratory pressures
      ii. May require high frequency oscillation ventilation, pulmonary vasodilators (e.g., nitric oxide), and extracorporeal membrane oxygenation (ECMO)
   c. NG tube to low suction (decompress stomach)
   d. Operative repair when hemodynamically stable on minimal ventilatory support

e. Postoperative management is complicated by pulmonary hypertension because of pulmonary hypoplasia (neither can be corrected surgically). Mortality is directly proportional to the degree of pulmonary hypoplasia.

> **! PITFALL**
>
> Ventilation with high positive pressures in cases of congenital diaphragmatic hernia can cause barotrauma to hypoplastic lung.

MORGAGNI HERNIA

1. **Definition and etiology**
   a. Herniation of bowel through anterior foramen of Morgagni; most commonly right-sided
   b. Accounts for <2% of all congenital diaphragmatic hernias
2. **Investigations**
   a. CXR: incidental finding in children with symptoms of intestinal obstruction/respiratory illness
3. **Management**
   a. Once identified, repair to avoid small risk of incarceration

GASTROSCHISIS AND OMPHALOCELE

See Table 17.1

Table 17.1	Characteristics of Gastroschisis and Omphalocele	
Factor	**Gastroschisis**	**Omphalocele**
Definition	Abdominal contents free on anterior abdominal wall; defect commonly to right of umbilical cord	Abdominal contents herniated onto anterior abdominal wall but are encased in sac (unless ruptured)
Umbilical cord	Separate	Included in defect
Size of defect	Small (2–3 cm)	Variable (2–15 cm)
Contents	Bowel; occasionally bladder; ovaries, testes	Bowel; frequently liver
Membrane	Never	Always (may rupture)
Rotational anomaly	Yes	Yes
Intestinal function	Prolonged ileus/dysmotility	Usually normal
Associated defects	Intestinal atresia (10%–15%)	Cardiac (20%–25%), chromosomal, e.g., Beckwith Wiedemann syndrome (5%–15%)

Continued

Table 17.1	Characteristics of Gastroschisis and Omphalocele—cont'd	
Factor	**Gastroschisis**	**Omphalocele**
Management	- Position in right lateral decubitus, NG to suction - Cover viscera with sterile saline soaked gauze and cellophane wrap - Generous IV fluids (goal: urine output ≥1 mL/kg/h) and antibiotics - OR for reduction (primary closure or staged closure with silastic silo)	- NG to suction - Sterile wrapping of bowel - Generous IV fluids (goal: urine output ≥1 mL/kg/h) and antibiotics - Small defects (2–3 cm): primary closure in OR - Larger defects: staged/delayed closure with use of silo, patch, eschar-inducing dressing

IV, Intravenous; *NG*, nasogastric; *OR*, operating room.

Modified from Holcombe GW, Murphy JP, Ostlie DJ. *Ashcraft's Pediatric Surgery*. 6th ed. Philadelphia: Elsevier; 2014.

HERNIAS AND THE GROIN

UMBILICAL HERNIA
1. Due to incomplete closure of umbilical ring after cord separation
2. Almost never incarcerate; majority close by 3 years of age
3. Unlikely to close spontaneously after 5 years of age; surgical repair required

INGUINAL HERNIA
1. **Definition and etiology**
   a. Protrusion of a portion of the abdominal contents into the scrotum or labia through an abnormal opening in the inguinal canal, usually secondary to a patent processus vaginalis. May contain omentum, bowel, and often ovary ± fallopian tube in infant females.
2. **Presentation**
   a. **Bulging in groin or scrotal sac**, increased with crying or straining
   b. **Incarceration:** herniated contents not reducible by manipulation, but contents are viable
      i. Occurs in 30% of inguinal hernias in the first year of life
      ii. Signs of incarceration: irritability, distension, vomiting, firm tender mass
   c. **Strangulation:** vascular compromise of the contents of an incarcerated hernia; can occur within 2 hours of incarceration. May lead to necrosis and perforation.
      i. Signs of strangulation: erythematous, hard, fixed, painful mass; fever

 PEARL

Risk of incarceration is higher in infants <4 months or history of prematurity; therefore these patients require early referral.

3. **Investigations**
   a. Physical examination: most important investigation
   b. Ultrasound can be helpful in diagnosis of incarcerated hernia
   c. AXR may reveal bowel loop in inguinal region
4. **Management**
   a. Incarceration and strangulation are surgical emergencies (unsuccessful reduction requires urgent surgical correction)
   b. If hernia is reducible, refer to surgeon for elective operative repair
   c. While awaiting surgery, counsel parents regarding need for medical attention should symptoms of incarceration/strangulation develop

HYDROCELE
1. **Definition and etiology**
   a. Fluid-filled collection around a testicle (or anywhere along the path of testicular descent) because of a persistently patent processus vaginalis (seen in approximately 10% of children). May be associated with an inguinal hernia.
2. **Presentation**
   a. Soft, nontender, transilluminating fluid-filled sac
   b. If fluid in hydrocele communicates with peritoneal cavity, size of hydrocele may fluctuate with changes in position

> **! PITFALL**
>
> Especially large hydroceles or hydroceles of the spermatic cord may be difficult to distinguish from an incarcerated inguinal hernia. Ultrasound may help clarify the diagnosis.

3. **Management**
   a. Noncommunicating hydroceles and small communicating hydroceles often involute in first 24 months of life
   b. Larger **communicating** hydroceles, or those that **persist beyond 24 months of life**, require surgical intervention

CRYPTORCHIDISM
1. **Definition and etiology**
   a. Testicle not present in normal intrascrotal position
   b. More common in premature boys; most often unilateral and right-sided
2. **Investigations**
   a. Physical examination: empty, and sometimes hypoplastic scrotum/hemiscrotum
   b. To determine location of testicle: physical exam, US, MRI, laparoscopy
   c. In cases of bilateral undescended testicles consider disorders of sexual development

3. **Management**
   a. Most testicles that are undescended at birth complete their descent by 6 months of age
   b. Testicles that have not descended by 6 months of age should be referred to surgeon to minimize risk of developing complications (testicular torsion or trauma, subfertility). Orchidopexy can improve fertility and facilitate monitoring for testicular malignancy (operative repair does *not* decrease lifetime risk of malignancy).

PREOPERATIVE FASTING GUIDELINES

See Table 17.2

Table 17.2	Preoprerative Fasting Recommendations
Ingested Material	**Minimum Fasting Period**
Clear fluids	2 h
Breast milk	4 h
Formula	6 h
Solid food	8 h

From American Society of Anesthesiologists. Practice guidelines for preoperative fasting and the use of pharmacologic agents to reduce the risk of pulmonary aspiration: application to healthy patients undergoing elective procedures. *Anesthesiology.* 2017;126:376–393.

General Surgery

17

Genetics and Teratology

Areej Mahjoub • Gregory Costain • Roberto Mendoza-Londono

COMMON ABBREVIATIONS

Also see page xviii for a list of other abbreviations used throughout this book

7-DHC	7-dehydrocholesterol
AD	autosomal dominant
ADHD	attention-deficit/hyperactivity disorder
AR	autosomal recessive
CMA	chromosomal microarray analysis
DNA	deoxyribonucleic acid
FISH	fluorescence in situ hybridization
FTT	failure to thrive
HC	head circumference
MLPA	multi-plex ligation dependent probe amplification
NF	neurofibromatosis
NGS	next-generation sequencing
NTD	neural tube defects
PCR	polymerase chain reaction
PKU	phenylketonuria
TSC	tuberous sclerosis complex
TOF	tetralogy of Fallot
UPD	uniparental disomy
VSD	ventricular septal defect

DEFINITIONS

1. **Anticipation:** worsening of disease severity and decreasing age of onset in successive generations; feature of a few AD conditions and characteristically occurs in triplet repeat disorders (e.g., myotonic dystrophy [maternal], Huntington disease [paternal])
2. **Association:** nonrandom group of developmental anomalies seen more frequently than expected by chance; not caused by a sequence or syndrome (e.g., vertebral defects, anorectal malformation, cardiac anomalies, tracheoesophageal fistula with esophageal atresia, renal anomalies, limb anomalies [VACTERL])
3. **Deformation:** extrinsic nondisruptive mechanical forces on a normal structure causing abnormalities
4. **Disruption:** extrinsic factors disrupt development of normal tissue causing destruction
5. **Dysplasia:** abnormal cellular organization of function affecting a single tissue type
6. **Genotype:** genetic makeup of an organism
7. **Malformation:** intrinsic defects in morphogenesis caused by disturbance in development or growth in embryogenesis
8. **Mosaicism:** presence of two or more genotypically different cell populations within an individual

9. **Penetrance:** proportion of individuals with a particular genetic change who exhibit any signs or symptoms of the associated genetic disorder; either complete or incomplete

10. **Phenotype:** clinical expression of the genotype

11. **Sequence:** series of developmental abnormalities caused by a single primary defect (e.g., Potter sequence)

12. **Syndrome:** recognizable pattern of developmental anomalies with a single etiology (e.g., Down syndrome)

13. **Uniparental disomy:** individual received two copies of a chromosome, or part of a chromosome, from one parent and no copy from the other parent

14. **Variable expressivity:** range of signs and symptoms in individuals with a particular genotype

 PEARL

Variable expression of phenotype is the norm for the majority of genetic conditions, even within a family.

MODES OF INHERITANCE

See Table 18.1

GENETIC TESTING

A. Approach to interpreting genetic tests

1. Pretest counselling and informed consent required before ordering genetic testing. Carrier testing or predictive testing for later onset disorders is discouraged until a patient is able to provide their own informed consent.

2. Potential outcomes of genetic testing

   a. **Normal or negative:** no abnormality identified. In most cases, this does not rule out a genetic contribution to the presenting phenotype.

   b. **(Likely) pathogenic variant or change:** this finding is (likely) associated with a specific pattern of health and/or developmental problems. An additional blood sample from the child and parents may be recommended to investigate the origin of the variant.

   c. **Variant of unknown significance:** this variant may or may not be associated with health and/or developmental problems. Testing of parents may be recommended to investigate the origin of the variant.

   d. **Unexpected finding:** this variant is unrelated to the reported health/developmental problems in the child but could be associated with risk for another disease

Table 18.1 Characteristics of Different Modes of Genetic Inheritance

Inheritance	Affected Sex	Transmission Risk	Typical Characteristics	Examples
Mendelian				
AD	M = F	- 50% if parent is affected - If de novo variant (parents are unaffected), low risk (<1%) in subsequent pregnancies	- Phenotype appears in every generation - Male-to-male transmission possible - Potential for incomplete penetrance and/or significant variable expressivity	Noonan syndrome, NF1, Marfan syndrome
AR	M = F	Unaffected (carrier) parents, risk of having: - Affected child: 25% - Unaffected (not carrier) child: 25% - Unaffected (carrier) child: 50%	- Parents are typically obligate carriers - If consanguinity or from same ethnic population, more likely to be carriers for the same genetic condition	Cystic fibrosis, sickle cell disease
X-linked	M > F	- Males transmit the variant to all their daughters and none of their sons - Females have a 50% chance of transmitting the variant - Female carrier's risk of disease depends on the underlying condition and the (random) pattern of X inactivation	- In general, more severe phenotype (including perinatal death) in males, compared with females - Heterozygous female carriers range from unaffected to less severely affected, based on X inactivation - No male-to-male transmission - Variant can be passed through multiple carrier females, so may appear to "skip" generations	Duchenne muscular dystrophy, fragile X syndrome, hemophilia A

Non-Mendelian

Multifactorial	Disease-specific	Risk of recurrence related to disease incidence, but typically lower than a Mendelian condition	- Multiple genetic and environmental factors - Occurs more often in first- and second-degree relatives than expected by chance	Nonsyndromic cleft lip and/or cleft palate, NTD, diabetes mellitus, asthma
Mitochondrial DNA	M = F	All maternal offspring can be affected	- Maternal inheritance of mitochondrial DNA - Phenotypic variability (threshold effect) - Males cannot transmit disease to offspring - Affects high-energy tissues (cardiac and skeletal muscle, brain, liver, optic tract)	MELAS (mitochondrial encephalomyopathy, lactic acidosis, and stroke-like episodes), mitochondrial DNA-associated Leigh syndrome

AD, Autosomal dominant; *AR*, autosomal recessive; *DNA*, deoxyribonucleic acid; *NF1*, neurofibromatosis 1; *NTD*, neural tube defects.

Genetics and Teratology

18

B. Types of genetic tests

1. **Fluorescence in situ hybridization (FISH)**
   a. Targeted test that requires selecting a probe for a specific chromosome region
   b. Quantifies the number of specific chromosomes or chromosomal regions through hybridization (attachment) of fluorescent-labeled DNA probes to denatured chromosomal DNA
   c. Used for rapid detection of microdeletion/microduplication syndromes (e.g., 22q11.2 deletion syndrome), chromosomal aneuploidy (e.g., trisomy 18), and sex chromosomes disorders (e.g., in the setting of ambiguous genitalia)

2. **Chromosomal microarray analysis (CMA)**
   a. Nontargeted, higher resolution test to detect genome-wide DNA copy number abnormalities (i.e., gains and losses of chromosomal material)
   b. First-line test for presentations such as global developmental delay, intellectual disability, autism spectrum disorder, multiple congenital anomalies

3. **Karyotype**
   a. Non-targeted, low-resolution test to determine number and gross microscopic structure of all chromosomes
   b. Uniquely informative for balanced chromosome rearrangements and low-level mosaicism

4. **Non-invasive prenatal testing (NIPT)**
   a. Screening (not diagnostic) test using a blood sample from a pregnant woman to deduce the presence or absence of trisomy 21 and limited number of additional chromosomal disorders in the fetus

5. **Single gene testing**
   a. Targeted technique used to detect variants in a gene of interest
   b. Used in the setting of a phenotype strongly suggestive of a specific single-gene disorder (e.g., frataxin gene in Friedreich ataxia)

6. **Gene panel testing**
   a. Semitargeted technique of sequencing multiple preselected genes in parallel via next-generation sequencing. Used in the setting of common phenotypes with a moderate degree of genetic heterogeneity (e.g., nonsyndromic epilepsy).

7. **Whole-exome sequencing (WES)**
   a. Nontargeted test that attempts to sequence the exome in a DNA sample
   b. Does not reliably detect all chromosomal disorders, so does not negate the need for CMA

c. Used in the setting of complex nonspecific phenotypes, or after negative targeted testing in an individual strongly suspected of having a genetic condition

8. **Whole-genome sequencing (WGS)**
   a. Nontargeted test that attempts to sequence the genome in a DNA sample
   b. Can detect both sequence variation (like WES) and chromosomal variation (like CMA)

9. Other disease-specific molecular tests that are not previously listed (e.g., fragile X syndrome [DNA repeat expansion analysis via polymerase chain reaction (PCR)], imprinting disorder [DNA methylation, multiplex ligation-dependent probe amplification (MLPA)], mitochondrial DNA disorders [mitochondrial/nuclear DNA])

CHILD WITH MULTIPLE CONGENITAL ANOMALIES

1. **History and physical examination**
   a. Comprehensive pregnancy/perinatal history (including infections, prenatal drug/other exposures), past medical history, developmental history
   b. Detailed family history
      i. At least three generations paying special attention to siblings, parents, maternal male relatives, first cousins
      ii. Consanguinity, ethnicity, similarly affected relatives, major congenital anomalies, global developmental delay/intellectual disability/autism spectrum disorder, recurrent miscarriages and/or infertility, early childhood death
   c. Growth parameters (weight, height, head circumference)
   d. Physical examination (Figure 18.1), tailored to phenotype and suspected genetic disease

2. **Diagnostic workup**
   a. Tailored to patient phenotype and suspected genetic disease
   b. Consider
      i. Midline workup—head ultrasound/brain magnetic resonance imaging (MRI), echocardiogram, abdominal ultrasound
      ii. Skeletal survey
      iii. Formal eye examination
      iv. Hearing test
      v. General and metabolic laboratory investigations based on presenting phenotype (e.g., serum cholesterol and 7-DHC for suspected Smith-Lemli-Opitz syndrome)
   c. Genetic testing should include pretest counselling
   d. First-tier test is CMA (may in the future be accompanied by WES, or superseded by WGS)

Figure 18.1 Physical Examination for Genetic Syndrome

Growth parameters: weight, length, head circumference
Microcephaly: HC < 2 standard deviations below mean
Macrocephaly: HC > 2 standard deviations above mean

Skull: symmetry, shape, fontanelle (size), sutures (patency), scalp
Hair: implantation (anterior and posterior hair line), texture pattern

Eyes: intercanthal distance, orientation, coloboma, eyelashes
Epicanthal fold: skin fold at the inner corner of the eye where upper and lower eyelids meet
Hypertelorism (hypotelorism): increased (decreased) distance between pupils
Palpebral fissures:
- **Upslanting:** lateral corner of eyelid above medial corner
- **Downslanting:** lateral corner of eyelid below medial corner
Low-set ears: positioning of ear below a hypothetical line between occiput and outer canthus
Mouth: cleft, shape of palate, lips, tongue (size, texture), teeth (eruption time, quality, number)
Philtrum: shape (smooth philtrum: flattening of the groove between nose and upper lip), length
Nose: shape of nasal root, bridge and tip, shape and position of nostrils
Ears: size, shape, placement, pits/tags
Retrognathia: posterior positioning of the mandible (micrognathia: small mandible)

Neck: length, shape, webbing, pits/fistulas

Thorax: shape, size, position of nipples, pectus deformities

Spine: curvature, vertebral anomalies, sacral dimple

Viscera: size, shape, localization, extra masses

Genitalia: hypoplasia, cryptorchidism, ambiguous genitalia, hypospadias
Anus: patency, localization

Hands and feet: creases, nails, digits (shape, number)
Arachnodactyly: abnormally thin, long fingers and toes
Clinodactyly: lateral or medial curvature of a digit
Camptodactyly: flexure contracture of a digit
Polydactyly: extra digit
- **Postaxial:** additional digit is on the ulnar margin of the hand, or lateral to the fifth toe
- **Preaxial:** additional digit is towards the first digit of the hand (radial side) or foot (medially)
Syndactyly: webbing/fusion of part/whole of two or more consecutive digits

Limbs: proportions, reductions/amputations, missing parts

HC, Head circumference.

SELECTED GENETIC CONDITIONS

1. Sequences and associations (Table 18.2)
2. Chromosomal aneuploidies (Table 18.3)
3. Single gene disorders (Table 18.4)
4. Microdeletion syndromes and imprinting disorders (Table 18.6)

> ✦ **PEARL**
>
> Use condition-specific standardized health supervision guidelines and/or growth charts, if available.

Table 18.2 Common Sequences and Associations

Type	Etiopathogenesis	Signs and Symptoms	Clinical Outcomes	Selected Investigations
(Pierre) Robin sequence	- Mandibular hypoplasia → posterior displacement of the tongue → incomplete closure of the palate - Isolated (66%), syndromic (33%, e.g., Stickler syndrome)	- Micrognathia - Glossoptosis - Airway obstruction and/or cleft palate	- Respiratory distress - Feeding difficulties - Favorable prognosis with expert surgical care	- Eye examination after 1 year of age (for signs of Stickler syndrome) - Consider CMA to rule out chromosomal disorder (e.g., 22q11.2 deletion syndrome)
Potter sequence (oligohydramnios)	- Renal anomaly → obstructive uropathy → oligohydramnios → deformation by constraint - Bilateral renal dysgenesis/agenesis (20%)	- Potter facies: flattened nose, wide-set eyes, retrognathia, large low-set ears - Bilateral pulmonary hypoplasia - Limb positioning defects - Growth deficiency	- Respiratory failure secondary to pulmonary hypoplasia - Acute renal failure - Later: chronic lung disease, chronic renal failure	- Renal ultrasound, pulmonary imaging, skeletal x-rays - Consider CMA to rule out chromosomal disorder and/or testing for specific genetic renal disorders
VACTERL association Typical diagnostic criteria: ≥3 anomalies (some suggest at least tracheoesophageal fistula/esophageal atresia or an anorectal anomaly must be present)	- Sporadic inheritance - Diagnosis of exclusion	V = vertebral defects A = anorectal malformation C = cardiac anomalies TE = tracheoesophageal fistula/esophageal atresia R = renal anomalies L = limb defects (particularly radial ray anomalies)	- Respiratory distress - Feeding/growth difficulties - Renal failure - Typical development - Favorable prognosis with expert surgical care - Later: scoliosis/back pain, constipation, nephrolithiasis/UTI	- Echocardiogram, renal ultrasound - Consider x-ray of the spine and upper extremities - CMA to rule out chromosomal disorder - Consider chromosome breakage studies for Fanconi anemia (particularly if radial defect)

CMA, Chromosomal microarray; *UTI,* urinary tract infection.

435

Table 18.3 Common Chromosomal Aneuploidies

Type	Inheritance	Early Clinical Features	Later Clinical Features	Selected Investigations	Attention
Trisomy 21 (Down syndrome)	- ~95%: three copies of chromosome 21 - ~3%: unbalanced translocation between chromosome 21 and another chromosome (often 14) - ~2%: mosaic - General recurrence risk: ~1% (higher with maternal age and translocation carrier)	- Brachycephaly, mild microcephaly, small ears with overfolded helices, epicanthal folds, upslanting palpebral fissures, protruding tongue - Hearing loss - Brushfield spots, myopia - Single palmar creases, fifth finger clinodactyly, sandal gap deformity - Hypotonia - Cardiac defects (~50% [e.g., ASD, VSD, AVSD]) - GI atresias (~12% [e.g., TEF, duodenal atresia/stenosis]), Hirschsprung disease - Congenital hypothyroidism (~1%) - Transient myeloproliferative disorder (~10%), polycythemia	- Developmental and intellectual disability - Asymptomatic atlantoaxial subluxation - Obstructive sleep apnea - Conductive hearing loss (otitis media) - Acute lymphoblastic leukemia (~1%–2%) - Obesity - Hip abnormalities: dislocation, slipped capital femoral epiphysis, avascular necrosis - Infertility (primary gonadal deficiency) - Cataracts - Early-onset Alzheimer disease	- FISH with chromosome 21 probe (for rapid diagnosis) - Karyotype (if unbalanced translocation, then test parents) - Echocardiogram - Eye examination - Hearing test - Thyroid function, CBC, differential - Cervical x-ray	- Careful neurologic examination: any change in bowel/bladder function, change in gait, neck pain/torticollis: rule out spinal cord compression - Increased risk of celiac disease - Follow Trisomy 21 health supervision guidelines and growth chart
Trisomy 13 (Patau syndrome)	- Majority have three copies of chromosome 13 - Rarely mosaic or partial trisomy 13 - General recurrence risk: <1%	- Microcephaly, depressed nasal bridge, low-set ears, cutis aplasia, micro/anophthalmia, hearing defects, holoprosencephaly, cleft lip/palate, omphalocele, polydactyly, clenched fist - Heart defects (~80% [ASD, VSD]) - Renal anomalies (PCKD, horseshoe kidney)	- Postnatal growth retardation - Severe to profound developmental and cognitive disability	- FISH with chromosome 13 probe (for rapid diagnosis) - Karyotype - Echocardiogram - Renal ultrasound - Head ultrasound	- Median survival is 1–2 weeks - Survival to 1 year ~20% in some studies - Long-term survival possible

Trisomy 18 (Edwards syndrome)	- Majority have three copies of chromosome 18 - Rarely mosaic or partial trisomy 18 - General recurrence risk: <1% (higher with maternal age)	- Prominent occiput, narrow bifrontal diameter, small mouth, micrognathia - Short sternum, overlapping fingers, rocker-bottom feet - Intrauterine growth restriction - Heart defects (90%: VSD ± polyvalvular dysplasia) - Renal anomalies (PCKD, horseshoe kidney) - Cryptorchidism	- Growth retardation - Apneic episodes - Feeding difficulties - Severe to profound developmental and cognitive disability	- FISH with chromosome 18 probe (for rapid diagnosis) - Karyotype - Echocardiogram - Renal ultrasound	- Median survival is 1–2 weeks - Survival to 1 year is ~13% in some studies - Long-term survival possible - Increased risk for Wilms tumor and hepatoblastoma
Monosomy X (Turner syndrome)	- ~50%: one X chromosome, no Y chromosome - Remainder are mosaic and/or have structural abnormalities involving the second X chromosome - General recurrence risk: low	- Cystic hygroma in utero, low posterior hairline, short webbed neck, puffiness of hands and feet (congenital lymphedema), broad chest, widely spaced nipples - Left-sided heart defects (15%–50% [bicuspid aortic valve, coarctation of aorta, mitral valve prolapse]) - Renal anomalies (horseshoe kidney)	- Short stature - Strabismus, glaucoma - Hypertension (40%), aortic root dilatation - Primary ovarian failure, no growth spurt, minimal breast development, ovarian dysgenesis (90%), infertility - Hypothyroidism, glucose intolerance, hyperlipidemia - Normal intelligence	- Karyotype (5%–10% will have Y chromosome in all/some cells) - FISH with X chromosome (± Y chromosome) probe - Echocardiogram - Renal ultrasound - Hearing test - Thyroid function	- Growth hormone therapy at early age - Later: estrogen therapy - Increased risk for autoimmune diseases - Increased risk for gonadoblastoma or dysgerminoma (7%–10%) - Follow Turner Syndrome health supervision guidelines and growth chart

ASD, Atrial septal defect; *AVSD*, atrioventricular septal defect; *CBC*, complete blood count; *FISH*, fluorescence in situ hybridization; *GI*, gastrointestinal; *PCKD*, polycystic kidney disease; *TEF*, tracheal esophageal fistula; *VSD*, ventricular septal defect.

Genetics and Teratology

18

Table 18.4 Selected Single Gene Disorders

Types	Inheritance	Clinical Features	Later Clinical Features	Selected Investigations	Attention
Achondroplasia	- AD - Most cases sporadic	- Macrocephaly, disproportionate short stature, low nasal bridge, prominent forehead, mild midfacial hypoplasia - Short vertebral pedicles, lumbar lordosis, short bones, trident hand, same-length fingers, short femoral neck; incomplete extension of elbow - Mild hypotonia	- Macrocephaly, hydrocephalus, short stature, bowing of legs, otitis media (short eustachian tubes); childhood obesity - Sleep apnea - Cervicomedullary junction compression (narrow foramen magnum) - Spinal stenosis	- Targeted variant testing in the *FGFR3* gene - X-ray of bones - MRI (assess foramen magnum size) in first year of life - Polysomnography in first year of life; repeat if apneas	- If large fontanelle, rapid ↑ in HC or symptoms of raised intracranial pressure: brain imaging - Discourage sitting positions where trunk curves anteriorly - Follow Achondroplasia health supervision guidelines and growth chart

CHARGE syndrome	- AD
	- Most cases sporadic
		C = coloboma, bilateral (80%)
		H = heart defects (50%–85% [conotruncal defects; ASD, VSD, coarctation])
		A = atresia choanae
		R = retarded growth and/or development delay (70%–80%)
		G = genital hypoplasia: micropenis, cryptorchidism (75%)
		E = ear anomalies and/or deafness (88%); abnormal semicircular canals
		- *Cranial nerves*:
		  I (hypo/anosmia)
		  VII (facial palsy)
		  VIII (hypoplasia of auditory nerve)
		  IX/X (swallowing difficulties and aspiration)
		- Cleft lip/palate: 15%–20%
		- T-cell deficiency
			- Short stature, delayed/absent puberty (hypogonadotropic hypogonadism), consider hormonal replacement
			- Mild to profound intellectual disability
			- Scoliosis
				- Molecular testing of the *CHD7* gene
				- CT temporal bones (semicircular canal hypoplasia)
				- Echocardiogram
				- Renal ultrasound
				- Eye examinations, audiologic evaluations
					- Aspiration risk
					- Postoperative airway problems
					- Venous malformations of temporal bone can lead to complications during otologic surgery

Syndrome	Inheritance/Frequency	Clinical features	Diagnosis/Testing	Management
Fragile X syndrome	- X-linked - M: 1:4000–5000 - F: 1:6000–8000	- Macrocephaly, prominent forehead, elongated face, large ears, pale blue irides, epicanthal folds, high arched palate, dental crowding, cataracts, strabismus, myopia - Hand flapping or biting (60%), poor eye contact (90%) - Autism spectrum disorder (60%) - Epilepsy *Infancy/childhood:* - Developmental disability, feeding difficulties/GERD, otitis media *Puberty:* - Intellectual disability (milder in females), anxiety - Macroorchidism *Adults:* - Mitral valve prolapse (50%)	- DNA molecular analysis for trinucleotide (CGG) repeat of the *FMR1* gene	- Developmental follow-up - Mothers obligate carriers for at least a "premutation" - Premutation carriers are at risk of premature ovarian failure and fragile X-associated tremor/ataxia syndrome - Follow Fragile X health supervision guidelines
Marfan syndrome	- AD - 25%–35% sporadic	- Ectopia lentis - Aortic root enlargement - See Table 18.5 for systemic score criteria (a score of ≥7 is considered positive) - Neonatal presentation rare - Learning disability and attention deficit disorder (42%)	- Molecular testing of the *FBN1* gene - Annual echocardiogram, eye examination - Monitor blood pressure, scoliosis	- Antibiotic prophylaxis should be used before dental procedures - Avoid isometric exercise, contact sports, scuba diving - Consider β-blocker as prophylaxis for aortic dilatation - Follow Marfan Syndrome health supervision guidelines

Continued

Table 18.4 Selected Single Gene Disorders—cont'd

Types	Inheritance	Clinical Features	Later Clinical Features	Selected Investigations	Attention
Noonan syndrome	- AD - Most cases sporadic	- Craniofacial: wool-like hair (curly), epicanthal folds, downslanting palpebral fissures, ptosis of eyelids, hypertelorism, low nasal bridge, low-set/abnormal ears, dental malocclusion, protruding upper lip, retrognathia, low posterior hairline, webbed neck - Pectus excavatum/carinatum, scoliosis/vertebral abnormalities - Cardiac (50%–80%): pulmonary valve stenosis, hypertrophic cardiomyopathy - Bilateral cryptorchidism (60%)	*Infancy:* - Short stature - FTT (poor feeding, vomiting, constipation) *Later:* - Mild-moderate cognitive disability - Strabismus, refractive errors - Bleeding diathesis (50%–89%): thrombocy-topenia, platelet dysfunction	- Molecular genetic test-ing with NGS panel for Noonan syndrome and related disorders - Echocardiogram - Eye examination - CBC, coagulation screen	- 20% with cardiomyopathy die in the first 2 years of life - Myelomonocytic leukemia in the first 2 months of life - Normal fertility in females and males with descended testes - Facial features change with age - Follow Noonan Syndrome health supervision guidelines

Smith–Lemli–Opitz syndrome	- AR	- Craniofacial: microcephaly, ptosis of eyelids, epicanthal folds, strabismus, broad nasal tip, micrognathia
		- 2–3 toe syndactyly, postaxial polydactyly
		- Cardiac defect (50%): endocardial cushion defect, hypoplastic left heart, ASD
		- Genital abnormalities (70%): hypospadias, cryptorchidism
		- Renal anomalies (57%): obstruction, agenesis
		- CNS: seizures, holoprosencephaly (5%)
		- Optic: cataract, optic atrophy, nystagmus
		- GI: rectal atresia, pyloric stenosis, intestinal malrotation, diaphragmatic hernia, Hirschsprung disease
		- Other: cleft palate, bifid tongue, hearing loss, thymus hypoplasia
			- Feeding difficulties (>50% require feeding tube in childhood)
			- Sleep disturbances in infancy
			- Moderate to severe intellectual disability
			- Behavioral: autism, self-injurious, aggressive, forceful backward arching
				- Clinical and biochemical diagnosis
				  - ↑ 7-DHC in blood
				  - ↑ Ratio of 7-DHC: cholesterol
				  - ± ↓Cholesterol (90% cases)
				- Molecular testing of the *DHCR7* gene
				- Echocardiogram
				- Renal ultrasound
					Life expectancy determined by severity of internal malformations and quality of general supportive care

7-DHC, 7-Dehydrocholesterol; *AD,* autosomal dominant; *AR,* autosomal recessive; *ASD,* atrial septal defect; *CBC,* complete blood count; *CNS,* central nervous system; *CT,* computed tomography; *DNA,* deoxyribonucleic acid; *FTT,* failure to thrive; *GERD,* gastroesophageal reflux disease; *GI,* gastrointestinal; *HC,* head circumference; *MRI,* magnetic resonance imaging; *NGS,* next-generation sequencing; *VSD,* ventricular septal defect.

Table 18.5 Systemic Score Criteria for Marfan Syndrome[a]

Feature	Score
Wrist (A) AND thumb (B) sign	+3

Feature	Score
Wrist OR thumb sign	+1
Pectus carinatum deformity	+2
Pectus excavatum or chest asymmetry	+1
Hindfoot deformity	+2
Pes planus	+1
Spontaneous pneumothorax	+2
Dural ectasia	+2
Protrusio acetabuli	+2
Scoliosis/thoracolumbar kyphosis	+1
Reduced elbow extension	+1
Facial features (3/5) - Dolichocephaly, enophthalmos, downslanting palpebral fissures, malar hypoplasia, retrognathia	+1
Skin striae	+1
Severe myopia (>3 diopters)	+1
Mitral valve prolapse	+1
Upper/lower segment ratio (<0.85 [Caucasian] or <0.78 [Black]) AND arm span/height >1.05 (Lower segment—distance from top of symphysis pubis to floor when standing)	+1

[a]Score of ≥7 is considered positive.

Data from www.marfan.org/dx/score. Images from McBride ART, Gargan M. Marfan syndrome. *Curr Orthop.* 2006;20:418–423.

Table 18.6

Selected Microdeletion Syndromes, Including Imprinting Disorders

Type	Inheritance	Early Clinical Features	Later Clinical Features	Selected Investigations	Attention
22q11.2 deletion syndrome (DiGeorge syndrome)	- >90% sporadic - AD	- Cleft palate - Congenital cardiac disease (e.g., conotruncal anomalies, VSD, right aortic arch) - Neonatal hypocalcemia (hypoparathyroidism) - T-cell immunodeficiency (thymus hypoplasia) - Renal tract anomalies - Structural brain defects	*Childhood:* - Delayed motor milestones: walking (16–24 months), speech and language - Hypotonia (70%–80%) leading to feeding difficulties, hypernasal speech - Learning difficulties (>90%), with or without intellectual disability *Adults:* - Schizophrenia, generalized anxiety disorder, other psychiatric conditions - Early-onset Parkinson disease	- CMA (or FISH with probe for 22q11.2 region if high index of suspicion) - Echocardiogram, renal ultrasound, audiogram - Monitor calcium, CBC - Immunologic studies (immunophenotyping, specific serologies)	- Obstructive sleep apnea following pharyngeal surgery to improve speech - No live vaccines until immune function checked - If transfusion necessary, CMV negative and irradiated if <6 months of age - Follow 22q11.2 health supervision guidelines and growth chart
Williams syndrome	- >90% sporadic - AD	- Mild microcephaly, premature gray hair, medial eyebrow flare, short palpebral fissures, depressed nasal bridge, epicanthal folds, blue eyes, stellate pattern in the iris, long philtrum, anodontia, microdontia - Cardiac: supravalvular aortic stenosis, ASD/VSD, peripheral pulmonary artery stenosis - Nephrocalcinosis, asymmetry in kidney size, bladder diverticula, urethral stenosis, vesicoureteral reflux	*Infancy:* - Feeding problems, frequent vomiting, colic *Childhood:* - ADHD, anxiety, average intelligence, hoarse voice *Adults:* - Hypertension, joint limitations, recurrent UTI, obesity, constipation, diverticulosis, cholelithiasis, hypercalcemia, hypercalciuria (30%), hypothyroidism (10%)	- CMA (or FISH with probe for 7q11.23 region if high index of suspicion) - Echocardiogram, renal ultrasound - Eye examination, hearing test - Urinalysis, calcium/creatinine ratio, renal function - Monitor serum calcium, thyroid function	- Increased incidence of celiac disease - Caution regarding vitamin D supplementation - Sudden death associated with anesthesia - Follow Williams Syndrome health supervision guidelines and growth chart

Continued

Table 18.6 Selected Microdeletion Syndromes, Including Imprinting Disorders—cont'd

Type	Inheritance	Early Clinical Features	Later Clinical Features	Selected Investigations	Attention
Angelman syndrome	- Sporadic deletion of maternal 15q11–15q13 (70%–75%) - Paternal UPD (3%–7%) - Imprinting defect (2%–3%) - Variants in the *UBE3A* gene in 10%	Microbrachycephaly, blond hair (65%), pale blue eyes (88%), maxillary hypoplasia, prognathia large mouth with tongue protrusion and widely spaced teeth	- Severe developmental/intellectual disability, speech impairment - Movement disorder (ataxia/tremors), seizures (86%), hypotonia, hyperreflexia, left hand preference - Frequent laughing/smiling, hand-flapping, drooling, excessive chewing - Strabismus (42%), refractive errors, nystagmus, scoliosis, hypopigmentation (39%)	- First-tier test: DNA methylation analysis of chromosome 15q11-q13 region - If negative, molecular testing of *UBE3A* gene - EEG, brain imaging as indicated	- Obesity and constipation in adolescence and adulthood
Prader-Willi syndrome	- Sporadic deletion of paternal chromosome 15q11–15q13 (70%) - Maternal UPD (25%–30%) - Imprinting defects <5%	- Severe central hypotonia at birth (improves with age) - Almond-shaped eyes with upslanting palpebral fissure, strabismus, thin upper lip - Small hands and feet - Genital hypoplasia, cryptorchidism	*Infancy:* - Respiratory and feeding difficulties (tube feeding) *Childhood:* - Rapid weight gain (2 years), increase interest in food (4.5 years), hyperphagia, inappropriate food seeking, binge eating (8 years), mild intellectual disability *Later:* - Obesity, diabetes, hypothyroidism, short stature, osteoporosis, scoliosis, temperature instability, high pain threshold, genital hypoplasia, amenorrhea	- DNA methylation analysis of chromosome 15q11-q13 region	- Early growth hormone therapy beneficial for body composition, even if growth is normal - Adolescents may require testosterone replacement therapy

| Beckwith–Wiedemann syndrome | - Mostly sporadic
- Aberrant methylation (50%–60%)
- Paternal UPD (~20%)
- Variants in the *CDKN1C* gene in 5% (more in familial cases) | - macrosomia, macroglossia, hemihyperplasia, prominent eyes with infraorbital hypoplasia, large fontanelles, underdeveloped maxilla
- Visceromegaly (cardiac, renal), omphalocele, diastasis recti, posterior diaphragmatic eventration, cryptorchidism, cardiovascular defects
- Polycythemia, hypoglycemia (30%–50%)
- Seizures | *Childhood:*
- Embryogenic malignancy (Wilms tumor, hepatoblastoma, neuroblastoma, rhabdomyosarcoma) present by 8 years (risk 4%–21%)
Adults:
- Hearing loss, aneurysmal arterial dilatations, male infertility, nephrocalcinosis, medullary sponge kidney disease | - DNA methylation analysis of chromosome 11p15 region
- X-ray bone: accelerated osseous maturation
- Renal ultrasound: nephrocalcinosis
- Malignancy surveillance: renal ultrasound, serum alpha-fetoprotein every 3 months until 4–8 years
- increased risk of malignancy highest if hemihypertrophy and nephromegaly |

AD, Autosomal dominant; *ADHD*, attention deficit hyperactivity disorder; *ASD*, atrial septal defect; *CBC*, complete blood count; *CMA*, chromosomal microarray analysis; *CMV*, cytomegalovirus; *DNA*, deoxyribonucleic acid; *EEG*, electroencephalogram; *FISH*, fluorescence in situ hybridization; *UPD*, uniparental disomy; *UTI*, urinary tract infection; *VSD*, ventricular septal defect.

TERATOLOGY

1. **Definition:** teratologic agents are chemical, physical, or biological agents that can damage embryonic tissue resulting in malformations
2. **Etiologies**
   a. **Maternal infections:** see Congenital/Perinatal Infections in Chapter 24 Infectious Diseases
   b. **Maternal disease (untreated or poorly controlled)**
      i. Diabetes mellitus (not gestational): wide spectrum of malformations (e.g., neural tube defects [NTDs], congenital cardiac defects, sacral agenesis) if poor glycemic control during early embryogenesis
      ii. Hypertension: growth restriction
      iii. Maternal phenylketonuria/hyperphenylalaninemia: intellectual disability, microcephaly, congenital heart disease
      iv. Thyroid disease: hyper—growth restriction; hypo—intellectual deficit
      v. Systemic lupus erythematosus: small for gestational age, neonatal lupus, congenital heart block (anti-Ro/SSA and/or anti-La/SSB antibodies)
   c. **Radiation:** exposure of about 25 rad can result in miscarriages, microcephaly, cognitive impairment, and skeletal malformations (exposure to the fetus from a two-view chest x-ray of the mother is <0.0001 rad)
   d. **Medications and chemicals**
      i. See Table 18.7 for selected medications and possible effects on the fetus
      ii. Alcohol consumption (>6 ounces/day): at risk of fetal alcohol spectrum disorder. Affects growth (height, weight <10%), facial features (microcephaly, epicanthal folds, small palpebral fissures, flat nasal bridge, upturned nose, smooth philtrum, thin upper lip), neurodevelopment.
      iii. Smoking: at risk of miscarriage, preterm labor, growth restriction, sudden infant death syndrome

Table 18.7	Selected Medications and Possible Effects
Medication	**Possible Effects on the Fetus**
ACE inhibitors	Renal tubular dysgenesis
Isotretinoin	Facial and ear anomalies, congenital heart disease
Lithium	Ebstein anomaly
NSAID	Premature closure of ductus arteriosus
Phenobarbital	Vitamin K deficiency
Phenytoin	IUGR, hypoplastic nails, facial and ear anomalies, microcephaly
Valproate/carbamazepine	Cognitive disability, NTD
Warfarin	Facial dysmorphisms, chondrodysplasia, developmental disability

ACE, Angiotensin converting enzyme; *IUGR*, intrauterine growth restriction; *NSAID*, nonsteroidal antiinflammatory drug; *NTD*, neural tube defects.

PERIMORTEM WORKUP IN CHILD WITH DYSMORPHISMS

1. **Indication:** undiagnosed child with dysmorphisms and/or multiple congenital anomalies, who is moribund or recently deceased
2. **Workup**
   a. Bank DNA
   b. Blood: two spots on filter paper
   c. Plasma: 5 mL (heparinized sample)
   d. Urine: 30 mL (to be frozen at $-20°C$)
   e. Cerebrospinal fluid (CSF): 1 mL (to be frozen)
   f. Skin biopsy (for fibroblast culture): 4-mm punch biopsy; place in cell culture medium or sterile saline (keep at room temperature if <24 hours or $+4°C$ if longer; do not freeze)
   g. Muscle and liver biopsies (frozen at $-70°C$)
   h. Clinical photographs
   i. Skeletal x-rays

Growth and Nutrition

Justin Lam • Laura Kinlin • Meta van den Heuvel

Dietitians: Mara Alexanian-Farr, Alisa Bar-Dayan, Kelsey Gallagher, Daina Kalnins, Alissa Steinberg, Lori Tuira, Laura Vresk, Kellie Welch, Jordan Beaulieu
Lactation Consultants: Caroline Currie, Laura McLean, Samantha Sullivan
Occupational Therapist: Ashley Graham

COMMON ABBREVIATIONS

Also see page xviii for a list of other abbreviations used throughout this book

BMI	body mass index
BMR	basal metabolic rate
CMPA	cow's milk protein allergy
DRI	dietary reference intake
EBM	expressed breast milk
EER	estimated energy requirement
FTT	failure to thrive
GER (D)	gastroesophageal reflux (disease)
HIV	human immunodeficiency virus
HTLV	human T-cell lymphotropic viruses
IBW	ideal body weight
PCOS	polycystic ovary syndrome
PN	parenteral nutrition
TEE	total energy expenditure
TFI	total fluid intake

ENERGY REQUIREMENTS

1. Energy requirements can be estimated to help establish goals for adequate calorie provision
2. Predictive equations provide only estimates for energy needs and should be used as a guideline only
3. A number of methods are used to estimate the energy needs of children in a clinical setting
   a. Assessing energy requirements using the World Health Organization (WHO) prediction equations estimate basal metabolic rate (BMR) and total energy expenditure (TEE)
      i. The WHO equation calculates BMR by gender, age, and weight (Table 19.1)
      ii. Total daily energy requirements are estimated by multiplying the calculated BMR by activity factor (AF) ± stress factor (SF) to adjust for physical activity, medical status and/or need for catch up growth ± tone factor (for patients with spasticity). See Table 19.2 for factors.
   b. Assessing energy requirements using dietary reference intakes (DRIs) for energy
      i. DRIs are a set of reference values used in Canada and the United States for both individuals and groups. DRIs are based on chronological age and not on developmental stage. DRI values are for healthy individuals, therefore adjustments for disease and nutritional status may be required. See Table 19.3 for estimated energy requirements based on DRIs for energy.

Table 19.1	Equations for Basal Metabolic Rate (FAO/WHO/UNU 1991)	
Age Range (Years)	**Males (kcal/day)**	**Females (kcal/day)**
0–3	60.9W − 54	61.0W − 51
3–10	22.7W + 495	22.5W + 499
10–18	17.5W + 651	12.2W + 746

FAO, Food and Agriculture Organization; *UNU,* United Nations University; *W,* weight in kg; *WHO,* World Health Organization.

Adapted from The Hospital for Sick Children Guidelines for the Administration of Enteral and Parenteral Nutrition in Paediatrics, 2018.

Table 19.2	Factors for Activity, Stress, and Muscle Tone in FAO/WHO/UNU Equations for Estimating Total Energy Expenditure (Institute of Medicine 2005)		
Situation	**Activity Factor**	**Situation**	**Activity Factor**
Paralyzed, comatose	0.8–1	Sepsis	1.2–1.4
Confined to bed	1.15	Elective surgery	1–1.1
Dependent	1.2	Starvation	0.7–0.85
Crawling	1.25	Cancer	1.1–1.45
Sedentary	1.3–1.5	Burns	1.2–2
Normal activity	1.7	Multiple trauma	1.4
Athlete	2	Multiple long bone fracture	1.1–1.3
Situation	**Stress factor**		
Fever	1.2 per 1°C >37°C	**Situation**	**Muscle tone factor**
		Decreased tone	0.9
Severe infection	1.2–1.6	Normal tone	1
Peritonitis	1.05–1.25	Increased tone	1.1

FAO, Food and Agriculture Organization; *UNU,* United Nations University; *WHO,* World Health Organization.

Adapted from The Hospital for Sick Children Guidelines for the Administration of Enteral and Parenteral Nutrition in Paediatrics, 2018.

 PEARL

Total energy expenditure = basal metabolic rate (× activity factor) (× stress factor) (× tone factor)

Brackets indicate to include if applicable

Table 19.3		Estimated Energy Requirement (EER) for Infants and Children as per Dietary Reference Intakes for Energy			
		EER[a] (kcal/kg/day)			
Age	Sex	Physical Activity Level (PAL)[a]			
Infants and Children (months)					
0–2	M	107			
	F	104–102			
3–6	M	95–82			
	F	95–82			
7–9	M	79–80			
	F	80			
10–20	M	79–82			
	F	82			
21–35	M	82–83			
	F	83			
		Sedentary	Low Active	Active	Very Active
Children (years)					
3–4	M	81–75	93–86	104–97	117–109
	F	78–72	89–83	100–94	118–111
5–6	M	69–64	80–74	90–84	103–97
	F	66–62	77–72	87–82	104–97
7–8	M	60–57	70–66	80–75	92–87
	F	57–53	67–62	75–71	90–85
9–10	M	54–50	63–59	71–67	83–78
	F	49–45	57–53	65–60	78–72
11–12	M	47–44	55–52	64–60	74–70
	F	41–39	49–46	56–53	67–64
13–14	M	42–41	50–48	57–56	67–64
	F	37–35	44–41	50–47	60–57
15–16	M	40–38	47–45	54–52	62–60
	F	33–32	40–38	45–44	55–54
17–18	M	37–36	43–42	50–49	58–57
	F	31–30	37–36	43–42	52–51

[a]PAL for infants not determined.

F, Female; M, male.

Adapted from The Hospital for Sick Children Guidelines for the Administration of Enteral and Parenteral Nutrition in Paediatrics, 2018.

ASSESSMENT OF GROWTH

1. Minimum parameters of growth assessment: weight, height/length, head circumference
2. Single measurements can be compared with normal population values by plotting on WHO growth charts (Figures 19.1–19.8)

Figure 19.1 Boys, Birth–24 Months: Length-for-Age and Weight-for-Age Percentiles

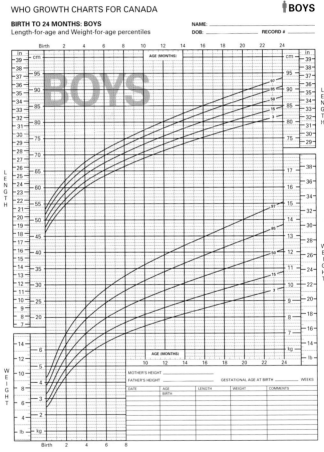

WHO GROWTH CHARTS FOR CANADA **♦BOYS**

BIRTH TO 24 MONTHS: BOYS
Length-for-age and Weight-for-age percentiles

NAME: _____
DOB: _____ RECORD # _____

SOURCE: Based on World Health Organization (WHO) Child Growth Standards (2006) and WHO Reference (2007) and adapted for Canada by Canadian Paediatric Society, Canadian Pediatric Endocrine Group, College of Family Physicians of Canada, Community Health Nurses of Canada, and Dietitians of Canada.

© Dietitians of Canada, 2014. Chart may be reproduced in its entirety (i.e., no changes) for non-commercial purposes only.

(From WHO Growth Charts Set 1, Dietitians of Canada. 2014. Accessed at: www.dietitians.ca/growthcharts.)

Figure 19.2 Girls, Birth–24 Months: Length-for-Age and Weight-for-Age Percentiles

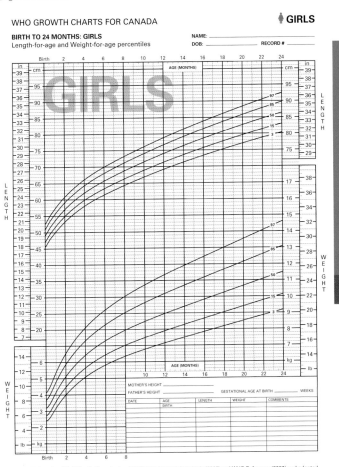

SOURCE: Based on World Health Organization (WHO) Child Growth Standards (2006) and WHO Reference (2007) and adapted for Canada by Canadian Paediatric Society, Canadian Pediatric Endocrine Group, College of Family Physicians of Canada, Community Health Nurses of Canada, and Dietitians of Canada.

© Dietitians of Canada, 2014. Chart may be reproduced in its entirety (i.e., no changes) for non-commercial purposes only.

(From WHO Growth Charts Set 1, Dietitians of Canada. 2014. Accessed at: www.dietitians.ca/growthcharts.)

Figure 19.3   Boys, Birth–24 Months: Head Circumference and Weight-for-Length Percentiles

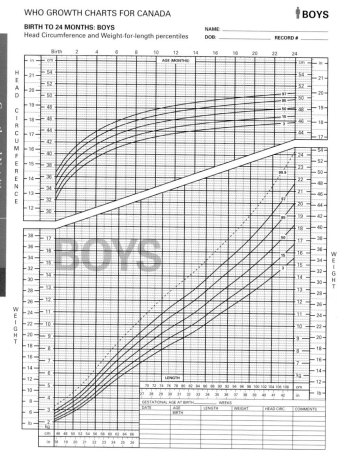

(From WHO Growth Charts Set 1, Dietitians of Canada. 2014. Accessed at: www.dietitians.ca/growthcharts.)

Figure 19.4 Girls, Birth–24 Months: Head Circumference and Weight-for-Length Percentiles

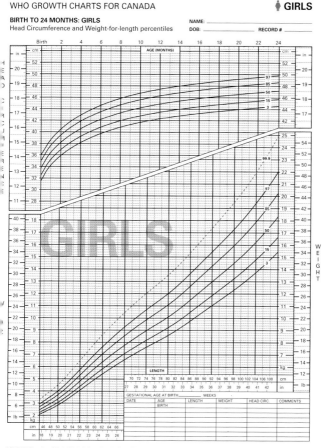

WHO GROWTH CHARTS FOR CANADA

GIRLS

BIRTH TO 24 MONTHS: GIRLS
Head Circumference and Weight-for-length percentiles

NAME: _____

DOB: _____   RECORD # _____

SOURCE: Based on World Health Organization (WHO) Child Growth Standards (2006) and WHO Reference (2007) and adapted for Canada by Canadian Paediatric Society, Canadian Pediatric Endocrine Group, College of Family Physicians of Canada, Community Health Nurses of Canada, and Dietitians of Canada.

© Dietitians of Canada, 2014. Chart may be reproduced in its entirety (i.e., no changes) for non-commercial purposes only.

From WHO Growth Charts Set 1, Dietitians of Canada. 2014. Accessed at: www.dietitians.ca/growthcharts.)

Growth and Nutrition

19

Figure 19.5 Boys, 2–19 Years: Height-for-Age and Weight-for-Age Percentiles

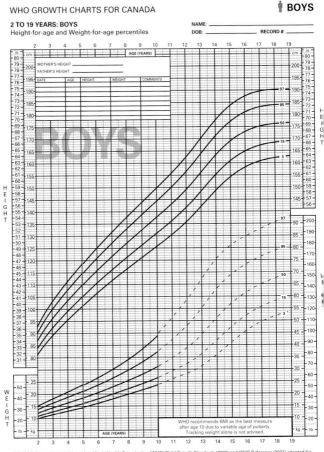

WHO GROWTH CHARTS FOR CANADA

BOYS

2 TO 19 YEARS: BOYS
Height-for-age and Weight-for-age percentiles

NAME: _____
DOB: _____ RECORD # _____

SOURCE: The main chart is based on World Health Organization (WHO) Child Growth Standards (2006) and WHO Reference (2007) adapted for Canada by Canadian Paediatric Society, Canadian Pediatric Endocrine Group (CPEG), College of Family Physicians of Canada, Community Health Nurses of Canada, and Dietitians of Canada. The weight-for-age 10 to 19 years section was developed by CPEG based on data from the US National Center for Health Statistics using the same procedures as the WHO growth charts.

© Dietitians of Canada, 2014. Chart may be reproduced in its entirety (i.e., no changes) for non-commercial purposes only.

(From WHO Growth Charts Set 1, Dietitians of Canada. 2014. Accessed at: www.dietitians.ca/growthcharts.)

Figure 19.6 Girls, 2–19 Years: Height-for-Age and Weight-for-Age Percentiles

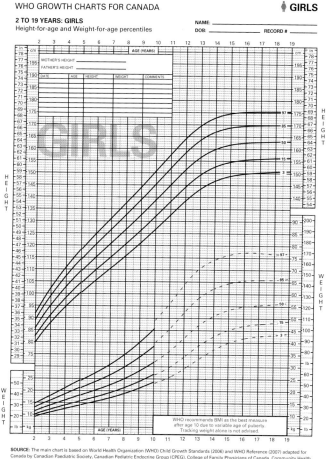

(From WHO Growth Charts Set 1, Dietitians of Canada. 2014. Accessed at: www.dietitians.ca/growthcharts.)

Figure 19.7 Boys, 2–19 Years: Body Mass Index-for-Age Percentiles

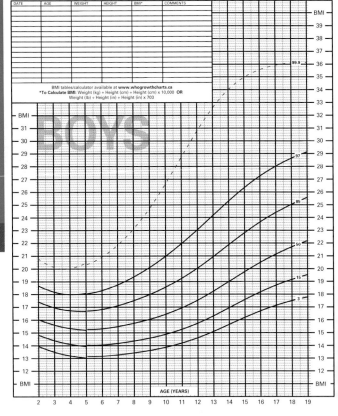

WHO GROWTH CHARTS FOR CANADA   👤 BOYS

2 TO 19 YEARS: BOYS
Body mass index-for-age percentiles

NAME: _____
DOB: _____ RECORD # _____

(From WHO Growth Charts Set 1, Dietitians of Canada. 2014. Accessed at: www.dietitians.ca/growthcharts.)

Figure 19.8 Girls, 2–19 Years: Body Mass Index-for-Age Percentiles

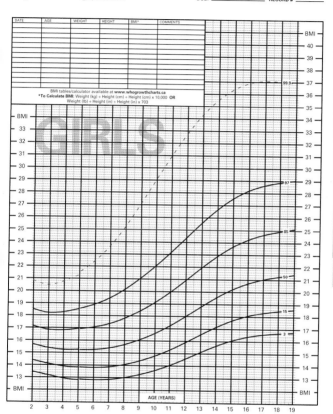

WHO GROWTH CHARTS FOR CANADA

2 TO 19 YEARS: GIRLS
Body mass index-for-age percentiles

NAME: _____
DOB: _____ RECORD # _____

🧍 **GIRLS**

SOURCE: Based on World Health Organization (WHO) Child Growth Standards (2006) and WHO Reference (2007) and adapted for Canada by Canadian Paediatric Society, Canadian Pediatric Endocrine Group, College of Family Physicians of Canada, Community Health Nurses of Canada and Dietitians of Canada.
© Dietitians of Canada, 2014. Chart may be reproduced in its entirety (i.e., no changes) for non-commercial purposes only. **www.whogrowthcharts.ca**

From WHO Growth Charts Set 1, Dietitians of Canada. 2014. Accessed at: www.dietitians.ca/
growthcharts.)

- Serial measurements provide information about a child's growth velocity and changes in growth pattern over time. See Table 19.4 for expected gain by day for infants and children.
- Premature infants (<37 weeks) should be plotted on the Fenton growth chart (see Figures 27.4 and 27.5 in Chapter 27 Neonatology) until

50 weeks gestational age; once term-corrected, growth parameters should be plotted on the WHO charts using corrected age until 2 years.

5. Specific growth charts are available for conditions with particular growth patterns (e.g., Trisomy 21, Prader-Willi syndrome, Turner syndrome, achondroplasia, cerebral palsy). When such charts are available, children should be plotted on both WHO and condition-specific charts.

6. Gains in weight, height and head circumference may be used to compare with predicted norms (Table 19.4 and Table 19.5)

WEIGHT

1. Weigh infants without clothes and diaper
2. Term neonates may lose up to 10% of birth weight in first week of life; should regain weight by at least 2 weeks of age, then gain approximately 20 to 30 g/day for first 3 months of life
3. Weight is a sensitive indicator of energy intake; however, nonnutritional causes (e.g., edema or dehydration) of weight changes should be considered

Table 19.4	Reference Gains in Weight, Length, and Head Circumference of Term Infants and Reference Gains in Weight and Height of Children					
	Boys			**Girls**		
Age	Weight (g/day)	Length/Height (mm/day)	Head Circumference (mm/day)	Weight (g/day)	Length/Height (mm/day)	Head Circumference (mm/day)
0–1 months	30	1.10	NA	26	1.03	NA
1–2 months	35	1.09	0.83	29	1.01	0.78
2–3 months	26	1.02	0.50	23	0.94	0.47
3–4 months	20	0.84	0.36	19	0.81	0.34
4–5 months	17	0.68	0.29	16	0.67	0.28
5–6 months	15	0.63	0.24	14	0.63	0.23
6–9 months	13	0.52	0.18	12	0.59	0.18
9–12 months	10	0.43	0.13	10	0.47	0.13
12–18 months	7.3	0.36	0.08	7.3	0.37	0.09
18–24 months	6.2	0.30	0.05	6.7	0.31	0.05
24–30 months	5.7	0.25	0.04	5.3	0.26	0.04
30–36 months	5.3	0.22	0.03	5.6	0.23	0.03
3.5 years	5.4	0.21		5.5	0.21	
4 years	5.2	0.20		5.4	0.20	
4.5 years	5.8	0.19		5.2	0.19	

	Boys			**Girls**		
Age	Weight (g/day)	Length/ Height (mm/ day)	Head Circumference (mm/day)	Weight (g/day)	Length/ Height (mm/ day)	Head Circumference (mm/day)
5 years	5.8	0.19		5.7	0.19	
5.5 years	6.4	0.19		5.3	0.19	
6 years	6.5	0.18		6.2	0.18	
6.5 years	6.4	0.18		6.5	0.17	
7 years	6.9	0.18		6.5	0.17	
7.5 years	7.6	0.16		7.3	0.17	
8 years	8.4	0.17		7.5	0.17	
8.5 years	7.9	0.16		8.1	0.16	
9 years	8.6	0.16		8.7	0.16	
9.5 years	8.5	0.15		8.4	0.15	
10 years	9.3	0.15		8.6	0.16	
10.5 years	8.9	0.14		10.8	0.15	
11 years	9.5	0.14		11.0	0.17	
11.5 years	10.5	0.14		13.6	0.18	
12 years	11.0	0.15		15.1	0.18	
12.5 years	13.5	0.15		15.2	0.18	
13 years	15.4	0.18		11.8	0.15	
13.5 years	16.8	0.19		12.7	0.11	
14 years	18.3	0.22		10.1	0.07	
14.5 years	20.2	0.20		8.2	0.05	
15 years	17.8	0.18		5.5	0.04	
15.5 years	14.2	0.11		5.1	0.03	
16 years	12.0	0.09		2.0	0.03	
16.5 years	9.3	0.05		4.1	0.01	
17 years	6.7	0.05		3.5	0.01	
17.5 years	6.0	0.02		2.2	0.00	
18 years	4.2	0.02		2.6	0.00	

Table 19.4 Reference Gains in Weight, Length and Head Circumference of Term Infants; Gains in Weight and Height of Children—cont'd

Adapted from The Hospital for Sick Children Guidelines for the Administration of Enteral and Parenteral Nutrition in Paediatrics, 2018.

Table 19.5	Average Growth Parameters and Rate of Growth	
	Birth	Rate of Growth
Weight	3–3.5 kg	2 × birth weight by 4–6 m 3 × birth weight by 1 year 4 × birth weight by 2 year
Height	50 cm	25 cm in first year 12 cm in second year 2 × birth height by age 4 year, then 5–8 cm/year until puberty
Head circumference	35 cm	2 cm/month until 3 months 1 cm/month from 3 to 6 months 0.5 cm/month from 6 to 12 months

LENGTH

1. Measure recumbent length until age 2 years with a length board, then standing height using a stadiometer
2. To estimate child's adult height from parental heights
   a. Boy's height: ([father's height in cm + mother's height in cm]/2) + 6.5 cm
   b. Girl's height: ([father's height in cm + mother's height in cm]/2) − 6.5 cm

HEAD CIRCUMFERENCE

1. Less sensitive indicator of short-term nutritional status; is closely related to brain growth and is influenced by nutritional status until 36 months of age
2. Measurement is taken using a flexible tape measure placed around the largest occipitofrontal circumference

WEIGHT FOR HEIGHT AND BODY MASS INDEX

1. Screening tool for wasting, overweight, and obesity (Table 19.6)
2. In children ≥2 years, use body mass index (BMI) for age
3. In children <2 years, use weight-for-height or percent ideal body weight (%IBW). To calculate %IBW:
   a. Plot height to determine height percentile
   b. Find the same percentile and determine weight (IBW)
   c. %IBW = Child's actual body weight/IBW × 100
4. If height plots <3rd percentile or >97th percentile, IBW can only be estimated
5. 90 to 110 %IBW indicates normal nutrition status, 80 to 89 %IBW mild risk of malnutrition, 70 to 79 %IBW moderate risk of malnutrition, <70 %IBW severe risk of malnutrition

Table 19.6

Growth Status	Indicator	BIRTH–5 YEARS		5–19 YEARS	
		Percentile	SD	Percentile	SD
Wasting	Weight-for-length[a]/BMI[b]	<3rd	<−2	<3rd	<−2
Severe wasting	Weight-for-length[a]/BMI[b]	<0.1st	<−3	<0.1st	<−3
Risk of overweight	Weight-for-length[a]/BMI[b]	>85th	>+1	N/A	N/A
Overweight	Weight-for-length[a]/BMI[b]	>97th	>+2	>85th	>+1
Obesity	Weight-for-length[a]/BMI[b]	>99.9th	>+3	>97th	>+2
Severe obesity	BMI[b]	N/A	N/A	>99.9th	>+3

Table 19.6 WHO Cut-Off Points for Wasting, Overweight and Obesity

[a]Weight-for-length in children <2 years.

[b]BMI in children ≥2 years.

BMI, Body mass index; *SD*, standard deviation; *N/A*, not applicable; *WHO*, World Health Organization.

Data from Promoting Optimal Monitoring of child growth in Canada. Using the new WHO growth charts. *Paediatr Child Health.* 2010;15(2):77–79.

MALNUTRITION INDICATORS

1. When only a single data point is available, use z-scores for weight-for-height/length, body mass index for age, or length/height for age or mid-upper arm circumference (Table 19.7)
2. When two or more data points are available, include weight gain velocity (<2 years of age), weight loss (2–20 years of age), decelerations in weight for length/height z-score, and inadequate nutrient intake (Table 19.8)

Table 19.7 Interpreting Malnutrition Risk With a Single Data Point

Indicator	Mild Malnutrition	Moderate Malnutrition	Severe Malnutrition
Weight for height (z-score)	−1 to −1.9	−2 to −2.9	−3 or less
Body mass index for age (z-score)	−1 to −1.9	−2 to −2.9	−3 or less
Length/height for age (z-score)	No data	No data	−3 or less
Mid-upper arm circumference (z-score)	−1 to −1.9	−2 to −2.9	−3 or less

Modified from Consensus Statement of the Academy of Nutrition and Dietetics/American Society for Parenteral and Enteral Nutrition: Indicators Recommended for the Identification and Documentation of Pediatric Malnutrition (Undernutrition). *Nutrition in Clinical Practice.* 2015;30(1):147–161.

Table 19.8	Interpreting Malnutrition Risk With Two or More Data Points		
Indicator	**Mild Malnutrition**	**Moderate Malnutrition**	**Severe Malnutrition**
Weight gain velocity (<2 years)	<75% of norm	<50% of norm	<25% of norm
Weight loss (2–20 years)	5% UBW	7.5% UBW	10% UBW
Decline in weight for length/height z-score	↓ of 1 z-score	↓ of 2 z-scores	↓ of 3 z-scores
Inadequate nutrient intake	51%–75% estimated energy/protein	26%–50% estimated energy/protein	≤25% estimated energy/protein

UBW, Usual body weight.

Modified from Consensus Statement of the Academy of Nutrition and Dietetics/American Society for Parenteral and Enteral Nutrition. Indicators recommended for the identification and documentation of pediatric malnutrition (undernutrition). *Nutr Clin Pract*. 2015;30(1):147–161.

ENTERAL FEEDING

BREASTFEEDING

1. **Counselling—the importance of breastfeeding**
   a. Breast milk is optimal for infants. Exclusive breastfeeding is recommended for the first 6 months of life. Continued breastfeeding with complementary foods is recommended for up to 2 years and beyond.
   b. **Infant benefits:** transfer of antibodies and immune factors, protection against respiratory and gastrointestinal (GI) infections, aids maturation of the GI tract, low allergenicity, supports neurodevelopment, decreases risk of obesity (infant intake is self-regulated at the breast), decreases risk of type 1 and 2 diabetes and is protective against sudden infant death syndrome
   c. **Maternal benefits:** decreases risk of type 2 diabetes, heart disease, osteoporosis, and cancers; convenient, economical, and environmentally friendly

2. **Counselling—practical support**
   a. In first few days of life, both breasts should be offered at each feeding, for a minimum of 10 minutes on each breast to establish a milk supply
   b. Milk usually comes in between day 3 and 5 postpartum, but can take up to 7 days, especially if the baby was born by cesarean section
   c. In the newborn period, average time at breast is 20 to 45 minutes per feed. Early frequent, unrestricted feeding establishes the milk supply.
   d. Once milk comes in, the first breast should be emptied before offering the second. Start each feed on opposite breast.

e. If there is interruption of breastfeeding or parent-infant separation for any length of time, parents need to be counselled on how to maintain milk supply with effective milk expression as many times a day as the infant would be feeding

3. **Markers of successful breastfeeding**
   a. Eight breastfeeding events in 24 hours
   b. Swallows evident during feeds
   c. Number of wet diapers matches day of age until day 5; after day 5 can expect six or more heavy wet diapers/day
   d. Return to birth weight by 2 weeks; 20 to 30 g/day weight gain during first 3 months of life

4. **Composition of breast milk**
   a. Colostrum for first 24 to 48 hours: yellow, small volume with increased electrolyte, high protein, immunoglobulin, and low-fat content; facilitates passage of meconium
   b. Breast milk energy: 0.67 kcal/mL; composed of carbohydrate (40% calories), fat (55%), protein (5%)

5. **Contraindications to breastfeeding**
   a. **Infant:** inborn errors of metabolism—in most cases of metabolic disorders (except galactosemia), infants can still breastfeed with close monitoring and a prescribed dose of specialized formula. Diet to be considered on a case-specific basis.
   b. **Mother**
      i. Infections: human immunodeficiency virus (HIV), human T-cell lymphotropic viruses (HTLV)-1/2, herpes in breast region, or active, untreated tuberculosis (these may not be absolute contraindications in some developing nations)
      ii. Most medications are safe to take while breastfeeding. Caution regarding certain medications, including chemotherapy, immuno-suppressants, lithium, ergot alkaloids, radiopharmaceuticals, bromocriptine, and iodides. Speak with a pharmacist.
      iii. Current maternal alcohol/drug abuse

6. **Problems associated with breastfeeding:** see Table 19.9

 PEARL

Maternal cytomegalovirus, hepatitis, and antibiotic-treated mastitis are not contraindications to breastfeeding.

Table 19.9	Onset, Characteristics and Management of Common Problems Associated With Breastfeeding		
	Onset	Characteristics	Management
Baby			
Breastfeeding jaundice	Usually in the first week of life		See Jaundice in Chapter 27 Neonatology
Breast milk jaundice	After the first week of life		
Oral candidiasis		White plaques on oral surfaces	Treat baby with antifungal Treat mother's nipples topically
Mother			
Sore/cracked nipples	Anytime	Normal nipple sensitivity typically subsides within 1 minute of suckling	Ensure proper positioning and good latch. Apply breast milk to nipples after each feed and allow to air dry. Avoid soap. May apply creams (e.g., lanolin).
Breast engorgement	Occurs most often in the first week	Caused by accumulated milk and edema in breast tissue; may be exaggerated by poor feeding	Encourage more frequent feeding; cold compresses between feeds, may require pumping
Mastitis	Anytime	Infection of the breast, usually because of *Staphylococcus aureus*. Typically presents as a hard, red, tender, swollen area of one breast associated with fever.	Continue breastfeeding, ensure adequate emptying of affected side. Treat mother with antibiotics, compresses. Monitor for abscess which may require drainage.

ALTERNATIVE CHOICE OF FEEDING SELECTION

1. If breast milk is unavailable, contraindicated, or mother chooses not to breastfeed, commercially available infant formula is to be used as an alternative (Figure 19.9)
2. Ensure parent's feeding choice is an informed one—refer to lifelong benefits of breast milk and breastfeeding

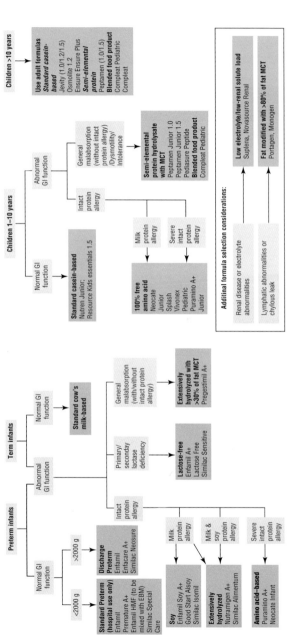

EBM, Expressed breast milk; *GI*, gastrointestinal; *HMF*, human milk fortifier; *MCT*, medium-chain triglycerides. (Provided with permission from Department of Dietetics, Hospital for Sick Children.)

3. If breast milk is unavailable because of a low milk supply, ensure parent is connected to appropriate lactation support (www.ontariobreastfeeds.ca)
4. See Table 19.10 for feeding frequency and volume
5. For children >1 year of age, Figure 19.9 helps determine appropriate formula selection for children requiring nutritional supplementation

Table 19.10	Infant Feeding Frequency and Volume	
Age	**Number of Feeds/Day**	**Approximate Quantity/Feed**
Birth–1 week	6–10	Day 1: 5 mL Day 2: 5–15 mL Day 3: 15–30 mL Day 4–7: 30–60 mL (1–2 oz)
1 week–1 month	6–8	90–120 mL (3–4 oz)
1–2 months	6–8	120–150 mL (4–5 oz)
2–6 months	5–6	150–210 mL (5–7 oz)
6–9 months	4–5	180–210 mL (6–7 oz)
7–12 months	3–4	210–240 mL (6–8 oz)

Data from Kalnins D, Saab J. *Better Baby Food: Your Essential Guide to Nutrition, Feeding and Cooking for All Babies and Toddlers.* Toronto, ON: Robert Rose Inc.; 2001:23.

COW'S MILK PROTEIN ALLERGY (CMPA)

1. **Definition:** immune reaction to cow's milk protein (immunoglobin [Ig]E [type 1 hypersensitivity, more immediate] or non-IgE mediated [type III hypersensitivity] or mixed)
2. **Clinical presentation**
   a. Immediate (urticaria, angioedema, vomiting, acute atopic dermatitis flare)
   b. Delayed (48 hours to 1 week—dysphagia, vomiting, regurgitation, dyspepsia, early satiety, diarrhea, rectal bleeding, failure to thrive (FTT), abdominal pain, severe colic, persistent constipation)
   c. Chronic iron-deficiency anemia
3. **Treatment, diagnostic approach and management:** see Figure 19.10
4. **Diagnostic elimination diet**
   a. Breastfed infants: continue breastfeeding; mothers should avoid all milk and milk products from their own diet
   b. Nonbreastfed infants: cow's milk-based formula should be avoided; first choice: extensively hydrolysed infant formula (eHF). For infants with extreme or life-threatening symptoms, an amino acid–based formula (AAF) may be considered as a first choice.
   c. Toddlers and older children: foods and liquids containing cow's milk protein or other unmodified animal milk proteins (e.g., goat's milk, sheep's milk) should be strictly avoided

d. Open or blind oral food challenge under medical supervision
e. If confirmed, elimination diet with reevaluation for cow's milk protein every 6 to 12 months (or 12–18 months for severe reactions) for tolerance

Figure 19.10 Treatment Diagnostic Approach and Management of Cow's Milk Protein Allergy

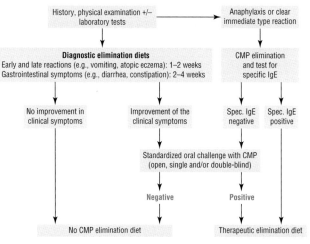

CMP, cow's milk protein; IgE, immunoglobulin E. (Modified from Koletzko S, Niggemann B, Arato A, et al. Diagnostic approach and management of cow's milk protein allergy in infants and children: ESPGHAN GI Committee Practical Guidelines. *J Pediatr Gastroenterol Nutr.* 2012;55(2):221–229.)

ENERGY/NUTRIENT DENSITY OF FEEDS AND THICKENING

1. **Energy/nutrient density of feeds**
   a. Energy density of breast milk and standard full-strength infant formulas = 0.68 kcal/mL = 20 kcal/oz = 2800 kJ/L
   b. Most standard pediatric enteral formulas for children >1 year of age are ready to feed = 1 kcal/mL = 30 kcal/oz = 4200 kJ/L
   c. Indications for increasing caloric content of feeds: fluid restriction, weight loss/poor weight gain, increased metabolic demands, impaired swallowing/oral aversion, impaired absorption/digestion
   d. Concentrating feeds increases energy density and provides additional nutrients; however, it also increases osmolality and renal solute load

e. Steps in fortification for expressed breast milk or infant formula
   i. Advance volume to full fluid allowance
   ii. Increase concentration in a stepwise fashion 0.67 kcal/mL →
      0.8 kcal/mL → 0.9 kcal/mL → 1.0 kcal/mL (Table 19.11). For
      breast milk, add infant formula, and for infant formula, mix with
      less water to obtain desired concentration.
f. Precaution: in infants <1 year, feeds should only be concentrated to
   a *maximum* of 4 g protein/kg (unless warranted by medical condition) because of risk of renal impairment from high solute load

Table 19.11	Stepwise Progression for Energy Density of Enteral Feedings	
kJ/L	**kcal/mL**	**kcal/oz**
2800	0.68	20
3300	0.8	24
3800	0.9	27
4200	1.0	30
4600	1.1	33
5000	1.2	36

Adapted from The Hospital for Sick Children Guidelines for the Administration of Enteral and
Parenteral Nutrition in Paediatrics, 2018.

2. **Thickening feeds**
   a. Indications to thicken feeds: known or suspected aspiration risk (as
      indicated by clinical assessment or video fluoroscopic feeding study,
      history of aspiration/suspected aspiration pneumonia, coughing/
      choking/gagging with feeds, severe neurological impairment)
   b. If aspiration suspected, feeding assessment by occupational therapist or
      speech language pathologist is recommended

SOLIDS
1. **Transition to solids**
   a. At around 6 months of age, solids can be introduced in the baby's
      diet. Follow the baby's cues on how much to feed. Try new foods
      many times. Infants may not always accept at initial offering.
   b. Offer iron-rich foods first (meat, poultry, fish, well-cooked egg, legumes,
      and iron-fortified infant cereals)
   c. Offer a variety of textures (Figure 19.11)
   d. Homogenized cow's milk may be introduced between 9 and 12 months
   e. An infant should be eating a wide variety of foods from all the food
      groups by 12 months of age

Figure 19.11 Introducing New Food Textures to Infants

Puréed
- Smooth, lump-free texture for baby's first introduction to solids
- Start with thin purée, gradually thicken when baby is ready
- Use infant cereal to thicken, breast milk or formula to thin
- Examples: smooth applesauce, rice cereal, sweet potato mash

Thin purée   **Thicker purée**

Minced
- Lumpy, fine chopped foods
- Helps teach baby about chewing and coordinating tongue movement
- Examples: cottage cheese, soft moist ground meats, small well-cooked pasta (pastina, stars)

Chopped
- Thicker, coarser texture of food
- Ideal when teeth start coming, but many babies can manage with their gums
- Baby can use pincer grasp (thumb and forefinger) to pick up food
- Examples: pieces of toast, elbow macaroni, chopped cubes of meat or cheese

(Courtesy of AboutKidsHealth at The Hospital for Sick Children.)

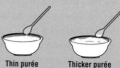

Growth and Nutrition

19

2. **Allergenic foods**
   a. Most common food allergens in children are cow's milk, egg, soy, wheat, peanut, tree nuts, and seafood (see Food Allergic Reactions in Chapter 7 Allergy)
   b. Do not restrict maternal diet during pregnancy or lactation

> ✳ **PEARL**
>
> Delaying introduction of these common allergenic foods beyond 6 months of age does not prevent allergy development.

3. **Other fluids**
   a. Water that meets safety standards including tap, commercially bottled water and well water, is safe to reconstitute powdered formula with. Do not use mineral or carbonated water.
   b. Bring water for feeding infants <4 months to boil for at least 2 minutes and let cool
   c. Limit juice intake to a maximum of 4 oz/day (from open cup)
4. **Food safety**
   a. Avoid hard, small, round, smooth, and sticky solid foods (e.g., hot dogs, grapes, peanuts, and raw vegetables and fruits not cut in small

471

pieces) in children <3 to 4 years of age, because of choking and aspiration risk
   b. Feed infants and children in an upright position with supervision
   c. Do not give honey to infants <1 year of age (risk of botulism)
5. **Vegetarian diet**
   a. A well-planned vegetarian diet with adequate nutrients and energy can meet growth and nutrition needs at any age
   b. Commercial soy-based formula is recommended until 2 years of age for vegan infants who are not breastfed; after 2 years of age fortified soy-based milk should be used
   c. Review intake of total calories, protein, iron, vitamin B12, zinc, calcium, and vitamin D to ensure child is growing well

VITAMIN AND MINERAL SUPPLEMENTATION

See Tables 19.12, 19.13, and 19.14 for daily reference intakes for macronutrients, vitamins and minerals

VITAMIN D

1. Vitamin D is found in a limited number of foods (e.g., egg yolks, fatty fish). Vitamin D deficiency is common in children in Canada.
2. Cow's milk, infant formula, and margarine have added vitamin D
3. There is a high level of vitamin D deficiency found in First Nations and Inuit peoples; special attention needs to be given to vitamin D supplementation in these populations
4. Supplementation
   a. Infants (<1 year): goal Vitamin D intake minimum 400 IU/day
   b. Toddlers and children (≥1 year): routine vitamin D supplementation not recommended
   c. Supplementation with 400 IU/day may be considered for children who do not regularly consume vitamin D-containing foods or have other risk factors for vitamin D deficiency

Table 19.12	Summary of Dietary Reference Intakes (DRIs) for Infants and Children: Macronutrients							
Age	Sex	Protein (g/day)	Carbohydrate (Digestible) (g/day)	Total Fat (g/day)	Linoleic Acid Omega-6 (g/day)	Alpha-Linolenic Acid Omega-3 (g/day)	Total Fiber (g/day)	Total Water (L/day)
Infants								
0–6 months	Both	*9.1*	*60*	*31*	*4.4*	*0.5*	ND	*0.7*
7–12 months	Both	**11**	*90*	*30*	*4.6*	*0.5*	ND	*0.8*
Children								
1–3 years	Both	**13**	**130**	ND	*7*	*0.7*	*19*	*1.3*
4–8 years	Both	**19**	**130**	ND	*10*	*0.9*	*25*	*1.7*
9–13 years	M	**34**	**130**	ND	*12*	*1.2*	*31*	*2.4*
	F	**52**	**130**	ND	*10*	*1*	*26*	*2.1*
14–18 years	M	**34**	**130**	ND	*16*	*1.6*	*38*	*3.3*
	F	**46**	**130**	ND	*11*	*1.1*	*26*	*2.3*

Recommended daily allowances (RDAs) in **bold** and adequate intakes (AIs) in *italics*. *F,* Female; *M,* male; *ND,* not determinable.

Adapted from Food and Nutrition Board, Institute of Medicine-National Academy of Sciences. Dietary Reference Intakes for Energy, Carbohydrate, Fiber, Fats, Fatty Acids, Cholesterol, Protein, and Amino Acids (Macronutrients), 2005. Available at www.nap.edu.

Growth and Nutrition

| | | Table 19.13 | | Summary of Dietary Reference Intakes (DRIs) for Infants and Children: Vitamins | | | | | | | | | | | |

Age	Sex	Vitamin A (mcg/ day)	Vitamin C (mg/ day)	Vitamin D (IU/ day)	Vitamin E (mg/ day)	Vitamin K (mcg/ day)	Thiamin (B1) (mg/ day)	Riboflavin (B2) (mg/day)	Niacin (B3) (mg/day)	Pyridoxine (B6) (mg/ day)	Folate (B9) (mcg/ day)	Vit B12 (mcg/ day)	Pantothenic Acid (B5) (mg/day)	Biotin (mcg/ day)	Choline (mg/ day)
Infants															
0–6 months	Both	*400*	*40*	*400*	*4*	*2*	*0.2*	*0.3*	*2*	*0.1*	*65*	*0.4*	*1.7*	*5*	*125*
7–12 months	Both	*500*	*50*	*400*	*5*	*2.5*	*0.3*	*0.4*	*4*	*0.3*	*80*	*0.5*	*1.8*	*6*	*150*
Children															
1–3 years	Both	**300**	**15**	*600*	**6**	*30*	**0.5**	**0.5**	**6**	**0.5**	**150**	**0.9**	*2*	*8*	*200*
4–8 years	Both	**400**	**25**	*600*	**7**	*55*	**0.6**	**0.6**	**8**	**0.6**	**200**	**1.2**	*3*	*12*	*250*
9–13 years	M	**600**	**45**	*600*	**11**	*60*	**0.9**	**0.9**	**12**	**1**	**300**	**1.8**	*4*	*20*	*375*
	F	**600**	**45**	*600*	**11**	*60*	**0.9**	**0.9**	**12**	**1**	**300**	**1.8**	*4*	*20*	*375*
14–18 years	M	**900**	**75**	*600*	**15**	*75*	**1.2**	**1.3**	**16**	**1.3**	**400**	**2.4**	*5*	*25*	*550*
	F	**700**	**65**	*600*	**15**	*75*	**1**	**1**	**14**	**1.2**	**400**	**2.4**	*5*	*25*	*400*

Recommended daily allowances (RDAs) in **bold** and adequate intakes (AIs) in *italics*. *F*, Female; *M*, male.

Modified from Food and Nutrition Board, Institute of Medicine-National Academy of Sciences. Available at: www.nap.edu.

Table 19.14		Summary of Dietary Reference Intakes (DRIs) for Infants and Children: Minerals															
Age	Sex	Cal-cium (mg/day)	Chromium (mcg/day)	Copper (mcg/day)	Flou-ride (mg/day)	Iodine (mcg/day)	Iron (mg/day)	Magne-sium (mg/day)	Manganese (mg/day)	Molybdenum (mcg/day)	Phos-phorus (mg/day)	Selenium (mcg/day)	Zinc (mg/day)	Potas-sium (g/day)	Sodium (g/day)	Chloride (g/day)
Infants																
0–6 months	Both	200	0.2	200	0.01	110	0.27	30	0.003	2	100	15	2	0.4	0.12	0.18
7–12 months	Both	260	5.5	220	0.5	130	**11**	75	0.6	3	275	20	**3**	0.7	0.37	0.57
Children																
1–3 years	Both	700	11	**340**	0.7	**90**	**7**	**80**	1.2	**17**	**460**	**20**	**3**	3	1	1.5
4–8 years	Both	1000	15	**440**	1	**90**	**10**	**130**	1.5	**22**	**500**	**30**	**5**	3.8	1.2	1.9
9–13 years	M	1300	25	**700**	2	**120**	**8**	**240**	1.9	**34**	**1250**	**40**	**8**	4.5	1.5	2.3
	F	1300	21	**700**	3	**120**	**8**	**240**	1.6	**34**	**1250**	**40**	**8**	4.7	1.5	2.3
14–18 years	M	1300	35	**890**	2	**150**	**11**	**410**	2.2	**43**	**1250**	**55**	**11**	4.5	1.5	2.3
	F	1300	24	**890**	3	**150**	**15**	**360**	1.6	**43**	**1250**	**55**	**9**	4.7	1.5	2.3

Recommended daily allowances (RDAs) in **bold** and adequate intakes (AIs) in *italics*. *F*, Female; *M*, male.

Modified from Food and Nutrition Board, Institute of Medicine-National Academy of Sciences. Available at: www.nap.edu.

Growth and Nutrition

19

IRON

1. Healthy terms infants have adequate iron stores for the first 6 months
2. At 6 months old, complementary iron-rich foods should be introduced
3. Preterm infants and small for gestational age infants (<2.5 kg) have a deficit of total body iron: preterm infants receiving breast milk should be started on an iron supplement by 1 month of age and small for gestational age infants by 2 weeks of age, continued until dietary sources are adequate. Additional information in Chapter 27 Neonatology.

✦ PEARL

An important risk factor for iron deficiency is the consumption of more than 500 mL/16 oz of milk per day in children >1 year of age.

VITAMIN B12

1. Vitamin B12 is only found naturally in animal products (meat, fish, dairy products, and eggs)
2. It is added to soy infant formula, cereals, yeasts, and fortified soy and nut beverages
3. Breastfed infants of vegan mothers, and children who follow a vegan diet are at high-risk for vitamin B12 deficiency
4. It is recommended that at least three servings of food rich in vitamin B12 be included in the daily diet or supplementation be provided at 5 to 10 mcg/day

FLUORIDE SUPPLEMENTATION

1. Fluoride has been shown to decrease dental caries, but excess fluoride can result in fluorosis
2. Fluoride supplementation recommended only for infants ≥6 months if water fluoride concentration <0.3 ppm, teeth not brushed at least twice a day, susceptibility to high caries activity (e.g., family history, geographic trends)

PARENTERAL NUTRITION (PN)

1. These guidelines are intended for the general inpatient pediatric population. Prescribers are encouraged to use clinical assessment and judgement of their patients' requirements when prescribing PN.
2. Parenteral nutrition in the neonatal period is covered in Chapter 27 Neonatology.
3. **Indications for PN:** PN is nutrition delivered intravenously to patients who are unable to ingest or absorb nutrients via the enteral tract for a significant period of time. Patients should not be without adequate nutrition longer than:
   a. Premature infants: 1 day
   b. Term infants and beyond: 3 to 7 days (consider withholding PN for 1 week in critically ill children)

4. Although the GI tract should be used whenever possible, PN may be used as a primary source of nutrition, providing full nutrition support, or as a partial source, providing nutrition repletion or augmentation in patients unable to tolerate full enteral nutrition
5. **Parenteral nutrition requirements**
    a. The energy cost of digestion of PN is minimal; therefore PN fed patients require approximately 7% to 15% (infants-children) to ~25% (neonates) fewer calories compared with when enterally fed
    b. To account for the decreased energy requirement when using PN, resting energy expenditure (REE) plus activity and/or stress factors are applied to estimate total caloric requirements, instead of the DRI (see Table 19.15)
    c. See Table 19.16 for amino acid (protein) rates, Table 19.17 for lipid (fat) rates, Table 19.18 for glucose rates, Table 19.19 for fluid rates, and Tables 19.20 and 19.21 for electrolyte recommendations

Table 19.15	Energy Requirements (kcal/kg/day) for Parenteral Nutrition in Different Phases of Disease		
	Acute Phase	**Stable Phase**	**Recovery Phase[a]**
0–1 years	45–50	60–65	75–85
1–7 years	40–45	55–60	65–75
7–12 years	30–40	40–55	55–65
12–18 years	20–30	25–40	30–55

[a]General adequate amounts to support growth. Higher or lower amounts may be required in specific patient populations.

Adapted from The Hospital for Sick Children Guidelines for the Administration of Enteral and Parenteral Nutrition in Paediatrics, 2018.

Table 19.16	Parenteral Amino Acid Recommendations for Stable Patients (g/kg/day)		
	Initiate	**Adequate[a]**	**Max[a]**
Term infants	1.5–2	1.5–3	3.5
2 months to 3 years	1.5–2	1.5–2.5	3.5
3–18 years	1.5–2	1.5–2	2

[a]Patients may require more protein to support growth and/or accommodate losses.

Adapted from The Hospital for Sick Children Guidelines for the Administration of Enteral and Parenteral Nutrition in Paediatrics, 2018.

Table 19.17	Parenteral Lipid Recommendations for Stable Patients (g/kg/day)			
	Initiate[a]	Min.[b]	Max.	Adequate Amount
Term infant	0.5–1.5	0.25	4	Intake of 25%–50% of nonprotein calories is recommended in fully parenterally fed patients
2 months–18 years		0.1	3	

[a]Lipid delivery range for ages between adolescents to neonates, respectively.
[b]Minimum lipid delivery required to prevent fatty acid deficiency.

Adapted from The Hospital for Sick Children Guidelines for the Administration of Enteral and Parenteral Nutrition in Paediatrics, 2018.

Table 19.18	Parenteral Glucose Recommendations (mg/kg/min)		
Patient	Acute Phase	Stable Phase	Recovery Phase[a]
<10 kg (>1 month of age)	2–4	4–6	6–10
11–30 kg	1.5–2.5	2–4	3–6
31–45 kg	1–1.5	1.5–3	3–4
>45 kg	0.5–1	1–2	2–3

[a]Adequate amounts to support growth in the average pediatric patient. Higher glucose amounts may be required to support medical needs. It is advisable to consider total macronutrient distribution within the total parenteral nutrition order.

Adapted from The Hospital for Sick Children Guidelines for the Administration of Enteral and Parenteral Nutrition in Paediatrics, 2018.

Table 19.19	Maintenance Fluid Requirements (Beyond the Neonatal Period)	
Weight	mL/kg/day	mL/kg/h
A: the first 10 kg	100	4
B: weight between 10 and 20 kg	+50 mL/extra kg/day	+2 mL/extra kg/hour
C: weight above 20 kg	+25 mL/extra kg/day	+1 mL/extra kg/hour
Sum total requirements	A+B+C	A+B+C

Adapted from The Hospital for Sick Children Guidelines for the Administration of Enteral and Parenteral Nutrition in Paediatrics, 2018.

Table 19.20	Parenteral Fluid and Electrolyte Recommendations[a]				
	28 Days–1 Year	1–2 Years	3–5 Years	6–12 Years	13–18 Years
Fluid (mL/kg/day)	120–150	80–120	80–100	60–80	50–70
Na (mmol/kg/day)	2–3		1–3		
K (mmol/kg/day)	1–3				
Cl (mmol/kg/day)			2–4		

[a]Adequate amounts to support the average pediatric patient. Higher or lower amounts may be required to support medical needs.

Adapted from The Hospital for Sick Children Guidelines for the Administration of Enteral and Parenteral Nutrition in Paediatrics, 2018.

Table 19.21	Recommended Parenteral Intake for Calcium, Phosphorus and Magnesium (mmol/kg/day)		
Age	Calcium	Phosphorus	Magnesium
0–6 months	0.8–1.5	0.7–1.3	0.1–0.2
7–12 months	0.3–0.8	0.3–0.8	0.1–0.2
1–18 years	0.25–0.4	0.2–0.7	0.05–0.15

Adapted from The Hospital for Sick Children Guidelines for the Administration of Enteral and Parenteral Nutrition in Paediatrics, 2018.

6. **Considerations in management**
   a. Ordering PN
      i. Amino acids (protein): standard solutions contain 20 g amino acids per 1000 mL (2%) for preterm or 30 g amino acids per 1000 mL (3%) for infants and children. Sample calculation for a 10-kg infant if starting at 1.5 g/kg/day of amino acids using 3% amino acid solution: 1.5 g/kg × 10 kg × 1000 mL/30 g ÷ 24 h/day = desired rate (mL/h).
      ii. Lipids: standard solutions are fat emulsion 20% (200 g lipids per 1000 mL) or fat emulsion 30% (300 g lipids per 1000 mL) if fluid restricted. Sample calculation for a 10-kg infant and if ordering separate lipid solution starting at 1 g/kg/day lipids using 20% lipid solution: 1 g/kg × 10 kg × 1000 mL/200 g ÷ 24 h/day = desired rate (mL/h).
   b. Weaning from PN
      i. Nonfluid restricted patients: rate of amino acid and dextrose solution should be tapered at a 1:1 ratio as enteral intake increases
      ii. Fluid restricted patients: incremental decreases in rate of amino acid and dextrose solution (i.e., 25%, 50%, etc.) based on enteral delivery. For example: enteral volume is 25% of goal, decrease PN solution by 25%.
      iii. Lipids may be stopped completely without tapering the rate

c. Cycling PN

   i. Cycling allows administration of incompatible medications, increases patient freedom for ambulation, and helps in weaning off PN

   ii. Sudden cessation of PN solution with high glucose concentration (>15% or GIR >8 mg/kg/min) may result in rebound hypoglycemia. Tapering PN should take place over 1 hour, with half the full PN rate given over the last 1 hour. Consider blood glucose check within 1 hour of abrupt decrease in PN rate.

7. See Table 19.22 for PN monitoring

Table 19.22	Sample Monitoring Schedule for Stable Patients on Parenteral Nutrition	
Parameter	**Monday**	**Thursday (×3 Weeks Only)**
Sodium, potassium, chloride	Yes	Yes
Glucose	Yes	Yes
Creatine, urea	Yes	Yes/no
Lipid level	Yes	Yes
ALT, GGT, ALP, conjugated bilirubin[a]	Yes	No
Ionized calcium, phosphate, magnesium	Yes	No

[a]Markers of hepatic injury (AST, ALT, conjugated bilirubin, ALP) can be followed periodically (once a week to twice a month) if known liver injury or other specific concerns.

ALP, Alkaline phosphatase; *ALT,* alanine aminotransferase; *AST,* aspartate aminotransferase; *GGT,* gamma-glutamyl transferase; *ICU,* intensive care unit.

Adapted from The Hospital for Sick Children Guidelines for the Administration of Enteral and Parenteral Nutrition in Paediatrics, 2018.

FAILURE TO THRIVE (FTT)

1. **Definition:** weight for age less than the third percentile, decrease in growth velocity resulting in weight and/or height crossing ≥2 percentiles, or weight <80% of ideal body weight. FTT is the result of interaction between the child's health, development, behavior, and the environment.

2. **Differential diagnosis:** see Table 19.23

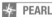 **PEARL**

Failure to thrive is a not a diagnosis but a sign of inadequate growth.

Table 19.23   Causes of Failure to Thrive

Inadequate Caloric Intake

Medical

- Gastroesophageal reflux
- Inadequate appetite (e.g., genetic syndromes; anorexia of chronic disease)
- Inadequate ability to eat large amounts (e.g., chronic constipation, intestinal tract obstruction)

Nutritional

- Insufficient lactation
- Inappropriate nutrition intake (e.g., excess milk, dilution of formula, excess fruit juice intake, restricted diet)

Feeding Skills

- Mechanical problems (e.g., cleft palate, nasal obstruction)
- Sucking or swallowing dysfunction (e.g., central nervous system disorders, neuromuscular)
- Oral aversion/hypersensitivity
- Neurodevelopmental delay (e.g., global development delay, autism spectrum disorder)

Psychosocial

- Food insecurity
- Disturbance of caregiver/child relation
- Force-feeding
- Inadequate knowledge about nutrition needs
- Failure to advance to age-appropriate feeding
- Caregiver mental health problems (e.g., anxiety, depression)
- Psychiatric disorders of child (e.g., mood disorders, eating disorders)
- Neglect/inadequate provisions of calories

Increased Expenditure of Calories

- Endocrine disorders: hyperthyroidism
- Chronic infections (e.g., congenital infections, urinary tract infections, tuberculosis, human immunodeficiency virus)
- Chronic inflammation (e.g., inflammatory bowel disease, juvenile idiopathic arthritis)
- Metabolic diseases (e.g., galactosemia, inborn errors of metabolism)
- Chronic respiratory insufficiency (e.g., chronic lung disease, cystic fibrosis)
- Congenital or acquired heart disease
- Hematological diseases (e.g., severe iron-deficiency anemia) or malignancy

Inadequate Nutrient Absorption or Increased Losses

- Malabsorption (e.g., cystic fibrosis, cow's milk protein allergy, celiac disease)
- Biliary atresia
- Vomiting (e.g., intestinal tract obstruction/atresia, infectious gastroenteritis, increased intracranial pressure)
- Diarrhea (e.g., infectious, inflammatory bowel disease)
- Renal diseases (e.g., renal tubular acidosis)
- Inborn errors of metabolism

3. **History**
   a. Detailed diet history: duration/quantity of feeds (sleep feeding, force-feeding, feeding regardless of hunger cues, distracting to feed), dilution of formula, other fluid intake (juice, water, etc.), dietary restrictions/beliefs
   b. Assessment of textures—feeding ability and appropriateness for age
   c. Past medical history, allergies, developmental milestones, detailed social history (i.e., caregivers, psychosocial stressors, parental mental illness/substance abuse, social services involvement, food insecurity)
   d. Pregnancy/birth history: small for gestational age, intrauterine growth restriction, prematurity, intrauterine infections, maternal substance abuse
4. **Physical examination**
   a. Plot all anthropometrics (length, weight, head circumference) and compare with prior measurements
   b. Hydration status, dysmorphic features, wasting, signs of chronic disease, development, signs of abuse/poor hygiene
   c. Observe parent–child interaction and child's temperament
5. **Investigations**
   a. Three-day food record
   b. Assessment by dietitian, occupational therapist, lactation consultant, social worker, as indicated
   c. Consider clinical observation to assess weight gain/observe feeding
   d. Basic laboratory assessment: complete blood count (CBC), electrolytes, blood gas, urinalysis, creatinine, urea, liver enzymes, albumin, ferritin, C-reactive protein (CRP)/erythrocyte sedimentation rate (ESR)
   e. Other tests, as indicated by history and physical examination
   f. Consider insulin-like growth factor 1 (IGF-1) and bone age (x-ray of left hand and wrist) if short stature (length less than the third percentile)
6. **Treatment**
   a. Energy-boosting strategies: use high fat foods such as butter, oils, margarine, creams (18%–35%), high fat yogurt and milk (≥3% milk fat) nut butters, sour cream, or mashed avocado added to foods to increase energy density
   b. Mealtime modifications: solids before liquids, no meals on the go or chasing, eliminate grazing between meals, encourage regular feeding

schedule (e.g., feed every 3–4 hours), encourage family mealtimes, avoid force feeding, eliminate distractions

   c. Involvement of psychologist/social worker to support parent–child interactions

   d. Assess the need for tube feeding if attempts at increasing energy intake orally are unsuccessful

OBESITY

1. **Definition:** see Table 19.6 for cut-offs
2. **Differential diagnosis**
   a. Idiopathic/familial
   b. Hormonal (hypothyroidism, growth hormone deficiency, Cushing syndrome, polycystic ovary syndrome, hypogonadism)
   c. Hypothalamic obesity (craniopharyngioma)
   d. Syndromic (Trisomy 21, Prader-Willi, Bardet-Biedl [retinal dystrophy, renal abnormalities, mitral regurgitation], Fragile X [macroorchidism, large ears], Albright hereditary osteodystrophy [short stature, skeletal defects])
   e. Genetic (melanocortin 4 receptor deficiency, congenital leptin deficiency, leptin receptor defect)
3. **History:** diet, physical activity (sedentary time, sleep), psychosocial factors (mental health, body image, depression, anxiety, binge eating disorder)
4. **Physical examination**
   a. Vital signs (heart rate [HR] increases with higher BMI, blood pressure [BP] by auscultation with cuff >80% of midarm circumference)
   b. Head and neck: papilledema, dental caries, wide neck, adenotonsillar hypertrophy
   c. Chest: gynecomastia (>2 cm breast tissue), cervicodorsal hump (Cushing syndrome)
   d. GI: hepatomegaly (nonalcoholic fatty liver disease [NAFLD])
   e. Genitourinary: inconspicuous penis (from enlarged suprapubic fat pad)
   f. Musculoskeletal: gait scoliosis, lordosis, slipped capital femoral epiphysis, genu valgum/varus, pes planus
   g. Skin: acanthosis nigricans, hirsutism, acne, striae, intertrigo, pannus
5. **Investigations:** directed by history and physical examination (Figure 19.12)
6. **Complications:** see Table 19.24

Figure 19.12   Evaluation of Child or Adolescent With Obesity

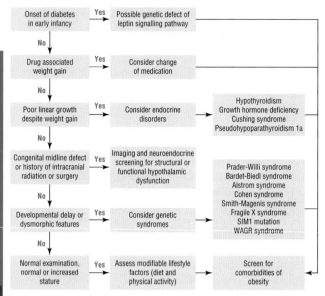

WAGR, Wilms tumour, anirida, genitourinary anomalies, intellectual disability. (From Han JC, Lawlor DA, Kimm SYS. Childhood obesity. *Lancet*, 2010;375(9727):1737–1748.)

Table 19.24	Complications of Childhood Obesity
CNS - Idiopathic intracranial hypertension **Psychosocial** - Depression - Anxiety **Cardiovascular** - Elevated blood pressure - Dyslipidemia - Atherosclerosis **Pulmonary** - Obstructive sleep apnea - Asthma - Exercise intolerance **Renal** - Glomerulopathy	**Endocrine** - Insulin resistance/T2DM - PCOS - Precocious puberty **Gastrointestinal/nutrition** - Fatty liver disease - Gastroesophageal reflux - Cholelithiasis - Iron deficiency - Vitamin D deficiency **Orthopedic** - Slipped capital femoral epiphysis - Osteoarthritis

CNS, Central nervous system; *PCOS*, polycystic ovary syndrome; *T2DM*, type 2 diabetes mellitus.

7. **Comorbidity screening**
   a. Children >2 years of age with BMI ≥85th percentile: lipid profile (total cholesterol, triglycerides, high density lipoprotein [HDL] cholesterol, non-HDL cholesterol) every 2 years
   b. Children with BMI ≥ 85th percentile with at least one risk factor: fasting plasma glucose, hemoglobin (Hb)A1C and oral glucose tolerance test every 3 years
      i. Risk factors: family history of type 2 diabetes, high risk ethnicity, signs of insulin resistance, or exposed to gestational diabetes mellitus in utero
   c. Children >10 years with BMI 85th to 94th percentile and metabolic risk factors or BMI ≥95th percentile: alanine aminotransferase (ALT)/aspartate aminotransferase (AST) every 2 years

8. **Management**
   a. Primary goal of pediatric obesity treatment is to improve health outcomes by increasing healthy behaviors (Table 19.25)
   b. Emphasize that weight loss in small increments (no more than 0.5 kg/week) can lead to large improved health outcomes
   c. Drastic weight loss with restrictive diets or extreme physical exercise should not be encouraged because it is not sustainable
   d. **Dietary:** establish normalized eating—eat as a family, decrease sugar-sweetened beverages, follow healthy portion sizes, increase consumption of vegetables and fruit, limit fast-food/restaurant meals
   e. **Physical activity:** integrate enjoyable activities to complete as family and/or with teams/programs, encourage active living (e.g., taking stairs vs. elevator), limit screen time appropriately, promote sleep hygiene
   f. **Pharmacotherapy:** minimal evidence for efficacy in weight loss
   g. **Surgery:** bariatric surgery rare in pediatric population

Table 19.25	Approach to Obesity Counselling
Step	**Actions**
Ask	Ask for permission to discuss weight Explore readiness for change
Assess	Assess obesity related risks and potential root causes of weight gain
Advise	Advise on obesity risks, discuss benefits and options
Agree	Agree on a realistic plan based on SMART[a] goals
Assist	Assist in addressing drivers and barriers, offer education and resources, refer to provider, and arrange follow-up

[a]A SMART goal is specific, measurable, achievable, realistic and timely.

Adapted from the Canadian Obesity Network. Accessible at: www.obesitynetwork.ca/5As-pediatrics.

19

9. **Counselling**
   a. Use phrases like "weight," "BMI," "weight issues," "excess weight"
   b. Focus on entire family, rather than the child alone
   c. Avoid conversations which are forced or shaming, create unrealistic expectations or practitioner driven goals

MICRONUTRIENT DEFICIENCIES

1. Micronutrients are vitamins and minerals that are obtained from the diet and are required in trace amounts to maintain physiological processes in the body and ensure normal growth and development
2. Micronutrient deficiencies other than iron deficiency are relatively rare in developed nations and often only seen in specific nutritional, medical, or developmental contexts, typically as a result of inadequate oral intake or malabsorption
3. Children with autism spectrum disorder are at risk of "rare" micronutrient deficiencies if restricted and repetitive behaviors manifest as restricted diet and limited food repertoire

XEROPHTHALMIA

1. Spectrum of eye disease caused by vitamin A deficiency
2. Characterized by pathological dryness of the cornea and conjunctiva: Bitot spots (abnormal keratinization of the conjunctiva), xerosis (dryness and keratinization) of cornea, keratomalacia (softening and liquefaction of cornea); also manifests as night blindness and retinopathy because of role of vitamin A in photoreception at the reception
3. Diagnosis usually made clinically, but may be supported by low serum retinol (vitamin A) level
4. May lead to permanent vision loss if not identified and treated promptly
5. Treat as per WHO guidelines with age-specific doses of vitamin A. Oral route of administration is strongly preferred.

SCURVY

1. Disease resulting from severe vitamin C deficiency
2. Clinical manifestations are dermatological (petechiae, ecchymosis, follicular hyperkeratosis, corkscrew hairs), gingival (bleeding, swelling, gingivitis), hematological (anemia), and musculoskeletal (arthralgias, subperiosteal hemorrhages)

3. Diagnosis is primarily clinical and is confirmed when symptoms resolve with vitamin C supplementation; plasma ascorbic acid level may be supportive (can be influenced by recent vitamin C intake)
4. Treatment: vitamin C replacement

RICKETS

1. Deficient mineralization of bone resulting in abnormalities at growth plate, usually classified based on underlying mineral deficiency: calcipenic versus phosphopenic
2. Calcipenic form caused by insufficient intake of vitamin D and/or calcium; rare genetic defects leading to vitamin D resistance do exist
3. Phosphopenic form almost exclusively caused by renal phosphate wasting (isolated or related to a tubular disorder [e.g., Fanconi syndrome])
4. Clinical findings similar in calcipenic and phosphopenic rickets (e.g., frontal bossing, delayed fontanelle closure, craniotabes, prominence of anterior ribs at costochondral junctions, wrist widening and bowing of legs; pattern of deformity depends on age and weight-bearing status of child)
5. Radiological findings include widening, cupping, and fraying of the metaphysis and an increase in thickness of the growth plate
6. Alkaline phosphatase is elevated in both forms of rickets; serum parathyroid hormone, calcium, and phosphorus levels help to distinguish between the two (Table 19.26)
7. In calcipenic rickets, serum 25-hydroxyvitamin D should be ordered to differentiate between vitamin D deficiency (most common) and other causes
8. Treatment involves vitamin and mineral supplementation, dependent on the underlying type of rickets

Table 19.26	Distinguishing Calcipenic Versus Phosphopenic Rickets	
	Calcipenic Rickets	**Phosphopenic Rickets**
Parathyroid hormone	Elevated	Usually normal, may be low or mildly elevated
Calcium	Normal or low	Normal
Phosphorus	Normal or low	Low

IRON DEFICIENCY

See Chapter 21 Hematology

FURTHER RESOURCES

1. Dietitians of Canada: www.dietitians.ca
2. Ontario Dieticians in Public Health: www.odph.ca
3. North American Society for Pediatric Gastroenterology, Hepatology and Nutrition: www.naspghan.org

Gynecology

Lauren Friedman • Heather Millar • Anjali Aggarwal

COMMON ABBREVIATIONS

Also see page xviii for a list of other abbreviations used throughout this book

AFP	alpha fetoprotein
AUB	abnormal uterine bleeding
β-hCG	β-human chorionic gonadotropin
BV	bacterial vaginosis
CHC	combined hormonal contraception
DHEAS	dehydroepiandrosterone
DMPA	depomedroxyprogesterone acetate
DUB	dysfunctional uterine bleeding
EUA	examination under anesthesia
FSH	follicle-stimulating hormone
FTA-ABS	fluorescent treponemal antibody absorption test
GU	genitourinary
IUD	intrauterine device
LDH	lactate dehydrogenase
LH	luteinizing hormone
NAAT	nucleic acid amplification testing
NAI	nonaccidental injury
OCP	oral contraceptive pill
PCOS	polycystic ovary syndrome
RPR	rapid plasma reagin
STI	sexually transmitted infection
TP-PA	*Treponema pallidum* particle agglutination
VDRL	venereal disease research laboratory

ANATOMY OF THE EXTERNAL GENITALIA

See Figure 20.1

Figure 20.1 Female External Genitalia

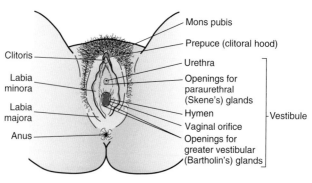

(Modified from Applegate E. *The Sectional Anatomy Learning System*. 3rd ed. Philadelphia: Saunders; 2001.)

GENITAL EXAMINATION OF PEDIATRIC AND ADOLESCENT FEMALES

A. Genital examination of the prepubertal child

1. **Preparation**
   a. Obtain assent from the patient and consent from the patient's caregiver with the child present
   b. Explain the reasoning for the examination and demonstrate the materials that will be used
   c. Put child at ease with caregiver visible and appropriate draping and lighting

2. **Examination techniques**
   a. Frog-leg position: child lays supine with feet together and knees apart either on examination table or caregiver's lap. First inspect the external genitalia and then apply gentle traction at 5 and 7 o'clock on the labia majora in a lateral and posterior direction. This allows visualization of the lower third of the vagina and the hymenal ring.
   b. Prone knee–chest position: patient kneels and leans forward to rest on forearms, which allows for inspection of the upper vagina and possibly the cervix

3. **Special considerations**
   a. *Never* force an examination
   b. Because of a lack of estrogen, prepubertal vaginal mucosa and hymenal tissue are thinner, redder, and more sensitive compared with postpubertal mucosa
   c. There are many hymenal variations. Certain congenital anomalies may require surgical consultation.
   d. Speculum examinations are not appropriate in prepubertal children. If better visibility is required, a cystoscope or vaginoscope may be used (under anaesthesia or conscious sedation).

PEARL

Gynecological examinations should be modified based on pubertal stage and history of sexual activity.

B. Genital examination of the adolescent

1. **Preparation**
   a. Review confidentiality and obtain consent
   b. Discuss and demonstrate the examination procedures and instruments
   c. Medical chaperone is strongly recommended for medicolegal reasons and to assist physician

2. **Examination techniques**
   a. Position the patient in lithotomy position in stirrups or in frog-leg position with appropriate draping
   b. First inspect external genitalia, noting Tanner stage (see Chapter 14 Endocrinology)

c. The examination should be modified based on sexual activity. In virginal patients, vaginal swabs, hymenal inspection, and abdominal (or rectoabdominal) palpation may be appropriate. Sexually active patients may require speculum and bimanual vaginal–abdominal examinations to palpate the adnexa and uterus.

3. **Special considerations**
   a. Adjust the size of the speculum based on age, hymenal status, and sexual activity
   b. Speculum and bimanual examinations are less often indicated in adolescent patients with the advent of the new vaginal swab (which patients can self-administer) and urine nucleic acid amplification testing (NAAT) STI tests, as well as new Canadian Pap smear guidelines (not recommended before age 21 years)

PREPUBERTAL GYNECOLOGICAL ISSUES

NEONATAL VAGINAL BLEEDING

1. **Definition:** Vaginal bleeding in a newborn female that usually occurs between day of life 5 and 10. Should not continue past 1 month of age.
2. **Etiology:** Maternal estrogens cross the placenta in utero and can cause various sequelae in the baby, including breast buds, nipple discharge, and vaginal discharge. Postdelivery, maternal estrogen withdrawal can lead to endometrial shedding and vaginal bleeding.
3. **Differential:** Other rare causes of neonatal vaginal bleeding include gynecological disease (infection, tumor), bleeding diathesis, urethral prolapse, and sexual abuse. Hematuria is often mistaken for vaginal bleeding.
4. **Treatment:** Observation and reassurance. Further workup is indicated only if persistent or if there are suspicions of another cause.

PREPUBERTAL VAGINAL BLEEDING

Definition: Acute or chronic vaginal bleeding in a child who has not yet passed through menarche. See Box 20.1 for differential diagnosis. Also see Chapter 14 Endocrinology.

A. Vulvar/vaginal trauma
1. **Etiology**
   a. Can be blunt straddle injury (force of body falling on an object, e.g., bike frame) or penetrating injury
2. **History**
   a. Inquire about method of injury: keep a high level of suspicion for nonaccidental injury (NAI) (see Chapter 9 Child Maltreatment) and ensure that mechanism of injury matches examination
   b. Inquire about sequelae of injury: amount of bleeding, degree of pain, dysuria, difficulty urinating, hematuria

Local Causes

- Trauma—straddle or penetrating injury
- Foreign body
- Sexual abuse
- Nonspecific vulvovaginitis
- Infections (group A strep, shigella), sexually transmitted infections (gonorrhea, chlamydia, etc.)
- Urethral mucosal prolapse
- Lichen sclerosis
- Hemangioma
- Uterine/vaginal pathology (benign or malignant)

Systemic Causes

- Endocrine conditions (e.g., precocious puberty, isolated precocious menarche)
- Exogenous estrogen exposure
- Hypothyroidism
- Blood dyscrasia
- Ovarian tumors (benign or malignant)

3. **Physical examination**
   a. May need analgesia before examination. Can apply ice pack for 15 to 20 minutes or use local anaesthetic. More severe injuries may require sedation or examination under anesthesia (EUA).
   b. Straddle injuries: examination may reveal ecchymoses/lacerations of the mons, clitoral hood, labia majora and minora, or periurethral areas, and/or vulvar hematomas. If there is evidence of trauma to the hymen or posterior fourchette consider NAI.
   c. Penetrating injuries: hymenal tear implies penetrating injury (accidental or abuse) and warrants investigation for vaginal or rectal tears. Deep tears (i.e., involving hymen and above, deep perineal, rectal) require EUA by a gynecologist to rule out more extensive injury

4. **Treatment**
   a. Superficial abrasion: treat with ice and compression
   b. Small laceration: often can be treated with topical anaesthetic and hygiene measures. Rarely requires suturing for cosmesis or hemostasis.
   c. Hematomas: conservative management with ice, compression, and sitz baths. Hemodynamic instability warrants surgical treatment.
   d. Referral to gynecology for: deep or penetrating lacerations, significant bleeding, inability to visualize extent of laceration, and uncooperative child
   e. If there is a true inability to void, may require Foley catheter or assessment by urology for urethral injury

B. Urethral prolapse

1. **Definition:** protrusion of the distal urethra through the urethral meatus
2. **Epidemiology:** more common in children of African ethnicity, age 2 to 10 years

3. **Clinical presentation:** vaginal bleeding, vaginal mass, dysuria, urinary frequency; may have history of recurrent Valsalva (constipation, acute/chronic cough)
4. **Examination:** friable red/purple annular mass with urethra at center
5. **Treatment:** treat precipitating factors. Conservative measures include stool softeners, topical estrogen creams (eg, Premarin cream applied twice daily for 2 weeks) and sitz baths, which often resolve the prolapse in a few weeks. Surgical excision may be required if the prolapse is large or persistent after medical treatment.

C. Foreign body
1. **Clinical manifestations:** vaginal discharge, foul odor, intermittent bleeding
2. **Etiology:** most common foreign body is toilet paper
3. **Examination:** attempt irrigation or direct visualization, ± rectoabdominal examination to palpate
4. **Treatment:** can irrigate vagina with warm water using catheter or feeding tube or use a calgi swab to remove toilet paper; EUA required if symptoms with no visualized foreign body despite irrigation

PREPUBERTAL VULVOVAGINITIS
1. **Definition:** Inflammation or irritation of the vaginal and vulvar tissue
2. **Epidemiology:** Most common gynecologic complaint in the prepubertal age group. Unestrogenized prepubertal vaginal tissue is thinner, alkaline and more sensitive to irritation.
3. **Clinical manifestations:** Pain, pruritus, vaginal discharge or bleeding, urinary frequency/dysuria, and vulvar erythema
4. **Differential:** 25% to 75% of cases are nonspecific. See Box 20.2 for an expanded differential.

Box 20.2 Differential Diagnosis of Prepubertal Vulvovaginitis

Nonspecific (25%–75%)
- Poor hygiene
- Chemical irritant
- Physiologic differences in prepubertal vaginal mucosa
- Tight clothing

Foreign Body
Trauma/Abuse
Infectious
- Respiratory (e.g., Group A strep, *Haemophilus influenza*) or enteric (e.g., *Shigella*) flora
- Pinworms
- Sexually transmitted infections (should raise flags for sexual abuse)
- *Candida* (rare in prepubertal girls who are no longer in diapers without predisposing factors [e.g., diabetes, recent antibiotic use]).

Systemic Conditions
- Viruses (e.g., Varicella, Epstein-Barr virus)
- Drug reactions (e.g., Stevens-Johnson syndrome)
- Dermatological conditions (e.g., atopic dermatitis, psoriasis, lichen sclerosis)

5. **Diagnosis**
   a. Clinical diagnosis
   b. A vaginal culture (see Table 20.1) may be indicated in select cases
   c. In cases of suspected sexual abuse, involve local child maltreatment experts (see Chapter 9 Child Maltreatment)
6. **Treatment**
   a. General measures: vulvar hygiene education and irritant avoidance (Box 20.3), Sitz baths, use of barrier creams (petroleum jelly, zinc oxide)
   b. Treat specific organisms, if identified
   c. For severe inflammation of nonspecific origin, consider steroid cream
   d. Referral to gynecology if unclear diagnosis, nonresponsive to therapy or if vaginoscopy is required for diagnosis or foreign body removal

---

Box 20.3 Maintaining Vulvar Hygiene

- No soap to labia
- Avoid scented products
- Avoid bubble baths
- Wear cotton underwear
- No underwear at night
- Avoid tight fitting clothing
- Avoid spending time in a wet bathing suit
- Avoid hair removal
- Appropriate voiding posture
- Wipe front to back
- Use gentle underwear detergent with no fabric softener
- Do not use pantiliners unless menstruating

✦ **PEARL**

Vulvar yeast infections are uncommon in the prepubertal age group without other risk factors (antibiotics, diabetes, etc.).

LABIAL ADHESIONS

1. **Definition:** Common acquired disorder in prepubertal children (typically 6 months to 6 years), where the labia adhere to each other in the midline
2. **Clinical presentation:** Asymptomatic or vulvovaginitis, urinary tract infection (UTI), urinary dribbling
3. **Treatment**
   a. Will often spontaneously resolve with endogenous estrogen (at puberty), therefore no treatment needed if asymptomatic
   b. General measures: vulvar hygiene (see Box 20.3), remove irritants, apply bland emollient cream (petroleum jelly or zinc oxide)
   c. If symptomatic, can apply estrogen cream to fused area for 2 to 6 weeks (e.g., Premarin cream applied twice daily using a fingertip) 495

d. If nonresponsive or acute urinary retention, experienced clinician can perform manual separation under topical anaesthetic or sedation

e. Recurrence is common until patient goes through puberty

GENITAL INFECTIONS

Infections of the female genitalia can result in various clinical syndromes and are caused by a wide variety of sexually transmitted and nonsexually transmitted infections. Primary care providers should review sexual history, risk factors and symptoms and consider testing for infections, as appropriate. "Reportable" STIs (e.g., chlamydia, gonorrhoea, syphilis, HIV) should be reported to the public health department for contact tracing and to ensure notification and treatment of sexual partners. The presence of one STI should raise suspicion for others. STIs in all prepubescent and nonsexually active children is a red flag for child abuse (see Chapter 9 Child Maltreatment).

POSTPUBERTAL VULVOVAGINITIS

1. **Definition:** Inflammation or infection of the vagina or vulva (external female genitalia)
2. **Clinical manifestations:** Vaginal or vulvar pain, itching, discharge, erythema, dyspareunia, dysuria, and spotting
3. **Differential**
   a. Infectious: *Candida albicans*, *Trichomonas vaginalis* and bacterial vaginosis. Also consider gonorrhea, chlamydia, herpes simplex virus (HSV), genital warts, and parasites (e.g., scabies)
   b. Noninfectious: contact dermatitis, retained tampon, poor hygiene and dermatologic disorders (e.g., psoriasis)
   c. Physiologic leukorrhea: normal vaginal discharge, seen in higher estrogen states (midcycle, pregnancy, patient taking OCP)
4. **Diagnosis**
   a. Physical examination: perineal and gynecologic examinations (adjusted based on sexual activity)
   b. Wet mount: pH, microscopy, potassium hydroxide (KOH) whiff test (Table 20.1)
   c. Other investigations: cervical or vaginal swabs for gonorrhea, chlamydia, trichomonas should be sent based on sexual activity
5. **Treatment:** Refer to Table 20.1. Ensure proper vulvar hygiene (see Box 20.3).

Clinical/Laboratory Features	Physiologic	Candida	Trichomonas	Bacterial Vaginosis
Appearance of discharge	White, grey, or clear	White, curd-like	Green-grey, frothy	Thin, homogeneous, grey
Vulvar/vaginal inflammation	None	Present (erythema, edema)	Often (erythema, strawberry cervix)	Rare
Other clinical signs and symptoms	None	Itching, dysuria, dyspareunia	Vulvar itching, burning, dysuria, pelvic discomfort	Fishy odor
Risk factors	Secretion of estrogen	Antibiotics, diabetes, heat/moisture, OCPs, pregnancy, obesity, immunodeficiency	Other STIs	Sexual activity, douching, previous BV
pH of discharge	≤4.5	≤4.5	>4.5	>4.5
Microscopy	Epithelial cells, many lactobacilli; few WBCs	Increased WBCs, pseudohyphae and buds	Increased WBCs, motile trichomonads	Increased WBCs, decreased lactobacilli, "clue cells"
Whiff test (fishy odor on addition of 10% KOH to sample)	Negative	Negative	Sometimes positive	Positive
Management	Reassurance	- Intravaginal Miconazole, Clotrimazole or Terconazole × 3–7 nights **OR** - PO Fluconazole 150 mg × 1 dose	- Metronidazole 500 mg PO bid × 7 days **OR** 2 g PO × 1 dose - Treat sexual partners	- Oral Metronidazole 500 mg bid × 7 days **OR** - Intravaginal Metronidazole gel (0.75%) 5 g gel daily × 5 days **OR** - Clindamycin cream 2%, 5 g gel daily × 7 days

KOH, Potassium hydroxide; *OCP*, oral contraceptive pill; *STI*, sexually transmitted infection; *WBC*, white blood cell.

Adapted from Zitelli BJ, Davis HW. *Atlas of Pediatric Physical Diagnosis*. 3rd ed. London: Mosby Wolfe; 1997.

ULCERATIVE DISORDERS

See Box 20.4 for list of infectious and noninfectious causes. It should be noted that aphthous ulcers are the most common cause of vulvar/vaginal ulcers in children.

> **Box 20.4   Differential Diagnosis of Genital Ulceration**
>
> **Venereal**
> - Painful
>   - Herpes (herpes simplex virus)
>   - Chancroid (*Haemophilus ducreyi*)
> - Painless
>   - Syphilis (*Treponema pallidum*)
>   - Granuloma inguinale (*Klebsiella granulomatis*)
>   - Lymphogranuloma venereum (*Chlamydia trachomatis* serotypes L1–L3)
>
> **Other**
> - Apthous ulcers (most common cause in children)
> - Viral (varicella, Epstein-Barr virus)
> - Trauma/Foreign body
> - Behçet's disease
> - Adverse drug reaction
> - Inflammatory bowel disease

A. Herpes simplex virus

1. **Etiology:** HSV-2, HSV-1
2. **Clinical manifestations:** nonprimary or recurrent disease presents with painful genital ulcers, radiculopathy, dysuria, and tender inguinal lymphadenopathy. Primary infection can have additional severe systemic symptoms (fever, malaise, aseptic meningitis).
3. **Investigations:** viral culture or PCR of lesion (must unroof lesion to swab). Type-specific serologies have limited utility given high carriage rates of virus.
4. **Treatment:** oral antivirals (acyclovir, valacyclovir, famciclovir). For recurrent episodes, can be treated episodically or with chronic suppressive therapy.

B. Syphilis

1. **Etiology:** caused by spirochetal bacteria, *Treponema pallidum*
2. **Clinical manifestations**
   a. Primary syphilis: painless ulcer (chancre) at inoculation site with inguinal lymphadenopathy
   b. Secondary syphilis: disseminated infection causes rash, fever, lymphadenopathy, mucous lesions, condyloma lata, alopecia, and aseptic meningitis

c. Latent syphilis: early (<1 year), late (>1 year); may last 10 to 30 years

d. Tertiary syphilis: presents with gummatous, cardiac or neurological disease

3. **Investigations:** Serologic testing to diagnose syphilis should include the use of *both* nontreponemal (RPR, VDRL) and treponemal (treponema pallidum particle agglutination, fluorescent treponemal antibody absorption) tests. The use of only one test is insufficient for diagnosis, because serologic testing (especially nontreponemal tests) can be associated with false positive results. False negative results can also occur in early disease or advanced immunosuppression.

4. **Treatment**

   a. Primary, secondary and early latent syphilis: one time IM dose of Benzathine penicillin G 2.4 million units

   b. Late latent and tertiary syphilis (excluding neurosyphilis): Benzathine penicillin G 2.4 million units IM weekly × 3 weeks

   c. RPR (quantitative assay) can be repeated at 3, 6, and 12 months for treatment response

CERVICITIS

Definition: Inflammation of the endocervix

A. Chlamydia trachomatis

1. **Epidemiology:** most commonly reported STI

2. **Clinical manifestations:** asymptomatic or can present with mucopurulent cervical discharge, intermenstrual bleeding, urethritis (dysuria, pyuria), vulvovaginitis (common in prepubertal patients), proctitis, pelvic inflammatory disease (PID; pelvic pain, systemic symptoms), and/or perihepatitis

3. **Diagnosis:** NAAT of first-catch urine, vaginal swabs, or endocervical swabs are the most sensitive tests

---

✦ **PEARL**

Urine samples submitted for nucleic acid amplification testing should be collected from the initial urine stream without precleansing the genital area.

---

4. **Treatment:** see Table 20.2 for antibiotics. Test of cure in 4 weeks recommended for prepubertal patients, pregnant patients, or suspected nonadherent patients.

5. **Complications:** chronic pelvic pain, infertility, ectopic pregnancy, reactive arthritis

B. Neisseria gonorrhea

1. **Clinical manifestations:** asymptomatic or can present with purulent cervical discharge, intermenstrual bleeding, urethritis (dysuria, pyuria), vaginitis (common in prepubertal patients), bartholinitis, proctitis, PID (pelvic pain, systemic symptoms), perihepatitis, pharyngitis, and/or conjunctivitis

2. **Diagnosis:** urine, vaginal, and endocervical NAAT is commonly used. Cultures can determine susceptibilities (may be negative if <48 hours from exposure). Cultures can be obtained from endocervical, vaginal, rectal, and pharyngeal locations, depending on the type of sexual activity.

3. **Treatment:** see Table 20.2 for antibiotics. Combination therapy recommended because of high resistance rates and for chlamydia cotreatment. Test of cure is recommended after 2 to 3 weeks in prepubertal children, pregnant patients, and when there is a high likelihood of resistance.

4. **Complications:** chronic pelvic pain, infertility, ectopic pregnancy, reactive arthritis, disseminated gonococcal infection (arthritis, dermatitis, endocarditis, and meningitis)

Table 20.2	Treatment of Uncomplicated Anogenital and Pharyngeal Sexually Transmitted Infections
Disease	**Treatment**
Chlamydia, ≥9 years and >45 kg	Azithromycin 1 g PO × 1 dose OR doxycycline 100 mg PO BID × 7 days
[a]Gonorrhea, <9 years OR ≤45 kg	Ceftriaxone[b] 50 mg/kg IM × 1 dose (max 250 mg) OR cefixime 8 mg/kg PO BID × 2 doses (max 400 mg/dose) PLUS azithromycin 20 mg/kg PO × 1 dose (max dose 1 g)
[a]Gonorrhea, ≥9 years OR >45 kg	Ceftriaxone[b] 250 mg IM × 1 dose OR cefixime 800 mg PO × 1 dose PLUS azithromycin 1g PO × 1 dose

[a]Dosing regimen also recommended for **postexposure prophylaxis**, as it covers for both chlamydia and gonorrhoea.

[b]Ceftriaxone is the preferred cephalosporin. Cefixime should only be used if ceftriaxone is unavailable.

IM, Intramuscular; *PO,* orally.

Adapted from The Hospital for Sick Children eFormulary, 2021.

PELVIC INFLAMMATORY DISEASE

1. **Definition:** Ascending infection of the female reproductive tract, which can include endometritis, salpingitis, oophoritis, perihepatitis, and pelvic peritonitis

2. **Etiology:** Polymicrobial infection with bacterial causes including STIs (*C. trachomatis, Neisseria gonorrhoeae*), endogenous genital organisms (*Mycoplasma genitalium, Ureaplasma urealyticum*), anaerobic organisms, and facultative bacteria. May be acquired sexually, postabortal, or postinstrumentation.

3. **Clinical manifestations:** May present with pelvic pain, abnormal uterine bleeding (postcoital, intermenstrual, menorrhagia), dyspareunia, vaginal discharge, and/or increased urinary frequency. More severe disease can be associated with systemic symptoms and peritoneal signs.

4. **Diagnosis:** Clinical diagnosis. See Box 20.5 for criteria. Pregnancy test and other STI tests may be helpful to rule out other diagnoses.

Box 20.5   Diagnostic Criteria for Pelvic Inflammatory Disease

Sexually active female with pelvic pain and no alternative cause with
- Cervical motion tenderness OR
- Uterine tenderness OR
- Adnexal tenderness

Supportive criteria
- Temperature >38.3°C
- Abnormal cervical or vaginal discharge
- WBCs on wet mount of vaginal discharge
- Elevated ESR/CRP
- Confirmed gonorrhea or chlamydia infection

CRP, C-reactive protein; *ESR*, erythrocyte sedimentation rate; *WBC*, white blood cell.
Data from Centers for Disease Control and Prevention: 2015 Sexually Transmitted Diseases Treatment Guidelines.

5. **Management**
   a. See Table 20.3 for antibiotic guidelines. Low threshold for treatment given the severity of the disease. Treat all sexual contacts.
   b. Consult gynecology
   c. Hospitalize if concerns about compliance, severe illness, immunosuppression, pregnancy, tuboovarian abscess, unable to tolerate oral medications, or failed oral therapy
   d. Patients treated in ambulatory setting must be followed up for improvement in 48 to 72 hours

Table 20.3	Treatment of Pelvic Inflammatory Disease	
Inpatient[a]	**Outpatient**	
• Preferred regimen: Cefoxitin 25 mg/kg/dose IV q6h (max 2 g/dose) <u>PLUS</u> doxycycline[b] 100 mg/dose PO q12h • Alternative regimen: Clindamycin 13 mg/kg/dose IV q8h (max 900 mg/dose) <u>PLUS</u> Tobramycin 5 mg/kg IV q24h (max 800 mg/dose)	• Preferred regimen: Ceftriaxone 250 mg IM as a single dose <u>PLUS</u> doxycycline[b] 100 mg PO BID × 14 days, ± metronidazole 500 mg PO BID × 14 days • Alternate regimen: Levofloxacin 500 mg PO daily × 14 days, ± metronidazole 500 mg PO BID × 14 days	

[a] IV therapy can be discontinued 24 h after clinical improvement. Oral therapy should consist of doxycycline 100 mg PO BID or clindamycin 450 mg/dose QID to complete a 14-day course.
[b] Doxycycline is not recommended in children under 8 years of age.

IM, Intramuscular; *IV*, intravenous; *PO*, orally.

Adapted from The Hospital for Sick Children eFormulary, 2020.

6. **Complications:** Chronic pelvic pain, infertility, ectopic pregnancy, or tuboovarian abscess

GENITAL WARTS (CONDYLOMATA ACUMINATA)

1. **Etiology:** Caused by HPV subtypes (e.g., 6, 11)
2. **Clinical manifestations:** Wide variety of appearances but are often flesh-colored and cauliflower-shaped or plaque-like. May be located on vulva, perineum, perianal area, vagina, cervix, or periurethral area. Often asymptomatic but may have mild symptoms (irritation, dysuria).
3. **Diagnosis:** Clinical; if uncertain, can do shave biopsy
4. **Treatment:** May defer treatment if asymptomatic as many will spontaneously regress. If symptomatic or distressing, can treat with topical (first-line) or procedural methods. Topical methods include trichloroacetic acid, imiquimod (3.75% or 5%) cream and Podophyllotoxin. Cryotherapy, laser ablation, and surgical excision reserved for large or recalcitrant warts. Treatment is often prolonged and warts may recur.
5. **Prevention:** Some formulations of the HPV vaccine prevent against genital warts

OVARIAN/ADNEXAL PATHOLOGY

OVARIAN MASSES
See Tables 20.4 and 20.5

Table 20.4	Simple Versus Complex Ovarian Mass on Ultrasound
Simple	**Complex**
• Unilateral • Thin walled • No septations • Cystic • No vascular flow	• Bilateral • Thick walls • Septations • Solid components • Vascular flow within walls • Associated ascites

Table 20.5 Ovarian Masses by Age

	Clinical Manifestations	Differential Diagnosis	Diagnosis	Management	Complications
Fetal/neonatal follicular cysts	- Detected on routine fetal US or as abdominal mass in neonatal period - Mostly unilateral	- GI and GU tract anomalies as well as other intraabdominal pathologies. - Ovarian malignancy is rare	Four US criteria: female sex, nonmidline regular cystic structure, normal GU tract, normal GI tract	- Observation with serial ultrasounds until 4–6 months. - Surgical management may be warranted for acute torsion, enlarging, complex or symptomatic cysts and for those that have not regressed by 4–6 months. - Potential role for postnatal aspiration of simple cysts >5 cm to reduce the risk of torsion. - 90% of simple cystic masses will have resolved on repeat US.	Ovarian torsion (higher risk with cysts >5 cm), intracystic hemorrhage, rupture, and GI/GU obstruction
Prepubertal ovarian masses	Varies: asymptomatic abdominal mass, chronic abdominal pain, sense of abdominal fullness, or acute abdominal pain	Broad: hormone-secreting cysts (McCune Albright syndrome), neoplasms, paraovarian/paratubal cysts, mesothelial cysts and true precocious puberty	US (plus Doppler if concern for torsion). Workup for precocious puberty if secondary sex characteristics present	- Varies: observation recommended for simple cystic masses with repeat US in 4–8 weeks (90% of simple cystic masses will have resolved on repeat US). - Surgery may be required for torsion or prevention of torsion. - Concerning US features (solid components, bilaterally, ascites, septations, metastases) mandate workup for malignancy: tumor markers (β-hCG, AFP, LDH, ± CA-125), MRI, or CT scan, surgical removal, and pathological examination	

Continued

Table 20.5 Ovarian Masses by Age—cont'd

	Clinical Manifestations	Differential Diagnosis	Diagnosis	Management	Complications
Postmenarchal ovarian masses	Varies: incidental finding, abdominal fullness/pain, menstrual irregularities or GI/GU obstruction	- Broad: functional cysts (follicular, corpus luteal), PCOS, as well as benign and malignant neoplasms - Nonovarian etiologies include tubal (tuboovarian abscess, paratubal cyst, ectopic pregnancy), GI (appendiceal abscess, Crohn's disease), and GU (pelvic kidney) causes	- US (plus Doppler if concern for torsion or malignancy) - Pregancy test - If complex or persistent cyst, can order tumor markers (β-hCG, AFP, LDH, CA-125), and CT/MRI	- Observation, analgesia, and repeat ultrasound in 4–8 weeks for asymptomatic simple cysts (most will involute spontaneously) - Combined hormonal contraception can be used to prevent new cyst formation. For cysts that are symptomatic, persistent, increasing in size or with features concerning for malignancy, surgical management may be warranted	

AFP, Alpha fetoprotein; β*-hCG,* β-human chorionic gonadotropin; *CA-125,* cancer antigen 125; *CT,* computed tomography; *GI,* gastrointestinal; *GU,* genitourinary; *LDH,* lactate dehydrogenase; *MRI,* magnetic resonance imaging; *PCOS,* polycystic ovary syndrome; *US,* ultrasound.

ADNEXAL TORSION

1. **Definition:** Twisting of the ovary/fallopian tube causing occlusion of the ovarian artery/vein. May be complete or intermittent.
2. **Etiology:** Infants and children may have torsion of normal adnexa. In postmenarchal patients, ovarian torsion is usually associated with adnexal mass (neoplasm or functional cysts).
3. **Clinical manifestations:** "Waves" of acute pelvic pain, often associated with nausea. Patients may have a palpable pelvic mass and may be febrile.
4. **Differential:** See Box 20.6 for a differential diagnosis of pelvic pain

> **Box 20.6   Differential Diagnosis of Pelvic Pain of Gynecological Origin**
>
> - Primary dysmenorrhea
> - Endometriosis
> - Anatomic obstructions (e.g., imperforate hymen, vaginal septum, mullerian anomalies)
> - Mittelschmerz (midcycle "ovulation pain")
> - Pelvic inflammatory disease/tuboovarian abscess
> - Ovarian cysts (ruptured, hemorrhagic)
> - Adnexal torsion
> - Pregnancy complications: ectopic pregnancy, spontaneous abortion

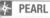

5. **Investigations**
   a. Laboratory studies: normal to mildly elevated WBC; β-hCG to rule out pregnancy
   b. Imaging: Doppler ultrasound may demonstrate enlargement and edema of the involved ovary, an ovarian mass, absence of Doppler flow to the ovary and/or peripheralization of ovarian follicles

> **! PITFALL**
>
> Adnexal torsion is a clinical diagnosis that is **not ruled out** by the presence of ovarian blood flow on Doppler ultrasound.

6. **Management:** Urgent laparoscopic detorsion ± ovarian cystectomy. Oophoropexy may be considered in select cases.

POLYCYSTIC OVARIAN SYNDROME

> **✦ PEARL**
>
> Since 30% of adolescents have polycystic ovaries, ultrasound is not required as part of the diagnostic evaluation of polycystic ovarian syndrome in this age group, unless there is a clinical concern for other causes of amenorrhea/oligomenorrhea/hyperandrogenism.

1. **Clinical presentation:** Hyperandrogenism (hirsutism, acne, or biochemical hyperandrogenism) and evidence of anovulation (infrequent and/or irregular menses); may also involve obesity and metabolic syndrome
2. **Diagnosis:** Evidence of anovulation (infrequent and/or irregular menses) AND clinical or biochemical hyperandrogenism. In adolescents, polycystic ovaries are not part of the diagnostic criteria.
3. **Treatment:** Often under the care of a gynecologist, treatment includes weight loss, cycle regulation with combination or progesterone-only contraceptives, and medications to reduce hirsutism (i.e., combined hormonal contraception [CHC], spironolactone) and protect the endometrium from long-term risk of endometrial hyperplasia and malignancy. PCOS is also associated with metabolic syndrome and patients should be screened for diabetes/glucose intolerance, dyslipidemia, and hypercholesterolemia.

DYSMENORRHEA AND PELVIC PAIN

1. **Etiology:** Can be primary (not caused by pelvic pathology) or secondary (as a result of pelvic pathology)
2. **History:** History of the pelvic/abdominal pain including associated symptoms (e.g., dysuria, dyschezia, pelvic pressure, dyspareunia if sexually active, other GI or GU symptoms), menstrual history, sexual history, history of contraceptive use, management to date (medications tried, etc.)
3. **Physical examination:** Should include musculoskeletal and abdominal examinations. If patient is sexually active, a gynecologic examination, including STI testing, may be appropriate. A rectoabdominal or bimanual examination may document cervical motion tenderness and/or adnexal tenderness masses.
4. **Differential:** See Box 20.6 for gynecological causes of pelvic pain and dysmenorrhea
5. **Investigations:** A β-hCG to rule out pregnancy. Consider urinalysis and culture to rule out UTI. If the patient is sexually active, cervical/vaginal swabs can be sent for gonorrhea, chlamydia, and trichomonas. If there is diagnostic uncertainty or a mass/uterine anomaly is suspected, a pelvic ultrasound should be ordered. If a patient fails medical management, a diagnostic laparoscopy may be warranted.

PRIMARY DYSMENORRHEA

1. **Definition:** Crampy pelvic pain that occurs during menstruation and is not a result of pathology. Generally occurs after the establishment of a regular menstrual cycle, which may occur 1 to 3 years after menarche. Dysmenorrhea that occurs at the onset of menarche is less common and should raise suspicion for an obstructive anomaly.

2. **Etiology:** Excess production and/or sensitivity to uterine prostaglandins, which causes uterine cramping, as well as other symptoms, including diarrhea, nausea, vomiting, and headache
3. **Management:** Pain management with NSAIDs. Combined hormonal contraception (pill, patch, ring), dienogest, depoprovera, progestin-containing IUD

ENDOMETRIOSIS

1. **Definition:** Presence of endometrial glands and stroma outside of uterus; usually early stage in adolescents but may be associated with significant pain; endometriomas less common at this age
2. **Clinical manifestations:** Dysmenorrhea (classically, may start just before menses), cyclic and/or non-cyclic pain, deep dyspareunia (pain during sexual intercourse), dyschezia (pain during defecation), dysuria, and abdominal tenderness. A bimanual examination may reveal cervical motion tenderness, a fixed retroverted uterus, uterosacral nodularity, and adnexal tenderness ± mass. Often no findings on bimanual exam in adolescents. It may eventually cause infertility and chronic pelvic pain.
3. **Diagnosis:** Diagnosed clinically based on symptoms and response to medical management. Definitive diagnosis requires laparoscopy with biopsy and histologic confirmation but this is not required for management.
4. **Management:** Conservative measures include NSAIDs, combined hormonal contraception (pill, patch, or ring), progesterone-only methods (norethindrone acetate, dienogest, DMPA, progestin-containing IUD) and suppression of the hypothalamic-pituitary-ovarian (HPO) axis with gonadotropin-releasing hormone agonists. Surgery may be required for treatment-resistant cases or for infertility. Involvement of multidisciplinary chronic pain teams should be considered on an individualized basis.

IMPERFORATE HYMEN/TRANSVERSE VAGINAL SEPTUM

1. **Definition:** An imperforate hymen is when the hymen lacks an opening and is obstructing the vaginal orifice. A transverse vaginal septum results from a failure of fusion and canalization of the upper and lower vagina.
2. **Clinical manifestations:** Both conditions may result in abdominal pain and hematocolpos (blood filled vagina). Vaginal distension may result in obstructive urinary symptoms, dyschezia, and back pain. On physical examination, an imperforate hymen may be seen as bluish bulge at the vaginal orifice. A transverse vaginal septum results in a shortened vagina and possible vaginal mass as a result of hematocolpos (Figure 20.2).
3. **Treatment:** Both conditions require surgical repair

Figure 20.2 Hematocolpos

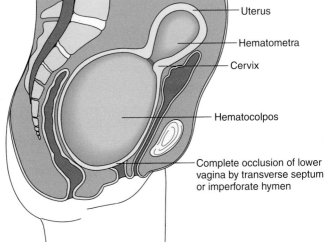

Uterus

Hematometra

Cervix

Hematocolpos

Complete occlusion of lower vagina by transverse septum or imperforate hymen

(Modified from Smith RP. *Netter's Obstetrics & Gynecology.* 3rd ed. Elsevier; 2018.)

ABNORMAL UTERINE BLEEDING

Abnormal uterine bleeding (AUB) refers to menstrual bleeding that occurs outside the normal range, and includes absence of menses, bleeding that is abnormal in frequency, duration, or volume

AMENORRHEA

Also see Chapter 14 Endocrinology

1. **Definition: Primary amenorrhea** (absence of menses by age 15 years, in the presence of secondary sex characteristics, or by age 13 years in the absence of secondary sex characteristics) or **secondary amenorrhea** (absence of menses for >6 months after documented menarche or for >3 consecutive cycles). Irregular menstrual bleeding is defined as menstrual cycle variation >20 days. All three conditions have a similar differential and workup.
2. **History:** Menstrual history, sexual history, pubertal history, growth, presence or absence of pain, medications, history of chronic or systemic illness, symptoms of other hormonal conditions (thyroid disease, hyperprolactinemia, hyperandrogenism, primary ovarian insufficiency, etc.), stressors (e.g., eating, exercise)
3. **Physical examination:** Tanner staging, signs of hirsutism, acne, acanthosis, signs of Cushing syndrome, thyroid examination, neurologic and gynecologic examinations for signs of virilization, and to assess patency of outflow tract

Table 20.6	Differential Diagnosis of Amenorrhea/Irregular Menstrual Bleeding
Hypothalamic	• Diet • Stress • Exercise • Chronic illness • Central nervous system lesion • Kallman syndrome • Constitutional
Anterior pituitary	• Thyroid • Prolactin • Neoplasm
Adrenal	• Neoplasm • Cushing • Congenital adrenal hyperplasia
Ovary/gonadal	• Anovulation • Polycystic ovarian syndrome • Neoplasm • Dysgenetic gonads • Premature ovarian insufficiency (genetic, autoimmune, idiopathic) • Cancer therapy
Uterus	• Pregnancy • Mullerian anomaly • Androgen insensitivity syndrome • Medications
Outflow tract	• Mullerian anomaly • Imperforate hymen • Transverse vaginal septum • Androgen insensitivity syndrome • Vaginal agenesis

4. **Differential diagnosis:** See Table 20.6 for differential diagnosis, and Figure 20.3 for diagnostic approach

5. **Investigations**
   a. Labs: CBC, β-hCG, LH, FSH, estradiol, testosterone, DHEAS, androstenedione, prolactin, TSH, and 17-OHP. Other investigations depending on clinical presentation and initial test results include karyotype, Fragile X, antiadrenal antibody, antithyroid Ab, AM cortisol, ACTH stimulation test, etc.
   b. If TSH is normal and prolactin is elevated, need to investigate for other causes of hyperprolactinemia (history, physical, ± MRI brain)
   c. Progesterone challenge (10 mg oral × 10–14 days to mimic luteal phase of menstrual cycle and attempt to induce withdrawal bleed): bleeding implies adequate endogenous estrogen and functional outflow tract. Amenorrhea is likely attributed to anovulation.

6. **Treatment:** Specific to underlying process

Figure 20.3 Diagnostic Approach to Amenorrhea

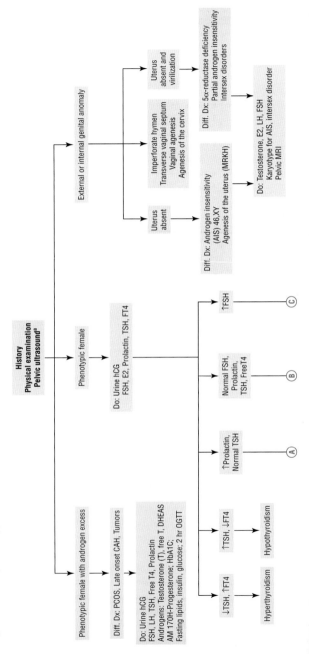

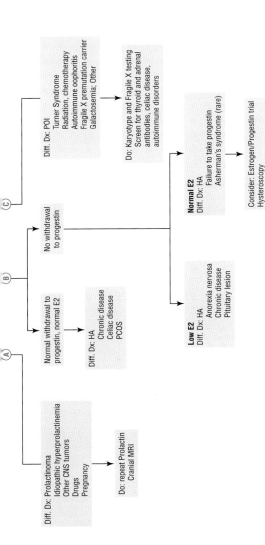

A

Diff. Dx: Prolactinoma
Idiopathic hyperprolactinemia
Other CNS tumors
Drugs
Pregnancy

Do: repeat Prolactin
Cranial MRI

B

Normal withdrawal to progestin, normal E2

Diff. Dx: HA
Chronic disease
Celiac disease
PCOS

No withdrawal to progestin

Low E2
Diff. Dx: HA
Anorexia nervosa
Chronic disease
Pituitary lesion

Normal E2
Diff. Dx: HA
Failure to take progestin
Asherman's syndrome (rare)

Consider: Estrogen/Progestin trial
Hysteroscopy

C

Diff. Dx: POI
Turner Syndrome
Radiation, chemotherapy
Autoimmune oophoritis
Fragile X premutation carrier
Galactosemia; Other

Do: Karyotype and Fragile X testing
Screen for thyroid and adrenal
antibodies, celiac disease,
autoimmune disorders

Gynecology

20

Pelvic ultrasound may not be needed in all cases of secondary amenorrhea.

AIS, Androgen insensitivity syndrome; *FT4,* free T4; *E2,* estradiol; *HA,* hypothalamic amenorrhea; *OGTT,* oral glucose tolerance test; *POI,* primary ovarian insufficiency; *MRKH,* Mayer–Rokitansky–Küster–Hauser syndrome. (Diagnostic Approach to Amenorrhea. Adapted from Emans, Laufer, *Goldstein's Pediatric & Adolescent Gynecology,* 6th ed. Lippincott Williams & Wilkins; 2011.)

511

HEAVY MENSTRUAL BLEEDING

1. **Pathophysiology:** Heavy menstrual bleeding refers to increased menstrual losses that interfere with quality of life. When this bleeding occurs at regular intervals but with excessive volume or duration, it is considered ovulatory in nature.

2. **Etiology:** See Box 20.7 for differential diagnosis

Box 20.7 Differential Diagnosis of Heavy Menstrual Bleeding

- Anovulatory bleeding (e.g., PCOS, immature HPO axis at onset of menarche)
- Pregnancy complications: (e.g., ectopic pregnancy, threatened/incomplete/complete abortion)
- Blood dyscrasia (e.g., ITP, von Willebrand disease, iatrogenic, liver disease)
- Infections (e.g., PID, endometritis)
- Endocrine disorders (e.g., hypothyroidism, PCOS)
- Structural lesions (e.g., polyp, fibroid)—rare in adolescents
- Trauma (accidental vs. abuse)
- Neoplasms (ovarian, vaginal, cervical)
- Copper IUD
- Medications
- Congenital (e.g., uterine vascular malformation)

HPO, Hypothalamic-pituitary-ovarian; *ITP,* immune thrombocytopenic purpura; *IUD,* intrauterine device; *PCOS,* polycystic ovary syndrome; *PID,* pelvic inflammatory disease.

---

3. **History:** Menstrual history (onset, timing/pattern, amount of bleeding), pubertal history, sexual and STI history, bleeding history (frequent epistaxis, easy bruising/bleeding, bleeding into joints, hematuria, family history of bleeding disorders), past medical history and medications, and associated symptoms/review of systems (bowel or bladder symptoms, symptoms of hypothyroidism)

4. **Physical examination:** Should include vital signs for assessment of hemodynamic stability, examination to look for stigmata of systemic illnesses (i.e., hypothyroidism, bleeding disorders), Tanner staging, examination to rule out other sources of bleeding (rectal, urethral, vaginal, cervical), consider a pelvic and bimanual/rectoabdominal examination to look for structural causes of bleeding, pregnancy, and malignancy based on history/clinical presentation

5. **Investigations:** Must do a β-hCG to rule out pregnancy. Other tests include a CBC, coagulation profile, TSH, prolactin. Consider tests for platelet function and Von Willebrand disease if severe bleeding, heavy menstrual bleeding present since menarche, and/or other features on history concerning for bleeding disorder. Testing for chlamydia, gonorrhea, and trichomonas should be done if the patient is sexually active. Although structural abnormalities (fibroids, polyps, etc.) are rare in adolescents, a pelvic US may be considered if first-line tests are negative.

6. **Treatment**
   a. Acute heavy menstrual bleeding: ensure hemodynamic stability. Treat bleed with tranexamic acid in conjunction with tapering course of hormonal therapy (for specific treatment regimens, see Tables 20.7 and 20.8). Follow acute treatment with maintenance therapy (see later).
   b. Chronic heavy menstrual bleeding: iron supplementation, NSAIDs, tranexamic acid, CHC (pill, patch, ring), dienogest (off-label for AUB), progesterone-only options (norethindrone, medroxyprogesterone acetate, progesterone-only IUD)

Table 20.7	Treatment for Acute Heavy Menstrual Bleeding
Mild	
Minimal drop in Hb, hemodynamically stable, mild bleeding on examination	• Provide reassurance • Consider NSAIDs, tranexamic acid, CHC, progesterone-only methods; depending on impact on quality of life and desire for contraception • Consider oral iron therapy
Moderate	
Significant drop in Hb, hemodynamically stable, moderate bleeding on examination	• Combined OCP or progesterone only taper • Tranexamic acid • Consider oral or IV iron therapy • Maintenance therapy following stabilization
Severe	
Significant drop in Hb, hemodynamic instability, severe bleeding on examination	• Hemodynamic stabilization • Combined OCP or progesterone only taper OR IV estrogen followed by OCP/progesterone taper • Antiemetic therapy • Tranexamic acid • Consider blood transfusion, IV iron infusion • In severe circumstances, dilation and curettage may be required and/or intrauterine balloon tamponade • Maintenance therapy following stabilization

CHC, Combined hormonal contraception; *Hb,* hemoglobin; *IV,* intravenous; *NSAID,* nonsteroidal anti-inflammatory drug; *OCP,* oral contraceptive pill.

Table 20.8	Hormonal Therapies for Acute Heavy Menstrual Bleeding		
Therapy	**Dose**	**Route**	**Initial Frequency**
Conjugated estrogen	25 mg	IV	Every 4–6 h
30–35 mcg ethinyl estradiol combined pill[a]	1 tablet	Oral	Every 6 h
Medroxyprogesterone[a]	10–20 mg (maximum 80 mg/day)	Oral	Every 6–12 h
Norethindrone acetate[a]	5–10 mg	Oral	Every 6 h

[a]Examples of tapering regimens (with plan for short-term follow-up to determine plan for longer-term therapy):

- **30–35 mcg ethinyl estradiol combined pill:**
  1 tablet q6h × 3 days, then 1 tablet q8h × 3 days, then 1 tablet q12h × 3 days, then continue 1 tablet daily
- **Progesterone-based pill (medroxyprogesterone or norethindrone acetate):**
  1 dose q6–12h × 3 days, then 1 dose q12h × 3 days, then 1 dose daily

IV, Intravenous.

Modified from Haamid F, Sass AE, Dietrich JE. Heavy menstrual bleeding in adolescents. NASPAG Committee Opinion. *J Pediatr Adolesc Gynecol.* 2017;30:335–340.

IRREGULAR MENSTRUAL BLEEDING

1. **Pathophysiology:** Excessive noncyclic (irregular) uterine bleeding is considered anovulatory (previously referred to as *dysfunctional uterine bleeding* [*DUB*]). Unopposed estrogen stimulation of the endometrium can lead to endometrial hypertrophy and uncoordinated shedding of the endometrial lining. This can lead to irregular and infrequent menstrual bleeding that is often heavy and prolonged.

2. **Etiology:** In the first 1 to 3 years postmenarche, this is most commonly because of an immature hypothalamic-pituitary-ovarian axis but can also be due to other etiologies (i.e., PCOS, pregnancy, stress, weight changes, endocrinopathies). Note overlap between etiology of amenorrhea (particularly secondary) and irregular/infrequent menstrual bleeding. See Table 20.6 for differential diagnosis.

3. **History:** Menstrual history (onset, timing/pattern, amount of bleeding), pubertal history, sexual history, past medical history and medications, associated symptoms/review of systems (i.e., symptoms of hypothyroidism, hyperprolactinemia/prolactinoma, hyperandrogenism), social history (stress, anxiety, disordered eating)

4. **Physical examination:** Assess hemodynamic stability, look for stigmata of systemic illnesses (e.g., acanthosis nigricans, hirsutism in PCOS, buffalo hump, abdominal striae), Tanner staging, examination to rule out other sources of bleeding (rectal, urethral, vaginal, cervical), consider a pelvic and bimanual/rectoabdominal examination to look for structural causes of bleeding or pregnancy
5. **Investigations:** β-hCG, CBC, coagulation profile, TSH, prolactin, FSH, LH, estradiol, testosterone, androstenedione, DHEAS, 17-OHP
6. **Treatment:** Management of acute bleeding as per Table 20.7; longer-term management with lifestyle changes (exercise, diet), CHC (pill, patch, ring), progesterone-only medications (norethindrone, medroxyprogesterone acetate, depo provera, progesterone-only IUD)

Hematology

Adam Yan • Vanja Cabric • Soumitra Tole • Michaela Cada

COMMON ABBREVIATIONS

Also see page xviii for a list of other abbreviations used throughout this book

ACS	acute chest syndrome	MCH	mean corpuscular hemoglobin
ANC	absolute neutrophil count		
BMA	bone marrow aspirate	MCV	mean corpuscular volume
BMT	bone marrow transplant	NAIT	neonatal alloimmune thrombocytopenia
DAT	direct antiglobulin test		
DIC	disseminated intravascular coagulation	NATP	neonatal autoimmune thrombocytopenia
DVT	deep vein thrombosis	NBS	newborn screen
EPO	erythropoietin	NTDT	non-transfusion dependent thalassemia
F	factor, e.g., FV = factor 5		
FFP	fresh frozen plasma	PE	pulmonary embolism
FVIII:C	factor VIII coagulant	PLT	platelets
G6PD	glucose-6-phosphate dehydrogenase	pRBC	packed red blood cell
		RDW	red blood cell distribution width
GH	growth hormone		
HIT	heparin-induced thrombocytopenia	SCD	sickle cell disease
		SLE	systemic lupus erythematosus
HU	hydroxyurea		
HUS	hemolytic uremic syndrome	TDT	transfusion dependent thalassemia
IGF-1	insulin-like growth factor 1	TIA	transient ischemic attack
		TIBC	total iron-binding capacity
ITP	immune thrombocytopenia (formerly idiopathic thrombocytopenic purpura)	TTP	thrombotic thrombocytopenic purpura
		UFH	unfractionated heparin
		VOC	vaso-occlusive crisis
IVF	intravenous fluids	V/Q	ventilation/perfusion
IVIG	intravenous immunoglobulin	VTE	venous thromboembolic event
LMWH	low-molecular-weight heparin	VWD	von Willebrand disease
		vWF	von Willebrand factor

ANEMIA

APPROACH TO ANEMIA

1. **Definition:** reduction in hemoglobin concentration, hematocrit, or red blood cell number. Normal Hb and hematocrit values vary with age
2. **Clinical presentation:** pallor, fatigue, weakness, irritability, decreased exercise tolerance, shortness of breath
3. **Diagnostic approach:** see Figure 21.1

Figure 21.1 Approach to Anemia

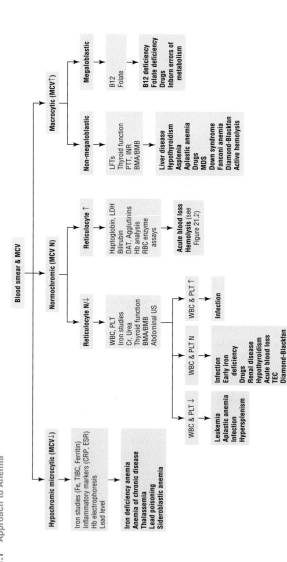

BMA, Bone marrow aspirate; BMB, bone marrow biopsy; Cr, creatinine; CRP, C-reactive protein; DAT, direct antiglobulin test; ESR, erythrocyte sedimentation rate; Hb, hemoglobin; INR, international normalized ratio; LDH, lactate dehydrogenase; LFTs, liver function tests; MCV, mean corpuscular volume; MDS, myelodysplastic syndrome; N, normal; PLT, platelets;

4. **Laboratory findings:** see Table 21.1

Table 21.1	Laboratory Features of Various Types of Anemia			
Test	**Aplastic Anemia**	**Thalassemia**	**Iron Deficiency Anemia**	**Anemia of Chronic Disease**
Hb	↓	↓	↓	↓
MCV	↑	↓	↓	N or ↓
MCH	N	↓	↓	N
RDW	N or ↑	N or ↑	↑	N
Iron	N	N or ↑	↓	N or ↓
TIBC	N	N or ↓	↑	↓
Ferritin	N	N or ↑	↓	N or ↑
Transferrin	N	N or ↓	↑	↓
Reticulocyte count	↓	N or ↑	↓	N or ↓

Hb, Hemoglobin; *MCH*, mean corpuscular hemoglobin; *MCV*, mean corpuscular volume; *N*, normal; *RDW*, red blood cell distribution width; *TIBC*, total iron-binding capacity.

PHYSIOLOGICAL ANEMIA OF INFANCY

1. **Healthy infants:** Hb is high at birth, then rapidly declines to nadir of 90 to 110 g/L at 8 to 12 weeks of age, because of decreased erythropoiesis
2. **Premature infants:** may have more rapid and extreme decline to 70 to 90 g/L at 4 to 8 weeks
3. Once at the nadir, EPO production is stimulated and Hb increases
4. **Exaggerated nadir:** can occur with RBC transfusions, mild hemolytic diseases and prematurity
5. **Treatment:** generally not required; iron supplementation may be beneficial

IRON DEFICIENCY ANEMIA

1. **Most common pediatric anemia, with two peaks**
   a. Toddlers: excessive milk intake, poor dietary iron intake
   b. Teenagers: rapid growth, poor dietary iron intake, menstrual losses in females
2. **Presentation:** pallor, irritability, anorexia, lethargy, pica, glossitis, angular stomatitis, koilonychia

3. **Prevention:** many cases preventable with nutritional counseling
   a. Breastfed infants: introduce iron-rich foods at 4 to 6 months of age
   b. Non-breastfed infants: iron-fortified formula
   c. Toddlers: limit milk intake to <450 mL/day, introduce iron-rich foods
4. **Treatment**
   a. Dietary counseling and education
   b. Trial of iron supplementation: in toddlers with hypochromic, microcytic anemia without further investigation, if typical history of nutritional deficiency
      i. Administer 1 hour before or 2 hours after dairy, eggs, tea, wholegrain bread, cereal
      ii. Vitamin C co-administration enhances absorption
   c. Monitoring: check Hb in 2 to 4 weeks to ensure response and adherence
   d. Duration: treat for 3 months after Hb normalizes to replenish iron stores
   e. Failed response to therapy: <10 g/L increase in 1 month
      i. Ensure correct dose and administration
      ii. If fully adherent, investigate for chronic inflammatory diseases, blood loss, thalassemia, concurrent B12 or folate deficiency

> **! PITFALL**
>
> Avoid transfusion in iron deficiency anemia unless patient is hemodynamically unstable

HEMOLYTIC ANEMIA

1. **Pathophysiology:** RBCs destroyed and removed from circulation, dropping Hb; EPO stimulates RBC production in bone marrow, increasing reticulocyte count
2. **History:** jaundice, anemia (fatigue, headaches, syncope), dark urine, recent infection, abdominal or back pain, gallstones, transfusions, fever, splenomegaly/splenectomy, family history, medications
3. **Physical:** tachycardia, dyspnea, pallor, jaundice, splenomegaly, growth retardation, thalassemic facies (e.g., frontal bossing), leg ulcers
4. **Diagnostic approach:** see Figure 21.2

Figure 21.2 Approach to Hemolytic Anemia

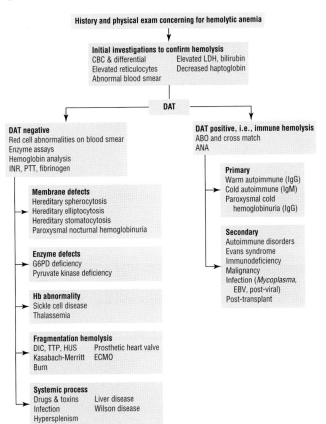

History and physical exam concerning for hemolytic anemia

Initial investigations to confirm hemolysis
CBC & differential   Elevated LDH, bilirubin
Elevated reticulocytes   Decreased haptoglobin
Abnormal blood smear

DAT

DAT negative
Red cell abnormalities on blood smear
Enzyme assays
Hemoglobin analysis
INR, PTT, fibrinogen

Membrane defects
Hereditary spherocytosis
Hereditary elliptocytosis
Hereditary stomatocytosis
Paroxysmal nocturnal hemoglobinuria

Enzyme defects
G6PD deficiency
Pyruvate kinase deficiency

Hb abnormality
Sickle cell disease
Thalassemia

Fragmentation hemolysis
DIC, TTP, HUS   Prosthetic heart valve
Kasabach-Merritt   ECMO
Burn

Systemic process
Drugs & toxins   Liver disease
Infection   Wilson disease
Hypersplenism

DAT positive, i.e., immune hemolysis
ABO and cross match
ANA

Primary
Warm autoimmune (IgG)
Cold autoimmune (IgM)
Paroxysmal cold
  hemoglobinuria (IgG)

Secondary
Autoimmune disorders
Evans syndrome
Immunodeficiency
Malignancy
Infection (*Mycoplasma*,
  EBV, post-viral)
Post-transplant

ANA, Antinuclear antibody; *CBC*, complete blood count; *DAT*, direct antiglobulin test; *DIC*, disseminated intravascular coagulation; *EBV,* Epstein-Barr virus; *ECMO*, extracorporeal membrane oxygenation; *G6PD*, glucose-6-phosphate dehydrogenase; *HUS*, hemolytic uremic syndrome; *Ig*, immunoglobin; *INR*, international normalized ratio; *LDH*, lactate dehydrogenase; *PTT*, partial thromboplastin time; *TTP*, thrombotic thrombocytopenic purpura.

HEMOGLOBINOPATHIES

SICKLE CELL DISEASE (SCD)

1. **Pathophysiology:** mutation in β-globin gene results in hemoglobin S (HbS) formation; deoxygenated HbS molecules form characteristic sickle shape
2. **Presentation:** often diagnosed during newborn screening
   a. If not, majority present with pain; infants commonly present with dactylitis

521

3. **Diagnosis:** suggested by anemia with sickle cells, target cells, polychromasia on blood smear
   a. Confirmed by Hb analysis: see Table 21.2

Table 21.2	Hemoglobin Analysis in Sickle Cell Disease							
				% Hb				
Hb Variant	**NBS**	**Hb (g/L)**	**MCV**	**HbA**	**HbS**	**HbA$_2$**	**HbF**	**HbC**
HbSA (sickle cell trait)	N	N	N	55–60	30–40	2–3	—	—
HbSS (sickle cell anemia)	FS	60–80	N or ↑	0	85–95	2–3	5–15	—
HbSβ°-thalassemia	FS	70–90	↓	0	70–80	3–5	10–20	—
HbSβ⁺-thalassemia	FSA	90–120	↓	10–20	60–75	3–5	10–20	—
HbSC disease	FSC	100–140	N	0	45–50	—	—	45–50

Hb, Hemoglobin; *MCV,* mean corpuscular volume; *NBS,* newborn screen.

Modified from Driscoll MC. Sickle cell disease. *Pediatr Rev.* 2007;28:259–268.

4. **Clinical manifestations and complications:** see Table 21.3

Table 21.3	Clinical Manifestations of Sickle Cell Disease		
Presentation	**Description**	**Screening**	**Management**
Acute chest syndrome (ACS)	New infiltrate(s) on CXR with ≥1 new respiratory symptom(s): fever, cough, dyspnea, sputum production, hypoxia May be secondary to infection, pulmonary infarct, hypoventilation, fat embolism, pulmonary edema, surgery, asthma, chronic hypoxemia or a combination of the aforementioned		See Figure 21.3 Consider pRBC transfusion if Hb 10–15 g/L below baseline Exchange transfusion if rapidly deteriorating
Anemia	Chronic, onset at 3–4 months of age	CBC with reticulocyte count every 3–6 months	Folic acid, hydroxyurea, chronic transfusion if complications or symptomatic
Aplastic crisis	Parvovirus infection causes RBC aplasia and reticulocytopenia Present with fever		Supportive care and transfusion as needed Monitor for complications (ACS, VOC, stroke, sequestration)

Table 21.3	Clinical Manifestations of Sickle Cell Disease—cont'd		
Presentation	**Description**	**Screening**	**Management**
Cardiomyo-pathy	Presents as heart failure. Rare, thought to be caused by fibrosis	Echo q2 yearly from age 12 years	
Cerebrovascular events	Ischemic stroke, TIA, silent infarct because of sickling and thrombosis in vessels. Hemorrhagic seen more in adults. Highest incidence 1–9 years of age	Transcranial Doppler yearly from 2–16 years of age, with initiation of chronic transfusions for abnormal results	Head MRI/MRA (or CT). Exchange transfusion, analgesia, hydration. Control seizures, BP, temperature
Chronic lung disease	Pulmonary fibrosis, restrictive lung disease, may lead to cor pulmonale	O_2 saturation at each visit. Consider baseline PFT at 12 years	
Dactylitis	Swelling of dorsal aspects of hands and feet <5 years of age (peak 6–12 months)		Analgesia, hydration
Gastrointestinal complications	Bilirubin stones, cholecystitis, hepatopathy, mesenteric vaso-occlusion	LFTs and bilirubin yearly	Elective cholecystectomy for recurrent cholecystitis and gallstones
Growth failure, pubertal delay		Anthropometrics yearly	Nutritional supplements
Infections	Abnormal immune function because of splenic infarcts. At risk for infection with encapsulated bacteria (pneumococcus, meningococcus, *Hemophilus influenza*) and osteomyelitis with *Salmonella* and *Staphylococcus aureus*		Prophylactic penicillin until at least 5 years of age. Routine immunizations including annual influenza vaccine. Additional pneumococcus, meningococcus, and *H. influenza* vaccines. Acute: see Figure 21.3
Leg ulceration	Unilateral or bilateral medial and lateral malleolar areas		
Ocular	Retinopathy, hyphema	Ophthalmological evaluation yearly from 10 years	

Continued

21

Table 21.3	Clinical Manifestations of Sickle Cell Disease—cont'd		
Presentation	**Description**	**Screening**	**Management**
Priapism	Prolonged erection >30 min Peak age 5–13 years Often in early morning, can be precipitated by sexual activity Eventual impotence if prolonged		Hydration, warm bath, exercise, masturbation, analgesia, O_2 and transfusions Urology consult for possible penile aspiration and irrigation, or surgical shunt α-Adrenergic agents (pseudoephedrine) orally or intracavernous)
Psychological	Anxiety, depression, neurocognitive impairment, poor school performance	Neuropsychometric testing if clinical concerns	Multidisciplinary care involving social work, psychiatry, psychology, school administration
Renal complications	Hematuria, renal papillary necrosis, nephrotic syndrome, renal infarcts, renal-concentrating defect (hyposthenuria), enuresis, renal medullary carcinoma	Serum creatinine and urinalysis yearly from 10 years	
Splenic sequestration	Pooling of large quantities of sickled RBCs in spleen Seen in HbSS (6 months–5 years) and HbSC, HbSβ (any age) Present with dyspnea, shock, fever (viral precipitant), abdominal pain, massive splenomegaly, Hb drop >20 g/L with reticulocytosis	Splenic palpation by caregivers at home	Volume expansion and transfusion Two-thirds recur within 6 months: consider chronic transfusions and splenectomy after >2 events
VOC affecting bone	Ischemic tissue injury from obstruction of blood flow by sickled RBCs Precipitated by infection, acidosis, hypoxia, dehydration, sleep apnea, exposure to extreme temperatures DDx: osteomyelitis, avascular necrosis		Analgesia (see Table 21.4), hydration Monitor for complications (e.g., ACS)

ACS, Acute chest syndrome; *BP,* blood pressure; *CBC,* complete blood count; *CT,* computed tomography; *CXR,* chest x-ray; *DDx,* differential diagnosis; *Hb,* hemoglobin; *LFTs,* liver function tests; *MRA,* magnetic resonance angiography; *MRI,* magnetic resonance imaging; *PFT,* pulmonary function test; *pRBC,* packed red blood cell; *TIA,* transient ischemic attack; *VOC,* vaso-occlusive crisis.

524 5. **Management:** see Figure 21.3, Table 21.4, and later for further details

Figure 21.3 Management of Ill Patients With Sickle Cell Disease

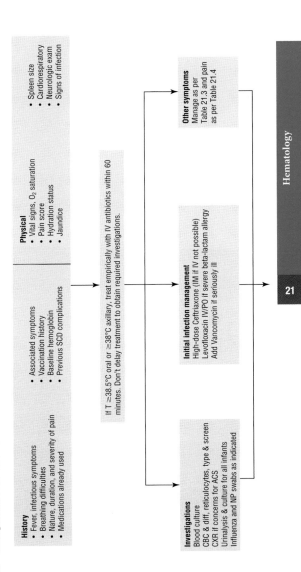

History
- Fever, infectious symptoms
- Breathing difficulties
- Nature, duration, and severity of pain
- Medications already used
- Associated symptoms
- Vaccination history
- Baseline hemoglobin
- Previous SCD complications

Physical
- Vital signs, O₂ saturation
- Pain score
- Hydration status
- Jaundice
- Spleen size
- Cardiorespiratory exam
- Neurologic exam
- Signs of infection

If T ≥38.5°C oral or ≥38°C axillary, treat empirically with IV antibiotics within 60 minutes. Don't delay treatment to obtain required investigations.

Investigations
Blood culture
CBC & diff, reticulocytes, type & screen
CXR if concerns for ACS
Urinalysis & culture for all infants
Influenza and NP swabs as indicated

Initial infection management
High-dose Ceftriaxone (IM if IV not possible)
Levofloxacin IV/PO if severe beta-lactam allergy
Add Vancomycin if seriously ill

Other symptoms
Manage as per Table 21.3 and pain as per Table 21.4

Hematology

21

Inpatient management

Analgesia, hydration, transfusions, and respiratory support as needed

Early mobilisation and incentive spirometry

Suspected Pneumococcal meningitis: high-dose Ceftriaxone

Seriously unwell: add Vancomycin

Concern for atypical pneumonia or positive Mycoplasma PCR: add Clarithromycin

Mild pneumonia: step down to Cefuroxime after 72 h

Positive blood culture: narrow antibiotic choice based on susceptibility

Negative blood culture at 48 h and no other bacterial source identified: stop antibioticss

Discharge

Tolerating PO fluids and medications

No respiratory distress, vitals stable

Follow-up arranged

Red flags?

Patient appears unwell

Suspected sepsis, meningitis, stroke, ACS, aplastic crisis, splenic sequestration

Shock, cardiovascular instability, or respiratory distress

T >40°C

Age <1 year

Previous severe sepsis or meningitis

WBC >30 or <5 × 10⁹/L or PLT <150 × 10⁹/L

Poor adherence (missed antibiotics or clinic visits)

2 return visits to ED for same episode

Uncertain follow-up or family coping

Yes

No

Outpatient management

Observe for 2–4 h in ED

PO analgesia with ibuprofen and acetaminophen

Encourage PO hydration

3 day course PO antibiotics with Cefuroxime or Levofloxacin

Adjust duration if source identified (AOM, UTI, etc.)

Review home fever management

Ensure follow-up arranged

Review when to return to ED

Provide procedure for notification of positive blood cultures

Provide clinic contact information

ACS, Acute chest syndrome; AOM, acute otitis media; CBC, complete blood count; CXR, chest x-ray; ED, emergency department; PCR, polymerase chain reaction; PLT, platelets; UTI, urinary tract infection; WBC, white blood cell. (© The Hospital for Sick Children. Adapted from Fever: Guidelines for Management in Children with Sickle Cell Disease. 3rd ed. Toronto, ON: Hospital for Sick Children; 2016)

Table 21.4	Pain Management in Vaso-occlusive Crisis		
Pain Severity	**Management**	**Comments**	**Discharge Planning**
Mild	**Acetaminophen** AND **ibuprofen** PO scheduled **Morphine**[a] 0.1–0.5 mg/kg PO q4–6h PRN (max. 15 mg/dose)	Give acetaminophen and ibuprofen regularly for 1–2 days, then switch to PRN	If pain control adequate within 60 min of medication administration, can discharge home
Moderate-severe	**Morphine**[a] 0.1–0.5 mg/kg PO q4–6h (max. 15 mg/dose) or 0.05–0.1 mg/kg IV q2–4h (max. 5 mg/dose) scheduled Consider intranasal **fentanyl** while establishing IV access if in severe pain	Start with IV if home PO management was not adequate If no pain relief from PO within 30–60 min, give IV bolus If pain relief within 2 h or with 1–2 IV doses, change to equivalent PO dose	Discharge when tolerating PO fluids and pain controlled on PO medications If pain uncontrolled on PO analgesics or if otherwise unwell, admit to hospital (consider if ≥3 IV doses required)
Severe (inpatient)	Start **morphine**[b] 0.1 mg/kg IV loading dose (max. 7.5 mg), followed by continuous IV infusion 40 mcg/kg/h **Morphine**[b] bolus 0.01–0.04 mg/kg IV q1–2 h PRN (max. 15 mg/dose) Consider patient controlled analgesia pump	Increase infusion rate in increments of 20 mcg/kg/h q8 h PRN (max. 100 mcg/kg/h) Decrease infusion by 10 mcg/kg/h as tolerated, once pain controlled	Discharge when tolerating PO fluids and pain controlled on PO medications
All patients	**Fluid management:** if not tolerating PO, start IVF at 1× maintenance TFI. If dehydrated, give 10 mL/kg bolus 0.9% NaCl (do not bolus if concerns for ACS). Monitor electrolytes. **Non-pharmacological pain management:** heating pads, warm baths, massage, structured activity, imagery/distraction techniques **ACS prevention:** incentive spirometry, physiotherapy, early mobilization **Managing opioid side effects:** PEG-3350 or docusate to prevent constipation. Antihistamines PRN for pruritus. **Follow-up:** arrange outpatient Hematology follow-up		

[a]Immediate-release form

[b]Alternatively can use hydromorphone

ACS, Acute chest syndrome; *IV,* intravenous; *IVF,* intravenous fluid; *PO,* orally; *PRN,* as needed; *TFI,* total fluid intake.

! PITFALL

Running IVF at 1.5× maintenance may increase the risk of ACS. Routine IVF for SCD patients should be run at 1× maintenance.

A. Hydroxyurea (HU)

1. **Mechanism:** increases production of fetal Hb, thereby decreasing HbS and sickling tendency
2. **Benefit:** decreases frequency of VOCs, dactylitis, ACS, blood transfusions, hospitalization, and death
3. **Side effects:** neutropenia, bone marrow suppression, macrocytosis, hepatic enzyme elevation, anorexia, nausea, vomiting, infertility; no proven increased risk of malignancy
4. **Monitoring:** monthly CBC, differential, reticulocytes, bilirubin, ALT, urea, creatinine while titrating dose

B. RBC transfusion

1. **Acute indications:** ACS, aplastic crisis, splenic sequestration, stroke
2. **Chronic indications:** splenic sequestration prevention, primary and secondary stroke prevention, treatment of symptomatic anemia
3. **Monitoring:** for side effects of repeat transfusions (Table 21.5)
   a. Alloantibody formation: extended cross-matching of pRBCs required
   b. Iron excess: consider iron chelation therapy after 100 mL/kg pRBCs, 15 transfusions or ferritin consistently above 1000 ng/mL (Table 21.6)

Table 21.5	Surveillance During Chronic Transfusion Therapy
System	**Specific Investigation(s) and Frequency**
Hematological	Ferritin q3 months
Renal	Cr and urea q6 months
Endocrine	GH, IGF-1, TSH, free T3/T4 annually
Hepatic	AST, ALT, GGT, ALP q6 months Ferriscan annually to assess liver iron concentration
Cardiac	Cardiac MRI annually
Hearing	Annual assessment
Ophthalmological	Annual assessment
Infectious	Hepatitis B, Hepatitis C, and HIV serology annually

Surveillance required because of risk of iron loading in the aforementioned organs and risk of infection transmission through blood. Ferritin is a general marker of iron loading.

ALP, Alkaline phosphatase; *ALT,* alanine aminotransferase; *ASP,* aspartate aminotransferase; *GGT,* gamma-glutamyl transferase; *GH,* growth hormone; *HIV,* human immunodeficiency syndrome; *IGF-1,* insulin-like growth factor 1; *MRI,* magnetic resonance imaging; *T3,* triiodothyronine; *T4,* thyroxine; *TSH,* thyroid stimulating hormone.

Table 21.6　Options for Iron Chelation Therapy

Agent (Trade Name)	Route	Side Effects	Monitoring	Comments
Deferoxamine (Desferal)	Given SC/IV 5–7 nights per week over 10–12 h	Ototoxicity, retinal changes, truncal shortening	Yearly hearing and eye examination	Fast for 30 min before administration
Deferasirox (Exjade, Jadenu)	Tablet taken daily	Nephrotoxicity, hepatotoxicity, ototoxicity, cataracts	Monthly renal function, ALT and urinalysis\nYearly hearing and eye examination	If transitioning from Exjade to Jadenu, the Jadenu dose should be 30% lower than the Exjade dose
Deferiprone (Ferriprox)	Tablet taken TID	Neutropenia, liver toxicity	Monthly CBC and ALT	Best for cardiac hemosiderosis

ALT, Alanine aminotransferase; *CBC,* complete blood count; *IV,* intravenous; *SC,* subcutaneous; *TID,* three times per day.

C. Peri-operative management of SCD

1. Patients with SCD are more likely to require surgical procedures than the general population, especially cholecystectomy, tonsillectomy, adenoidectomy, splenectomy
2. Increased risk of post-operative complications, e.g., VOC, ACS, post-operative fever, stroke, splenic sequestration, death
3. **Pre-operative management**
   a. Hematologist should review 2 weeks before procedure
   b. Consider correcting anemia and reducing % HbS pre-operatively via simple transfusion
   c. Admit 1 day pre-operatively for CBC, reticulocytes, extended cross-match; request blood on hold for surgery and post-operatively
   d. Ensure adequate hydration with IVF for at least 8 hours pre-procedure
   e. Pre-oxygenate with O_2 at 2 L/min for 15 minutes pre-procedure
4. **Post-operative management**
   a. Optimize respiratory supports and bedside spirometry; target O_2 saturation $\geq 95\%$
   b. Maintain hydration with IVF at maintenance rate
   c. Provide adequate analgesia
   d. Encourage early mobilization
   e. Avoid hypothermia

THALASSEMIA

1. **Pathophysiology:** imbalance in α-globin and β-globin chain synthesis; un-paired globin chains precipitate, with hemolysis and ineffective erythropoiesis
2. **Classification:** historically based on genetic abnormality; now also classified based on transfusion requirement, because of phenotypic variability
3. **Clinical features and treatment:** see Table 21.7

Table 21.7	**Features of Thalassemia Syndromes**					
	% Hb					
Genetics	**HbA**	**HbA$_2$**	**HbF**	**Other**	**Clinical Syndrome**	**Treatment**
Normal $\alpha_2\beta_2$	96–98	2–3	<1	—	None	
β-Thalassemias						
β°/β°	0	2–5	95	—	Diagnosed in late infancy (↓ γ-chain)	Regular transfusions
					Severe anemia, pallor, failure to thrive, hepatosplenomegaly	Iron chelation BMT Family counseling
β⁺/β⁺	20–40	—	60–80	—	Moderate-severe anemia beyond infancy	No or irregular transfusions
					Anisocytosis, poikilocytosis	± Iron chelation Family counseling
β/β° or β/β⁺	90–95	5–7	2–10	↑ RBC count	Asymptomatic mild anemia	Family counseling
					Hypochromic/microcytic smear, basophilic stippling	
α-Thalassemias						
Homozygous α-thalassemia --/--	—	—	—	HbH (β$_4$) Hb Bart (γ$_4$) 80%–90%	Hydrops fetalis, majority stillborn	Antenatal and regular transfusions Iron chelation BMT Family counseling
HbH disease --/-α	60–90	2–5	2–5	HbH 30%–40%	Neonatal microcytic anemia (Hb 70–100 g/L), Heinz bodies	Transfusion in hemolytic or aplastic crisis ± splenectomy Folic acid Family counseling
α-Thalassemia trait -α/-α αα/--	90–98	2–3	2–3	—	Hypochromic/microcytic smear, no anemia	Family counseling
Silent carrier -α/αα	90–98	2–3	2–3	—	Normal	Family counseling

°Denotes alleles that make no globulin chains

⁺Denotes alleles that make reduced globulin chains

BMT, Bone marrow transplant; *Hb,* hemoglobin; *RBC,* red blood cell.

4. **Transfusion-dependent thalassemia (TDT):** require regular pRBC transfusions
   a. Require regular monitoring (see Table 21.5) and iron chelation therapy (see Table 21.6)
5. **Non-transfusion-dependent thalassemia (NTDT):** do not require regular pRBC transfusions; may require occasional transfusions

THROMBOCYTOPENIA

1. **Diagnostic approach:** see Figure 21.4

Figure 21.4 Approach to Thrombocytopenia

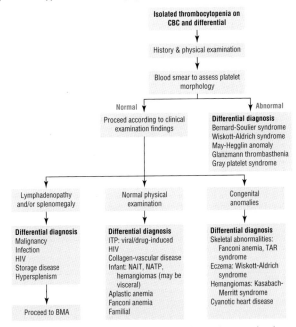

CBC, Complete blood count; HIV, human immunodeficiency syndrome; ITP, immune thrombocytopenia, NAIT, neonatal alloimmune thrombocytopenia; NATP, neonatal autoimmune thrombocytopenia; TAR, thrombocytopenia and absent radius. (Modified from Hastings CA, Lubin BH. Blood. In: Rudolph AM, Kamel RK, eds., *Rudolph's Fundamentals of Pediatrics.* 2nd ed. Norwalk, CT: Appleton & Lange; 1998:441–490. Reprinted with permission of The McGraw-Hill Companies, Inc.)

IMMUNE THROMBOCYTOPENIA (ITP)

1. **Definition:** antibody-mediated platelet destruction, resulting in isolated thrombocytopenia (platelet count $<100 \times 10^9$/L)
2. **Classification:** newly diagnosed (0–3 months), persistent (3–12 months) or chronic (>12 months)
3. **Peak incidence:** 1 to 4 years of age
4. **Presentation:** minor bleeding, such as epistaxis, bruising, petechial rash
   a. No history of constitutional symptoms, bony or joint pain, lymphadenopathy, hepatosplenomegaly, dysmorphism, congenital anomalies, developmental or growth delay, family history of hematological malignancy or thrombocytopenia
   b. Approximately half of cases occur 1 to 4 weeks following a viral illness
5. **Investigations**
   a. CBC and differential: normal apart from low platelet count; low Hb if significant blood loss
   b. Blood smear: platelets of varying sizes, many large platelets
   c. Bone marrow examination: not recommended in children with typical features of ITP
6. **Treatment**
   a. Very low risk of major bleeding (<1% develop intracranial hemorrhage) with high rates of spontaneous remission
   b. Conservative management: children with no or mild bleeding (e.g., petechiae) can be observed, regardless of platelet count
   c. Active management: see Table 21.8 for options
   d. Management of major bleeding episodes: intravenous immunoglobulin (IVIG) + high-dose IV steroids + platelet transfusion
   e. Management of chronic ITP: includes thrombopoietin receptor agonists, rituximab, low dose corticosteroids, splenectomy

---

⚛ PEARL

Treatment decisions in ITP should be guided by clinical symptoms and take into account family preference. There is no platelet count threshold for decision to treat.

Table 21.8	Management Options for Immune Thrombocytopenia		
Drug	**Dose**	**Benefits**	**Side Effects**
IVIG	Single dose of 0.8–1 g/kg	Rapid response in platelet count	Infusion reaction, aseptic meningitis, renal impairment, thromboembolic events, hemolysis
Corticosteroids	Prednisone 4 mg/kg/day divided BID-QID (max. 150 mg/day) × 4 days, no taper required	No IV treatment required, no admission required	Sleep disturbance, hypertension, hyperglycemia

BID, Twice per day; *ITP*, immune thrombocytopenia; *IV*, intravenous; *IVIG*, intravenous immunoglobulin; *QID*, four times per day.

NEONATAL ALLOIMMUNE THROMBOCYTOPENIA (NAIT)

1. **Pathophysiology:** maternal IgG alloantibodies against fetal platelets expressing paternal platelet antigens
2. Most common cause in Caucasians is materno-fetal incompatibility of human platelet antigen 1a (HPA-1a)
3. **Presentation:** well-appearing neonate with petechiae/purpura and isolated, usually severe thrombocytopenia (platelets <10–20×10^9/L) at 0 to 72 hours of life
   a. No history of maternal thrombocytopenia
4. **Complications:** high risk of prenatal or perinatal intracranial hemorrhage
5. **Investigations**
   a. Serological testing demonstrates the presence of maternal anti-HPA IgG antibodies which react with neonatal platelets
   b. Check maternal CBC for thrombocytopenia (consider neonatal autoimmune thrombocytopenia [NATP] if maternal platelets low)
   c. Screening head ultrasound (US) for intracranial hemorrhage
6. **Treatment**
   a. Reduce risk of fetal hemorrhage with antenatal IVIG and planned cesarean section delivery
   b. Gold standard: transfusion of washed maternal platelets; often not practical or easily obtained
   c. Second-best option: transfusion of HPA-matched (or HPA-1a negative) platelets
   d. Random donor platelets often given as a reasonable and practical alternative
   e. Consider IVIG to improve response to random donor platelets, or if severely thrombocytopenic despite matched platelets
7. **Prognosis:** resolves spontaneously in 2 to 4 months
   a. Need to counsel for future pregnancies

NEONATAL AUTOIMMUNE THROMBOCYTOPENIA (NATP)

1. **Pathophysiology:** transplacental transfer of maternal IgG anti-platelet antibodies, resulting in maternal AND neonatal ITP
2. **Presentation:** neonatal thrombocytopenia with maternal history of ITP, systemic lupus erythematosus (SLE), or autoimmune disease and maternal thrombocytopenia before delivery
3. **Treatment**
   a. Treat maternal ITP antenatally with IVIG $\pm$ corticosteroids
   b. Treat neonatal thrombocytopenia with IVIG $\pm$ corticosteroids
   c. Maternal and random donor platelets destroyed if transfused
4. **Prognosis:** resolves spontaneously in 2 to 4 months

NEUTROPENIA

1. **Absolute neutrophil count (ANC):** (total WBC count) $\times$ (% of segmented neutrophils + bands)
2. **Neutropenia:** decrease in ANC below expected range for age and ethnicity
3. **Classification:** acute (<3 months) or chronic (lasting >3 months)
4. **Clinical features**
   a. Systemic: high fever, chills, irritability because of infection
   b. Mucocutaneous: necrotic and ulcerative lesions of oropharyngeal and nasal mucosa, skin, gastrointestinal (GI) tract, vagina, uterus
   c. Risk of infection inversely proportional to ANC, particularly when ANC <0.5 $\times$ 10^9/L
   d. Risk of infection proportional to the duration of neutropenia
5. **Diagnostic approach**
   a. Acute neutropenia: see Figure 21.5
   b. Chronic neutropenia: see Figure 21.6

ANC, Absolute neutrophil count; CBC, complete blood count. (Adapted from Boxer IA. Neutropenia. In Sills RH, ed. *Protocol Algorithms on Pediatric Hematology and Oncology*. Albany, NY: Karger; 2003:42.)

Hematology

21

536

Figure 21.6 Approach to Chronic Neutropenia

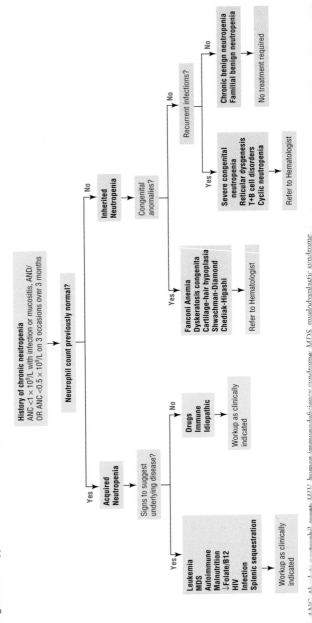

History of chronic neutropenia
ANC <1 × 10⁹/L with infection or mucositis, AND/
OR ANC <0.5 × 10⁹/L on 3 occasions over 3 months

Neutrophil count previously normal?

Yes

Acquired Neutropenia

Signs to suggest underlying disease?

Yes

Leukemia
MDS
Autoimmune
Malnutrition
↓Folate/B12
HIV
Infection
Splenic sequestration

Workup as clinically indicated

No

Drugs
Immune
Idiopathic

Workup as clinically indicated

No

Inherited Neutropenia

Congenital anomalies?

Yes

Fanconi Anemia
Dyskeratosis congenita
Cartilage-hair hypoplasia
Shwachman-Diamond
Chediak-Higashi

Refer to Hematologist

No

Recurrent infections?

Yes

Severe congenital neutropenia
Reticular dysgenesis
T+B cell disorders
Cyclic neutropenia

Refer to Hematologist

No

Chronic benign neutropenia
Familial benign neutropenia

No treatment required

ANC, Absolute neutrophil count; HIV, human immunodeficiency syndrome; MDS, myelodysplastic syndrome.

6. **Treatment**
   a. Treat underlying condition
   b. Granulocyte colony-stimulating factor: consider to increase ANC
   c. Management of fever and neutropenia: see Chapter 30 Oncology

BLEEDING DISORDERS

1. **Coagulation pathway:** see Figure 21.7

Figure 21.7 Simplified Pathway of Blood Coagulation

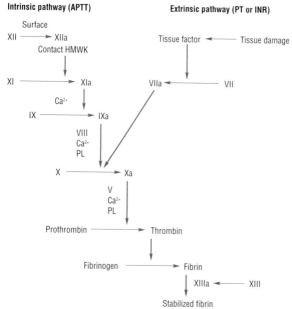

APTT, Activated partial thromboplastin time; HMWK, high molecular weight kininogen; INR, international normalized ratio; PL, phospholipid; PT, prothrombin time.

2. **History**
   a. Easy bruising, petechiae, mucosal bleeding (epistaxis, menorrhagia), surgical bleeding (dental extraction, tonsillectomy, post-circumcision), bleeding from umbilical stump, bleeding into joints and muscles, post-immunization hematomas; ask duration of bleed, amount of blood loss
   b. Previous blood transfusions
   c. Underlying medical conditions that can affect coagulation
   d. Drugs, including non-steroidal anti-inflammatory drug (NSAID) use
   e. Family history of bleeding disorders

3. **Diagnosis:** see Table 21.9
   a. Mucosal bleeding and skin manifestations suggest primary hemostatic disorder (Table 21.10)
   b. Bleeding into joints and deep hematomas suggest secondary hemostatic disorder (Table 21.11)
   c. Non-accidental injury should be considered in the differential diagnosis

Table 21.9	Screening Tests for Bleeding Disorders	
Investigation	Measure/Process Assessed	Diagnosis
CBC and peripheral blood smear	Platelet number and morphology, RBC morphology	Large platelets: peripheral destruction (e.g., ITP), congenital platelet disorders Small platelets: Wiskott-Aldrich syndrome Fragmented RBCs: microangiopathic process (e.g., HUS, TTP, DIC)
Platelet function analysis (PFA)	Primary hemostasis and platelet function	Quantitative platelet defect (thrombocytopenia), platelet dysfunction, VWD, drugs (NSAIDs), uremia
PT, INR	Extrinsic (FVII) and common pathways (FX, FV, prothrombin, fibrinogen)	Defect in vitamin K-dependent factors, hemorrhagic disease of the newborn, malabsorption, liver disease, DIC, warfarin
APTT, PTT	Intrinsic (FVIII, FIX, FXI, FXII) and common pathways (FX, FV, prothrombin, fibrinogen)	Hemophilia A and B, VWD, heparin, DIC, lupus anticoagulant
Thrombin time (TT)	Fibrinogen-to-fibrin conversion	Decreased plasma fibrinogen (hypo/afibrinogenemia), dysfunctional fibrinogen (dysfibrinogenemia), heparin, DIC
Fibrinogen	Quantitative fibrinogen level	Decreased plasma fibrinogen (hypo/afibrinogenemia), DIC
D-Dimer	Fibrin breakdown product	Increased in DIC and thrombosis
Factor assays	Quantitative factor level	Vitamin K-dependent: FII, FVII, FIX, FX, protein C, protein S All factors are made in the liver except FVIII FXIII does not affect PTT or INR FVII has the shortest half life FXII deficiency does not cause clinical bleeding
1:1 Mixing study (mix of patient's plasma and normal pooled plasma)	Cause of prolonged PTT	PTT remains prolonged: presence of factor inhibitor (heparin, lupus anticoagulant) PTT normalizes: factor deficiency

APTT, Activated partial thromboplastin time; *CBC,* complete blood count; *DIC,* disseminated intravascular coagulation; *HUS,* hemolytic uremic syndrome; *INR,* international normalized ratio; *ITP,* immune thrombocytopenia; *NSAID,* non-steroidal anti-inflammatory drug; *PT,* prothrombin time; *PTT,* partial thromboplastin time; *RBC,* red blood cell; *TTP,* thrombotic thrombocytopenic purpura; *VWD,* von Willebrand disease.

Table 21.10	Primary Hemostasis Disorders		
Type	**Description**	**Investigations**	**Management**
Type 1 von Willebrand disease	Quantitative deficiency of vWF Inheritance: AD Most common subtype	vWF:Ag <30 IU/dL Reduced vWF:RCo	Desmopressin IV or intranasal vWF concentrate Tranexamic acid[a] or aminocaproic acid for bleeding
Type 2 von Willebrand disease	Dysfunctional vWF Four subtypes: 2A, 2B, 2M, 2N Inheritance: AD or AR	vWF activity:antigen ratio <0.6	Desmopressin in 2A and 2M – Contraindicated in 2B – Limited benefit in 2N Tranexamic acid or aminocaproic acid for bleeding
Type 3 von Willebrand disease	Quantitative absence of vWF Inheritance: AR Most severe form, no vWF made. Patients may present with deep bleeding into joints/tissues	vWF:Ag <5 IU/dL Reduced/absent vWF:RCo Decreased FVIII	vWF concentrate Tranexamic acid or aminocaproic acid for bleeding
Qualitative platelet abnormalities	Bernard-Soulier syndrome, Glanzmann thrombasthenia, storage pool deficiency, uremia, drug effect	Increased bleeding time CBC shows low/normal platelet count Blood smear may show abnormal platelet morphology Platelet functional analysis may be abnormal	Varies based on etiology Most disorders are mild; however, for significant bleeds, consider platelet transfusion, tranexamic acid, and rFVIIa

[a]Tranexamic acid is contraindicated for hematuria

AD, Autosomal dominant; *AR*, autosomal recessive; *IV*, intravenous; *RCo*, ristocetin cofactor; *vWF*, von Willebrand factor; *vWF:Ag*, von Willebrand factor antigen.

Table 21.11	Secondary Hemostasis Disorders		
Type	**Description**	**Investigations**	**Management**
FVIII deficiency (Hemophilia A)	X-linked deficiency, 30% spontaneous Severity related to degree of residual FVIII procoagulant activity Mild and moderate types present with bleeding after minor trauma Severe disease presents with spontaneous bleeding into joints, muscles or deep tissues	Prolonged PTT, normal PT/INR Decreased FVIII:C DNA analysis	Mild: consider desmopressin (responders achieve FVIII:C ~30%) For bleed management or prophylaxis give rFVIII
FIX deficiency (Hemophilia B, Christmas disease)	X-linked deficiency FIX is vitamin K-dependent Levels are lower at birth, making early diagnosis difficult	DNA analysis Prolonged PTT, normal PT/INR Decreased FIX	For bleed management or prophylaxis, give rFIX

Table 21.11	Secondary Hemostasis Disorders—cont'd		
FXIII deficiency	Often presents with bleeding from umbilical stump	Normal PTT/INR	Monthly FXIII concentrate, or FFP if unavailable
DIC	Characterized by hemorrhage and microthrombi, resulting in microangiopathic hemolytic anemia Underlying etiology varies, e.g., sepsis, malignancy, trauma	Increased INR and PTT Increased D-Dimer Increased thrombin time Decreased fibrinogen Decreased platelets	Treat underlying cause Supportive management with replacement of pRBC, PLT, FFP, cryo-precipitate or fibrinogen concentrate
Vitamin K deficiency	Results in decreased levels of vitamin K-dependent factors (FII, FVII, FIX, FX, protein C, protein S) Causes of vitamin K deficiency include cystic fibrosis, biliary atresia, malabsorption caused by intestinal disease, e.g., celiac or IBD, liver failure	Increased INR and PTT (INR> PTT) Decreased FII, FVII, FIX, FX	Vitamin K prophylaxis at birth Vitamin K supplementation FFP if bleeding
Lupus anti-coagulant	Transient antiphospholipid antibodies acquired in children, often following a recent infection (usually viral)	Increased PTT	Typically transient and do not cause bleeding Rare cases of anti-phospholipid antibody syndrome reported

DIC, Disseminated intravascular coagulation; *DNA*, deoxyribonucleic acid; *FFP*, fresh frozen plasma; *IBD*, inflammatory bowel disease; *INR*, international normalized ratio; *ITP*, immune thrombocytopenia; *PLT*, platelets; *pRBC*, packed red blood cell; *PT*, prothrombin time; *PTT*, partial thromboplastin time.

THROMBOSIS

VENOUS THROMBOEMBOLIC EVENT (VTE)

1. Rare in children, particularly in the absence of risk factors (Table 21.12)
2. **Imaging**
   a. Suspected DVT: Doppler US
      i. High false-negative rate for intrathoracic VTE may require MRV, CT, or contrast venography
      ii. If normal and high clinical suspicion for lower limb proximal DVT, repeat after 1 week
   b. Suspected PE: CT pulmonary angiography
      i. CXR, echocardiogram, V/Q scan may be useful
      ii. D-dimer and Wells score lack utility for diagnosis in children

Table 21.12

	Inherited Thrombophilias	**Acquired Disorders**
More common	FV Leiden mutation Prothrombin gene mutation	CVL (most common cause)
Less common	Antithrombin deficiency	Antiphospholipid antibody syndrome
	Dysfibrinogenemia/ hypofibrinogenemia	Chemotherapy (e.g., tamoxifen, thalidomide, L-asparaginase)
	Heparin cofactor II deficiency	Congenital heart disease, heart failure
	Homocystinuria	Estrogen (oral contraceptive or hormone replacement therapy)
	Protein S or C deficiency	Hemolytic anemia
		Immobilization
		Inflammatory bowel disease
		Leukocytosis in acute leukemia
		Malignancy
		Myeloproliferative disorders
		Nephrotic syndrome
		Paroxysmal nocturnal hemoglobinuria
		Pregnancy
		Surgery, especially orthopedic
		Trauma

CVL, Central venous line.

Modified from Albisetti M, Chan AKC. Venous thrombosis and thromboembolism in children: Risk factors, clinical manifestations and diagnosis. *UpToDate.* https://www.uptodate-com.uml. idm.oclc.org/contents/venous-thrombosis-and-thromboembolism-in-children-risk-factors-clinical-manifestations-and-diagnosis. Accessed December 29, 2017.

3. **Thrombotic work-up:** CBC, INR, PTT, fibrinogen, D-dimer, creatinine
   a. Further prothrombotic workup not recommended routinely
   b. Refer to Hematology if non-CVL-related VTE, recurrent VTEs, or purpura fulminans
4. **Initial management:** start anticoagulation before imaging if suspicion of thrombosis is high or if life/limb-threatening
   a. Initial therapy with UFH or LMWH for a minimum of 5 days or 10 to 14 days if extensive clot
5. **Maintenance therapy:** therapeutic dosing of LMWH or warfarin
   a. Duration: dependent on the clinical circumstance; generally
      i. DVT after acquired insult: 6 weeks to 3 months
      ii. Idiopathic DVT: 6 to 12 months
      iii. Recurrent idiopathic DVT: indefinite

6. **Prevention:** consider for teenagers, patients with immobility and other risk factors, with guidance from Hematology
   a. Non-pharmacological: early ambulation and mechanical prophylaxis (pneumatic inflation device and/or graduated compression stockings)
   b. Pharmacological: LMWH or UFH

 PEARL

Consult Hematology before initiating anticoagulation therapy if high-risk bleeding surgery performed in preceding 7 to 10 days (e.g., intraocular, intracranial, retroperitoneal, GI/GU, or bleeding requiring blood products)

UNFRACTIONATED HEPARIN (UFH)

1. **Administration:** SC or via a dedicated IV line
   a. Obtain CBC, aPTT, INR, fibrinogen, D-dimer before initiation
   b. Do not bolus in neonates, children with stroke, or children at high risk of bleeding
   c. Avoid ASA, other anti-platelet medications, IM injections, and arterial punctures
   d. Patient may be transitioned to warfarin or LMWH for ongoing management
2. **Monitoring:** aPTT and/or heparin anti-factor Xa
   a. Check 4 hours after bolus or 6 hours after starting infusion if no bolus given
   b. Take peripheral samples to avoid contamination
   c. Can use aPTT to monitor if >12 months of age and results correlate with anti-factor Xa level
   d. Monitor platelets daily for 10 days, then every 3 to 5 days, to monitor for heparin-induced thrombocytopenia (HIT) (fall of >50% from baseline)
3. **Reversal:** termination of the infusion for an hour usually suffices
   a. Protamine sulfate reverses 60% of antifactor Xa activity—consult Hematology for guidance

LOW-MOLECULAR-WEIGHT HEPARIN (LMWH)

1. **Indication:** consider LMWH in most patients requiring therapeutic or prophylactic anticoagulation
2. **Administration:** obtain CBC, INR, aPTT, fibrinogen, D-dimer, creatinine before initiation
   a. Do not administer to damaged or edematous skin
3. **Monitoring**
   a. Send peripheral sample for antifactor Xa level 4 hours after second dose

b. Adjust dosing as per Table 21.13; therapeutic level usually 0.5 to 1 unit/mL

c. Once therapeutic, monitor antifactor Xa level weekly (inpatient) or monthly (outpatient)

d. Monitor CBC: consider HIT if platelets decrease ≥50% from baseline

e. Monitor renal function: renally excreted; may need dose reduction if GFR <30 mL/min/1.73 m^2 (see Table 21.13)

f. Consider bone densitometry at baseline and annually for osteoporosis screening if taking LMWH >3 months

4. **LMWH prophylaxis:** can give SC as once daily or BID dose (see formulary)

   a. Antifactor Xa, CBC, and renal function monitoring not required unless in renal failure

5. **Precautions:** avoid trauma, contact sports, ASA and other anti-platelet medications, IM injections, and arterial punctures while on LMWH

6. **Converting therapeutic LMWH to UFH:** do not initiate until at least 8 hours after last dose of LMWH; do not bolus until at least 12 hours after last dose of LMWH

7. **LMWH reversal:** as with UFH

Table 21.13	**Nomogram for Adjusting Low-Molecular-Weight Heparin Treatment Doses**		
Anti-FXa Level	**Hold Next Dose**	**Dose Change**	**Repeat Anti-FXa Level**
<0.35 units/mL	No	↑ by 25%	4 h post next AM dose
0.35–0.49 units/mL	No	↑ by 10%	4 h post next AM dose
0.5–1 units/mL	No	0	4 h post AM dose once weekly
1.01–1.6 units/mL	No	↓ by 20%	4 h post next AM dose
>1.6 units/mL	Yes (until level <0.5 units/mL)	↓ by 40%	Trough level before next dose, and if not <0.5 units/mL, repeat before each dose is due

© The Hospital for Sick Children. Modified from *Antithrombotic Therapy—Low Molecular Weight Heparin (LMWH) Use in Children and Neonates.* Toronto, ON: Hospital for Sick Children; 2016.

WARFARIN

1. Most commonly used oral anticoagulant

2. **Administration:** consult Hematology for initiation and monitoring

   a. Obtain CBC, aPTT, INR before initiation; review patient's medications to ensure no interactions (Box 21.1)

   b. Must be taking full oral intake to prevent INR rising to dangerously high levels

      i. If formula-fed, give formula with low vitamin K content

ii. If exclusively breastfed, consider supplementing with small amount of formula for constant vitamin K intake (require 1 mcg/kg/day; i.e., ~120 mL of standard formula)

Box 21.1	Drugs Interacting With Warfarin			
Acetaminophen	Chloral hydrate	Levofloxacin	Piperacillin	Spironolactone
Allopurinol	Ciprofloxacin	Levothyroxine	PPIs	SSRIs
Amiodarone	Cisapride	Macrolides	Prednisone	Valproate
Amitriptyline	Cyclophosphamide	Metronidazole	Propafenone	Vitamin C
Aspirin	Doxycycline	NSAIDs	Ranitidine	Vitamin E
Carbamazepine	Fluconazole	Penicillins	Rifampicin	Vitamin K
Celecoxib	Heparin	Phenobarbital	Tetracycline	Voriconazole
Cephalosporins	Lactulose	Phenytoin	TMP-SMX	

NSAID, Non-steroidal anti-inflammatory drug; *PPI*, proton-pump inhibitor; *SSRI*, selective serotonin reuptake inhibitor; *TMP-SMX*, trimethoprim-sulfamethoxazole.

© The Hospital for Sick Children. Modified from *Antithrombotic Therapy: Warfarin*. Toronto, ON: Hospital for Sick Children; 2016.

3. **Contraindications:** generally avoided in children <12 months unless a mechanical heart valve is present
   a. Teratogenic: females of reproductive age require reliable birth control
4. **Initiation:** dosing adjusted based on INR (Table 21.14)
   a. Takes 3 to 5 days before stable maintenance dosing is achieved
   b. Target INR usually 2 to 3, or 2.5 to 3.5 with mechanical heart valves, recurrent VTEs on warfarin, ongoing risk factors for VTE
   c. Can discontinue heparin once INR is >2 for 2 consecutive days

Table 21.14	Nomogram for Adjusting Warfarin Loading Doses
INR	**Action**
1.1–1.3	Repeat initial loading dose
1.4–3	Give 50% of initial loading dose
3.1–3.5	Give 25% of initial loading dose
>3.5	Hold until INR <3.5, then restart at 50% less than previous dose

If INR >3 on day 1, hold the next dose, repeat INR and restart at 50% of loading dose.
INR, International normalized ratio.

© The Hospital for Sick Children. Modified from *Antithrombotic Therapy: Warfarin*. Toronto, ON: Hospital for Sick Children; 2016.

5. **Maintenance:** can discharge home once INR is therapeutic for 2 consecutive days
   a. Give prescription for Vitamin K 10 mg PO, to be used if INR >9
   b. Maintenance dose adjustment as per Table 21.15

Table 21.15	Nomogram for Adjusting Warfarin Maintenance Doses
INR	**Action**
1.1–1.4	Check adherence. If adherent, increase dose by 20%
1.5–1.7	Increase dose by 10%
1.8–3.2	No change
3.2–3.5	Decrease dose by 10%
3.6–4	Administer 1 dose at 50% less than maintenance, then restart at 20% less than maintenance dose
4.1–5	Hold × 1 dose, then restart at 20% less than maintenance dose
>5	Contact expert

INR, International normalized ratio.
© The Hospital for Sick Children. Modified from *Antithrombotic Therapy Warfarin*. Toronto, ON: Hospital for Sick Children; 2016.

6. **Monitoring:** check INR
   a. 3 to 4 days after discharge
   b. 5 to 7 days after any change in dose
   c. Once patient has two INRs in therapeutic range 7 days apart, the interval for monitoring can be gradually increased to once a month if stable
7. **Reversal:** should only be performed with Hematology input
   a. Indications: include hemorrhage and surgery
   b. Low-dose warfarin (INR 1.4–1.9) and low-risk bleeding surgeries (non-neurosurgical, non-intraorbital): no reversal usually necessary; hold warfarin for approximately 72 hours before surgery
   c. Full-dose warfarin (INR >2) or high-risk bleeding surgeries: full reversal usually required pre-operatively because of risk of hemorrhage
   d. Consider bridging with heparin for patients with high risk of thrombosis (mechanical valve, recurrent stroke)
   e. Reversal agents: Vitamin K is antidote for warfarin
   i. Concurrent use of FFP or factor VIIa concentrate dependent on clinical situation

TRANSFUSION MEDICINE

OBTAINING CONSENT

1. It is the responsibility of the physician ordering the transfusion to obtain informed consent
2. **Describe:** role of the blood product, benefits, risks, and alternatives to transfusion
3. **Adverse transfusion effects:** see Table 21.16

Table 21.16	Adverse Transfusion Reactions
Adverse Transfusion Effects	**Frequency**
Urticaria	1:100
Transfusion-associated circulatory overload (TACO)	1:100
Fever	1:300
Delayed hemolytic reaction	1:7,000
Transfusion-related acute lung injury (TRALI)	1:10,000
Bacterial sepsis from platelet transfusion	1:10,000
Anaphylaxis	1:40,000
Bacterial sepsis from RBC transfusion	1:250,000
Hepatitis B	1:7,500,000
Hepatitis C	1:13,000,000
HIV	1:21,000,000

HIV, Human immunodeficiency virus; *RBC,* red blood cell.

BLOOD PRODUCTS

PEARL

The volume of pRBC or platelets transfused is generally capped at 1 unit, unless the patient is unwell or other extenuating circumstances exist

1. **Common blood products:** see Table 21.17

Table 21.17	Common Blood Products		
Blood Product	**Indications**	**Considerations**	**Dosage**
pRBCs	To maintain adequate tissue oxygenation by increasing oxygen-carrying capacity of blood Transfusion threshold depends on acuity of anemia, Hb value, baseline Hb, clinical symptoms, etc.	ABO/Rh: pRBCs should always be cross-matched unless in the case of an emergency CMV status: in Canada, all blood products are leukoreduced and considered CMV-safe. The evidence for additional benefits of CMV-negative blood products is limited; they are used in exceptional circumstances only Irradiated pRBCs: required for immunosuppressed patients, particularly – T-cell immunodeficiency – Undergoing hematopoietic stem cell transplantation	10–15 mL/kg (raises Hb by 20–30 g/L) 1 unit = approx. 300 mL, HCT 0.65 Transfuse over 1–4 h – More rapidly if there is acute blood loss compromising tissue perfusion

Table 21.17	Common Blood Products—cont'd		
Blood Product	**Indications**	**Considerations**	**Dosage**
		– Intrauterine transfusions – Directed donations – HLA-matched platelet transfusions – Malignancy on active chemotherapy	– More slowly if patient at risk for circulatory overload, e.g., congenital heart disease
PLT	Bleeding from thrombocytopenia or platelet function abnormality	<6 months of age: give ABO-identical platelets >6 months of age: ABO-identical platelets preferred; can give non-ABO-identical platelets in certain circumstances	5–10 mL/kg (raises PLT count by 30–60 ×10⁹/L) Transfuse over 30–60 min
Fresh frozen plasma (FFP)	Contains all coagulation factors and complement Management of – DIC – Warfarin reversal – Vitamin K deficiency – Severe liver disease with coagulopathy		10–15 mL/kg Transfuse over 30–60 min
Cryoprecipitate	Contains concentrated fibrinogen, FVIII, FXIII, Von Willebrand factor For patients with known factor deficiency, use of recombinant product is recommended where available Management of hypo/dysfibrinogenemia		1 unit/10 kg (increases fibrinogen by 0.5 g)
IVIG	Management of – ITP – Hypogammaglobulinemia – Kawasaki disease – BMT – Guillain-Barré syndrome – Juvenile rheumatoid arthritis	Monitor for side effects, including – Flu-like symptoms – Rash – Hypotension – TRALI – Aseptic meningitis – Hemolysis	Varies depending on pathology

BMT, Bone marrow transplant; *CMV,* cytomegalovirus; *DIC,* disseminated intravascular coagulation; *Hb,* hemoglobin; *HCT,* hematocrit; *HLA,* human leukocyte antigen; *ITP,* immune thrombocytopenia; *IVIG,* intravenous immunoglobulin; *PLT*; platelets; *pRBC,* packed red blood cell; *TRALI,* transfusion-related acute lung injury.

MANAGING TRANSFUSION REACTIONS

1. See Figure 21.8

Figure 21.8 Management of Suspected Transfusion Reactions

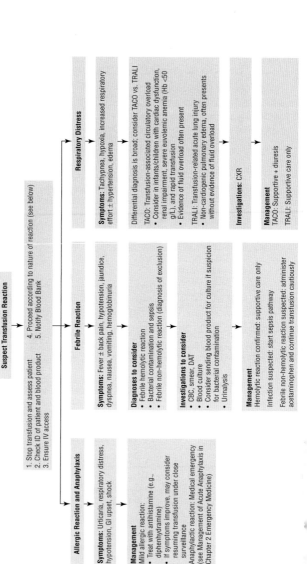

Suspect Transfusion Reaction

1. Stop transfusion and assess patient
2. Check ID of patient and blood product
3. Ensure IV access
4. Proceed according to nature of reaction (see below)
5. Notify Blood Bank

Allergic Reaction and Anaphylaxis

Symptoms: Urticaria, respiratory distress, hypotension, GI upset, shock

Management
Mild allergic reaction:
• Treat with antihistamine (e.g., diphenhydramine)
• If symptoms improve, may consider resuming transfusion under close surveillance
Anaphylactic reaction: Medical emergency (see Management of Acute Anaphylaxis in Chapter 2 Emergency Medicine)

Febrile Reaction

Symptoms: Fever ± back pain, hypotension, jaundice, dyspnea, nausea, vomiting, hemoglobinuria

Diagnoses to consider
• Febrile hemolytic reaction
• Bacterial contamination and sepsis
• Febrile non-hemolytic reaction (diagnosis of exclusion)

Investigations to consider
• CBC, smear, DAT
• Blood culture
• Consider sending blood product for culture if suspicion for bacterial contamination
• Urinalysis

Management
Hemolytic reaction confirmed: supportive care only
Infection suspected: start sepsis pathway
Febrile non-hemolytic reaction suspected: administer acetaminophen and continue transfusion cautiously

Respiratory Distress

Symptoms: Tachypnea, hypoxia, increased respiratory effort ± hypertension, edema

Differential diagnosis is broad; consider TACO vs. TRALI

TACO: Transfusion-associated circulatory overload
• Consider in infants/children with cardiac dysfunction, renal impairment, severe euvolemic anemia (Hb <50 g/L), and rapid transfusion
• Evidence of fluid overload often present

TRALI: Transfusion-related acute lung injury
• Non-cardiogenic pulmonary edema, often presents without evidence of fluid overload

Investigations: CXR

Management
TACO: Supportive + diuresis
TRALI: Supportive care only

TRANSFUSION-ASSOCIATED GRAFT-VERSUS-HOST DISEASE

1. Very rare complication of transfusion
2. **Pathophysiology:** transfused donor lymphocytes attack (engraft) recipient tissues that are seen as expressing foreign antigen
3. **Highest risk:** immunocompromised patients
   a. Immunocompetent patients' immune systems are able to fight off donor lymphocytes before they are able to attack recipient tissues in the large majority of cases
4. **Presentation:** often 5 to 14 days after transfusion; rash, fever, liver dysfunction, diarrhea, nausea, vomiting, followed by pancytopenia
5. **Mortality:** >90%
6. **Prevention:** irradiate blood products for immunocompromised patients

FURTHER READING

McCavit TL. Sickle cell disease. *Pediatr Rev.* 2012:33:195–206.

Walkovich K, Boxer LA. How to approach neutropenia in childhood. *Pediatr Rev.* 2013;34:173-184.

Vilmarie R, Warad D. Pediatric coagulation disorders. *Pediatr Rev.* 2016;37:41–45.

Sharathkumar AA, Pipe SW. Bleeding disorders. *Pediatr Rev.* 2008;29: 121–129.

Neunert C, Lim W, Crowther M, et al. The American Society of Hematology 2011 evidence-based practice guideline for immune thrombocytopenia. *Blood.* 2011;117:4190–4207.

Leebeek FWG, Eikenboom JCJ. Von Willebrand's disease. *N Engl J Med.* 2016;375:2067–2080.

USEFUL SITES

American Society of Hematology. www.hematology.org
Journal of Pediatric Hematology/Oncology. www.jpho-online.com/
Medeiros N. Atlas of Hematology. www.hematologyatlas.com/
Ontario Regional Blood Coordinating Network. transfusionontario.org/en/documents/?cat=bloody_easy

Immunology

Ori Scott • Amiirah Aujnarain • Vy Kim

COMMON ABBREVIATIONS

Also see page xviii for a list of other abbreviations used throughout this book

ADA	adenosine deaminase
AFP	alpha-fetoprotein
ALPS	autoimmune lymphoproliferative syndrome
APECED	autoimmune polyendocrinopathy candidiasis ectodermal dystrophy
AT	ataxia telangiectasia
CHS	Chediak-Higashi syndrome
CGD	chronic granulomatous disease
CID	combined immunodeficiency
CMV	cytomegalovirus
CVID	common variable immunodeficiency
DGS	DiGeorge syndrome
EBV	Epstein-Barr virus
GVHD	graft-versus-host disease
HLH	hemophagocytic lymphohistiocytosis
HSCT	hematopoietic stem cell transplant
Ig	immunoglobulin
IPEX	immunodysregulation polyendocrinopathy enteropathy x-linked
LAD	leukocyte adhesion deficiency
NK	natural killer cells
NOBI	neutrophil oxidative burst index
PHA	phytohemagglutinin
PID	primary immunodeficiency
PJP	*Pneumocystis jirovecii*
PNP	purine nucleoside phosphorylase
SCID	severe combined immunodeficiency
SCN	severe chronic neutropenia
SIGAD	selective immunoglobin (Ig)A deficiency
STAT	signal transducer and activator of transcription
TNF	tumour-necrosis factor
TLR	toll-like receptor
TREC	T-cell receptor excision circles
THI	transient hypogammaglobulinemia of infancy
Treg	T-regulatory cells
WAS	Wiskott-Aldrich syndrome
WHIM	warts, hypogammaglobulinemia, immunodeficiency, and myelokathexis
XL	X-linked

Immunology

22

SCREENING TESTS AND INTERPRETATION

1. **Newborn screen:** T-cell receptor excision circles (TREC) levels to screen for thymic output and T-cell production; if low will be flagged indicating low T-cell production (e.g., severe combined immunodeficiency [SCID])
2. **Complete blood count (CBC) with differential:** screen for abnormal production/release of cells from the bone marrow or sign of autoimmunity
3. **Quantitative immunoglobulins (IgG, IgA, IgM):** first 6 months of life represent maternal IgG values. If low, may indicate humoral/combined immunodeficiency.
4. **Antibody titers to protein vaccines if previously immunized** (e.g., diphtheria, tetanus, measles, mumps, rubella, and varicella): protective values indicate B-cells can mount a response to an antigen. Interpret in relation to timing of vaccine administration.

SPECIFIC TESTS FOR SUSPECTED IMMUNODEFICIENCIES
See Table 22.1

Table 22.1	Specific Tests for Suspected Immunodeficiencies	
	Initial Tests That Can Be Done by General Practitioners	**Specialized Tests**
Suspected humoral immunodeficiency	1. Quantitative immunoglobulins 2. Antibody response to protein vaccines	1. **B-cell quantitation by flow cytometry:** provides total count of B-cells by identifying cells expressing CD19 and/or CD20 2. **Antibody response to pneumococcal polysaccharide vaccine:** measure IgG antibodies to pneumococcal polysaccharide before giving vaccine, again 4–6 weeks post-vaccination and compare pre-/post-levels 3. **Isohemagglutinins (if child >1 year):** assesses IgM antibodies toward non-self blood group antigens via response to carbohydrate antigens on gut microbes. Can be falsely low with recent gut pathology (e.g., diarrhea) or antibiotic use.
Suspected cellular immunodeficiency	1. **Lymphocyte count (on differential):** reduced in many cases of SCID or profound CID. Normal count does not rule out PID. 2. **Chest x-ray:** thymic shadow absent in SCID (helpful in children <1 year of age)	1. **T-cell quantitation by flow cytometry:** provides total count of T-cells by identifying cells expressing CD3. May also look at T-cell subpopulations (CD4/T-helper, CD8/T-cytotoxic cells). 2. **In vitro T-cell proliferative responses to mitogens and antigens:** demonstrates T-cell function and ability to proliferate in response to stimulation 3. **ADA and PNP enzyme levels:** low in specific subtypes of SCID

Immunology

22

	Initial Tests That Can Be Done by General Practitioners	Specialized Tests
		4. **TREC:** if initial TREC on newborn screen is abnormal, repeat test to ensure accuracy of results (results can be falsely abnormal in premature babies or in those receiving steroids)
		5. **T-cell repertoire analysis:** examines the diversity and/or degree of clonality of T-cell receptors
		6. **Thymic biopsy**
Suspected phagocytic defects	1. **Neutrophil count (on differential):** reduced number may represent bone marrow production issue, inability for neutrophil to leave the bone marrow (as found in WHIM) or increased neutrophil destruction 2. **NOBI by flow cytometry:** measures oxidative burst of neutrophils, sensitive test for CGD	1. **Adhesion antigens (CD11/CD18) by flow cytometry:** examines presence of adhesion molecules that allow neutrophil to migrate to the site of infection (decreased or absent in LAD type I)
Suspected complement deficiency		1. **Total hemolytic complement for classical pathway (CH50) and alternate pathway (AH50):** if abnormal, demonstrates inability of complement system to lyse at least 50% of presented cells, suggesting deficiency of a complement protein in the pathway
Miscellaneous tests	1. **AFP:** embryonically derived protein, elevated in AT	1. **NK cell cytotoxicity:** looks at the ability of NK cells to respond to stimulation

Table 22.1 **Specific Tests for Suspected Immunodeficiencies—cont'd**

ADA, Adenosine deaminase; *AFP,* alpha-fetoprotein; *AT,* ataxia telangiectasia; *CGD,* chronic granulomatous disease; *CID,* combined immunodeficiency; *LAD,* leukocyte adhesion deficiency; *NK,* natural killer; *NOBI,* neutrophil oxidative burst index; *PID,* primary immunodeficiency; *PNP,* purine nucleoside phosphorylase; *SCID,* severe combined immunodeficiency; *TREC,* T-cell receptor excision circles; *WHIM,* warts, hypogammaglobulinemia, immunodeficiency, and myelokathexis.

1. **Consider immunodeficiency if two or more "red flags" are present** (Box 22.1)
   a. May display various forms of immune dysfunction, including autoimmunity, exaggerated or abnormal inflammatory response, malignant predisposition
   b. May have multiorgan involvement

Box 22.1   Immunodeficiency "Red Flags"

Consider the diagnosis of an immunodeficiency if two or more of the criteria below are met:
1. Four or more new ear infections in 1 year
2. Two or more serious sinus infections in 1 year
3. Two or more months on antibiotics with little effect
4. Two or more pneumonias within 1 year
5. Failure of infant to gain weight or grow normally
6. Recurrent deep skin or organ abscesses
7. Persistent oral thrush or fungal skin infection
8. Need for intravenous antibiotics to clear infections
9. Two or more deep-seated infections, including septicemia
10. A family history of primary immunodeficiency

Data from Jeffrey Modell Foundation, 10 Warning Signs of Primary Immunodeficiency.

---

2. **History**
   a. **Characterize the infections:** age at onset of infections, type of infection(s), presenting features and illness severity, frequency of infections, total number of infections, causative pathogen(s) (if identified), treatment and response to therapy—antibiotics (oral vs. intravenous), antivirals, antifungals
   b. **Pregnancy, delivery, and neonatal history**
   c. **Past medical history:** genetic diagnoses, autoimmunity, cardiac defects, chronic lung disease/bronchiectasis, malignancy, development
   d. **Immunizations**
   e. **Family history:** parental ethnicity, consanguinity, recurrent or severe infections, neonatal or childhood deaths, frequent hospital admissions, autoimmunity, malignancy
3. **Signs and symptoms**
   a. **Growth:** failure to thrive
   b. **Gastrointestinal:** feeding intolerance, recurrent ulcers, diarrhea, malabsorption
   c. **Integument:** skin rashes, poor wound healing, abnormal hair, nails and/or teeth, heat intolerance/poor sweating
   d. **Musculoskeletal:** skeletal deformities

4. **Physical examination:** see Figure 22.1

Figure 22.1 Physical Examination for Immunodeficiency

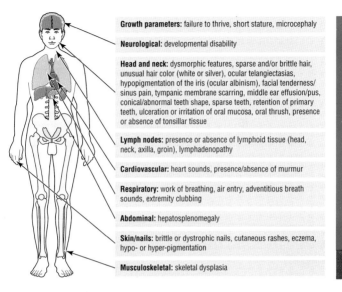

Growth parameters: failure to thrive, short stature, microcephaly

Neurological: developmental disability

Head and neck: dysmorphic features, sparse and/or brittle hair, unusual hair color (white or silver), ocular telangiectasias, hypopigmentation of the iris (ocular albinism), facial tenderness/sinus pain, tympanic membrane scarring, middle ear effusion/pus, conical/abnormal teeth shape, sparse teeth, retention of primary teeth, ulceration or irritation of oral mucosa, oral thrush, presence or absence of tonsillar tissue

Lymph nodes: presence or absence of lymphoid tissue (head, neck, axilla, groin), lymphadenopathy

Cardiovascular: heart sounds, presence/absence of murmur

Respiratory: work of breathing, air entry, adventitious breath sounds, extremity clubbing

Abdominal: hepatosplenomegaly

Skin/nails: brittle or dystrophic nails, cutaneous rashes, eczema, hypo- or hyper-pigmentation

Musculoskeletal: skeletal dysplasia

Immunology

22

PRIMARY IMMUNODEFICIENCIES

1. **Definition:** genetic defects in one or more components of the immune system
2. **Innate immunity**
   a. Activated minutes to hours following antigen exposure
   b. Uses pattern recognition that identify and mount a reaction against pathogens
   c. Components include
      i. Phagocytes (macrophages, neutrophils), which engulf and eliminate pathogens
      ii. NK cells, which act against cells affected by viruses or tumors
      iii. Complement proteins, which induce an inflammatory response and render antigens more susceptible to phagocytosis
   d. Characterized by low antigen specificity and no immunologic memory

3. **Adaptive immunity**
   a. Activated in an antigen-specific manner, resulting in a longer onset of action following antigen exposure (days)
   b. Primary cells
      i. T-cells—cellular-mediated responses
      ii. B-cells—humoral (antibody)-mediated responses
   c. Intact T-cell function is required for costimulatory B-cell activation and antibody production
   d. Has immunologic memory, resulting in faster and more robust reaction upon future exposure to the same antigen
4. **Classification:** primary immunodeficiencies (PIDs) can be classified as
   a. Affecting cellular and humoral immunity
   b. Predominantly antibody deficiencies
   c. Immune dysregulatory disorders
   d. Phagocyte defects
   e. Complement deficiencies
   f. Defects in innate immunity other than phagocyte and complement
   g. Autoinflammatory disorders

IMMUNODEFICIENCIES AFFECTING CELLULAR AND HUMORAL IMMUNITY

1. Primarily from T-cell dysfunction, leading to aberrant B-cell response
   a. Classified as either SCID or the less severe combined immunodeficiency (CID)
   b. T-cell defects typically begin to manifest in infancy or early childhood with recurrent opportunistic, viral, and fungal infections. Severity depends on extent of defect. May have failure to thrive, protracted diarrhea, persistent oral candidiasis, viral or PJP pneumonitis.
   c. B-cell defects typically begin to manifest once maternal antibodies are no longer present (approximately 6 months of age), with recurrent sinopulmonary infections (pneumonia, otitis media, sinusitis) from encapsulated organisms
2. See Table 22.2 for selected SCID
3. See Table 22.3 for selected CID

Table 22.2	Severe Combined Immunodeficiencies		
Clinical Manifestations	**Laboratory Features**	**Treatment**	**Complications**
Severe Combined Immunodeficiency (SCID)			
1. Recurrent, severe and opportunistic infections, candidiasis/oral thrush, intractable diarrhea, and failure to thrive since early infancy 2. Infections often poorly responsive to oral antimicrobials 3. Asymptomatic patients can be identified via newborn screen	**CBC:** lymphopenia **Quantitation by flow cytometry:** ↓ T-cell numbers. B-cell and NK-cell numbers ↓ or normal. **In vitro T-cell proliferative responses to mitogens and antigens:** absent **T-cell repertoire analysis:** decreased diversity **Chest x-ray:** absent thymic shadow	1. HSCT 2. Before transplant: PJP prophylaxis, Ig replacement, avoid live vaccines 3. Keep isolated 4. Discontinue breastfeeding if CMV-positive mother 5. Use irradiated and CMV-negative blood products	1. High mortality if untreated within 1st year of life 2. Toxicity from HSCT conditioning regimens 3. GvHD following transplant 4. Hematologic malignancies, both before and after HSCT
Omenn Syndrome			
1. Similar to SCID. May also have features of T-cell infiltration, including severe erythroderma and desquamating skin rash, lymphadenopathy, hepatosplenomegaly, diarrhea.	**CBC:** normal or ↑ total lymphocyte count. Eosinophilia may be seen. **Quantitation by flow cytometry:** ↑ T-cell numbers, B- and NK-cell numbers vary **T-cell repertoire analysis:** expansion (proliferation) of a single or small number of clones, which are typically self-reactive	1. Similar to classic SCID but may also require immunosuppressive therapy to treat uncontrolled T-cell proliferation	1. Similar to classic SCID

CBC, Complete blood count; *CMV*, cytomegalovirus; *GvHD*, graft-vs-host disease; *HSCT*, hematopoietic stem cell transplant; Ig, immunoglobulin; *NK*, natural killer; *PJP*, *Pneumocystis jirovecii*.

✦ PEARL

Recurrent sinopulmonary infections (ear, lungs, sinuses)—think humoral immunodeficiency. Infant with viral, fungal, invasive, or opportunistic infections—think T-cell or combined immunodeficiency.

Table 22.3 Combined Immunodeficiencies

Clinical Manifestations	Laboratory Features	Treatment	Complications
22q11.2 Deletion (Digeorge Syndrome [DGS])			
1. Conotruncal cardiac anomalies 2. Cleft palate and facial dysmorphism 3. Thymic hypoplasia (abnormal T-cell production) 4. Hypoparathyroidism, causing hypocalcemia 5. Range of immunodeficiency depends on the degree of thymic disruption	**Calcium:** hypocalcemia depending on hypoparathyroidism **Immunoglobulins:** ↓ or normal IgG/IgA **Quantitation by flow cytometry:** ↓ T-cell numbers (may improve over time), normal B-cell numbers **T-cell proliferation assay:** usually normal **TREC screen:** may be abnormal	**Complete DGS:** HSCT or thymic transplant **Partial DGS:** often require no treatment 1. Ig replacement and prophylactic antibiotics (in some) 2. Avoid live vaccines until cleared by Immunology 3. Calcium and activated Vitamin D supplementation (if hypocalcemic)	1. Increased incidence of autoimmunity, atopic disease, behavioral concerns, learning disabilities, schizophrenia
Ataxia Telangiectasia (AT)			
1. Prone to sinopulmonary infections 2. Progressive cerebellar ataxia develops by the second year of life 3. Other neurologic symptoms include oculomotor apraxia, dysarthria, dysphagia 4. Oculocutaneous telangiectasias start appearing at age 3–5 years 5. Cafe-au-lait spots and skin nevi are common	**AFP:** ↑ **CBC:** ↓ or normal lymphocytes **Immunoglobulins:** ↓ IgG/IgA (sometimes) **Quantitation by flow cytometry:** ↓ T-cell numbers, normal B-cell numbers **T-cell proliferative responses:** ↓ **Specific antibody responses:** ↓ (sometimes) **TREC:** ↓ (sometimes)	1. Prophylactic antibiotics and/or Ig replacement 2. Radiation sensitive—avoid ionizing radiation if possible 3. No curative treatment available, HSCT contraindicated	1. Growth retardation 2. Diabetes mellitus because of insulin resistance 3. Radiation sensitivity 4. Progressive pulmonary disease 5. Risk of aspiration because of progressive oropharyngeal dysphagia 6. Increased risk of malignancy

1. Recurrent bacterial infections—soft tissue and deep-seated "cold" abscesses (*Staphylococcus aureus* common), sinopulmonary infections, fungal infections 2. Lung pneumatoceles 3. Coarse facial features, delayed primary teeth shedding, severe eczema, fractures, scoliosis, joint hypermobility, coronary artery aneurysms	**CBC:** eosinophilia **Immunoglobulins:** ↑ IgE, ↓ or normal IgG **Antibody response to protein and polysaccharide vaccines:** normal or ↓ **Quantitation by flow cytometry:** T- and B-cell counts normal, ↓ Th17 subset **NOBI:** normal	1. Antibiotic prophylaxis against *S. aureus* 2. Skin hygiene to prevent infections 3. May require fungal prophylaxis 4. Close follow-up of lung pneumatoceles 5. May require Ig replacement	1. Pneumatoceles may become superinfected or bleed 2. Vascular damage may result in myocardial infarction because of coronary aneurysms and ruptured intracranial aneurysms 3. Lymphoma

Wiskott-Aldrich Syndrome (WAS)

1. Recurrent sinopulmonary and invasive infections with encapsulated bacteria, viral and opportunistic infections 2. Thrombocytopenia 3. Eczema 4. Autoimmune manifestations (hemolytic anemia, vasculitis, colitis, nephritis)	**CBC:** thrombocytopenia with small platelets **Immunoglobulins:** ↓ or normal IgG/IgM, ↑ IgA/IgE **Quantitation by flow cytometry:** B- and T- cell counts initially normal in infancy then decrease, NK counts usually normal **NK cell cytotoxicity:** ↓ **Antibody response:** impaired to some vaccines **T-cell proliferative responses:** ↓	**Supportive:** prophylactic antimicrobials for opportunistic infections, Ig replacement, platelet transfusions, immunosuppression for autoimmune manifestations **Curative:** HSCT	1. Life-threatening hemorrhages because of thrombocytopenia 2. Increased risk of malignancy (B-cell lymphoma most common)

AFP, Alpha-fetoprotein; *HSCT*, hematopoietic stem cell transplant; *Ig*, immunoglobulin; *NK*, natural killer; *NOBI*, neutrophil oxidative burst index; *Th*, t-helper; *TREC*, T-cell receptor excision circles.

PREDOMINANTLY ANTIBODY DEFICIENCY DISORDERS

1. Primarily affect B-cell formation, maturation and/or immunoglobulin production
   a. Typically, later onset (later childhood to adulthood) and less severe compared with T-cell defects
   b. Associated with sinopulmonary infections, chronic gastrointestinal (GI) symptoms, malabsorption, mycoplasma arthritis, enteroviral meningoencephalitis
   c. Can have increased risk of autoimmunity and malignancy
2. See Table 22.4 for selected antibody deficiency disorders

Table 22.4	Predominantly Antibody Deficiency Disorders		
Clinical Manifestations	**Laboratory Features**	**Treatment**	**Complications**
X-Linked Agammaglobulinemia (XLA)			
1. Present after maternal antibodies wane (3–6 months of age) 2. Sinopulmonary infections caused by encapsulated bacteria. Infections from Enteroviruses, *Salmonella, Campylobacter,* and *Helicobacter.* 3. Tonsils and lymph nodes usually absent	**CBC:** ↓ or normal lymphocytes **Immunoglobulins:** ↓ IgG/IgA/IgM **Quantitation by flow cytometry:** mature B-cells ↓ or absent, normal T-cell numbers **Antibody responses to protein and polysaccharide vaccines:** ↓↓ **T-cell proliferation:** normal	1. Ig replacement	1. Chronic lung disease/ bronchiectasis (if recurrent chest infections)
Common Variable Immunodeficiency (CVID)			
1. Usually present between the second and third decade of life 2. Sinopulmonary or other invasive infections 3. Autoimmune disorders (hemolytic/pernicious anemia, thrombocytopenia, arthritis, thyroiditis)	**CBC:** autoimmune cytopenias (anemia, thrombocytopenia) **Immunoglobulins:** ↓ IgG, ↓ levels of IgA ± IgM **Quantitation by flow cytometry:** normal B-cell counts **Antibody responses to protein and polysaccharide vaccines:** ↓↓	1. Ig replacement 2. Antibiotic prophylaxis if ongoing respiratory infections 3. Immunosuppression for autoimmune manifestations	1. Systemic complications include chronic lung disease/ bronchiectasis, infiltrative granulomatous disease 2. Autoimmune manifestations 3. Increased risk of malignancy (B-cell lymphoma)

Table 22.4   Predominantly Antibody Deficiency Disorders—cont'd

Clinical Manifestations	Laboratory Features	Treatment	Complications
Selective IgA Deficiency (SIGAD)			
1. Most are asymptomatic, picked up incidentally 2. May develop recurrent sinopulmonary infections, gastrointestinal disorders (giardiasis, IBD, celiac disease), autoimmune disorders, atopic disease, anaphylaxis to plasma-containing blood products	**Immunoglobulins:** ↓ IgA levels, normal IgG/IgM **Quantitation by flow cytometry:** normal B- and T-cell counts **Antibody responses to vaccines:** normal	1. Asymptomatic: no treatment 2. Immunosuppressive agents for autoimmune manifestations 3. Ig replacement not indicated 4. If history of anaphylaxis to blood product, test for anti-IgA antibodies (if present, minimize blood product transfusions, premedicate with steroids, antihistamines)	1. Symptomatic individuals should be retested periodically to ensure they have not developed CVID NOTE: When testing for specific IgA antibodies, such as anti-tissue transglutaminase IgA in suspected celiac disease, results will be falsely negative
Transient Hypogammaglobulinemia of Infancy (THI)			
1. Most are asymptomatic and may be picked up incidentally 2. If symptomatic, may have sinopulmonary infections	**Immunoglobulins:** ↓ IgG levels with or without a decrease in IgA/IgM levels **Quantitation by flow cytometry:** B- and T-cell counts normal **Vaccine responses:** typically normal Repeat above tests, especially in symptomatic patients, to exclude other PIDs	1. Most do not require treatment 2. Antibiotic prophylaxis if recurrent infections 3. Ig replacement typically not required	1. Spontaneous resolution of infections usually by early childhood 2. IgG level typically normalizes by 2–4 years of age

CBC, Complete blood count; *IBD,* inflammatory bowel disease; *PIDs,* primary immunodeficiency.

IMMUNE DYSREGULATORY DISORDERS

1. Robust inflammatory, autoimmune, or infiltrative manifestations, with or without infectious susceptibility
2. See Table 22.5 for selected immune dysregulatory disorders

Table 22.5 Immune Dysregulatory Disorders

Clinical Manifestations	Laboratory Features	Treatment	Complications
Chediak-Higashi Syndrome (CHS)			
1. Present in infancy or early childhood with oculocutaneous albinism, recurrent pyogenic infections, soft tissues abscesses, bacterial pneumonias, gingival/oral ulcers 2. May have mild bleeding/bruising 3. After childhood, development of severe progressive neurologic abnormalities (neuropathy, ataxia, tremors, cranial nerve palsies, intellectual decline, seizures)	**CBC:** neutropenia **Quantitation by flow cytometry:** NK-, B-, and T-cell counts normal **NK cell cytotoxicity assay:** diminished, B-cells usually normal in number and function **Platelet aggregation:** abnormal	1. Aggressive treatment of infections, prophylactic antibiotics, G-CSF for neutropenia 2. Treatment of HLH 3. HSCT may prevent infections but not neurologic deterioration	1. Most patients eventually enter "accelerated" phase, often triggered by EBV infection (HLH-like features—fever, hepatosplenomegaly, lymphadenopathy, pancytopenia, hemophagocytosis)
Immune Dysregulation Polyendocrinopathy Enteropathy X-Linked (IPEX)			
1. Present in infancy with refractory diarrhea because of autoimmune enteropathy, severe dermatitis, autoimmune endocrinopathies (neonatal type I diabetes mellitus or thyroiditis) 2. May have cytopenias, nephritis, severe atopy, invasive infections	**CBC:** autoimmune cytopenias, eosinophilia **Immunoglobulins:** ↑ IgE **Quantitation by flow cytometry:** total T-, B-, and NK-cell counts are typically normal, Tregs (CD4+CD25+Foxp3+) absent **T-cell proliferation:** normal **Vaccine responses:** normal	1. Supportive nutritional care 2. Treatment of autoimmunity with immunosuppressive agents 3. HSCT may be considered, autoimmunity may persist following transplant	1. Failure to thrive from severe enteropathy, recurrent infections, food allergies 2. Periods of bowel rest may be required 3. Prolonged use of immunosuppression may have adverse effects

Autoimmune Polyendocrinopathy with Candidiasis and Ectodermal Dystrophy (APECED)

1. Wide clinical variability, presentation ranging from early infancy to adulthood
2. Classic triad includes candidiasis, hypoparathyroidism, adrenal insufficiency
3. Other endocrinopathies and autoimmune features less common

Quantitation by flow cytometry: total T-, B-, and NK-cell counts normal

T-cell proliferation responses: may be abnormal to fungal antigens

Vaccine responses: may show inadequate antibody response to polysaccharide vaccines because of acquired asplenia

Other: features of endocrinopathies and autoimmunity

1. Treat fungal infections, some may require antifungal prophylaxis
2. Treat endocrinopathies
3. Autoimmune manifestations may require immunosuppressive therapy

1. Autoimmune fulminant necrotizing hepatitis, obstructive lung disease, interstitial nephritis
2. If long-lasting oral candidiasis, increased risk of esophageal squamous cell carcinoma

Autoimmune Lymphoproliferative Syndrome (ALPS)

1. Symptom onset typically between 2 and 5 years
2. Clinical manifestations include chronic lymphoproliferation (lymphadenopathy, hepatosplenomegaly), autoimmune cytopenias (Coombs-positive hemolytic anemia, thrombocytopenia)
3. Autoimmune features, including glomerulonephritis, hepatitis, uveitis
4. Skin manifestations (urticaria, eczema)

CBC: anemia, thrombocytopenia, neutropenia

Quantitation by flow cytometry: T-, B-, NK-cell numbers and function typically normal, double-negative T-cells (CD4-/CD8-) greater than 2.5% of CD3+ T-cells

Other: elevated levels of vitamin B12

1. Management of autoimmunity with immunosuppression
2. HSCT may be offered to patients with homozygous Fas mutations

1. Increased risk of malignancy (lymphoma)
2. Prone to complications from prolonged immunosuppressive therapy

CBC, Complete blood count; *EBV,* Epstein-Barr virus; *G-CSF,* granulocyte colony-stimulating factor; *HLH,* hemophagocytic lymphohistiocytosis; *HSCT,* hematopoietic stem cell transplant; *Ig,* immunoglobulin; *NK,* natural killer; *Tregs,* T-regulatory cells.

Immunology

22

PHAGOCYTE DEFECTS

1. Present as recurrent skin and respiratory tract infections because of either bacteria or fungi (especially *Candida* and *Aspergillus*)
2. Phagocyte defects caused by decreased production, impairments of chemotaxis/mobilization, dysfunction of the phagocytes' ability to kill pathogens, which manifests as poor wound healing, abscesses, ulcers
3. See Table 22.6 for selected phagocyte defect disorders

> **! PITFALL**
>
> Infant with incidental neutropenia? Do not assume viral suppression or benign neutropenia of childhood. Repeat a CBC periodically to ensure they do not have an immunodeficiency.

Table 22.6 Phagocyte Defects

Clinical Manifestations	Laboratory Features	Treatment	Complications
Chronic Granulomatous Disease (CGD)			
1. Recurrent fungal and bacterial infections (pneumonia, skin abscess, lymphadenitis, liver abscess, osteomyelitis) 2. Caused by catalase-positive microorganisms (especially *Staphylococcus aureus, Burkholderia cepacia, Serratia, Nocardia, Aspergillus*) 3. Abnormal wound healing, diarrhea, infected dermatitis, autoimmunity 4. Growth failure, hepatomegaly, splenomegaly, lymphadenopathy	**CBC:** typically normal **NOBI:** ↓↓	1. Daily antimicrobial prophylaxis against *S. aureus* and *Aspergillus* 2. Prompt aggressive treatment of infections 3. Immune suppression for management of inflammatory sequelae (colitis or granulomata) 4. Avoid all live bacterial vaccines and probiotics 5. HSCT as a curative option	1. Granulomata of various organs 2. Gastrointestinal complications (colitis, proctitis, strictures, fistulae, obstruction) 3. Growth failure 4. Chronic pulmonary disease 5. Autoimmune disorders (SLE, JIA, ITP)
Leukocyte Adhesion Deficiency (LAD)			
1. Delayed (>4 weeks) separation of the umbilical cord (often accompanied with acute omphalitis) 2. Recurrent serious bacterial infections 3. Poor wound healing, lack of pus 4. Periodontitis later in life	**CBC:** neutrophilia **Quantitation by flow cytometry:** normal B- and T-cell numbers. In LAD1, reduced expression of CD18.	1. Avoid live vaccines 2. Consider antimicrobial prophylaxis 3. Mild-to-moderate disease: antibiotic therapy 4. Severe disease: HSCT	1. Resulting complications from poor wound healing

Table 22.6 Phagocyte Defects—cont'd

Clinical Manifestations	Laboratory Features	Treatment	Complications
Severe Chronic Neutropenia			
1. Fever and malaise 2. Common infections include: pharyngitis with lymphadenopathy, pneumonia, mastoiditis, cellulitis 3. Periodontitis with oral ulceration and gingivitis 4. Vaginal and rectal mucosal ulcers 5. Cyclic neutropenia (milder form) presents with less severe infections	**CBC:** ANC (neutrophils and bands) $<0.5 \times 10^9$/L Serial neutrophil measurements to distinguish between cyclic and chronic neutropenia. Obtain CBC 2–3 times weekly for 6–8 weeks. Periodicity of cyclic neutropenia is about 21 days (range 14–36 days)	1. Avoid all live bacterial vaccines 2. G-CSF 3. Antimicrobial prophylaxis 4. Consider HSCT if no response to G-CSF or if severe infections continue despite increased counts 5. Symptoms tend to decrease in severity with age	1. Infections occur only during the nadirs of the neutrophil count (lag between nadir and the onset of clinical symptoms)

ANC, Absolute neutrophil count; *CBC*, complete blood count; *G-CSF*, granulocyte colony-stimulating factor; *HSCT*, hematopoietic stem cell transplant; *ITP*, immune thrombocytopenia; *JIA*, juvenile idiopathic arthritis; *LAD*, leukocyte adhesion deficiency; *NOBI*, neutrophil oxidative burst index, *SLE*, systemic lupus erythematosus.

Immunology

22

COMPLEMENT DEFICIENCIES

1. Complement system is responsible for control of bacterial infection and clearance of immune complexes generated during immune responses
2. Present with recurrent bacterial infections from *Neisseria* organisms, pneumococcus (meningitis, arthritis, septicemia, recurrent sinopulmonary infections)
3. Complement levels can also be low because of consumption from infection or autoimmune disease
4. See Table 22.7 for description of complement deficiency

Table 22.7	Complement Deficiency		
Clinical Manifestations	**Laboratory Features**	**Treatment**	**Complications**
Complement Deficiency			
1. Deficiency in **early** complement pathway components: SLE-like syndrome, rheumatoid disease, multiple autoimmune diseases, infections 2. Deficiency in **late** complement pathway components: Neisserial infections, SLE-like syndrome	**Quantitation by flow cytometry:** normal T- and B-cell numbers **Vaccine responses:** normal **Low CH50 only:** Deficiency in classical complement pathway components: C1q, C1r, C2, C4 **Low AH50 only:** Deficiency in alternate complement pathway components: factor B, factor D or properidin **Both CH50 and AH50 are low:** Deficiency in shared components (late complement pathway): C5, C6, C7, C8, C9	1. Immunizations (including live viral and bacterial vaccines) 2. Antibiotic therapy 3. Meningococcal and pneumococcal vaccines	1. Recurrent infections

SLE, Systemic lupus erythematosus.

DEFECTS IN INNATE IMMUNITY (OTHER THAN PHAGOCYTES AND COMPLEMENT)

1. Result from dysfunction of the signaling pathways that recognize common patterns on pathogens and/or the cells involved in mounting an immune response
2. Signalling may be appropriate to attract innate immune cells, such as neutrophils or NK cells, but the cells themselves are unable to phagocytose
3. See Table 22.8 for selected disorders of the innate immune system

Table 22.8	Defects in Innate Immunity (other than phagocytes and complement)		
Clinical Manifestations	**Laboratory Features**	**Treatment**	**Complications**
Warts, Hypogammaglobulinemia, Infections, and Myelokathexis (WHIM) Syndrome			
1. Susceptibility to HPV-induced warts 2. Recurrent bacterial sinopulmonary infections with encapsulated organisms 3. Skin abscesses and periodontitis because of neutropenia (retained in bone marrow)	**CBC:** leukopenia primarily because of neutropenia (ANC [neutrophils and bands] <0.5 × 10⁹/L) **Immunoglobulins:** ↓ IgG **Vaccine responses:** initially normal, but tend to wane over time **Neutrophil function:** normal	1. Ig replacement if low immunoglobulin levels and poor vaccine responses	1. Treat refractory warts 2. Increased risk of congenital cardiac manifestations 3. Increased risk of malignancy
Chronic Mucocutaneous Candidiasis (CMCC)			
1. Noninvasive recurrent infections of the skin, nails, and mucosa by *Candida albicans* 2. Autoimmune manifestations (commonly endocrinopathies)	**Quantitation by flow cytometry:** normal T- and B-cell number, ↓ Th17 numbers, ↓ or normal NK-cell numbers **T-cell proliferation responses:** defective cutaneous or in vitro T-cell response to *Candida* species. **NK-cell cytotoxicity:** ↓ or normal	1. Prolonged treatment with antifungal agents 2. Treat associated endocrine or autoimmune abnormalities	1. Fungal infections 2. Esophageal complications from recurrent fungal candidiasis

ANC, Absolute neutrophil count; *CBC,* complete blood count; *HPV,* human papilloma virus; *Ig,* immunoglobulin; *NK,* natural killer; *Th,* T-helper.

AUTOINFLAMMATORY DISORDERS

1. Overactivation of the innate system, marked by excessive inflammation
2. Characteristics include episodic fever and other systemic manifestations resulting from inflammatory tissue injury
3. Inflammasome-related disorders (e.g., Familial Mediterranean fever, Muckle-Wells syndrome) or noninflammasome-related disorders (e.g., tumor necrosis factor [TNF]-receptor associated periodic syndrome, Blau syndrome)
4. See Autoinflammatory Syndromes in Chapter 36 Rheumatology

1. **Causes of secondary immunodeficiency**
   a. **Infections:** human immunodeficiency virus (HIV), Epstein-Barr virus (EBV), cytomegalovirus (CMV), varicella zoster virus (VZV), herpes simplex virus (HSV)-1, mycobacteria, severe bacterial infections
   b. **Nutritional deficiencies:** malnutrition secondary to protein, calories, vitamin, or mineral deficiency
   c. **Protein-losing states:** nephrotic syndrome, hepatic failure/cirrhosis, protein-losing enteropathy, intestinal lymphangiectasia
   d. **Malignancy**
   e. **Immune-modulating/immunosuppressive agents:** corticosteroids, chemotherapy, myeloablative agents, biologics
   f. **Adverse drug reactions:** anticonvulsants, sulfonamides, hydroxyurea
   g. **Asplenia/functional asplenia:** right/left atrial isomerism, sickle cell disease, post-splenectomy
   h. **Metabolic disorders:** galactosemia
   i. **Autoimmune/inflammatory diseases:** systemic lupus erythematosus (SLE), sarcoidosis
   j. **Loss of skin barrier:** burns, trauma
   k. **Toxic environmental exposures:** radiation, chemical exposure
   l. **Prematurity**

2. **Management of secondary immunodeficiency**
   a. Correction, to the extent possible, of the underlying cause
   b. Encapsulated organism prophylaxis in patients with asplenia (physical or functional)
   c. PJP prophylaxis in individuals with malignancies undergoing chemotherapy or in those with HIV
   d. Infectious precautions in patients with extensive burns
   e. Screening for and treatment of tuberculosis before administration of biologics
   f. Avoid probiotics
   g. Consider Immunology consultation

Immunoprophylaxis

Ana C. Blanchard • Shama Sud • Shaun K. Morris

Also see page xviii for a list of other abbreviations used throughout this book

anti-HBs	hepatitis B surface antibody
BCG	Bacille Calmette-Guérin vaccine
CHD	congenital heart disease
CLD	chronic lung disease
CMV	cytomegalovirus
DTaP-IPV	diphtheria, tetanus, acellular pertussis, and inactivated polio vaccine
GBS	Guillain-Barré syndrome
HAV	hepatitis A virus
HB	hepatitis B virus vaccine
HBIg	hepatitis B immune globulin
HBsAg	hepatitis B surface antigen
HBV	hepatitis B virus
HCV	hepatitis C virus
Hib	*Haemophilus influenzae* type B
HIV	human immunodeficiency virus
HPV	human papillomavirus
HTLV	human T-lymphotropic virus
ID	intradermal
IMD	invasive meningococcal disease
Ig	immune globulin
IM	intramuscular
IVIg	intravenous immunoglobulin
LAIV	live attenuated influenza vaccine
Men-C-ACYW	meningococcal conjugate A, C, Y, W vaccine
Men-C-ACYW-CRM	Menveo
Men-C-ACYW-DT	Menactra
Men-C-ACYW-TT	Nimenrix
4CMenB	Bexsero
MenB-fHBP	Trumenba®
Men-C-C	meningococcal conjugate C vaccine
MMR	measles, mumps, and rubella, vaccine
MMRV	measles, mumps, rubella, and varicella vaccine
OPV	oral poliovirus vaccine
PCV-13	pneumococcal-13-valent conjugate vaccine
PEP	post-exposure prophylaxis
PPV23	pneumococcal 23-valent polysaccharide vaccine
RIg	rabies immune globulin
RSV	respiratory syncytial virus
SC	subcutaneous
Tdap	tetanus, diphtheria, acellular pertussis vaccine
TIg	tetanus immune globulin
VAR	varicella vaccine
VarIg	varicella zoster immune globulin

IMMUNIZATIONS

1. See Tables 23.1, 23.2, and 23.3 for routine immunization schedules in Canada

Table 23.1	Routine Childhood Immunization Schedule, Infants and Children (Birth–17 Years of Age)																			
									AGE											
Vaccine	Birth	2 Months	4 Months	6 Months	12 Months	15 Months	18 Months	23 Months	2 Years	4 Years	5 Years	6 Years	9 Years	12 Years	14 Years	15 Years	16 Years	17 Years
DTaP-IPV-Hib or DTaP-HB-IPV-Hib	—	A or B first dose	A or B second dose	A or B third dose	A or fourth dose Generally at 18 months of age				—									
DTaP-IPV or Tdap-IPV	—	—	—	—	—	F			—	C		—						
Tdap	—	—	—	—	—				—	—	—	—	—	—	D	—	—	—
Rot	—	E 2 or 3 doses Complete series before 8 months																
Pneu-C-13	—	F According to regional schedule	F	F														
Men-C-C	—	G	G	Generally at 12 months	G													

Continued

Table 23.1 Routine Childhood Immunization Schedule, Infants and Children (Birth–17 Years of Age)—cont'd

Vaccine	Birth	2 Months	4 Months	6 Months	12 Months	15 Months	18 Months	23 Months	2 Years	4 Years	5 Years	6 Years	9 Years	12 Years	14 Years	15 Years	16 Years	17 Years
Men-C-C or Men-C-ACYW	—	—	—	—	—	—	—	—	—	—	—	—	—	H	—	—	—	—
MMR and Var or MMRV	—	—	—	—	I + J	I + J	—	—	I + J		—	—	—	—	—	—	—	—
						K			K — Generally at 4–6 years									
HB	—	L — 3 doses			—	—	—	—	—	—	—	—	—	—	—	—	—	—
or HB	—	—	—	—	—	—	—	—	—	—	—	—	—	—	—	—	—	—
HPV	—	—	—	—	—	—	—	—	—	—	—	—	N — 2 or 3 doses		—	—	—	—
or HPV	—	—	—	—	—	—	—	—	—	—	—	—		M — 2 or 3 doses			P — 3 doses	—
Inf	—	—	—	—	Q — 1 or 2 doses — Recommended annually						Q — 1 dose — Recommended annually							

A. **DTaP-IPV-Hib,** Diphtheria toxoid-tetanus toxoid-acellular pertussis-inactivated polio-*Haemophilus influenzae* type b: for infants and children beginning primary immunization at 7 months of age and older, the number of doses of Hib vaccine required varies by age.

B. **DTaP-HB-IPV-Hib,** Diphtheria toxoid-tetanus toxoid-acellular pertussis-hepatitis B-inactivated polio-*Haemophilus influenzae* type b: Alternative schedules may be used: DTaP-HB-IPV-Hib at 2, 4, and 12–23 months of age with DTaP-IPV-Hib vaccine at 6 months of age; or DTaP-HB-IPV-Hib at 2, 4, and 6 months of age with DTaP-IPV-Hib vaccine at 12–23 months of age.

C. **DTap-IPV,** Diphtheria toxoid-tetanus toxoid-acellular pertussis-inactivated polio or *Tdap-IPV,* tetanus toxoid-reduced diphtheria toxoid-reduced acellular pertussis-inactivated polio.

D. **Tdap,** Tetanus toxoid-reduced diphtheria toxoid-reduced acellular pertussis: 10 years after last dose of DTaP- or Tdap-containing vaccine.

E. **Rotavirus:** Rotavirus pentavalent vaccine: 3 doses, 4 to 10 weeks apart; Rotavirus monovalent vaccine: 2 doses, at least 4 weeks apart. Give the first dose starting at 6 weeks and before 15 weeks of age. Administer all doses before 8 months of age.

F. **Pneu-C-13, Pneumococcal conjugate 13-valent:** healthy infants beginning primary immunization at 2–6 months of age: 3 or 4 dose schedule. For a 3 dose schedule: 2, 4 months of age, followed by a booster dose at 12 months of age. For a 4 dose schedule: minimum of 8 weeks interval between doses beginning at 2 months of age, followed by a booster dose at 12–15 months of age. Healthy infants beginning primary immunization at 7–11 months of age: 2 doses, at least 8 weeks apart followed by a booster dose at 12–15 months of age, at least 8 weeks after the second dose. Children who have received age-appropriate pneumococcal vaccination with a pneumococcal conjugate vaccine but not Pneu-C-13 vaccine: 12–35 months of age: 1 dose; 36–59 months of age and of aboriginal origin or attend group childcare: 1 dose; other healthy children 36–59 months of age: consider 1 dose.

G. **Men-C-C, Meningococcal conjugate monovalent:** children 12–48 months of age: 1 dose routinely provided at 12 months of age, regardless of any doses given during the first year of life. Immunization may be considered for unimmunized children 5–11 years of age.

H. **Men-C-C, Meningococcal conjugate monovalent** or *Men-C-ACYW,* **meningococcal conjugate quadrivalent:** early adolescence (around 12 years of age): 1 dose, even if meningococcal conjugate vaccine received at a younger age. Vaccine chosen depends on local epidemiology and programmatic considerations.

I. *MMR,* Measles-mumps-rubella: first dose at 12–15 months of age; second dose at 18 months of age or anytime thereafter, but should be given no later than around school entry.

J. *Var,* Varicella (chickenpox): first dose at 12–15 months of age; second dose at 18 months of age or anytime thereafter, but should be given no later than around school entry.

Immunoprophylaxis

23

573

K. *MMR*, **Measles-mumps-rubella-varicella:** first dose at 12–15 months of age; second dose at 18 months of age or anytime thereafter, but should be given no later than around school entry.

L. *HB*, **Hepatitis B:** months 0, 1, and 6 (first dose = month 0) with at least 4 weeks between the first and second dose, at least 2 months between the second and third dose, and at least 4 months between the first and third dose. Alternatively, can be administered as DTaP-HB-IPV-Hib vaccine, with first dose at 2 months of age.

M. *HB*, **Hepatitis B:** 9–17 years of age: months 0, 1, and 6 (first dose = month 0) with at least 4 weeks between the first and second dose, at least 2 months between the second and third dose, and at least 4 months between the first and third dose; 11–15 years of age: 2 doses; schedule depends on the product used.

N. *HPV*, **Human papillomavirus:** Girls, 9–14 years of age: HPV bivalent (HPV2) or HPV quadrivalent (HPV4) vaccine or HPV nonavalent (HPV9) vaccine: months 0 and 6–12 (first dose = month 0). Alternatively, a 3 dose schedule may be used for HPV2 vaccine: months 0, 1, and 6 (first dose = month 0), for HPV4 vaccine: months 0, 2, and 6 (first dose = month 0), and HPV nonavalent (HPV9) vaccine: months 0, 2, and 6 (first dose = month 0). Boys, 9–14 years of age: HPV4 or HPV9 vaccine: months 0 and 6–12 (first dose = month 0). Alternatively, a 3 dose schedule may be used for HPV4 vaccine: months 0, 2, and 6 (first dose = month 0), and HPV9 vaccine: months 0, 2, and 6 (first dose = month 0). For a 2 or 3 dose schedule, the minimum interval between first and last doses is 6 months.

P. *HPV*, **Human papillomavirus:** Girls, 15–17 years of age: HPV2 vaccine: months 0, 1, and 6 (first dose = month 0), HPV4 vaccine: months 0, 2, and 6 (first dose = month 0) or HPV9 vaccine: months 0, 2, and 6 (first dose = month 0). Boys, 15–17 years of age: HPV4 vaccine: months 0, 2, and 6 (first dose = month 0) or HPV9 vaccine: months 0, 2, and 6 (first dose = month 0). In individuals who received the first dose of HPV2 or HPV4 or HPV9 vaccine between 9 and 14 years of age, a 2 dose schedule can be used with the second dose administered at least 6 months after the first dose.

Q. *Inf*, **Influenza:** recommended annually for anyone >6 months of age without contraindications. Children 6 months to <9 years of age, receiving influenza vaccine for the first time: 2 doses, at least 4 weeks apart. Children 6 months–8 years of age, previously immunized with influenza vaccine and children ≥9 years of age: 1 dose.

From Public Health Agency of Canada. *Canadian Immunization Guide: Part 1—Key Immunization Information*. Recommended immunization schedules: Canadian Immunization Guide, Table 1. © All rights reserved. Canadian Immunization Guide. Public Health Agency of Canada. Adapted and reproduced with permission from the Minister of Health, 2020.

	Table 23.2	**Routine Immunization Schedule for Children <7 Years of Age Not Immunized Before 12 Months of Age**					
		TIME AFTER FIRST VISIT					**6–12 Months After Last Dose**
Vaccine	**First Visit**	**4 Weeks**	**8 Weeks**	**3 Months**	**4 Months**	**6 Months**	
DTaP-IPV-Hib or DTaP-IPV	A	—	A	—	A	—	A [B]
Pneu-C-13	[C]	—	[C]	—	—	—	
Men-C-C	D	—	—	—	—	—	
MMR	E	E	—	—	—	—	
Var or MMRV	F	—	—	F	—	—	
	G	—	—	G	—	—	
HB	[H]	[H]	—	—	—	[H]	
Inf	I	I	—	—	—	—	

[ ] = dose(s) may not be required depending upon age of child or vaccine used or both

A. ***DTaP-IPV-Hib,*** **Diphtheria toxoid-tetanus toxoid-acellular pertussis-inactivated polio-*Haemophilus influenzae* type b or *DTaP-IPV,* diphtheria toxoid-tetanus toxoid-acellular pertussis-inactivated polio:** 4 doses of DTaP-IPV-containing vaccine. The number of doses of Hib-containing vaccine required varies by age at first dose. If first visit at 12–14 months of age: 1 dose of Hib-containing vaccine at first visit and booster dose at least 2 months after the previous dose. If first visit between 15–59 months of age: 1 dose of Hib-containing vaccine. If first visit at 60 months of age or older, Hib-containing vaccine is not required.

B. ***DTaP-IPV,*** **Diphtheria toxoid-tetanus toxoid-acellular pertussis-inactivated polio or *Tdap-IPV,* tetanus toxoid-reduced diphtheria toxoid-reduced acellular pertussis-inactivated polio:** if the fourth dose of DTaP-IPV vaccine was given before the fourth birthday, a booster dose of DTaP-IPV or Tdap-IPV vaccine should be provided at 4–6 years of age.

C. ***Pneu-C-13,*** **Pneumococcal conjugate 13-valent:** 12–23 months of age: 2 doses, at least 8 weeks apart; 24–59 months of age: 1 dose.

D. ***Men-C-C,*** **Meningococcal conjugate monovalent:** 12–59 months of age: 1 dose; 5–11 years of age: consider 1 dose.

E. ***MMR,*** **Measles-mumps-rubella:** 2 doses, at least 4 weeks apart; second dose after 18 months of age, but should be given no later than around school entry.

F. ***Var,*** **Varicella:** 2 doses, at least 3 months apart; second dose after 18 months of age, but should be given no later than around school entry. A minimum interval of 4 weeks between doses may be used if rapid, complete protection is required.

G. ***MMRV,*** **Measles-mumps-rubella-varicella:** 2 doses, at least 3 months apart; second dose after 18 months of age, but should be given no later than around school entry. A minimum interval of 4 weeks between doses may be used if rapid, complete protection is required.

H. ***HB,*** **Hepatitis B:** 3 doses: months 0, 1, and 6 (first dose = month 0) with at least 4 weeks between the first and second dose, 2 months between the second and third dose, and 4 months between the first and third dose.

I. ***Inf,*** **Influenza:** 2 doses, at least 4 weeks apart.

From Public Health Agency of Canada. *Canadian Immunization Guide: Part 1—Key Immunization Information.* Recommended immunization schedules: Canadian Immunization Guide, Table 2. © All rights reserved. Canadian Immunization Guide. Public Health Agency of Canada. Adapted and reproduced with permission from the Minister of Health, 2020.

Table 23.3	Routine Immunization Schedule for Children 7–17 Years of Age Not Previously Immunized						
		TIME AFTER FIRST VISIT				6–12 Months After Last Dose	10 Years After Last Dose
Vaccine	**First Visit**	**4 Weeks**	**8 Weeks**	**3 Months**	**6 Months**		
Tdap-IPV Tdap	A	—	A	—	—	A	B
Men-C-C	[C] 7–11 years of age	—	—	—	—	—	—
or Men-C-C or Men-C-ACYW	D 12–17 years of age	—	—	—	—	—	—
MMR	E	E	—	—	—	—	—
Var	F	—	—	—	F	—	—
or MMRV	G 7–12 years of age	—	—	G	—	—	—
HB	H	[H]	—	—	H	—	—
HPV	I 9–14 years of age	—	—	—	I	—	—
or HPV	I 9–14 years of age 3 doses					—	—
or HPV	J 15–17 years of age 3 doses					—	—
Inf	K 7–8 years of age	K	—	—	—	—	—
or Inf	K 9–17 years of age	—	—	—	—	—	—

A. *Tdap-IPV,* **Tetanus toxoid-reduced diphtheria toxoid-reduced acellular pertussis-inactivated polio:** 2 doses, 8 weeks apart; third dose 6–12 months after second dose.

B. *Tdap,* **Tetanus toxoid-reduced diphtheria toxoid-reduced acellular pertussis:** 10 years after last dose of Tdap-IPV.

C. *Men-C-C,* **Meningococcal conjugate monovalent:** 7–11 years of age: consider 1 dose.

D. *Men-C-C or Men-C-ACYW,* **Meningococcal conjugate monovalent or quadrivalent:** 12–17 years of age: 1 dose, even if meningococcal conjugate vaccine received at a younger age. Vaccine chosen depends on local epidemiology and programmatic considerations.

E. *MMR,* **Measles-mumps-rubella:** 2 doses, at least 4 weeks apart.

F. *Var,* **Varicella (chickenpox):** 7–12 years of age: 2 doses, at least 3 months apart. 13 years of age and older: 2 doses, at least 6 weeks apart. A minimum interval of 4 weeks between doses may be used if rapid, complete protection is required.

G. *MMRV,* **Measles-mumps-rubella-varicella:** 7–12 years of age: 2 doses, at least 3 months apart. A minimum interval of 4 weeks between doses may be used if rapid, complete protection is required.

H. *HB,* **Hepatitis B:** 7–17 years of age: 3 doses, months 0, 1, and 6 (first dose = month 0) with at least 4 weeks between the first and second dose, 2 months between the second and third dose, and 4 months between the first and third dose; 11–15 years of age: two doses; schedule depends on the product used.

I. *HPV,* **Human papillomavirus:** Girls, 9–14 years of age: HPV bivalent (HPV2) or HPV quadrivalent (HPV4) vaccine or HPV nonavalent (HPV9): months 0 and 6–12 (first dose = month 0). Alternatively, a 3 dose schedule may be used for HPV2 vaccine: months 0, 1, and 6 (first dose = month 0), for HPV4 vaccine: months 0, 2, and 6 (first dose = month 0), and for HPV nonavalent (HPV9) vaccine: months 0, 2, and 6 (first dose = month 0). Boys, 9–14 years of age HPV4 vaccine or HPV9: months 0 and 6–12 years (first dose = month 0). Alternatively, a 3 dose schedule may be used for HPV4 or HPV9 vaccine: months 0, 2, and 6 (first dose = month 0). For a 2 or 3 dose schedule, the minimum interval between first and last doses is 6 months.

J. *HPV,* **Human papillomavirus:** Girls, 15–17 years of age: HPV2 vaccine—months 0, 1, and 6 (first dose = month 0), HPV4 vaccine—months 0, 2, and 6 (first dose = month 0) or HPV9 vaccine: months 0, 2, and 6 (first dose = month 0). Boys, 15–17 years of age: HPV4 vaccine - months 0, 2, and 6 (first dose = month 0) or HPV9 vaccine—months 0, 2, and 6 (first dose = month 0). In individuals who received the first dose of HPV2 or HPV4 or HPV9 vaccine between 9 and 14 years of age, a 2 dose schedule can be used with the second dose administered at least 6 months after the first dose.

K. *Inf,* **Influenza:** children <9 years of age: 2 doses, at least 4 weeks apart. Children ≥9 years of age: 1 dose.

2. See Box 23.1 for conditions that are not contraindications to immunization
3. See Table 23.4 for immunization contraindications and considerations
4. Report through local public health officials any serious or unexpected adverse event felt to be temporally related to vaccination
5. Visit a travel health clinic for travel related vaccinations and prophylaxis recommendations

Box 23.1 Conditions That Are Not Contraindications to Immunization

1. Minor acute illness, regardless of fever
2. Neurological disorder
3. Prematurity
4. Immunocompromised (may usually receive inactivated vaccines)
5. Antimicrobial therapy, except live oral typhoid (delay until 48 h after last dose of antibiotics)
6. Tuberculin skin testing (TST)
   a. Although co-administration of live vaccines and TST is not contraindicated, TST should be implanted on the same day as live vaccines are administered, or TST implantation should be delayed for at least 28 days after live vaccine administration

Table 23.4 Immunization Contraindications and Considerations

| Conditions | TYPE OF VACCINE | | Comments |
	Inactivated	Live	
Anaphylaxis: after a previous dose of a vaccine	Contraindicated if receiving the same vaccine		
Anaphylaxis: proven immediate or anaphylactic hypersensitivity to any vaccine component or its container (e.g., latex)	Contraindicated if receiving vaccine containing the same component		Except for administration of influenza, MMR, or MMRV vaccines to egg-allergic persons
Asthma (on oral or inhaled high dose steroids, or active wheezing requiring medical attention)	No contraindication	LAIV contraindicated if severe asthma or recent exacerbation 7 days prior	Asthma control should be optimized before any vaccine
Congenital malformation of the gastrointestinal tract, uncorrected	No contraindication or precaution	Rotavirus vaccine contraindicated (increased risk of intussusception)	
Guillain-Barré syndrome (GBS) within 6 weeks of receiving a vaccine	In general, contraindicated if receiving the same vaccine		Balance risk of GBS associated with influenza vaccination vs. risk of GBS associated with influenza infection
Immunocompromised individuals because of underlying condition	In general, no contraindication	In general, contraindicated if severely immunocompromised	Referral to a physician with expertise in immunization and/or immunodeficiency

Table 23.4 | Immunization Contraindications and Considerations—cont'd

| Conditions | TYPE OF VACCINE | | Comments |
	Inactivated	Live	
Immunosuppressive therapy (e.g., chemotherapy, monoclonal antibodies)	No contraindication; may need to delay inactivated vaccines up to 3 months after completion of therapy	Contraindicated in most cases	Referral to a physician with expertise in immunization and/or immunodeficiency
Intussusception, past history	No contraindication or precaution	Rotavirus vaccine contraindicated	
Pregnancy	In general, no contraindications for routine vaccines	In general, contraindicated	
Tuberculosis, active	No contraindications for routine vaccines	Contraindicated: MMR, MMRV, varicella, herpes zoster and BCG vaccines	Referral to a physician with expertise in immunization and/or tuberculosis

BCG, Bacille Calmette-Guérin vaccine; *LAIV*, live attenuated influenza vaccine; *MMR*, measles, mumps, and rubella vaccine; *MMRV*, measles, mumps, rubella, and varicella vaccine.

Adapted from Public Health Agency of Canada. *Canadian Immunization Guide: Part 2—Contraindications, Precautions and Concerns.* Canadian Immunization Guide, Table 1.
Adapted from Public Health Agency of Canada. Canadian Immunization Guide: Part 2–Contraindications, precautions and concerns: Canadian Immunization Guide, Table 1. © All rights reserved. Canadian Immunization Guide. Public Health Agency of Canada. Adapted and reproduced with permission from the Minister of Health, 2020.

Immunoprophylaxis

23

SELECTED INFECTIONS AND PROPHYLAXIS

HEPATITIS A

Hepatitis A vaccine

1. **Typical dosing and administration:** 0.5 mL intramuscularly (IM) (check product monograph)
2. **Adverse reactions:** pain, induration at injection site, fever, headache
3. Complete vaccine series according to schedule (≥12 months) for long-term protection
4. Available for children >6 months of age who are traveling to endemic zones; a dose before 12 months of age should not count in the completion of primary vaccine series

Pre-exposure prophylaxis

1. Hepatitis A virus (HAV) vaccine, unless contraindicated, in those at increased risk of infection or severe HAV
   a. Travelers to endemic countries
   b. Residents of endemic areas or areas at risk of outbreaks
   c. Living in a household with someone at increased risk of infection or severe HAV
   d. Chronic liver disease (including idiopathic, metabolic, infectious [hepatitis C virus (HCV)] causes or cholestasis), recipients (or likely recipients) of hepatotoxic medications
   e. Hemophilia patients receiving plasma-derived replacement clotting factors
2. IM immune globulin (Ig) (see Table 39.10 Immune Globulins for dosing in travelers aged <6 months, HAV is contraindicated, or elect not to receive vaccine

Post-exposure prophylaxis

1. Healthy children aged >12 months who have been exposed to HAV within the prior 14 days and have not previously completed the 2-dose HAV vaccine series should receive a single dose of monovalent HAV vaccine (complete HAV vaccine series with a second dose at least 6 months after the first dose). Protection occurs within 2 weeks of immunization.
2. Use IMIg in infants <6 months if vaccine unavailable or if vaccine is contraindicated
3. If chronic liver disease or immunocompromised, within 14 days of exposure, use monovalent HAV vaccine and IMIg

HEPATITIS B

Hepatitis B vaccine

1. **Typical dosing and administration:** IM, see Table 23.5 for dosing and schedule
2. **Adverse reactions:** irritability, headache, fatigue, injection site reactions
3. Complete vaccine series according to schedule for long-term protection

Table 23.5 Recommended Dosages and Schedules for Hepatitis B-Containing Vaccines

| | MONOVALENT HEPATITIS B | | | | | | DTAP-HB-IPV-HIB | | | TWINRIX® | | | TWINRIX® JUNIOR | | |
| | RECOMBIVAX HB® | | | ENGERIX®-B | | | INFANRIX HEXA™ | | | | | | HAHB | | |
Recipients	mcg HBsAg[a]	mL[b]	Schedule[c]	mcg HBsAg[a]	mL[b]	Schedule[c]	mcg HBsAg[a]	mL[b]	Schedule[c]	mcg HBsAg[a]	mL[b]	Schedule[c]	mcg HBsAg[a]	mL[b]	Schedule[c]
Infants <6 months of age born to HBV-negative mothers	5	0.5[d]	0, 1, 6[e]	10	0.5	0, 1, 6 or 0, 1, 2, 12	10	0.5	Months of age: 2, 4, 6, 12–23 or 2, 4, 6 or 2, 4, 12–23	Not indicated			Not indicated		
Infants of HBV-positive mothers[f]	5	0.5[d]	0, 1, 6[e]	10	0.5	0, 1, 6 or 0, 1, 2, 12	Not indicated before 6 weeks of age			Not indicated			Not indicated		
6 months to <24 months of age[g]	5	0.5[d]	0, 1, 6[e]	10	0.5	0, 1, 6 or 0, 1, 2, 12	10	0.5	Months: (1st dose= month 0) 0, 2, 4, 10–21 or 0, 2, 4 or 0, 2, 10–21	20	1.0	0, 6–12	10	0.5	0, 1, 6

Continued

Immunoprophylaxis

23

581

Table 23.5 Recommended Dosages and Schedules for Hepatitis B-Containing Vaccines—cont'd

	VACCINE														
	MONOVALENT HEPATITIS B						DTAP-HB-IPV-HIB			HAHB					
	RECOMBIVAX HB®			ENGERIX®-B			INFANRIX HEXA™			TWINRIX®			TWINRIX® JUNIOR		
Recipients	mcg HBsAg[a]	mL[b]	Schedule[c]	mcg HBsAg[a]	mL[b]	Schedule[c]	mcg HBsAg[a]	mL[b]	Schedule[c]	mcg HBsAg[a]	mL[b]	Schedule[c]	mcg HBsAg[a]	mL[b]	Schedule[c]
24 months to <11 years of age	5	0.5[d]	0, 1, 6[e]	10	0.5	0, 1, 6 or 0, 1, 2, 12	May be given to children aged 24 months to <7 years, if necessary			20	1.0	0, 6–12	10	0.5	0, 1, 6
11 to <16 years of age	10 5	1.0 0.5	0, 4–6[e] 0, 1, 6[e]	20 10[h]	1.0 0.5	0, 6 0, 1, 6 or 0, 1, 2, 12	Not indicated			20	1.0	0, 6–12	10	0.5	0, 1, 6
16 to <19 years of age	5	0.5	0, 1, 6[e]	10	0.5	0, 1, 6 or 0, 1, 2, 12	Not indicated			Not indicated			10	0.5	0, 1, 6
Dialysis, chronic renal failure, and some immunocompromised[i] children, <16 years of age	double the mcg dose for healthy child of same age	0.5	0, 1, 6 or 0, 1, 2, 12	double the mcg dose for healthy child of same age	0.5	0, 1, 6 or 0, 1, 2, 12	Not indicated			Not indicated			Not indicated		

| Dialysis, chronic renal failure, and some immunocompromised[i] people, 16 to <20 years of age | double the mcg dose for healthy individual of same age | 0, 1, 6 or 0, 1, 2, 12 | 40 | 2.0 | 0, 1, 2, 6 | Not indicated | Not indicated | Not indicated |

[a]Micrograms (mcg) of HBsAg per dose.

[b]Milliliters (mL) per dose.

[c]Months: 1st dose = month 0.

[d]Following the review of Recombivax HB® vaccine immunogenicity and safety data, the National Advisory Committee on Immunization (NACI) is now recommending the provision of a full dose (0.5 mL/5 mcg) to all children of HB-negative mothers who are <11 years of age. This change will harmonize dosing schedules and reduce vaccine wastage. Infants and children <11 years of age who were immunized with a complete series using the previously recommended 0.25 mL dosage do not require revaccination.

[e]Although a schedule of months 0, 1, and at least 2 is authorized, the preferred schedule is months 0, 1, and 6.

[f]For post-exposure immunization of infants born to HB-infected mothers, refer to Post-exposure immunization. Premature infants (<37 weeks and weighing <2000 grams) of HB-infected mothers, require 4 doses of HB vaccine.

[g]For pre-exposure immunization, persons 6 months of age and older may be immunized with HAHB vaccine, if indicated.

[h]The manufacturer recommends the standard adult dosage (20 mcg/1.0 mL) using a 2 dose schedule if it is unlikely that there will be compliance with the 3 or 4 dose schedule.

[i]Immunocompromised defined as: congenital immunodeficiency, hematopoietic stem cell transplant, solid organ transplant recipients, HIV-infected.

DTAP-HB-IPV-HIB, diphtheria toxoid-tetanus toxoid-acellular pertussis-hepatitis B-inactivated polio-*Haemophilus influenzae* type b vaccine; *HAHB*, combined hepatitis A hepatitis B vaccine; *HBaAg*, hepatitis B surface antigen.

Immunoprophylaxis

23

Pre-exposure immunization

1. Most effective means to prevent HBV transmission
   a. Recommended for
      i. all infants, children and adolescents <18 years of age
      ii. susceptible individuals if household contact of an acute case or chronic carrier
      iii. susceptible individuals traveling to areas with intermediate to high prevalence of chronic hepatitis B virus (HBV) infection (HbsAg prevalence ≥2%) or all international travelers, depending on individual risk
2. Initiate ≥6 months before travel to complete 3 dose series before departure
   a. Some protection with 2 doses so series should at least be initiated before departure

Post-exposure prophylaxis

1. **Infants born to HbsAg positive mothers**
   a. HBIg IM as soon as possible after birth, preferably within 12 hours
      i. See Table 39.10 for dosing
      ii. Significantly decreased efficacy after 48 hours
      iii. May be given up to 7 days after birth
   b. HBV vaccine within 12 hours of birth
      i. Second and third dose of HBV vaccine series at 1 and 6 months of age
      ii. 6 month dose can be given as DTaP-HB-IPV-Hib
   c. Post-immunization serological testing
2. **Maternal HBsAg status is unknown**
   a. Test mother at delivery
   b. If the results are not available within 12 hours of delivery, consider administering HBV vaccine and HBIg, considering maternal risk factors, erring on the side of providing prophylaxis
3. **If birth weight <2 kg**
   a. If first dose is routinely given at birth and mother is HBsAg negative, delay immunization until weight >2000 g or >1 month
   b. If mother is HBsAg positive, administer HBV vaccine and HBIg within 12 hours of birth
      i. Administer 3 additional HBV vaccine doses at ages 1, 2, and 6 months
      ii. DTaP-HB-IPV-Hib vaccine may be given for the 2 and 6 month doses

Post-immunization serological testing

1. Infants born to HBsAg positive mothers should not have HBV serological testing before 9 months of age

2. Conduct serological testing (HBsAg and anti-HBs) between 1 and 4 months after vaccine series is complete
3. If HbsAg is present, child will likely become a chronic carrier
4. If HBsAg is negative and anti-HBs titers <10 IU/L after 3 dose series, give additional dose of vaccine and repeat serological testing 1 to 2 months after

INFLUENZA

Influenza vaccine
1. Available as intramuscular inactivated influenza vaccine, or intranasal live attenuated vaccine
2. Efficacy of each specific vaccine formulation varies, refer to annually updated guidelines
3. Previously unvaccinated children <9 years require two doses at least 4 weeks apart
   a. Second dose within the same season is not required if the child received a dose during the previous influenza season
4. Egg allergy not a contraindication to influenza vaccine

Pre-exposure immunization
1. All children >6 months of age should receive influenza vaccine annually

Post-exposure prophylaxis
1. Use oseltamivir for treatment and prophylaxis (see Table 40.1 for dosing)
2. Early therapy preferred over prophylaxis because of concerns about drug resistance
3. Consider prophylaxis in individuals who cannot reliably be protected by immunization (vaccine contradicted, age <6 months, immunocompromised)

MEASLES

Measles vaccine
1. **Administration:** SC (check product monograph)
2. **Preparations**
   a. MMR
   b. MMRV (children >12 months)
3. **Adverse reactions:** injection site reactions, fever after ~7 days, headache, rash

Pre-exposure immunization
1. Measles vaccine recommended as part of routine immunization series (see Table 23.1)

2. International travelers who are not measles immune should receive the MMR/MMRV vaccine before travel
   a. Infants 6 to 11 months: 1 dose of MMR before travel and repeat vaccination after 1 year of age according to routine immunization series
   b. Children >12 months: 2 doses of MMR or MMRV with a minimum of 28 days between

Post-exposure prophylaxis
1. See Table 23.6

Table 23.6	Summary of Measles Post-Exposure Prophylaxis Recommendations for Susceptible Contacts	
	TIME SINCE EXPOSURE TO MEASLES	
Population	**≤72 h**	**73 h–6 days**
Infants 0–6 months-old	IMIg (0.5 mL/kg)	
Susceptible immunocompetent infants 6–12 months old	MMR vaccine then complete routine vaccine series	IMIg (0.5 mL/kg)
Susceptible immunocompetent individuals >12 months	MMR vaccine series	

IMIg, Intramuscular immune globulin; *MMR,* measles, mumps, and rubella vaccine.

Adapted from Public Health Agency of Canada. *Canadian Immunization Guide: Part 4—Active Vaccines.* Measles vaccine: Canadian Immunization Guide, Table 2. © Adapted from Public Health Agency of Canada. Canadian Immunization Guide: Part 4–Active Vaccines. Measles vaccine: Canadian Immunization Guide, Table 2. © All rights reserved. Canadian Immunization Guide. Public Health Agency of Canada. Adapted and reproduced with permission from the Minister of Health, 2020.

MENINGOCOCCAL DISEASE
Meningococcal vaccine
1. **Typical dosing and administration:** 0.5 mL IM (check product monograph)
2. **Preparations**
   a. Monovalent conjugate meningococcal vaccine (Men-C-C)
   b. Quadrivalent conjugate meningococcal vaccine (Men-C-ACYW)
   c. Serogroup B meningococcal vaccine (4CMenB, MenB-fHBP)
3. **Adverse reactions:** injection site reactions, fever, irritability, headache

Pre-exposure immunization
1. Meningococcal vaccine recommended as part of routine immunization series (see Table 23.1)
2. **Invasive meningococcal disease (IMD):** if at increased risk for IMD, schedule depends on age and previously received meningococcal

immunizations (see Table 23.7 for recommendations for high risk individuals not previously immunized)

a. Increased risk for IMD because of underlying medical conditions
   i. Functional or anatomic asplenia, including sickle cell anemia, or combined T and B cell immunodeficiencies
   ii. Properdin, factor D, or complement deficiency (or acquired complement deficiency from eculizumab), primary antibody deficiency
   iii. Human immunodeficiency virus (HIV)

Table 23.7	Recommended Immunization for High Risk Groups Because of Underlying Medical Conditions Not Previously Immunized With Men-C-ACYW or Serogroup B Meningococcal Vaccine[a]	
Age	Recommended Vaccine(s)	Schedule
2–11 months of age	Men-C-ACYW-CRM[b] and 4CMenB	2 or 3 doses[c] given 8 weeks apart (with another dose between 12 and 23 months of age that is at least 8 weeks from the previous dose)
12–23 months of age	Men-C-ACYW-CRM[b] and 4CMenB	2 doses (given at least 8 weeks apart)[d]
24 months–9 years of age	Men-C-ACYW[b] and 4CMenB	2 doses (given at least 8 weeks apart)[d]
≥10 years of age	Men-C-ACYW[b] and 4CMenB or MenB-fHBP	2 doses of Men-C-ACYW (given 8 weeks apart)[d]; 2 doses of 4CMenB (given at least 4 weeks apart) or 3 doses of MenB-fHBP (given 4 weeks apart, with another dose at least 4 months after dose two and at least 6 months after dose one)

[a]A serogroup B meningococcal vaccine should be offered for the active immunization of individuals with underlying medical conditions that would put them at higher risk of meningococcal disease. 4CMenB vaccine is indicated for immunization of high-risk individuals greater than or equal to 2 months of age; MenB-fHBP vaccine may be considered as an option for use in high-risk individuals 10 years of age and older.

[b]A booster dose should be given every 3 to 5 years if vaccinated at 6 years of age or younger and every 5 years for those vaccinated at 7 years of age and older.

[c]Depending on the age at which immunization is initiated, the manufacturer of 4CMenB recommends three doses for infants who begin primary immunization between the ages of 2 and 5 months, and two doses when the first dose is received between ages of 6 and 11 months.

[d]Men-C-ACYW vaccines may be given a minimum of 4 weeks apart if accelerated immunization is needed.

From Public Health Agency of Canada. *Canadian Immunization Guide: Part 4—Active Vaccines.* Meningococcal vaccine: Canadian Immunization Guide, Table 1.

© All rights reserved. Canadian Immunization Guide. Public Health Agency of Canada. Adapted and reproduced with permission from the Minister of Health, 2020.

b. Increased risk for IMD because of potential for exposure
  i. Travelers to endemic areas (e.g., sub-Saharan Africa and Hajj pilgrims)
  ii. Close contact of someone with invasive meningococcal disease
3. **Travel:** for travel to sub-Saharan Africa ("meningitis belt") from December to June, one dose of quadrivalent (ACYW) meningococcal vaccine before travel
  a. **Infants ≥2 months and <24 months of age:** use Men-C-ACYW-CRM
  b. **Initiating vaccination ≥24 months of age:** use any Men-C-ACYW
  c. Serogroup B is rare in this region
4. **Revaccination:** recommended in individuals at high risk of developing IMD or traveling to areas where meningococcal vaccine is recommended or required

Post-exposure prophylaxis

1. **Exposure (7 days before symptom onset in the case to 24 hours after onset of effective treatment) to a case of IMD:** regardless of immunization status, prescribe chemoprophylaxis to
  a. Household contacts
  b. Persons who share sleeping arrangements with a case of IMD
  c. Persons who have direct nose or mouth contamination with oral or nasal secretions of a case of IMD (e.g., kissing on the mouth, sharing bottles)
  d. Children and staff in contact with a case of IMD in childcare facilities
2. Chemoprophylaxis consists of: oral rifampin (infants, children, adults), IM ceftriaxone (older children, adults), or ciprofloxacin (nonpregnant adults)
3. If identified meningococcal serogroup identified is vaccine preventable, consider immunoprophylaxis (Table 23.8)

Table 23.8	Recommended Vaccination of Close Contacts for Post-Exposure Management and for Outbreak Control for Meningococcal Disease	
Group	**Recommended Vaccine(s)**	**Schedule**
Close contacts and outbreak control of serogroup C invasive meningococcal disease		
2 months to <12 months of age	Men-C-C	**Unvaccinated:** 1 dose immediately after exposure then complete the routine series of Men-C-C **Previously vaccinated:** If previously vaccinated then revaccinate with Men-C-C if at least 4 weeks have elapsed since last dose, then complete the routine series of Men-C-C if necessary

Group	Recommended Vaccine(s)	Schedule
12 months– 10 years of age	Men-C-C	**Unvaccinated:** 1 dose immediately after exposure **Previously vaccinated:** If previously vaccinated at <1 year of age OR person is at high risk for IMD because of underlying medical conditions, then revaccinate with one dose of Men-C-C if at least 4 weeks since last dose; otherwise revaccinate if at least 1 year since last dose
≥11 years of age	Men-C-C OR Men-C-ACYW	**Unvaccinated:** 1 dose immediately after exposure **Previously vaccinated:** If previously vaccinated at <1 year of age OR person is at high risk for IMD because of underlying medical conditions, then revaccinate with one dose of vaccine of choice if at least 4 weeks since last dose; otherwise revaccinate if at least 1 year since last dose

Close contacts and outbreak control of serogroup A, Y, or W-135 invasive meningococcal disease

Group	Recommended Vaccine(s)	Schedule
2 months to <12 months of age	Men-C-ACYW-CRM	**Unvaccinated:** 2 or 3 doses given 8 weeks apart with another dose between 12 and 23 months and at least 8 weeks from the previous dose **Previously vaccinated:** - If previously vaccinated with only Men C-C, give Men-C-ACYW-CRM as for unvaccinated persons, regardless of when Men-C-C was previously given[a] - If previously vaccinated with Men-C-ACYW, then revaccinate with one dose of Men-C-ACYW-CRM if at least 4 weeks since last dose of Men-C-ACYW vaccine; then complete series
12–23 months of age	Men-C-ACYW-CRM	**Unvaccinated:** 2 doses at least 8 weeks apart **Previously vaccinated:** - If previously vaccinated with only Men C-C, give Men-C-ACYW-CRM as for unvaccinated persons, regardless of when Men-C-C was previously given[a] - If previously vaccinated with Men-C-ACYW at <1 year of age OR person is at high risk for IMD because of underlying medical conditions, then revaccinate with one dose of Men-C-ACYW-CRM if at least 4 weeks since last dose of Men-C-ACYW; otherwise revaccinate with one dose of Men-C-ACYW-CRM if at least 1 year since last dose of Men-C-ACYW

Immunoprophylaxis

23

Continued

Table 23.8	Recommended Vaccination of Close Contacts for Post-Exposure Management and for Outbreak Control for Meningococcal Disease—cont'd	
Group	**Recommended Vaccine(s)**	**Schedule**
≥2 years	Men-C-ACYW	**Unvaccinated:** 1 dose immediately after exposure[b] **Previously vaccinated:** - If previously vaccinated with only Men C-C, give Men-C-ACYW as for unvaccinated persons, regardless of when Men-C-C was previously given[a] - If previously vaccinated with Men-C-ACYW at <1 year of age OR person is at high risk for IMD because of underlying medical conditions, then revaccinate with one dose of Men-C-ACYW if at least 4 weeks since last dose of Men-C-ACYW; otherwise revaccinate if at least 1 year since last dose
Close contacts and outbreak control of serogroup B invasive meningococcal disease[c]		
2 months to <6 months	4CMenB	**Unvaccinated:** 1 dose immediately after exposure[d]; then revaccinate with 2 more doses with at least a 4 week interval between doses **Previously vaccinated:** 1 dose immediately after exposure[d]
6 months to <10 years	4CMenB	**Unvaccinated:** 1 dose immediately after exposure[d]; then revaccinate with a single dose after at least 8 weeks **Previously vaccinated:** 1 dose immediately after exposure[d]
≥10 years	4CMenB or MenB-fHBP	**Unvaccinated:** 1 dose immediately after exposure[d]; then revaccinate with a single dose after at least 4 weeks with 4CMenB or MenB-fHBP **Previously vaccinated:** 1 dose immediately after exposure[d]

[a]In general, a minimum 4 week interval is recommended between doses of conjugate meningococcal vaccines; however, in an outbreak or to manage a close contact of a case of IMD, the second dose of conjugate meningococcal vaccine may be given as soon as indicated to provide protection to a close contact who is unvaccinated for the implicated serogroup.

[b]Individuals at high risk because of underlying medical conditions routinely need two doses of Men-C-ACYW.

[c]Only for outbreak control of IMD caused by serogroup B strains that are predicted to be susceptible to the vaccine. Consultation with public health officials, experts in communicable disease, or both is required for optimal management of meningococcal disease outbreaks.

[d]During an outbreak, the vaccine should be provided as soon as possible after the identification of a serogroup B strain that is predicted to be susceptible to the vaccine.

IMD, Invasive meningococcal disease.

PERTUSSIS

Pertussis vaccine

1. **Administration:** IM
2. **Preparations**
   a. Acellular preparation in a combination vaccine
   b. "aP" component: higher concentrations of acellular pertussis antigen for primary immunization of infants and young children; booster for children 4 to 7 years old
   c. "ap" component: reduced concentration of acellular pertussis antigen for older children, adolescents and adults; can be used as booster for children 4 to 7 years old
3. **Adverse reactions:** redness at injection site, extensive limb swelling, fever, drowsiness

Pre-exposure immunization

1. Pertussis vaccine recommended as part of routine immunization series (see Table 23.1)

Post-exposure prophylaxis

1. **Vaccination:** all unimmunized or partially immunized close contacts <7 years old
   a. Fourth dose of DTaP if third dose was given >6 months before
   b. Booster dose of DTaP if last dose >3 years before and child <7 years old
2. **Chemoprophylaxis:** for all close contacts (household, childcare)
   a. <1 month of age: azithromycin
   b. >1 month of age: azithromycin, erythromycin, or clarithromycin

RABIES

Rabies vaccine

1. **Administration:** 1 mL IM or 0.1 mL ID
   a. <2 years: administer vaccine IM in the anterolateral area of the thigh
   b. >2 years: administer vaccine IM in the deltoid area of the arm
   c. Do not administer into gluteal muscles
   d. Use IM route for persons who are immunocompromised or on chloroquine
   e. ID route will require postimmunization antibody titers 2 weeks after completion of vaccine series or after booster doses
2. **Adverse reactions**
   a. Common: pain, erythema, swelling, pruritis, induration at injection site
   b. Less common: myalgia, arthralgia, headache, fever

Pre-exposure immunization

1. Offer to individuals at high risk for rabies exposure
   a. Close contact with rabies virus or rapid animals (laboratory workers, wildlife workers)
   b. Travel to rabies-endemic settings (especially if limited access to rabies serological testing, rabies biologicals in a timely fashion, and access to booster doses)
2. Pre-exposure immunization makes administration of rabies immune globulin (RIg) unnecessary after a bite
3. Pre-exposure immunization rabies regimens for all ages, either
   a. 1-site IM vaccine administrations on days 0 and 7
   b. 2-sites ID vaccine administration on days 0 and 7
4. If immunodeficiency, evaluate on an individual basis

Post-exposure prophylaxis

1. Rabies vaccine and RIg administration depends on type of exposure
   a. Category I (no exposure): touching or feeding animals, animal licks on intact skin
   b. Category II (exposure): nibbling of uncovered skin, minor scratches, or abrasions without bleeding
   c. Category III (severe exposure): single or multiple transdermal bites or scratches, contamination of mucous membrane or broken skin with saliva from animal licks, exposures because of direct contact with bats
2. See Table 23.9 for vaccine and RIg recommendations

Table 23.9	Post-Exposure Prophylaxis Recommendations by Category of Exposure to Rabies		
	Category I Exposure	Category II Exposure	Category III Exposure
Immunologically naive individuals of all age groups	Wash exposed skin surfaces. No PEP required.	Wound washing and immediate vaccination: - 2-sites ID on days 0, 3, and 7[a] OR - 1-site IM on days 0, 3, 7 and between day 14–28[b] OR - 2-sites IM on day 0 and 1-site IM on days 7, 21[c] RIg is not indicated	Wound washing and immediate vaccination: - 2-sites ID on days 0, 3 and 7[a] OR - 1-site IM on days 0, 3, 7 and between day 14–28[b] OR - 2-sites IM on day 0 and 1-site IM on days 7, 21[c] RIg administration is recommended

Table 23.9

Table 23.9	Post-Exposure Prophylaxis Recommendations by Category of Exposure to Rabies—cont'd		
	Category I Exposure	**Category II Exposure**	**Category III Exposure**
Previously immunized individuals of all age groups	Wash exposed skin surfaces. No PEP required.	Wound washing and immediate vaccination[d]: - 1-site ID on days 0 and 3 OR - at 4-sites ID on day 0 OR - at 1-site IM on days 0 and 3 RIg is not indicated	Wound washing and immediate vaccination[d]: - 1-site ID on days 0 and 3 OR - at 4-sites ID on day 0 OR - at 1-site IM on days 0 and 3 RIg is not indicated

[a]1 week, 2-site ID regimen/Institut Pasteur du Cambodge (IPC) regimen/2-2-2-0-0; duration of entire PEP course: 7 days.

[b]2 week IM PEP regimen/4-dose Essen regimen/1-1-1-1-0; duration of entire PEP course: between 14 and 28 days.

[c]3 week IM PEP regimen/Zagreb regimen/2-0-1-0-1; duration of entire PEP course: 21 days.

[d]Except if complete PEP already received within <3 months previously.

ID, Intradermal; *IM*, intramuscular; *PEP*, post-exposure prophylaxis; *RIg*, rabies immune globulin.

From World Health Organization. Rabies vaccines and immunoglobulins. April 2018 (Table 1).

RESPIRATORY SYNCYTIAL VIRUS

1. No available vaccine
2. Palivizumab immune globulin (respiratory syncytial virus [RSV]-Ig) used for prevention of RSV hospitalizations in specific populations (see Box 23.2 for indications)
3. RSV-Ig is not indicated for the treatment of active RSV infection

---

Box 23.2   Indications for use of Respiratory Syncytial Virus Immune Globulin

1. Offer to infants with hemodynamically significant CHD or CLD (oxygen need after 36 weeks postmenstrual age) on diuretics, bronchodilators, supplemental oxygen or steroids if <12 months of age when RSV season begins
2. Consider offering to preterm infants without CLD born <30 weeks of gestation who are <6 months when RSV season begins
3. Offer to infants who live in remote areas who depend on air transportation for hospitalization, born <36 weeks' gestation and are <6 months of age when RSV begins (consider incidence of RSV hospitalization from members of the community in previous years)
4. Children with immunodeficiencies, cystic fibrosis, trisomy 21, chronic pulmonary disease (other than CLD), or upper airway obstruction should not routinely be offered RSV-Ig
5. Discontinue RSV-Ig in children who develop an RSV infection while on monthly RSV-Ig

---

CHD, Congenital heart disease; *CLD*, chronic lung disease; *RSV*, respiratory syncytial virus.

Adapted from Robinson J and Le Saux N. Preventing hospitalizations for respiratory syncytial virus infection. *Paediatr Child Health*. 2015;20(6):321–326.

TETANUS

Tetanus vaccine

1. **Administration:** IM
2. **Preparations**
   a. Combination vaccine in multiple different formulations
3. **Adverse reactions:** redness, limb swelling, pain at injection site, nodule at injection site
   a. Large injection site reaction to a previous dose is not a contraindication to continuing the recommended schedule

Pre-exposure immunization

1. Tetanus vaccine recommended as part of routine immunization series (see Table 23.1)

Post-exposure prophylaxis

1. See Table 23.10
2. If indicated, give tetanus immune globulin (TIg) and tetanus-toxoid containing vaccines at different injection sites using separate needles and syringes

Table 23.10	Tetanus Post-Exposure Prophylaxis				
	CLEAN, MINOR WOUNDS		**ALL OTHER WOUNDS**	
History of Tetanus Immunization	**Tetanus Toxoid-Containing Vaccine**	**TIg**	**Tetanus Toxoid-Containing Vaccine**	**TIg[a]**
Unknown or <3 doses in a vaccine series	Yes	No	Yes	Yes
≥3 doses in a vaccine series and <5 years since last booster dose	No	No	No	No[b]
≥3 doses in a vaccine series and 5–9 years since last booster dose	No	No	Yes	No[b]
≥3 doses in a vaccine series and ≥10 years since last booster dose	Yes	No	Yes	No[b]

[a]Given at different injection sites using separate needles and syringes.
[b]Yes, if known to have a humoral immune deficiency state.

TIg, Tetanus immune globulin.

From Public Health Agency of Canada. *Canadian Immunization Guide: Part 4—Active Vaccines.* Tetanus toxoid: Canadian Immunization Guide, Table 1. © All rights reserved. Canadian Immunization Guide. Public Health Agency of Canada. Adapted and reproduced with permission from the Minister of Health, 2020.

VARICELLA

Varicella vaccine

1. **Administration:** SC
2. **Preparations**
   a. Univalent varicella vaccine (VAR)
   b. Combined with MMR as MMRV
3. **Adverse reactions:** injection site pain, swelling and redness, varicella-like rash 5 to 26 days after immunization
   a. If varicella-like rash appears within first 2 weeks after immunization, obtain specimens to determine if rash is caused by a natural varicella infection or vaccine-derived strain

Pre-exposure immunization

1. Administration of VAR is recommended as part of routine immunization series (see Table 23.1)
2. Children with history of varicella <1 year of age should receive VAR as per routine immunization series
3. Offer VAR to susceptible older children who are close contacts of immuno-compromised patients
4. Individualize plan for VAR in persons with chronic diseases at high risk of severe varicella
   a. Asplenic or hypersplenic patients
   b. Chronic renal disease or on dialysis
   c. Chronic salicylic acid therapy (avoid ASA for 6 weeks after VAR because of increased risk of Reye syndrome)
   d. Chronic lung disease including cystic fibrosis
   e. Immunocompromised children

Post-exposure prophylaxis

1. In susceptible, healthy, nonpregnant individuals, give VAR within 5 days of exposure (preferably within 72 hours)
2. See Box 23.3 for considerations for use of varicella zoster immune globulin (VarIg)
   a. Maximal benefit if administered within 96 hours after first exposure, but can be given up to 10 days after exposure
3. For high-risk patients who have additional exposures to varicella zoster virus ≥3 weeks after initial VarIg administration, another dose of VarIg should be considered
4. VarIg in special populations
   a. Newborns of mothers who develop varicella 5 days before or 48 hours after delivery
   b. Hospitalized premature infants (<28 weeks of GA or ≤1000 g) with exposure, regardless of maternal immunity
   c. Hospitalized premature infants (≥28 weeks of GA) born to susceptible mothers

Box 23.3   Considerations for Varicella Zoster Immune Globulin Administration

Decision to administer varicella zoster immune globulin based on fulfilling all four criteria:
1. Exposed person is susceptible to varicella
2. Significant exposure to a person with varicella or herpes zoster
3. Exposed person is at increased risk of severe varicella
4. Post-exposure immunization with univalent varicella vaccine is contraindicated

Data from Public Health Agency of Canada. *Canadian Immunization Guide: Part 4—Active Vaccines.* Varicella (chickenpox) vaccine: Canadian Immunization Guide. © All rights reserved. Canadian Immunization Guide. Public Health Agency of Canada. Adapted and reproduced with permission from the Minister of Health, 2020.

Considerations

1. Concurrent antivirals used against *Herpesviridae* may reduce efficacy of VAR; discontinue, if possible, for at least 24 hours before and 14 days after vaccination

ASPLENIC PATIENTS

1. See Table 23.11 for vaccine recommendations
2. See Table 23.12 for chemoprophylaxis recommendations

Table 23.11	Vaccine Recommendations in Asplenic (Anatomic or Functional) Patients[a]

Streptococcus pneumoniae	1. PCV13
	  a. Administer four doses at 2, 4, 6, 12–15 months of age
	  b. If 12–24 months of age with no previous doses of PCV13, two doses 8 weeks apart
	  c. If >24 months, one dose if no prior PCV vaccine or only prior PCV7 or PCV10
	2. PPV23
	  a. Administer as soon as possible after 24 months and at least 8 weeks after all doses of PCV for age have been given
	  b. Booster 5 years after first dose
	  c. No more than 2 lifetime doses

Neisseria meningitidis	1. If >2 months of age, give two or three doses of both Men-C-ACYW and 4CMenB beginning at time of diagnosis a. Men-C-ACYW-CRM is the preferred Men-C-ACYW vaccine before 2 years of age 2. Each dose of Men-C-ACYW and 4CMenB vaccine should be administered a minimum of 8 weeks apart (except 4CMenB doses can be given 4 weeks apart if the child is at least 11 years old). Administer these vaccines even if the child has already received Men-C-C. 3. Periodic booster doses with Men-C-ACYW and 4CMenB vaccines are also recommended with a dose of each vaccine at 12–23 months, every 3–5 years until 7 years of age and every 5 years thereafter

Table 23.11	Vaccine Recommendations in Asplenic (Anatomic or Functional) Patients—cont'd
Haemophilus influenzae type b	1. Primary series of 3 doses given at 2, 4, 6 months of age with a booster at 18 months 2. One dose for patients ≥5 years who have never received Hib vaccine or have missed one or more doses 3. If asplenic and presents with Hib infection, give Hib vaccine (infection does not provide lifelong protection)
Influenza virus	1. Annually, beginning at 6 months of age
Other	1. If traveling to areas with risk of *Salmonella*, pre-travel clinic for *S. typhi* vaccine
Splenectomy	1. Give vaccines minimum of 2 weeks before surgery if possible 2. Otherwise, start immunizations at least 2 weeks after splenectomy

[a]All patients should receive the standard childhood and adolescent immunizations at the recommended age. Supplementary immunizations as listed in this table should be ensured and may be administered on an earlier schedule than is routine. Household contacts of asplenic patients should receive all age-appropriate vaccines and the annual influenza vaccine.

4CMenB, Meningococcal B vaccine; *Men-C-C*, meningococcal conjugate C vaccine; *Men-C-ACYW*, meningococcal conjugate A, C, Y, W vaccine; *Men-C-ACYW-CRM*, Menveo; *PCV 13*, pneumococcal-13-valent conjugate vaccine; *PPV 23*, pneumococcal 23-valent polysaccharide vaccine.

Data from Salvadori et al. Preventing and treating infections in children with asplenia or hyposplenia. *Paediatr Child Health*. 2014 May; 19(5): 271–274. Updated Nov 6, 2019.

Table 23.12	Chemoprophylaxis in Asplenic Patients	
	Oral Prophylaxis	**Comments**
Birth–5 years	Amoxicillin 10 mg/kg/dose two times per day	Penicillin V suspension is not available
>5 years	Penicillin V 300 mg per dose two times per day OR amoxicillin 250 mg per dose two times per day	

Data from Salvadori et al. Preventing and treating infections in children with asplenia or hyposplenia. *Paediatr Child Health*. 2014 May; 19(5): 271–274. Updated Nov 6, 2019.

NEEDLESTICK INJURIES

1. Risk of seroconversion after percutaneous needlestick injury from known infected source
   a. HBV: up to 30% (if HBeAg positive)
   b. HCV: 3%
   c. HIV: 0.3%
2. **Management**
   a. **Local wound care:** immediately cleanse site with water and soap, allow wound to bleed freely, do not squeeze the area

b. **Baseline blood tests**
   i. Exposed patient: serology for HBV, HCV, HIV
   ii. Source patient (if available): serology for HBV, HCV, HIV (with consent)
c. **Immunization status for HBV and tetanus** (exposed patient)
   i. If child did not receive complete HBV immunization series, give HBIg and first HBV dose immediately; continue vaccination series if no antibodies present and HBsAg negative
   ii. If child received complete HBV immunization and is anti-HBs positive, no prophylaxis indicated
   iii. If child received complete HBV immunization and is HBsAg positive, refer to infectious disease and/or hepatology specialist
d. **HIV prophylaxis:** consult infectious disease specialist to discuss indications
   i. Usually not recommended >72 hours after exposure
   ii. Risk of acquiring HIV from discarded needles in the community is extremely low
   iii. If initiating post-exposure prophylaxis, check complete blood count (CBC), liver enzymes
e. **Follow-up counseling and testing:** 6 weeks, 3 months, and 6 months

EXPRESSED BREAST MILK: ADMINISTRATION ERRORS

See Table 23.13

Table 23.13	Pathogens Potentially Transmissible by Breast Milk		
Pathogen	**Transmission**	**Laboratory Tests**[a]	**Post-Exposure Prophylaxis**
CMV	Excreted in breast milk; main risk is to premature newborns who lack protective antibody (<28 week GA or seronegative mother)	CMV IgM and IgG serology	Usually not indicated
HIV	Estimated probability of transmission 0.00064/L of EBM	HIV serology (stat)	Decision based on donor's HIV status and HIV risk factors in consultation with infectious disease specialist and infant caregivers

Table 23.13	Pathogens Potentially Transmissible by Breast Milk—cont'd		
Pathogen	Transmission	Laboratory Tests[a]	Post-Exposure Prophylaxis
HTLV I/II	Transmitted primarily by breast milk; risk from single exposure unknown	HTLV serology	Not available
HBV	Theoretical	HBsAg (stat), anti-HBs IgG	Where indicated, HBIg and vaccine within 48 h of incident
HCV	Theoretical	Anti-HCV IgG serology	Not available

[a]Laboratory testing of donor mother, recipient mother, and recipient infant.

Anti-HBs, Hepatitis B surface antibody; *anti-HCV,* hepatitis C antibody; *CMV*, cytomegalovirus; *EBM*, expressed breast milk; *GA*, gestational age; *HBIg*, hepatitis B immune globulin; *HBsAg*, hepatitis B surface antigen; *HBV*, hepatitis B virus; *HCV*, hepatitis C virus; *HIV*, human immunodeficiency virus; *HTLV*, human T-lymphotropic virus; *Ig*, immune globulin.

Adapted from The Hospital for Sick Children Policy: Expressed Breast Milk—Errors in Administration, 2017.

Immunoprophylaxis

23

Infectious Diseases

Ryan Giroux • Jennifer Tam • Ari Bitnun

COMMON ABBREVIATIONS

Also see page xviii for a list of other abbreviations used throughout this book

ADEM	acute disseminated encephalomyelitis
ARDS	acute respiratory distress syndrome
BAL	bronchoalveolar lavage
CFU	colony forming units
CMV	cytomegalovirus
CoNS	coagulase-negative Staphylococci
CSF	cerebrospinal fluid
CVL	central venous line
CXR	chest x-ray
EBV	Epstein-Barr virus
ELISA	enzyme-linked immunosorbent assay
EM	electron microscopy
FSWU	full septic workup
GAS	group A streptococcus
GBS	group B streptococcus
GVHD	graft-versus-host disease
HCV	hepatitis C virus
HHV	human herpes virus
HIV	human immunodeficiency virus
HSCT	hematopoietic stem cell transplant
HSV	herpes simplex virus
ICP	intracranial pressure
IGRA	interferon gamma release assay
INH	isoniazid
LIP	lymphoid interstitial pneumonitis
LOC	level of consciousness
LP	lumbar puncture
LTBI	latent tuberculosis infection
PBP	penicillin-binding protein
PCR	polymerase chain reaction
PJP	*Pneumocystis jiroveci* pneumonia
PMN	polymorphonuclear cells (neutrophils)
PPD	purified protein derivative
PTLD	posttransplant lymphoproliferative disorder
RBC	red blood cell
SBI	serious bacterial infection
SCID	severe combined immunodeficiency
SNHL	sensorineural hearing loss
STI	sexually transmitted infection
TB	tuberculosis

Infectious Diseases

24

TMP/SMX	trimethoprim/sulfamethoxazole
TST	tuberculin skin test
UTI	urinary tract infection
VP	ventriculoperitoneal shunt

CLASSIFICATION OF BACTERIA

See Figures 24.1 and 24.2 for classification of bacteria

Figure 24.1 Classification of Gram-Positive Bacteria

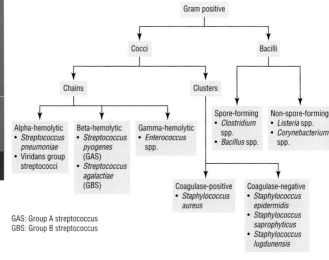

GAS: Group A streptococcus
GBS: Group B streptococcus

Figure 24.2 Classification of Gram-Negative Bacteria

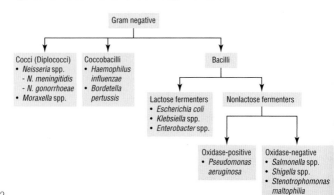

1. First-line therapy should be based on local susceptibility patterns
2. Duration of antimicrobial therapy should be used as a guideline only and may need to be extended on a case-by-case basis. Duration is *total* duration from all routes (IV ± PO, where applicable).
3. General approach to duration of antibiotic therapy and time to switch from intravenous to oral antibiotics is discussed by the Australasian Society for Infectious Disease and can be found at www.asid.net.au/documents/item/1243

FOCAL BACTERIAL INFECTIONS
See Tables 24.1 to 24.7

Infectious Diseases

24

Table 24.1 Central Nervous System Infections

Disease Process	Common Physical Examination Findings	Suspected Pathogens	Empiric Antimicrobial Therapy	Usual Duration of Treatment[a]	Additional Comments
Bacterial meningitis					
Neonates (up to 4 weeks)	Irritability, reduced responsiveness, fever, apnea, bulging fontanelle, focal neurological signs, seizures	Group B *Streptococcus* (GBS), gram-negative enteric bacilli (e.g., *Escherichia coli*), *Listeria monocytogenes*	Ampicillin + cefotaxime ± vancomycin	*E. coli*: 21 days GBS/*L. monocytogenes*: 14–21 days	If viral encephalitis suspected, consider addition of acyclovir for HSV coverage
4 weeks to 3 months	Same as neonatal age range; nonblanchable hemorrhagic rash (meningococcemia)	Organisms from both neonatal and older age range	Ceftriaxone + vancomycin	Gram-negative enteric bacilli: minimum 21 days GBS/*L. monocytogenes*: 14–21 days *Streptococcus pneumoniae*: 10–14 days *Haemophilus influenzae*: 7–10 days *Neisseria meningitidis*: 5–7 days	Add ampicillin if immunocompromised (risk of *L. monocytogenes*)
≥3 months	Fever, nuchal rigidity, altered LOC, nonblanchable hemorrhagic rash (meningococcemia), Kernig/	*S. pneumoniae, N. meningitidis, H. influenzae*	Ceftriaxone + vancomycin	*S. pneumoniae*: 10–14 days *H. influenzae*: 7–10 days *N. meningitidis*: 5–7 days	

VP shunt infection	Neurological symptoms (dependent on underlying neurological status of child); hydrocephalus, signs of increased ICP (if blockage); similar examination findings to bacterial meningitis	Coagulase negative staphylococci, *Staphylococcus aureus*, gram negative enteric bacilli	Vancomycin + ceftriaxone (vancomycin + ceftazidime if concern for *Pseudomonas aeruginosa*)	If GNB, minimum 21 days from time of CSF clearance; all other organisms, minimum 10–14 days from time of CSF clearance	May require shunt revision
Brain abscess (excluding neonates or patients with CSF shunts)	Focal or generalized seizure activity, focal neurological symptoms, signs of extension from adjacent infections (e.g., otitis externa, mastoiditis, cranial surgery site infections)	*Streptococcus* spp., *S. aureus*, oral anaerobic gram-negative and gram-positive bacteria	Ceftriaxone + cloxacillin + metronidazole	Minimum 6 weeks, depending on response to therapy	Consider vancomycin instead of cloxacillin if MRSA suspected. Consider ceftazidime instead of ceftriaxone if chronic otitis externa.

[a]Usual duration of treatment reflects total duration of therapy (IV ± PO, where applicable).

CSF, Cerebrospinal fluid; *GNB*, gram negative bacilli; *HSV*, herpes simplex virus; *ICP*, intracranial pressure; *LOC*, level of consciousness; *MRSA*, methicillin-resistant *S. aureus*.

Adapted from The Hospital for Sick Children eFormulary Antimicrobial Guidelines—Empiric Antibiotic Therapy in Children, 2021.

Table 24.2 Respiratory Infections

Disease Process	Common Physical Examination Findings	Suspected Pathogens	Empiric Antimicrobial Therapy	Usual Duration of Treatment[a]	Additional Comments
Epiglottitis	Tripod position, muffled voice, drooling	Group A *Streptococcus*, *Staphylococcus aureus*, *Haemophilus influenzae* (type b)	Cefuroxime (Ceftriaxone + vancomycin if severely ill)	7–10 days	Vaccination against *H. influenzae* (type b) has significantly reduced incidence
Bacterial tracheitis	Fever, toxic appearance, stridor, cough	*S. aureus*, group A *Streptococcus*, *H. influenzae*	Cefuroxime (Ceftriaxone + vancomycin if severely ill)	7–10 days	
Neonatal bacterial pneumonia (up to 4 weeks)	Respiratory distress, tachypnea, crackles, decreased breath sounds, apnea, fever	Group B *Streptococcus*, gram-negative enteric bacilli (e.g., *Escherichia coli*), *Chlamydia trachomatis*, *S. aureus*, *Listeria monocytogenes*	Ampicillin + tobramycin[b]	7–10 days	Add IV erythromycin or PO azithromycin if *C. trachomatis* suspected. If unwell, use neonatal sepsis/meningitis guidelines.
Community acquired pneumonia					
4 weeks to 3 months	Respiratory distress, tachypnea, crackles, decreased breath sounds, hypoxia	*Streptococcus pneumoniae*, *C. trachomatis*, *S. aureus*, *H. influenzae*	Nonsevere: ampicillin or cefuroxime Severe: ceftriaxone (if >44 weeks PMA), cefotaxime (if ≤44 weeks PMA)	7–10 days; minimum, 2–4 weeks if complicated pneumonia	- Add vancomycin if rapidly progressing multilobar disease or pneumatoceles for presumed MRSA - Add macrolide if *C. trachomatis* or atypical pneumonia suspected - Presence of large effusions or empyema may lengthen therapy

≥3 months	Fever, respiratory distress, tachypnea, crackles, decreased breath sounds, hypoxia	S. pneumoniae, H. influenzae, S. aureus, group A Streptococcus, Mycoplasma pneumoniae, Chlamydia pneumoniae	Outpatient: amoxicillin (high dose) Nonsevere inpatient: ampicillin or cefuroxime Severe inpatient: ceftriaxone	7–10 days; minimum 2–4 weeks if complicated pneumonia	- Add vancomycin if rapidly progressing multilobar disease or pneumatoceles for presumed MRSA - Add macrolide or levofloxacin if Mycoplasma/Chlamydia suspected (e.g., subacute onset, prominent cough, minimal leukocytosis, nonlobar infiltrate) - Presence of large effusions or empyema may lengthen therapy
Ventilator associated pneumonia					
Neonates	Fever, apneas, bradycardias, increasing pressure or oxygen requirements	S. aureus, gram-negative enteric bacilli, Pseudomonas aeruginosa	Vancomycin + tobramycin[b]	7 days (assuming good clinical response)	
Infants and children	Fever, increasing pressure or oxygen requirements, increased oral secretions, new consolidation on CXR	S. pneumoniae, S. aureus, H. influenzae, gram-negative enteric bacilli, P. aeruginosa	Piperacillin-tazobactam + tobramycin[b] ± vancomycin (if MRSA suspected, ≥7 days on ventilator or recent antibiotics)	7 days (assuming good clinical response)	S. pneumoniae, H. influenzae less common if recent antibiotics or ≥7 days on ventilator. Pneumonia presenting within 72 h of admission may represent community acquired pneumonia.

Continued

Infectious Diseases

24

Infectious Diseases

24

Table 24.2 Respiratory Infections—cont'd

Disease Process	Common Physical Examination Findings	Suspected Pathogens	Empiric Antimicrobial Therapy	Usual Duration of Treatment[a]	Additional Comments
Aspiration pneumonia					
Neonates	Respiratory distress, oxygen requirements, pressure support	Same pathogens as neonatal sepsis	Ampicillin + tobramycin[b] (empiric therapy for presumed neonatal sepsis)		Empiric therapy not recommended for mild aspiration events or meconium aspiration
Infants and children	Similar signs to community-acquired pneumonia. RML and RLL most common (gravity dependent)	Same pathogens as community-acquired and hospital-acquired pneumonias ± oral anaerobes	Ceftriaxone ± clindamycin if risk of anaerobic infection or severe Consider piperacillin-tazobactam if *P. aeruginosa* or severe	7 days assuming good clinical response	Oral stepdown therapy with amoxicillin-clavulanate, cefuroxime, or cefprozil
Pertussis	*Catarrhal Stage* (1–2 weeks): URTI symptoms *Paroxysmal Stage* (2–8 weeks): paroxysmal cough, inspiratory whoop, posttussive vomiting *Convalescent Stage* (1–4 weeks): improvement	*Bordetella pertussis*	Azithromycin (PO)	Duration 5 days (7–14 days if erythromycin or clarithromycin)	

[a]Usual duration of treatment reflects total duration of therapy (IV ± PO, where applicable).
[b]Tobramycin or other aminoglycoside, such as gentamicin, depending on local availability.

CXR, chest x-ray; *MRSA*, methicillin-resistant *S. aureus*; *PMA*, postmenstrual age; *RML*, right middle lobe; *RLL*, right lower lobe; *URTI*, upper respiratory tract infection.

Table 24.3 **Head and Neck Infections**

Disease Process	Common Physical Examination Findings	Suspected Pathogens	Empiric Antimicrobial Therapy	Usual Duration of Treatment[a]	Additional Comments
Otitis media (acute)	Acute onset of otalgia, middle ear fluid, inflammation of the middle ear	Streptococcus pneumoniae, non-typeable Haemophilus influenzae, Moraxella catarrhalis, group A Streptococcus	Amoxicillin (high dose)	Children 6–24 months: 10 days; ≥ 2 years: 5 days	Additional detail available in Chapter 33 Otolaryngology
Otitis externa	Tenderness of tragus/pinna, ear canal edema/erythema, otorrhea, lymphadenitis	Pseudomonas aeruginosa, Staphylococcus aureus, multiple aerobes and anaerobes	Mild-severe: topical antibiotic and corticosteroid (e.g., CiproDex) Extension beyond ear canal: topical + oral ciprofloxacin	7–10 days	Additional detail available in Chapter 33 Otolaryngology
Mastoiditis (acute)	Postauricular erythema and tenderness, protrusion of the auricle, fever, headache, tympanic membrane erythema	S. pneumoniae, S. aureus, M. catarrhalis, H. influenzae, group A Streptococcus	Cefuroxime (IV), oral PO stepdown: cefuroxime/cefprozil or amoxicillin-clavulanate	3–4 weeks	Additional detail available in Chapter 33 Otolaryngology, consider surgical drainage
Bacterial sinusitis (acute and subacute)	Persistent nasal discharge, cough	S. pneumoniae, M. catarrhalis, H. influenzae, group A Streptococcus	Amoxicillin (PO) or cefuroxime (IV)	10–14 days	Amoxicillin-clavulanate is an alternative option
Orbital cellulitis	Pain with eye movements, proptosis, vision changes, ophthalmoplegia	S. pneumoniae, group A Streptococcus, S. aureus, H. influenzae, M. catarrhalis, anaerobes	Cloxacillin + ceftriaxone + metronidazole (IV)	3 weeks	Consider vancomycin if MRSA suspected, failed first-line treatment, or systemically unwell

Continued

Infectious Diseases

24

609

Table 24.3 Head and Neck Infections—cont'd

Disease Process	Common Physical Examination Findings	Suspected Pathogens	Empiric Antimicrobial Therapy	Usual Duration of Treatment[a]	Additional Comments
Periorbital cellulitis (nontraumatic)	Periorbital erythema, edema, eyelid swelling	S. pneumoniae, group A Streptococcus, S. aureus, H. influenzae, M. catarrhalis	Mild-moderate: cefuroxime (PO or IV) Moderate-severe: ceftriaxone (IV)	7–10 days	Consider vancomycin if MRSA suspected, failed first-line treatment, or systemically unwell If orbital cellulitis cannot be ruled out, treat as moderate-severe
Periorbital cellulitis (traumatic)	Same as earlier but with evidence of trauma (abrasion, laceration)	S. aureus, group A Streptococcus	Mild: Cephalexin Moderate-severe: cefazolin or cloxacillin (IV)	7–10 days	
Bacterial conjunctivitis					
Neonates	Unilateral or bilateral eye redness and discharge	Neisseria gonorrhoeae, Chlamydia trachomatis, P. aeruginosa Other (including skin flora)	N. gonorrhoeae: cefotaxime (IV) C. trachomatis: azithromycin PO HSV: acyclovir IV P. aeruginosa: piperacillin-tazobactam + tobramycin[b] (IV) Other: polytrim or polysporin ophthalmic solution		

Infants and children	Unilateral or bilateral redness and discharge	Nontypeable *H. influenzae*, *S. pneumoniae*, *S. aureus*, *N. gonorrhoeae*	Polytrim or polysporin ophthalmic solutions; Ceftriaxone (IV) if severe	Eye drops: 7–10 days	Viral causes (EBV, CMV) are more common
Bacterial cervical adenitis	Unilateral, enlarged painful node, fever	*S. aureus*, group A *Streptococcus*	Mild-moderate: cephalexin (PO); Moderate-severe: cefazolin (IV)	7–10 days	
Facial cellulitis of dental origin/dental abscess	Facial swelling, dental/gum pain	*Viridans* group streptococci, *S. aureus*, oral anaerobes	Clindamycin (IV/PO)	7–10 days	Use antibiotics as an adjunct to surgical intervention
Bacterial pharyngitis and tonsillitis	Tonsillar exudate, palatal petechiae, tender cervical LNs, scarlet fever rash (fine, red, diffuse)	Group A *Streptococcus*	Amoxicillin or penicillin V (PO)	10 days	Majority of pharyngitis episodes are viral and self-resolving
Retropharyngeal abscess	Neck stiffness, anterior neck pain, stridor, drooling, croup-like cough	Group A *Streptococcus*, *S. aureus*, oral anaerobes	Clindamycin ± cloxacillin (IV)	10–14 days	ENT consultation for drainage

aUsual duration of treatment reflects total duration of therapy (IV ± PO, where applicable).

bTobramycin or other aminoglycoside, such as gentamicin, depending on local availability.

CMV, Cytomegalovirus; *EBV,* Epstein-Barr virus; *ENT,* ear, nose and throat; *HSV,* herpes simplex virus; *LNs,* lymph nodes; *MRSA,* methicillin-resistant *S. aureus*; *STI,* sexually transmitted infection.

Adapted from The Hospital for Sick Children eFormulary Antimicrobial Guidelines—Empiric Antibiotic Therapy in Children, 2021.

Infectious Diseases

24

Table 24.4 Skin and Soft Tissue Infections

Disease Process	Common Physical Examination Findings	Suspected Pathogens	Empiric Antimicrobial Therapy	Usual Duration of Treatment[a]	Additional Comments
Superficial cutaneous and soft tissue abscesses	**Furuncle:** superficial purulent collection within a single hair follicle, surrounding erythema **Carbuncle:** clusters of furuncles connected subcutaneously **Abscess:** purulent collection in any tissue, surrounding erythema, pain	*Staphylococcus aureus* (including MRSA), group A *Streptococcus*	Incision and drainage Cephalexin or cloxacillin (PO) if outpatient Cefazolin (IV) if inpatient Vancomycin (IV) if severe TMP/SMX or clindamycin if MRSA suspected	5–7 days	All patients should have incision and drainage, consider I+D alone if mild and no cellulitis
Cellulitis (without drainable abscess)					
Neonates	Erythematous, poorly demarcated warm patch, painful, but nonpurulent	Gram-negative enteric bacilli, *S. aureus*, group B *Streptococcus*	Cloxacillin + tobramycin[b] IV	7–10 days	
Infants and children	Same as earlier	*S. aureus*, group A *Streptococcus*	Mild: cephalexin or cloxacillin (PO) Moderate-severe: cefazolin or cloxacillin (IV)	7–10 days	Consider vancomycin if MRSA risk factors If facial cellulitis with dental origin, consider clindamycin
Impetigo	Yellow or honey- coloured crusted sores, sometimes on erythematous base	Group A *Streptococcus*, *S. aureus*	Mild: mupirocin (topical) Moderate-severe: cephalexin (PO)	Mild: 5 days Moderate-severe: 7 days	

Deep soft tissue abscesses	Can involve any layer of skin, fascia, and underlying muscle Erythema, edema extending beyond erythema, severe pain, fever	S. aureus (including MRSA), group A Streptococcus	Vancomycin (IV)	Drainage and culture recommended in consultation with surgery Risk of developing necrotizing fasciitis if untreated
Necrotizing fasciitis	Appears as cellulitis in early stage Edema, severe pain out of keeping with physical exam, fever, crepitus, and skin changes (bullae, bruising, necrosis)	Group A Streptococcus, S. aureus (incl. MRSA)	Clindamycin + cloxacillin (IV) ± vancomycin (if MRSA risk)	Immediate consultation with plastic surgery and infectious diseases Selected severe cases of invasive group A streptococcus may benefit from IVIG

^aUsual duration of treatment reflects total duration of therapy (IV ± PO, where applicable).

^bTobramycin or other aminoglycoside, such as gentamicin, depending on local availability.

IVIG, intravenous immune globulin; MRSA, methicillin-resistant S. aureus; TMP/SMX, trimethoprim/sulfamethoxazole.

Adapted from The Hospital for Sick Children eFormulary Antimicrobial Guidelines—Empiric Antibiotic Therapy in Children, 2021.

Table 24.5 Skin and Soft Tissue Infections (Caused by Bites)

Disease Process	Common Physical Examination Findings	Suspected Pathogens	Empiric Antimicrobial Therapy	Usual Duration of Treatment[a]	Additional Comments
Infected dog or cat bite	Dog bites tend to be larger and may look more serious superficially Cat bites tend to puncture and introduce bacteria further into the tissues	*Pasteurella multocida, Streptococcus* spp., *Eikenella corrodens,* anaerobes, many other organisms	Amoxicillin/clavulanate (IV/PO) Piperacillin/Tazobactam (IV) In cases where anaerobic coverage is not required, cloxacillin + penicillin	Prophylaxis: 5 days Treatment: 7–14 days	Assess need for tetanus vaccine ± tetanus immune globulin, and rabies prophylaxis If infection, consider I+D
Human bite	Teeth marks	*Streptococcus* spp., *Staphylococcus aureus, E. corrodens,* anaerobes	Oral: Amoxicillin-clavulanate IV: Cloxacillin + penicillin	Prophylaxis: 5 days Treatment: 7–14 days	Assess need for tetanus vaccine ± tetanus immune globulin If infection, consider I+D

[a]Usual duration of treatment reflects total duration of therapy (IV ± PO, where applicable).

Adapted from The Hospital for Sick Children eFormulary Antimicrobial Guidelines—Empiric Antibiotic Therapy in Children, 2021.

Table 24.6 Musculoskeletal Infections

Disease Process	Common Physical Examination Findings	Suspected Pathogens	Empiric Antimicrobial Therapy	Usual Duration of Treatment[a]	Additional Comments
Septic arthritis					
Neonates (up to 4 weeks)	Septicemia, cellulitis, swelling, fever. Pain or irritability with mobilization affected joint or handling.	Group B *Streptococcus*, *Staphylococcus aureus*, gram-negative enteric bacilli	Cloxacillin + tobramycin[b]	Acute, uncomplicated septic arthritis (for all age groups): 3–4 weeks, 4–6 weeks for hip septic arthritis	Neonates and young infants may have more than one joint involved
4 weeks to 3 months	Same as earlier	*S. aureus*, group A or group B streptococci, *Streptococcus pneumoniae*, *Haemophilus influenzae* type b	Cloxacillin + tobramycin[b]		If possible, therapeutic and diagnostic drainage of fluid essential before antibiotics for all age groups
≥3 months	Swelling, tenderness at joint, limited range of motion of affected joint, limitation of function (e.g., limp), fever	Group A *Streptococcus*, *S. aureus*, *S. pneumoniae*, *Kingella kingae*	Cefazolin or cloxacillin or clindamycin if MRSA suspected or beta-lacam allergy		Consider *Neisserie gonorrhoeae* in adolescents
Osteomyelitis (acute)					
Neonates (up to 4 weeks)	Irritability, with or without fever. Focal warmth, swelling, pain.	*S. aureus*, group B *Streptococcus*, gram-negative enteric bacilli	Cloxacillin + tobramycin[b]	Acute, uncomplicated osteomyelitis (for all age groups): 3–6 weeks	If possible, therapeutic and diagnostic drainage of fluid essential for all age groups

Continued

Table 24.6	Musculoskeletal Infections—cont'd			
Disease Process	Common Physical Examination Findings	Suspected Pathogens	Empiric Antimicrobial Therapy	Usual Duration of Treatment[a]	Additional Comments
4 weeks to 3 months	Same as earlier	S. aureus, group A or group B streptococci, S. pneumoniae, H. influenzae type b, gram-negative enteric bacilli	Cefotaxime + cloxacillin		For all age groups, antibiotic therapy duration may be lengthened if ESR/CRP remain elevated
≥3 months	Same as earlier, limitation of function (refusal to walk, crawl, sit, weight bear)	S. aureus, S. pneumoniae, group A Streptococcus, Kingella kingae (consider in 6 months to 4 years)	Cefazolin or cloxacillin (IV) or clindamycin if MRSA suspected or beta-lactam allergy		Oral stepdown: Cephalexin (high dose) or clindamycin
Puncture wound (foot)	Wound on dorsal aspect of foot ± ventral aspect of foot, bleeding, erythema, discharge, pain, refusal to bear weight	Pseudomonas aeruginosa (with sneakers), S. aureus (without sneakers)	With sneakers: piperacillin-tazobactam Without sneakers: cephalexin (PO) or cefazolin (IV)	Prophylaxis: 5–7 days Infection: 10–14 days	Assess if soft tissue or bone involvement; consider I + D

[a]Usual duration of treatment reflects total duration of therapy (IV ± PO, where applicable).

[b]Tobramycin or other aminoglycoside, such as gentamicin, depending on local availability.

CRP, C-reactive protein; ESR, erythrocyte sedimentation rate; MRSA, methicillin-resistant S. aureus.

Adapted from The Hospital for Sick Children eFormulary Antimicrobial Guidelines—Empiric Antibiotic Therapy in Children, 2021.

Table 24.7 Gastrointestinal/Genitourinary Infections

Disease Process	Common Physical Examination Findings	Suspected Pathogens	Empiric Antimicrobial Therapy	Usual Duration of Treatment[a]	Additional Comments
Necrotizing enterocolitis (neonates)	Abdominal distention, bilious vomiting/aspirates, bloody stools, peritonitis, vital sign instability	Enteric gram-negative bacilli, *Enterococcus* spp., anaerobes	Ampicillin + tobramycin[b] ± metronidazole	7–14 days	Add metronidazole for perforation, peritonitis, or rapidly advancing sepsis
Perforated appendix or bowel (non-neonates)	Diffuse abdominal pain, peritonitis, rebound tenderness, vital sign instability	Enteric gram-negative bacilli, *Enterococcus* spp., anaerobes	Ceftriaxone + metronidazole	7–10 days	Oral stepdown: ciprofloxacin + metronidazole, OR amoxicillin-clavulanate May require surgical drainage of collections
Bacterial enteritis	Bloody diarrhea, abdominal pain, dehydration	*Salmonella* spp., *Shigella* spp., *Campylobacter jejuni/coli*, *Escherichia coli* (Verotoxin-producing), *Yersinia enterocolitica*, *Clostridium difficile*, *Entamoeba hystolytica*	Empiric therapy generally not indicated, infectious diseases consultation recommended for specific therapy		Empiric antibiotics indicated for: all *Shigella* and *E. histolytica* infections; *Salmonella* in severe infections or at-risk patients (immunocompromised or <3 months old); *Yersinia* infections in presence of terminal ileitis or mesenteric adenitis; toxin-producing *C. difficile*; enteric infection with sepsis

Continued

Table 24.7 Gastrointestinal/Genitourinary Infections—cont'd

Disease Process	Common Physical Examination Findings	Suspected Pathogens	Empiric Antimicrobial Therapy	Usual Duration of Treatment[a]	Additional Comments
Helicobacter pylori infection					
<8 years old	Epigastric abdominal pain, hematemesis, melena	H. pylori	Amoxicillin + metronidazole + PPI + bismuth subsalicylate	14 days	
≥8 years old	Same as earlier	H. pylori	Tetracycline + metronidazole + PPI + bismuth subsalicylate	14 days	
Urinary tract infection and pyelonephritis					
<2 months	Poor feeding, lethargy, fever, cloudy urine	E. coli, Enterococcus spp., Proteus mirabilis, Klebsiella spp., Pseudomonas aeruginosa	Ampicillin + tobramycin[b]	7–14 days	Prophylactic antibiotics for recurrent UTIs are no longer routinely recommended, unless high-grade vesicoureteral reflux or urological abnormality
≥2 months	Cloudy urine, hematuria, suprapubic or flank pain, fever	Same as earlier, Enterococcus spp. unlikely in pyelonephritis	Outpatient[c]: amoxillin-clavulanate or cephalexin Inpatient: ampicillin + tobramycin[b]	Febrile infant/child with UTI/pyelonephritis: 7 days Older children, cystitis, no fever: 2–4 days	Complicated UTIs may require different antimicrobials and/or duration

[a]Usual duration of treatment reflects total duration of therapy (IV ± PO, where applicable).

[b]Tobramycin or other aminoglycoside, such as gentamicin, depending on local availability.

[c]Outpatient therapy applies to patients WITHOUT any of the following risk factors: age <12 weeks, genitourinary abnormalities, current antibiotic use, pyelonephritis or critical illness/hospitalization.

PPI, Proton-pump inhibitor; UTIs, urinary tract infections.

Adapted from The Hospital for Sick Children eFormulary Antimicrobial Guidelines—Empiric Antibiotic Therapy in Children, 2021.

MULTISYSTEM BACTERIAL INFECTIONS

See Table 24.8

Table 24.8	Septicemia/Bacteremia		
Disease Process	**Suspected Pathogens**	**Empiric Antimicrobial Therapy**	**Additional Comments**
Septicemia and bacteremia			
Neonate (0–28 days)	Group B *Streptococcus*, gram-negative enteric bacilli (*E. coli*, *Listeria monocytogenes*, coagulase-negative staphylococci	Ampicillin + tobramycin[a]	Add vancomycin if: colonized with MRSA, or sepsis presents >48 h after admission and have a CVL or >4 vascular access attempts in preceding 48 h
1–3 months	Organisms seen in both neonates and older children	Ceftriaxone + vancomycin ± tobramycin[a]	Add tobramycin[a] for sepsis acquired in the ICU, or for recent post-surgical patients. Consideration should also be made for patients with a tracheostomy or urinary catheter/stent.
≥3 months	*Streptococcus pneumoniae*, *Neisseria meningitidis*, *Staphylococcus aureus*, *Haemophilia influenzae*	Ceftriaxone + vancomycin ± tobramycin[a]	Add tobramycin[a] for sepsis acquired in the ICU, or for recent post-surgical patients. Consideration should also be made for patients with a tracheostomy or urinary catheter/stent.
Central line-associated infections	Coagulase-negative staphylococci, *S. aureus*, gram-negative enteric bacilli	Vancomycin ± gram-negative coverage	Add gram-negative coverage in immunocompromised or hospital acquired infection Urgent line removal in CVL tunnel infections and uncontrolled sepsis

Continued

Table 24.8 Septicemia/Bacteremia—cont'd

Disease Process	Suspected Pathogens	Empiric Antimicrobial Therapy	Additional Comments
Sickle cell disease with fever	*S. pneumoniae, H. influenzae, Salmonella* spp.	Ceftriaxone ± vancomycin	Add vancomycin if clinically septic
Typhoid fever	*Salmonella typhi*	Ceftriaxone	Because of the emergence of ceftriaxone resistance to *Salmonella typhi* in Pakistan, empiric therapy with meropenem is recommended for hospitalized patients with suspected or confirmed typhoid fever who recently returned from Pakistan; azithromycin is an alternative option for uncomplicated cases

ᵃTobramycin or other aminoglycoside, such as gentamicin, depending on local availability. For Febrile Neutropenia, see Chapter 30 Oncology.

CVL, Central venous line; *ICU,* intensive care unit.

Adapted from The Hospital for Sick Children eFormulary Antimicrobial Guidelines—Empiric Antibiotic Therapy in Children, 2021.

TUBERCULOSIS

1. **Epidemiology and transmission**
   a. At risk populations in Canada: foreign-born children, children of foreign-born parents, First Nations or Inuit children, children who travel to endemic countries
   b. Transmission is primarily by the airborne route
   c. Children <4 years of age less able to contain infection than adults and are at higher risk of developing pulmonary, as well as extrapulmonary disease

2. **Definitions**
   a. **Latent tuberculosis (TB) infection (LTBI):** an individual infected with *Mycobacterium tuberculosis* (as demonstrated by a positive TB skin test or interferon gamma release assay [IGRA]) and is asymptomatic with normal physical examination and has a normal chest x-ray (CXR)
   b. **Active TB disease:** an individual infected with *M. tuberculosis* with symptoms/signs of TB (pulmonary/extrapulmonary) or abnormal CXR suggestive of TB or microbiological/pathological evidence of active TB

3. **History**
   a. Exposure (duration, proximity), including disease site and severity of source patient, and susceptibility of source isolate if available
   b. Patient symptoms and duration
   c. Prior anti-TB therapy
   d. Prior investigations (particularly culture results and susceptibility of isolates)
   e. Immunocompromised state: human immunodeficiency virus (HIV) status, immunosuppressant therapy
   f. Previous Bacille Calmette-Guerin (BCG) vaccination

4. **Investigations**
   a. Immunological evidence of exposure
      i. TST/Mantoux test (Table 24.9): a positive reaction can be caused by infection with *M. tuberculosis,* nontuberculous mycobacteria, or prior receipt of BCG
      ii. Interferon gamma release assay (IGRA) preferable for children who have received BCG vaccine. Pros: more specific than TB skin test; no need for two visits. Cons: reduced sensitivity in young children (<5 years) and immunocompromised patients; more expensive

> ✴ **PEARL**
>
> Negative TST or IGRA does not rule out TB disease, particularly in immunocompromised children. Can use both TST and IGRA to increase sensitivity.

b. Chest x-ray (two-view)
   i. Hilar lymphadenopathy
   ii. Parencyhmal consolidation, particularly in lung apex. Cavitary lesions may not appear in young children.
   iii. Ghon complex: calcified parenchymal focus ("tuberculoma") with adjacent hilar lymphadenopathy
c. Microbiological samples (acid-fast bacillus [AFB] smear, mycobacterial culture, TB polymerase chain reaction [PCR])
   i. Induced sputum: children <8 years of age usually cannot expectorate enough bacilli for testing; can attempt induced sputum × 3; taken a minimum of 1 hour apart
   ii. Gastric aspirates × 3 in the early morning before ambulation or feeding (if respiratory involvement)
   iii. Cerebrospinal fluid (CSF, if suspected meningitis)
   iv. Body fluid or tissue biopsy depending on suspected extraparenchymal involvement

Table 24.9	Definition of Positive Tuberculin Skin Test
Induration	**Group**
0–4 mm	In general, considered negative Child <5 years of age and high risk of TB infection

≥5 mm	Immunosuppressed:
	  HIV Infection
	  Immunosuppressive therapy
	  TNF Alpha inhibitors
	  End-stage renal disease
	Higher likelihood of TB:
	  Contact with infectious TB case within past 2 years
	  Presence of fibronodular disease on CXR (healed TB, not previously treated)

≥10 mm	In general, considered positive (sensitivity of 90% and specificity of >95%)

CXR, Chest x-ray; *HIV*, human immunodeficiency virus; *TB*, tuberculosis; *TNF*, tumor necrosis factor.

Adapted from Public Health Agency of Canada. *Canadian Tuberculosis Standards.* 7th ed. 2014. Available at: www.canada.ca/content/dam/phac-aspc/migration/phac-aspc/tbpc-latb/pubs/tb-canada-7/assets/pdf/tb-standards-tb-normes-pref-eng.pdf.

! PITFALL

A tuberculin skin test (TST)/Mantoux test does not differentiate between latent or active TB and therefore should not be used to diagnose active TB.

Treatment

a. Involve a TB expert

b. Anti-TB therapy should be individualized based on known isolate or presumed susceptibility

c. LTBI

   i. Standard regimen: daily isoniazid (INH) for 9 months

   ii. Other options include rifampin for 4 months or rifampin + INH for 3 months

d. Active pulmonary TB and non-central nervous system (CNS) extra-pulmonary TB

   i. Pulmonary TB: 6 months of combination therapy, preferably with directly observed therapy (DOT); extrapulmonary TB: 9 to 12 months

   ii. For cases with unknown susceptibility: INH, rifampin, pyrazinamide, and ethambutol

   iii. Step down to three drugs if fully sensitive for 2 months, then complete course with INH and rifampin

   iv. Pyridoxine (vitamin B6) supplementation with INH regimens (prevention of peripheral neuropathy)

   v. Consider vitamin D deficiency

e. CNS-involved or disseminated/extensive TB

   i. Longer duration of therapy, often 12 to 24 months

   ii. Adjunctive corticosteroid therapy may be warranted in CNS-involved cases, pericardial TB, or immune reconstitution inflammatory syndrome (IRIS)

LYME DISEASE

1. **Epidemiology and transmission:** caused by *Borrelia burdorferi*

   a. Tick vector: *Ixodes scapularis* (Eastern and Central Canada), *Ixodes pacificus* (British Columbia)

   b. Greatest risk in late spring and summer

✦ PEARL

Tick needs to be attached for >24 to 36 h for transmission of bacteria to occur. If the tick is removed within 24 h, there is almost zero chance of transmission.

2. **Clinical manifestations:** See Table 24.10

Table 24.10	Clinical Manifestations of Lyme Disease in Children
Clinical Stage (Post-tick Bite)	**Clinical Manifestation**

Early, localized (cutaneous) disease
 Commonly 7–14 days
 (Range 3–30 days)
	Erythema migrans (71%)
	   i. Erythematous "bulls eye" lesion
	   ii. >5 cm in diameter
	   iii. Usually single, at site of bite
	 Flu-like symptoms

Later (extracutaneous) disease	Neurological signs
	   i. Bell palsy (9%)
	   ii. Radiculoneuropathy (4%)
	   iii. Meningitis/encephalitis (1%)
	 Carditis (1%)
	 Large joint pauciarticular arthritis (31%), often involving the knees

Data from Onyett H. Canadian Paediatric Society Practice Point: Lyme disease in Canada: focus on children. Posted: July 28, 2020.

3. **Diagnosis**
   a. Early localized disease: clinical diagnosis; serology has poor sensitivity at this stage and is not recommended
   b. Later (extracutaneous) disease: laboratory confirmed (two-tiered serological testing)
      i. ELISA: screening test; good sensitivity, less specific (false positive with other spirochetes, viral infections, autoimmune disease)
      ii. Western blot: confirmatory test; specific; if positive, suggests Lyme disease; if negative, is not Lyme disease even if ELISA was positive; may get false negatives with European strains of Lyme disease (speak with a microbiologist if this is suspected on history)
      iii. Repeat serology in 3 to 5 weeks if highly suspicious of Lyme with initial negative result
4. **Treatment:** see Table 24.11

Table 24.11	Antibiotic Therapy for Lyme Disease in Children and Adolescents		
Clinical Presentation	**Antibiotic of Choice**	**Route**	**Duration**
Erythema migrans[a]	Doxycycline	PO	10 days
	Amoxicillin	PO	14 days
	Cefuroxime	PO	14 days
Isolated facial palsy	Doxycycline	PO	14 days
Arthritis[b]	Doxycycline	PO	28 days
	Amoxicillin	PO	28 days
	Cefuroxime	PO	28 days
Heart block/carditis[c]	Doxycycline	PO	14–21 days
	Amoxicillin	PO	14–21 days
	Cefuroxime	PO	14–21 days
	Ceftriaxone	IV	14–21 days
Meningitis/encephalitis	Doxycycline	PO	14 days
	Ceftriaxone	IV	14 days

[a]Azithromycin is an alternative agent for the treatment of erythema migrans in children unable to take a beta-lactam or doxycycline.

[b]Persistent arthritis after first course of antibiotics can be retreated with oral agent for 28 days or IV ceftriaxone for 14–28 days.

[c]Can stepdown to oral therapy once discharged.

Modified from American Academy of Pediatrics. Lyme disease. In: Kimberlin DW, Brady MT, Jackson MA, Long SS, eds., *Red Book: 2018 Report of the Committee on Infectious Diseases.* 31st ed. Itasca, IL: American Academy of Pediatrics; 2018:515–523.

5. **Postexposure prophylaxis**
   a. Indications (need all criteria to be met)
      i. *Ixodes* tick estimated to have been attached for ≥36 hours
      ii. Prophylaxis started within 72 hours of time that the tick was removed
      iii. Local rate of infection of ticks with *B. burgdorferi* is ≥20%
      iv. Doxycycline treatment is not contraindicated (such as in pregnancy, younger children)
   b. Regimens
      i. <45 kg: doxycycline 4.4 mg/kg × 1 dose
      ii. ≥45 kg: doxycycline 200 mg × 1 dose
      iii. No evidence for amoxicillin prophylaxis

VIRAL INFECTIONS

HERPES SIMPLEX VIRUS (HSV)

1. Two types: HSV 1 and HSV 2
2. Transmission via direct contact with infected secretions or lesions

3. Patients with primary infection shed virus for at least 1 week; patients with recurrent infection for 3 to 4 days

A. Neonatal herpes simplex virus

1. Risk of transmission varies according to maternal infection type, highest with first episode primary maternal genital infection (60%) and lowest with recurrent maternal genital disease (<3%)

2. **Clinical manifestations**
   a. **Localized to skin, eyes, mouth (SEM) (40%):** usually 1 to 2 weeks of life; if untreated can progress to disseminated or CNS disease
   b. **Localized CNS disease (35%):** usually 2 to 3 weeks of life; fever, seizures, altered consciousness
   c. **Disseminated disease (25%):** usually 1 to 2 weeks of life, sepsis-like presentation with multiorgan involvement (commonly lung, liver)
   d. Initial symptoms may occur up to 6 weeks of age
   e. High morbidity and mortality rates for CNS and disseminated disease despite treatment

3. **Management**
   a. Asymptomatic infants: see Table 24.12
   b. Symptomatic infants (includes those with both local lesions and suspected systemic disease): full workup that includes a complete blood count (CBC), liver enzymes, creatinine, and lumbar puncture; HSV PCR should be done on CSF, blood, vesicular lesions, and mucous membrane/surface swabs
   c. Treatment: intravenous (IV) acyclovir
      i. SEM: 14 days (+1% triluridine topically if eye involved)
      ii. Disseminated: 21 days
      iii. CNS: 21 days; repeat lumbar puncture (LP) toward end of treatment course and continue treatment if PCR positive, repeat LP weekly until PCR negative
      iv. Suppressive oral acyclovir 300 mg/m^2/dose 3 times daily for 6 months following IV treatment for CNS and disseminated disease (may consider for mucocutaneous disease); monthly CBC, creatinine, liver enzymes while on oral acyclovir

Table 24.12	**Management of Asymptomatic Term Infants With Suspected Maternal Genital HSV at or Near Delivery[a]**		
Maternal Status	**Delivery Type**	**Investigations**	**Treatment**
First Episode HSV	- C-section before membrane rupture	- 24-h swabs[b] - Clinical monitoring for symptoms	- No empiric treatment - If swabs positive, complete full workup and treat as if symptomatic
First episode HSV	- Vaginal delivery - C-section after membrane rupture	- 24-h swabs[b] - Clinical monitoring for symptoms	- Empiric acyclovir pending swab results - If swabs negative, complete 10 days of IV acyclovir - If swabs positive, complete full workup and treat as if symptomatic
Recurrent HSV	- Any delivery type	- 24-h swabs[b] - Clinical monitoring for symptoms	- No empiric treatment - If swabs positive, complete full workup and treat as if symptomatic

[a]Swabs or empiric treatment are not indicated for infants born to mothers without active genital herpes lesions

[b]24-h swabs entails "mucous membrane/surface swabs" taken from the conjunctivae, mouth, nasopharynx, any skin lesions (e.g., sites of scalp electrodes, if present), and rectum for HSV PCR. Some experts also recommend blood PCR.

HSV, Herpes simplex virus; *IV,* intravenous; *PCR,* polymerase chain reaction.

Data from Allen UD, et al. Canadian Paediatric Society Position Statement: Prevention and management of neonatal herpes simplex virus infection. Posted: March 6, 2020.

B. Herpes simplex virus infants and children beyond the neonatal period

1. **Clinical presentation**
   a. **Mucocutaneous disease**
      i. Gingivostomatitis: ulcerative exanthema of gingival and oral mucous membranes
      ii. Herpes labialis: vesicles, usually on vermilion border of the lips
      iii. Herpetic whitlow: single or multiple vesicular lesions on distal finger
      iv. Eczema herpeticum: emergency; widespread vesicular eruption
   b. **Genital herpes**
   c. **Ocular disease:** conjunctivitis, keratitis usually secondary to autoinoculation
   d. **CNS disease**
      i. Encephalitis: fever, altered level of consciousness, personality changes, seizures, focal neurological findings, coma, death
      ii. Meningitis: nonspecific clinical signs; mild and self-limited presentation often occurs with primary HSV 2 infections in sexually active adolescents

2. **Diagnosis**
   a. PCR testing of vesicular fluid from skin lesions, mucosal lesions, CSF, blood, or tissue
   b. Electron microscopy (EM)/direct fluorescent antibody staining, and culture can be diagnostic, but rarely used
   c. Repeat LP should be considered if strongly suspect HSV as cause of encephalitis and initial LP negative, or if ongoing active viral replication is a concern

3. **Treatment**
   a. Urgent ophthalmology consultation if any ocular involvement
   b. Mucocutaneous disease
      i. IV acyclovir necessary for severe or complicated infections, including eczema herpeticum
      ii. Oral acyclovir or valacyclovir may be effective if initiated early in primary gingivostomatitis or genital herpes
      iii. Prophylactic oral acyclovir or valacyclovir may be of benefit in those with frequent recurrence
   c. CNS disease (encephalitis): IV acyclovir for 21 days

EBV

1. **Clinical manifestations**
   a. Wide spectrum: asymptomatic (infants and young children) to fulminant infection (immunocompromised)
   b. Infectious mononucleosis: fever, exudative pharyngitis, lymphadenopathy, hepatosplenomegaly, atypical lymphocytosis, morbilliform rash (most frequent in those treated with ampicillin or penicillin)
   c. Amoxicillin associated with rash in approximately 80% of patients with primary EBV

2. **Diagnosis**
   a. See Figure 24.3 for EBV antibody progression

Figure 24.3 Epstein-Barr Virus Antibody Progression

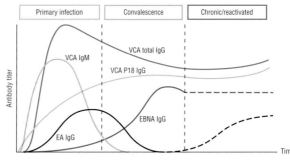

EA, Early antigen; *EBNA*, Epstein-Barr nuclear antigen; *Ig*, immunoglobulin; *VCA*, viral capsid antigen. (Modified from Jaap M. Middeldorp at Cyto-Barr BV, The Netherlands. With permission.)

b. Nonspecific tests for heterophile antibody (e.g., monospot) often negative in children <4 years of age

c. >10% atypical lymphocytes and positive monospot highly suggestive of acute infection

3. **Treatment**

a. Supportive; rest during acute phase

b. Avoid contact sports if splenomegaly present

c. Corticosteroids considered in select cases (impending airway obstruction, massive splenomegaly, myocarditis, hemolytic anemia, hemophagocytic syndrome)

d. Antiviral treatment required in immunocompromised host or in presence of severe disease (encephalitis)

4. **Complications**

a. Hematological: thrombocytopenia, agranulocytosis, hemolytic anemia, hemophagocytic syndrome

b. CNS: aseptic meningitis, encephalitis, Guillain-Barré syndrome, transverse myelitis, optic neuritis, cranial nerve palsies

c. Others: orchitis, pneumonia, myocarditis, splenic rupture

VARICELLA-ZOSTER VIRUS

1. **Transmission**

a. Airborne, direct contact of chickenpox or zoster lesions, transplacental

b. Contagious 2 days before onset of rash until vesicles have crusted over

c. Incubation period: 10 to 21 days (28 days if varicella zoster immune globulin given)

2. **Clinical manifestations**

a. Primary infection (chickenpox): generalized pruritic vesicular rash, mild fever, pharyngitis

   i. Complications: bacterial superinfection of skin lesions including invasive group A streptococcus, thrombocytopenia, arthritis, hepatitis, cerebellar ataxia, encephalitis, meningitis, stroke, glomerulonephritis, pneumonia

b. Reactivation (zoster) of latent virus in dorsal root ganglion: grouped vesicular lesions in distribution of one to three dermatomes, sometimes with localized pain

3. **Diagnosis**

a. Typically clinical

b. Direct detection by PCR, antigen detection, or EM of lesion scraping for confirmation in select cases

4. **Treatment**

a. Therapy not routinely recommended in healthy children <12 years unless severe disease and/or complications present

b. Acyclovir or valacyclovir recommended:
  i. Children ≥12 years of age
  ii. Chronic cutaneous or pulmonary disorders
  iii. Long-term salicylate therapy
  iv. Recent corticosteroid use
  v. Immunocompromised patients
c. Avoid acetyl salicylic acid (ASA) because of risk of Reye syndrome; avoid use of other nonsteroidal antiinflammatory drugs (NSAIDs)
d. Perinatal varicella infection: see Table 24.17

HIV

1. **Epidemiology**
   a. Vertical transmission (in utero 5%, intrapartum 20%, breast milk 14%)
   b. Factors affecting the risk of vertical transmission of HIV include maternal factors (viral load, CD4 count, poor adherence to antiretrovirals [ARVs]), obstetric factors (premature rupture of membranes [PROM], chorioamnionitis, other sexually transmitted infection [STIs], vaginal delivery), and fetal/infant factors (prematurity, breastfeeding)

2. **Clinical manifestations**
   a. Mild: generalized lymphadenopathy, hepatosplenomegaly, parotitis, dermatitis, recurrent sinusitis, otitis media
   b. Moderate: bacterial meningitis, sepsis or pneumonia, recurrent or chronic diarrhea, cardiomyopathy, nephropathy, CMV or toxoplasmosis with onset before 1 month of age, complicated chickenpox, persistent fever (>1 month), lymphoid interstitial pneumonitis, nocardiosis
   c. Severe: opportunistic infections (*Pneumocystis jiroveci* pneumonia [PJP], esophageal candidiasis, disseminated CMV, cryptococcal meningitis, CNS toxoplasmosis, *M. tuberculosis* disease, *Mycobacterium avium* complex infection, chronic enteritis [*Cryptosporidium, Isospora*]), malignancies (Kaposi sarcoma, lymphomas, smooth-muscle tumors), HIV encephalopathy (global developmental disability), HIV-associated wasting (failure to thrive)

3. **Treatment:** antiretroviral therapy
   a. Recommended for all HIV-infected children regardless of symptoms or CD4 count
   b. Selection of initial regimen individualized based on patient characteristics (age, weight, sexual maturity), viral resistance testing, characteristics of the proposed regiment (potential adverse events, formulation, tolerability, dosing frequency)
   c. For treatment-naïve children with fully susceptible virus, initial treatment should consist of a dual-nucleoside/nucleotide reverse transcriptase inhibitor (NRTI, such as zidovudine plus lamivudine

or abacavir, abacavir plus lamivudine or tenofovir alafenamide plus emtricitabine) and either an integrase strand transfer inhibitor (INSTI, such as raltegravir, elvitegravir or dolutegravir), a nonnucleoside reverse transcriptase inhibitor (NNRTI, such as nevirapine), or a boosted protease inhibitor (PI, such as atazanavir or darunavir)

4. **Care of the infant vertically exposed to HIV**
   a. HIV testing during pregnancy
      i. Recommended routine prenatal HIV testing for all pregnant women
      ii. Repeat serological testing in third trimester and at delivery for higher-risk women
      iii. Rapid HIV antibody testing for women with unknown status at the time of delivery; consider STAT viral load if in labor and high-risk activities in month before delivery
   b. Management/prevention of vertical transmission in HIV-positive mothers
      i. Maternal antenatal management: involvement of HIV experts, initiation of antiretroviral therapy as soon as possible and viral load monitoring to determine adequacy of treatment
      ii. Maternal intrapartum and postpartum management: intravenous zidovudine during labor, maternal counselling on infant management, including recommending exclusive formula feeding
      iii. Infant of mother who was treated effectively and has undetectable viral load before delivery: exclusive formula feeding, zidovudine for 4 weeks, CBC (for trending hemoglobin) and alanine aminotransferase (ALT) at birth, 1 month and 2 months; HIV testing: HIV PCR within 48 hours of birth, 1 to 2 months of life and 2 to 4 months of life, and serology at 18 months of life
      iv. Infant of mother who was not effectively treated (e.g., has detectable viral load, poor adherence in the absence of documented virological suppression): consultation with HIV experts
      v. Long-term follow-up into adulthood of all HIV-exposed uninfected children who were exposed in utero to antiretroviral medications is recommended

FUNGAL INFECTIONS

1. **Selected fungal infections in the immunocompetent host**: see Table 24.13
2. **Selected invasive fungal infections in the immunocompromised host:** see Table 24.14

Table 24.13	Selected Fungal Infections in the Immunocompetent Host			
Pathogen	**Risk Factors**	**Organ Involvement**	**Diagnostic Tests**	**Antifungal Agents**
Candida spp.	Prematurity, antibiotic therapy	Oropharyngeal (thrush) Diaper dermatitis	Clinically diagnosed, stain and culture	Topical nystatin (low-risk mucocutaneous disease)
		Congenital Candidiasis (preterm infants) Candidemia and acute disseminated candidiasis (preterm infants): chorioretinitis, skin lesions, muscle abscesses Renal, CNS, bone involvement	Stains and cultures of specimens (including CSF, biopsies), lesion scrapings	Amphotericin B
Dermatophytes	Direct or indirect contact with human or animal cases	Skin, nails	Tissue stain and culture	Terbinafine, itraconazole, fluconazole
Blastomycosis	Travel to Northern Ontario, Great Lakes region, St. Lawrence River; Midwest, Southeast, and South-Central United States	Lung, skin, bone, brain	Tissue stain and culture (BAL, biopsy), serology, antigen tests	Amphotericin B, itraconazole
Histoplasmosis	Travel to Ohio, Mississippi River, or St. Lawrence River basins; spelunking; bird and bat guano; soil upheaval	Lung, disseminates to multiple organs	Tissue stain and culture (BAL, biopsy), urine or serum antigen, serology	Amphotericin B, itraconazole
Coccidioidomycosis	Travel to Southwestern United States, Mexico, Central and South America	Lung, rarely disseminates	Tissue stain and culture (BAL, biopsy), serology	Fluconazole, itraconazole, amphotericin B

Table 24.13	Selected Fungal Infections in the Immunocompetent Host—cont'd			
Pathogen	Risk Factors	Organ Involvement	Diagnostic Tests	Antifungal Agents
Cryptococcosis	Travel to Vancouver Island, British Columbia lower mainland	Brain, lung, skin	CSF, blood antigen; CSF India ink stain, CSF culture	Amphotericin B ± 5-FC, fluconazole

5-FC, 5-Fluorocytosine (flucytosine); *BAL*, bronchoalveolar lavage; *CNS*, central nervous system; *CSF*, cerebrospinal fluid.

Table 24.14	Selected Invasive Fungal Infections in the Immunocompromised Host				
Pathogen	Prevalence	Risk Factors	Organ Involvement	Diagnostic Tests	Potential Antifungal Agents
Candida spp.	+ + + +	Indwelling lines, prematurity, malignancy, transplantation, prolonged antibiotics, HIV	Blood, liver, spleen, CNS	Stains and culture of specimens	Amphotericin B, fluconazole, caspofungin
Aspergillus spp.	+ +	Malignancy, transplantation, SCID	Lung, sinuses, brain, bone	Stains and culture of aspirates, tissue samples	Voriconazole, amphotericin B, caspofungin
Mucormycosis	+	Malignancy, transplantation, SCID	Sinuses, lung, brain	Stains and culture of aspirates, tissue samples	Posaconazole, amphotericin B
Cryptococcosis	+	HIV, corticosteroids, malignancy, transplantation, diabetes mellitus	Brain, lung, skin	CSF India ink stain; CSF, blood antigen detection	Amphotericin B, fluconazole

CNS, Central nervous system; *CSF*, cerebrospinal fluid; *HIV*, human immunodeficiency virus; *SCID*, severe combined immunodeficiency.

PARASITIC INFECTIONS

See Table 24.15 for selected parasitic infections

Table 24.15	Selected Parasitic Infections			
Parasite	**Geographic Distribution and Epidemiology[a]**	**Common Sources**	**Common Symptoms**	**Treatment Drug of Choice (alternatives in brackets)**
Helminths				
Roundworm (*Ascaris lumbricoides*)	Worldwide (common in tropics and subtropics)	Fecal–oral (ingestion of infective Ascaris eggs)	- Most asymptomatic - Acute transient pneumonitis with fever (Löffler syndrome) during larva migration - May cause bowel or biliary tree obstruction	Albendazole (mebendazole or ivermectin)
Hookworm (*Ancylostoma duodenale, Necator americanus*)	Worldwide (most common in moist warm climates); S. Europe, N. Africa, N. Asia, S. America, SE United States	Soil (skin contact); walking in bare feet/sandals (filariform larva penetrate skin)	- Most are asymptomatic - Hypochromic normocytic anemia - Protein energy malnutrition	Albendazole (mebendazole or pyrantel pamoate)
Pinworm (*Enterobius vermicularis*)	Worldwide	Fecal–oral (human to human)	- Pruritis ani or pruritis vulvae	Mebendazole (pyrantel pamoate or albendazole); if recurs, consider treating family
Strongyloides stercoralis	Tropics/ subtropics	Soil (skin contact); walking in bare feet/sandals; direct contact (human-to-human, lab setting); autoinfection	- Most asymptomatic - Pneumonitis (Löffler-like syndrome) during larval migration - Disseminated hyperinfection in immunocompromised patients	Ivermectin (albendazole)
Whipworm (*Trichuris trichiura*)	Worldwide; common in tropical regions with poor sanitation	Fecal–oral (ingestion of eggs)	- Most asymptomatic - Dysentery syndrome: abdominal pain, tenesmus, bloody diarrhea - Recurrent rectal prolapse	Mebendazole (albendazole or ivermectin)

Table 24.15 Selected Parasitic Infections—cont'd

Parasite	Geographic Distribution and Epidemiology[a]	Common Sources	Common Symptoms	Treatment Drug of Choice (alternatives in brackets)
Pork tapeworm (Taenia solium)	Worldwide; ↑ risk if close contact with pigs; high prevalence in Mexico, Central and South America, Africa, India, SE Asia, Philippines, S. Europe	Ingestion of raw/undercooked pork; cysticercosis occurs if Taenia solium eggs ingested (contaminated food or water)	- Asymptomatic or mild GI symptoms; passage (passive) of proglottids - Neurocysticercosis usually presents with seizures	Praziquantel (niclosamide); cysticercosis: consult infectious diseases specialist
Beef tapeworm (Taenia saginata)	Worldwide; cattle-breeding areas; high prevalence in central Asia, Near East, central and E. Africa	Ingestion of raw or undercooked beef	- Mild GI symptoms, passage (active and passive) of proglottids	Praziquantel (niclosamide)
Fish tapeworm (Diphyllobothrium latum)	Siberia, Northern Europe, North America, Japan, Chile	Ingestion of raw or undercooked freshwater fish (smoked or dried fish)	- Most asymptomatic; mild GI symptoms; pernicious anemia	Praziquantel (niclosamide)
Protozoa				
Entamoeba histolytica (symptomatic)	Worldwide, highest risk in developing countries; risk groups: travel, recent immigrants, institutionalized populations	Fecal–oral	- May be asymptomatic - Amebic dysentery (bloody diarrhea); liver abscess (rarely at other sites)	Metronidazole or tinidazole (followed by lumicidal agent iodoquinol or paromomycin)
Blastocystis hominis[b] (symptomatic)	Worldwide	Fecal–oral	- Most asymptomatic - Bloating, flatulence, diarrhea, abdominal pain, nausea	Metronidazole (iodoquinol or TMP/SMX)
Dientamoeba fragilis (symptomatic)	Worldwide; associated with pinworm infections	Fecal–oral	- Most asymptomatic - Mild-moderate GI symptoms (cramping, diarrhea, weight loss, nausea)	Metronidazole or paromomycin or iodoquinol; consider treating for pinworm as well

Continued

Infectious Diseases

24

Table 24.15	Selected Parasitic Infections—cont'd			
Parasite	Geographic Distribution and Epidemiology[a]	Common Sources	Common Symptoms	Treatment Drug of Choice (alternatives in brackets)
Giardia lamblia (symptomatic)	Worldwide, more prevalent in warm climates	Fecal–oral	GI tract symptoms: abdominal pain, diarrhea, flatulence	Metronidazole (nitazoxanide or tinidazole)

[a]For more detailed geographic distribution, visit the Center for Disease Control and Prevention Web site (www.cdc.gov).

[b]Role as pathogen controversial.

GI, Gastrointestinal; *TMP/SMX,* trimethoprim/sulfamethoxazole.

MALARIA

1. Canadian recommendations for the prevention and treatment of malaria (CATMAT Guidelines): www.canada.ca/en/public-health/services/catmat/canadian-recommendations-prevention-treatment-malaria.html
2. **Epidemiology:** Table 24.16 compares *Plasmodium* species
3. **Clinical manifestations**
   a. General incubation rule: 2 weeks to 2 months
      i. Relapses caused by persistent liver forms of *Plasmodium vivax* and *Plasmodium ovale* can appear months later (up to 5 years)
      ii. *P. malariae* can persist for many years (not life-threatening)
   b. Symptoms: high fevers, severe chills, profuse sweating, fatigue
   c. Signs: hepatosplenomegaly, anemia, acute respiratory distress syndrome may occur on day 3 or 4 (immune phenomenon), monitor for respiratory decompensation
4. **Diagnosis and management:** see Figure 24.4 and consult an infectious diseases specialist

PEARL

Severe malaria is a serious multisystem infection that can involve the CNS, respiratory, cardiovascular, renal, and hematopoietic systems. Laboratory evidence includes severe anemia, hypoglycemia, acidosis, elevated creatinine, hyperlactatemia, and hyperparasitemia ($\geq 2\%$).

Table 24.16	Malaria Species	
Species	**Key Epidemiology**	**Clinical Pearls**

Plasmodium falciparum	- Found in most malarious areas, especially Africa, Haiti, New Guinea, SE Asia, South America, Oceania
	- In Africa, malaria most often caused by *P. falciparum*
		- q36–48h fever cycles (less regular, almost continuous)
		- Medical emergency
		  - Up to 60% parasitemia possible
		  - Severe infection mortality ≥20%
		- 98% will present within the first month of exposure
		- Infects both mature and immature RBCs

Plasmodium vivax	- Predominant malaria species in countries outside of sub-Saharan Africa; found in Bangladesh, India, Pakistan, Sri Lanka, southeast Asia, Oceania, Central and South America	- q48h fever cycle (tertian malaria) - Has hypnozoite (dormant) liver stage - Can occasionally lead to severe disease - Incubation can be up to a year - Only infects immature RBCs
Plasmodium ovale	- Mostly in Africa	- q48h fever cycle (tertian malaria) - Has hypnozoite (dormant) liver stage - Only infects immature RBCs
Plasmodium malariae	- South America, Asia, and Africa - Most common malaria in blood transfusions	- q72h fever cycle (quartan malaria) - Mildest form of malaria - Can manifest up to 40 years after infection - Only infects mature RBCs
Plasmodium knowlesi	- SE Asia: Brunei, Myanmar, Indonesia, Malaysia, the Philippines, Singapore, Thailand, and Vietnam - Primate malaria species shown to cause human disease in 2004	- Can cause severe and fatal infection similar to *P. falciparum* → requires close monitoring and careful management - May be confused with *P. malariae* under the microscope, but has higher (>1%) parasitemia levels

Note: fever cycles are less observed in practice and should not be relied upon to make a species diagnosis.

RBC, Red blood cell.

Figure 24.4   Diagnosis and Management of Malaria

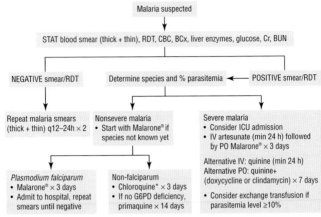

*Chloroquine-resistant *Plasmodium vivax* highly prevalent in New Guinea, Indonesia, and East Timor, so consider alternative

Malarone® = Atovaquone/proguanil. *BCx*, Blood cultures; *BUN*, blood urea nitrogen; *CBC*, complete blood count; *Cr*, creatinine; *G6PD*, glucose-6-phosphate dehydrogenase; *RDT*, rapid diagnostic test.
© All rights reserved. CCDR: Volume 40-7, April 3, 2014: Malaria—Summary of recommendations for the diagnosis and treatment of malaria by the Committee to Advise on Tropical Medicine and Travel (CATMAT) by Boggild A, Brophy J, Charlebois P, Crockett M, Geduld J, Ghesquiere W, McDonald P, Plourde P, Teitelbaum P, Tepper M, Schofield S and McCarthy A (Chair). Public Health Agency of Canada, 2014. Adapted and reproduced with permission from the Minister of Health, 2020.)

CONGENITAL/PERINATAL INFECTIONS

1. See Box 24.1 for a list of congenitally acquired infections
2. See Table 24.17 for clinical features of common congenital infections
3. See Table 24.18 for transmission, diagnosis, and treatment
4. See Table 24.18 for approach to gonococcal and chlamydial infections

Box 24.1	**CHEAP TORCHES Congenital Infection Acronym**		
C	Chickenpox	**T**	Toxoplasmosis
H	Hepatitis viruses (hepatitis B, hepatitis C)	**O**	Other (Zika, lymphocytic choriomeningitis virus, malaria, TB, Chagas)
E	Enteroviruses		
A	AIDS (HIV)	**R**	Rubella
P	Parvovirus B19	**C**	CMV
		H	HSV
		E	Every other STI (human papillomavirus)
		S	Syphilis

AIDS, Acquired immunodeficiency syndrome; *CMV,* cytomegalovirus; *HIV,* human immunodeficiency virus; *HSV,* herpes simplex virus; *STI,* sexually transmitted infection; *TB,* tuberculosis.

Table 24.17 Selected Clinical Features of Common Congenital Infections

Infection	General	CNS	Eye	Ear	Cardiac	Hematologic	Reticuloendothelial System	Skin	Musculoskeletal
Chagas	Low birth weight (<2500 g)	Meningoencephalitis (rare)	—	—	Early: congestive heart failure Late: myocarditis, pericardial effusion, cardiac arrythmias	Anemia	HSM	—	—
CMV	IUGR	Early: microcephaly, periventricular calcifications Late: speech and language delay, developmental disability	Chorioretinitis	SNHL	Hydrops	Cytopenias	HSM	Petechiae, blueberry muffin rash	—
HSV	IUGR	Microcephaly, hydranencephaly, cerebral calcifications	Chorioretinitis, microphthalmia	—	Hydrops	Cytopenias	HSM	Skin lesions and scars	—
Rubella	IUGR Late: endocrinopathies (diabetes mellitus, thyroid disorders), typically later childhood/adulthood	Microcephaly, meningoencephalitis Late: intellectual disability, panencephalitis	Cataracts Late: salt and pepper retinitis	SNHL	PDA, pulmonary stenosis	—	HSM	Blueberry muffin rash	Bony lucencies

Continued

Infectious Diseases

24

Table 24.17 Selected Clinical Features of Common Congenital Infections—cont'd

Infection	General	CNS	Eye	Ear	Cardiac	Hematologic	Reticuloendothelial System	Skin	Musculoskeletal
Syphilis	IUGR, snuffles Late: frontal bossing, saddle nose, Hutchinson teeth, mulberry molars	Aseptic meningitis, cranial nerve palsies Late: intellectual disability, cranial nerve palsies, hydrocephalus	Chorioretinitis, cataracts Late: interstitial keratitis	SNHL	Hydrops	Hemolytic anemia, thrombocytopenia	HSM	Desquamating or maculopapular rash involving palms and soles	Pseudoparalysis, osteitis Late: saber shins, Clutton joints
Toxoplasmosis	IUGR	Hydrocephalus, macrocephaly (or microcephaly), parenchymal calcifications Late: seizures, psychomotor delay	Chorioretinitis	SNHL	Hydrops	Cytopenias	HSM	Maculopapular rash	—
VZV	Esophageal dilatation and reflux, hydronephrosis, hydroureter	—	Microphthalmia, chorioretinitis	—	—	—	Cicatricial scars	—	Limb hypoplasia
Zika	Severe microcephaly with partially collapsed skull	Thin cerebral cortex with subcortical calcifications, early hypotonia	Macular scarring, focal pigmentary retinal mottling	—	—	—	—	—	Congenital limb contractures

CMV, Cytomegalovirus; *CNS,* central nervous system; *HSV,* herpes simplex virus; *HSM,* hepatosplenomegaly; *IUGR,* intrauterine growth retardation; *PDA,* patent ductus arteriosus; *SNHL,* sensorineural hearing loss; *VZV,* varicella zoster virus.

Congenital Infection	Transmission and Key Points	Microbiological Diagnosis	Treatment
CMV	- Most common congenital infection (0.5% live births) - Vertical transmission risk 30%–40% with primary maternal infection - 85%–90% asymptomatic at birth - Neurological sequelae develop in ~20% of cases - Late-onset hearing loss most common adverse outcome in asymptomatic newborns	- Detection of CMV by PCR from amniotic fluid, or urine, saliva and/or blood within 2–3 weeks of birth - PCR of birth dried blood spot can be helpful for retrospective diagnosis (a positive result confirms congenital infection) - Presence of CMV-specific IgM suggestive but not diagnostic of congenital CMV infection	- Treatment not routinely indicated for asymptomatic or mildly symptomatic newborns - Valganciclovir (PO) × 6 months for moderate to severely symptomatic children (multiple systemic manifestations or central nervous system involvement) - Ganciclovir (IV) for hospitalized patients
Parvovirus B19	- Transmission risk: 30% - Potential adverse outcomes include fetal loss and nonimmune hydrops fetalis	- Maternal serology: IgM indicates infection within previous 2–4 months, IgG appears on day 7 of the illness and persists for life - Fetal US monitoring for hydrops recommended if mother diagnosed with acute infection in pregnancy - Detection of virus by PCR in amniotic fluid or fetal blood confirms fetal infection	- Supportive - Intrauterine blood transfusions for hydrop fetalis
Rubella	- Congenital defects almost exclusively with infections acquired during first trimester	- Isolation of virus (or detection by PCR) in throat swab, urine, blood, CSF samples - IgM indicates recent postnatal or congenital infection	- Supportive
Syphilis (*Treponema pallidum*)	- Transplacental transmission at any time during pregnancy/delivery, any stage of disease (highest risk during untreated primary or secondary syphilis)	- Serological diagnosis: infant nontreponemal titer fourfold higher than maternal titer at birth, titer increases after birth, infant treponemal test remains positive at 12–18 months	- Penicillin G (IV) for 10–14 days - See Figure 24.5 for management of infant born to a mother with reactive syphilis serology during pregnancy

Continued

Table 24.18	Transmission, Diagnosis, and Treatment of Selected Congenital Infections—cont'd		
Congenital Infection	Transmission and Key Points	Microbiological Diagnosis	Treatment
	- Most asymptomatic at birth	- Direct detection (dark-field microscopy, direct fluorescent antibody) of organism in samples from active lesions (snuffles, ulcers) - Full evaluation of infant with suspected syphilis includes: serological testing, CBC, CSF studies (including VDRL), long-bone x-rays, ophthalmological assessment, audiological assessment	
Toxoplasmosis	- Risk of transmission greatest in third trimester but higher risk of severe infection if transmitted in first or second trimester - 70%–90% asymptomatic at birth - Prevention: routine handwashing after handing food, avoid consumption of undercooked meat, avoid handing cat feces	- Serology: IgM or IgA antibodies in first 6 months of life or persistence of IgG antibodies beyond 12–18 months of life - Detection of organism by PCR in amniotic fluid, CSF, vitreous fluid, tissue samples - Histological demonstration of organism	- Pyrimethamine + sulfadiazine (or clindamycin) and leucovorin if congenital infection is confirmed
Zika	- Mosquito-borne (most commonly *Aedes aegypti*) - Endemic regions: Southern United States, Central America and Caribbean, most of South America, sub-Saharan Africa, Indian Subcontinent, Southeast Asia, and Polynesia - Majority of children and adults are asymptomatic (~80%) or have non-specific febrile illness - Vertical transmission to the neonate in approximately 5%–10% and more likely when maternal infection is during the first trimester	Antenatal diagnosis - Maternal serology (IgM and IgG ELISA followed by PRNT) - Maternal PCR of blood/urine - Fetal amniocentesis with PCR and imaging Postnatal diagnosis - Serology: IgM and IgG ELISA followed by PRNT - PCR: placental tissue, umbilical cord tissue, blood, urine, or CSF	- Supportive

CBC, Complete blood count; *CMV*, cytomegalovirus; *CSF*, cerebrospinal fluid; *ELISA*, enzyme-linked immunosorbent assay; *Ig*, immunoglobulin; *PCR*, polymerase chain reaction; *PRNT*, plaque reduction neutralization test; *US*, ultrasound; *VDRL*, Venereal Disease Research Laboratory.

Figure 24.5 Management of Infant Born to a Mother With Reactive Syphilis Serology During Pregnancy

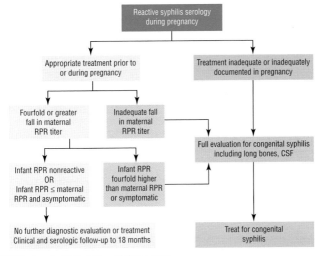

CSF, Cerebrospinal fluid; RPR, rapid plasma reagin.

Table 24.19	Approach to Gonococcal and Chlamydial Infections		
Infection	**Prenatal Screening and Prophylaxis**	**Manifestations**	**Workup and Immediate Treatment**
Gonococcal Infection (*Neisseria gonorrhoeae*)	- Screening recommended for all pregnant women - 0.5% erythromycin ocular prophylaxis no longer recommended by the Canadian Pediatric Society, but may still be medicolegally required in many jurisdictions	- Ophthalmia neonatorum: hyperpurulent conjunctivitis, eyelid swelling; often 2–5 days after birth. Risk of blindness. - Disseminated infections, sepsis, septic arthritis, scalp abscesses	- If unknown maternal infection: immediate maternal testing and education on symptoms of neonatal gonococcal infections. Consider single dose of ceftriaxone if infant unwell or high risk with follow-up concerns. - If known untreated maternal infection: Ceftriaxone 50 mg/kg (max 125 mg) IM/IV and conjunctival culture. If baby unwell, complete blood and CSF cultures, consult infectious diseases specialist.

Continued

Table 24.19	Manifestations and Treatment of Sexually Transmitted Infection Exposed Neonates—cont'd		
Infection	**Prenatal Screening and Prophylaxis**	**Manifestations**	**Workup and Immediate Treatment**
Chlamydial Infection (*C. trachomatis*)	- Screening recommended for all pregnant women - No prophylaxis	- Conjunctivitis: watery followed by mucopurulent discharge with eyelid swelling; often 5–14 days after birth - Pneumonia: usually afebrile, cough, and tachypnea; often 4–12 weeks of age	- All infants should be monitored for signs and symptoms of conjunctivitis and pneumonia - Conjunctival and nasopharyngeal cultures recommended only if infant is symptomatic

CSF, Cerebrospinal fluid; *STI*, sexually transmitted infection.

Data from Moore DL, MacDonald NE, Canadian Paediatric Society, et al. Preventing ophthalmia neonatorum. *Paediatr Child Health*. 2015;20(2):93–96.

> **!** **PITFALL**
>
> Before administering a blood transfusion to an infant suspected of having a congenital infection, save blood for possible serological testing later.

CNS INFECTIONS

ENCEPHALITIS

1. **Definition:** encephalopathy persisting for 24 hours and two of: fever, seizures, new onset focal neurological deficits, CSF pleocytosis, electroencephalogram (EEG) suggesting encephalopathy and imaging suggesting diffuse brain inflammation
2. **History:** season, travel, camping, insect bites, animal contact (cats, horses, mice, hamsters), unpasteurized milk, TB exposures, history of flu-like illness, varicella, rash, seizures, vomiting, diarrhea, lymphadenopathy, mononucleosis-like illness, neurological defects, recent immunizations
3. **Diagnosis**
   a. CSF examination: typically see elevated levels of protein, normal glucose, pleocytosis with predominant monocytosis. Send bacterial culture and PCR for enteroviruses, parechoviruses, HSV 1/2 and selectively for EBV, CMV, varicella-zoster virus (VZV), HHV-6, HHV-7, adenovirus, *Mycoplasma pneumoniae*.
   b. NP swab (influenza A and B, parainfluenza, adenovirus)
   c. Throat swab for *M. pneumoniae* PCR (viral culture medium needed)
   d. Serology should be done selectively depending on clinical presentation, exposure history and other risk factors; is of most utility for arboviruses (e.g., West Nile virus), EBV, *Bartonella henselae*, syphilis, and Lyme disease

e. Noninfectious causes: consider anti-N-methyl-D aspartic acid (NMDA) and other autoantibody testing on CSF and serum

f. Brain magnetic resonance imaging (MRI) usually indicated as it can be helpful both diagnostically and in determining the extent of disease

g. EEG can be done selectively to aid in the diagnosis of encephalopathy and assess for seizure foci

4. **Treatment**

a. Empiric IV acyclovir warranted for all children with acute encephalitis without clear cause

b. Tailor antiviral or antibiotic therapy to isolated organism

c. Steroid treatment, intravenous immune globulin (IVIG), or plasmapheresis for acute disseminated encephalomyelitis, vasculitis, or other inflammatory brain diseases

MENINGITIS

1. **Etiology**

a. Universal vaccination against *Haemophilus influenzae* type b, *Neisseria meningitidis,* and *Streptococcus pneumoniae*, as well as universal prenatal screening for group B *Streptococcus* has reduced incidence of bacterial meningitis

b. Aseptic meningitis (routine bacterial cultures are negative), partially treated bacterial meningitis, viruses, unusual or slow-growing pathogens (*M. tuberculosis, Cryptococcus neoformans*), or noninfectious causes (ruptured dermoid cyst, drugs, such as cotrimoxazole, IVIG)

2. **Initial management:** assessment of hydration, weight, electrolytes (risk of syndrome of inappropriate antidiuretic hormone secretion [SIADH]), head circumference in neonates/young infants, metastatic foci of infection

3. **Investigations**

a. Urgent neuroimaging required before LP if focal neurological findings or suspicion of increase intracranial pressure (ICP)

b. LP for cell count, chemistry (protein, glucose), Gram stain, and bacterial culture. Consider additional tube for viral PCR or culture. See Table 24.20 for CSF reference values. Boxes 24.2 and 24.3 demonstrate strategies for correction of CSF white blood cell count and protein.

c. Gram stain interpretation: gram-positive diplococci (*S. pneumoniae*), gram-negative diplococci (*N. meningitidis*), or small pleomorphic gram-negative coccobacilli (*H. influenzae*)

d. Consider bacterial deoxyribonucleic acid (DNA) PCR or 16s ribonucleic acid (RNA) PCR on CSF if LP done after empiric antibiotics given and culture is negative

e. Blood cultures and other investigations (urine culture, throat swab, chest x-ray) as clinically indicated

Table 24.20	Cerebrospinal Fluid Findings Based on Infection Type				
	NORMAL VALUES		**ABNORMAL VALUES**		
Component	**Neonate**	**>1 month**	**Bacterial**	**Viral**	**TB**
WBC ($\times 10^6$/L)	0–20	<5	50–5000	20–2000	100–500
%PMN	<60	0	95	<30[a]	<30[a]
Protein (g/L)[b]	<1.7	<0.3	>0.6	0.3–0.8	0.5–0.8
Glucose (mmol/L)	1.7–6.4	>2.8	<2.8	<3.3	<2.8
Glucose (% of serum glucose)	45–125	>50	<40	<50	<40

[a]Early in course, PMN predominance may be seen.

[b]Increased protein seen in meningitis, encephalitis, abscess, leukemia, or other intracranial malignancy.

PMN, Polymorphonuclear leukocyte; *TB*, tuberculosis; *WBC*, white blood cell.

From Crain EF, Gershel JC. *Clinical Manual of Emergency Pediatrics.* 3rd ed. New York, NY: McGraw-Hill; 1997.

Box 24.2   Cerebrospinal Fluid White Blood Cell Correction Strategies[a]

Option 1: For every 500 RBC in the CSF sample, reduce WBC count in the CSF sample by 1 to get adjusted WBC count

Option 2: Observed:Predicted WBC ratio
- Predicted CSF WBC = CSF RBC $\times$ (blood WBC/blood RBC)
- If Observed:Predicted WBC ratio ≥1, concerning for meningitis

Traumatic LPs are very difficult to interpret

[a]Supported by limited evidence.

CSF, Cerebrospinal fluid; *LPs*, lumbar punctures; *RBC*, red blood cell; *WBC*, white blood cell.

Box 24.3   Cerebrospinal Fluid Protein Correction Strategy

For every 1000 red blood cell in the cerebrospinal fluid (CSF) sample, reduce protein in the CSF sample by 0.01–0.02 g/L to get adjusted CSF protein

---

4. **Treatment**
   a. Empiric therapy (see Table 24.1)
      i. Should be initiated immediately, do not delay antibiotics in favor of LP if high clinical suspicion
      ii. Tailor antibiotic therapy based on culture and susceptibility results
      iii. Corticosteroids: have been shown to reduce hearing loss in children with HiB meningitis and adults with *S. pneumoniae* meningitis. Consider administration of steroids within 4 hours of first antibiotic dose and continue for 2 days if bacteria found to be *H. influenzae* type b or *S. pneumoniae*.

   b. Additional management
      i. Notification of public health if reportable in region (for
         H. influenzae type b or *N. meningitidis*)
      ii. Prophylactic antibiotics (rifampin) for close contacts with
          persons who have meningococcal disease or HiB meningitis
      iii. Audiological assessment before discharge from hospital
      iv. Neurocognitive follow-up

⚡ PITFALL

Antibiotic therapy for bacterial meningitis should not be narrowed based on Gram stain alone;
wait until organism and resistance pattern is confirmed.

MANAGEMENT OF INFANT WITH FEVER OF UNCERTAIN SOURCE

. **Definitions**
   a. Fever (>38°C [rectal]) in an infant aged 1 to 90 days with uncertain
      source and who is otherwise well appearing
   b. Full septic workup (FSWU): CBC, cultures of blood, urine, and CSF
      with CXR and stool cultures, if clinically indicated
. **Management**
   a. Infants (≤28 days) are at high risk of serious bacterial infection
      (SBI): require admission, FSWU, and empiric antibiotic therapy
   b. Infants (29–90 days) require careful assessment, with workup and
      commencement dependent on assessment of risk factors (Box 24.4),
      clinical presentation. Observation can be key.
   c. Potential HSV infection should be considered (see Box 24.5 for risk factors)

Box 24.4   Perinatal High-Risk Factors

History of prematurity (<37 weeks)
Current or previous antibiotics
Previous hospitalization
Chronic illness
Not discharged with mother

Box 24.5   Risk Factors for Herpes Simplex Virus infection

Maternal herpes simplex virus (HSV) infection before delivery
Intrapartum genital HSV lesions
Postnatal HSV contact
Vesicular skin rash
Eye and/or mouth manifestations, hepatosplenomegaly
Seizures

24

FEVER IN THE RETURNING TRAVELER

1. **Key points**
   a. Differential diagnosis can be narrowed down based on travel itinerary (regions visited), exposure history, and incubation periods
   b. Most infections acquired during travel present within first month of return. Malaria (most commonly *P. vivax*), tuberculosis, typhoid fever, brucellosis, leishmaniasis, hepatitis viruses, and amebic liver abscess may have incubation periods >4 weeks.
   c. Life-threatening travel-related infections: malaria, typhoid fever, meningococcemia, viral hemorrhagic fevers
   d. Malaria must be excluded in all people returning from endemic area
   e. Infection control considerations paramount; some pathogens may pose substantial public health risk (e.g., viral hemorrhagic fevers)
2. **History:** see Table 24.21

Table 24.21	Key Points on History for Fever in the Returning Traveler
Travel itinerary	Exact dates and countries visited; rural vs. urban areas
Immunizations	Routine childhood vaccines plus additional vaccines given pretravel Proof of vaccination insufficient to exclude pathogen; travel-related vaccine efficacy varies (e.g., typhoid vaccines 50%–70% effective)
Malaria prophylaxis	Agent and adherence, use after return, if appropriate Use of bed nets, mosquito repellents
Exposure history	Sick contacts, animal contacts, freshwater exposure (swimming), walking barefoot, consumption of unpasteurized milk products, undercooked meat, fish or seafood or unusual foods; bloodborne pathogen exposure (needles, tattoos, transfusions), sexual contacts, insect bites (ticks)

3. **Investigations**
   a. All cases: CBC and differential, liver function tests, electrolytes, creatinine, urinalysis, blood cultures
   b. If returning from malaria endemic areas: see Malaria section
   c. Other investigations such as CXR, TST, stool examination (EM, culture ova and parasites, *C. difficile* toxin), serology for various pathogens, should be considered on selective basis
   d. Acute serology tube can be saved in lab and paired with convalescent sera if no diagnosis in 10 to 14 days

4. **Management**
   a. High suspicion of malaria should prompt admission for observation, irrespective of malaria smear results; empiric therapy considered selectively
   b. Empiric therapy for typhoid fever should be considered if returning from high-prevalence regions (e.g., South Asia) and no cause of fever identified after initial investigations

IMMIGRANT AND REFUGEE CHILDREN

See Caring for Kids New to Canada: Canadian Pediatric Society's guide for immigrant and refugee children and youth: www.kidsnewtocanada.ca

IMMUNOCOMPROMISED PATIENTS

1. Considerations prior to commencement of immunosuppression: see Box 24.6
2. **Opportunistic infections**
   a. Post-hematopoietic stem cell transplant opportunistic infections (Table 24.22)
   b. Post-solid organ transplant opportunistic infections (Table 24.23)
   c. Presentation and management of select opportunistic infections (Table 24.24)

Box 24.6 Considerations Before Commencement of Immunosuppression

1. Screening tests
   a. TB: TST or IGRA if ≥5 years old, CXR
   b. Other infections to consider screening for: histoplasmosis, toxoplasmosis, strongyloidiasis, hepatitis B, VZV, EBV, CMV
2. Counselling
   a. Food safety (avoid undercooked meats, raw eggs, unpasteurized dairy)
   b. Dental hygiene
   c. Avoid heavy exposure to garden soil, pets, animals
   d. Caution with high-risk activities (e.g., excavation sites and Histo)
   e. Caution with travel to endemic areas for fungi (e.g., southwest United States and coccidiodes) or TB

CXR, Chest x-ray; *CMV*, cytomegalovirus; *EBV*, Epstein-Barr virus; *IGRA*, interferon gamma release assay; *TB*, tuberculosis; *TST*, TB skin test; *VZV*, varicella zoster virus.

Table 24.22	Post-Hematopoietic Stem Cell Transplant Opportunistic Infections		
	Pre-engraftment (<30 Days)	**Post-engraftment (30–100 Days)**	**Late (>100 Days)**
Bacteria	Gram-positive organisms (e.g., *Staphylococcus aureus*, CoNS), GI streptococcal species (e.g., *Viridans* group streptococci), gram-negative bacilli	CoNS (especially if CVL still in situ), *S. aureus*, gram-negative bacilli	Encapsulated bacteria (can give antibiotic prophylaxis if chronic GVHD)
Viruses	HSV (reactivation), seasonal respiratory and enteric, HHV6 (@~2 weeks), adenovirus *In general, too early for CMV and EBV*	CMV, EBV (@~6 weeks; caution PTLD), seasonal respiratory and enteric	CMV, EBV, VZV, seasonal respiratory and enteric
Fungi	Candida, Aspergillus, Mucormycosis	Candida, Aspergillus, PJP	Aspergillus, PJP

CMV, Cytomegalovirus; *CoNS*, coagulase-negative staphylococci; *CVL*, central venous line; *EBV*, Epstein-Barr virus; *GI*, gastrointestinal; *GVHD*, graft-versus-host disease; *HHV6*, human herpes virus 6; *HSCT*, hematopoietic stem cell transplant; *HSV*, herpes simplex virus; *PJP*, Pneumocystis jiroveci pneumonia; *PTLD*, posttransplant lymphoproliferative disorder; *VZV*, varicella zoster virus.

Data from Tomblyn M, et al. Guidelines for preventing infectious complications among hematopoietic cell transplantation recipients: a global perspective. *Biol Blood Marrow Transplant.* 2009; 15(10):1143–1238.

Table 24.23	Post-Solid Organ Transplant Opportunistic Infections		
	<1 Month	**1–6 Months**	**>6 Months**
Main risk factors	Pretransplant infections, donor infection, postoperative infections, central venous access devices	Activation of latent infections; relapsed, residual, opportunistic infections	Community-acquired infections
Bacteria	Postoperative wound infections, anastamotic leaks/ischemia, CVL infections (e.g., CoNS), antimicrobial-resistant organisms (e.g., MRSA, VRE), *Clostridium difficile* colitis, aspiration pneumonia, *Pseudomonas aeruginosa* (recipient-derived colonization)	*C. difficile*, *Mycobacterium tuberculosis*, Listeria, Nocardia	Pneumonia, UTI *Nocardia, Rhodococcus*
Viruses	HSV (donor-derived)	BK virus, hepatitis B, hepatitis C, influenza, adenovirus HSV, CMV, EBV, VZV	CMV (colitis, retinitis), hepatitis B, hepatitis C, HSV encephalitis, seasonal respiratory, JC virus
Fungi	*Candida, Aspergillus* (recipient-derived colonization)	*Cryptococcus*, PJP	*Aspergillus, mucor, Candida*, endemic fungi

Table 24.23	Post-solid Organ Transplant Opportunistic Infections—cont'd		
	<1 Month	1–6 Months	>6 Months
Parasites		*Strongyloides, Toxoplasma* (especially with heart transplant), *Leishmania, Tripanozoma cruzi*	*Toxoplasma* (especially with heart transplant)

CMV, Cytomegalovirus; *CoNS*, coagulase-negative staphylococci; *CVL*, central venous line; *EBV*, Epstein-Barr virus; *HSV*, herpes simplex virus; *MRSA*, methicillin-resistant *S. aureus*; *PJP*, *Pneumocystis jiroveci* pneumonia; *UTI*, urinary tract infection; *VRE*, vancomycin-resistant enterococcus; *VZV*, varicella zoster virus.

Data from Fishman JA and the AST Infectious Diseases Community of Practice. Introduction: infection in solid organ transplant recipients. *Am J Transplant.* 2009;9(suppl 4):S3–S6.

Table 24.24	Select Opportunistic Infections in Immunocompromised Hosts		
Infection	**Clinical Presentation**	**Prophylaxis (Alternatives)**	**Treatment (Alternatives)**
Adenovirus	- Upper respiratory infection, pharyngitis, conjunctivitis, pneumonia, gastroenteritis/colitis, hemorrhagic cystitis, fulminant hepatitis/pancreatitis (less common), encephalitis (rare) - Disseminated (≥ 2 sites)	—	Cidofovir (brincidofovir)
BK virus	- Hemorrhagic cystitis - Tubulointerstitial nephritis (may mimic renal transplant rejection), nephropathy	—	Key is to reduce immunosuppression; Cidofovir (brincidofovir)
Cytomegalovirus	- Tissue invasive disease: pneumonitis, colitis, retinitis, encephalitis, esophagitis, hepatitis, encephalitis (HIV > transplant) - Viral syndrome: fever, malaise, cytopenias	Ganciclovir/valganciclovir (foscarnet if neutropenia)	Ganciclovir/valganciclovir (foscarnet, cidofovir, brincidofvir, letermovir); consider Cytogram as adjunctive therapy
Pneumocystis jiroveci	- Pneumonia - May have classic ground-glass appearance on CXR	Trimethoprim-sulfamethoxazole (dapsone, pentamidine [aerosolized monthly or IV q2wk], atovaquone)	Trimethoprim-sulfamethoxazole × 21 days (pentamidine IV); steroids within 72 h if moderate-severe infection

CXR, Chest x-ray; *HIV*, human immunodeficiency virus; *IV*, intravenous.

Mental Health

Gabrielle Salmers • Daphne Korczak

Also see page xviii for a list of other abbreviations used throughout this book

ACE	adverse childhood experience
ADHD	attention deficit/hyperactivity disorder
APA	American Psychiatric Association
CBT	cognitive–behavioral therapy
CD	conduct disorder
DSM-5	*Diagnostic and Statistical Manual of Mental Disorders*, 5th Edition
GAD	generalized anxiety disorder
HEADSSS	home, education, activities/employment, drugs, suicidality, safety, sex
MDD	major depressive disorder
LD	learning disability
NMDA	*N*-methyl-d-aspartate
NMS	neuroleptic malignant syndrome
OCD	obsessive–compulsive disorder
ODD	oppositional defiant disorder
PTSD	post-traumatic stress disorder
SAD	separation anxiety disorder
SNRI	serotonin-norepinephrine reuptake inhibitor
SSRI	selective serotonin reuptake inhibitor

Mental Health

25

PRINCIPLES OF ASSESSMENT AND DIAGNOSIS

- **Importance of a mental health assessment:** pediatric assessment can present an opportunity to identify mental health concerns and initiate early intervention. Mental health problems are common and undertreated in children and adolescents. Over 70% of lifelong mental illness presents before the age of 14 years. Most disorders are sensitive to treatment early in the course of illness.

- **Components of assessment:** detailed history of the primary present-ing complaint including timeline, review of systems (with a focus on ruling-out possible physical causes of psychiatric presentation), thor-ough developmental history, mental status examination, neurologic ex-amination, safety assessment, social history, and HEADSSS assessment in adolescents looking for social context and possible precipitants of the current presentation (see Interviewing the Adolescent in Chapter 6 Adolescent Medicine)

- **Mental status examination:** consider the following aspects of the patient: appearance, attitude, behavior, speech, affect, mood, thought process, thought content, perception, orientation, memory and concen-tration, and insight and judgment

4. **Safety assessment:** assessment of the risk the patient currently poses to themselves and to others including:
   a. Current and past thoughts of death, suicide, or deliberate self-harm
   b. Whether or not the patient acted on these thoughts in the past
   c. Intent to act on thoughts of suicide and specific plans for suicide or self-harm
   d. Details of any past suicide attempts or self-harm
   e. Protective factors, such as parental involvement, good social suppor
   f. Consider the use of a standardized tool, such as the Columbia-Suicide Severity Rating Scale (C-SSRS), when conducting a safety assessment
5. **DSM-5 and diagnosis:** the DSM-5 is a manual published by the APA that defines and classifies all well-recognized mental disorders.

✦ PEARL

Two criteria are common to nearly all DSM-5 diagnoses—the disorder cannot be attributed by another cause (e.g., primary organic causes of the disorder, medications or substance use, or other mental disorder) AND the symptoms must be causing a significant functional impairment (e.g., poor school performance, poor relationships)

COMMON MANAGEMENT PRINCIPLES

1. **Address modifiable lifestyle and environmental factors first**
   a. **Sleep hygiene**
      i. Minimize caffeine intake during the day, and eliminate caffeine in the afternoon if possible
      ii. Develop a consistent bedtime routine incorporating relaxation
      iii. No screen time for 2 hours before bedtime
      iv. Maintain consistent bedtimes and wake-up times. For teenagers they should sleep-in no more than 1 hour on the weekends.
      v. Maintain an environment conducive to good sleep: cool temperature, dark, quiet
      vi. Bed should be used for sleep only
      vii. If sleep latency is the issue: after staying awake in bed for 20 to 30 minutes, get up, do a quiet activity until feeling tired again, then return to bed. Melatonin can reduce sleep latency.
   b. **Physical activity:** thirty minutes of aerobic physical activity daily can improve a variety of symptoms of mental disorders (e.g., mood, anxiety, energy, and concentration)
   c. Regular balanced meals and snacks

- Professional self-care
- **Provide psychoeducation:** parents and youth need to understand why you think they have the diagnosis that you have made, and how you understand the problem

ADVERSE CHILDHOOD EXPERIENCES

1. **Definition:** adverse childhood experiences (ACEs) are potentially traumatic events that can have negative, lasting effects on health and wellbeing
   a. Examples include chronic poverty (most common), physical, sexual, or emotional abuse, physical or emotional neglect, exposure to domestic violence, household substance abuse, household mental illness, parental separation or divorce, incarcerated household member, violence in a community, and racism
2. **Impact:** there is a correlation between ACEs and increased risk of heart disease, type 2 diabetes, obesity, depression, substance abuse, smoking, poor academic achievement underemployment, and early death. The effects of these experiences are thought to be the result of a chronic activation of the body's stress-response system.
3. **Mitigating factors:** strong positive relationships between children and parents or caregivers
4. https://developingchild.harvard.edu/guide/a-guide-to-toxic-stress/ explores ACEs and childhood development

DEPRESSION

1. Definitions
   a. **Depression:** a state of low mood
   b. **Depressive disorder:** persistent low mood and associated symptoms, that inhibits one's ability to function as they normally would by affecting thoughts, behavior, feelings, sense of self, and sense of wellbeing

MAJOR DEPRESSIVE DISORDER

1. **Epidemiology**
   a. Prevalence: increases with age, 5% to 8% by adolescence
   b. Female to male ratio increases from 1:1 prepuberty to 2:1 following puberty
   c. Box 25.1 illustrates risk factors for Major Depressive Episodes
   d. Comorbidities: anxiety disorders, eating disorders, ADHD, LD, substance use, and substance use disorders
2. **Presentation and DSM-5 criteria**
   a. ≥5 of the following symptoms (remembered by the mnemonic M-SIG-E-CAPS) must be present in the same 2-week period for most of the day every day (Box 25.2)

Box 25.1 Risk Factors for Major Depressive Episodes

First-degree relative with anxiety or depression (heritability is ~40%)
Family dysfunction or caregiver-child conflict
Psychosocial stressors (academic failure, bullying)
History of anxiety, LD, ADHD, ODD, trauma
Gender dysphoria, distress regarding sexual orientation
Chronic illness

ADHD, Attention deficit/hyperactivity disorder; *LD*, learning disability; *ODD*, oppositional defiant disorder.

Box 25.2 Symptoms of a Major Depressive Episode

[a]**Mood:** depressed mood
Sleep: insomnia or hypersomnia
[a]**Interest:** loss of interest or pleasure in almost all activities (i.e., anhedonia)
Guilt: feelings of worthlessness or excessive/inappropriate guilt
Energy: fatigue or loss of energy
Concentration: true or perceived diminished ability to think, concentrate, or make decisions
Appetite: poor appetite, >5% weight loss in 1 month, or failure to gain weight
Psychomotor changes: either agitation or slowing
Suicidal ideation

---

[a] At least 1 of these must be present.

 PEARL

Presentation is culturally dependent—some cultures may express symptoms differently.

3. Management is determined by symptom severity and assessment of suicide risk and safety
   a. **Non-pharmacological:** lifestyle management should be part of management. Cognitive–behavioral therapy (CBT) has the most evidence for efficacy in mild-moderate cases of major depressive disorder (MDD).
   b. **Pharmacotherapy:** selective serotonin reuptake inhibitor (SSRIs) are the first-line in pharmacotherapy (see Table 25.1). Fluoxetine has the greatest evidence for efficacy based on randomized control trials.
4. **Course**
   a. Variable, mean duration is 8 months
   b. Chronicity: common, consider other untreated comorbid mental illness

c Remission: no significant signs and symptoms for >2 months

d **Recurrence:** more likely when symptoms are severe, do not completely resolve between episodes, or multiple episodes have already occurred

Table 25.1	Pharmacological Options in the Management of Depression		
Medication	**Indication**	**Side Effects**	**Monitoring Parameters**
All SSRIs (e.g., fluoxetine)	MDD	GI upset, sleep disturbance, increased suicidality on initiation, restlessness, appetite change, headaches, sexual dysfunction	Weeks 1–4: weekly, weeks 5–8: biweekly, then every 4 weeks until stable, and then every 3 months after that Monitor in particular for suicidality, unmasking of mania/hypomania
Citalopram/ escitalopram	MDD	QT prolongation	Pre-initiation ECG in high-risk children: long QT syndrome Note: avoid in children with congenital heart disease

ECG, Electrocardiogram; *GI*, gastrointestinal; *MDD*, major depressive disorder; *SSRIs*, selective serotonin reuptake inhibitors.

PEARL

Bipolar disorder (BD) can present with a depressive episode. Differentiating BD from MDD is important as SSRIs may precipitate manic or hypomanic episodes. Distinguishing factors include family history of BD, psychotic features, history of hypomania, and severe psychomotor retardation.

PEARL

As depression is associated with high rates of suicidal ideation, behavior, and death by suicide, untreated depression may be more harmful than appropriate use of SSRI medication.

EXTERNALIZING DISORDERS (DISRUPTIVE BEHAVIORAL DISORDERS)

1. Definitions

   a. **Behavior:** the way in which a person conducts themselves in response to various situations or stimuli

   b. **Behavioral disorder:** a pattern of behavior that is disruptive to the person exhibiting the behavior, for example in their social, work, or family lives, and to those around them

OPPOSITIONAL DEFIANT DISORDER

1. **Epidemiology**
   a. More common in males before adolescence; equal thereafter
   b. Risk factors
      i. Inconsistent/chaotic primary caregiving
      ii. Harsh/punitive parenting
      iii. Emotional regulation difficulties (e.g., high emotional reactivity, poor frustration tolerance)
   c. Comorbidities include attention deficit/hyperactivity disorder (ADHD), conduct disorder (CD) and learning disability (LD)

2. **Presentation and DSM-5 criteria**
   a. Symptoms include angry or irritable mood, argumentative or defiant behavior, and vindictiveness
   b. The behavioral disturbance is associated with distress in the individual or in others, or the symptoms must negatively impact functioning (e.g., social, educational)
   c. Symptoms must be present on many days for ≥6 months
   d. Symptoms usually begin in preschool (rarely later than early-adolescence) and may be present in one or multiple settings

---

PEARL

Some features (e.g., tantrums) can be typical of certain developmental stages, so it is important to consider the functional impairment when making a diagnosis.

---

3. **Management**
   a. Treatment usually consists of a combination of Parent-Management Training Programs, therapy to support the parent-child interaction, and individual child therapy focusing on development of coping and social skills.
   b. Identify and manage comorbidities and environmental stressors
   c. Pharmacologic measures are only used to treat comorbidities (e.g., ADHD)

4. **Prognosis**
   a. Can infrequently evolve into conduct disorder. Risk of developing anxiety and depressive disorders along with antisocial behavior and substance abuse.
   b. Potential impairments/consequences
      i. Conflicts with parents, teachers, supervisors, peers, and romantic partners
      ii. Impact on emotional, social, academic, and occupational functioning

CONDUCT DISORDER

Epidemiology
a. Increases from childhood to adolescence, more common in males
b. Risk factors: cognitive deficits, family (inconsistent caregiving and discipline, abuse and neglect, large family, parental criminality, parental substance-related disorders, certain parental mental health disorders), social (peer rejection, delinquent peer group) and comorbidities (at risk for mood, anxiety, impulse-control, psychotic, substance-related, and somatic symptom disorders, as well as post-traumatic stress disorder [PTSD])

Presentation and DSM-5 criteria
a. A repetitive and persistent pattern of behavior, which results in the violation of basic rights of others or societal norms/rules (e.g., aggression toward people and animals, destruction of property, and deceitfulness or theft)
b. Behavior must cause clinically significant impairment in social, academic, or occupational functioning
c. Commonly preceded by ODD

Management
a. Support network and professional mental health service (care coordination)
b. Pharmacologic therapies are used only for treatment of comorbid disorders

Prognosis
a. The majority will remit in adulthood and achieve adequate social and occupational adjustment
b. Potential impairment/consequences
   i. Poor self-control and frustration tolerance, insensitive to punishment, thrill seeking, and recklessness
   ii. Earlier onset of sexual behavior and substance use
   iii. School suspension or expulsion, work problems, legal problems, sexually transmitted infections (STIs), unplanned pregnancy, and injury

ANXIETY

Definitions
a. **Anxiety:** feeling of fear, worry, nervousness, or unease that may or may not be an appropriate response to a stressor
b. **Anxiety disorder:** pathological anxiety that interferes with daily living, social interactions, typical development, and/or achievement of goals

GENERALIZED ANXIETY DISORDER

1. **Epidemiology**
   a. Prevalence: very common (10% among children and adolescents), more common in females
   b. Risk factors: sensitive personality or negative affect, social stressors (e.g., bullying, life changes)
2. **Presentation and DSM 5 criteria**
   a. Excessive anxiety or worry that is difficult to control about a number of events or activities occurring most days for at least 6 months
   b. Must be associated with physical symptoms (≥ 1 in children and ≥ 3 in adolescents); for example, restlessness or feeling "keyed up" or "on edge," easy fatiguability, difficulty concentrating, irritability, muscle tension, sleep disturbance
3. **Management**
   a. Patient and family education around the condition and addressing stressors
   b. Psychotherapy is first line; CBT has the most evidence
   c. Pharmacotherapy: SSRIs depending on level of severity. Benzodiazepines may be used, but sparingly because of potential for tolerance and withdrawal.
4. **Prognosis**
   a. Children tend to remain anxious lifelong, but treatment can decrease symptom severity and degree of impairment
   b. Severity varies in relation to stressors, comorbidities
   c. Comorbidities: other anxiety disorders, depression (more common with earlier symptom onset)

SEPARATION ANXIETY DISORDER

1. **Epidemiology**
   a. Risk factors: life stressors (e.g., loss), family history
   b. Comorbidities: GAD, specific phobias
2. **Presentation:** developmentally inappropriate and excessive fear or anxiety concerning separation from attachment figures
3. **Management**
   a. Therapy (CBT) is the mainstay
   b. Pharmacotherapy: SSRIs if symptoms are severe, therapy alone is insufficient, or comorbidities are present. Benzodiazepines not preferred because of risk of dependence.
4. **Prognosis**
   a. Most will not develop significant anxiety disorders as adults. Periods of exacerbation and remission tend to occur.
   b. Potential impairments/consequences: limited independence (e.g., not sleeping alone)

OBSESSIVE–COMPULSIVE DISORDER

1. **Definitions**
   a. **Obsessions:** recurrent, disturbing, intrusive thoughts or images that cause marked anxiety and distress
   b. **Compulsions:** repetitive behaviors or mental acts that are performed in response to an obsession or according to rigidly applied rules to neutralize the thought or minimize distress

2. **Epidemiology**
   a. Prevalence: 1% to 2% (disorder), 10% (traits)
   b. Risk factors: family history of obsessive–compulsive disorder (OCD), presence of anxiety disorder
   c. Comorbidities
      i. Tics are most common
      ii. Triad of tics, OCD, and ADHD is common in males
      iii. ADHD, anxiety, depression, other obsessive–compulsive and related disorders (e.g., trichotillomania, skin picking, body dysmorphic disorder), eating disorders, Tourette Syndrome, schizophrenia, and schizoaffective disorders

3. **Presentation**
   a. Patient must have either obsessions OR compulsions, although most have both
   b. Symptom content can change with developmental stage (e.g., sexual obsessions more common in adolescents than children)

4. **Management**
   a. Exposure response prevention (ERP) is the primary therapy modality although CBT specific to OCD can also be effective
   b. SSRIs are the first-line pharmacotherapy. Atypical antipsychotics can be used to augment SSRIs in refractory cases.

5. **Prognosis**
   a. 40% will experience symptom remission in early adulthood
   b. Potential impairments/consequences
      i. Avoidance of situations that exacerbate obsessions
      ii. Compulsions can be significantly time consuming or even physically harmful
      iii. Mental distress and anxiety if obsessions are felt to be sensitive or offensive

PEARL

Obsessive–compulsive symptoms are common, whereas obsessive–compulsive disorder is much less common.

POST-TRAUMATIC STRESS DISORDER

1. **Epidemiology**
   a. Prevalence: 11% of refugee children
   b. Risk factors
      i. Child-related: female, presence of another mental disorder, type of response to event (e.g., high level of anger or rumination)
      ii. Family or environmental: poor family functioning, presence of parental PTSD symptoms, limited social support, lack of a supportive response from caregivers
      iii. More likely to develop with a larger number of events or events that are more life threatening
      iv. Single session debriefings of events without follow-up increases risk of PTSD and MDD
   c. Comorbidities: mood and anxiety disorders
2. **Presentation:** occurs after experiencing a traumatic event where either their own life is threatened or a life-threatening event is witnessed
3. **Management**
   a. Consider if report to child protective services is appropriate
   b. Therapy should be tailored to the age of the child and modalities include trauma-focused CBT, exposure therapy (if avoidance of triggering stimuli is a concern), and Eye Movement Desensitization and Reprocessing (EMDR)
   c. Manage any associated symptoms (e.g., sleep disturbance)
   d. Pharmacotherapy is only used to manage comorbidities, if present
4. **Prognosis**
   a. One-third experience chronic symptoms
   b. Potential impairments/consequences: up to 50% experience major depression, substance abuse, anxiety, and/or behavioral disorders

SOMATIC SYMPTOM AND RELATED DISORDERS

1. Definitions
   a. **Somatic symptom:** emotion expressed as a physical symptom. Up to 44% of children and adolescents will experience somatic symptoms at some time in their life. Examples include headaches, abdominal pain, fatigue, or dizziness.
   b. **Conversion:** emotion expressed as a motor/sensory deficit that is not explained by an underlying medical condition

b0110

p1585

 PEARL

Multiple terms are used across various specialties to describe the same—medically unexplained symptoms, functional symptoms, non-organic, psychosomatic.

Etiology: not fully understood and varies based on the presentation; considered to be rooted in the mind-body connection and involve the fight-or-flight response

OMATIC SYMPTOM DISORDER

1. **Epidemiology**
   a. Prevalence: female to male ratio increases from 1:1 prepuberty to 2:1 following puberty
   b. Table 25.2 illustrates risk factors for the development of somatic symptom disorder

Table 25.2	Risk Factors for Development of Somatic Symptom Disorder

Individual Factors

- Perfectionistic
- Minimizes impact of stressors on self
- Difficulty labeling feelings
- Preceding medical illness or injury (often more complicated in these cases)
- Learning disability
- Depression and/or anxiety
- Somatosensory amplification and sensitivity to pain
- Psychosocial stressors (e.g., family, death)

Family Factors

- Perception of illness (e.g., as scary, life threatening)
- Perception of child/teen (e.g., as vulnerable, fragile)
- Relatives with illness, disability, chronic pain, somatization (model of communicating distress)
- Communication breakdown
- Parents' response to symptoms may determine level of associated distress and functional impairment

Community Factors

- Comfort given for "sick role"
- Altered expectations and interactions

Medical System Factors

- Biomedical approach reinforces mind-body split
- Focus on physical complaints resulting in overinvestigation and medicalization

2. **Presentation and DSM-5 criteria**
   a. One or more somatic symptoms that are distressing or result in significant disruption of daily life
   b. The patient will be disproportionately worried about the symptoms, have a high level of anxiety about their health or the symptoms, and/or devote an excessive amount of time and energy to the symptoms or their health
   c. Typically, the patient is symptomatic for more than 6 months, although the specific symptom or set of symptoms may change over this period

Features suggestive of somatic symptoms and/or conversion disorder:
a. History and physical examination does not correlate with degree of impairment
b. School avoidance
c. Descriptive language of pain
d. *La belle indifference* or overly dramatic presentation

Somatic symptom disorder should be considered and presented to the patient as part of your initial differential diagnosis and not only a diagnosis of exclusion. Investigations should be used judiciously, and excessive investigation with the aim of ruling out all other causes can serve to over-medicalize patients.

3. **Management:** the **VEER** (validate, educate, empathize, rehabilitate) approach is commonly used and recommended in the management of patients with somatic symptoms (see Box 25.3)

4. **Prognosis**
   a. The majority of symptoms will resolve spontaneously or with simple strategies over months
   b. Longer duration of symptoms is associated with greater treatment difficulty

Box 25.3 The VEER Approach to Management of Patients With Somatic Symptoms

Validate that the symptoms are real and not under voluntary control
Educate about the natural history of the condition and the positive prognosis
Empathize that the symptoms are distressing and about the stigma of a mental health diagnosis
Patients worry that future concerns will be attributed to this diagnosis. Reassure them you will continue to follow-up and be available if there are any new or changed concerns, or arrange for another provider to follow them closely.
Rehabilitate: Focus on improving function and development of coping strategies using goal setting and planned ignoring of symptoms. This includes lifestyle changes, normalizing routine, developing a return-to-school plan, and involving allied health services, such as occupational and/or physical therapy where necessary. Identify stressors and address comorbidities. Psychotherapy can include individual CBT and/or mindfulness techniques, family or group therapy.

CBT, Cognitive–behavioral therapy.
Data from Krasnik CE, Meaney B, Grant C. A clinical approach to paediatric conversion disord VEER in the right direction. *Canadian Paediatric Surveillance Program*, 2011.

Be aware to not attribute all symptoms of these patients to somatization. Close attention must be paid to new or changed symptoms with medical reassessment and/or investigations to be done as deemed appropriate by the clinician.

1. Definitions
   a. **Psychosis:** a break with reality, constituted by either hallucinations, delusions, or both
   b. **Hallucination:** a sensory perception/experience in the absence of an external stimulus
   c. **Delusion:** a fixed, false belief
   d. **Delirium:** an acute, fluctuating, reversible abnormal mental state

PSYCHOSIS

1. **Etiology**
   a. Primary psychosis
      i. The result of an underlying psychotic disorder
      ii. Not initiated by or occurring in the context of another illness, metabolic derangement, or substance use
      iii. Uncommon in children
   b. Psychosis secondary to another condition (see Table 25.3)

Table 25.3	Psychosis Secondary to Another Condition
Neurologic	Cerebral hypoxia
	Post-ictal state
	Space occupying lesion
	CNS infection
	Anti-NMDA encephalitis
	SLE
Metabolic	Hypocalcemia
	Hypercalcemia
	Hepatic encephalopathy
	Wilson's disease
	Urea cycle defect
	Acute intermittent porphyria
Substance	Drugs of abuse
	Medications—anticholinergics, benzodiazepines, corticosteroids, anesthetic agents
	Polypharmacy
	Ingestion (including withdrawal)

CNS, Central nervous system; *NMDA,* N-methyl-D-aspartate; *SLE,* systemic lupus erythematosus.

2. **Clinical assessment**
   a. **History**
      i. Key points: nature of onset, prodromal phase, substance use/ingestions, associated physical symptoms, mental health history, past medical history, allergies

      ii. Attempt to rule out reversible causes before treating with an antipsychotic and to assess for any possible risks of pharmacologic management

      iii. Safety assessment (see Principles of Assessment and Diagnosis section)

  b. **Examination:** mental status, signs and symptoms of secondary causes of psychosis, and possible self-inflicted injury including overdose ingestion, substance use/intoxication

3. **Investigations**

  a. Blood tests: blood glucose, electrolytes, liver enzymes, creatinine, urea, blood alcohol level, lupus workup (antinuclear antibodies [ANA], double-stranded DNA [dsDNA], complement), ceruloplasmin, serum anti-N-methyl-D-aspartate (NMDA)

  b. Urine tests: urine toxicology screen, urine porphyrins

  c. Imaging: MRI brain with contrast

  d. Other: lumbar puncture (protein, glucose, cell count, and CSF anti-NMDA), EEG, ECG (if concerned about ingestion)

4. **Management**

  a. Ensure safety, call for assistance if necessary

  b. Stabilization: airway, breathing, circulation (ABCs)

  c. Only in extreme cases where patient is at risk of harm to themselves or others should this stage include chemical or physical restraints

  d. Verbal de-escalation

  e. Consider continuous observation (individual with knowledge, skill, and judgment to contact healthcare professional if needs are increasing)

  f. Consider safety of environment (e.g., sharps, medical equipment or furniture not in use or needed)

  g. Consider clothing (avoid long cords) and content of personal belongings

  h. Treat reversible causes

      i. Environmental adjustments: orient patient by ensuring a clock and calendar are easily visible, gentle reminders of time/place, presence of family members/friends, ensure room is light during the day and dark at night

      ii. Remove offending pharmaceuticals/substances

      iii. Correct metabolic and electrolyte derangements

      iv. Reversal agents (e.g., naloxone for opioids)

      v. Treatment of identified cause

  i. Pharmacologic agents (see Box 25.4)

      i. Sedation: benzodiazepines—first-line: lorazepam; other options: midazolam, diazepam

      ii. Antipsychotics: first-line: olanzapine; other options: loxapine, risperidone, quetiapine, haloperidol

| Box 25.4 | Acute Psychosis Medication Considerations |

Caution

Medications (e.g., loxapine) can cause dystonic reactions (dyskinesias), which are characterized by intermittent spasmodic or sustained involuntary contractions of muscles. Can occur within hours–minutes of administration of a neuroleptic. Treatment: Benztropine.

Contraindications

Loxapine with opiates and dopamine agonists
Lorazepam with Olanzapine

DELIRIUM

1. **Presentation**
   a. Fluctuating hallucinations, delusions, decreased cognitive ability, and disorientation to person/place/time with a rapid onset (and offset) and in the context of an underlying illness or treatment regimen
   b. Usually temporary and reversible
2. **Causes**
   a. Pharmaceuticals: anticholinergics, benzodiazepines, steroids, sedation, anesthetics
   b. Acute systemic illness or severe traumatic injury
   c. Post-operative
3. **Management:** consider environmental modifications as outlined under treatment of psychosis, along with medication review

FURTHER RESOURCES

Mental Health: Screening Tools and Rating Scales from the Canadian Pediatric Society, cps.ca/mental-health-screening-tools.

Metabolic Disease

Carsten Krueger • Resham Ejaz • Neal Sondheimer

COMMON ABBREVIATIONS

Also see page xviii for a list of other abbreviations used throughout this book

AG	anion gap
BMT	bone marrow transplant
CDG	congenital disorders of glycosylation
CPS	carbamoyl phosphate synthetase
CK	creatine kinase
CPT II	carnitine palmitoyltransferase II deficiency
ERT	enzyme replacement therapy
FAOD	fatty acid oxidation defect
FFA	free fatty acid
GALT	galactose-1-phosphate uridyltransferase
GIR	glucose infusion rate
GSD	glycogen storage disease
HCC	hepatocellular carcinoma
HFI	hereditary fructose intolerance
HSM	hepatosplenomegaly
ID	intellectual disability
IEM	inborn errors of metabolism
IVA	isovaleric acidemia
LCHAD	long chain 3-hydroxyacyl-coenzyme A dehydrogenase
LVH	left ventricular hypertrophy
MCAD	medium chain acyl-coenzyme A dehydrogenase
MELAS	mitochondrial encephalomyopathy, lactic acidosis, stroke-like episodes
MMA	methylmalonic aciduria
MPS	mucopolysaccharidosis
MSUD	maple syrup urine disease
NAGS	N-acetylglutamate synthase
NH_4	ammonium
OA	organic acidopathy
OTC	ornithine transcarbamylase
PA	propionic aciduria
PDH	pyruvate dehydrogenase
Phe	phenylalanine
PKU	phenylketonuria
qAA	quantitative amino acids
RTA	renal tubular acidosis
SLO	Smith-Lemli-Opitz syndrome
UCD	urea cycle defect
UOA	urine organic acids

Metabolic Disease

26

VLCAD	very long chain acyl-coenzyme A dehydrogenase
VLCFA	very long chain fatty acid
X-ALD	X-linked adrenoleukodystrophy

USEFUL CALCULATIONS

1. Anion gap = $Na^+ - (Cl^- + HCO_3^-)$ (normal is <16 mmol/L)
2. Glucose infusion rate (mg/kg/min) =

$$\frac{Infusate\ rate\left(\dfrac{mL}{h}\right) \times Dextrose\ content\ (\%)}{6 \times Weight\ (kg)}$$

GENERAL METABOLIC CONCEPTS

1. Inborn errors of metabolism (IEMs) are caused by defects in metabolic pathways
2. Most are autosomal recessive disorders, although dominant or X-linked inheritance occurs
3. Rare individually (some <1 in 500,000 live births); relatively common collectively (1 in 2500)
4. Can present from birth to old age, affecting any or all body systems
5. Vast majority of metabolic disorders occur because of enzyme defects resulting in
   a. Substrate accumulation (e.g., ↑Phe in phenylketonuria [PKU], ↑NH_4 in urea cycle defect [UCD])
   b. Lack of product (e.g., ↓ glucose in glycogen storage disease [GSD] type I)
   c. Accumulation of alternative product (e.g., succinylacetone in hepatorenal tyrosinemia)

CLASSIFICATION OF INBORN ERRORS OF METABOLISM

1. Two main groups: small molecule disorders and organelle disorders
2. For classification, see Figure 26.1 and for clinical differentiation, see Table 26.1

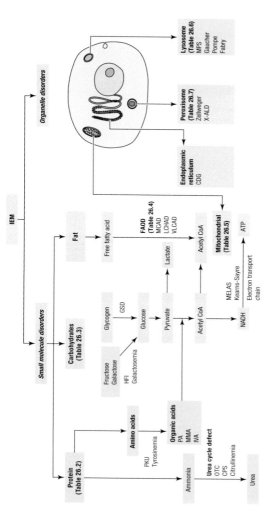

ATP, Adenosine triphosphate; *CoA*, coenzyme A; *CPS*, carbamoyl phosphate synthetase; *GSD*, glycogen storage disease; *HFI*, hereditary fructose intolerance; *IEM*, inborn errors of metabolism; *IVA*, isovaleric acidemia; *LCHAD*, long chain 3-hydroxyacyl-coenzyme A dehydrogenase; *MCAD*, medium chain acyl-coenzyme A dehydrogenase; *MELAS*, mitochondrial encephalomyopathy, lactic acidosis, stroke-like episodes; *MMA*, methylmalonic aciduria; *MPS*, mucopolysaccharidosis; *OTC*, ornithine transcarbamylase; *PA*, propionic aciduria; *PKU*, phenylketonuria; *VLCAD*, very long chain acyl-coenzyme A dehydrogenase; *X-ALD*, X-linked adrenoleukodystrophy.

Metabolic Disease

26

Table 26.1	Clinical Differentiation of Small Molecule Disorders and Organelle Disorders	
Feature	**Small Molecule Disorder**	**Organelle Disorder**
Definition	Disorders of intermediary metabolism (fat, protein, carbohydrates)	Disorders within specific subcellular organelles (e.g., lysosomes, peroxisomes, mitochondria)
Onset	Often sudden, even catastrophic	Gradual
Course	Relapsing and remitting	Slowly progressive
Physical findings	Nonspecific	Characteristic features
Histopathology	Generally nonspecific changes	Often characteristic changes
Response to supportive therapy	Brisk	Poor

Adapted from Clarke JTR. *A Clinical Guide to Inherited Metabolic Diseases*. 3rd ed. Cambridge, England: Cambridge University Press; 2006:243.

SMALL MOLECULE DISORDERS

1. Classified as disorders of protein (Table 26.2), carbohydrate (Table 26.3), or fat metabolism (Table 26.4)
2. Usually present with intoxication when toxic metabolites build up (e.g., aminoacidopathies, organic acidopathy [OA], UCD) or because of interference in energy generation (e.g., medium chain acyl-coenzyme A dehydrogenase [MCAD] deficiency, GSD)

Table 26.2 Selected Disorders of Amino Acid (Protein) Metabolism

Disorder (Enzyme)	Clinical Features	Investigation/Diagnosis[a]	Treatment
Aminoacidopathies			
Phenylketonuria *(phenylalanine hydroxylase)*	1. **Poor control:** risk of IQ loss, late neurologic signs 2. **Untreated:** severe ID, hypopigmentation, eczema, musty smell	1. Plasma amino acids: ↑Phe 2. Urine pterins to exclude biopterin defects	1. Diet therapy: low Phe 2. Intake titrated to plasma levels
Tyrosinemia type I *(fumarylacetoacetate hydrolase)*	1. **Untreated:** hepatic dysfunction, coagulopathy, RTA, boiled cabbage odor 2. Secondary porphyria (inhibition of porphobilinogen synthase) 3. Risk of HCC	1. Plasma amino acid: ↑tyrosine 2. Urine: ↑ urinary succinylacetone 3. Other: high alpha-fetoprotein	1. NTBC (substrate inhibitor) 2. Diet therapy: low tyrosine/Phe 3. Liver transplantation: NTBC nonresponders; HCC
Homocystinuria *(cystathionine β-synthase)*	1. **Untreated:** Marfanoid habitus, ID, osteoporosis, lens dislocation, myopia, thrombosis, stroke	1. ↑ Total plasma homocysteine level 2. Plasma amino acid: ↑ methionine	1. Vitamin B₆ (cofactor, 50% responsive) 2. Folate; betaine (alternative pathway) 3. Diet therapy: low Methionine 4. Aspirin (post-thrombosis)
MSUD *(branched-chain keto acid dehydrogenase complex)*	1. **Severe/neonatal:** acute neonatal encephalopathy and seizures; maple syrup odor 2. **Mild/intermittent:** ketoacidosis during catabolic stress	1. Normal blood gas, NH₄, lactate 2. Ketonuria 3. Plasma amino acid: ↑ branched-chain amino acids (Valine, Leucine, Isoleucine) 4. UOA: ↑ keto acids	1. Diet therapy: branched-chain amino acid–restricted diet
Nonketotic hyperglycinemia *(glycine cleavage enzyme)*	1. ↑ Fetal movements (in utero seizures), intractable seizures, hypotonia, severe developmental disability	1. CSF and plasma amino acid: ↑glycine 2. CSF-plasma glycine ratio >0.08	1. Supportive

Continued

Table 26.2   Selected Disorders of Amino Acid (Protein) Metabolism—cont'd

Disorder (Enzyme)	Clinical Features	Investigation/Diagnosis[a]	Treatment
Organic Acidopathies			
PA (propionyl-CoA carboxylase)	1. Hepatomegaly, seizures, vomiting, FTT, protein intolerance, developmental disability, hypotonia, acidosis, and ↑NH₄ with decompensation 2. **Complications:** cardiomyopathy, bone marrow suppression, renal disease, pancreatitis	1. Metabolic acidosis with ↑AG, ↑NH₄ 2. UOA: metabolites of propionyl-CoA 3. Plasma acylcarnitine: ↑ propionylcarnitine 4. ↓ Free carnitine level	1. Diet therapy: reduce intake of target amino acids 2. L-carnitine, metronidazole (gut sterilization) 3. Carbamyl glutamate if ↑NH₄
MMA (methylmalonyl-CoA mutase)	1. Hepatomegaly, seizures, vomiting, FTT, protein intolerance, developmental disability, hypotonia, acidosis, and ↑NH₄ with decompensation 2. **Complications:** renal disease, pancreatitis, dystonia	1. Metabolic acidosis with ↑AG, ↑NH₄ 2. UOA: large methylmalonic acid 3. Plasma acylcarnitine: ↑propionylcarnitine 4. ↓ Free carnitine level	1. As for PA 2. ~15% vitamin B12 responsive
Glutaric aciduria type I (glutaryl-CoA dehydrogenase)	1. Encephalopathy, dystonia, macrocephaly, subdural hemorrhages	1. UOA: glutaric acid, 3-OH glutaric acid 2. Plasma acylcarnitine: ↑ glutarylcarnitine 3. ↓ Free carnitine level	1. Diet therapy: low lysine 2. Riboflavin, carnitine 3. Prevent febrile decompensation
Urea Cycle Defect			
Ornithine transcarbamylase deficiency (OTC)	1. **Neonatal onset:** males (X-linked), present at 24–48 h with sepsis-like presentation; ↓ feeding, vomiting, lethargy, coma 2. **Female carriers/late-onset males (~20%):** recurrent metabolic decompensations associated with catabolic stress	1. Respiratory alkalosis, ↑NH₄, ↑AST/ALT, ↑INR 2. Plasma amino acid: ↓ citrulline, ↑ glutamine 3. UOA: ↑ urine orotic acid	1. Diet therapy: low protein diet 2. Sodium benzoate/sodium phenylbutyrate and citrulline 3. Liver transplantation

[a]Final diagnosis requires specific enzyme assay/molecular testing.

AG, Anion gap; ALT, alanine transaminase; AST, aspartate transaminase; CSF, cerebrospinal fluid; FTT, failure to thrive; HCC, hepatocellular carcinoma; ID, intellectual disability; INR, international normalized ratio; MSUD, maple syrup urine disease; NTBC, 2-(2-nitro-4-trifluoromethylbenzoyl)-1,3-cyclohexanedione; PTA, renal tubular acidosis; UOA, urine organic acids.

Table 26.3 Selected Disorders of Carbohydrate Metabolism

Disorder (Enzyme)	Clinical Features	Investigation/Diagnosis[a]	Treatment
Galactosemia (*GALT*)	1. **Untreated:** hepatomegaly, jaundice, FTT, cataracts 2. Risk of *Escherichia coli* urosepsis 3. Speech difficulties, ovarian insufficiency despite treatment	1. ↑ Conjugated bilirubin, ↑INR, RTA, hemolytic anemia 2. RBC GALT before blood transfusion	1. Diet therapy: restriction of galactose and lactose 2. Calcium supplements
HFI (*aldolase B*)	1. On fructose/sucrose/sorbitol ingestion: variable symptoms; seizures, colic, vomiting, diarrhea, jaundice	1. Blood: ↓ glucose, lactic acidosis, ↑ urate 2. RTA: generalized amino aciduria	1. Diet therapy: restriction of fructose, sucrose, sorbitol
GSD			
GSD I (1a: *glucose-6-phosphatase*; 1b: *glucose-6-phosphate translocase*)	1. Characteristic facies, massive hepatomegaly, seizures, short stature, bleeding diathesis, nephromegaly 2. Recurrent infection (1b) 3. Crohn's-like bowel disease (1b)	1. ↓ Glucose, ↑ lactate, ↑ urate, ↑ triglycerides 2. Neutropenia (1b)	1. Frequent daytime feedings 2. Overnight glucose, uncooked cornstarch 3. Allopurinol 4. G-CSF (1b)
GSD III (*glycogen debranching enzyme*)	1. Similar to type I but typically milder ± muscle (skeletal/cardiac) involvement	1. ↓ Glucose, ↑AST, ↑ALT, ↑CK 2. ↑ Urine myoglobin	
Disorders of Gluconeogenesis			
Fructose-1,6-biphosphatase deficiency	1. Episodic hypoglycemia, lactic acidosis, hepatomegaly, seizures	1. ↑ Lactate, ketones, marked hypoglycemia, metabolic acidosis, RTA	1. Treat hypoglycemia (D10W) 2. Treat acidosis (saline ± bicarbonate)

[a]Final diagnosis requires specific enzyme assay/molecular testing.

ALT, Alanine transaminase; *AST*, aspartate transaminase; *CK*, creatine kinase; *FTT*, failure to thrive; *G-CSF*, granulocyte colony-stimulating factor; *GSD*, glycogen storage disease; *HFI*, hereditary fructose intolerance; *INR*, international normalized ratio; *RBC*, red blood cell; *RTA*, renal tubular acidosis.

Metabolic Disease

26

Table 26.4	Selected Fatty Acid Oxidation Defects		
Defect	**Clinical Features**	**Investigation/Diagnosis[a]**	**Treatment**
MCAD deficiency	1. Acute encephalopathy 2. Hypoketotic hypo-glycemia	1. ↓ Blood glucose, ↓ urine ketones 2. Plasma acylcarnitine: ↑C8 3. ↑ Plasma FFA: 3-hydroxybutyrate 4. UOA: dicarboxylic aciduria	1. Avoid fasting 2. Do not give IV lipids
VLCAD, LCHAD deficiency	1. Cardiac/skeletal myopathy 2. Liver dysfunction 3. Retinopathy (LCHAD)	1. Abnormal LFTs, ↑CK 2. Abnormal echocardio-gram 3. Plasma acylcarnitine: ↑C14:1 in VLCAD, ↑C14:OH in LCHAD	1. Fat-restricted diet, medium chain triglyc-erides/essential fatty acid supplementation 2. Do not give IV lipids

[a]Final diagnosis requires specific enzyme assay/molecular testing.

CK, Creatine kinase; *FFA*, free fatty acid; *IV*, intravenous; *LCHAD*, long chain 3-hydroxyacyl-coenzyme A dehydrogenase; *LFTs*, liver function tests; *MCAD*, medium chain acyl-coenzyme A dehydrogenase; *UOA*, urine organic acids; *VLCAD*, very long chain acyl-coenzyme A dehydrogenase.

ORGANELLE DISORDERS

1. **Mitochondrial disorders** (Table 26.5): features similar to small molecule disorders as energy production is affected

Table 26.5	Selected Mitochondrial Disorders		
Disorder	**Clinical Features**	**Investigation/ Diagnosis[a]**	**Treatment**
MELAS	Encephalomyopathy, lactic acidosis, stroke-like episodes	1. ↑ blood and CSF lactate 2. **UOA:** ↑ lactate, ketones 3. **MRI/MRS:** lactate peak, hyperintense lesion in basal ganglia, brainstem 4. Skin and muscle biopsy 5. DNA depletion studies	1. Supportive therapy 2. Avoid sodium valproate 3. Consider L-arginine in MELAS for stroke-like episode
Kearns-Sayre syndrome	Triad (onset <20 years, ophthalmoplegia, retinopathy) ± ataxia, heart block, ↑CSF protein		
Leigh	Subacute necrotizing encepha-lomyopathy, extrapyramidal symptoms, leukodystrophy, necrotic lesions in thalamus and brainstem		

[a]Final diagnosis requires molecular testing.

CSF, Cerebrospinal fluid; *DNA*, deoxyribonucleic acid; *MELAS*, mitochondrial encephalomyopathy, lactic acidosis, stroke-like episodes; *MRI*, magnetic resonance imaging; *MRS*, magnetic resonance spectroscopy; *UOA*, urine organic acids.

26

2. **Lysosomal storage disorders** (Table 26.6): appearance is typically normal at birth; features progress as substrates accumulate

Table 26.6	Selected Lysosomal Storage Disorders		
Disorder (*Enzyme*)	**Clinical Features**	**Investigation/ Diagnosis**[a]	**Treatment**
Pompe disease/ GSD II (*α-glucosidase*)	1. Cardiomyopathy, profound hypotonia, hyporeflexia, large tongue	1. **Blood:** ↑ALT, ↑AST, ↑CK 2. **ECG changes:** ↓PR, ↑QRS, LVH 3. Atypical urine oligosaccharides	1. Supportive 2. ERT
Mucopolysaccharidoses			
Hurler/MPS I (*α-L-iduronidase*)	1. Coarse facial features, HSM, macrocephaly, cardiac disease, recurrent ear infections, joint restriction, restrictive airway disease, cardiac disease 2. ID 3. Corneal clouding	1. Urine MPS 2. Blood film (vacuolation) 3. Skeletal survey (dysostosis multiplex) 4. Enzyme testing	1. Severe type: BMT for patients <18 months 2. Attenuated type: ERT
Hunter/MPS II (*iduronate-2-sulfatase—X linked*)	1. Features similar to Hurler, but without corneal clouding	1. Similar to Hurler	1. Attenuated type: ERT 2. Supportive
Sphingolipidoses			
Gaucher (*glucocerebrosidase*)	1. Type I: HSM, bleeding tendency, thrombocytopenia, osteopenia, pain 2. Type II: CNS involvement, rapidly progressive in infancy 3. Type III: CNS involvement, ophthalmoplegia, spasticity	1. Gaucher cells in bone marrow 2. Enzyme testing	1. ERT, excluding Type II where supportive management is used
Fabry (*α-galactosidase A*)	1. Limb pain/paresthesia, angiokeratoma, renal failure, cardiomyopathy	1. Urine glycolipid (↑Gb3) 2. Enzyme analysis 3. Mutation analysis	1. ERT
GM2 gangliosidosis Tay-Sachs/ Sandhoff (*β-hexosaminidase*)	1. Macrocephaly, hypotonia, developmental regression, cherry-red spot	1. Enzyme testing on WBC	1. Supportive

[a]Final diagnosis requires specific enzyme assay/molecular testing.

ALT, Alanine transaminase; *AST*, aspartate transaminase; *BMT*, bone marrow transplant; *CK*, creatine kinase; *CNS*, central nervous system; *ECG*, electrocardiogram; *ERT*, enzyme replacement therapy; *HSM*, hepatosplenomegaly; *ID*, intellectual disability; *LVH*, left ventricular hypertrophy; *MPS*, mucopolysaccharidosis; *WBC*, white blood cell.

3. **Peroxisomal disorders** (Table 26.7): may be dysmorphic and have involvement of brain, liver and other systems

Table 26.7	Selected Peroxisomal Disorders		
Disorder (Enzyme/Protein)	**Clinical Features**	**Investigation/Diagnosis**[a]	**Treatment**
X-ALD	1. ADHD, adrenal insufficiency, developmental regression	1. Blood: ↑VLCFA 2. Brain MRI: leukodystrophy	1. Symptomatic: early BMT 2. Steroids for adrenal insufficiency
Zellweger (*peroxins*)	1. Severe hypotonia, seizures, cataracts, dysmorphic features, epiphyseal stippling, renal cysts, liver dysfunction	1. Blood: liver dysfunction, ↑ conjugated bilirubin, ↑VLCFA 2. X-ray of long bones, renal US	1. Supportive

[a]Final diagnosis requires specific enzyme assay/molecular testing.

ADHD, Attention deficit hyperactivity disorder; *BMT*, bone marrow transplant; *MRI*, magnetic resonance imaging; *US*, ultrasound; *VLCFA*, very long chain fatty acid; *X-ALD*, X-linked adreno-leukodystrophy.

DIAGNOSTIC TESTS

1. **Basic metabolic investigations**
   a. **Blood glucose:** hypoglycemia seen in disorders of carbohydrate, fatty acid, and energy metabolism
   b. **Ammonia:** hyperammonemia seen in UCD, and some OA and fatty acid oxidation defect (FAOD)

> **! PITFALL**
>
> Blood ammonia can be falsely elevated if sample taken with tourniquet, not kept on ice, or not processed immediately.

   c. **Blood gas:** metabolic acidosis: OA, mitochondrial diseases; alkalosis: UCD
   d. **Lactate:** ↑ lactate seen in IEM (mitochondrial disease, disorders of carbohydrate metabolism) and non-IEM (intercurrent illnesses, hypoxia, hypoperfusion). Collect without a tourniquet.
   e. **Urine ketones:** ketosis is a physiological response to fasting or catabolism. Abnormal in the fed state or in the neonatal period (<1 month). ↑ urine ketones: OA, disorders of carbohydrate

metabolism and ketolysis. ↓ urine ketones in a fasting state are seen in FAOD. ↑ urine ketones can be the only abnormal basic laboratory finding in maple syrup urine disease (MSUD).

f. **Liver enzymes/function tests:** hepatic dysfunction is seen in various IEM

> ⁂ **PEARL**
>
> Unexpected abnormal values for glucose, ammonia, and acid/base status (bicarbonate or pH) are helpful in establishing the possibility of inborn errors of metabolism.

2. **Specialized metabolic investigations**
   a. **Plasma amino acids:** aminoacidopathies (e.g., PKU and tyrosinemia), UCD
   b. **Acylcarnitine profile:** diagnostic test for FAOD and some OA
   c. **Urine organic acids:** diagnostic urine metabolites can be seen in OAs and FAODs
   d. **Urine orotic acid:** used to differentiate various types of UCD
   e. **Carbohydrate-deficient transferrin:** screen for some congenital disorders of glycosylation (CDG)
   f. **Very long chain fatty acids (VLCFA):** elevated VLCFA are seen with some peroxisomal disorders
   g. **CK:** elevated CK can be seen with some GSD, FAOD, and mitochondrial disorders specifically affecting muscle
   h. **Urine oligosaccharides and mucopolysaccharides:** screening tests for lysosomal storage disorders

APPROACH TO INBORN ERRORS OF METABOLISM

1. **History**
   a. **Consider IEM in the following presentations**
      i. Neonates presenting with unexplained, progressive decompensation with symptoms, such as lethargy, poor feeding, refractory seizures with no obvious triggers/perinatal causes
      ii. Unexplained lethargy, recurrent vomiting, or neurologic deterioration at any age
      iii. Hypoglycemia or acidosis without obvious etiology
      iv. Developmental delay, history of regression or coarsening of facial features
      v. Multiorgan dysfunction, particularly involving the heart, liver, or muscle with no clear environmental cause
      vi. Exaggerated response to metabolic stress (intercurrent illnesses, fasting, fever, surgery, puberty)

b. **Age of presentation:** "intoxication defects" display no symptoms in first hours of life but present later with nonspecific and rapidly progressive symptoms

2. **Prenatal and perinatal history**
   a. Maternal acute fatty liver of pregnancy or HELLP (hemolytic anemia, elevated liver enzymes, and low platelet count) syndrome (increased when fetus affected by LCHAD [long chain 3-hydroxyacyl-coenzyme A dehydrogenase] or other FAOD)
   b. Abnormal or increased fetal movement or hiccups, which may indicate seizures in utero
   c. Prenatal screening or carrier testing
   d. Newborn screening results

3. **Diet history**
   a. Relationship between new food introduction and development of symptoms (e.g., galactosemia after introduction of milk; hereditary fructose intolerance [HFI] after introduction of solids)
   b. FAOD or GSD presents when children lengthen interval between feedings (e.g., overnight fasting around 6−8 months) but can present earlier based on severity and intercurrent stressers.
   c. Aversion to protein in UCDs

4. **Development**
   a. Global developmental delay/disability or regression without obvious cause
   b. Behavioral problems: aggressive and destructive behavior (e.g., Sanfilippo disease), self-mutilation (e.g., Lesch–Nyhan), irritability, hyperactivity, nocturnal restlessness

5. **Medication history**
   a. Adverse response to drug exposure
      i. Rifampin, progesterone, and barbiturates in porphyria
      ii. Valproic acid in mitochondrial disorders, such as *POLG*-related disorders

6. **Family history**
   a. Three generation pedigree
   b. Determine consanguinity, ethnic/geographic background, sibling death from unexplained disease, previous multiple miscarriages

7. **Physical examination**
   a. See Figure 26.2
   b. See Table 26.8 for IEM causing dysmorphism

Figure 26.2 Selected Physical Examination Findings in Inborn Errors of Metabolism

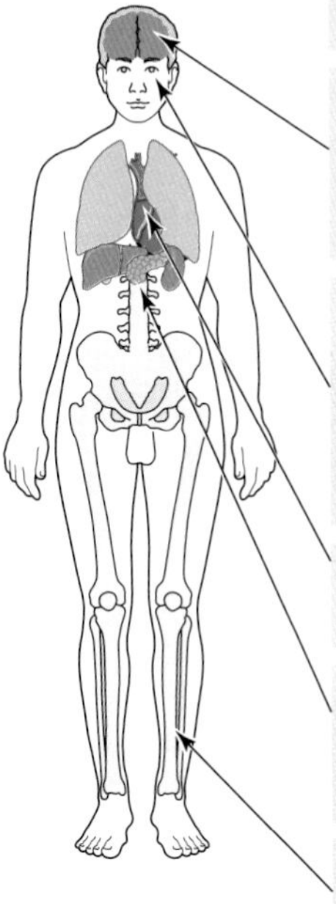

Growth Parameters
Weight: FTT (e.g., small molecule disorder)
Macrocephaly: GA1, Canavan, Alexander, Hunter disease

Dysmorphic Features
Coarse facial features: MPS
Inverted nipples and abnormal fat distribution: CDG
2–3 toe syndactyly, genital abnormalities: SLO

Skin and Hair
Alopecia or kinky hair: Menkes, arginosuccinic aciduria
Hirsutism: MPS
Ichthyosis: Sjögren-Larsson

Neurologic Examination
Supranuclear paralysis: Gaucher, Niemann–Pick type C
Hypotonia: Pompe, Zellweger
Spasticity: nonketotic hyperglycinemia, Menkes
Ataxia, peripheral neuropathy and dystonia: GA1, neurotransmitter defects, PDH deficiency

Eye Examination
Cataracts: galactosemia, peroxisomal disorders
Corneal clouding: Hurler syndrome
Lens dislocation: homocystinuria
Macular cherry-red spot: GM1 and GM2 gangliosidosis, sialidosis, Niemann–Pick disease
Pigmentary retinopathy: FAOD, mitochondrial, peroxisomal disorders

Cardiovascular Disease
Heart failure signs: Pompe disease
Valvular heart diseases: MPS

Abdominal Examination
HSM: MPS, GSD, GM1, Niemann–Pick, Wolman, tyrosinemia
Splenomegaly: Gaucher disease
Hepatomegaly: GSD, FDPase, CDG
Inguinal and umbilical hernia: MPS

Skeletal Examination
Limitation in joint movements: MPS I, II, IV, VI
Scoliosis: homocystinuria

Unusual Odor
Burnt sugar (MSUD), sweaty feet (isovaleric acidemia), musty (PKU), cabbage (tyrosinemia type I), fish (trimethylaminuria)
Absence of these odors does not exclude disease

CDG, Congenital disorders of glycosylation; *FAOD*, fatty acid oxidation defect; *FDPase*, fructose 1,6-diphosphatase; *FTT*, failure to thrive; *GA1*, glutaric acidemia type I; *GSD*, glycogen storage disease; *HSM*, hepatosplenomegaly; *MPS*, mucopolysaccharidosis; *MSUD*, maple syrup urine disease; *PDH*, pyruvate dehydrogenase; *PKU*, phenylketonuria; *SLO*, Smith-Lemli-Opitz syndrome.

Table 26.8	Metabolic Disorders Causing Dysmorphic Features
Organelle Metabolism	**Investigations**
Lysosomal disorders (e.g., MPS, I-cell disease, mannosidosis)	Urine MPS screening Urine oligosaccharide screening
Peroxisomal disorders (e.g., Zellweger, rhizomelic chondrodysplasia punctata)	Plasma VLCFA, phytanic acid, and plasmalogens
PDH	Plasma lactate and pyruvate
Biosynthetic Defects	
SLO	Serum 7-dehydrocholesterol
CDG	Plasma isoelectric focusing of transferrin
Menkes	Copper, ceruloplasmin
Homocystinuria	Plasma qAA, plasma total homocysteine

CDG, Congenital disorders of glycosylation; *MPS*, Mucopolysaccharidosis; *PDH*, pyruvate dehydrogenase; *qAA*, quantitative amino acid; *SLO*, Smith-Lemli-Opitz syndrome; *VLCFA*, very long chain fatty acid.

MANAGEMENT OF INBORN ERRORS OF METABOLISM

1. **Control of accumulated substrate**
   a. **Restrict dietary intake**
      i. UCD and OA: stop/restrict exogenous protein intake
      ii. Amino acid disorders: restrict specific amino acids (e.g., Phe in PKU, tyrosine in tyrosinemia)
      iii. Galactosemia and HFI: stop galactose and fructose/sucrose intake, respectively
2. **Control endogenous production of substrate**
   a. UCD, amino acidopathies and OA: provide sufficient calories to prevent the breakdown of endogenous protein using
      i. Intravenous (IV) D10 with appropriate saline at glucose infusion rate (GIR) of 10 mg/kg/min or 1.5 times maintenance
      ii. Intralipid (1–2 g/kg/day), except in FAOD
      iii. Reintroduce protein into diet after 24 to 48 hour of exclusion

> **! PITFALL**
>
> Prolonged restriction of protein can worsen amino acidopathies or urea cycle defects because it can trigger catabolism.

3. **Clear toxic metabolites**
   a. Severe hyperammonemia or hyperleucinemia (MSUD): hemodialysis
   b. Organic acidopathies: carnitine to aid toxic metabolite elimination and restore acylcarnitine shuttle
   c. UCD: ammonia scavengers, such as sodium benzoate and sodium phenylbutyrate to allow nitrogen excretion through alternative pathway
4. **Supply deficient product:** FAOD, GSD: provide glucose

5. **Enzyme replacement therapy:** beneficial in Gaucher disease, Fabry disease, MPS I, II, IV, VI, VII, Pompe disease
6. **Cofactor replacement therapy**
   a. Multiple carboxylase deficiency/biotinidase deficiency: biotin
   b. Pyridoxine-responsive homocystinuria and pyridoxine-dependent epilepsy: pyridoxine
   c. Vitamin B_{12}–responsive MMA: vitamin B_{12}
7. **Organ transplantation**
   a. MPS I and X-ALD: BMT
   b. UCD/MSUD (considered in other OA): liver transplantation
8. **Supportive management:** control seizures and relieve spasticity, facilitate feeding, prevent constipation
9. **Genetic counseling:** recurrence risk, prenatal diagnosis for future pregnancies, sibling screening

HYPOGLYCEMIA

1. **Definition:** blood glucose ≤ 2.6 mmol/L
2. **Diagnostic approach**
   a. For neonatal hypoglycemia, see Chapter 27 Neonatology
   b. See Figure 26.3 for approach

Figure 26.3 Approach to Hypoglycemia

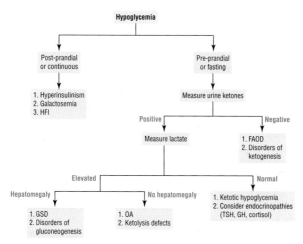

FAOD, Fatty acid oxidation defect; *GH*, growth hormone; *GSD*, glycogen storage disease; *HFI*, hereditary fructose intolerance; *OA*, organic acidopathy; *TSH*, thyroid stimulating hormone.

3. **Management**
   a. **Critical blood work (collect at time of hypoglycemia):** glucose, free fatty acids (FFAs), ketone bodies (3-hydroxybutyrate), insulin, IGF-1, cortisol, TSH, T_4, acylcarnitine profile, qAA, NH_4, lactate, UOAs, urine dip for ketones
   b. For neonates, see Figure 27.6
   c. For non-neonates, glucose bolus (5 mL/kg D10W) followed by continuous infusion GIR 7 to 10 mg/kg/min
   d. Rule out severe systemic illness, liver disease, sepsis
4. **Other clues to diagnosis**
   a. **Timing of hypoglycemia:** within minutes of feeding (hyperinsulinism), within 1 to 6 hours (GSD), after 8 to 24 hours fasting (FAOD)
   b. **Response to glucagon administration:** absent in GSD type I (glucagon may precipitate lactic acidosis in GSD I patients)
   c. **Endocrinologic causes:** vary with age
      i. <1 year old: hyperinsulinemic hypoglycemia
      ii. >1 year old: ketotic hypoglycemia
   d. **Calculate GIR:** requiring a GIR over 10 mg/kg/min suggests an endocrine cause (usually hyperinsulinism)
   e. If BG does not fall to <2.7 mmol/L spontaneously, consider provocative fast

To provide 0.5 g/kg (treatment for symptomatic hypoglycemia), the concentration of dextrose in the fluid to be given multiplied by the volume to be given should equal 50, i.e., D10W = 5 mL/kg (10 × 5 = 50), D25W = 2 mL/kg (25 × 2 = 50), D50W = 1 mL/kg (50 × 1 = 50).

HYPERAMMONEMIA

1. **Background**
   a. Severe hyperammonemia is a medical emergency because of the risk of cerebral edema
   b. **May present at any age:** neonates often present with poor feeding and encephalopathy, whereas older children and adults may present with behavioural changes and confusion
   c. **Upper limit of normal varies by age:** up to 180 μmol/L in sick neonates without an underlying metabolic disease. NH_4 >200 μmol/L (neonates) and >100 μmol/L (after the first month) raise suspicion of a metabolic disorder.
   d. Include plasma NH_4 in investigation of encephalopathy of unclear cause
2. **Diagnostic approach:** see Figure 26.4

26

684

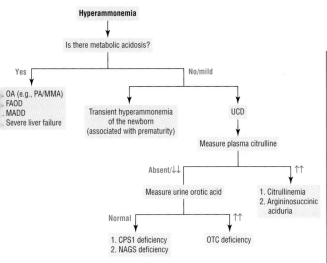

Hyperammonemia

Is there metabolic acidosis?

Yes → OA (e.g., PA/MMA), FAOD, MADD, Severe liver failure

No/mild →
- Transient hyperammonemia of the newborn (associated with prematurity)
- UCD → Measure plasma citrulline

Absent/↓↓ → Measure urine orotic acid
- Normal → 1. CPS1 deficiency 2. NAGS deficiency
- ↑↑ → OTC deficiency

↑↑ → 1. Citrullinemia 2. Argininosuccinic aciduria

PS, Carbamoyl phosphate synthetase; *OA*, organic acidopathy; *FAOD*, fatty acid oxidation defect; *ADD*, multiple acyl-coenzyme A dehydrogenase deficiency; *NAGS*, N-acetylglutamate synthase; *TC*, ornithine transcarbamylase; *UCD*, urea cycle defect.

Metabolic Disease

26

Management

a. **Consult a metabolics specialist**

b. **Limit catabolism**

   i. Make nil per mouth (NPO) and cease protein intake

   ii. Start IV D10 with appropriate saline and 20 mmol of KCl/L (if voiding) at 1.5 × maintenance, aiming for GIR 8-10 mg/kg/min

   iii. Consider IV Intralipid 1 to 2 g/kg/day

c. **Clear toxic metabolites**

   i. Alternative pathway for nitrogen excretion: sodium benzoate/sodium phenylacetate

   ii. Replenish urea cycle intermediates with arginine hydrochloride

   iii. Consider hemodialysis immediately for NH_4 level >500 μmol/L or if patient deteriorating (e.g., encephalopathy)

   iv. Consider carglumic acid for unknown disease or known N-acetylglutamate synthase (NAGS) deficiency

v. Consider supplemental carnitine in case of suspected or confirmed organic acidopathies

d. **Monitoring and supportive management**

   i. Supportive care: antiseizure medication, antibiotics for sepsis, adequate ventilation, transfer to intensive care for close monitoring

   ii. Neurovitals q2–4h; if patient deteriorates ($\downarrow$LOC), NH_4 level stat

   iii. Accurate ins/outs, daily weight (look for signs of fluid overload)

   iv. Repeat NH_4 level, blood gas, and electrolytes q2–4h initially while monitoring response to emergent therapy, then as needed

---

✦ PEARL

Sodium benzoate/phenyl acetate and arginine administration can be associated with hypotension and hypernatremia. Closely monitor blood pressure and serum sodium levels.

METABOLIC ACIDOSIS

1. See Figure 26.5 for approach.
2. **Calculate anion gap (AG):** if high AG—blood lactate, urine organic acids, and ketones are useful in identifying lactic acidosis or OA
3. Marked ketosis unusual in neonates, indicates primary metabolic disease

Figure 26.5 Approach to Metabolic Acidosis

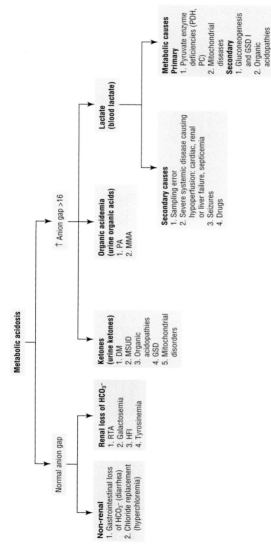

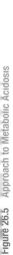

Metabolic Disease

26

DM, Diabetes mellitus; *GSD*, glycogen storage disease; *HFI*, hereditary fructose intolerance; *MMA*, methylmalonic aciduria; *MSUD*, maple syrup urine disease; *PA*, propionic aciduria; *PC*, pyruvate carboxylase; *PDH*, pyruvate dehydrogenase; *RTA*, renal tubular acidosis.

687

LACTIC ACIDOSIS

1. **Metabolic causes:** gluconeogenesis and mitochondrial disorders, GSD type 1
2. See Figure 26.6 for approach

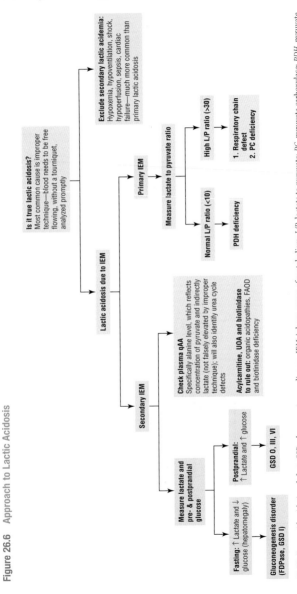

Figure 26.6 Approach to Lactic Acidosis

FAOD, Fatty acid oxidation defect; *GSD,* glycogen storage disease; *IEM,* inborn errors of metabolism; *L/P,* lactate to pyruvate; *PC,* pyruvate carboxylase; *PDH,* pyruvate dehydrogenase; *qAA,* quantitative amino acid; *UOA,* urine organic acids.

HEPATOCELLULAR DYSFUNCTION

See Table 26.9 for IEM causing hepatocellular dysfunction

Table 26.9	Metabolic Disorders Causing Hepatocellular Dysfunction	
Small-Molecule Disorder	**Organelle Disorder**	
Amino acid disorders (Tyrosinemia type I)	Mitochondrial disorder (MtDNA depletion)	
Carbohydrate disorders (galactosemia, HFI, GSD IV)	Lysosomal storage disorder (Niemann–Pick type C)	
UCD	Peroxisomal disorders (Zellweger)	
FAODs (CPTII, LCHAD)	CDG	

CDG, Congenital disorders of glycosylation; *CPTII*, carnitine palmitoyltransferase II deficiency; *FAOD*, fatty acid oxidation defect; *GSD*, glycogen storage disease; *HFI*, hereditary fructose intolerance; *LCHAD*, long chain 3-hydroxyacyl-coenzyme A dehydrogenase; *MtDNA*, mitochondrial deoxyribonucleic acid; *UCD*, urea cycle defect.

CARDIOMYOPATHY

See Table 26.10 for IEM causing cardiomyopathy

Table 26.10	Metabolic Disorders Causing Cardiomyopathy			
Small-Molecule Disorder		**Organelle Disorder**		
FAOD	- Primary systemic carnitine deficiency - LCHAD	**Mitochondrial syndromes**	- Kearns-Sayre syndrome - Barth syndrome - MELAS	
Organic acidopathies	- PA - MMA - HMG-CoA lyase deficiency	**Lysosomal storage disorders**	- Pompe disease - Fabry disease - Hurler syndrome - Hunter syndrome	
Carbohydrate	- GSD III			

FAOD, Fatty acid oxidation defect; *GSD*, glycogen storage disease; *HMG-CoA*, 3-hydroxy-3-methylglutaryl-coenzyme A; *LCHAD*, long chain 3-hydroxyacyl-coenzyme A dehydrogenase; *MELAS*, mitochondrial encephalomyopathy, lactic acidosis, stroke-like episodes; *MMA*, methylmalonic aciduria; *PA*, propionic aciduria.

STORAGE DISORDERS

1. Disorder in which a substance (e.g., glycogen, glycosaminoglycans, sphingolipids) accumulates within organelles or organ tissue and disrupts function
2. Examples include glycogen storage diseases (GSD) and lysosomal storage diseases, such as mucopolysaccharidoses and sphingolipidoses. See Tables 26.3 and 26.6.

3. In general, have multisystem involvement, often including the brain, and characteristic dysmorphology
4. Enzyme replacement therapy (ERT) and hematopoietic stem cell transplant halt disease progression. Preventing neurodevelopmental deterioration remains challenging because of difficulty of ERT crossing the blood-brain barrier.

PERIMORTEM/POSTMORTEM INVESTIGATIONS

1. In cases of death without known etiology, helpful to investigate for IEM (to establish or confirm diagnosis for future genetic counseling)
2. Try collecting blood and urine samples before expected death
3. Skin fibroblasts may remain viable for 2 days after death (earlier is better)

Neonatology

Julia DiLabio • Amy Zipursky • Tapas Kulkarni • Aideen Moore

COMMON ABBREVIATIONS

Also see page xviii for a list of other abbreviations used throughout this book

AXR	abdominal x-ray
BD	base deficit
BE	base excess
BW	birth weight
CAH	congenital adrenal hyperplasia
CHD	congenital heart disease
CHF	congestive heart failure
CPAP	continuous positive airway pressure
DAT	direct antiglobulin test
EBM	expressed breast milk
ECMO	extracorporeal membrane oxygenation
ELBW	extremely low birth weight
ETT	endotracheal tube
FiO_2	fraction of inspired oxygen
FSWU	full septic workup
GA	gestational age
GBS	group B streptococcus
GIR	glucose infusion rate
HBR	hyperbilirubinemia
HCT	hematocrit
HFO	high-frequency oscillation
HIE	hypoxic ischemic encephalopathy
HMF	human milk fortifier
IDM	infant of diabetic mother
iNO	inhaled nitric oxide
IPPV	intermittent positive pressure ventilation
IUGR	intrauterine growth restriction
IVH	intraventricular hemorrhage
LBW	low birth weight
LGA	large for gestational age (BW >90th percentile for GA)
MAP	mean airway pressure
MCA	middle cerebral artery
NAS	neonatal abstinence syndrome
NEC	necrotizing enterocolitis
NPT	nasopharyngeal tube
OI	oxygenation index
$PaCO_2$	arterial partial pressure of carbon dioxide
PaO_2	arterial partial pressure of oxygen
PDA	patent ductus arteriosus
PEEP	positive end expiratory pressure
PFO	patient foramen ovale
PIP	peak inspiratory pressure

PPHN	persistent pulmonary hypertension of the newborn
PROM	premature rupture of membranes
PVL	periventricular leukomalacia
RDS	respiratory distress syndrome
ROP	retinopathy of prematurity
SEH	subependymal hemorrhage
SGA	small for gestational age (BW <10th percentile for GA)
SpO$_2$	oxygen saturation
TcB	transcutaneous bilirubin
(T)PN	(total) parenteral nutrition
TSB	total serum bilirubin
TTN	transient tachypnea of the newborn
UAC	umbilical artery catheter
UVC	umbilical vein catheter
VLBW	very low birth weight
V/Q	ventilation/perfusion

CLASSIFICATION OF THE NEONATE

1. Term: 37 weeks and 0 days to 41 weeks and 6 days
2. Premature: <37 weeks
3. Late Preterm: 34 to <37 weeks
4. Postterm: ≥42 weeks
5. Low birth weight (LBW): <2500 g
6. Very low birth weight (VLBW): <1500 g
7. Extremely low birth weight (ELBW): <1000 g

NEWBORN RESUSCITATION

CASE ROOM EQUIPMENT

1. Gloves, barrier precautions
2. Clean warm towels
3. Radiant warmer turned on
4. Suction equipment turned on
5. Stethoscope
6. Oxygen saturation probe and monitor
7. O$_2$ bagging equipment with masks (sizes 0, 1, 2)
8. Temperature probe
9. Laryngoscope
10. Uncuffed endotracheal tubes (ETTs) (sizes 2.5, 3.0, 3.5, 4.0) (Table 27.1)
11. Magill forceps
12. Gastric tubes (size 5, 8 F)

13. Polyethylene plastic wrap for newborns <32 weeks gestational age (GA)
14. Electrocardiogram (ECG) leads and monitor (if available)
15. Meconium aspirator
16. Umbilical catheterization tray (catheter sizes 3.5, 5.0 F) (Box 27.1)
17. Emergency drugs/fluids: epinephrine 1:10,000, 0.9% NaCl, D10W

Table 27.1	Endotracheal Tube Size		
GA (Week)	**Weight (kg)**	**ETT Size (mm)**	**Depth of Insertion[a] (cm)**
<28	<1.0	2.5	6–7
28–34	1.0–2.0	3.0	7–8
35–38	2.0–3.0	3.0–3.5	8–9
>38	>3.0	3.5–4.0	9–10

[a]Depth of insertion (cm from lips) for oral tubes: 6 + weight (kg) or nasal-tragus length (in cm) + 1 cm; nasal tubes: 7 + weight (kg) or nasal-tragus length (in cm) + 2 cm.

ETT, Endotracheal tube; *GA*, gestational age.

Data from Weiner, GM. *Textbook of Neonatal Resuscitation.* 7th ed. IL: American Academy of Pediatrics; 2016.

Box 27.1	**Calculations for Umbilical Artery Catheter and Umbilical Vein Catheter Placement**

UAC insertion depth: weight (kg) × 3 + 9 (for T6–T9 position)
UVC insertion depth: (UAC depth/2) + 1 (for T8–T9, in IVC, above diaphragm)

IVC, Inferior vena cava; *UAC*, umbilical artery catheter; *UVC*, umbilical vein catheter.

NEONATAL RESUSCITATION ALGORITHM

1. Normal sequence of response to resuscitation: increased heart rate (HR) → reflex activity → improved color → spontaneous breathing → improved tone and responsiveness
2. See Figure 27.1 for resuscitation algorithm and Box 27.2 for resuscitation interventions
3. See Table 27.2 for Apgar score

Figure 27.1 Neonatal Resuscitation Algorithm

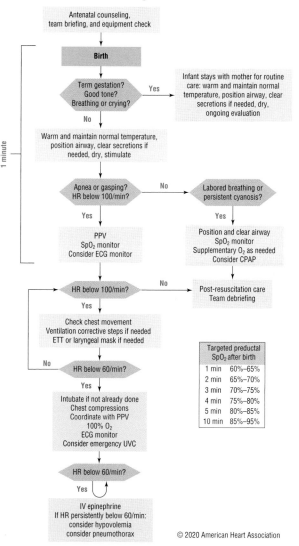

CPAP, Continuous positive airway pressure; *ECG*, electrocardiogram; *ETT*, endotracheal tube; *HR*, heart rate; *IV*, intravenous; *PPV*, positive pressure ventilation; *UVC*, umbilical vein catheter. (Adapted from Aziz K, Lee HC, Escobedo MB, Hoover AV, Kamath-Rayne BD, Kapadia VS, Magid DJ, Niermeyer S, Schmölzer GM, Szyld E, Weiner GM, Wyckoff MH, Yamada NK, Zaichkin J. Part 5: neonatal resuscitation: 2020 American Heart Association Guidelines for Cardiopulmonary Resuscitation and Emergency Cardiovascular Care. *Circulation.* 2020;142(suppl 2):S524–S550. doi: 10.1161/CIR.0000000000000902)

Box 27.2 ABCD of Newborn Resuscitation

Airway
1. Put baby's head in sniffing position
2. Suction mouth, then nose

Breathing
1. PPV: start at 21% FiO_2 (or 30% if <35 weeks) for apnea, gasping, or pulse <100 beats/min
2. Assess for rising HR, breath sounds, chest rise. If no response within 15 s, MR. SOPA (Figure 27.2) corrective measures. If no change in HR, see Table 27.3.
3. Intubate if no response to maneuvers or if chest compressions required; use CO_2 detector if intubated. Increase FiO_2 to 100%.
4. Ventilate at rate of 40–60 breaths/min, initial PIP 20–25 cmH_2O, initial PEEP for preterm 5 cmH_2O

Circulation
1. Compressions if HR <60 after 30 s of effective PPV
2. Give 3 compressions:1 breath every 2 s
3. Compress $\frac{1}{3}$ AP diameter of the chest

Drugs
1. Epinephrine: if HR <60 after 60 s of compressions; 1:10,000 solution 0.2 mL/kg IV/IO (or 1 mL/kg ETT, max 3 mL, while IV access being obtained)
2. Volume expanders: 0.9% NaCl 10 mL/kg; other: O Rh-negative blood— give over 5–10 min

AP, Anteroposterior; *ETT,* endotracheal tube; *HR,* heart rate; *IO,* intraosseus; *IV,* intravenous; *PEEP,* positive end expiratory pressure; *PIP,* peak inspiratory pressure; *PPV,* positive pressure ventilation.

Table 27.2 Apgar Score[a]

Sign	0	1	2
Activity (muscle tone)	Limp, flaccid	Some flexion of extremities	Active, well flexed
Pulse (heart rate)	Absent	<100 beats/min	>100 beats/min
Grimace (reflex irritability)	No response	Minimal response to stimulation	Prompt response to stimulation
Appearance (skin color)	Blue, pale	Body pink; extremities blue	Completely pink
Respiratory effort	Absent	Gasping, slow, irregular	Regular, good cry

[a]Apgar scoring system should not be used to determine need for resuscitation. Scoring should be done at 1 and 5 min and thereafter at 5-min intervals until score of 7 is achieved.

Data from Apgar V. Proposal for a new method of evaluation of the newborn infant. *Anesth Analg* 1953;32:260.

Figure 27.2 Ventilation Corrective Steps

6 Ventilation Corrective Steps: MR. SOPA

	Corrective Steps	Actions
M	Mask adjustment	Reapply the mask, consider the two-hand technique
R	Reposition airway	Place head neutral or slighlty extended
	Try PPV and reassess chest movement	
S	Suction mouth and nose	Use a bulb syringe or suction catheter
O	Open mouth	Open the mouth and lift the jaw forward
	Try PPV and reassess chest movement	
P	Pressure increase	Increase pressure in 5–10 cmH₂O increments, max 40 cmH₂O
	Try PPV and reassess chest movement	
A	Alternative airway	Place an endotracheal tube or largyngeal mask
	Try PPV and assess chest movement and breath sounds	

PPV, Positive pressure ventilation. (From Weiner GM. *Textbook of Neonatal Resuscitation.* 7th ed. IL: American Academy of Pediatrics; 2016.)

ADDITIONAL FACTORS IN INITIAL MANAGEMENT

1. **Small for gestational age (SGA) infants:** risk of hypothermia, hypoglycemia, polycythemia
2. **Large for gestational age (LGA) infants:** risk of birth trauma, asphyxia, hypoglycemia
3. **Premature infants**
   a. Avoid hypothermia at <32 weeks GA (do not dry, wrapping body in clear polyethylene wrap may reduce heat loss/evaporation in preterm infants)
   b. Low threshold for intubation at <29 weeks GA if born outside of a tertiary care center, early use of surfactant beneficial
   c. Avoid hyperoxia (i.e., saturation >95%)
   d. Initiate positive pressure ventilation (PPV) with FiO_2 0.21 to 0.30 and supplemental O_2 should be used if HR < 100 beats/min or remains cyanotic; provide positive end expiratory pressure (PEEP) of 5 to 8 cmH₂O during resuscitation

Table 27.3	Management of Poor Response to Positive Pressure Ventilation After MR. SOPA	
Cause of Nonresponse	**Diagnostic Considerations**	**Action**
ETT not in correct location	Observe chest movement; auscultate for symmetric air entry; CXR	Pull back ETT if in right main stem bronchus; reintubate if uncertain and reassess
Tension pneumothorax	Displaced apex beat $\pm$ hemodynamic compromise; decreased or unequal air entry; CXR or transillumination to confirm	Urgent drain with butterfly needle if unstable; insert chest tube
Diaphragmatic hernia	Scaphoid abdomen noted at birth $\pm$ respiratory distress; bowel sounds heard over chest; CXR diagnostic; $\uparrow$ risk of PPHN	Pass NG tube and connect to low Gomco; intubate; IPPV; sedate and paralyze
Hypoplastic lungs	History of oligohydramnios $\pm$ PROM $\pm$ Potter facies; bell-shaped chest; CXR	Urgent intubation; ventilatory support; requires high peak pressures
Sepsis or congenital pneumonia	History of PROM, GBS, or maternal fever; hemodynamic compromise; CXR (may look like RDS); cultures may be positive	Antibiotics; ventilatory support $\pm$ volume expanders $\pm$ inotropes
Severe RDS	Prematurity, stiff lungs, "ground glass" CXR	Higher pressures required; early surfactant via ETT
Cyanotic CHD	Persistent cyanosis despite adequate ventilation	Investigate for CHD
Acute blood loss	History of abruption, previa; asystole, bradycardia, pallor after oxygenation; subgaleal hemorrhage	Volume resuscitation: 0.9% NaCl 10 mL/kg, repeat; transfuse blood if large volume loss
Severe HIE	Agonal respirations, gasping, bradycardia, asystole, low Apgar scores, ongoing need for ventilation	Cord and blood gases; discontinuation of resuscitation after 20 min of asystole despite adequate resuscitation

CHD, Congenital heart disease; *CXR,* chest x-ray; *ETT,* endotracheal tube; *GBS,* group B streptococcus; *HIE,* hypoxic ischemic encephalopathy; *IPPV,* intermittent positive pressure ventilation; *PPHN,* persistent pulmonary hypertension of the newborn; *PROM,* premature rupture of membranes; *RDS,* respiratory distress syndrome.

NEWBORN CARE

NEWBORN PHYSICAL EXAMINATION
1. See Table 27.4 for key physical examination findings
2. Use postnatal maturational examination (New Ballard Score) to estimate GA if unknown (see Figure 27.3)

Table 27.4	Pertinent Findings on Newborn Examination		
System	**Finding**	**Diagnosis**	**Management**
Head	Small head circumference (<2 or 3 SD below the mean)	Microcephaly	Examine for signs of associated syndromes and possible etiology
Skin	White papules	Milia	Self-resolves
	Pustules over hyperpigmented macules	Transient pustular melanosis	Pustules resolve with bath
	Small white papules on erythematous macules; body>face; spare palms and soles	Erythema toxicum	Self-resolves, can take up to 7 days
	Red patch identified at birth; commonly around eyes, between eyebrows or on back of neck	Nevus simplex	Self-resolves, can take up to 2 years
Eyes	Absent red reflex	Retinoblastoma, cataracts, persistent fetal vasculature, Coats disease	Refer to Ophthalmology
Ears	Preauricular pits or tags	Isolated finding or associated with syndrome	Hearing test Examination for features of associated syndromes
Mouth	Natal teeth	Isolated finding or associated with syndrome	Can be observed or require further intervention with dentistry if affecting feeding or causing discomfort
	Cleft lip and/or palate	Isolated finding or associated with syndrome	Examine for signs of associated syndromes Refer for surgical repair Support or refer for feeding assistance Hearing test
Neck	Tenderness or crepitus on palpation of clavicle, decreased range of motion or shoulder or asymmetry	Clavicle fracture	Clavicle x-ray
Heart	Murmur and/or cyanosis	CHD	Consider 4-limb blood pressure, pre/postductal oxygen saturations, echocardiography, CXR, ECG, hyperoxia test if cyanosis, Cardiology consult
	Absent/decreased femoral pulses	Coarctation of the aorta	4-limb blood pressure, pre/postductal oxygen saturation, echocardiography, Cardiology consult
	Bounding femoral pulses	PDA	Echocardiography

Continued 699

Table 27.4	Pertinent Findings on Newborn Examination—cont'd		
System	**Finding**	**Diagnosis**	**Management**
Lungs	Work of breathing		See Table 27.12
Abdomen	Erythema or discharge around umbilical stump	Omphalitis	Swab and culture of discharge If systemic signs, consider blood and CSF cultures Consider antibiotics
	Imperforate anus	VACTERL or isolated finding	Consult General Surgery Examine for signs of VACTERL May require antibiotics Assess for imperforate anus if meconium has not passed by 48 h
Genitalia	Atypical or ambiguous Undescended testicle		Endocrinology consult Referral to General Surgery or Urology prior to 6 months of age
	Hypospadias, hooded foreskin or other peno-scrotal abnormalities		Urology referral Ensure void prior to discharge Avoid circumcision until assessed by Urology
Spine	Soft tissue mass, tuft of hair, hemangioma, skin change or sacral dimple (>0.5 cm, with overlying skin changes or located above the gluteal creases)	Vertebral or spinal cord pathology	Spine ultrasound If other systemic symptoms or neurological abnormalities, spine MRI and consider Neurosurgery referral
Limbs	Polydactyly	Isolated finding or associated with syndrome	Examine for signs of associated syndromes Consider Plastic Surgery referral
Hips	Positive Barlow/Ortolani tests (hip click is not clinically meaningful)	Developmental dysplasia of the hip	Hip ultrasound at 4–6 weeks of age (also consider hip ultrasound if risk factors: breech position, positive family history)

CHD, Congenital heart disease; *CSF,* cerebrospinal fluid; *MRI,* magnetic resonance imaging; *PDA,* patent ductus arteriosus; *VACTERL,* vertebral defects, anal atresia, cardiac defects, tracheo-esophageal fistula, renal anomalies, and limb abnormalities.

Neuromuscular maturity

Neuromuscular maturity sign	Score							Record score here
	−1	0	1	2	3	4	5	
Posture								
Square window (wrist)	>90°	90°	60°	45°	30°	0°		
Arm recoil		180°	140°–180°	110°–140°	90°–110°	<90°		
Popliteal angle	180°	160°	140°	120°	100°	90°	<90°	
Scarf sign								
Heel to ear								
							Total neuromuscular maturity score	

Total Score _____

Continued

Physical maturity

Physical maturity sign		Score							Record score here
	-1	0	1	2	3	4	5		
Skin	Sticky, friable, transparent	Gelatinous, red, translucent	Smooth, pink, visible veins	Superficial peeling &/or rash, few veins	Cracking pale areas, rare veins	Parchment, deep cracking, no vessels	Leathery, cracked, wrinkled		
Lanugo	None	Sparse	Abundant	Thinning	Bald areas	Mostly bald			
Plantar surface	Heel-toe 40–50 mm: –1 <40 mm: –2	>50 mm no crease	Faint red marks	Anterior transverse crease only	Creases anterior 2/3	Creases over entire sole			
Breast	Imperceptible	Barely perceptible	Flat areola, no bud	Stippled areola 1–2 mm bud	Raised areola 3–4 mm bud	Full areola 5–10 mm bud			
Eye/ear	Lids fused Loosely: –1 Tightly: –2	Lids open, pinna flat, stays folded	Slightly curved pinna; soft; slow recoil	Well-curved pinna; soft but ready recoil	Formed & firm, instant recoil	Thick cartilage, ear stiff			
Genitals, (Male)	Scrotum flat, smooth	Scrotum empty, faint rugae	Testes in upper canal, rare rugae	Testes descending, few rugae	Testes down, good rugae	Testes pendulous, deep rugae			
Genitals, (Female)	Clitoris prominent, labia flat	Prominent clitoris, small labia minora	Prominent clitoris, enlarging minora	Majora & minora equally prominent	Majora large, minora small	Majora covers clitoris & minora			

Total physical maturity score

Maturity Rating

Score	Weeks
-10	20
-5	22
0	24
5	26
10	28
15	30
20	32
25	34
30	36
35	38
40	40
45	42
50	44

Gestational age (weeks) _____

By exam _____

Adapted from Ballard JL, Khoury JC, Wedig K, et al. New Ballard score, expanded to include extremely premature infants. *J Pediatr.* 1991;119(3):417–423; used with permission from Mosby

Medications

a. Vitamin K as a single intramuscular dose of 0.5 mg (BW ≤1500 g) or 1 mg (BW >1500 g) within the first 6 hours after birth to prevent hemorrhagic disease of the newborn

   i. If intramuscular (IM) injection declined, vitamin K 2 mg PO given at the first feed, with repeat doses at 2–4 weeks and at 6–8 weeks of age

b. Ocular prophylaxis with 0.5% erythromycin ointment can be considered for prevention of gonorrhea infection

Screening

a. Newborn screen (conditions screened vary based on local protocol)

   i. Collect between 24 hours and 7 days after birth on all infants (ideally between 24 and 48 hours)

   ii. If sample is collected before 24 hours, repeat within 5 days

   iii. Ideally, collect before any packed red cell transfusions. If has received blood transfusion, repeat sample should be collected 4 months after the most recent transfusion.

   iv. For premature infants <33 weeks GA or VLBW <1500 g, collect screen between 24 and 48 hours and a second screen should be collected at 3 weeks (or earlier if the infant is discharged before 3 weeks of age)

b. Critical congenital heart disease screening

c. Hearing screen

RENATAL COUNSELING AND SCREENING

Genetic screening: see Table 27.5 for genetic screening options and interpretation of findings

Ultrasound abnormalities: see Table 27.6 for common ultrasound findings and recommended follow-up

Maternal conditions: see Table 27.7 for maternal conditions that may have manifestations in the newborn

Neonatology

27

Table 27.5	Antenatal Testing and Interpretation of Findings		
Screening Test	**Timing**	**Disorders Screened**	**Components**
First trimester screen (FTS)	11–13+6/7 weeks	Trisomy 18/21	Nuchal translucency, PAPP-A, free B-hCG, maternal age
Maternal serum screen (MSS)	15–20+6/7 weeks	Trisomy 18/21, neural tube defects	Alpha-fetoprotein, unconjugated estriol, free B-hCG, inhibin A, maternal age
Integrated prenatal screen (IPS)	11–13+6/7 weeks AND 15–20+6/7 weeks	Trisomy 18/21, neural tube defects	Nuchal translucency, PAPP-A, alpha-fetoprotein, unconjugated estriol, free B-hCG, inhibin A, maternal age
Noninvasive prenatal testing (NIPT) using cell-free fetal DNA in maternal blood	As early as 9 weeks following a positive screening test, or first line test in high risk women	Trisomy 13/18/21, Turners	Offer referral to genetics and diagnostic testing (CVS or amniocentesis) if positive screen

DNA, Deoxyribonucleic acid; *CVS*, chorionic villus sampling; *hCG*, human chorionic gonadotropin; *PAPP-A*, pregnancy-associated plasma protein A.

Table 27.6	Ultrasound Abnormalities and Interpretation of Findings	
Ultrasound Finding	**Clinical Significance**	**Recommended Follow-Up**
Echogenic cardiac focus	Isolated finding, or associated with aneuploidy	If isolated finding, no further workup. If other risk factors for aneuploidy present, consider further workup
Pelviectasis	Transient, or represents a congenital anomaly of the kidney/urinary tract	See Chapter 28 Nephrology and Urology
Single kidney, multicystic kidney	Congenital anomaly of the kidney/urinary tract	Postnatal renal ultrasound
Echogenic bowel	Associated with aneuploidy, cystic fibrosis, congenital infection, and congenital malformation of bowel	Consider fetal genetic screening and testing for maternal infection
Choroid plexus cyst	Isolated finding, or associated with trisomy 18 and 21	If isolated finding, no further workup. If other risk factors for aneuploidy present, consider further workup for aneuploidy
Cerebral ventriculomegaly	Isolated finding, or associated with infection, genetic abnormalities	Assess for macrocephaly. Postnatal head ultrasound. Referral to Neurosurgery for moderate-severe ventriculomegaly

Table 27.7 Maternal Conditions and Manifestations in the Newborn

Condition	Potential Manifestations in the Newborn	Mechanism	Recommended Monitoring
Maternal immune thrombocytopenia	Thrombocytopenia (autoimmune)	Autoimmune reaction; maternal antibodies react with maternal and fetal platelets	Routine CBC and monitoring for petechiae and bleeding
Maternal diabetes	1. Hypoglycemia 2. Large for gestational age 3. Anatomic anomalies (e.g., sacral agenesis, cardiac anomalies)		Monitor for hypoglycemia after birth

Maternal lupus (anti-Ro and/or anti-La antibody positive mothers with or without a diagnosis of lupus)	Neonatal lupus
	1. Cardiac
	  a. Congenital 1st, 2nd or 3rd degree heart block with bradycardia
	  b. Endocardial fibroelastosis or cardiomyopathy
	2. Dermatological
	  a. Erythematous plaques with scale
	  b. Can present anywhere, but typically on face and scalp
	3. Hematological
	  a. anemia
	  b. thrombocytopenia
	  c. neutropenia
			1. Fetal echocardiogram (serial between 18 and 24 weeks GA if high maternal anti-Ro/La antibodies)
			2. ECG at birth (if any abnormalities, Cardiology consult)
			3. Monitor for rash (if rash appears, typically will resolve without intervention)
			4. Rheumatology referral

Maternal Graves	Neonatal Graves disease	TSH receptor antibodies (TRAb) can cross the placenta	If positive or unknown maternal TRAb level in 2nd or 3rd trimester in setting of maternal Graves disease: check TRAb in cord blood or after birth. If positive or unknown, check thyroid function at 3–5 days and at 10–14 days of life
Hypertension/ preeclampsia	1. Hypoxia 2. Growth restriction	Placental insufficiency can lead to hypoxia and growth restriction of the developing fetus	Regular antenatal ultrasound monitoring, including umbilical and MCA dopplers

CBC, Complete blood count; *ECG,* electrocardiogram; *GA,* gestational age; *MCA,* middle cerebral artery; *TSH,* thyroid stimulating hormone.

Neonatology

27

PLANNING FOR PRETERM BIRTH

1. If there is a risk of extremely preterm delivery, the mother should be transferred to a tertiary care center. Find up-to-date outcome data from the Canadian Neonatal Network (www.canadianneonatalnetwork.org).
2. Recommend antenatal corticosteroids within 7 days to all women expected to deliver a premature infant ≤34+6 weeks GA (and between 35+0 and 36+6 weeks GA in select situations) for lung development
3. Consider magnesium sulphate for all women experiencing imminent preterm delivery (≤33+6 weeks GA) for neuroprotection

NUTRITION AND GROWTH

1. **Key principles:** depending on BW and GA, feeding may be initiated enterally and/or parenterally
2. **Enteral nutrition:** see Table 27.8

Table 27.8	Guidelines for Initiating and Advancing Enteral Feeds in Stable Infants			
Weight (g)[a]	Initiation of Feeds[b]	**INCREASE FEEDS**		Days to Full Feeds (TFI ~150 mL/kg/day)[c]
		Bolus	Continuous	
500–749	1 mL q4h × 72h 1 mL q2h × 48h	1 mL q24h	0.5 mL q24h	10–13
750–999	1 mL q2h × 96h	1.5 mL q24h	0.75 mL q24h	10–12
1000–1249	1 mL q2h × 72h	1 mL q12h	0.5 mL q12h	9–10
1250–1499	2 mL q2h × 24h	1 mL q8h	0.5 mL q8h	6–7
1500–1749	3 mL q3h × 24h	1.5 mL q6h	0.5 mL q6h	6
1749–1999	4 mL q3h × 24h	1 mL q3h	0.3 mL q3h	5–6
2000–2499	5 mL q3h × 24h	2 mL q3h	0.7 mL q3h	4
>2500[d]	6 mL q3h × 24h	3 mL q3h	1 mL q3h	3

[a]Special considerations: For IUGR/SGA infants, use birth weight to guide feeding. Trophic feed duration may be extended and may need to slow advances (especially if born <29 weeks). For high-risk infants (significant congenital heart disease/PDA, intestinal ischemia concerns, polycythemia, exchange transfusion), use one to two weight categories below weight to guide feeding.

[b]Start feeds either as regular/slow bolus or continuous. Initiate feeds within the first 24 h with mother's own milk unless contraindicated.

[c]For EBM fed preterm infants, fortify with HMF to 0.74 kCal/mL at enteral TFI 120 mL/kg/day for 24–48 h and after 24–48 h, fortify to 0.8 kCal/mL. For formula fed preterm infants, change from 0.68 to 0.8 kCal/mL at enteral TFI 120–140 mL/kg/day. Term infants do not routinely require fortification.

[d]For infants >48 hours of age AND born ≥37 weeks gestational age AND birth weight ≥2500 g, if there are no identified risk factors, may individualize feeding advancement (e.g., start at 5–10 mL q3h and increase 5–8 mL q3h OR ad lib feeds with a minimum TFI).

EBM, Expressed breast milk; *HMF,* human milk fortifier; *IUGR,* intrauterine growth retardation; *PDA,* patent ductus arteriosus; *SGA,* small for gestational age; *TFI,* total fluid intake.

Adapted from The Hospital for Sick Children NICU Nutrition Guidelines, July 2020.

3. Parenteral nutrition: see Table 27.9

Table 27.9	Parenteral Nutrition Guidelines for Infants			
	PN FOR PRETERM INFANTS[a]		**PN FOR TERM INFANTS[a]**	
Timing	**Protein**	**Lipid**	**Protein**	**Lipid**
Initial Dose	1.5–2 g/kg/day	0.5–1 g/kg/day	1.5–2 g/kg/day	0.5–1 g/kg/day
Advance Daily	1 g/kg/day	1 g/kg/day	1 g/kg/day	1 g/kg/day
Goal	3.5–4 g/kg/day	2.5–3 g/kg/day[b]	2.5–3 g/kg/day	3 g/kg/day[b]
>Week 3–4	Discontinue PN once full enteral feeds reached			

[a]Add electrolytes based on clinical and laboratory assessment
[b]Monitor lipid levels when at 2 g fat/kg/day before increasing

PN, Parenteral nutrition.

Adapted from The Hospital for Sick Children Guidelines for the Administration of Enteral and Parenteral Nutrition in Paediatrics, 2018.

4. Nutritional supplements
  a. Human milk fortifier (HMF)
      i. Indicated for premature infants once full enteral feeds established
      ii. Continue until 2000 g or beyond in special circumstances
      iii. Further supplementation may be necessary (e.g., transitional formula, Polycose, Microlipid)
  b. Supplemental vitamin D 400 IU/day for premature infants receiving fortified human milk or preterm formula, and term infants fed exclusively human milk
  c. Oral iron supplementation
      i. Preterm infants: 3 to 4 mg/kg/day elemental iron for BW<1000 g or 2 to 3 mg/kg/day for BW ≥1000 g starting at 2 to 4 weeks postnatal age and once full enteral feeds reached
      ii. Term infants <2500 g BW, if breastfed: 2 mg/kg/day elemental iron starting at 2 weeks postnatal age

5. Growth charts
  a. See Figures 27.4 and 27.5 for growth charts for female and male infants 22 to 50 weeks gestation
  b. Target growth
      i. Weight: preterm 15 to 20/kg/day, term 20 to 30 g/day
      ii. Head circumference: preterm (23–30 weeks) 1 cm/week, preterm (≥30 weeks) 0.5 cm/week; term (first 3 months) 0.5 to 1 cm/week
      iii. Length: preterm 1 cm/week, term 0.69 to 0.75 cm/week

Neonatology

27

Figure 27.4 Fetal-Infant Growth Chart for Preterm Infants—Females

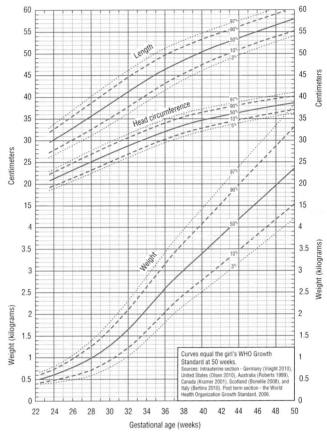

Curves equal the girl's WHO Growth
Standard at 50 weeks.
Sources: Intrauterine section - Germany (Voight 2010),
United States (Olsen 2010), Australia (Roberts 1999),
Canada (Kramer 2001), Scotland (Bonellie 2008), and
Italy (Bertino 2010). Post term section - the World
Health Organization Growth Standard, 2006.

WHO, World, Health Organization. (From Fenton TR, Kim JH. A systematic review and meta-analysis to revise the Fenton growth chart for preterm infants. *BMC Pediatr.* 2013;13:59.)

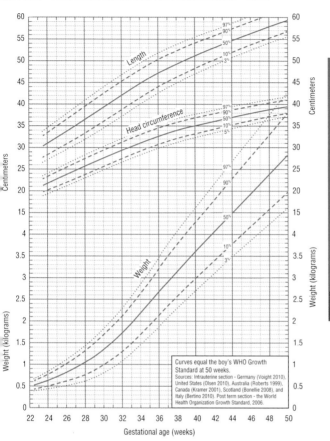

Figure 27.5 Fetal-Infant Growth Chart for Preterm Infants—Males

Curves equal the boy's WHO Growth Standard at 50 weeks.
Sources: Intrauterine section - Germany (Voight 2010), United States (Olsen 2010), Australia (Roberts 1999), Canada (Kramer 2001), Scotland (Bonellie 2008), and Italy (Bertino 2010). Post term section - the World Health Organization Growth Standard, 2006.

WHO, World, Health Organization. (From Fenton TR, Kim JH. A systematic review and meta-analysis to revise the Fenton growth chart for preterm infants. *BMC Pediatr.* 2013;13:59.)

FLUIDS AND ELECTROLYTES

Key points

a. High surface area:weight ratio

b. Immature renal function

c. Immature skin; higher losses in premature infants

d. See Table 27.10 for fluid guidelines

Table 27.10	Guidelines for Neonatal Fluid Therapy		
	FLUID REQUIREMENTS (mL/kg/DAY) BY AGE		
BW (g)	**1–2 days**	**3–7 days**	**7–30 days**
<750	100–200	150–200	160–180
750–1000	80–150	100–150	120–180
1000–1500	60–100	100–150	120–180
>1500	60–80	100–150	120–180

BW, Birth weight.

Modified from Kirpalani HM, Moore AM, Perlman M. *Residents Handbook of Neonatology*. 3rd ed. Hamilton, ON: BC Decker; 2007:85, Table 3.

2. **Goals of therapy**
    a. Achieve balance between input and output
        i. Weigh daily as weight is most useful indicator of fluid status
        ii. Use BW for fluid calculations until return to BW
    b. Meet normal metabolic and growth requirements
    c. Replace necessary losses
        i. Insensible fluid losses: 70% through skin, 30% through respirator tract
            <1500 g: 30 to 60 mL/kg/day
            1500 to 2500 g: 15 to 35 mL/kg/day
            >2500 g: 10 to 15 mL/kg/day
        ii. Urinary output: 50 to 100 mL/kg/day
        iii. Fecal losses: 5 to 10 mL/kg/day, usually minimal during first week
    d. Assess fluid balance: q8-12h for 2 to 3 days, then as clinically indicated but minimum daily
        i. Prediuretic phase: ~day 1 to 2—urine output <1 to 2 mL/kg/h
        ii. Diuretic phase: ~day 2 to 3—urine output >1 to 2 mL/kg/h, negative balance
        iii. Postdiuretic phase: after day 2 to 4—fluid balance stabilizes, then becomes positive
3. **Approach**
    a. **Minimum fluid requirements:** adjust by monitoring urine output weight, serum Na^+. In first 2 days, Na^+ and K^+ replacement not usually required.
    b. **Glucose:** start concentration of 10% to maintain caloric requirement and osmolarity
        i. Normal glucose infusion rate (GIR) is 4 to 6 mg/kg/min, may increase to 10 to 12 mg/kg/min if hypoglycemic
        ii. GIR (mg/kg/min) = carbohydrate (mg/mL) × infusion rate (mL/h) ÷ weight (kg) ÷ 60 minutes

Sample glucose infusion rate calculation: 0.8 kg infant infusing D10W at 3 mL/h = (100 mg/mL × 3 mL/h) ÷ 0.8 kg ÷ 60 min = 6.2 mg/kg/min

Note: DxW = x × 10 mg/mL of carbohydrate (e.g., D5W = 50 mg/mL of carbohydrate)

  c. **Electrolytes**

    i. Add Na^+ (2–3 mmol/kg/day) and K^+ (1–2 mmol/kg/day) once diuretic phase is established. If K^+ required, usually added to TPN.

    ii. Larger doses of Na^+ may be required in postdiuretic phase in infants <750 g because of high urinary Na^+ losses

  d. **Nutrition:** in all infants <1000 g BW and infants 1000 to 1500 g not expected to be taking full oral feeds within 4 to 7 days, start parenteral nutrition. Avoid glucose-only regimens beyond 24 hours of age, unless in prediuretic phase.

HYPONATREMIA

1. **Definition:** Na^+ <130 mmol/L
2. **Etiology and management:** see Table 27.11
3. Early hyponatremia (in the first few days of life, Na^+ < 127 mmol/L) is often caused by increased fluid intake or syndrome of inappropriate antidiuretic hormone secretion (SIADH). Treatment involves fluid restriction.

Table 27.11	**Hyponatremia Etiology and Management**	
Etiology	**Examples**	**Management**

Excess Na^+ loss	1. Renal tubular immaturity: high urinary Na^+ losses (up to 10–12 mmol/kg/day in premature infants <30 week)
	2. Hypoxic injury
	3. Diuretics
	4. GI losses
	5. CAH
	6. "Late hyponatremia of prematurity" (>1 week): inadequate intake in addition to excess loss
		1. Calculate deficit: [Na^+ (desired) − Na^+ (actual)] × 0.6 × weight (kg)
		  a. Replace over 24–48 h in addition to providing maintenance and insensible losses
		  b. Monitor serum and urinary Na^+ q6–12h
		2. Consider oral Na^+ supplements in LBW infants once enteral feeds established

Continued

Table 27.11	Hyponatremia Etiology and Management—cont'd	
Etiology	**Examples**	**Management**
Water retention	1. Iatrogenic overload (excess dextrose solutions) 2. SIADH (low urine output, urine osmolality>serum osmolality, low serum sodium, low serum osmolality, high urine sodium, high urine specific gravity) 3. CHF 4. Renal failure	1. Fluid restriction (½–⅔ of maintenance requirement) 2. If symptomatic: 3% NaCl (with caution) to correct to 125 mmol/L ± diuretics 3. Monitor serum Na⁺ q6–12h

CAH, Congenital adrenal hyperplasia; *CHF,* congestive heart failure; *GI,* gastrointestinal; *LBW,* low birth weight; *SIADH,* syndrome of inappropriate antidiuretic hormone secretion.

HYPERNATREMIA

1. **Definition:** $Na^+ > 150$ mmol/L
2. **Etiology**
   a. Dehydration from ↑ insensible losses (mostly <30 weeks GA, under radiant warmer or phototherapy)
   b. Renal or gastrointestinal (GI) losses
   c. Iatrogenic (excess Na^+ administration [e.g., 0.9% NaCl])
3. **Management**
   a. Based on etiology, severity of symptoms, timing (acute or chronic)
   b. Dehydration (most common cause)
      i. Assume fluid deficit of 10% to 15% (100–150 mL/kg)
      ii. Aim to correct over 24 to 48 hours to avoid too rapid decrease in Na^+
   c. Calculate water deficit (L), P_{Na^+} is current plasma Na^+ concentration:

$$\text{Water deficit} = 0.6 \times \text{body weight} \times \left[1 - \frac{P_{Na^+}}{140} \right]$$

   d. If patient hypotensive, resuscitate with 10 to 20 mL/kg 0.9% NaCl, subtracting volume from total deficit to be replaced
   e. If initial $Na^+ > 160$, use 0.9% NaCl with D5W or D10W to replace water deficit, then 0.45% NaCl with D5W or D10W as maintenance fluid
   f. If initial $Na^+ < 160$, use 0.45% NaCl or 0.2% NaCl with D5W or D10W for deficit
   g. For infants <1.5 kg, deficits may be 20% to 25% of body weight
      i. Initially use 0.2% NaCl, D5W or D10W for replacement of deficit
      ii. Monitor and adjust further based on Na^+, weight, urine output, urine Na^+
   h. In hypervolemic hypernatremia: goal is to remove Na^+
      i. Restrict Na^+
      ii. Restrict water if congestive heart failure (CHF) present
      iii. Diuretics (furosemide)

See Chapter 15 Fluids, Electrolytes, and Acid-Base

HYPOCALCEMIA

1. **Definition**
   a. Full term: Ca^{2+} <1.75 mmol/L
   b. Premature: Ca^{2+} <1.5 mmol/L (because of lower albumin levels)
   c. Ionized Ca^{2+} <1.1 mmol/L (preferred method of measurement)

2. **Clinical presentation**
   a. Usually asymptomatic
   b. May have tremors, seizures, lethargy, apnea, irritability, stridor, ↑ reflexes
   c. Prolonged QT interval

3. **Etiology**
   a. Early hypocalcemia (day 1–2): prematurity, infant of diabetic mother (IDM), asphyxia, shock, sepsis
   b. Late hypocalcemia: hypoparathyroidism, hypomagnesemia, maternal hyperparathyroidism, cow's milk–based formula (because of poor bioavailability)
   c. Iatrogenic: bicarbonate administration, furosemide

4. **Management**
   a. Identify high-risk infants: premature, SGA, sepsis, cardiovascular compromise
   b. Prevention: maintenance Ca^{2+} as continuous infusion for 48 to 72 hours starting at 6 to 48 hours of age: 8.3 to 33.3 mg/kg/h calcium **gluconate** intravenous (IV) (=0.02–0.08 mmol/kg/h elemental Ca^{2+})
   c. Acute symptomatic hypocalcemia: 50 to 100 mg/kg/dose of calcium **gluconate** IV (=0.12–0.23 mmol/kg/dose of elemental Ca^{2+}) with ECG monitoring (bradycardias, asystole can occur) followed by maintenance infusion as above; observe IV sites closely for extravasation
   d. Asymptomatic infants: variable, may treat when Ca^{2+} <1.8 mmol/L with oral supplementation or IV infusion
   e. Vitamin D
   f. Treat hypomagnesemia as may be associated with hypocalcemia

ACID-BASE STATUS

1. **Respiratory acidosis**
   a. Corrected by adjusting ventilation (e.g., increasing tidal volume or rate)
   b. "Permissive hypercapnia" accepted to minimize lung damage (pH 7.22–7.25 and PCO_2 55–65 mmHg)

2. **Respiratory alkalosis**
   a. In general occurs in infants receiving ventilation
   b. Correct by adjusting ventilation (e.g., consider decreasing PEEP)

Neonatology

27

3. **Metabolic acidosis**
   a. See Box 27.3 for common causes of metabolic acidosis in neonates
   b. See Chapter 15 Fluids, Electrolytes, and Acid-Base for approach and management
4. **Metabolic alkalosis**
   a. See Chapter 15 Fluids, Electrolytes, and Acid-Base for approach and management

---

Box 27.3 Causes of Metabolic Acidosis in Neonates

1. Sepsis (consider septic workup)
2. Hypoxia, shock, severe anemia
3. PDA with CHF
4. HCO_3^- losses (renal tubular acidosis, diarrhea)
5. Metabolic (amino acidemia, organic acidemia, congenital lactic acidosis)
6. Excess protein load
7. SEH, IVH

CHF, Congestive heart failure; *IVH,* intraventricular hemorrhage; *PDA,* patent ductus arteriosus; *SEH,* subependymal hemorrhage.

GLUCOSE DYSREGULATION

HYPOGLYCEMIA

1. **Definition:** blood glucose <2.6 mmol/L
2. **Etiology**
   a. **Decreased carbohydrate stores:** SGA, premature, respiratory distress syndrome (RDS), maternal hypertension
   b. **Endocrine:** excess insulin: LGA, IDM; hormonal deficiencies (e.g., growth hormone, cortisol)
   c. **Miscellaneous mechanisms:** shock, asphyxia, sepsis, hypothermia, polycythemia, hemolytic disease, genetic or metabolic conditions, maternal labetalol use, late preterm exposure to antenatal steroids, rapid weaning of IV glucose
3. **Clinical presentation**
   a. May present with lethargy, apnea, cyanosis, tremor, tachypnea, seizures
   b. Many are asymptomatic
4. **Screening and management**
   a. See Figure 27.6
   b. Bolus of 2 mL/kg of D10W if symptomatic (uncertain benefit of bolus before starting infusion in asymptomatic babies). Repeated boluses without an increase in the infusion rate not recommended.
   c. If previous management inadequate with IV fluids, perform critical sample (see Hypoglycemia in Chapter 26 Metabolic Disease) and consider
      i. Glucagon: 0.01 to 0.02 mg/kg/h IV via continuous infusion; if IV access not available, may give 0.1 mg/kg/dose IM q3–4h to maximum total dose of 1.5 mg/day
      ii. Diazoxide, octreotide, or hydrocortisone for refractory cases (consult endocrinologist)

Figure 27.6 Algorithm for the Screening and Immediate Management of Infants at Risk of Neonatal Hypoglycemia

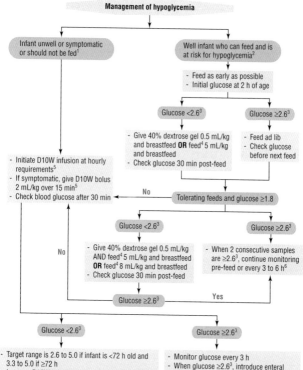

Management of hypoglycemia

Infant unwell or symptomatic or should not be fed[1]

Well infant who can feed and is at risk for hypoglycemia[2]
- Feed as early as possible
- Initial glucose at 2 h of age

Glucose <2.6[3]
- Give 40% dextrose gel 0.5 mL/kg and breastfeed **OR** feed[4] 5 mL/kg and breastfeed
- Check glucose 30 min post-feed

Glucose ≥2.6[3]
- Feed ad lib
- Check glucose before next feed

- Initiate D10W infusion at hourly requirements[5]
- If symptomatic, give D10W bolus 2 mL/kg over 15 min[5]
- Check blood glucose after 30 min

Tolerating feeds and glucose ≥1.8 — No

Glucose <2.6[3]
- Give 40% dextrose gel 0.5 mL/kg AND feed[4] 5 mL/kg and breastfeed **OR** feed[4] 8 mL/kg and breastfeed
- Check glucose 30 min post-feed

Glucose ≥2.6[3]
- When 2 consecutive samples are ≥2.6[3], continue monitoring pre-feed or every 3 to 6 h[6]

Glucose ≥2.6[3] — Yes

Glucose <2.6[3]
- Target range is 2.6 to 5.0 if infant is <72 h old and 3.3 to 5.0 if ≥72 h
- Increase D10W infusion every 30 min by 1 mL/kg/h; repeat glucose every 30 min until within target range
- Calculate the lowest GIR at which blood glucose is within target range[7]
- Calculate D%W concentration needed to stay within the maximum daily fluid intake[8]
- Check electrolytes in 8 to 12 h

- If GIR >8 to 10 mg/kg/min, central access[8] and tertiary care should be considered
- If GIR >10 to 12 mg/kg/min, consider medication
- If GIR >10 to 12 mg/kg/min and infant is >72 h old, further investigation is required

Glucose ≥2.6[3]
- Monitor glucose every 3 h
- When glucose ≥2.6[3], introduce enteral feeds as tolerated and wean IV stepwise
- Continue pre-feed glucose monitoring until on full enteral feeds and 2 consecutive samples within normal range

1. Infants who are unwell, symptomatic, or cannot feed should have their glucose checked at first encounter
2. At-risk for hypoglycemia: SGA, IUGR, LGA, IDM, GA <37 weeks, asphyxia, maternal exposure to labetalol, late preterm antenatal steroids
3. Low glucose threshold is 3.3 after 72 h of age or with known congenital hypoglycemia disorder (e.g., hyperinsulinemia) or GIR >10 to 12 mg/kg/min. All glucose values are in mmol/L
4. Feed (in order of preference) mother's expressed milk, donor milk or formula, and record intake
5. If delay in starting IV, give 40% dextrose gel 0.5 mL/kg
6. Duration of surveillance for well IDM or LGA: 12 h; for SGA or IUGR or well premature infants: 24 h
7. GIR calculation: GIR = dextrose concentration (in %) × infusion rate (in mL/kg/h) / 6 (Example: If D10W at 4 mL/kg/h, then GIR = 6.7 mg/kg/min)
8. Can give up to D20W by peripheral IV until central access is obtained

IDM, Infant of diabetic mother; *IUGR*, intrauterine growth restriction; *IV*, intravenous; *GIR*, glucose infusion rate; *LGA*, large for gestational age; *SGA*, small for gestational age. (Adapted from Narvey et al. The screening and management of newborns at risk for low blood glucose. *Paediatr Child Health*. 2019;24(8):536–544.)

Neonatology

27

HYPERGLYCEMIA

1. **Definition**
   a. Glucose >10 mmol/L $\pm$ glycosuria (prefeeding, postfeeding, or random)
2. **Etiology**
   a. Iatrogenic: TPN, dextrose solutions, steroids
   b. Stress: exclude sepsis
   c. Endocrine: neonatal diabetes mellitus
3. **Management**
   a. Decrease glucose concentration: wean dextrose by 2.5% in stages
   b. Monitor: urine, blood glucose, weight, fluid balance
   c. Investigate: consider sepsis workup
   d. Insulin: therapy rarely required unless blood glucose persistently >12 mmol/L

RESPIRATORY CONDITIONS

RESPIRATORY DISTRESS

1. Etiology: see Table 27.12

Table 27.12	Differential Diagnosis of Respiratory Distress in Newborns	
Pulmonary Disorders		
Common	**Less Common**	
RDS	Pulmonary hypoplasia	
TTN	Upper airway obstruction (e.g., choanal atresia)	
Meconium aspiration	Rib cage anomalies	
Pneumonia	Diaphragmatic hernia	
Pneumothorax	Pulmonary hemorrhage	
	Immature lung syndrome	
Extrapulmonary Disorders		
Vascular	**Metabolic**	**Neurological**
PPHN	Acidosis	Cerebral hypertension
CHD	Hypoglycemia	Cerebral hemorrhage
Hypovolemia	Hypothermia	Muscle or NMJ disorders
Polycythemia		Spinal cord pathology
Anemia		Encephalopathy (HIE, others)
		Phrenic nerve palsy
		Drugs: morphine, phenobarbital

CHD, Congenital heart disease; *HIE*, hypoxic ischemic encephalopathy; *NMJ*, neuromuscular junction; *PPHN*, persistent pulmonary hypertension of the newborn; *RDS*, respiratory distress syndrome; *TTN*, transient tachypnea of the newborn.

Adapted from Klaus MH, Fanaroff AA, eds. *Care of the High-Risk Neonate*. Philadelphia, PA: WB Saunders; 2001.

2. Management
   a. See Box 27.4 for goals of therapy
   b. All term neonates with respiratory distress should be treated with empiric antibiotics (ampicillin + aminoglycoside) for at least 36 to 48 hours until sepsis ruled out

---

Box 27.4   Goals of Therapy for Neonatal Respiratory Distress

- Maintain arterial values: PCO_2, <50 mmHg; PO_2, 50–70 mmHg; pH >7.25
- Maintain O_2 saturation levels: term infants >94%; premature infants 88%–92%

RESPIRATORY DISTRESS SYNDROME

1. **Etiology:** caused by surfactant deficiency in preterm neonates, IDM also at risk
2. **Presentation:** respiratory distress, tachypnea, hypoxia, cyanosis, increasing ventilator/oxygen requirements
3. **Investigations:** chest x-ray (CXR) shows bilateral ground-glass opacities, air bronchograms, small lung volumes
4. **Management**
   a. See Figure 27.7 for initial management
   b. Indications for surfactant therapy
      i. Intubated infants with RDS whose oxygen requirements exceed FiO_2 of 0.5
      ii. Can consider replacement surfactant in infants with meconium aspiration syndrome or pulmonary hemorrhage
      iii. Intubated infants with RDS should receive surfactant prior to inter-facility transport
   c. For spontaneously breathing infants on CPAP with RDS, non-invasive methods of surfactant administration are preferable
   d. Additional dosing of surfactant should be provided to infants only when there is evidence of ongoing moderate to severe RDS
   e. Rapid sequence intubation medications should be used for all nonemergency intubations: atropine 0.01 to 0.02 mg/kg IV + fentanyl 1 to 2 mcg/kg IV slowly + succinylcholine 2 mg/kg IV

Figure 27.7 Initial Management of Respiratory Distress Syndrome

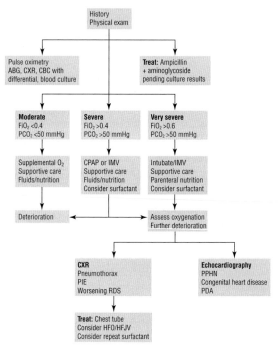

ABG, arterial blood gas; *CBC*, complete blood count; *CPAP*, continuous positive airway pressure; *CXR*, chest x-ray; HFJV, high-frequency jet ventilation; *HFO*, high-frequency oscillation; *IMV*, invasive mechanical ventilation; *PDA*, patent ductus arteriosus; *PIE*, pulmonary interstitial emphysema; *PPHN*, persistent pulmonary hypertension of the newborn; *RDS*, respiratory distress syndrome.

TRANSIENT TACHYPNEA OF THE NEWBORN

1. **Etiology:** persistent fluid in lungs postnatally; common after caesarean deliveries
2. **Presentation:** tachypnea often without hypoxia/cyanosis
3. **Investigations:** CXR shows parenchymal infiltrates and fluid in fissures
4. **Management:** supportive care, may require supplemental oxygen/ continuous positive airway pressure (CPAP) support, typically resolves in 72 hours

APNEA

1. **Definition:** no respiration for >20 seconds duration, or >10 seconds with bradycardia or oxygen desaturation

2. **Management:** immediate resuscitation by surface stimulation, gentle nasopharyngeal suction, ventilation with inflating bag and mask, intubation with intermittent positive pressure ventilation (IPPV) as needed
    a. See Table 27.13 for causes and management
    b. Drug therapy: caffeine for apnea of prematurity (consider other causes if new apneas in an infant >30 weeks)
    c. Persistent apnea: consider short-term assisted ventilation, nasopharyngeal tube or nasal-prong CPAP, or IPPV with slow backup rate (i.e., ~6–10/min)

Table 27.13	Causes and Management of Apnea	
Cause	**Details**	**Action**
Infection	Neonatal sepsis, meningitis, NEC	FSWU including LP; antibiotics; NPO for NEC
Thermal instability	Hypo-/hyperthermia	Assess body and isolate temperature
Metabolic disorders	Hypoglycemia	See section on Hypoglycemia
	Hypocalcemia	Serum Ca^{2+}, ECG
	Hypo/hypernatremia	Electrolytes, fluid balance, weight
	Hyperammonemia	Serum NH_4, amino acids, blood gas, liver enzymes, urine organic acids
CNS problems	Asphyxia	Observation, intubation, mechanical ventilation
	Intracranial hemorrhage	EEG, head US, CT/MRI
	Cerebral malformation	Head US, CT/MRI
	Seizures	EEG, consider anticonvulsants
Decreased O_2 delivery	Hypoxemia	Check ETT, adjust FiO_2 and MAP
	Worsening RDS ± complications	CXR
	Anemia/shock	CBC, electrolytes, ABG
	Left-to-right shunt (e.g., PDA)	ECG, echocardiography
	Pneumothorax	Needle decompression + chest tube
Upper airway	Choanal atresia, macroglossia, Pierre Robin sequence, GERD (vagal stimulation, aspiration)	Attempt passage of NG tube, oropharyngeal airway, CXR for aspiration
Drugs	Prenatal or postnatal exposure	Drug/toxin screen, depending on history and clinical findings

ABG, Arterial blood gas; *CBC,* complete blood count; *CNS,* central nervous system; *CT,* computed tomography; *CXR,* chest x-ray; *ECG,* electrocardiogram; *EEG,* electroencephalogram; *ETT,* endotracheal tube; *FSWU,* full septic workup; *GERD,* gastroesophageal reflux disease; *LP,* lumbar puncture; *MAP,* mean airway pressure; *MRI,* magnetic resonance imaging; *NEC,* necrotizing enterocolitis; *NG,* nasogastric; *US,* ultrasound; *PDA,* patent ductus arteriosus; *RDS,* respiratory distress syndrome.

Adapted from Forfar JL, Arneil GC. *Textbook of Paediatrics.* 2nd ed. New York, NY: Churchill Livingstone; 2003.

BRONCHOPULMONARY DYSPLASIA

1. **Definition**
    a. Persistent O_2 ± ventilator support needs at 36 weeks PMA with respiratory symptoms and compatible CXR changes

719

b. Also known as chronic lung disease (CLD)

c. **Risk factors:** prematurity, neonatal respiratory distress, O_2 supplementation, mechanical ventilation

d. **Association:** poor neurodevelopmental outcomes at 18 to 24 months

e. **Management**

   i. No definitive treatment

   ii. Improved outcomes with certain measures in specific situations (supplemental oxygen, diuretics)

   iii. An echocardiogram at term for infants dependent on oxygen is recommended to assess for pulmonary hypertension

MECHANICAL VENTILATION

1. **Basic principles of ventilation**

a. **Oxygenation:** indications for oxygen therapy: PaO_2 <50 mmHg and/or SpO_2 levels <88%. Factors affecting oxygenation include MAP, PEEP, and FiO_2.

b. **Ventilation:** CO_2 elimination is directly proportional to minute ventilation. Factors affecting ventilation include respiratory rate and tidal volume (affected by ΔP or difference between peak inspiratory pressure (PIP)-PEEP and inspiratory time).

2. **Modes of ventilation:** see Table 27.14 for description of selected modes of noninvasive and invasive ventilation

Table 27.14	Neonatal Mechanical Ventilation		
Modes of Ventilation	**Description**	**Advantages**	**Disadvantages**
Noninvasive Modes			
HFNC	1. Start at 2 L/kg/min up to max flows on cannula specifications 2. Minimum of 3 L/min	1. Able to provide consistent FiO_2 of warm, humidified gases	1. Skin breakdown from nasal mask/prongs 2. Minimal effect on CO_2 clearance 3. Contraindicated in CDH
nCPAP	1. Continuous PEEP (start at 5–8 cmH$_2$O) 2. Relies on spontaneous respiratory effort	1. May decrease risk of BPD	1. Skin breakdown from nasal mask/prongs 2. May have abdominal distension—OG to vent 3. Contraindicated in CDH
NiPPV	1. Two levels of pressure with PIP and PEEP, delta pressure of at least 10–15 cmH$_2$O 2. Set unsynchronized rate of 30–40	1. Indicated in CPAP failure or as way to prevent extubation failure 2. Improved CO_2 clearance compared with CPAP	1. Can cause gastric distention

Continued

Table 27.14   Neonatal Mechanical Ventilation—cont'd

Modes of Ventilation	Description	Advantages	Disadvantages
Invasive Modes			
PC/AC +VG	1. Fully assisted breaths with background rate 2. VG is used to deliver a set Vt (4–6 mL/kg)	1. Synchronizes with respiratory effort 2. VG varies PIP according to lung compliance, resistance, and patient effort (reduces lung injury) 3. Pressures vary and often auto wean as lung condition improves	1. Can deliver excessive volumes if VG not used 2. VG is limited by ETT leaks
Pressure-support	1. Weaning mode 2. Provides preset pressure for spontaneous breaths	1. Helpful to assess readiness for extubation using a spontaneous breathing trial	1. Contraindicated if sedated, no respiratory drive, or large ETT leak
HFOV	1. Pressure variations oscillate around set MAP at high frequency (10 Hz) with *active* exhalation	1. Indicated in failure of conventional modes or as a lung protective strategy 2. Improved CO_2 clearance	1. Used with caution in air leaks and MAS
HFJV	1. Rapid pulses of gas (iT 0.02 s) at high rate (240–420/min) with *passive* exhalation	1. Indicated for air leaks, secretion clearance, MAS, pulmonary hemorrhage/hypoplasia, or failure of other modes 2. Lung-protective	1. Not readily available at all centers 2. Requires companion ventilator to deliver PEEP

CLD, Chronic lung disease; *CPAP*, continuous positive airway pressure; *ETT*, endotracheal tube; *HFNC*, high flow nasal cannula; *HFOV*, high-frequency oscillatory ventilation; *HFJV*, high-frequency jet ventilation; *iT*, inspiratory time; *MAP*, mean airway pressure; *nCPAP*, nasal continuous positive airway pressure; *NiPPV*, noninvasive positive pressure ventilation; *PC/AC*, pressure-control/assist-control; *PEEP*, positive end expiratory pressure; *PIP*, peak inspiratory pressure; *VG*, volume guarantee; *Vt*, tidal volume.

Neonatology

27

CARDIAC CONDITIONS

PERSISTENT PULMONARY HYPERTENSION

1. **Definition:** severe hypoxemia because of elevated pulmonary vascular resistance and pulmonary artery hypertension

2. **Associations:** may be associated with right-to-left shunting through patent ductus arteriosus/patient foramen ovale (PDA/PFO)
3. **Clinical manifestations:** present at birth or within a few hours after birth with marked cyanosis, acidosis, right ventricular (RV) heave
4. **Investigations**
   a. CXR: oligemic lung fields or consistent with underlying disease; cardiomegaly; may look normal
   b. Oxygen saturation
      i. Pre-/postductal O_2 saturation: difference of >5% to 10% are suggestive of persistent pulmonary hypertension of the newborn (PPHN) (preductal saturation probe on right arm, postductal saturation probe on either leg)
      ii. If no significant ductal shunt and atrial right-left shunting, right arm and leg saturations may be low
      iii. Oxygen saturation is often labile, oxygen saturation in cyanotic congenital heart disease (CHD) is often fixed
   c. Hyperoxia test to exclude CHD (see Congenital Heart Disease in Chapter 8 Cardiology)
   d. ECG: RV strain pattern
   e. Echocardiogram: pulmonary pressures, cardiac anatomy, function, presence/level of shunt (PFO or PDA)

> ### ✦ PEARL
>
> Rule out cyanotic congenital heart disease before diagnosing persistent pulmonary hypertension of the newborn.

5. **Management**
   a. Prevention is critical: treat hypothermia, respiratory distress, hypoxia, acidosis
   b. Goal of treatment: oxygenation and pulmonary vasodilatation
   c. Calculate oxygenation index (OI): OI >15 needs aggressive therapy

$$OI = MAP \times FiO_2 \times 100 / PaO_2$$

   d. Conventional ventilation: aim to keep PaO_2 >80 mmHg, $PaCO_2$ 35 to 45 mmHg
   e. Maintain normal systemic blood pressure (BP) to limit right-to-left shunting—use volume priming (10 mL/kg 0.9% NaCl) and inotropes/pulmonary vasodilators (e.g., dobutamine, milrinone)
   f. Sedate (morphine 0.05–0.1 mg IV bolus, then start at 10 mcg/kg/h, consider fentanyl if systemic hypotension) and muscle relax, especially in severe hypoxemia

g. Consider HFO ventilation

h. Pulmonary vasodilation: inhaled nitric oxide (iNO) for hypoxia, OI >20 (start iNO at 20 ppm with gradual reduction following improvement in oxygenation)

i. Correct metabolic acidosis with bicarbonate infusion

j. Consider extracorporeal membrane oxygenation (ECMO) if multiple OI values >40

PATENT DUCTUS ARTERIOSUS

1. **Clinical signs:** harsh systolic or continuous murmur, hyperactive precordium, bounding pulses, wide pulse pressure >25 mmHg, hypotension, worsening respiratory status, tachycardia, CHF, pulmonary hemorrhage (*emergency*)

2. **Diagnosis:** echocardiogram to confirm presence, size, direction of shunting

3. **Treatment:** decision to treat depends on clinical significance

   a. **Fluid restriction:** two-thirds of maintenance fluids

   b. **Indomethacin**

      i. Adverse effects: platelet dysfunction, decreased renal artery flow leading to decreased glomerular filtration rate (GFR) and urine output, fluid retention ± hyponatremia, increased creatinine, bowel perforation (rare)

      ii. Contraindications: duct-dependent cardiac lesions, ↑ creatinine, oliguria <0.5 mL/kg/h, necrotizing enterocolitis (NEC), thrombocytopenia <80,000 or clinical bleeding, intraventricular hemorrhage (IVH) grade III or IV

      iii. Can use acetaminophen for PDA closure after failure of two courses of indomethacin and/or absolute contraindications to indomethacin

   c. **Surgical ligation**

      i. Indication: hemodynamically significant PDA despite two courses of indomethacin

      ii. Complications: thrombus, interruption of thoracic duct with chylothorax, damage to recurrent laryngeal nerve, ligation of wrong vessel

HEART FAILURE

See Table 27.15 for causes of heart failure in neonates

Table 27.15	Causes of Heart Failure in Neonates	
Birth	**1–2 Weeks**	**>2 Weeks**
Decreased cardiac function	**Congenital heart disease**	**Congenital heart disease**
Asphyxia	Critical AS	Systemic outflow tract obstruction
Sepsis	Coarctation	PDA
Electrolyte disorders	HLHS	AVSD
	TAPVD	TAPVD
Hematological disorders	**Decreased cardiac function**	**Decreased cardiac function**
Anemia	Asphyxia	Myocarditis
Hyperviscosity disorders	Sepsis	Cardiomyopathy
	Arrhythmias	Anomalous coronary artery
Heart rhythm disorders	**Renal disorders**	**Renal/endocrine**
SVT	Renal failure	Renal failure
Complete AV block	Systemic hypertension	Thyroid/adrenal disease
Congenital heart disease	**Endocrine disorders**	**Pulmonary**
Severe TR (Ebstein)	Hyperthyroidism	Bronchopulmonary dysplasia
AV malformation	Adrenal insufficiency	Hypoventilation syndrome

AS, Aortic stenosis; *AVSD,* atrioventricular septal defect; *HLHS,* hypoplastic left heart syndrome; *PDA,* patent ductus arteriosus; *SVT,* supraventricular tachycardia; *TAPVD,* total anomalous pulmonary venous drainage; *TR,* tricuspid regurgitation.

27   NEUROLOGICAL CONDITIONS

NEONATAL ENCEPHALOPATHY

1. **Definition**
   a. **Encephalopathy**
      i. Brain dysfunction including altered consciousness, irritability or seizures
      ii. May be temporary or permanent
   b. **Hypoxic ischemic encephalopathy (HIE):** brain injury because of impaired cerebral blood flow in the setting of hypoxia-ischemia, typically associated with an intrapartum hypoxic event
   c. See Table 27.16 for classification of encephalopathy
2. **Etiology**
   a. **Neurological:** perinatal asphyxia, stroke, intracranial hemorrhage (risk factors include birth trauma, bleeding tendency)
   b. **Infection:** bacterial meningitis or viral encephalitis (e.g., herpes simplex virus [HSV])
   c. **Metabolic:** hypoglycemia, inborn errors of metabolism, kernicterus
3. **Presentation of HIE**
   a. **Clinical**
      i. Intrapartum: fetal bradycardia, nonreassuring tracing, meconium, uterine rupture, cord prolapse

Table 27.16 Classification of Encephalopathy

Modified Sarnat Score

Category	Mild Encephalopathy	Moderate Encephalopathy	Severe Encephalopathy
Level of consciousness	Hyperalert	Lethargic	Stupor/coma
Spontaneous activity	Normal	Decreased	No activity
Posture	Mild distal flexion	Strong distal flexion, truncal extension	Decerebate (arms extended and internally rotated, legs extended with feet in forced plantar flexion)
Tone	Normal	Mild hypotonia	Flaccid tone
Primitive reflexes			
Moro	Weak	Weak	Absent
Suck	Strong	Incomplete	Absent
Autonomic system			
Pupils	Dilated, responsive	Constricted	Skew deviation, dilated/non-reactive to light
Heart rate	Tachycardia	Bradycardia	Variable heart rate
Respirations	Normal	Periodic breathing	Apnea

Thompson Score[a]

Sign	0	1	2	3
Tone	Normal	Hypertonic	Hypotonic	Flaccid
Level of consciousness	Normal	Hyper alert stare	Lethargic	Comatose
Seizures	None	Infrequent (<3/day)	Frequent (≥3/day)	
Posture	Normal	Fisting/cycling	Strong distal flexion	Decerebrate
Moro reflex	Normal	Partial	Absent	
Grasp	Normal	Poor	Absent	
Sucking reflex	Normal	Poor	Absent ± bites	
Respiration	Normal	Hyperventilation	Brief apnea	Apnea (requiring IPPV)
Fontanel	Normal	Full, not tense	Tense	

[a]Final score sums the individual points.

IPPV, Intermittent positive pressure ventilation.

Adapted from The Hospital for Sick Children Hypoxic Ischemic Encephalopathy Clinical Pathway, 2020.

ii. Postpartum: metabolic acidosis, Apgar <5 at 10 minutes, at least 10 minutes of PPV

b. **Multiorgan involvement**

   i. Respiratory: PPHN, meconium aspiration, pulmonary hemorrhage
   ii. Renal: oliguria, acute tubular necrosis, SIADH, urinary retention
   iii. Cardiovascular: myocardial ischemia, cardiogenic shock, tricuspid regurgitation
   iv. Metabolic: acidosis, hypoglycemia, hypocalcemia, hypomagnesemia
   v. Hematological: thrombocytopenia, disseminated intravascular coagulation (DIC)
   vi. GI: liver dysfunction, ileus, bowel ischemia, NEC

4. **Investigations**

a. **Laboratory studies**

   i. Serum tests: blood gas, lactate, complete blood count (CBC), glucose, calcium, creatinine, urea, liver enzymes, partial thromboplastin time (PTT)/international normalized ratio (INR)
   ii. Depending on presentation, consider full septic workup (FSWU) and metabolic screen
   iii. Urinalysis

b. **Neurological imaging:** brain ultrasound (US), computed tomography (CT) head (rule out hemorrhage/trauma), magnetic resonance imaging (MRI) brain (edema, diffusion restriction, lactate peak)

5. **Management of HIE**

a. **Neuroprotective strategies:** resuscitation in room air, prevention of hyperthermia

b. **Therapeutic hypothermia:** whole-body cooling (34°C ± 0.5°C) performed for 72 hours, under sedation while NPO

   i. Initiate therapeutic hypothermia for infants who meet the criteria in Box 27.5 (may require transfer to tertiary care NICU).

Box 27.5   Criteria for Initiating Therapeutic Hypothermia

Infants should fulfill all 4 criteria:

1. GA greater than or equal to 35 weeks
2. Less than 6 hours post-delivery
3. Evidence of intrapartum hypoxia defined as **EITHER:** cord or postnatal blood gas within one hour of birth with pH less than or equal to 7.00 OR base deficit of greater than or equal to −16 **OR** If pH 7.01–7.15 or BD −10 to 15.9, or if no blood gas available then must have evidence of an acute perinatal event (abruption, uterine rupture, maternal trauma or cardio-pulmonary arrest, late or variable decelerations) and Apgar score 5 or less at 10 min or need for continued ventilation or resuscitation at 10 min
4. Signs of moderate or severe encephalopathy defined as the presence of clinical seizures, or 3 or more of the items in the moderate or severe categories using the modified Sarnat score, or a Thompson score of >8 (Table 27.16).

---

ii. **Monitoring:** monitor end-organ function and neurological status; MRI/evoked potentials after rewarming (MRI brain at 3–5 days once rewarmed, repeat MRI can be considered at 10–14 days)

iii. **Side effects:** bradycardia, hypotension, arrhythmias, hyponatremia, edema, impaired glucose homeostasis, coagulopathy, NEC, altered drug metabolism, subcutaneous fat necrosis

iv. **Outcomes:** therapeutic hypothermia decreases mortality and significant long-term neurodevelopmental disabilities in infants with moderate HIE

c. **Long-term complications of HIE**

i. Brain damage: cerebral palsy (spastic, dystonic, athetoid), microcephaly, epilepsy, cortical blindness, sensorineural hearing loss, cognitive impairment

ii. End-organ damage: renal failure, myocardial damage, liver failure (rare)

NEONATAL SEIZURES

. **Clinical presentation**

a. May be difficult to distinguish from normal neonatal movements (e.g., jitteriness, yawning, sucking, chewing)

b. Suspicious if movements are focal, asymmetric, rhythmic, nonsuppressible, accompanied by autonomic phenomena (changes in heart rate and blood pressure, apnea, pallor, blotchy or flushed skin, altered pupils, drooling) or associated with abnormal eye movements

. **Etiology**

a. Metabolic (decreased glucose, Ca^{2+}, Mg^{2+}, or Na^+ levels)

b. Central nervous system (CNS): perinatal asphyxia (HIE), infections, bleeding, stroke, structural brain anomaly, seizure disorder

c. Inborn errors of metabolism (if intractable seizures with other neurological signs)

d. Drug withdrawal

. **Investigations**

a. **Laboratory studies**

i. Serum tests: glucose, electrolytes, calcium, magnesium, CBC, metabolic screen, ammonium, lactate, blood gas

ii. Septic workup: blood/cerebrospinal fluid (CSF)/urine cultures, HSV, enterovirus and parechovirus polymerase chain reaction (PCR), CXR, consider workup for congenital infection

b. **Neuroimaging:** head US, CT, or MRI

c. **Other studies:** electroencephalogram (EEG)

. **Management:** see Figure 27.8

Figure 27.8 Neonatal Seizure Guidelines

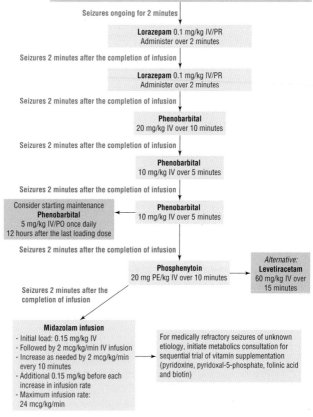

Guidelines for the management of seizures in late pre-term and term neonates (gestational age ≥34 weeks and postmenstrual age <44 weeks)

Seizure Onset

- Support ABCs
- Establish IV access
- Check glucose, eletrolytes, and blood gas
- Bedside aEEG, if available
- Early referral to tertiary care NICU, consider initiation of therapeutic hypothermia for HIE when indicated
- Plan brain US, CT, or MRI, monitor closely for loss of airway reflexes and respiratory depression, hypotension, or cardiac arrhythmias. Consider need for intubation.

Seizures ongoing for 2 minutes

Lorazepam 0.1 mg/kg IV/PR
Administer over 2 minutes

Seizures 2 minutes after the completion of infusion

Lorazepam 0.1 mg/kg IV/PR
Administer over 2 minutes

Seizures 2 minutes after the completion of infusion

Phenobarbital
20 mg/kg IV over 10 minutes

Seizures 2 minutes after the completion of infusion

Phenobarbital
10 mg/kg IV over 5 minutes

Seizures 2 minutes after the completion of infusion

Consider starting maintenance
Phenobarbital
5 mg/kg IV/PO once daily
12 hours after the last loading dose

Phenobarbital
10 mg/kg IV over 5 minutes

Seizures 2 minutes after the completion of infusion

Phosphenytoin
20 mg PE/kg IV over 10 minutes

Alternative:
Levetiracetam
60 mg/kg IV over
15 minutes

Seizures 2 minutes after the completion of infusion

Midazolam infusion
- Initial load: 0.15 mg/kg IV
- Followed by 2 mcg/kg/min IV infusion
- Increase as needed by 2 mcg/kg/min every 10 minutes
- Additional 0.15 mg/kg before each increase in infusion rate
- Maximum infusion rate: 24 mcg/kg/min

For medically refractory seizures of unknown etiology, initiate metabolics consultation for sequential trial of vitamin supplementation (pyridoxine, pyridoxal-5-phosphate, folinic acid and biotin)

ABC, Airway, breathing and circulation; *aEEG,* amplitude integrated electroencephalography; *IV,* intravenous; *NICU,* neonatal intensive care unit; *PE,* phenytoin equivalents; *PO,* per os; *PR,* per rectum. (Adapted from The Hospital for Sick Children eFormulary Neonatal Seizure Guidelines, 2020.)

Neonatology

27

INTRAVENTRICULAR HEMORRHAGE

1. **IVH:** bleeding from germinal matrix lining ventricles, especially 24 to 32 week GA. See Box 27.6 for grading of IVH.

Box 27.6	Grading of Intraventricular Hemorrhage
Grade 1	Germinal matrix/SEH
Grade 2	IVH: small (filling <½ of lateral ventricle ± slight dilation) ± SEH
Grade 3	IVH: large (filling >½ of lateral ventricle with ventricular dilation)
Grade 4	IVH + intraparenchymal hemorrhage

IVH, Intraventricular hemorrhage; *SEH*, subependymal hemorrhage.

2. **Etiology:** increased risk with systemic hypertension or hypotension, hypoxia, asphyxia, traumatic birth, acidosis, volume expansion, hypercarbia, hypoglycemia, anemia, seizures, ECMO
3. **Presentation**
   a. **Clinical:** asymptomatic or subtle neurological signs, apneas, respiratory distress, pallor, poor perfusion, hemorrhagic shock, increasing head circumference, altered mental status, seizures
   b. **Metabolic:** drop in hemoglobin/hematocrit levels, metabolic/respiratory acidosis, glucose instability
   c. **Long-term:** may lead to periventricular leukomalacia (PVL), communicating hydrocephalus, CP, developmental disability
4. **Investigations**
   a. Routine head US for all infants <32 week GA and selected high-risk infants >32 week GA
   b. Repeat US at regular intervals until ventricular size stabilized
   c. Early US for hemorrhagic lesions
   d. Later US for cystic lesions, PVL, or ventriculomegaly
   e. Consider MRI at term for ELBW infants
5. **Management**
   a. **Prevention**
      i. **Environmental:** infants at high risk (<30 weeks) should receive minimal handling/procedures, head in midline position, head of bed elevated
      ii. **Medical:** consider maternal antenatal corticosteroids and magnesium sulfate, prophylactic indomethacin (if BW <1000 g, unless intrauterine growth restriction [IUGR])
   b. **Surgical:** neurosurgical intervention rarely required; Ommaya reservoir or VP shunt for enlarging ventriculomegaly
   c. **Surveillance:** neonatal follow-up required to monitor neurodevelopment because of risk of developmental disability, CP, and seizures

NEONATAL DRUG WITHDRAWAL

1. **Etiology**
   a. Multiple pharmacological classes, including opiates, alcohol, sedatives, antidepressants
   b. Usually incomplete history
   c. High index of suspicion for multiple drug use
   d. Neonatal abstinence syndrome refers to findings associated with opioid withdrawal

2. **Clinical presentation**
   a. **Clinical signs:** changes in vital signs, CNS, GI, or vasomotor manifestations
   b. **Onset:** see Table 27.17
   c. **Duration:** ranges from 1 to 8 weeks, may last up to several months

3. **Laboratory studies**
   a. Urine toxicology: detects recent drug use by mother; many false-negative results
   b. Meconium toxicology: detects longitudinal exposure during last two trimesters

Table 27.17	Onset of Withdrawal Symptoms by Drug
Drug	**Approximate Time to Onset of Withdrawal Symptoms**
Barbituates	4–7 days, but can range from 1–14 days
Cocaine	Usually no withdrawal signs, but sometimes neurobehavioral abnormalities (decreased arousal and physiological stress) occur at 48–60 h
Alcohol	3–12 h
Heroin	Within 24 h
Marijuana	Usually no clinical withdrawal signs
Methadone	3 days, but up to 5–7 days; rate of severity of withdrawal cannot be correlated to dose of maternal methadone
Methamphetamines	Usually no withdrawal signs, but sometimes neurobehavioral abnormalities (decreased arousal, increased physiological stress, and poor quality of movement) occur at 48–60 h
Opioids	24–36 h, but can be up to 5–7 days
Sedatives	1–3 days
Selective serotonin reuptake inhibitors (SSRIs)	Usually second day of life, ranges from 5 to 48 h

From University of Iowa Children's Hospital. Identifying Neonatal Abstinence Syndrome (NAS) and Treatment Guidelines; 2013. uichildrens.org/sites/default/files/neonatal_abstinence_syndrome_treatment_guidelines_feb2013_revision-1.pdf.

4. **Management of neonatal abstinence syndrome from opioid withdrawal**
   a. **Confirm diagnosis:** rule out alternative causes of infant's symptoms (e.g., hypoglycemia, hypocalcemia, central nervous system injury, hyperthyroidism, infection)

b. **Monitor:** see Figure 27.9 for assessment of risk newborns and Table 27.18 for a sample neonatal abstinence syndrome scoring tool

Figure 27.9 Assessment and Care for Newborns at Risk of Neonatal Abstinence Syndrome From Opioid Withdrawal

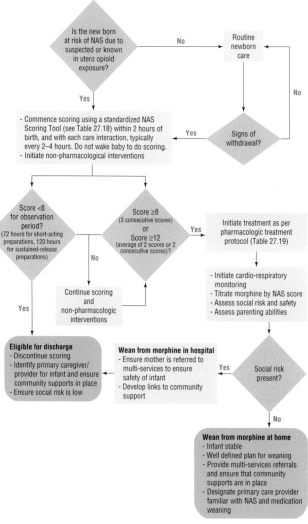

Neonatology

27

NAS, Neonatal abstinence syndrome. (Modified from Provincial Council for Maternal and Child Health. Neonatal Abstinence Syndrome Clinical Practice Guidelines (revised November 25, 2016).)

Table 27.18	Sample Neonatal Abstinence Scoring Tool	
System	**Signs and Symptoms**	**Score**
Central Nervous System Disturbances	Excessive cry	2
	Excessive cry (inconsolable)	3
	Sleeps <1 h after feeding	3
	Sleeps 1–2 h after feeding	2
	Sleeps 2–3 h after feeding	1
	Hyperactive Moro reflex	2
	Markedly hyperactive Moro reflex	3
	Mild tremors when disturbed	1
	Moderate-severe tremors when disturbed	2
	Mild tremors when undisturbed	1
	Moderate-severe tremors when undisturbed	2
	Increased muscle tone	1–2
	Excoriation: skin red, intact	1
	Excoriation: skin broken	2
	Generalized convulsions	8
	Excessive irritability	1–3
Metabolic/Vasomotor/ Respiratory Disturbances	Sweating	1
	Hyperthermia ≥37.3°C (axilla)	1
	Frequent yawning (≥4 times/scoring interval)	1
	Nasal stuffiness	1
	Sneezing (≥4 times/scoring interval)	1
	Respiratory rate >60/min	1
Gastrointestinal Disturbances	Poor feeding	2
	Vomiting	2
	Loose stools	2
	Weight loss/failure to thrive	2
	Total Score	

Modified from Jansson L, Velez M, Harrow C. The opioid-exposed newborn: assessment and pharmacologic management. *J Opioid Manag.* 2009;5(1):47–55.

5. **Treatment**
   a. Non-pharmacological interventions: support rooming-in, swaddling, breastfeeding (if no contraindications), soothing behaviors, positional support, modify baby's environment to reduce sensory stimulation, and frequent, hypercaloric, smaller volume feedings
   b. Pharmacological measures for NAS: see Table 27.19

Table 27.19 Neonatal Abstinence Syndrome Pharmacological Treatment Dosing Guidelines[a]

Medication	Dosing Guidelines		
Morphine			
Morphine is indicated when three consecutive scores are ≥8 according to the Standardized NAS Scoring tool or when the average of two scores or the score for two consecutive intervals is ≥12	**Score**	**Oral Morphine Dose**	
	8–10	0.32 mg/kg/day divided q4–6h	
	11–13	0.48 mg/kg/day divided q4–6h	
	14–16	0.64 mg/kg/day divided q4–6h	
If the scores remain ≥8 for three consecutive scores or ≥12 on two occasions, the morphine dose is increased to the next range. If 0.80 mg/kg/day fails to control signs of withdrawal, morphine may be increased to 0.96–1 mg/kg/day. Consider Clonidine at this point.	17+	0.80 mg/kg/day divided q4–6h	
Weaning			
Initiate weaning when scores are <8 for 24–48 h. Wean by 10% of the total daily dose or 0.05 mg/kg/day every 48–96 h as tolerated. Discontinue morphine when scores are stable for 48–72 h on a dose of 0.05–0.1 mg/kg/day.			
Clonidine			
Clonidine has been explored as a possible therapeutic option in combination with morphine. Clonidine may be considered as an adjunct to morphine when high doses fail to control withdrawal symptoms.	**Clonidine Dose**		
Some studies gradually increase doses over 1–2 days to begin therapy, and taper doses by 0.25 mcg/kg every 6 h to discontinue (or by 25% of the total daily dose every other day)	0.5–1 mcg/kg[b], given orally every 4–6 h	Much higher doses (0.5–3 mcg/kg/h) have been used as a continuous infusion	
Phenobarbital			
Phenobarbital may be used in combination with morphine in infants exposed to polydrug abuse (sedatives, alcohol, or barbiturates in addition to opiates).	**Score**	**Oral Morphine Dose in Combination With Phenobarbital**	
	8–10	0.16 mg/kg/day divided q4–6h	
	11–13	0.32 mg/kg/day divided q4–6h	
	14–16	0.48 mg/kg/day divided q4–6h	
Phenobarbital 10 mg/kg is given every 12 h for 3 doses, then 5 mg/kg/day is continued as a maintenance dose. The doses of morphine used in combination with phenobarbital are lower than those given when morphine is used alone.	17+	0.62 mg/kg/day divided q4–6h	

[a]Some countries also use methadone and buprenorphine.
[b]Adequate clinical trials to establish an efficacious and safe dose still are required.

From Provincial Council for Maternal and Child Health. Neonatal Abstinence Syndrome Clinical Practice Guidelines; revised November 25, 2016.

JAUNDICE

1. **Etiology**
   a. **Risk factors:** prematurity, sepsis, asphyxia, glucose-6-phosphate dehydrogenase (G6PD) deficiency, maternal blood group O or Rh negative, sibling with severe hyperbilirubinemia (HBR) requiring phototherapy, cephalohematoma, ethnic origin
   b. **Physiological jaundice:** peaks day 3 to 5, recedes by day 10; persists in some breastfed infants
   c. **Differential diagnosis:** see Table 27.20 for differential diagnosis by age
2. **Complications**
   a. **Untreated severe unconjugated HBR:** may result in acute bilirubin encephalopathy (lethargy, hypotonia, high-pitched cry, seizures) and kernicterus
3. **Laboratory studies**
   a. Total serum bilirubin (TSB) and other investigations as necessary based on history and physical examination
   b. If prolonged jaundice in an infant >2 weeks, check conjugated bilirubin

Table 27.20	Differential Diagnosis of Jaundice by Age	
Timing of Onset of HBR[a]	**Diagnosis**	**Tests to Consider**
First 24 h	Hemolytic disease	Blood group ± direct Coombs/DAT, CBC with blood smear (spherocytes, elliptocytes), G6PD assay, rule out sepsis
1–10 days	Enclosed hemorrhage Polycythemia Breastfeeding	Head/abdomen US Venous hematocrit Weight
1–10+ days	Infections	Increased conjugated bilirubin, septic workup, virology, serology for TORCH
3–10+ days	Crigler-Najjar syndrome, Gilbert syndrome	By exclusion, liver biopsy, and genetic testing
>7–10 days	Breast milk jaundice Hypothyroidism Galactosemia Cystic fibrosis Urinary tract infection	Diagnosis of exclusion Thyroid function tests, Newborn Screen Urine for reducing substances, Newborn Screen Sweat chloride test Urinalysis and culture
>14 days	Neonatal biliary atresia	Conjugated bilirubin (refer if conjugated bilirubin >20% of total bilirubin)

[a]Timing of onset of HBR suggests possible diagnoses, but exceptions occur

CBC, Complete blood count; *DAT,* direct antiglobulin test; *G6PD,* glucose-6-phosphate dehydrogenase; *HBR,* hyperbilirubinemia; *TORCH,* toxoplasmosis, rubella cytomegalovirus, herpes simplex, HIV; *US,* ultrasound.

Neonatology

27

4. **Phototherapy**
   a. Phototherapy is first line of therapy, independent of etiology
   b. **Term and late preterm infants (≥35 weeks):** see Figure 27.10 for clinical pathway for hyperbilirubinemia management
      i. See Figure 27.11 for phototherapy graph
      ii. See Figure 27.12 for exchange transfusion graph
      iii. See Figure 27.13 for hour specific nomogram to determine risk zone
      iv. See Figure 27.14 for follow-up algorithm based on hour specific nomogram
   c. **Preterm infants (<35 weeks):** see Figure 27.15 for phototherapy and exchange transfusion guidelines
5. **Feeding**
   a. Breastfeeding should continue
   b. Phototherapy more effective when combined with feeding
   c. Supplemental fluids (oral or IV) with phototherapy if risk of exchange transfusion
6. **Intravenous immune globulin (IVIG):** infants with positive DAT with predicted severe disease
7. **Exchange transfusion**
   a. Controversy about safe/critical levels of unconjugated bilirubin
   b. Threshold for intervention in "sick" or very premature infants should be low
   c. Consultation and transfer to tertiary care NICU
   d. Indications
      i. Rise of TSB above exchange threshold despite phototherapy and supplemental fluids
      ii. Hydrops or severe anemia (cord Hb <120 g/L)
      iii. Acute bilirubin encephalopathy
   e. Emergency cases: use group O Rh-negative blood

Figure 27.10 Clinical Pathway for the Management of Hyperbilirubinemia in Term and Late Preterm Infants (≥35 Weeks)

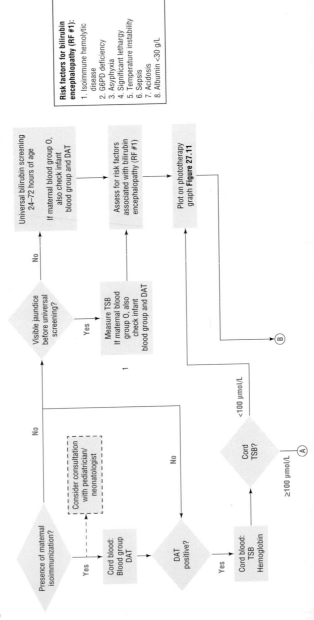

Risk factors for bilirubin encephalopathy (RF #1):
1. Isoimmune hemolytic disease
2. G6PD deficiency
3. Asphyxia
4. Significant lethargy
5. Temperature instability
6. Sepsis
7. Acidosis
8. Albumin <30 g/L

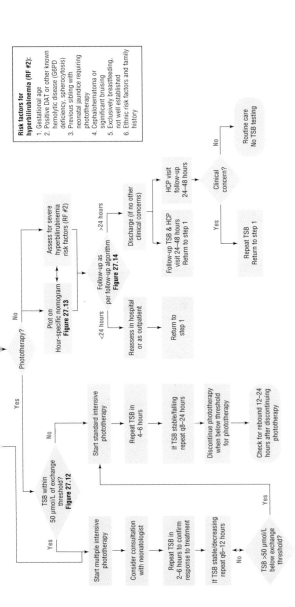

Yes — Phototherapy? — No

Yes branch:

TSB within 50 µmol/L of exchange threshold? **Figure 27.12**

No:
Start standard intensive phototherapy → Repeat TSB in 4–6 hours → If TSB stable/falling repeat q8–24 hours → Discontinue phototherapy when below threshold for phototherapy → Check for rebound 12–24 hours after discontinuing phototherapy

Yes:
Start multiple intensive phototherapy → Consider consultation with neonatologist → Repeat TSB in 2–6 hours to confirm response to treatment → If TSB stable/decreasing repeat q6–12 hours → TSB >50 µmol/L below exchange threshold?
- No → (return to Repeat TSB)
- Yes → (to Start standard intensive phototherapy)

No branch (Phototherapy? No):

Plot on Hour-specific nomogram **Figure 27.13** → Assess for severe hyperbilirubinemia risk factors (RF #2)

Follow-up as per follow-up algorithm **Figure 27.14**

- <24 hours → Reassess in hospital or as outpatient → Return to step 1
- >24 hours → Discharge (if no other clinical concerns) → HCP visit follow-up 24–48 hours → Clinical concern?
  - Yes → Repeat TSB Return to step 1
  - No → Routine care No TSB testing

Follow-up TSB & HCP visit 24–48 hours Return to step 1

Risk factors for hyperbilirubinemia (RF #2):
1. Gestational age
2. Positive DAT or other known hemolytic disease (G6PD deficiency, spherocytosis)
3. Previous sibling with neonatal jaundice requiring phototherapy
4. Cephalohematoma or significant bruising
5. Exclusively breastfeeding, not well established
6. Ethnic risk factors and family history

DAT, Direct antibody test; *G6PD,* glucose-6-phosphate dehydrogenase; *HCP,* health care provider; *TSB,* total serum bilirubin. (From Provincial Council for Maternal & Child Health & Ministry of Health and Long-Term Care. Clinical Pathway Handbook for Hyperbilirubinemia in Term and Late PreTerm Infants (≥35 weeks); 2018.)

Neonatology

27

737

Figure 27.11 Phototherapy Graph for Term and Late Preterm Infants (≥35 Weeks)

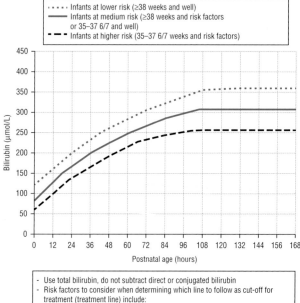

····· Infants at lower risk (≥38 weeks and well)
── Infants at medium risk (≥38 weeks and risk factors or 35–37 6/7 and well)
╍╍ Infants at higher risk (35–37 6/7 weeks and risk factors)

- Use total bilirubin, do not subtract direct or conjugated bilirubin
- Risk factors to consider when determining which line to follow as cut-off for treatment (treatment line) include:
  - Isoimmune hemolytic disease, G6PD deficiency
  - Asphyxia
  - Current and significant lethargy
  - Unresolved temperature instability (requiring current, active treatment)
  - Sepsis currently being treated
  - Ongoing acidosis (not just low cord pH)
  - Albumin <30 g/L (if measured)
  Exclusive breast feeding DOES NOT affect treatment line

G6PD, Glucose-6-phosphate dehydrogenase. (From Provincial Council for Maternal & Child Health & Ministry of Health and Long-Term Care. Clinical Pathway Handbook for Hyperbilirubinemia in Term and Late Pre-Term Infants (≥35 weeks); 2018.)

Figure 27.12 Exchange Transfusion Graph for Term and Late Preterm Infants (≥35 Weeks)

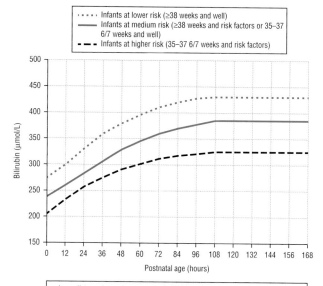

····· Infants at lower risk (≥38 weeks and well)
─── Infants at medium risk (≥38 weeks and risk factors or 35–37 6/7 weeks and well)
▬ ▬ Infants at higher risk (35–37 6/7 weeks and risk factors)

- Immediate exchange is recommended if infant shows signs of acute bilirubin encephalopathy (hypertonic, arching, retrocollis, opisthotonos, fever, high pitched cry).
- Risk factors: isoimmune hemolytic disease, G6PD deficiency, asphyxia, respiratory distress, significant lethargy, temperature instability, sepsis, acidosis.
- Use total bilirubin. Do not subtract direct or conjugated bilirubin.
- If infant is well and 35–37 6/7 wks (medium risk) can individualize levels for exchange based on actual gestational age.

(From Provincial Council for Maternal & Child Health & Ministry of Health and Long-Term Care. Clinical Pathway Handbook for Hyperbilirubinemia in Term and Late Pre-Term Infants (≥35 weeks); 2018.)

Figure 27.13 Hour Specific Nomogram for Term and Late Preterm Infants (≥35 Weeks)

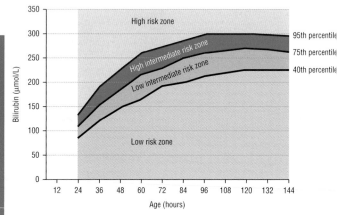

(From Provincial Council for Maternal & Child Health & Ministry of Health and Long-Term Care. Clinical Pathway Handbook for Hyperbilirubinemia in Term and Late Pre-Term Infants (≥35 weeks); 2018.)

Figure 27.14 Follow-Up Algorithm Based on Hour Specific Nomogram

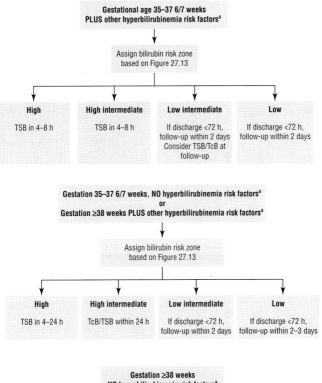

**Gestational age 35–37 6/7 weeks
PLUS other hyperbilirubinemia risk factors[a]**

Assign bilirubin risk zone
based on Figure 27.13

| **High** | **High intermediate** | **Low intermediate** | **Low** |
| TSB in 4–8 h | TSB in 4–8 h | If discharge <72 h, follow-up within 2 days Consider TSB/TcB at follow-up | If discharge <72 h, follow-up within 2 days |

**Gestation 35–37 6/7 weeks, NO hyperbilirubinemia risk factors[a]
or
Gestation ≥38 weeks PLUS other hyperbilirubinemia risk factors[a]**

Assign bilirubin risk zone
based on Figure 27.13

| **High** | **High intermediate** | **Low intermediate** | **Low** |
| TSB in 4–24 h | TcB/TSB within 24 h | If discharge <72 h, follow-up within 2 days | If discharge <72 h, follow-up within 2–3 days |

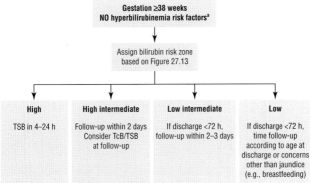

**Gestation ≥38 weeks
NO hyperbilirubinemia risk factors[a]**

Assign bilirubin risk zone
based on Figure 27.13

| **High** | **High intermediate** | **Low intermediate** | **Low** |
| TSB in 4–24 h | Follow-up within 2 days Consider TcB/TSB at follow-up | If discharge <72 h, follow-up within 2–3 days | If discharge <72 h, time follow-up according to age at discharge or concerns other than jaundice (e.g., breastfeeding) |

Modeled on Maisels' Algorithm (Maisels MJ, 2009), reflecting the findings of the Clinical Expert Advisory Group.

[a]Risk factors for hyperbilirubinemia (RF #2) from Figure 27.10. *TcB,* Transcutaneous bilirubin; *TSB,* total serum bilirubin. (From Provincial Council for Maternal & Child Health & Ministry of Health and Long-Term Care. Clinical Pathway Handbook for Hyperbilirubinemia in Term and Late Pre-Term Infants (≥35 weeks); 2018.)

Neonatology

27

Figure 27.15 Phototherapy and Exchange Transfusion Guidelines for Preterm Infants <35 Weeks Gestational Age

Use total bilirubin (add conjugated and unconjugated bilirubin). If conjugated bilirubin is > 50% of total serum bilirubin, consult tertiary care centre.

PHOTOTHERAPY INITIATION LEVELS
Total serum bilirubin (TSB) (μmol/L)

- **For infants >1000 grams use INTENSIVE phototherapy (irradiance ~30 μW/cm²/nm)**
- **For infants ≤1000 grams use STANDARD phototherapy (irradiance ~10 μW/cm²/nm) unless TSB is rapidly rising or TBS continues to rise while receiving phototherapy** (less irradiance used to reduce risk of oxidative tissue injury by phototherapy in extremely immature infants)

	Age in hours	<24 hours	24–48 hours	49–72 hours	>72 hours
Post menstrual age (weeks)	<28 0/7 and at risk*	70	80	80	90
	<28 0/7	80	90	90	100
	28 0/7 to 29 6/7 and at risk*	80	90	90	100
	28 0/7 to 29 6/7	90	100	120	140
	30 0/7 to 31 6/7 and at risk*	90	100	120	140
	30 0/7 to 31 6/7	100	120	140	170
	32 0/7 to 33 6/7 and at risk*	100	120	140	170
	32 0/7 to 33 6/7	100	130	170	200
	34 0/7 to 34 6/7 and at risk*	110	140	170	200
	34 0/7 to 34 6/7	110	160	210	230

EXCHANGE TRANSFUSION LEVELS
Total serum bilirubin (TSB) (μmol/L)

- Exchange transfusion is recommended for infants whose TSB levels continue to rise to exchange levels despite receiving intensive phototherapy to the maximal surface area
- Exchange transfusion is recommended if infant shows signs of acute bilirubin encephalopathy (hypertonia, arching, retrocollis, opisthotonos, high-pitched cry); even if below exchange levels (these signs can be subtle in very low birth weight infants and may be difficult to detect)

	Age in hours	<24 hours	24–48 hours	49–72 hours	>72 hours
Post menstrual age (weeks)	<28 0/7 and at risk*	190	190	210	220
	<28 0/7	190	200	210	240
	28 0/7 to 29 6/7 and at risk*	200	200	210	220
	28 0/7 to 29 6/7	200	210	220	240
	30 0/7 to 31 6/7 and at risk*	220	220	230	260
	30 0/7 to 31 6/7	220	230	260	270
	32 0/7 to 33 6/7 and at risk*	240	240	260	300
	32 0/7 to 33 6/7	240	250	290	300
	34 0/7 to 34 6/7 and at risk*	250	260	290	310
	34 0/7 to 34 6/7	260	270	310	320

*INFANTS AT GREATER RISK for BILIRUBIN TOXICITY

Risk factors for bilirubin toxicity include:
- Serum albumin level <25 g/L
- Rapidly rising TSB levels, greater than 8.5 μmol/L/hour suggesting hemolytic disease
- Clinically unstable infants#

#Clinically unstable infants:
If one or more of the following in the preceding 24 hours:
- Blood ph <7.15
- Blood culture positive sepsis
- Apnea and bradycardia requiring cardio-respiratory resuscitation (bagging and/or intubation)
- Hypotension requiring pressor treatment
- Mechanical ventilation at time of blood sampling

Providing and discontinuing phototherapy
- The purpose of phototherapy is to prevent the need for exchange transfusion
- With phototherapy, the serum bilirubin should decrease by ~20–35 μmol/L in 4–6 hours
- **Use postmenstrual age for phototherapy:** i.e. when a 29 0/7 week infant is 7 days old, use the TSB level for 30 0/7 weeks
- **Discontinuing phototherapy:** discontinue phototherapy when the TSB is 20–35 μmol/L below the initiation level. Check TSB 6–12 hours after discontinuing phototherapy to assess for rebound.

(Adapted from The Hospital for Sick Children Phototherapy and Exchange Transfusion Guidelines for Preterm Infants <35 weeks gestational age, 2019.)

POLYCYTHEMIA

1. **Definition:** venous hematocrit (HCT) ≥ 0.65
2. **Clinical presentation:** signs and symptoms include plethora, hyperbilirubinemia, hypoglycemia, lethargy, cyanosis, respiratory distress, seizures
3. **Complications**
   a. Decreased cerebral blood flow with risk of ischemic stroke
   b. End organ dysfunction
   c. Hyperbilirubinemia
   d. Thrombocytopenia
   e. Hypoglycemia, hypomagnesemia, hypocalcemia
4. **Management**
   a. IV fluids
   b. If infant symptomatic or HCT >0.75 despite IV fluids, consider partial exchange transfusion (controversial)

PLATELET DISORDERS

See Thrombocytopenia in Chapter 21 Hematology

NEONATAL SEPSIS

1. **Etiology**
   a. **High-risk infants:** maternal group B streptococcal (GBS) colonization, <37 weeks GA, prolonged rupture of membranes (>18 hours), maternal fever ($>38^\circ$C), instrumented vaginal delivery, indwelling catheters, maternal urinary tract infection
   b. See Figure 27.16 for the approach to management of term infants at risk for early onset bacterial sepsis

Figure 27.16 Management of Term Infants at Risk for Early Onset Bacterial Sepsis

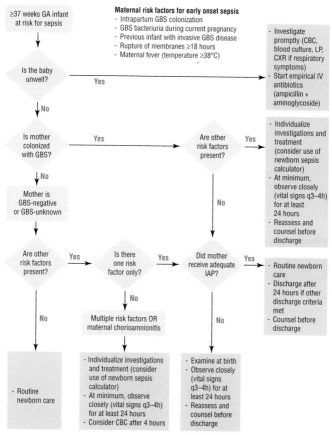

CBC, Complete blood count; CXR, chest x-ray; GA, gestational age; GBS, group B streptococcus; IAP, intrapartum antibiotic prophylaxis; LP, lumbar puncture. (Modified from Jefferies AL; Canadian Paediatric Society, Fetus and Newborn Committee. Management of term infants at increased risk for early onset bacterial sepsis. *Paediatr Child Health.* 2017;22(4):223–228.)

2. **Clinical presentation:** see Box 27.7 for signs and symptoms of neonatal infection
3. **Investigations**
   a. **Laboratory studies**
      i. Serum tests: CBC, blood culture, C-reactive protein (CRP)

ii. Urine tests: urinalysis, urine culture (catheter sample)

iii. CSF tests: Gram stain, protein, glucose, cell count, culture (defer LP if cardiorespiratory instability); bacterial PCR may be useful if antibiotics already initiated; viral PCR (HSV, enterovirus)

b. **Imaging studies:** CXR if respiratory symptoms

Box 27.7   Signs and Symptoms of Neonatal Infection

1. Apnea
2. Respiratory distress, increasing O_2 or ventilation requirements
3. Feeding intolerance, abdominal distension, or ileus
4. Temperature instability
5. Jaundice
6. Lethargy
7. Seizures
8. Metabolic: hyperglycemia, hypoglycemia, acidosis
9. Obvious focus: skin, bones, joints, omphalitis

---

4. **Management**
   a. **Organisms:** GBS, coliforms, *Listeria*, coagulase-negative *Staphylococcus* (in infants >7 days with IV catheters)
      i. Consider *Staphylococcus aureus* in skin, bone, and joint disease
      ii. Consider *Shigella* or *Salmonella* in gastroenteritis
      iii. Consider superinfection with *Candida*, other fungi in prolonged or recurrent illness, high white blood cells (WBCs), indwelling shunt or IV catheter
      iv. *Ureaplasma urealyticum* sometimes implicated in chronic lung disease
   b. **Empiric coverage:** depends on clinical presentation, timing, and local sensitivity/resistance patterns:
      i. Ampicillin + aminoglycoside (i.e., gentamycin, tobramycin), if sepsis is suspected
      ii. Ampicillin + cefotaxime, if meningitis is suspected
   c. **Specific coverage**
      i. Consider cloxacillin if *Staphylococcus* is suspected
      ii. Vancomycin for late-onset sepsis (>7 days), recurrent illness, recent indwelling shunt or catheter (or coagulase-negative *S. aureus*)
      iii. *Pseudomonas* requires coverage with ceftazidime or piperacillin-tazobactam
      iv. For NEC, use ampicillin + aminoglycoside + metronidazole
      v. For *Candida* sepsis, treat with amphotericin B or IV fluconazole

NECROTIZING ENTEROCOLITIS

1. **Definition:** severe disorder of the intestine, involving inflammation, bacterial overgrowth $\pm$ necrosis of the bowel wall
2. **Risk factors**
   a. Prematurity (90%), IUGR, perinatal asphyxia, hypoglycemia, polycythemia, PDA, CHD, formula feeding
   b. Breast milk feeding (expressed breast milk [EBM] or donor milk) is protective
3. **Clinical presentation** (typically presents at 2–3 weeks, range 1–12 weeks)
   a. **GI signs:** abdominal distension, abdominal wall tenderness and discoloration, hematochezia, bile-stained gastric aspirates
   b. **Systemic signs:** lethargy, temperature instability, apnea and bradycardia, poor perfusion, shock
   c. **Bowel necrosis:** persistent thrombocytopenia, metabolic acidosis, shock, GI bleeding, abdominal wall erythema, right lower quadrant mass
4. **Diagnosis**
   a. Based on presenting signs, laboratory tests, radiological or surgical findings
   b. Features on abdominal x-ray (AXR) (AP and lateral decubitus) include pneumatosis intestinalis (intramural gas) usually in terminal ileum and ascending colon, portal venous gas, free intraperitoneal air (if perforated NEC)
   c. Increasing role of abdominal ultrasonography to detect radiograph findings not seen on AXR
5. **Management**
   a. **Investigations**
      i. Septic workup: CBC, blood culture, urine, stool (bacterial and viral), CSF (when stable)
      ii. Serial AXRs q6 to 12h for 24 hour or while clinically unstable
      iii. Monitor blood gas, lactate, glucose, electrolytes, creatinine
   b. **Feeding/fluid management**
      i. Strictly NPO
      ii. Nasogastric (NG) tube to straight drainage
      iii. IV fluid resuscitation, correct acidosis and hypoperfusion, anticipate increased fluid requirements because of third spacing
      iv. Ensure good vascular access, start parenteral nutrition (PN)
   c. **Antibiotics**
      i. Broad-spectrum antibiotics initially (IV ampicillin + aminoglycoside + metronidazole), then change based on culture results
      ii. In area with higher prevalence of methicillin-resistant *Staphylococcus aureus* or existing indwelling catheter, consider vancomycin instead of ampicillin
      iii. Consider adding antifungal therapy if patient not responding
      iv. Duration of NEC treatment based on clinical staging (Table 27.21)

Neonatology

27

d. **Surgery:** urgent surgical consultation required for definitive NEC or perforation

6. **Complications**
   a. Strictures (10%), usually large bowel
   b. Recurrent NEC
   c. Post-NEC bleeding because of strictures
   d. Short-bowel syndrome likely if >50% to 75% of small intestine lost
   e. Liver cirrhosis secondary to prolonged TPN

Table 27.21	Duration of Necrotizing Enterocolitis Treatment Regimen According to Modified Bell's Staging Criteria	
Manifestation	**Treatment**
Suspected NEC (stage I)	
"Suspected sepsis" plus mild GI symptoms but no blood in stool or intramural gas	NPO, antibiotics × 3 days, pending cultures
AXR may be normal or show mild ileus	
Definite NEC (stage II)	
Presence of intramural gas (pneumatosis intestinalis); intestinal dilatation, ileus	NPO, antibiotics × 7–14 days, depending on severity of illness
Advanced NEC (stage III)	
Definite NEC plus complication (e.g., acidosis, shock, thrombocytopenia, coagulopathy, portal vein gas, evidence of localized or early peritonitis, ascites)	NPO, antibiotics × 10–14 days Likely to require fluid resuscitation, blood products, inotropic and ventilatory support
Perforated NEC	Same as earlier, minimum 14 days antibiotics plus surgical intervention

AXR, Abdominal x-ray; *GI,* gastrointestinal; *NEC,* necrotizing enterocolitis.

Data from Necrotizing enterocolitis: treatment based on staging criteria MC Walsh, RM Kliegman–Pediatric clinics of North America, 1986–Elsevier.

ABDOMINAL WALL DEFECTS
See Gastroschisis and Omphalocele in Chapter 17 General Surgery

OBSTRUCTION
See Obstruction—Neonatal in Chapter 17 General Surgery

RETINOPATHY OF PREMATURITY
1. **Definition:** proliferative disorder of developing retinal blood vessels in preterm infants that may lead to reduced visual acuity or blindness
2. **Retinal zones:** see Figure 27.17
3. **Staging:** see Box 27.8

Figure 27.17 Retina of the Right and Left Eye, Showing Zone Borders and Clock Hours Used to Describe the Location and Extent of Retinopathy of Prematurity

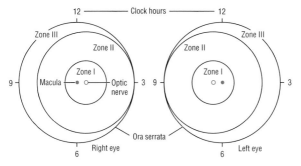

(From the International Committee for the Classification of ROP. The international classification of retinopathy of prematurity revisited. *Arch Ophthalmol.* 2005;123:992, Figure 1.)

Box 27.8	Stages (1–5) and Description of Retinopathy of Prematurity
Stage 1	Demarcation line separating avascular from vascularized retina
Stage 2	Ridge arising in region of demarcation line
Stage 3	Extraretinal fibrovascular proliferation/neovascularization extending into the vitreous
Stage 4	Partial retinal detachment
Stage 5	Total retinal detachment
Plus disease	Increased vascular dilatation and tortuosity of posterior retinal vessels in at least two quadrants of the retina
Pre-plus disease	More vascular dilatation and tortuosity than normal but insufficient to make the diagnosis of plus disease
Type 1 ROP (requires treatment)	Zone I—any stage ROP with plus disease OR stage 3 ROP without plus disease Zone II—stage 2 or 3 ROP with plus disease
Type 2 ROP (careful monitoring)	Zone I—stage 1 or 2 ROP without plus disease Zone II—stage 3 ROP without plus disease

ROP, Retinopathy of prematurity. Adapted from Jefferies AL, Fetus and Newborn Committee, Canadian Paediatric Society. Retinopathy of prematurity: recommendations for screening. *Paediatr Child Health.* 2010;15(10):667–674.

4. **Screening:** dilated eye examinations for all infants ≤1250 g BW OR <31 week GA at 4 weeks postnatally or 31 weeks (whichever is later), then 2 to 4 weeks thereafter if retinopathy of prematurity (ROP) does not exist or more frequently if present
5. **Prevention:** avoidance of hyperoxia with lower oxygen saturation targets to reduce reactive oxygen species toxic to the retina
6. **Treatment:** laser photocoagulation of avascular retina or intravitreal injection of antivascular endothelial growth factor (bevacizumab)
7. **Surveillance:** ongoing follow-up of vision in infancy

Magdalena Riedl • Mallory L. Downie • Joana Dos Santos • Anne Sophie Blais
Seetha Radhakrishnan

COMMON ABBREVIATIONS

Also see page xviii for a list of other abbreviations used throughout this book

ABPM	ambulatory blood pressure monitoring
ACE	angiotensin-converting enzyme
ACR	albumin-to-creatinine ratio
AKI	acute kidney injury
ANH	antenatal hydronephrosis
APD	anteroposterior diameter of the renal pelvis
ARB	angiotensin receptor blocker
ASOT	anti-streptolysin O titre
ATN	acute tubular necrosis
BBD	bladder and bowel dysfunction
BXO	balanitis xerotica obliterans
C3G	C3 glomerulopathy
CAKUT	congenital abnormalities of the kidney and urinary tract
CFU	colony-forming units
CIC	clean intermittent catheterization
CKD	chronic kidney disease
CMV	cytomegalovirus
CRRT	continuous renal replacement therapy
DAT	direct antiglobulin test
DDAVP	desmopressin
DMSA	dimercaptosuccinic acid
DTPA	diethylene triamine pentaacetic acid
FSGS	focal segmental glomerulosclerosis
FTT	failure to thrive
G6PD	glucose-6-phosphate dehydrogenase
GFR	glomerular filtration rate
GN	glomerulonephritis
HEADSS	home, education/employment, activities, drugs, sexuality, suicide
HSP	Henoch-Schönlein purpura
HTN	hypertension
HVA	homovanillic acid
HUS	hemolytic uremic syndrome
MPGN	membranoproliferative glomerulonephritis
PCR	protein-to-creatinine ratio
PIGN	post-infectious glomerulonephritis
PKD	polycystic kidney disease
PSGN	post-streptococcal glomerulonephritis
PUV	posterior urethral valves
RNC	radiopharmaceutical nuclear cystography
RTA	renal tubular acidosis
SBE	subacute bacterial endocarditis
SLE	systemic lupus erythematosus

SNHL	sensorineural hearing loss
STEC	Shiga toxin-producing *Escherichia coli*
TB	tuberculosis
UNC	urinary net charge
UPJ	ureteropelvic junction
UVJ	ureterovesical junction
VACTERL	vertebral anomalies, anorectal malformation, cardiac defects, tracheoesophageal fistula, esophageal atresia, renal and limb anomalies
VCUG	voiding cystourethrogram
VDRL	venereal disease research laboratory test
VMA	vanillylmandelic acid
VUR	vesicoureteral reflux

CLINICAL EVALUATION OF RENAL FUNCTION

1. **History**
   a. **Urinary symptoms:** change in urine color, odor, volume or frequency, dysuria, incontinence, post-void dribbling, abdominal or flank pain
   b. **Renal failure:** anorexia, fatigue, nausea, vomiting, failure to thrive (FTT)
   c. **Hypertension (HTN):** headaches, seizures, flushing, visual changes, chest pain
   d. **Fluid overload:** dyspnea, edema
   e. **Renal osteodystrophy:** bony pain, skeletal deformities
   f. Symptoms associated with underlying cause of renal dysfunction
      i. **Infectious:** sore throat, URTI, fever, bloody diarrhea, rash
      ii. **Autoimmune/vasculitic:** eye symptoms, rash, joint pain, abdominal pain, aphthous ulcers, sinusitis, hemoptysis, epistaxis
      iii. **Genetic:** dysmorphic features, hearing loss, retinal changes, glaucoma, cataract, other organ defects
   g. **Nephrotoxic medications:** antibiotics, antivirals, antifungals, NSAIDs, chemotherapy, radiocontrast dye, calcineurin inhibitors
   h. **Birth history:** antenatal US findings, polyhydramnios, oligohydramnios, single umbilical artery, umbilical catheterization
   i. **Family history:** HTN, renal failure/dialysis, renal cystic disease, hematuria, proteinuria, deafness (Alport syndrome)
2. **Physical examination**
   a. **General:** pallor, fluid overload or volume depletion, evidence of FTT
   b. **Head and neck:** fundoscopy (e.g., exudates, cotton-wool spots, flame-shaped hemorrhages), preauricular pits or tags, external ear deformities, branchial fistulae
   c. **Respiratory:** signs of pulmonary edema, pleural effusions

d. **CVS:** evidence of congestive heart failure, HTN, peripheral pulses, perfusion
e. **Abdominal:** bruits, costovertebral angle tenderness, palpable kidney/mass, prune-belly, ascites
f. **GU:** balanitis, hypospadias, undescended testicles, ambiguous genitalia
g. **MSK:** bony deformities, arthritis
h. **Skin:** rash, café-au-lait spots, ash leaf macules (tuberous sclerosis), purpura, petechiae

3. **Investigations**
   a. **Urine dipstick:** evaluate within 1 hour of voiding; Table 28.1
   b. **Quantification of urinary protein:** ideally first-morning void; Table 28.2
   c. **Urine microscopy:** Table 28.3
   d. **Bloodwork:** extended electrolytes (Na, K, Cl, Ca, PO_4, Mg, tCO_2), Cr, urea, albumin, CBC
   e. **Renal imaging:** Table 28.4

> ✱ **PEARL**
>
> Send protein-to-creatine and albumin-to-creatinine ratios when proteinuria is noted on urine dipstick, to confirm and quantify amount.

28

Table 28.1	Interpreting Urine Dipsticks	
Test	**Normal Values**	**Comment**
Specific gravity	1.010–1.025	↑ in dehydration, glycosuria; ↓ in diabetes insipidus
pH	4.6–8.0	Influenced by diet, medications, tubular disorders
Glucose	Negative	Positive in hyperglycemia, isolated glucosuria, proximal tubular disorders
Protein	Negative or trace	Tests for albumin
Blood	Negative or "trace non-hemolyzed"	Positive from intact RBCs, hemoglobin, myoglobin
Bilirubin	Negative or small amounts	May be caused by hepatitis or biliary obstruction
Urobilinogen	Negative or positive	Present in normal urine but may be increased in hepatic dysfunction
Ketones	Negative or trace	Positive in starvation, diabetic ketoacidosis, metabolic disorders
Leukocyte esterase	Negative	Positive in presence of significant leukocytes in urine
Nitrites	Negative	Some bacteria (urea-splitting organisms) convert nitrate to nitrite; negative result does *not* rule out infection

RBC, Red blood cell.

Table 28.2 Quantification of Proteinuria

	Normal	Significant	Nephrotic
PCR			
6–24 months of age	<50 mg/mmol	50–200 mg/mmol	>200 mg/mmol
>24 months of age	<20 mg/mmol	20–200 mg/mmol	>200 mg/mmol
ACR	<3 mg/mmol	>30 mg/mmol	>250 mg/mmol
24 h urinary protein	<4 mg/m²/h	>4 mg/m²/h	>40 mg/m²/h

ACR, Albumin-to-creatinine ratio; *PCR*, protein-to-creatinine ratio.

Table 28.3 Findings on Urine Microscopy

Category	Type	Significance
Cells	White blood cells	>2/high-power field may signify infection or inflammation
	Red blood cells	>3–5/high-power field is abnormal Normal shape: suggests lower urinary tract source Dysmorphic: likely glomerular source Also used to differentiate between hematuria and hemoglobinuria
	Epithelial cells	Tubular, squamous or transitional. Normal finding
	Oval fat bodies	Usually seen in context of heavy proteinuria but may be normal
Casts	Hyaline matrix casts	Most frequent type. Considered physiologic
	White blood cell casts	Seen in inflammatory and infectious conditions
	Red blood cell casts	Indicative of glomerular disease
	Renal tubuloepithelial cell casts	Found in conditions primarily affecting tubules
	Fatty casts	Frequently seen in nephrotic syndrome
	Granular casts	May be found with proteinuria or under normal conditions. Dark brown granular casts can be seen in ATN
Crystals	Calcium oxalate	Envelope-shaped. Most common cause for kidney stones
	Uric acid	Several shapes (rhomboid, hexagonal, needle-shaped); yellow-brown
	Calcium phosphate	Granular precipitate
	Struvite	Pyramid shape. Associated with infections
	Cystine	Colorless, hexagonal. Always pathologic
	Calcium carbonate	Small spheres, alone or in groups of four
	Drug crystals	Sulfamethoxazole, ampicillin, contrast dye

ATN, Acute tubular necrosis.

Table 28.4	Renal Imaging Modalities	
Modality	**Indication**	**Findings**
Renal US	First febrile UTI <2 years of age Follow-up of congenital anomalies Workup of hematuria and renal pathology	Renal size/position, hydronephrosis, hydroureter, corticomedullary differentiation, signs of renal scarring
VCUG	Evidence of hydronephrosis or renal reflux on US Second febrile UTI <2 years Suspected PUV Urogenital abnormalities	Presence/grade of VUR, bladder and urethral abnormalities (e.g., uretero-cele, PUV), post-void residual urine (not precise)
DMSA	Assess for renal scarring Confirm presence of functional renal tissue	Absent uptake correlated with non-functional tissue, e.g., scars, infarcts, masses Differential renal function
MAG3 or DTPA	Assess for urinary tract obstruction Evaluate differential renal function	Uptake, excretion and drainage Percentage contribution of each kidney to global renal function
Diuretic renography	Suspected UPJ obstruction	Excretion/drainage from kidney
RNC	Follow-up of VUR Less radiation exposure than VCUG	Presence of VUR Does not provide grade or delineate urethral anatomy
MRI	Detailed evaluation of congenital anomalies	Obstruction, duplications, abnormal ureteral insertion, cysts, angiomyolipomas
CT angiogram	Suspected renal artery stenosis	Renal artery stenosis

CT, Computed tomography; *DMSA*, dimercaptosuccinic acid; *DTPA*, diethylene triamine pentaacetic acid; *MAG3*, mercaptoacetyltriglycine; *MRI*, magnetic resonance imaging; *PUV*, posterior urethral valves; *RNC*, radiopharmaceutical nuclear cystography; *UPJ*, ureteropelvic junction; *US*, ultrasound; *UTI*, urinary tract infection; *VCUG*, voiding cystourethrogram; *VUR*, vesicoureteral reflux.

USEFUL CALCULATIONS AND VALUES

1. **Estimated bladder volume (mL)** = $[2 + \text{age (years)}] \times 30$ (to a max. of 500–700 mL)
2. **Renal length:** see Figure 28.1
3. **Schwartz formula for estimated glomerular filtration rate (eGFR)** = $36.5 \text{ (constant)} \times \text{length (cm)} \div \text{serum Cr } (\mu\text{mol/L})$
4. **Body surface area (BSA):** $\sqrt{\{\text{height (cm)} \times \text{weight (kg)} \div 3600\}}$
5. **Insensible losses**
   a. Neonate = $500 \times \text{BSA (m}^2)$
   b. Infant–adult = $400 \times \text{BSA (m}^2)$
6. **Urinary Ca:Cr ratio:** see Table 28.5
7. **Urinary net charge/anion gap (UNC)** = $[U_{Na}] + [U_K] - [U_{Cl}]$
   a. Negative UNC: appropriate response to chronic metabolic acidosis
   b. Positive UNC: suggests absence of urinary ammonium and defect in distal urinary acidification

Figure 28.1 Renal Length

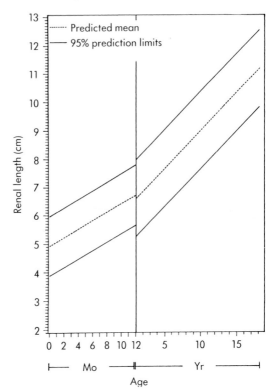

(From Zale KE. Neonatal and pediatric adrenal and urinary system. In: Hagen-Ansert SL, ed. *Textbook of Diagnostic Sonography*. 8th ed., Vol. 1–2. St Louis, MO: Elsevier Inc.; 2018.)

Table 28.5	Normal Values for Ca:Cr Ratio
Age	**Normal Value (mmol/mmol)**
<12 months	<2.2
1–3 years	<1.5
3–5 years	<1.1
5–7 years	<0.8
>7 years	<0.7

CONGENITAL ABNORMALITIES OF THE KIDNEYS AND URINARY TRACT (CAKUT)

A. Unilateral renal agenesis
1. Sporadic failure of formation of one kidney
2. One-third have additional CAKUT
3. One-third have extra-renal defects, e.g., cleft lip/palate, preauricular pits, cardiac and vertebral defects
4. **Evaluation:** consider VCUG to rule out vesicoureteral reflux (VUR) if abnormal contralateral kidney on US or history of febrile UTI
5. **Monitoring**
   a. Annual BP (to detect HTN), urine dipstick (to detect proteinuria) and renal US (to monitor compensatory growth of normal kidney)
   b. Check serum creatinine to document normal renal function; frequency determined by clinical presentation
6. **Prognosis:** overall good with adequate growth and hypertrophy of solitary kidney

B. Hypoplastic kidney(s)
1. Small kidney(s) because of reduced number of otherwise normal nephrons
2. **Monitoring:** as with unilateral renal agenesis
3. **Prognosis:** clinically significant if both kidneys affected; can progress to CKD

C. Dysplastic kidney(s)
1. Kidney lacks normally developed nephrons
2. **Monitoring:** as with unilateral renal agenesis
3. **Prognosis:** extent of renal dysfunction depends on degree of morphological abnormalities

D. Multicystic dysplastic kidney
1. Second most common cause of flank mass in newborn, after antenatal hydronephrosis (ANH)
2. Nonfunctional; normal tissue replaced by multiple cysts of varying size
3. Contralateral kidney may have limited dysplasia and/or VUR
4. **Monitoring:** as earlier, US to monitor involution of multicystic dysplastic kidney and compensatory growth of contralateral kidney
5. **Prognosis:** good, similar to solitary kidney

E. Abnormalities of position
1. Includes ectopic kidney, horseshoe kidney, crossed fused renal ectopia
2. Few long-term consequences unless associated with dysplasia, reflux, or obstruction

F. Cystic kidney disease

1. **Polycystic kidney disease:** autosomal dominant or recessive (Table 28.6)
2. **Syndromes associated with renal cysts:** tuberous sclerosis, von Hippel-Lindau disease, VACTERL association, Smith-Lemli-Opitz, branchio-oto-renal, and renal cysts and diabetes (RCAD) syndromes, nephronophthisis

Table 28.6	Polycystic Kidney Disease	
	AR PKD	**AD PKD**
Definition	Polycystic kidneys and congenital hepatic fibrosis May have severe liver disease with bile duct dilatation (Caroli disease) Cysts often smaller, sometimes difficult to discern on US	Renal cysts throughout nephron Often larger, macroscopic cysts
Epidemiology	1 in 20,000	1 in 500
Presentation	Majority present in infancy; may present in childhood Often presents as large, palpable flank masses	Renal function usually normal throughout childhood Found on US screening in family known to have disease or presents in adulthood with HTN and renal failure
Features	Renal: HTN, hyponatremia, renal insufficiency, flank masses Extrarenal: respiratory insufficiency, hepatosplenomegaly, esophageal varices, hypersplenism, signs of liver failure	Renal: HTN, UTI/pyuria, gross or microscopic hematuria, flank masses, urolithiasis, renal insufficiency Extrarenal: mitral valve prolapse, GI diverticuli, cerebral aneurysms, hepatic, pancreatic, ovarian and seminal vesicle cysts
Diagnosis	Based on clinical findings, imaging and family history (absence of cysts in both parents but may have an affected sibling) Genetic testing: *PKHD1*	Based on clinical findings, imaging and family history (gene mutation in one parent) Genetic testing: *PKD1* (Type 1) or *PKD2* (Type 2)
Management	Renal US as needed Supportive treatment: BP control, management of CKD	

AD, Autosomal dominant; *AR*, autosomal recessive; *BP*, blood pressure; *CKD*, chronic kidney disease; *GI*, gastrointestinal; *HTN*, hypertension; *PKD*, polycystic kidney disease; *US*, ultrasound; *UTI*, urinary tract infection.

ANTENATAL HYDRONEPHROSIS

1. **Antenatal hydronephrosis:** renal pelvic anteroposterior diameter (APD) >4 mm in second trimester and/or >7 mm in third trimester (Table 28.7)
2. **Pelviectasis:** dilated renal pelvis
3. **Pelvicaliectasis:** dilated renal pelvis and calyces, associated with parenchymal thinning if severe
4. **Etiology:** see Table 28.8

Table 28.7	Definition of Antenatal Hydronephrosis	
	Renal Pelvic Anteroposterior Diameter (APD)	
Classification	**Second Trimester**	**Third Trimester**
Mild	4–6 mm	7–9 mm
Moderate	7–10 mm	10–15 mm
Severe	>10	>15 mm

From Nguyen HT, Herndon CD, Cooper C, et al. The Society for Fetal Urology consensus statement on the evaluation and management of antenatal hydronephrosis. *J Ped Urol.* 2010;6(3):212–231.

Table 28.8	Etiology of Antenatal Hydronephrosis
Cause of Antenatal Hydronephrosis	**Frequency**
Transient hydronephrosis	41%–88%
UPJ obstruction	10%–30%
VUR	10%–20%
UVJ obstruction/megaureters	5%–10%
Ureterocele/ectopic ureter/duplex system	5%–7%
Multicystic dysplastic kidney	4%–6%
PUV/urethral atresia	1%–2%
Others: Prune-belly syndrome, cystic kidney disease, congenital ureteric stricture, megalourethra	Uncommoh

PUV, Posterior urethral valves; *UPJ*, ureteropelvic junction; *UVJ*; ureterovesical junction; *VUR*, vesicoureteral reflux.

Modified from Nguyen HT, Herndon CD, Cooper C, et al. The Society for Fetal Urology consensus statement on the evaluation and management of antenatal hydronephrosis. *J Ped Urol.* 2010;6(3):212–231.

5. **Investigation and management**
   a. **Renal US:** all neonates with isolated ANH (third trimester APD ≥9 mm) and/or any urinary tract abnormalities (ureteral dilatation, abnormal bladder)
      i. Should not be done in the first 48 to 72 hours of life, because of low urine output
      ii. Bilateral severe ANH or ANH in solitary kidney: US before hospital discharge
      iii. All other patients: US between 7 and 30 days of life
   b. **VCUG before hospital discharge:** any infant with concern for bladder outlet obstruction (PUV)
   c. **Other indications for VCUG in ANH:** severe bilateral hydronephrosis, suspected infravesical obstruction, dilated ureter, duplex kidney, abnormal renal echogenicity, abnormal bladder

d. **Prophylactic antibiotics:** use from birth is controversial; consider if APD >10 mm, until postnatal US performed

VESICOURETERAL REFLUX

1. **VUR:** retrograde flow of urine from the bladder into upper urinary tract
   a. Classified into five grades of severity on contrast VCUG (Figure 28.2)

Figure 28.2   Classification of Vesicoureteral Reflux

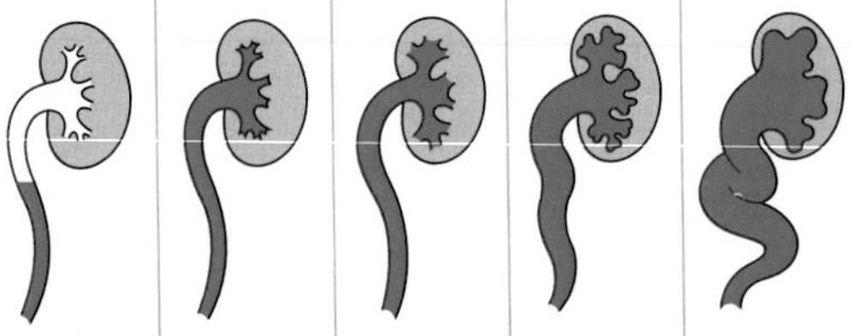

Grade	I	II	III	IV	V
Appearance on VCUG	Contrast in ureter, not reaching renal pelvis, no ureteral dilatation	Contrast up to pelvis, no ureteral dilatation	Contrast up to pelvis, mild dilatation of ureter and pelvis, no/slight blunting of calyces	Moderate dilatation of ureter and pelvicalyceal system, mild tortuosity and blunting of calyces	Significant dilatation and tortuosity of ureter, severe dilatation of pelvis, significant blunting of calyces
Resolution at 5 years of age	90%	80%	60%	30%	Rarely

(From Shaw K. Nephrology. In: Laubisch J, Engorn B, eds. *The Johns Hopkins Hospital, The Harriet Lane Handbook: A Manual for Pediatric House Officers.* 20th ed. Philadelphia, PA: Elsevier Inc.; 2015.)

2. **Primary VUR:** reflux with no bladder dysfunction or obstruction
   a. Usually caused by deficient ureterovesical junction (UVJ) anti-reflux mechanism
3. **Secondary VUR:** high bladder pressures caused by functional or anatomic obstruction
   a. Bladder dysfunction caused by a congenital, acquired, or behavioral pathology
4. **History**
   a. **Usually asymptomatic:** often diagnosed during workup of hydronephrosis or febrile UTI

b. **Antenatal history:** including hydronephrosis on US
c. **Patient age:** relevant to likelihood of resolution
d. **UTIs:** presence of fever, method of urine specimen collection and storage, culture result
e. **Antibiotic prophylaxis**
f. **Circumcision status**
g. **Family history:** prevalence of VUR higher in siblings

5. **Investigations:** see Table 28.4
   a. **VCUG:** provides anatomic details; preferred for diagnosis
   b. **RNC:** can be used for follow-up; less radiation exposure but does not provide grade
   c. **DMSA:** assess for cortical defects from congenital renal dysmorphism or acquired renal scarring
      i. About half of children with grade IV–V reflux have cortical defects at diagnosis, often from congenital renal dysmorphism

6. **Management**
   a. **Goals of treatment:** prevent renal injury, prevent febrile UTI, minimize the morbidity of treatment and follow-up
   b. **Majority spontaneously resolve:** high-grade VUR in adolescence or adulthood less likely to disappear
   c. Sterile reflux not associated with renal damage
   d. **Antibiotic prophylaxis:** safe
      i. No longer routinely recommended for VUR grades I–III
      ii. Consider prophylaxis for children with high-grade reflux after discussion with Urology/Nephrology: preferably trimethoprim alone; alternatively trimethoprim/sulfamethoxazole or nitrofurantoin (unless contraindicated or previously resistant)
      iii. Usually discontinued after 1 year of age or after toilet training
   e. Prompt full-dose treatment of UTIs
   f. If secondary VUR, treat underlying cause: bladder training, constipation management, biofeedback
   g. Ensure good voiding patterns (see Enuresis), maintain hydration
   h. **Surgical management:** high success rate, see Box 28.1 for indications
      i. Endoscopic injection of bulking agent or surgical ureteral reimplantation
   i. **Follow-up US:** for renal growth, hydronephrosis and scarring

---

Box 28.1 Indications for Surgical Correction of Vesicoureteral Reflux

Breakthrough febrile UTI despite prophylactic antibiotics
Non-adherence to antibiotic prophylaxis (relative indication)
Reflux that persists into puberty in the presence of breakthrough UTIs
Evidence of new verified renal scarring, not confounded by existing renal dysmorphism

OBSTRUCTIVE UROPATHY

1. May occur anywhere between urethral meatus and calyceal infundibula
2. **Classification:** congenital, acquired, or functional; see Table 28.9 for causes

Table 28.9	Causes of Obstructive Uropathy	
Congenital	**Acquired**	**Functional**
Congenital infundibulopelvic stenosis	Obstruction anywhere in urinary tract, secondary to	Neurogenic bladder
UPJ obstruction	- Calculi	- Neurospinal dysraphism
Congenital obstructive megaureter	- Trauma	(myelomeningocele)
Ureteral ectopia	- Inflammation, e.g., IBD	- Degenerative diseases
Ureterocele	- Infection e.g., TB	- Guillain-Barré
Posterior urethral valves	- Post-surgical	- Post-myelitis
Anterior urethral valves	- Neoplasm	- Anatomic
Urethral atresia		- Myopathic
		- Endocrine
		- Toxic

IBD, Inflammatory bowel disease; *TB*, tuberculosis; *UPJ*, ureteropelvic junction.

URETEROPELVIC JUNCTION OBSTRUCTION

1. Functionally significant impairment of urinary flow from renal pelvis to ureter
2. **Congenital:** majority, e.g., intrinsic narrowing of UPJ (most common in newborns and infants), external compression from aberrant vessels or muscular bands (present later in childhood)
3. **Acquired:** e.g., stones, post-operative or inflammatory stricture, urothelial cancer, external compression
4. **Clinical presentation**
   a. 75% unilateral, left > right; M:F 2:1
   b. Symptoms can manifest at any time in life, even in congenital cases
   c. **Neonates:** asymptomatic or flank mass; increased number diagnosed because of ANH screening
   d. **Older children:** intermittent acute flank/abdominal pain ± nausea/vomiting ± hematuria
   e. Increased risk of febrile UTI
   f. Up to 50% have another urological anomaly, e.g., contralateral UPJ, multicystic dysplastic kidneys, renal agenesis, horseshoe kidney, VUR
5. **Investigations**
   a. **Goal:** identify anatomic site and functional significance of the obstruction
   b. **Renal US:** usually shows hydronephrosis
      i. May show thinning of renal cortex in high-grade obstruction
      ii. Rules out other causes of obstruction, e.g., stone, and other differential diagnoses, e.g., multicystic kidney

   c. **Diuretic renography:** may use to assess differential renal function and degree of obstruction

      i. Can be used to follow patients for functional loss (indication for surgery)

. **Management**

   a. Approximately one-third will need surgery

   b. **Indications for intervention:** worsening symptoms or hydronephrosis on serial US, impaired renal function, stones, infection, hypertension

   c. **Goal:** preservation/improvement of renal function, relief of symptoms

   d. **Treatment:** surgical removal of obstructed segment and re-anastomosis of ureter to renal pelvis (pyeloplasty)

   e. Other options include endopyelotomy (endoscopic incision of the obstructed proximal ureter) and stent insertion (double J ureteral stent, nephrostomy)

PRUNE-BELLY SYNDROME

. **Triad:** absent abdominal wall musculature, urinary tract anomalies and bilateral intra-abdominal cryptorchidism

. **Wide spectrum of clinical presentation:** urological anomalies range from mild (urinary tract dilatation) to severe (renal failure)

   a. Renal dysplasia present in half

   b. Ureters usually dilated, redundant and tortuous

   c. Bladder usually massively enlarged with pseudodiverticula

   d. Posterior urethra usually dilated

. Most cases are sporadic and have normal karyotype

. **Management**

   a. Management of cardiac and pulmonary issues

   b. Monitoring of urine output and renal function

   c. Renal and bladder US

   d. UTI prevention: circumcision, antibiotic prophylaxis

POSTERIOR URETHRAL VALVES

1. Valves in posterior urethra obstruct urine outflow from bladder

2. **Spectrum of presentations**

   a. **Mild:** straining to urinate, weak urinary stream, frequent UTIs

   b. **Severe:** can cause bilateral renal dysplasia in utero, may present as oligohydramnios; common congenital cause of chronic kidney disease with approximately 50% of patients progressing to ESRD over time

3. Boys with PUV may develop bladder failure over time (incontinence, poor bladder emptying/urinary retention, recurrent UTIs)

4. Early detection on antenatal US and early surgical intervention significantly improve prognosis

5. **Investigations**
   a. **Antenatal US:** thick dilated bladder, bilateral hydroureters and hydronephrosis
   b. **VCUG:** bilateral VUR, thickened and trabeculated bladder, bladder diverticuli, hypertrophied bladder neck, dilated posterior urethra
   c. Diagnosis can also be made on urethroscopy
   d. Laboratory evaluation of renal function
6. **Management**
   a. **Immediate treatment:** ensure adequate urine drainage via bladder catheter, feeding tube, or stent
   b. **Definitive treatment:** surgical ablation of valves, or vesicostomy when ablation is not possible
   c. Long-term pediatric urological follow-up of bladder and renal function required

URINARY TRACT INFECTION

1. **UTI:** infection involving the kidneys, ureters, bladder, or urethra
2. **Cystitis:** infection involving the bladder or lower urinary tract
   a. No fever, commonest in post-pubertal girls
3. **Pyelonephritis:** infection involving the kidneys
   a. Fever present, most common in infants and children with renal malformations
4. **Complicated UTI:** obstruction or abscess
   a. Consider if hemodynamically unstable, elevated creatinine, bladder/abdominal mass, poor urine flow, not clinically improving within 24 hours or fever not trending down within 48 hours of adequate antibiotic treatment
5. **Clinical presentation**
   a. **<2 months of age:** always consider UTI if unwell or febrile, even if URTI symptoms present
   b. **<3 years of age:** send urine culture if fever (>39°C rectal) and no apparent source
   c. **>3 years of age**
      i. Cystitis: dysuria, urgency, frequency, suprapubic pain, incontinence, malodorous urine
      ii. Pyelonephritis: fever, flank pain, malaise, nausea, vomiting
   d. **Risk factors:** female sex (>1 year), uncircumcised male (<1 year), voiding dysfunction, constipation, neurogenic bladder, obstructive uropathy, VUR, urethral instrumentation
6. **Investigations:** see Table 28.4
   a. **Urine culture:** obtain before initiating antibiotic treatment
      i. Midstream urine sample considered positive if single pathogen $\geq 10^5$ CFU/mL

ii. Catheter specimen considered positive if single pathogen $\geq 5 \times 10^4$ CFU/mL

iii. Suprapubic aspiration gold standard but rarely performed—any growth is indicative of UTI

b. **Renal US:** every child <2 years with first febrile UTI during or within 2 weeks of episode; or if suspecting pyelonephritis (enlarged kidney) or complicated UTI

c. **VCUG:** if US suggestive of renal abnormality, obstruction or high grade reflux; or after second well-documented UTI in child <2 years of age

d. **DMSA:** to diagnose pyelonephritis during acute episode (not routinely done); or to identify scarring and determine split renal function (months after clinical episode) in patients with abnormal US, renal function, or proteinuria after UTI has resolved

7. **Management**

a. Treat constipation and/or other underlying cause of voiding dysfunction, if applicable

b. **Symptomatic and positive urinalysis:** empiric antibiotics in keeping with local sensitivities (see Chapter 24 Infectious Diseases, Table 24.7 for details); modify if appropriate once culture results available

   i. **Duration:** 2 to 4 days for acute cystitis; 10 to 14 days for pyelonephritis

   ii. **Route:** PO unless <2 months of age, appears toxic, complicated UTI, positive blood culture, known urological abnormality, or not tolerating oral treatment

c. **Antibiotic prophylaxis:** not routine, except in VUR grade IV–V

   i. Use before VCUG is controversial

d. **Refer to Urology:** if VUR grade IV–V or any grade VUR with breakthrough UTIs

e. **Refer to Nephrology:** if abnormal renal US, impaired renal function, or recurrent UTIs despite normal imaging

> **! PITFALL**
>
> Urine bag samples have a high rate of contamination, making culture reports unreliable for diagnosis of UTI. However, a bag can be used as an initial screen and, if negative, makes a UTI unlikely.

HYPERTENSION

1. **<13 years:** BP $\geq$95th percentile for age, height and sex on $\geq$3 occasions
2. **$\geq$13 years:** >130/80 mmHg on $\geq$3 occasions
3. Abnormal ambulatory blood pressure monitoring (ABPM) in any age
4. See Table 28.10 for BP norms in boys and girls

> **PEARL**
>
> Pediatric blood pressure percentiles are determined by age, sex, and height. Weight is not a determining factor.

28

Table 28.10 Blood Pressure Levels for Boys and Girls by Age and Height Percentile

BOYS

Age (Years)	BP Percentile	SBP (mmHg)							DBP (mmHg)						
		HEIGHT PERCENTILE OR MEASURED HEIGHT							HEIGHT PERCENTILE OR MEASURED HEIGHT						
		5%	10%	25%	50%	75%	90%	95%	5%	10%	25%	50%	75%	90%	95%
1	Height (cm)	77.2	78.3	80.2	82.4	84.6	86.7	87.9	77.2	78.3	80.2	82.4	84.6	86.7	87.9
	50th	85	85	86	86	87	88	88	40	40	40	41	41	42	42
	90th	98	99	99	100	100	101	101	52	52	53	53	54	54	54
	95th	102	102	103	103	104	105	105	54	54	55	55	56	57	57
	95th + 12 mmHg	114	114	115	115	116	117	117	66	66	67	67	68	69	69
2	Height (cm)	86.1	87.4	89.6	92.1	94.7	97.1	98.5	86.1	87.4	89.6	92.1	94.7	97.1	98.5
	50th	87	87	88	89	89	90	91	43	43	44	44	45	46	46
	90th	100	100	101	102	103	103	104	55	55	56	56	57	58	58
	95th	104	105	105	106	107	107	108	57	58	58	59	60	61	61
	95th + 12 mmHg	116	117	117	118	119	119	120	69	70	70	71	72	73	73
3	Height (cm)	92.5	93.9	96.3	99	101.8	104.3	105.8	92.5	93.9	96.3	99	101.8	104.3	105.8
	50th	88	89	89	90	91	92	92	45	46	46	47	48	49	49
	90th	101	102	102	103	104	105	105	58	58	59	59	60	61	61
	95th	106	106	107	107	108	109	109	60	61	61	62	63	64	64
	95th + 12 mmHg	118	118	119	119	120	121	121	72	73	73	74	75	76	76

4 Height (cm)	98.5	100.2	102.9	105.9	108.9	111.5	113.2	98.5	100.2	102.9	105.9	108.9	111.5	113.2
50th	90	90	91	92	93	94	94	48	49	49	50	51	52	52
90th	102	103	104	105	105	106	107	60	61	62	62	63	64	64
95th	107	107	108	108	109	110	110	63	64	65	66	67	67	68
95th + 12 mmHg	119	119	120	120	121	122	122	75	76	77	78	79	79	80
5 Height (cm)	104.4	106.2	109.1	112.4	115.7	118.6	120.3	104.4	106.2	109.1	112.4	115.7	118.6	120.3
50th	91	92	93	94	95	96	96	51	51	52	53	54	55	55
90th	103	104	105	106	107	108	108	63	64	65	65	66	67	67
95th	107	108	109	109	110	111	112	66	67	68	69	70	70	71
95th + 12 mmHg	119	120	121	121	122	123	124	78	79	80	81	82	82	83
6 Height (cm)	110.3	112.2	115.3	118.9	122.4	125.6	127.5	110.3	112.2	115.3	118.9	122.4	125.6	127.5
50th	93	93	94	95	96	97	98	54	54	55	56	57	57	58
90th	105	105	106	107	109	110	110	66	66	67	68	68	69	69
95th	108	109	110	111	112	113	114	69	70	70	71	72	72	73
95th + 12 mmHg	120	121	122	123	124	125	126	81	82	82	83	84	84	85
7 Height (cm)	116.1	118	121.4	125.1	128.9	132.4	134.5	116.1	118	121.4	125.1	128.9	132.4	134.5
50th	94	94	95	97	98	98	99	56	56	57	58	58	59	59
90th	106	107	108	109	110	111	111	68	68	69	70	70	71	71
95th	110	110	111	112	114	115	116	71	71	72	73	73	74	74
95th + 12 mmHg	122	122	123	124	126	127	128	83	83	84	85	85	86	86

Continued

Table 28.10 Blood Pressure Levels for Boys and Girls by Age and Height Percentile—cont'd

BOYS

Age (Years)	BP Percentile	SBP (mmHg) HEIGHT PERCENTILE OR MEASURED HEIGHT							DBP (mmHg) HEIGHT PERCENTILE OR MEASURED HEIGHT						
		5%	10%	25%	50%	75%	90%	95%	5%	10%	25%	50%	75%	90%	95%
8	Height (cm)	121.4	123.5	127	131	135.1	138.8	141	121.4	123.5	127	131	135.1	138.8	141
	50th	95	96	97	98	99	99	100	57	57	58	59	59	60	60
	90th	107	108	109	110	111	112	112	69	70	70	71	72	72	73
	95th	111	112	112	114	115	116	117	72	73	73	74	75	75	75
	95th + 12 mmHg	123	124	124	126	127	128	129	84	85	85	86	87	87	87
9	Height (cm)	126	128.3	132.1	136.3	140.7	144.7	147.1	126	128.3	132.1	136.3	140.7	144.7	147.1
	50th	96	97	98	99	100	101	101	57	58	59	60	61	62	62
	90th	107	108	109	110	112	113	114	70	71	72	73	74	74	74
	95th	112	112	113	115	116	118	119	74	74	75	76	76	77	77
	95th + 12 mmHg	124	124	125	127	128	130	131	86	86	87	88	88	89	89
10	Height (cm)	130.2	132.7	136.7	141.3	145.9	150.1	152.7	130.2	132.7	136.7	141.3	145.9	150.1	152.7
	50th	97	98	99	100	101	102	103	59	60	61	62	63	63	64
	90th	108	109	111	112	113	115	116	72	73	74	74	75	75	76
	95th	112	113	114	116	118	120	121	76	76	77	77	78	78	78
	95th + 12 mmHg	124	125	126	128	130	132	133	88	88	89	90	90	90	90

		|| Systolic BP (mmHg) ||						|| Diastolic BP (mmHg) ||					
11	Height (cm)	134.7	137.3	141.5	146.4	151.3	155.8	158.6	134.7	137.3	141.5	146.4	151.3	155.8	158.6
	50th	99	99	101	102	103	104	106	61	61	62	63	63	63	63
	90th	110	111	112	114	116	117	118	74	74	75	75	75	76	76
	95th	114	114	116	118	120	123	124	77	78	78	78	78	78	78
	95th + 12 mmHg	126	126	128	130	132	135	136	89	90	90	90	90	90	90
12	Height (cm)	140.3	143	147.5	152.7	157.9	162.6	165.5	140.3	143	147.5	152.7	157.9	162.6	165.5
	50th	101	101	102	104	106	108	109	61	62	62	62	62	63	63
	90th	113	114	115	117	119	121	122	75	75	75	75	75	76	76
	95th	116	117	118	121	124	126	128	78	78	78	78	78	79	79
	95th + 12 mmHg	128	129	130	133	136	138	140	90	90	90	90	90	91	91
13	Height (cm)	147	150	154.9	160.3	165.7	170.5	173.4	147	150	154.9	160.3	165.7	170.5	173.4
	50th	103	104	105	108	110	111	112	61	60	61	62	63	64	65
	90th	115	116	118	121	124	126	126	74	74	74	75	76	77	77
	95th	119	120	122	125	128	130	131	78	78	78	78	80	81	81
	95th + 12 mmHg	131	132	134	137	140	142	143	90	90	90	90	92	93	93
14	Height (cm)	153.8	156.9	162	167.5	172.7	177.4	180.1	153.8	156.9	162	167.5	172.7	177.4	180.1
	50th	105	106	109	111	112	113	113	60	60	62	64	65	66	67
	90th	119	120	123	126	127	128	129	74	74	75	77	78	79	80
	95th	123	125	127	130	132	133	134	77	78	79	81	82	83	84
	95th + 12 mmHg	135	137	139	142	144	145	146	89	90	91	93	94	95	96

Continued

Table 28.10 Blood Pressure Levels for Boys and Girls by Age and Height Percentile—cont'd

BOYS

Age (Years)	BP Percentile	SBP (mmHg)							DBP (mmHg)						
		HEIGHT PERCENTILE OR MEASURED HEIGHT							HEIGHT PERCENTILE OR MEASURED HEIGHT						
		5%	10%	25%	50%	75%	90%	95%	5%	10%	25%	50%	75%	90%	95%
15	Height (cm)	159	162	166.9	172.2	177.2	181.6	184.2	159	162	166.9	172.2	177.2	181.6	184.2
	50th	108	110	112	113	114	114	114	61	62	64	65	66	67	68
	90th	123	124	126	128	129	130	130	75	76	78	79	80	81	81
	95th	127	129	131	132	134	135	135	78	79	81	83	84	85	85
	95th + 12 mmHg	139	141	143	144	146	147	147	90	91	93	95	96	97	97
16	Height (cm)	162.1	165	169.6	174.6	179.5	183.8	186.4	162.1	165	169.6	174.6	179.5	183.8	186.4
	50th	111	112	114	115	115	116	116	63	64	66	67	68	69	69
	90th	126	127	128	129	131	131	132	77	78	79	80	81	82	82
	95th	130	131	133	134	135	136	137	80	81	83	84	85	86	86
	95th + 12 mmHg	142	143	145	146	147	148	149	92	93	95	96	97	98	98
17	Height (cm)	163.8	166.5	170.9	175.8	180.7	184.9	187.5	163.8	166.5	170.9	175.8	180.7	184.9	187.5
	50th	114	115	116	117	117	118	118	65	66	67	68	69	70	70
	90th	128	129	130	131	132	133	134	78	79	80	81	82	82	83
	95th	132	133	134	135	137	138	138	81	82	84	85	86	86	87
	95th + 12 mmHg	144	145	146	147	149	150	150	93	94	96	97	98	98	99

Age (Years)	BP Percentile	SBP (mmHg) HEIGHT PERCENTILE OR MEASURED HEIGHT							DBP (mmHg) HEIGHT PERCENTILE OR MEASURED HEIGHT						
		5%	10%	25%	50%	75%	90%	95%	5%	10%	25%	50%	75%	90%	95%
1	Height (cm)	75.4	76.6	78.6	80.8	83	84.9	86.1	75.4	76.6	78.6	80.8	83	84.9	86.1
	50th	84	85	86	86	87	88	88	41	42	42	43	44	45	46
	90th	98	99	99	100	101	102	102	54	55	56	56	57	58	58
	95th	101	102	102	103	104	105	105	59	59	60	60	61	62	62
	95th + 12 mmHg	113	114	114	115	116	117	117	71	71	72	72	73	74	74
2	Height (cm)	84.9	86.3	88.6	91.1	93.7	96	97.4	84.9	86.3	88.6	91.1	93.7	96	97.4
	50th	87	87	88	89	90	91	91	45	46	47	48	49	50	51
	90th	101	101	102	103	104	105	106	58	58	59	60	61	62	62
	95th	104	105	106	106	107	108	109	62	63	63	64	65	66	66
	95th + 12 mmHg	116	117	118	118	119	120	121	74	75	75	76	77	78	78
3	Height (cm)	91	92.4	94.9	97.6	100.5	103.1	104.6	91	92.4	94.9	97.6	100.5	103.1	104.6
	50th	88	89	89	90	91	92	93	48	48	49	50	51	53	53
	90th	102	103	104	104	105	106	107	60	61	61	62	63	64	65
	95th	106	106	107	108	109	110	110	64	65	65	66	67	68	69
	95th + 12 mmHg	118	118	119	120	121	122	122	76	77	77	78	79	80	81

Continued

Nephrology and Urology

28

Table 28.10 Blood Pressure Levels for Boys and Girls by Age and Height Percentile—cont'd

GIRLS

Age (Years)	BP Percentile	SBP (mmHg) HEIGHT PERCENTILE OR MEASURED HEIGHT							DBP (mmHg) HEIGHT PERCENTILE OR MEASURED HEIGHT						
		5%	10%	25%	50%	75%	90%	95%	5%	10%	25%	50%	75%	90%	95%
4	Height (cm)	97.2	98.8	101.4	104.5	107.6	110.5	112.2	97.2	98.8	101.4	104.5	107.6	110.5	112.2
	50th	89	90	91	92	93	94	94	50	51	51	53	54	55	55
	90th	103	104	105	106	107	108	108	62	63	64	65	66	67	67
	95th	107	108	109	109	110	111	112	66	67	68	69	70	70	71
	95th + 12 mmHg	119	120	121	121	122	123	124	78	79	80	81	82	82	83
5	Height (cm)	103.6	105.3	108.2	111.5	114.9	118.1	120	103.6	105.3	108.2	111.5	114.9	118.1	120
	50th	90	91	92	93	94	95	96	52	52	53	55	56	57	57
	90th	104	105	106	107	108	109	110	64	65	66	67	68	69	70
	95th	108	109	109	110	111	112	113	68	69	70	71	72	73	73
	95th + 12 mmHg	120	121	121	122	123	124	125	80	81	82	83	84	85	85
6	Height (cm)	110	111.8	114.9	118.4	122.1	125.6	127.7	110	111.8	114.9	118.4	122.1	125.6	127.7
	50th	92	92	93	94	96	97	97	54	54	55	56	57	58	59
	90th	105	106	107	108	109	110	111	67	67	68	69	70	71	71
	95th	109	109	110	111	112	113	114	70	71	72	72	73	74	74
	95th + 12 mmHg	121	121	122	123	124	125	126	82	83	84	84	85	86	86

Age (Year)		115.9	117.8	121.1	124.9	128.8	132.5	134.7	115.9	117.8	121.1	124.9	128.8	132.5	134.7
7	Height (cm)	115.9	117.8	121.1	124.9	128.8	132.5	134.7	115.9	117.8	121.1	124.9	128.8	132.5	134.7
	50th	92	93	94	95	97	98	99	55	55	56	57	58	59	60
	90th	106	106	107	109	110	111	112	68	68	69	70	71	72	72
	95th	109	110	111	112	113	114	115	72	72	73	73	74	74	75
	95th + 12 mmHg	121	122	123	124	125	126	127	84	84	85	85	86	86	87
8	Height (cm)	121	123	126.5	130.6	134.7	138.5	140.9	121	123	126.5	130.6	134.7	138.5	140.9
	50th	93	94	95	97	98	99	100	56	56	57	59	60	61	61
	90th	107	107	108	110	111	112	113	69	70	71	72	72	73	73
	95th	110	111	112	113	115	116	117	73	73	74	74	75	75	75
	95th + 12 mmHg	122	123	124	125	127	128	129	85	85	86	86	87	87	87
9	Height (cm)	125.3	127.6	131.3	135.6	140.1	144.1	146.6	125.3	127.6	131.3	135.6	140.1	144.1	146.6
	50th	95	95	97	98	99	100	101	57	58	59	60	60	61	61
	90th	108	108	109	111	112	113	114	71	71	72	73	73	73	73
	95th	112	112	113	114	116	117	118	74	74	75	75	75	75	75
	95th + 12 mmHg	124	124	125	126	128	129	130	86	86	87	87	87	87	87
10	Height (cm)	129.7	132.2	136.3	141	145.8	150.2	152.8	129.7	132.2	136.3	141	145.8	150.2	152.8
	50th	96	97	98	99	101	102	103	58	59	59	60	61	61	62
	90th	109	110	111	112	113	115	116	72	73	73	73	73	73	73
	95th	113	114	114	116	117	119	120	75	75	76	76	76	76	76
	95th + 12 mmHg	125	126	126	128	129	131	132	87	87	88	88	88	88	88
11	Height (cm)	135.6	138.3	142.8	147.8	152.8	157.3	160	135.6	138.3	142.8	147.8	152.8	157.3	160
	50th	98	99	101	102	104	105	106	60	60	60	61	62	63	64
	90th	111	112	113	114	116	118	120	74	74	74	74	74	75	75
	95th	115	116	117	118	120	123	124	76	77	77	77	77	77	77
	95th + 12 mmHg	127	128	129	130	132	135	136	88	89	89	89	89	89	89

Continued

Table 28.10 | Blood Pressure Levels for Boys and Girls by Age and Height Percentile—cont'd

GIRLS

Age (Years)	BP Percentile	SBP (mmHg) HEIGHT PERCENTILE OR MEASURED HEIGHT							DBP (mmHg) HEIGHT PERCENTILE OR MEASURED HEIGHT						
		5%	10%	25%	50%	75%	90%	95%	5%	10%	25%	50%	75%	90%	95%
12	Height (cm)	142.8	145.5	149.9	154.8	159.6	163.8	166.4	142.8	145.5	149.9	154.8	159.6	163.8	166.4
	50th	102	102	104	105	107	108	108	61	61	61	62	64	65	65
	90th	114	115	116	118	120	122	122	75	75	75	75	76	76	76
	95th	118	119	120	122	124	125	126	78	78	78	78	79	79	79
	95th + 12 mmHg	130	131	132	134	136	137	138	90	90	90	90	91	91	91
13	Height (cm)	148.1	150.6	154.7	159.2	163.7	167.8	170.2	148.1	150.6	154.7	159.2	163.7	167.8	170.2
	50th	104	105	106	107	108	108	109	62	62	63	64	65	65	66
	90th	116	117	119	121	122	123	123	75	75	75	76	76	76	76
	95th	121	122	123	124	126	126	127	79	79	79	79	80	80	81
	95th + 12 mmHg	133	134	135	136	138	138	139	91	91	91	91	92	92	93
14	Height (cm)	150.6	153	156.9	161.3	165.7	169.7	172.1	150.6	153	156.9	161.3	165.7	169.7	172.1
	50th	105	106	107	108	109	109	109	63	63	64	65	66	66	66
	90th	118	118	120	122	123	123	123	76	76	76	76	77	77	77
	95th	123	123	124	125	126	127	127	80	80	80	80	81	81	82
	95th + 12 mmHg	135	135	136	137	138	139	139	92	92	92	92	93	93	94

Age		SBP (mmHg) Height percentile							DBP (mmHg) Height percentile						
15	Height (cm)	151.7	154	157.9	162.3	166.7	170.6	173	151.7	154	157.9	162.3	166.7	170.6	173
	50th	105	106	107	108	109	109	109	64	64	64	65	66	67	67
	90th	118	119	121	122	123	123	124	76	76	76	77	77	78	78
	95th	124	124	125	126	127	127	128	80	80	80	81	82	82	82
	95th + 12 mmHg	136	136	137	138	139	139	140	92	92	92	93	94	94	94
16	Height (cm)	152.1	154.5	158.4	162.8	167.1	171.1	173.4	152.1	154.5	158.4	162.8	167.1	171.1	173.4
	50th	106	107	108	109	109	110	110	64	64	65	66	66	67	67
	90th	119	120	122	123	124	124	124	76	76	76	77	78	78	78
	95th	124	125	125	127	127	128	128	80	80	80	81	82	82	82
	95th + 12 mmHg	136	137	137	139	139	140	140	92	92	92	93	94	94	94
17	Height (cm)	152.4	154.7	158.7	163.0	167.4	171.3	173.7	152.4	154.7	158.7	163.0	167.4	171.3	173.7
	50th	107	108	109	110	110	110	111	64	64	65	66	66	66	67
	90th	120	121	123	124	124	125	125	76	76	76	77	78	78	78
	95th	125	125	126	127	128	128	128	80	80	80	81	82	82	82
	95th + 12 mmHg	137	137	138	139	140	140	140	92	92	92	93	94	94	94

BP, Blood pressure; DBP, diastolic blood pressure; SBP, systolic blood pressure.

From Flynn JT, Kaelber BC, Baker-Smith CM, et al. Clinical practice guideline for screening and management of high blood pressure in children and adolescents. *Pediatrics*. 2017;140(3): 1–72 (Tables 4 and 5).

Nephrology and Urology

28

A. Blood pressure measurement

1. Annual BP measurements are recommended in children >3 years of age
2. Monitor BP <3 years of age if renal or cardiac disease, recurrent UTIs, prematurity (<32 weeks), solid organ transplant, malignancy, systemic illnesses or drugs associated with HTN
3. **Technique:** measure in the right arm, held at the level of the heart, in a calm patient
   a. Oscillometric (automated) readings must be confirmed by auscultatory measurements
   b. Neonates: use oscillometric method in supine position
4. **Correct cuff size:** inflatable bladder width at least 45% to 55% of arm circumference; bladder length should cover 80% to 100% of arm circumference (if too small, will overestimate BP)
5. **If elevated:** measure twice more and average the three measurements
6. **ABPM:** use to confirm diagnosis of HTN in children with height >120 cm

B. Etiology of hypertension

1. **Primary HTN**
   a. Predominant form in children ≥6 years of age
   b. Associated with overweight/obesity or family history of HTN
   c. No extensive workup needed if a) and b) are present and no findings on history or examination to suggest a secondary cause
2. **Secondary HTN**
   a. **Intrinsic renal:** glomerulonephritis (GN), acute tubular necrosis (ATN), chronic kidney disease (CKD), hemolytic uremic syndrome (HUS), Henoch-Schönlein purpura (HSP) nephritis, tumor, cystic kidney disease
   b. **Renal vascular:** renal artery stenosis (common in neurofibromatosis 1 Williams syndrome), renal artery/vein thrombosis, fibromuscular dysplasia, vasculitis
   c. **Cardiovascular:** coarctation of aorta, mid-aortic syndrome
   d. **Endocrine:** hyperthyroidism, hyperparathyroidism, congenital adrenal hyperplasia, Cushing syndrome, primary hyperaldosteronism, pheochromocytoma, neuroblastoma
   e. **CNS:** intracranial mass/hemorrhage, increased intracranial pressure, Guillain-Barré syndrome
   f. **Medications/toxins:** corticosteroids, oral contraceptives, nasal decongestants, cocaine, sympathomimetic agents, vitamin D intoxication, stimulants
   g. **Monogenic hypertension:** Liddle and Gordon syndromes, apparent mineralocorticoid excess

h. **Miscellaneous:** sleep apnea, pain, anxiety, iatrogenic fluid and salt overload (from TPN or IV fluids)

C. Investigating hypertension

1. **History:** symptomatology; perinatal; nutritional; psychosocial; home, education/employment, activities, drugs, sexuality, suicide (HEADSS) assessment (adolescents); physical activity; family history
2. **Physical examination:** calculate BMI, four-limb BP measurements, peripheral pulses, signs of secondary HTN and end-organ damage
3. **Urine:** urinalysis
4. **Serum:** CBC, Cr, urea, electrolytes, lipid profile
5. **Imaging:** Renal US with doppler, echocardiogram
6. **Additional studies for underlying disorder:** as guided by history and physical examination
   a. Obese patients: transaminases (fatty liver), fasting glucose and HbA1c (diabetes screen)
   b. Depending on history: plasma renin, cortisol, aldosterone, urine VMA and HVA, plasma and urine metanephrines, drug screen, TSH, polysomnography
7. **Evaluation for target-organ damage:** echocardiogram, retinal examination, urine albumin-to-creatinine ratio

D. Management of hypertension

1. **Acute hypertensive crisis:** see Hypertensive Crisis in Chapter 2 Emergency Medicine for management
2. **Long-term treatment goal:** reduce systolic (S)BP and diastolic (D)BP to <90th percentile or <130/80 mmHg, whichever is lower
3. **Initial approach**
   a. **Primary HTN:** weight reduction, exercise, dietary modification
   b. **Secondary HTN:** treat underlying cause
4. **Pharmacological agents:** indicated for secondary or symptomatic HTN, HTN associated with CKD or diabetes, or where insufficient response to lifestyle changes in primary HTN
   a. Begin with monotherapy, targeting the underlying mechanism
   b. **First-line:** calcium channel blocker, angiotensin-converting enzyme (ACE) inhibitor, angiotensin receptor blocker (ARB)
   c. **Second-line:** β-blocker, diuretics, α_1-blocker

PROTEINURIA

1. Defined on spot urine or 24-hour collection; see Table 28.2
2. **Types:** may be glomerular (loss of albumin) or tubular (loss of low molecular weight proteins, e.g., β_2-microglobulin)—urine dipstick will only detect glomerular proteinuria
3. **Differential diagnosis:** see Box 28.2

Box 28.2 Differential Diagnosis of Proteinuria

Benign

Orthostatic

Transient: fever, exercise, cold exposure, stress, epinephrine infusion

Pathological: Glomerular

Congenital: congenital nephrosis (Finnish), diffuse mesangial sclerosis, CMV, syphilis

Primary: idiopathic nephrotic syndrome (see Box 28.4)

Secondary:

- Infection, e.g., PSGN, shunt nephritis, SBE, hepatitis B and C, HIV, malaria, syphilis
- Multisystem, e.g., Alport, SLE, HUS, HSP, sickle cell disease, granulomatosis with polyangiitis, Goodpasture disease
- Drugs, e.g., penicillamine, NSAIDs, captopril, gold, mercury, lithium
- Neoplasm, e.g., leukemia, lymphoma, renal tumors
- Renovascular, e.g., renal vein thrombosis, renal artery stenosis, HTN
- Metabolic, e.g., diabetes mellitus
- CKD

Pathological: Tubular

Congenital/genetic: Fanconi syndrome, cystic/dysplastic renal disease

Acquired: interstitial nephritis, pyelonephritis, ATN, transplant rejection, reflux nephropathy, drugs (e.g., aminoglycosides, analgesics, cyclosporine, cisplatin)

ATN, Acute tubular necrosis; *CKD*, chronic kidney disease; *CMV*, cytomegalovirus; *HIV*, human immunodeficiency virus; *HSP*, Henoch-Schönlein purpura; *HTN*, hypertension; *HUS*, hemolytic uremic syndrome; *NSAIDs*, non-steroidal anti-inflammatory drugs; *PSGN*, post-streptococcal glomerulonephritis; *SBE*, subacute bacterial endocarditis, *SLE*, systemic lupus erythematosus.

4. **Investigations**
   a. **Confirm diagnosis:** for asymptomatic patients with proteinuria, repeat first morning urinalysis and quantify proteinuria before extensive investigation
   b. **Laboratory studies:** Box 28.3

Box 28.3 Investigation of Proteinuria

Urine microscopy and culture

Morning urine for ACR/PCR

Split 24-h urine collection to rule out orthostatic proteinuria: overnight (supine) urine sample collected separately from daytime (upright) sample

Serum: CBC, electrolytes, urea, Cr, albumin, C3, C4, cholesterol

Consider: ANA, ASOT, hepatitis serology, HIV, VDRL, abdominal US, renal biopsy (guided by history and physical examination)

ACR, Albumin-to-creatinine ratio; *ANA*, antinuclear antibody; *ASOT*, anti-streptolysin O titre; *CBC*, complete blood count; *Cr*, creatinine; *HIV*, human immunodeficiency virus; *PCR*, protein-to-creatinine ratio; *US*, ultrasound; *VDRL*, venereal disease research laboratory test.

NEPHROTIC SYNDROME

1. **Nephrotic syndrome:** nephrotic-range proteinuria, hypoalbuminemia, edema
2. **Nephrotic range proteinuria:** see Table 28.2
3. **Etiology:** see Box 28.4

Box 28.4 Etiology of Nephrotic Syndrome

Primary

Idiopathic (90% of pediatric patients)
- Minimal change disease (77%)
- MPGN/C3G
- FSGS
- Proliferative GN, mesangial proliferation, glomerulosclerosis
- Membranous nephropathy

Congenital

Secondary

Infections: syphilis, HIV, hepatitis B or C, leprosy, malaria, schistosomiasis, toxoplasmosis

Malignancy: leukemia, lymphoma

Drugs: penicillamine, captopril, NSAIDs, mercury, gold, lithium, pamidronate, heroin

C3G, C3 glomerulopathy; *FSGS*, focal segmental glomerulosclerosis; *GN*, glomerulonephritis; *HIV*, human immunodeficiency virus; *MPGN*, membranoproliferative glomerulonephritis; *NSAID*, non-steroidal anti-inflammatory drug.

PRIMARY IDIOPATHIC NEPHROTIC SYNDROME

1. Common between 2 and 6 years of age; M:F ratio 2:1
2. **Clinical presentation**
   a. Decreased urine output
   b. Periorbital and lower limb edema progressing to generalized edema, ascites, pleural effusions
   c. Anorexia, irritability, abdominal pain, diarrhea
3. **Investigations:** see Box 28.3
   a. **Urine:** nephrotic-range proteinuria (see Table 28.2), microscopic hematuria (20% of patients)
   b. **Blood**
      i. Cr usually normal (may be increased if intravascularly depleted)
      ii. Albumin <25 g/L
      iii. Elevated serum cholesterol and triglycerides
   c. **Renal biopsy:** if age <1 or >12 years, elevated Cr, gross hematuria, low C3, infection with HIV, TB, hepatitis B/C, or steroid resistance
4. **Treatment**
   a. **Initial presentation**
      i. Prednisone 60 mg/m^2/dose once daily for 6 weeks
      ii. Reduce to 40 mg/m^2/dose every other day for 6 weeks
      iii. Then taper prednisone off over 4 subsequent weeks

b. Consider 25% albumin infusion if symptomatic edema or volume-depleted
c. Low-salt diet
d. Monitor fluid balance, may require fluid restriction; cautious use of diuretics
e. **Second-line agents:** cyclophosphamide, cyclosporine, tacrolimus, mycophenolate mofetil/mycophenolic acid or rituximab for steroid-resistant, steroid-dependent or frequently relapsing nephrotic syndrome

5. **Complications**
   a. Intravascular depletion, pulmonary edema/respiratory distress caused by hypoalbuminemia
   b. Increased susceptibility to infection with encapsulated bacteria, caused by decreased concentrations of IgG and factor B, e.g., spontaneous bacterial peritonitis (2%–6%)
   c. Increased risk of thromboembolic events, caused by decreased levels of antithrombin III, increased platelet aggregation, volume depletion, hyperviscosity, immobilization, use of diuretics and corticosteroids (2%–5%)

6. **Prognosis**
   a. **Remission:** defined as urine showing negative or trace protein for 3 consecutive days
      i. Median time to remission: 10 days
      ii. 85% to 90% respond to steroids
      iii. Two-thirds relapse
   b. **Steroid-resistant:** persistent proteinuria after 6–8 weeks of steroid therapy
   c. **Steroid-dependent:** relapse on alternate-day prednisone dosing, or relapse within 14 days of prednisone discontinuation
   d. **Frequent relapser:** ≥4 relapses in 1 year, or 2 relapses in 6 months

HEMATURIA

1. **Definition:** >3 to 5 red blood cells (RBCs) per high-power field in spun urine
2. Prevalence of isolated microscopic hematuria in children and adolescents is about 1.5%
3. Majority asymptomatic, do not develop significant renal disease
4. Persistent microscopic hematuria (on 3 samples) should prompt further investigation
5. **Diagnostic approach:** see Figure 28.3

> **! PITFALL**
>
> Dark urine may be mistaken for hematuria caused by drugs (e.g., rifampin, nitrofurantoin, methyldopa, levodopa, metronidazole) or pigments (e.g., hemoglobin, myoglobin, bilirubin, beets, blackberries, urates).

Figure 28.3   Diagnostic Approach to Hematuria

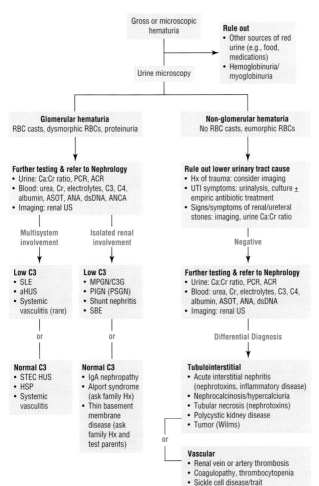

ACR, Albumin-to-creatinine ratio; aHUS, atypical hemolytic uremic syndrome; ANA, Antinuclear antibody; ANCA, antineutrophil cytoplasmic antibodies; ASOT, anti-streptolysin O titre; C3G, C3 glomerulopathy; Cr, creatinine; dsDNA, double-stranded deoxyribonucleic acid; HSP, Henoch-Schönlein purpura; HUS, hemolytic uremic syndrome; Hx, history; IgA, immunoglobulin A; MPGN, membranoproliferative glomerulonephritis; PCR, protein-to-creatinine ratio; PIGN, post-infectious glomerulonephritis; PSGN, post-streptococcal glomerulonephritis; RBC, red blood cell; SBE, subacute bacterial endocarditis, SLE, systemic lupus erythematosus; STEC, Shiga toxin-producing E. coli; US, ultrasound; UTI, urinary tract infection.

NEPHRITIC SYNDROME

1. **Definition:** hematuria, proteinuria, impaired renal function, oliguria, and HTN
2. **Etiology:** see Figure 28.3 for differential diagnosis

> ### ✦ PEARL
>
> The two most important considerations for guiding the differential diagnosis of glomerulonephritis are:
> 1. C3 level (low or normal)
> 2. Whether the disease is renal-limited or systemic

ALPORT SYNDROME

1. Hereditary disease affecting the glomerular basement membrane, caused by abnormality in type IV collagen
2. Majority demonstrate X-linked dominant inheritance
3. Female carriers develop milder symptoms
4. Enquire about family history of CKD, renal transplantation, sensorineural hearing loss
5. **Clinical manifestations**
   a. **Renal:** hematuria, proteinuria, HTN, renal insufficiency
   b. **Ocular:** anterior lenticonus, perimacular flecks
   c. **Cochlear:** high-frequency sensorineural hearing loss (50% patients)
   d. **Smooth muscle:** leiomyomas of esophagus, trachea, and female genital tract
   e. Progress to kidney failure in fourth to sixth decade of life with ACE inhibition, earlier if untreated
6. **Investigations**
   a. **Basic investigations:** see Figure 28.3
   b. **Renal US:** to rule out other pathology
   c. **Renal biopsy:** to confirm diagnosis
   d. Genetic testing, audiology and ophthalmology assessments
7. **Treatment**
   a. **ACE inhibitors:** early initiation slows progression to kidney failure
   b. **Supportive measures:** as renal function declines

HENOCH-SCHÖNLEIN PURPURA NEPHRITIS

1. See section on Henoch-Schonlein Purpura in Chapter 36 Rheumatology

IgA NEPHROPATHY (BERGER DISEASE)

1. Immune-complex disease with deposition of IgA in glomerular mesangium
2. Most common cause of GN in children
3. More common in adolescents, Asian population; M:F ratio 2:1

4. Usually manifests as episodic gross hematuria during intercurrent illness
5. May also be detected incidentally as asymptomatic proteinuria and microscopic hematuria
6. Rarely associated with HTN or edema in the pediatric population
7. 25% progress to chronic renal insufficiency
8. **Investigations**
   a. Exclude other causes of GN
   b. C3, C4 normal
   c. IgA elevated in only one-third of cases
   d. Renal biopsy is diagnostic
9. **Management**
   a. **Immunosuppression:** consider based on biopsy findings
   b. **ACE inhibitors:** consider if significant proteinuria and/or HTN

POST-INFECTIOUS GLOMERULONEPHRITIS

1. All age groups; majority between 3 and 15 years
2. Presents 7 to 14 days after a URTI or 3 to 8 weeks following a skin infection
3. Most common infection is group A β-hemolytic Streptococci; can also occur after other bacterial, viral, or parasitic infections
4. **Clinical manifestations**
   a. Cola-colored urine, edema, HTN
   b. Mild to moderate impairment of renal function, hyperkalemia
   c. May present with isolated hematuria if symptoms of nephritis are subclinical or missed
5. **Investigations**
   a. Anti-streptolysin O titre initially elevated in post-streptococcal GN
   b. Low serum C3, returns to normal within 6 to 8 weeks
   c. If C3 does not normalize by 8 to 12 weeks, consider renal biopsy to establish diagnosis
6. **Management**
   a. **Acute phase:** fluid and salt restriction, with diuretics and antihypertensives as indicated
   b. **Antibiotic treatment:** will not prevent development of nephritis but should be prescribed if positive streptococcal throat culture
   c. **Excellent prognosis:** microscopic hematuria generally resolves within 6 to 12 months; may persist for up to 2 years but does not reoccur

HEMOLYTIC UREMIC SYNDROME

1. **Triad:** microangiopathic hemolytic anemia (DAT-negative), thrombocytopenia, and renal insufficiency
2. Leading cause of acute renal failure in North America in otherwise healthy children

3. Subdivided into Shiga toxin-producing *Escherichia coli* (STEC) HUS (90%) and atypical HUS (aHUS)
4. Most common between 9 months and 4 years of age
5. aHUS can occur at any age

A. Shiga toxin-producing *E. coli* hemolytic uremic syndrome

1. Caused by Shiga toxin-producing strains of *E. coli*, e.g., O157:H7
2. Presents with abdominal pain followed by diarrhea (often bloody)
3. Renal symptoms develop 2 to 7 days after onset of diarrhea
4. Other organ involvement includes CNS, pulmonary, cardiac, pancreatic, and hepatic (elevated transaminases)
5. **Treatment:** supportive; 60% require dialysis
6. **Prognosis:** varies, long-term follow-up required
   a. 2% to 4% mortality; 5% CKD with possible need for renal replacement therapy
   b. 20% proteinuria/HTN, can occur up to 5 years after HUS
   c. No recurrence after transplant

B. Atypical hemolytic uremic syndrome

1. Due to genetic mutations in complement components, majority are sporadic
2. Presents similarly to STEC HUS–usually triggered by infection e.g., URTI, gastroenteritis including non-bloody diarrhea
3. **Treatment:** eculizumab (anti-C5 antibody) if available, otherwise plasma exchange
4. **Prognosis:** long-term outcome dependent on genetic mutation and treatment response
   a. 6% to 8% mortality
   b. Good long-term renal function with eculizumab
   c. High risk of disease recurrence—continue eculizumab post-transplant

C. Other causes of hemolytic uremic syndrome

1. Infection e.g., *Streptococcus pneumoniae* (DAT-positive), HIV, influenza
2. Cobalamin C deficiency impairing vitamin B12 metabolism
3. Pregnancy and postpartum
4. Solid organ or stem cell/bone marrow transplantation
5. Drugs, e.g., calcineurin inhibitors

ACUTE KIDNEY INJURY

1. **Definition:** decrease in GFR as per KDIGO criteria (Box 28.5)
2. **Etiology and staging:** see Box 28.6 and Table 28.11

Box 28.5 KDIGO Criteria for Acute Kidney Injury

Increase in creatinine by 26.5 µmol/L from baseline within 48 h, OR
Increase in creatinine to ≥1.5 times baseline within the prior 7 days, OR
Urine volume ≤0.5 mL/kg/h for 6 h

KDIGO, Kidney Disease: Improving Global Outcomes.

Taken from https://kdigo.org/wp-content/uploads/2016/10/KDIGO-2012-AKI-Guideline-English.pdf.

Box 28.6 Etiology of Acute Kidney Injury

Prerenal
Volume depletion: diarrhea, vomiting, osmotic diuresis, burns, hemorrhage
↓ Effective circulating volume: septic shock, anaphylactic shock, nephrotic syndrome
Cardiac: ↓ function, ↓ systemic blood flow (anatomic malformation), arrhythmia, tamponade

Intrinsic Renal
Glomerular: PSGN, lupus nephritis, HSP, IgA nephropathy, crescentic GN, SBE, MPGN/C3G
Vascular/hemodynamic: HUS, renal vein thrombosis, vasculitis, malignant HTN, NSAIDs, ACE inhibitors
Tubular (ATN): uncorrected prerenal or postrenal acute kidney injury, hypoxemia, obstruction by
  crystals, medications, toxins, tumor lysis syndrome
Interstitial nephritis: allergic interstitial nephritis, malignant infiltrates, pyelonephritis, sarcoidosis

Postrenal
UPJ/UVJ obstruction, obstructive nephrolithiasis, neoplasm, PUV, urolithiasis

ACE, Angiotensin-converting enzyme; *ATN*, acute tubular necrosis; *C3G*, C3 glomerulopathy;
FSGS, focal segmental glomerulosclerosis; *GN*, glomerulonephritis; *HSP*, Henoch-Schönlein
purpura; *HTN*, hypertension; *HUS*, hemolytic uremic syndrome; *IgA*, immunoglobulin A;
MPGN, membranoproliferative glomerulonephritis; *NSAIDs*, non-steroidal anti-inflammatory
drugs; *PSGN*, post-streptococcal glomerulonephritis; *PUV*, posterior urethral valves; *SBE*, subacute
bacterial endocarditis; *UPJ*, ureteropelvic junction; *UVJ*, ureterovesical junction.

Table 28.11 KDIGO Staging of Acute Kidney Injury

Stage	Serum Creatinine	Urine Output
1	1.5–1.9 times baseline, OR ≥26.5 µmol/L increase	<0.5 mL/kg/h for 6–12 h
2	2–2.9 times baseline	<0.5 mL/kg/h for ≥12 h
3	3 times baseline, OR Increase in serum creatinine to ≥353.6 µmol/L, OR Initiation of renal replacement therapy, OR Decrease in eGFR to <35 mL/min/1.73 m^2	<0.3 mL/kg/h for ≥24 h, OR Anuria for ≥12 h

eGFR, Estimated glomerular filtration rate.

Source: https://kdigo.org/wp-content/uploads/2016/10/KDIGO-2012-AKI-Guideline-English.pdf.

3. **Clinical presentation**
   a. Fluid overload or dehydration, altered perfusion, HTN, altered
      mental status

b. Anorexia, nausea, vomiting, abdominal pain, flank pain, urinary symptoms
c. Rash, joint involvement
d. Anemia, platelet dysfunction
e. Hyperkalemia, metabolic acidosis, hyperphosphatemia, hypocalcemia, uremia

4. **Investigations**
   a. **Urine:** urinalysis, Na, Cr
   b. **Blood:** Cr, urea, extended electrolytes, bicarbonate, albumin, CBC
   c. **Imaging:** renal Doppler US
   d. If glomerular origin of AKI, refer to previous sections (Proteinuria, Hematuria) for further workup of underlying disease

5. **Management**
   a. Largely consists of management of underlying condition, fluid and metabolic derangements
   b. **Treat metabolic acidosis:** oral sodium citrate, oral or IV sodium bicarbonate, consider dialysis if persistent
   c. **Treat hyperkalemia and hyperphosphatemia:** see relevant sections in Chapter 15 Fluids, Electrolytes, and Acid-Base
   d. **Treat hypocalcemia:** resolves with correction of hyperphosphatemia and oral/dietary calcium supplementation; give IV calcium gluconate or calcium chloride if evidence of tetany
   e. Adjust medications for degree of renal failure
   f. Avoid further injury from nephrotoxins and contrast agents
   g. Careful fluid management
      i. **Euvolemia:** give insensible losses + urine output + other losses
      ii. **Dehydration:** give deficit + insensible losses + urine output + other losses
      iii. **Fluid overload:** give insensible losses + urine output – estimated volume of fluid to be deficited over given time period

CHRONIC KIDNEY DISEASE

1. Abnormalities of kidney structure or function, present for >3 months, with implications for health
2. **Classification:** based on cause, GFR category (G1–G5) and albuminuria category (A1–A3) (Table 28.12)
3. **Clinical presentation**
   a. Often insidious, highly variable
   b. **Antenatal:** oligohydramnios or polyhydramnios
   c. **Childhood:** FTT, fatigue, headache, anorexia, nausea, vomiting, pallor, rickets, edema, HTN
   d. **Adolescent:** as for childhood ± delayed puberty, anemia
   e. **Less common:** pruritus, peripheral neuropathy

Table 28.12	**KDIGO Classification of Chronic Kidney Disease**	
Stage	Description	GFR (mL/min/1.73 m²)
1	Kidney damage with normal or ↑ GFR	≥90
2	Kidney damage with mildly ↓ GFR	60–89
3a	Mild to moderately ↓ GFR	45–59
3b	Moderate to severely ↓ GFR	30–44
4	Severely ↓ GFR	15–29
5	Kidney failure	≤15, or patient on dialysis

GFR, Glomerular filtration rate; *KDIGO*, Kidney Disease: Improving Global Outcome.

Data from Levin A, Stevens PE. Summary of KDIGO 2012 CKD Guideline: behind the scenes, need for guidance, and a framework for moving forward. *Kidney Int.* 2014;85(1):49–61.

4. **Complications**
   a. **Renal osteodystrophy**
      i. **Etiology:** osteitis fibrosa (high bone turnover) or adynamic bone disease (low turnover)
      ii. **Monitor:** ionized calcium, phosphate, ALP, PTH, Vitamin D
      iii. **Treatment:** low-phosphate diet, phosphate binders (calcium carbonate, calcium acetate, sevelamer), cholecalciferol, and activated vitamin D
   b. **Growth failure**
      i. **Multifactorial etiology:** inadequate calorie and protein intake, renal osteodystrophy, metabolic acidosis, anemia, deranged growth hormone–insulin-like growth factor axis
   c. **Anemia**
      i. Normochromic, normocytic anemia with low reticulocyte count
      ii. **Etiology:** reduced erythropoietin production, bone marrow inhibition, iron/B12/folate deficiency, osteitis fibrosa
      iii. **Treatment:** iron supplementation ± erythropoietin replacement
5. **Management**
   a. **Monitor bloodwork:** Hb, extended electrolytes, Cr, urea, albumin, bicarbonate, iron studies
      i. PTH, vitamin D levels to detect renal osteodystrophy
   b. **Monitor urine:** for proteinuria; may consider ACE inhibitors in early stages
   c. **CVS:** serial echocardiograms, ABPM, manage HTN as indicated
   d. **Nutrition:** optimize intake; may require enteral tube feeding if unable to meet recommended calories
   e. **Medications:** adjust for degree of renal impairment, avoid nephrotoxic drugs, e.g., NSAIDs
   f. Growth hormone, erythropoietin if required

RENAL REPLACEMENT THERAPY

1. See Table 28.13 for indications and Table 28.14 for modalities

Table 28.13	Indications for Renal Replacement Therapy
Short-Term	**Long-Term**
Refractory hyperkalemia with ECG abnormalities HTN or congestive heart failure secondary to fluid overload Severe uremic pericarditis Uremic encephalopathy Toxins, poisons Refractory acidosis Inborn errors of metabolism	GFR <15 mL/min/1.73 m^2 Fluid overload Symptomatic uremia (nausea, anorexia, lethargy) Uncontrolled biochemical abnormalities

ECG, Electrocardiogram; *GFR*, glomerular filtration rate; *HTN*, hypertension.

Table 28.14	Modalities for Renal Replacement Therapy		
	Hemodialysis	**Peritoneal Dialysis**	**CRRT**
Advantages	Rapid ultrafiltration and solute clearance	Easy access and technically simple Better option for infants Continuous and gradual ultrafiltration and solute clearance No need for systemic anticoagulation	Continuous ultrafiltration and solute clearance Usually tolerated even with cardiac instability
Technical aspects	Double-lumen venous catheters used for short-term dialysis Arteriovenous fistula preferred in children and teenagers receiving long-term dialysis	Continuous ambulatory peritoneal dialysis (CAPD): manual process of exchange Automated peritoneal dialysis (APD): use of cycler	Used in an ICU setting Continuous venovenous hemofiltration (CVVH) Continuous venovenous hemodialysis (CVVHD) Continuous venovenous hemodiafiltration (CVVHDF)
Complications	Vascular access dysfunction Clotting of extracorporeal circuit Hypotension Infection Bleeding	Exit site and tunnel infections Peritonitis Leakage Hernia, lower back pain Anorexia Caregiver burnout	Similar to hemodialysis

CRRT, Continuous renal replacement therapy; *ICU*, intensive care unit.

RENAL TRANSPLANT

1. Treatment of choice for kidney failure as improves patient survival and quality of life compared with dialysis

. Patients must remain on immunosuppressive medications for the duration of life of the graft (average 10 years)
. **Complications:** see section on Post-transplant Complications in Chapter 38 Transplantation
    a. **Delayed graft function:** need for dialysis during the first post-transplant week
        i. **Risk factors:** deceased donor transplant, increased cold ischemia time, surgical complications
    b. **Graft vascular thrombosis:** occlusion of the vascular anastamoses by blood clot
    c. **Recurrence of primary disease:** monitor patients with nephrotic syndrome, atypical HUS, membranous nephropathy
    d. **Infection:** see section on Infection in Chapter 38 Transplantation
    e. **Rejection:** marked by increased Cr, confirmed by renal biopsy (gold standard)
    f. **Malignancy:** chronic immunosuppressive medications increase the risk of cancer, particularly post-transplant lymphoproliferative disorders (see relevant section in Chapter 38 Transplantation)
    g. **Chronic allograft nephropathy:** gradual worsening of graft function over time; factors include subclinical immunological damage, calcineurin inhibitor toxicity, non-adherence to medications, fluid mismanagement, HTN

RENAL STONES

. **Clinical presentation:** UTI, dysuria; abdominal/flank pain; microscopic or macroscopic hematuria
    a. May be asymptomatic, incidental finding
2. **Etiology**
    a. See Box 28.7

Box 28.7   Etiology of Renal Stones
Idiopathic (25%)	Ketogenic diet
Underlying metabolic disease	Stasis or obstruction
Medications, e.g., anticonvulsants, diuretics, adrenocorticotropin hormone, corticosteroids, antibiotics, calcineurin inhibitors	Infection

3. **Investigations**
    a. **Compositional analysis:** of passed stone or sediment from strained urine
    b. **Abdominal x-ray:** calcium oxalate and calcium phosphate stones are densely opaque; struvite and cystine stones have intermediate density; uric acid stones are radiolucent

c. **US:** assess size and location of stones, renal parenchyma, urinary tract anatomy, signs of obstruction, nephrocalcinosis

d. **Blood:** extended electrolytes, Cr, urea, Ca, albumin, uric acid, bicarbonate, ALP

e. **Urine:** urinalysis, pH, culture, Ca, PO_4, oxalate, citrate, uric acid, cystine/amino acids, Cr; 24-hour collection most accurate

4. **Treatment**

a. **High fluid intake:** >2 L/1.73 m^2/day, preferably as water

b. **Low salt diet:** reduces urinary calcium excretion

c. **Specific therapies:** based on underlying disorder and stone type (see below)

d. **Surgical correction:** of anatomic abnormalities predisposing to stones or infection

e. **Lithotripsy:** for large stones, refractory cases

NEPHROCALCINOSIS

1. Calcium deposition in renal tubules and interstitium

2. Most commonly associated with idiopathic hypercalciuria, furosemide use, prematurity, tubular disorders (e.g., distal renal tubular acidosis [RTA], Bartter syndrome)

3. **Clinical presentation:** hematuria, nephrolithiasis, renal tubular acidosis, CKD

4. **Treatment:** hydration, citrate, thiazide diuretics

DIFFERENTIAL DIAGNOSIS BY STONE COMPOSITION
A. Calcium

1. Majority of urinary calculi in children

2. **Types:** calcium phosphate (precipitates in alkaline urine), calcium oxalate (precipitates in acidic urine)

3. Laboratory findings indicate pathogenesis

a. **Hypercalcemia:** hyperparathyroidism, hyperthyroidism, hypervitaminosis D, immobilization

b. **Normocalcemic hypercalciuria:** familial, sporadic, tubular disorders, drugs (e.g., furosemide, antiepileptics), ketogenic diet

c. **Hyperoxaluria:** intestinal malabsorption, pyridoxine deficiency, increased vitamin C intake, increased oxalate intake or inherited metabolic disorder

d. **Hypocitraturia:** dietary, renal tubular acidosis, idiopathic

e. **Treatment:** as above, and

i. **Thiazide diuretics:** reduce urinary calcium excretion by increasing tubular calcium reabsorption

ii. **Potassium citrate:** inhibits calcium stone formation

B. Cystine

1. Cystinuria characterized by autosomal recessive inherited defect in renal tubular reabsorptive transport of cystine and dibasic amino acids (ornithine, arginine, lysine)

2. **Treatment:** increased fluid intake, urine alkalinization, chelating agents

C. Magnesium ammonium phosphate (struvite)

1. Precipitates in alkaline urine

2. Associated with UTI because of urea-splitting organisms (commonly *Proteus*)

D. Uric acid

1. Precipitates in acidic urine

2. Uncommon in childhood

3. **Causes:** tumor lysis syndrome, lymphoproliferative or myeloproliferative disorders, gout, Lesch-Nyhan syndrome, G6PD deficiency, short gut

4. **Treatment:** increased fluid intake, dietary purine restriction, urinary alkalinization, allopurinol trial

TUBULAR DISORDERS

A. Renal tubular acidosis

1. Heterogeneous group of disorders presenting with normal anion gap metabolic acidosis, hyperchloremia, and tubular dysfunction; see Table 28.15

Table 28.15	Types of Renal Tubular Acidosis		
	Type 1: Distal RTA	**Type 2: Proximal RTA**	**Type 4: Hyperkalemic RTA**
Pathogenesis	Impaired acid excretion in the distal tubule	Impaired bicarbonate reabsorption in the proximal tubule	Reduced production or response to aldosterone, causing impaired ammoniagenesis
Etiology	Genetic Acquired: drugs, renal disease, sickle cell disease, autoimmune (e.g., Sjögren)	Genetic Drugs (e.g., acetazolamide, topiramate)	Primary hypoaldosteronism Pseudohypoaldosteronism: aldosterone resistance caused by drugs (e.g., NSAIDs, ACE inhibitors, ARBs, spironolactone, trimethoprim) or obstructive uropathy
Clinical presentation	Rickets/osteomalacia Nephrocalcinosis/stones	Failure to thrive	Hyperkalemia

Continued 791

Table 28.15	Types of Renal Tubular Acidosis—cont'd		
	Type 1: Distal RTA	**Type 2: Proximal RTA**	**Type 4: Hyperkalemic RTA**
Lab findings	Urine pH > 5.5 Positive UNC Low serum K	Urine pH < 5.5 Negative UNC Low serum K	Urine pH < 5.5 Negative UNC High serum K
Treatment	Alkali therapy with sodium or potassium salts	Alkali therapy with potassium supplementation	Treat hyperkalemia Potassium restriction Sodium supplementation Alkali therapy Fludrocortisone

ACE, Angiotensin-converting enzyme; *ARB,* angiotensin receptor blocker; *NSAID,* non-steroidal anti-inflammatory drug; *RTA,* renal tubular acidosis; *UNC,* urine net charge.

B. Renal Fanconi syndrome

1. Proximal RTA with glycosuria, phosphaturia, aminoaciduria, and low-molecular-weight proteinuria
2. **Primary genetic or metabolic causes:** Dent or Lowe syndrome, cystinosis, Wilson disease, galactosemia, mitochondrial disorders
3. **Acquired causes:** myeloma, drugs (e.g., ifosfamide, cisplatin, antiretrovirals, aminoglycosides), heavy metals
4. **Lab findings:** urine pH < 5.5, low serum bicarbonate, low potassium, elevated chloride

C. Bartter syndrome

1. Autosomal recessive genetic disorder
2. Failure of Na and Cl reabsorption leads to salt wasting, urinary Mg and Ca loss, polyuria, and volume depletion, causing activation of aldosterone
3. **Clinical presentation:** hypochloremic metabolic alkalosis, hypokalemia hypercalciuria
4. **Treatment:** electrolyte replacement, potassium-sparing diuretic, NSAID

D. Gitelman syndrome

1. Mutation in thiazide-sensitive apical NaCl co-transporter causes mild salt loss
2. Often asymptomatic, diagnosed incidentally in late childhood or adulthood
3. **Clinical presentation:** hypokalemia and metabolic alkalosis with hypomagnesemia, hypocalciuria
4. **Treatment:** electrolyte replacement

E. Hereditary nephrogenic diabetes insipidus

1. Genetic mutations cause resistance to vasopressin

2. Acquired form caused by lithium
3. See section on Diabetes Insipidus in Chapter 14 Endocrinology for presentation, workup, and management

SCROTAL DISORDERS

1. **The acute scrotum:** new onset pain, swelling and/or tenderness of intrascrotal contents
2. **Physical examination**
   a. General and abdominal examination: important for referred and systemic causes of pain
   b. Always examine normal testis first
   c. Identify erythema, swelling, skin integrity, discharge, position of testes
   d. Changes in scrotal size with position or Valsalva
      i. Swelling may increase with Valsalva in inguinal hernia, communicating hydrocele or varicocele
      ii. Swelling may decrease when supine in varicocele
      iii. Varicoele in pre-pubertal males and right-sided varicocele in any age should prompt an abdominal US to rule out intra-abdominal mass
   e. Cremasteric reflex: stroking medial thigh should cause elevation of ipsilateral testicle
      i. Intact reflex makes testicular torsion highly unlikely
   f. Transilluminate any masses
      i. Hydrocele and spermatocele will transilluminate
      ii. Tumors and varicocele will not
3. **Investigations**
   a. Testicular torsion can be diagnosed presumptively on the basis of history and examination
   b. **Scrotal Doppler US:** to evaluate perfusion of testis (Table 28.16)
   c. **Sexually transmitted infection screening:** if sexually active; gram stain, culture, nucleic acid amplification testing of urine or urethral discharge; see section on Genital Infections in Chapter 20 Gynecology
   d. **Urinalysis and urine culture:** pyuria in epididymitis
   e. Bloodwork, including CBC, not routinely recommended; may detect leucocytosis in torsion or epididymitis
4. **Differential diagnosis:** see Table 28.16

> ### ✳ PEARL
>
> Patients with suspected testicular torsion should be referred urgently for evaluation and Urology consult, as extended periods of ischemia (>6 h) may cause infarction of the testis requiring orchidectomy. Obtaining imaging should not delay surgical exploration if clinical findings are in keeping with testicular torsion.

Table 28.16	Approach to the Acute Scrotum by Diagnosis			
Diagnosis	**Etiology**	**History**	**Physical Examination**	**Investigations**
Testicular torsion	Torsion of spermatic cord	Perinatal/pubertal Sudden onset severe pain Usually no preceding trauma	High-riding testis with transverse lie ("bell-clapper") Cremasteric reflex usually absent	Doppler US: decreased/ absent parenchymal perfusion compared to normal testis
Appendage torsion	Torsion of the appendix testis or epididymis	Prepubertal Abrupt or gradual onset of pain, usually at superior pole of testis	Blue dot (rare) Cremasteric reflex usually present Tender nodule at upper pole	Doppler US: normal or increased perfusion
Epididymitis	UTI, STI, viral, chemical, traumatic	Infant/ postpubertal Gradual onset of symptoms Fever common Urinary symptoms	Swelling Erythema	Pyuria common ± positive urine culture CBC: leukocytosis Doppler US: normal or increased perfusion
Orchitis	Viral, STI, vasculitis May be associated with epididymitis	Recent viral infection ± fever New testicular pain and swelling	Testis tenderness Swelling Erythema Normal cremasteric reflex	Doppler US: may show increased vascularity, scrotal wall thickening, enlarged testicle, hydrocele
Trauma	Hematocele, testicular fracture	Preceding trauma	Hematocele Swelling	Doppler US: may show hematocele, abnormal testicular contour/ vascularity
Inguinal hernia	Patent processus vaginalis (before puberty)	Intermittent bulge Incarceration: irritability, persistent bulge, symptoms/signs of bowel obstruction	May be normal if hernia is reduced Bulge along inguinal canal with Valsalva	Clinical diagnosis US: may show omentum or bowel in hernial sac, hydrocele
Musculoskeletal or referred pain	Varied, e.g., inguinal tendonitis or muscle strain, ureteral calculus, lumbar pathologies	Based on differential diagnosis	Testicular/scrotal examination normal	Based on differential diagnosis Testicular US: normal

CBC, Complete blood count; *STI*, sexually transmitted infection; *US*, ultrasound; *UTI*, urinary tract infection.

PHIMOSIS

1. Narrowed opening of the prepuce that results in non-retractile foreskin

A. Physiological phimosis

1. Present at birth because of adhesions between the glans and inner preputial skin
2. Foreskin may balloon with voiding but urine drains spontaneously
3. Separation of the glans and foreskin occurs gradually, usually by the onset of puberty; does not require medical attention

B. Pathological phimosis

1. White, scarred ring at preputial outlet: may crack and bleed; no response to topical steroid
   a. May be caused by balanitis xerotica obliterans (BXO): chronic infiltrative and cicatrizing skin condition (lichen sclerosus of the penis)
   b. Enquire about obstructive urinary symptoms to outrule urethral stricture
2. Severe ballooning of the foreskin with voiding, need to milk foreskin to pass urine: rare, most likely to occur in infants
3. Urine stream changes: thin stream, spraying, dribbling, straining to urinate
4. Recurrent balanoposthitis requiring oral antibiotics
5. Recurrent UTIs
6. May be secondary to forceful/traumatic retraction, complications from previous circumcision or penile surgery

C. Management of phimosis

1. Parents should not attempt to manually retract the foreskin at any age
   a. Only retract as much as easily possible without force
   b. Clean accessible areas during bathing
2. **Indications for treatment:** primary pathological phimosis, secondary phimosis, recurrent balanitis/posthitis, BXO, recurrent UTI in patients <1 year old
3. **Topical corticosteroid creams:** few side effects
   a. Use for 6 weeks only; can repeat course 2 to 6 weeks later if no or only partial improvement seen
   b. Apply within the preputial outlet and not externally (squeezable tube prescription or with a cotton swab)
4. **Circumcision:** irreversible; risk of complications, particularly bleeding in older boys

PARAPHIMOSIS

1. Trapping of foreskin in retracted position causes ischemia, swelling and pain of foreskin and glans, requiring prompt reduction or surgical release
2. Usually iatrogenic (foreskin left retracted after manipulation) or caused by phimosis
3. **Management**
   a. Decrease edema and facilitate reduction using manual compression of the glans between fingers (Figure 28.4) or a compressive elastic dressing
   b. Sedation and pre-emptive analgesia may help (local, e.g., EMLA; systemic, e.g., midazolam, ketamine)
   c. Dorsal slit can be performed under local analgesia (penile block) if manual reduction is unsuccessful
   d. Patient should be offered circumcision after the acute phase has resolved (questionable if iatrogenic)

Figure 28.4   Manual Reduction of Paraphimosis

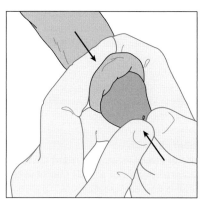

(From Buttaravoli P, Leffler SM, eds. *Minor Emergencies.* 3rd ed. Philadelphia, PA: Elsevier Inc.; 2012.)

PENILE INFECTION AND INFLAMMATION

1. **Balanoposthitis:** inflammation of both glans (balanitis) and preputial skin (posthitis)
   a. Mostly self-limiting, local hygiene recommendations
   b. Occasionally require topical antibiotics
   c. True infection (i.e., cellulitis) is painful, requires oral antibiotics
2. **Smegma:** whitish discharge from under foreskin caused by normal desquamated skin cells and mucus; often misinterpreted as pus/infection
   a. Need reassurance only

3. **Reddened foreskin:** minimal inflammation at tip of foreskin, common in infants wearing diapers; usually not worrisome
   a. Local measures: barrier ointment (e.g., petroleum jelly), dry after voiding

HYPOSPADIAS

1. Congenital termination of the urethra on the ventral penile surface, proximal to the normal glanular location (Figure 28.5)

Figure 28.5   Classification of Hypospadias

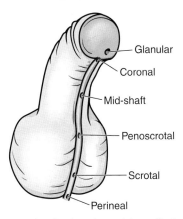

- Glanular
- Coronal
- Mid-shaft
- Penoscrotal
- Scrotal
- Perineal

(Modified from Fraser D. Hemolytic disorders and congenital anomalies. In: Lowdermilk DL, Perry SE, Cashion K, Alden KR, eds. *Maternity & Women's Health Care.* 11th ed. Fig. 36.12.)

2. **Clinical presentation**
   a. Usually an isolated anomaly
   b. **Recurrence risk in first-degree relatives:** enquire about family history
   c. **Common associations:** dorsal hooded foreskin and ventral skin deficiency
   d. **Other associations:** ventral curvature, downward tilt of the glans, deviation of the penile median raphe, scrotal webbing, penoscrotal transposition

3. **Management**
   a. **Karyotype:** to rule out a disorder of sexual development if hypospadias associated with at least one undescended testis (particularly if non-palpable)

b. **Surgical repair after 6 months of age:** non-mandatory—discuss thoroughly with family

c. Inform families not to circumcise newborns with hypospadias, as preputial skin often used to reconstruct urethra or skin coverage

BLADDER DISORDERS

ENURESIS

1. **Monosymptomatic enuresis:** urinary incontinence during sleep in children >5 years of age, in the absence of a neurological disorder
2. **Nonmonosymptomatic enuresis:** wets during day and night-time, i.e., daytime urinary incontinence and enuresis
3. **Primary enuresis:** child has never been dry at night for >6 months
4. **Secondary enuresis:** previously dry for >6 months
5. **Etiology**
   a. Multifactorial pathophysiology with strong genetic component
   b. Maturational delay in development of bladder control
6. **Investigation**
   a. **History:** including voiding diary, thorough physical examination
   b. **Urinalysis:** glycosuria, proteinuria, rule out infection
   c. **Secondary enuresis:** rule out bladder and bowel dysfunction, underlying medical conditions, e.g., diabetes, spinal dysraphism, neurological disease
7. **Management**
   a. **Two categories of treatment:** behavioral and pharmacotherapy
   b. Base decision to treat or not on the degree of concern and motivation of the child
   c. **Optimize bladder and bowel habits**
      i. Regular voids (q2h), void before bedtime
      ii. Avoid sugary and caffeinated drinks
      iii. Optimise daily fluid intake during day, reduce fluid intake after dinner (80% before 4 pm, 20% after)
      iv. Prevent/manage constipation
   d. **Enuresis alarm:** most effective long-term treatment in monosymptomatic enuresis
      i. Only effective if child is motivated
      ii. Caregiver will need to wake child when alarm goes off for first few weeks of treatment
      iii. Discontinue if no improvement after 6 weeks
   e. **Desmopressin:** desmopressin (DDAVP) melts
      i. Most efficient in children with nocturnal polyuria and normal bladder capacity
      ii. High rates of recurrence, but helpful for short-term use in special situations, e.g., camp, sleepovers

iii. Recommend taking 1 hour before bed, no fluid intake up to 8 hours after ingestion to decrease risk of hyponatremia

iv. Hold treatment during episodes of fluid/electrolyte imbalance, e.g., gastroenteritis

f. **Anticholinergics:** e.g., oxybutynin; usually second-line therapy after failure of alarm and DDAVP

g. **Tricyclic antidepressants:** rarely used because of poor results and significant side effects

ADDER AND BOWEL DYSFUNCTION

Spectrum includes

a. **Lower urinary tract conditions:** e.g., overactive bladder and urge incontinence, voiding postponement, underactive bladder, and voiding dysfunction

b. **Bowel issues:** e.g., constipation and encopresis

The stool-loaded rectum compresses the bladder and decreases its capacity, leading to urgency, frequency, or incomplete bladder emptying

Children who voluntarily hold urine for longer periods will gradually present with decreased sensation of the urge to evacuate, thus establishing the bladder and bowel dysfunction (BBD) cycle pattern

Investigations: see Figure 28.6

a. **History:** voiding schedule and symptomatology, bowel habit, medical and family history, antenatal history, developmental milestones, toilet training, neuropsychiatric comorbidities, social history, diet, previous UTIs

b. **Bladder diary:** fluid intake, frequency and volume of each void over 48 hours

c. **Physical examination:** genitourinary anatomy (meatal stenosis, labial adhesions, vaginal reflux), neurological (including lower back for spinal dysraphism, power, reflexes), abdominal (constipation)

d. **Urine:** urinalysis and culture

e. **US:** anatomic details of the kidneys, bladder, and rectum (hydronephrosis, bladder wall thickness, constipation); can be used for post-void residual

f. **Uroflowmetry and urodynamics:** rarely indicated

Management: see Figure 28.6

a. Tailor treatment to individual patient

b. **Urotherapy:** as with enuresis management, optimal voiding posture, treatment of constipation, support and encourage patient

c. **Rarely needed:** biofeedback, anticholinergics, α-adrenergic receptor antagonists, Botox, neuromodulation, clean intermittent catheterization (CIC)

Figure 28.6 Approach to Managing Bladder and Bowel Dysfunction

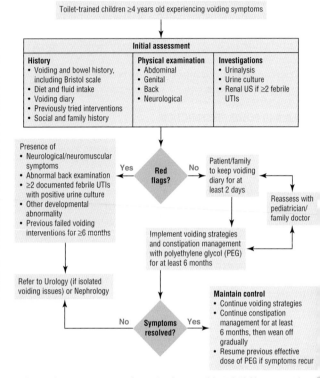

US, Ultrasound; *UTI,* urinary tract infection. (© The Hospital for Sick Children, 2012. Adapted from The Hospital for Sick Children Management of Bladder and Bowel Dysfunction in Children Over 4 Years Clinical Practice Guideline.)

NEUROGENIC BLADDER

1. **Congenital:** e.g., neural tube defect, sacral agenesis, anorectal malformations
2. **Acquired:** e.g., pelvic surgery, central nervous system insults, spinal cord insults
3. Most common cause in children is abnormal development of the spinal canal and spinal cord
4. **Investigations**
   a. **Post-void residual:** measure by renal US or catheterization after 48 to 72 hours of life
   b. **Urinalysis and Cr:** send after first week of life if abnormal upper tracts, to document the infant's, rather than mother's, renal function
   c. **Renal US**

d. **Urodynamic studies:** usually delayed

e. **VCUG:** recommended if hydronephrosis seen on ultrasound

5. **Management**

   a. **Early management with CIC and anticholinergics:** proven to improve outcomes

   b. **Low sphincter tone:** α-adrenergic medication (e.g., pseudoephedrine) or surgery

   c. **Unstable detrusor muscle function:** oxybutynin (anticholinergic) ± CIC ± detrusor botox ± surgery if refractory to medical/CIC therapy

   d. Approximately half of those requiring CIC develop latex allergy (acquired IgE-mediated, secondary to repeated exposure); all myelomeningocele patients should follow latex precautions

   e. Control concomitant constipation

6. **Follow-up**

   a. Urological history (continence, UTIs), physical examination

   b. **US:** renal growth and hydronephrosis, bladder stones

   c. **VCUG:** bladder capacity, new trabeculation, diverticulae, VUR

   d. **Urodynamic studies:** capacity, compliance (filling at low pressure to protect upper tract), detrusor stability (uninhibited contractions), adequate emptying

---

✳ PEARL

These red flags for voiding dysfunction warrant urgent specialist review

- **Central nervous system:** recent onset seizures, developmental delay or regression, focal neurological signs or symptoms
- **Neurogenic bladder:** suggested by abnormal back or lower limb examination
- **Endocrine/renal:** headache, visual change, acromegaly, vomiting, polyuria, polydipsia, weight loss, deranged renal function, proteinuria, hypertension, abnormal renal US (hydronephrosis, renal scarring, cortical scarring, trabeculated bladder)
- **Functional:** Hinman syndrome, i.e., severe non-neurogenic voiding dysfunction with dilated upper tracts on US
- **Neuromuscular:** e.g., proximal muscle weakness

FURTHER READING

Wein AJ, Kavoussi LR, Campbell MF, Walsh PC. *Campbell-Walsh Urology*. Philadelphia, PA: Elsevier Saunders; 2012.

Geary D, Schaefer F. *Pediatric Kidney Disease.* 2nd ed. Berlin, Germany: Springer-Verlag Berlin Heidelberg; 2016.

USEFUL WEBSITES

The National Kidney Foundation, Kidney Disease Outcomes Quality Initiative. Available at: www.kidney.org/professionals/KDOQI

Kidney Disease: Improving Global Outcome (KDIGO). Available at: www.kdigo.org

CUA Guidelines. Available at: https://www.cua.org/en/guidelines

Neurology and Neurosurgery

Djurdja Djordjevic • Nurin Chatur • Tina Go • Abhaya Kulkarni • Liza Pulcine

COMMON ABBREVIATIONS

Also see page xviii for a list of other abbreviations used throughout this book

ACTH	adrenocorticotropic hormone
ADEM	acute disseminated encephalomyelitis
AED	antiepileptic drug
AVM	arteriovenous malformation
CSF	cerebrospinal fluid
CK	creatine kinase
CSVT	cerebral sinovenous thrombosis
CTA	computed tomography angiogram
CTV	computed tomography venogram
EEG	electroencephalography
EMG	electromyography
GCS	Glasgow Coma Scale
ICH	intracranial hemorrhage
ICP	intracranial pressure
IEM	inborn errors of metabolism
LOC	level of consciousness
LMN	lower motor neuron
LP	lumbar puncture
MRA	magnetic resonance angiogram
MRI	magnetic resonance imaging
MRV	magnetic resonance venogram
MS	multiple sclerosis
NCS	nerve conduction studies
SJS	Stevens-Johnson syndrome
TIA	transient ischemic attack
TMJ	temporomandibular joint
TS	tuberous sclerosis
VP	ventriculoperitoneal
UMN	upper motor neuron

NEUROLOGICAL EXAMINATION

1. **Physical examination:** see Table 29.1
2. **Dermatomes:** see Figures 29.1A and 29.1B
3. **Primative and secondary reflexes:** see Box 29.1

Table 29.1	Neurological Examination
Components	**Description**
Mental status	Mini-mental State Examination (MMSE) Montreal Cognitive Assessment (MOCA)
Language	Fluency, comprehension, repetition, naming, reading, and writing
Cranial nerves	I: Smell
	II: Visual acuity with Snellen chart, color vision, visual fields, optokinetic nystagmus, fundoscopy, pupillary light reflex (afferent limb)
	III, IV, VI: Extraocular movements, pupillary light reflex (efferent limb III)
	V: Light touch (V_1, V_2, V_3), corneal reflex (afferent limb), sneeze reflex, muscles of mastication: masseter, temporalis, medial, and lateral pterygoids, jaw jerk reflex
	VII: Salivation, lacrimation, taste (anterior 2/3 of tongue); muscles of facial expression: show teeth, raise eyebrows, and squeeze eyes shut; upper motor neuron lesion (forehead sparing) vs. lower motor neuron lesion (involving all muscles of facial expression on one side); corneal reflex (efferent limb), blink reflex, hyperacusis
	VIII: Nystagmus (vestibular), hearing—Rinne/Weber (auditory)
	IX, X: Swallowing, gag reflex, movements of the uvula and palate, phonation, articulation, taste (posterior 1/3 tongue—IX)
	XI: Trapezius (shoulder shrug) and sternocleidomastoid (contralateral cervical rotation)
	XII: Tongue protrusion and lateral movements
Motor	Muscle bulk, tone, power, deep tendon reflexes, pronator drift, involuntary movements
Sensory	Primary modalities: light touch, pain/temperature, vibration, and proprioception Secondary modalities: two-point discrimination, graphesthesia, stereognosis Romberg testing for proprioception/vibration
Coordination	Posture, titubation, nystagmus, dysarthria, finger-to-nose, heel-to-shin, rapid alternating movements
Gait	Heel, toe, tandem gait, balance on each foot independently

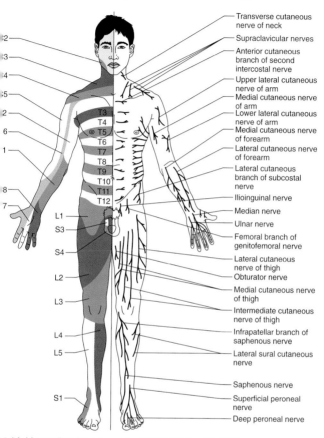

Figure 29.1A Anterior Aspect of the Body Showing the Distribution of Cutaneous Nerves on the Right and Dermatomes on the Left

- Transverse cutaneous nerve of neck
- Supraclavicular nerves
- Anterior cutaneous branch of second intercostal nerve
- Upper lateral cutaneous nerve of arm
- Medial cutaneous nerve of arm
- Lower lateral cutaneous nerve of arm
- Medial cutaneous nerve of forearm
- Lateral cutaneous nerve of forearm
- Lateral cutaneous branch of subcostal nerve
- Ilioinguinal nerve
- Median nerve
- Ulnar nerve
- Femoral branch of genitofemoral nerve
- Lateral cutaneous nerve of thigh
- Obturator nerve
- Medial cutaneous nerve of thigh
- Intermediate cutaneous nerve of thigh
- Infrapatellar branch of saphenous nerve
- Lateral sural cutaneous nerve
- Saphenous nerve
- Superficial peroneal nerve
- Deep peroneal nerve

(Modified from Snell R. *Clinical Neuroanatomy for Medical Students*. 5th ed. Baltimore, MD: Lippincott Williams and Wilkins; 2001. Reprinted by permission of Lippincott Williams and Wilkins.)

Neurology and Neurosurgery

29

Figure 29.1B Posterior Aspect of the Body Showing the Distribution of Cutaneous Nerves on the Left and Dermatomes on the Right

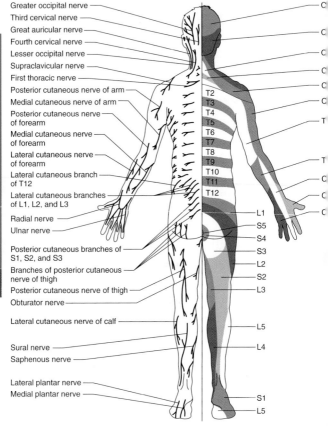

Greater occipital nerve
Third cervical nerve
Great auricular nerve
Fourth cervical nerve
Lesser occipital nerve
Supraclavicular nerve
First thoracic nerve
Posterior cutaneous nerve of arm
Medial cutaneous nerve of arm
Posterior cutaneous nerve of forearm
Medial cutaneous nerve of forearm
Lateral cutaneous nerve of forearm
Lateral cutaneous branch of T12
Lateral cutaneous branches of L1, L2, and L3
Radial nerve
Ulnar nerve
Posterior cutaneous branches of S1, S2, and S3
Branches of posterior cutaneous nerve of thigh
Posterior cutaneous nerve of thigh
Obturator nerve
Lateral cutaneous nerve of calf
Sural nerve
Saphenous nerve
Lateral plantar nerve
Medial plantar nerve

T2
T3
T4
T5
T6
T7
T8
T9
T10
T11
T12
L1
S5
S4
S3
L2
S2
L3
L5
L4
S1
L5

C
C
C
C
C
C
T
T
C
C
C

(Modified from Snell R. *Clinical Neuroanatomy for Medical Students.* 5th ed. Baltimore, MD: Lippincott Williams and Wilkins; 2001. Reprinted by permission of Lippincott Williams and Wilkins.)

Box 29.1   Primitive and Secondary Reflexes[a]

Primitive Reflexes (present at birth; disappear between 3 and 5 months)
Local
- Head: rooting, righting response
- Upper limbs: palmar grasp
- Lower limbs: plantar grasp, placing, stepping

General
- Asymmetric tonic neck reflex
- Moro reflex

Secondary Reflexes (appear between 4 and 10 months and persist)
- Balancing
- Protective: parachute, lateral propping

[a]Abnormalities include absent or asymmetric reflexes, and persistence beyond expected time period

NEUROLOGY TESTS

See Table 29.2

Table 29.2	Neurology Tests
Test Name	**Description**
Opening pressure	Obtained during a lumbar puncture while the patient is in the lateral decubitus position, preferably with the legs straight out Normal range (1–18 years): <28 cm H_2O or <25 cm H_2O if unsedated or non-obese
CSF analysis	CSF appearance, cell count, glucose, protein, gram stain, culture; can also be sent for specific antibody and PCR tests
EEG	Evaluation of the brain's electrical activity obtained by placing leads on the scalp Indications: suspicion of seizure, comatose patient receiving neuromuscular blockade, post-ictal versus subclinical seizures, assessment of prognosis and before weaning an AED
EMG and NCS	Evaluation of the electrical activity of muscle fibers and the motor neurons which innervate them. Distinguishes between disorders of nerve and/or muscle.
MRI brain and spine	High resolution, radiation-free imaging modality that provides information regarding the anatomy of the brain, spine, and detailed soft tissue imaging Gadolinium is used to show enhancement. Indications: infection, tumor, demyelinating disease.
CT brain and spine	Rapid imaging technique of lower resolution that provides good anatomic images of the brain and spine using radiation. Used in acute situations, such as head trauma, suspected stroke or hemorrhage, unexplained loss of consciousness.

AED, Antiepileptic drug; *CSF*, cerebrospinal fluid; *CT*, computed tomography; *EEG*, electroencephalogram; *EMG*, electromyogram; *MRI*, magnetic resonance imaging; *NCS*, nerve conduction studies; *PCR*, polymerase chain reaction.

SEIZURES

1. **Definition:** transient occurrence because of abnormal excessive or synchronous neuronal activity in the brain
2. **Risk of seizure recurrence:** 33% after first unprovoked seizure, 76% after second unprovoked seizure
3. **Epilepsy:** may be diagnosed after either
   a. ≥2 or more unprovoked seizures (absence of concurrent illness/fever or acute brain injury) OR
   b. a single unprovoked seizure if the risk of a second unprovoked seizure is significant
4. **Seizure imitators**
   a. Breath-holding spells (precipitated by trauma, anger, frustration, emotional stress)
   b. Nightmares/night terror
   c. Benign myoclonus of infancy
   d. Migraine
   e. Syncope
   f. Gastroesophageal reflux/Sandifer syndrome
   g. Pseudoseizures (confirmed by normal EEG during an event)
   h. Self-stimulation/stereotypies
5. See Figure 29.2 for classification of seizure types, Table 29.3 for description of seizure types, Figure 29.3 for epilepsy syndromes by age and Table 29.4 for descriptions of selected main seizure syndromes

Figure 29.2   Classification of Seizure Types

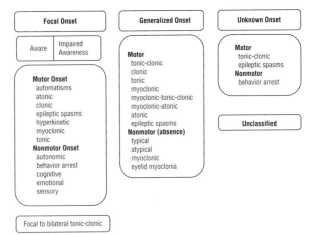

(Adapted from Fisher RS, et al. Instruction Manual for the ILAE 2017 Operational Classification of Seizure Types. *Epilepsia.* 2017;58(4):531–542.)

Table 29.3	Descriptions of Seizure Types (2017 International League Against Epilepsy Classification)	
Seizure Type	**Clinical Features**	**Comments**
Generalized Onset		
Nonmotor: typical absence	Brief, abrupt cessation of activity, changes in facial expressions	Treatment: ethosuximide
	Childhood absence epilepsy: peak age 5–7 years	
	Juvenile absence epilepsy: 10–12 years	
Motor: tonic-clonic	Most common; tonic phase: stiff limbs for 10–30 s; clonic phase: rapid, rhythmic jerks of limbs and trunk	
Motor: clonic	Rhythmic and symmetric contractions of muscle groups	
Motor: tonic	Increased tone in extension; high-pitched cry; <60 s	
Motor: atonic	Sudden loss of muscle tone; rare	Corpus callosotomy for intractable drop seizures
Motor: myoclonic	Brief involuntary muscle contractions; generalized or focal; single or repetitive; rhythmic or irregular	AVOID: oxcarbazepine, carbamazepine, phenytoin, vigabatrin
Focal Onset		
Aware motor onset	Tongue, lips, hands commonly involved; may have spreading to involve other body parts (Jacksonian march)	Treatment: oxcarbazepine or carbamazepine
Aware nonmotor onset: sensory	Numbness or dysesthesias in any body part; abnormal proprioception	Treatment: oxcarbazepine or carbamazepine
Aware nonmotor onset: autonomic	Abdominal discomfort; sweating; dilated pupils; behavioral arrest	Treatment: oxcarbazepine or carbamazepine
Focal onset, impaired awareness	Any focal onset seizure with loss of consciousness	

Figure 29.3 Epilepsy Syndromes by Age

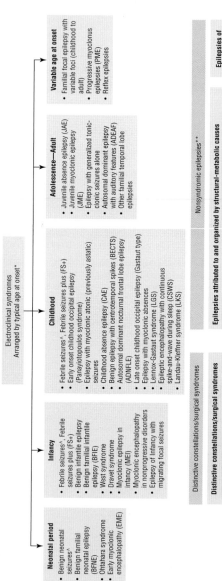

Electroclinical Syndromes and Other Epilepsies Grouped by Specificity of Diagnosis

Electroclinical syndromes
Arranged by typical age at onset*

Neonatal period
- Benign neonatal seizures^
- Benign familial neonatal epilepsy (BFNE)
- Ohtahara syndrome
- Early myoclonic encephalopathy (EME)

Infancy
- Febrile seizures^, Febrile seizures plus (FS+)
- Benign infantile epilepsy
- Benign familial infantile epilepsy (BFIE)
- West syndrome
- Dravet syndrome
- Myoclonic epilepsy in infancy (MEI)
- Myoclonic encephalopathy in nonprogressive disorders
- Epilepsy of Infancy with migrating focal seizures

Childhood
- Febrile seizures^, Febrile seizures plus (FS+)
- Early onset childhood occipital epilepsy (Panayiotopoulos syndrome)
- Epilepsy with myoclonic atonic (previously astatic) seizures
- Childhood absence epilepsy (CAE)
- Benign epilepsy with centrotemporal spikes (BECTS)
- Autosomal dominant nocturnal frontal lobe epilepsy (ADNFLE)
- Late onset childhood occipital epilepsy (Gastaut type)
- Epilepsy with myoclonic absences
- Lennox-Gastaut syndrome (LGS)
- Epileptic encephalopathy with continuous spike-and-wave during sleep (CSWS)
- Landau-Kleffner syndrome (LKS)

Adolescence—Adult
- Juvenile absence epilepsy (JAE)
- Juvenile myoclonic epilepsy (JME)
- Epilepsy with generalized tonic-clonic seizures alone
- Autosomal dominant epilepsy with auditory features (ADEAF)
- Other familial temporal lobe epilepsies

Variable age at onset
- Familial focal epilepsy with variable foci (childhood to adult)
- Progressive myoclonus epilepsies (PME)
- Reflex epilepsies

Nonsyndromic epilepsies**

Epilepsies of unknown cause

Distinctive constellations/surgical syndromes

Distinctive constellations/surgical syndromes
- Mesial temporal lobe epilepsy with hippocampal sclerosis (MTLE with HS)
- Rasmussen syndrome
- Gelastic seizures with hypothalamic hamartoma
- Hemiconvulsion-hemiplegia-epilepsy

Epilepsies attributed to and organized by structural-metabolic causes
- Malformations of cortical development (hemimegalencephaly, heterotopias, etc.)
- Neurocutaneous syndromes (tuberous sclerosis complex, Sturge-Weber, etc.)
- Tumor, infection, trauma, angioma, antenatal and perinatal insults, stroke, etc.

*The arrangement of electroclinical syndromes does not reflct etiology
^Not traditionally diagnosed as epilepsy
**Forms of epilepsies not meeting criteria for specific syndrome or constellations

Table 29.4 **Main Seizure Syndromes**

Seizure Syndrome	Age at Onset	Type of Seizures	Investigations	Treatment
Benign neonatal seizures	First week of life (4–6 days of life)	- Unifocal clonic and rarely focal tonic seizures - Self-limited disorder presenting with seizures within the first week of life; otherwise asymptomatic with normal neurological status between events and family history is negative for early-life seizures	- EEG: normal or *theta pointu alternant*	- Tends to be initiated for acute seizure management and does not have to be continued for long once diagnosis established and hypoglycemia, sepsis, and meningitis excluded
Benign familial neonatal epilepsy	2–3 days of life	- Seizure semiology—hypertonia, apnea, facial movements, clonus, myoclonus, spasms, GTCS - Brief duration, but may cluster and be very frequent - Positive family history	- Causative gene: *KCNQ2* - Transmission by autosomal dominant inheritance with high penetrance with mutation in potassium channel	- Treatment: phenobarbital, levetiracetam - Seizure remission is expected by 6 months of age
Early-onset epileptic encephalopathies—early infantile epileptic encephalopathy (Ohtahara syndrome) and early myoclonic encephalopathy (EME)	First 10 days of life	- Tonic (Ohtahara) - Myoclonic (EME) - Profound neurodevelopmental impairment	- EEG: burst suppression (more prominent in sleep in early myoclonic encephalopathy) - MRI: structural malformations - Genetic epilepsy panel	- Refractory to treatment - Can progress to infantile spasms → Lennox-Gastaut syndrome
Infantile spasms	3–12 months	- Sudden flexion, extension, or mixed flexion-extension movements in proximal and trunk muscles, last 1–2 s, occur in clusters lasting minutes - May have history of seizures, perinatal complications, developmental disability, neurocutaneous disorder - Usually evolve to different seizure disorder by 18 months	- EEG: hypsarrhythmia (most prominent during quiet sleep) - Wood's lamp: neurocutaneous disorders	- First line: ACTH, prednisolone, vigabatrin (treatment of choice in TS) - Majority develop intellectual disability - Underlying etiology most critical predictor of developmental outcome

Continued

Neurology and Neurosurgery

29

Table 29.4 Main Seizure Syndromes—cont'd

Seizure Syndrome	Age at Onset	Type of Seizures	Investigations	Treatment
Early onset childhood occipital epilepsy (Panayiotopoulos syndrome)	3–10 years	- Autonomic symptoms include vomiting, pallor, eye deviation, sweating, ±tonic-clonic movements, nocturnal seizures at sleep onset	- Interictal EEG: multifocal shifting spikes, often occipital, accentuated by sleep	- Treatment not always necessary - If frequent seizures, levetiracetam or oxcarbazepine
Childhood absence epilepsy (CAE)	Peak age 5–7 years	- Typically absence seizures are the only seizure type at presentation, occur very frequently (10–50 times/day) - GTCS can develop but not before adolescence - Brief 20–30 s, triggered by hyperventilation, mild facial myoclonus is common	- EEG: normal background, generalized 3 Hz spike and wave - MRI: normal	- First line: ethosuximide - Second line: valproic acid and lamotrigine - 2/3 achieve seizure control on first or second AED - A minority evolve to juvenile myoclonic epilepsy
Benign epilepsy with centrotemporal spikes (BECTS)	6–13 years	- Nocturnal seizures, hemisensory or motor phenomena of the face, motor findings in limbs	- Interictal EEG: characteristic pattern of centrotemporal spikes	- Treatment not always necessary; avoid sleep deprivation - If frequent seizures, levetiracetam or oxcarbazepine - Most patients outgrow by age 16–18 years
Juvenile absence epilepsy (JAE)	10–12 years	- Healthy children 10–12 years with infrequent absences - 80% of patients have GTCS, usually after onset of absence - 20% minor myoclonic jerks	- EEG: similar to childhood absence epilepsy - MRI: normal	- First line: valproic acid and lamotrigine - Ethosuximide may be efficacious for absence, monotherapy not advised as ineffective for GTCS - Lifelong condition
Juvenile myoclonic epilepsy (JME)	12–18 years	- Neurodevelopmentally typical individuals, slight female predilection - GTCS provoked by sleep deprivation, alcohol ingestion, exposure to flashing lights - Early morning myoclonic jerks triggered by sleep deprivation often attributed to "nervousness" or "clumsiness"	- Interictal EEG: paroxysmal generalized 4–6 Hz polyspike and wave discharges on a normal background, photosensitivity - MRI: normal	- Pharmacoresponsive, but lifelong therapy needed - First line: valproic acid (avoid in females of child-bearing age), lamotrigine, and levetiracetam - AVOID: carbamazepine, phenytoin, and vigabatrin

ACTH, Adrenocorticotropic hormone; *AED*, antiepileptic drug; *EEG*, electroencephalogram; *EMG*, electromyogram; *GTCS*, generalized tonic-clonic seizures; *MRI*, magnetic resonance imaging;

Management

a. **Status epilepticus:** see Neurological Emergencies in Chapter 2 Emergency Medicine
b. **Parental education:** first-aid training, administration of rescue medications
c. **Lifestyle advice:** avoidance of sleep deprivation, alcohol and drug use, baths, high-risk activities, including swimming in deep water, scuba diving, rock climbing. Report to local ministry of transportation if driving.
d. **Anticonvulsants:** balance seizure control with drug side effects, monitor side effects and drug-drug interactions (Table 29.5), wean gradually when seizure free for a minimum of 2 years
e. **Ketogenic diet:** special high fat, low carbohydrate diet that can help seizure control
    i. **Diet candidates:** medically intractable seizures, poor tolerance to antiepileptic drugs (AEDs), certain neurometabolic or neurological syndromes (e.g., Dravet syndrome, Lennox-Gastaut)
    ii. Started in hospital under supervision of neurologist and dietician
    iii. **Adverse effects:** constipation, exacerbation of gastroesophageal reflux, poor growth, kidney stones, dyslipidemia, prolonged corrected QT interval (QTc) interval, cardiomyopathy, optic neuropathy, elevated very-long-chain fatty acids, vitamin D and trace mineral deficiencies
    iv. Avoid dextrose containing intravenous (IV) fluids, oral and IV steroids, and all liquid suspension medications that contain carbohydrates
f. **Surgery:** intractable seizures with a definite seizure focus; consider early for medical refractory epilepsy

Table 29.5	Side Effects of Selected Antiepileptic Drugs		
AED	**Side Effects**	**Monitor**	**Drug Interaction**
Carbamazepine	Leukopenia, hyponatremia (less than with oxcarbazepine), lethargy, ataxia, SJS especially in Han Chinese, hepatic dysfunction, brittle bones in long-term use	AED levels, CBC, sodium, LFTs	Erythromycin, cimetidine, fluoxetine, warfarin, cyclosporine, oral contraceptives, theophylline
Clonazepam	Tolerance, drowsiness, excess salivation, cognitive impairment	—	—
Ethosuximide	Nausea, dizziness, abdominal discomfort	AED levels	—
Gabapentin	Lethargy, dizziness, weight gain	—	—
Lamotrigine	SJS, oral contraceptive failure (decreased levels), but relatively safe (compared with other AEDs) in pregnancy	—	High risk of SJS with concurrent valproic acid

Continued

Table 29.5	Side Effects of Selected Antiepileptic Drugs—cont'd		
AED	**Side Effects**	**Monitor**	**Drug Interaction**
Levetiracetam	Behavioral changes "Kepprage"	—	—
Oxcarbazepine	Drowsiness, hyponatremia	Sodium	—
Phenobarbital	SJS, drowsiness, impaired cognition with long-term use	AED levels	Opiates, benzodiaz-epines, cough preparations, anti-histamines, steroids, warfarin
Phenytoin	Hypersensitivity, gingival hypertrophy, hirsutism, ataxia, lymphadenopathy, SJS, lupus-like illness, blood dyscra-sias, brittle bones, cerebellar atrophy with long-term use	AED levels	Cimetidine, isoniazid, estrogen, trime-thoprim, steroids, cyclosporine, rifampin, warfarin
Topiramate	Lethargy, mental clouding, acute angle closure glaucoma, low appetite, renal stones, sensory paresthesias, terato-genic	—	—
Valproate	Hepatotoxicity, fatal liver necrosis, weight gain, thrombocytopenia, pancreatitis, dose-dependent tremor, hyperammonemia, encephalopathy, ter-atogenic, brittle bones with long-term use, lowers carnitine levels	AED levels, lipase, am-monia, CBC, LFTs, serum total and free carnitine	ASA, higher rate of SJS with concurrent use of lamotrigine
Vigabatrin	Short-term: hypotonia, GI discomfort, fatigue	Ophthalmo-logical examination	—
	Long-term: permanent concentric visual field defects, movement disorder	Electroretino-gram	—
Zonisamide	↓ Sweating, hyperthermia, drowsiness, anorexia	—	—

AED, Antiepileptic drug; *ASA,* acetyl salicylic acid; *CBC,* complete blood count; *GI,* gastrointestinal; *LFT,* liver function test; *SJS,* Stevens-Johnson syndrome.

NEONATAL SEIZURES

See Neonatal Seizures in Chapter 27 Neonatology

FEBRILE SEIZURES

1. **Epidemiology:** usual first presentation 6 months to 3 years of age
   a. Risk factors: positive family history
2. **Clinical manifestations and investigations:** see Figure 29.4
3. **Treatment:** prophylactic anticonvulsants not indicated, prophylactic antipyretics not effective to prevent febrile seizures

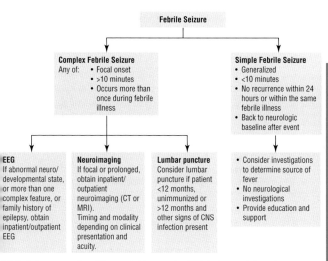

CNS, Central nervous system; *CT*, computed tomography; *EEG*, electroencephalography; *MRI*, magnetic resonance imaging.

3. **Prognosis**: if simple febrile seizure, typical resolution of seizures by 5 to 6 years of age
    a. Risk of febrile seizure recurrence: age <12 months at time of first febrile seizure, history of febrile seizures in first-degree relatives, relative low-grade fever during seizure, seizure at onset of fever
    b. Risk of developing epilepsy with febrile seizures 2% to 5%: increases with developmental disability, abnormal neurological examination, first-degree relative with epilepsy

FIRST UNPROVOKED AFEBRILE SEIZURE

1. **Definition:** first seizure without any clear precipitating factor
2. **Etiology**
    a. Rule out provoked seizure: hypoglycemia, electrolyte imbalances, toxic ingestion, intracranial infection, mass or trauma
    b. Unprovoked seizures may be linked with genetic cause or preexisting brain abnormality or injury
3. **Investigations:** consider more immediate investigations in neonates and children who have not returned to baseline or have seizure focality
    a. **Laboratory tests:** CBC, differential, glucose, creatinine, sodium, calcium, magnesium, blood gas, toxicology screen

   b. **Other tests**
      i. **LP:** if clinical concerns of meningitis or encephalitis
      ii. **EEG:** for all patients with first unprovoked seizure to determine recurrence risk and rule out known epilepsy syndromes; can be done as an outpatient
      iii. **Neuroimaging:** if lateralizing seizure or abnormality on examination or EEG, will require imaging more urgently. If obtained, 3 Tesla MRI preferred to look for subtle focal cortical dysplasia.

✦ PEARL

The decision whether to treat a child with an AED after first unprovoked seizure should be individualized, weighing the risks of recurrent seizure against the potential risks and benefits of AED therapy, and incorporating patient values and preferences.

HEADACHE

1. **History**
   a. **Symptoms:** onset (sudden, episodic, daily, mixture), location, pattern/quality (pounding, stabbing, squeezing), duration, frequency, severity, associated symptoms (nausea, vomiting, photophobia, phonophobia, osmophobia, neck stiffness), preceding symptoms/aura (visual, sensory, speech, motor, brainstem)
   b. **Alleviating and aggravating factors:** drugs, sleep, Valsalva maneuvers
   c. **Past medical history:** meningitis, encephalitis, concussion, traumatic brain injury, aneurysm, arteriovenous malformation (AVM)
   d. **Medications:** prophylactic, abortive
   e. **Family history:** migraine, aneurysm, AVM, polycystic kidney disease, brain tumor
2. **Red flags for secondary causes**
   a. Systemic symptoms and signs, behavior changes, academic deterioration
   b. Abnormal neurological examination, focal neurological signs, seizures
   c. Occipital location
   d. Previous history (worse or different), progressive/persistent, postural (worse supine, waking at night, worse in morning), worsens with increased pressure (Valsalva, cough)
   e. Younger age (<3 years)

3. **Physical examination**
   a. **General:** growth parameters, blood pressure
   b. **Neurological:** full neurological examination, fundoscopy (papilledema), cranial bruits
   c. **Dermatological:** neurocutaneous features
   d. **Head, eyes, ears, nose, and throat (HEENT):** evidence of sinusitis, otitis media, mastoiditis, temporomandibular joint (TMJ) dysfunction, neck stiffness
4. **Causes of secondary headaches:** idiopathic intracranial hypertension (positional, pulsatile tinnitus, transient visual obscurations, recent weight gain), central nervous system (CNS) tumors, stroke, demyelination, vasculitis, hypertension, drug-induced, eye strain, sinusitis, TMJ arthritis
5. **Investigations**
   a. **Indications:** no neuroimaging if no red flags and normal neurological examination
   b. **Imaging:** CT or MRI with MRA/MRV if red flags
   c. **Other tests:** LP if encephalopathy or focal neurological deficits on examination—MUST perform neuroimaging before LP
      i. Measure opening pressure in lateral decubitus position with legs extended
      ii. Cerebrospinal fluid (CSF) for cell count, culture, microscopy, virology, special tests (antibodies, PCR as indicated)
6. **Management:** see Table 29.6

Table 29.6	Features and Management of Selected Primary Headache Disorders	
Headache Type	**Clinical Features**	**Management**
Tension	- Chronic, low-grade with long duration, bilateral, diffuse/band-like, dull/aching - Not aggravated by routine exercise - Associated with anxiety or depression - Normal neurological examination	**Lifestyle modifications** - High-protein breakfast (12–15 g) - Sleep hygiene - Adequate hydration - Avoid caffeinated beverages - Exercise - Stress management/avoiding triggers - Headache diary - Ibuprofen or acetaminophen

Continued

Table 29.6	Features and Management of Selected Primary Headache Disorders—cont'd	
Headache Type	**Clinical Features**	**Management**
Migraine	May be with or without aura Associated with 1. Any TWO of: unilateral or bilateral (frontal/temporal), pulsating, moderate to severe intensity, aggravated by routine physical activities 2. At least ONE of: nausea/vomiting, photophobia/phonophobia Triggers: stress, exercise, head trauma, menstrual cycle, food	**Non-pharmacological:** lifestyle modifications **Pharmacological: acute treatment** - Goal: abort the headaches within 1–2 h - Nonsteroidal antiinflammatory drugs: ibuprofen, ketorolac - Analgesics: acetaminophen - Dopamine antagonists: metoclopramide, prochlorperazine - Other antiemetics: dimenhydrinate, promethazine - Triptans: sumatriptan, rizatriptan **Pharmacological: preventive treatment** - Goals: ↓ headaches by >50%, ↓ acute medication use, ↑ acute medication effectiveness, prevent chronic symptoms - Neutraceuticals: magnesium citrate 150 mg at night increase as tolerated to 300 mg/day (may cause loose stools on higher doses), riboflavin (vitamin B2) 100 mg twice daily up to 400 mg/day, Coenzyme Q10 100 mg daily up to 200 mg/day, MigreLief for kids (magnesium, riboflavin, and feverfew) 1 tablet at night, up to 2 tablets/day - Beta-blockers: propranolol - Antidepressants: amitriptyline - Antiepileptics: topiramate (first line), divalproex sodium, gabapentin, levetiracetam - Calcium channel blockers: flunarizine (first line) - Other: botulinum toxin A (chronic migraine)

RAISED INTRACRANIAL PRESSURE

1. **Signs, symptoms, and acute management:** see Neurological Emergencies in Chapter 2 Emergency Medicine
2. **Pseudotumor cerebri syndrome** (idiopathic intracranial hypertension)
   a. See Figure 29.5 for diagnostic approach
   b. Neurology consultation for management

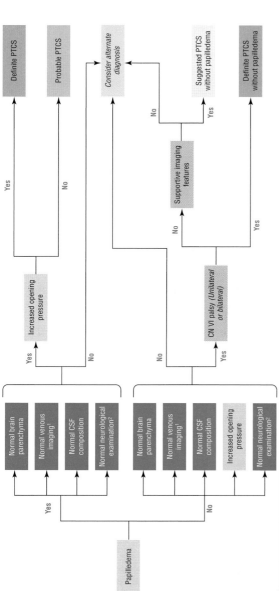

CN, Cranial nerve; CSF, cerebrospinal fluid; PTCS, pseudotumor cerebri syndrome. (Adapted from Barmherzig R, Szperka CA. Pseudotumor cerebri syndrome in children. *Curr Pain Headache Rep.* 2019;23(8):58.)

[1]Venous imaging only required in select cases
[2]Except for cranial nerve abnormalites

1. **Definitions**
   a. **Acute hemiparesis:** sudden, acute onset of focal neurological weakness
   b. **Stroke:** focal cerebral, spinal, or retinal infarction in a defined vascular distribution
   c. **Transient ischemic attack (TIA):** a transient episode of neurological dysfunction caused by focal brain, spinal cord, or retinal ischemia, without acute infarction on CT or MRI

2. **History**
   a. **Current history:** last seen well, symptom onset and current residual symptoms, duration and location, triggers (i.e., movement with vertigo) symptoms suggestive of migraine or seizures (e.g., Todd's paralysis), encephalopathy, drug use, trauma, preceding/concurrent infections
   b. **Past medical history:** systemic diseases, vascular and congenital malformations, coagulopathies, cardiac disease

3. **Differential diagnosis**
   a. **Neurological:** stroke, TIA, migraine with/without aura, seizure/postictal state, periodic paralysis/episodic ataxia, demyelinating disease (e.g., multiple sclerosis)
   b. **Infectious:** meningitis, focal-presenting encephalitis (e.g., herpes simplex)
   c. **Oncologic:** brain tumor
   d. **Trauma/toxin:** head injury, fractures, toxic encephalopathy

4. **Risk factors**
   a. **Arterial ischemic stroke:** congenital/acquired heart disease, sickle cell disease, vasculopathy (transient cerebral arteriopathy, primary CNS vasculitis), trauma (e.g., dissection), prothrombotic state, oral contraceptives
   b. **Hemorrhagic stroke:** coagulopathies, AVM, aneurysm, brain tumor, cerebral sinovenous thrombosis (CSVT), connective tissue disease
   c. **CSVT:** recent infection of head and neck, dehydration, prothrombotic states (inflammatory bowel disease, iron deficiency anemia, nephrotic syndrome, systemic lupus erythematosus (SLE), hematological malignancy, chemotherapy)

5. **Clinical presentation and management:** see Neurological Emergencies in Chapter 2 Emergency Medicine

WEAKNESS

See Table 29.7 for approach to generalized weakness

Table 29.7 Neurological Signs and Differential Diagnosis of Weakness by Anatomic Localization

Localization	Power	Muscle Bulk	Deep Tendon Reflexes	Plantar Response	Differential Diagnosis	Investigations
Central	N	N	↑	Extensor	Perinatal asphyxia, ICH, IEM, genetic disorder, brain dysgenesis, benign congenital hypotonia, cervical spinal cord injury	MRI/CT, genetic testing, metabolic testing
Anterior horn cell	→	Proximal atrophy	↓ to absent	Flexor to nonreactive	SMA, poliomyelitis	EMG/NCS, genetic testing
Peripheral nerve	↓	Distal atrophy	→	Flexor to nonreactive	Congenital neuropathy, Charcot-Marie-Tooth, toxins, trauma, vitamin deficiency (B12, E)	EMG/NCS, genetic testing
Neuromuscular junction	Weakness fluctuates	N	N →	Flexor	Myasthenia gravis, botulism	EMG/NCS, Tensilon test
Muscle	→	↓ (pattern depends on disease type)	N →	Flexor	Congenital myopathy, metabolic or mitochondrial myopathy; congenital muscular dystrophy; myotonic dystrophy; inflammatory (polymyositis, dermatomyositis); infectious (viral myositis, parasitic, bacterial); electrolyte disturbances (hypophosphatemia, hypokalemia, hypocalcemia); endocrine (hypothyroidism, Cushing); toxins (steroids, statins)	CK, EMG/NCS, muscle biopsy, genetic tests, metabolic tests

CK, Creatine kinase; CT, computed tomography; EMG, electromyogram; Extensor, upgoing toe; Flexor, downgoing toe; ICH, intracranial hemorrhage; IEM, inborn errors of metabolism; MRI, magnetic resonance imaging; N, normal; NCS, nerve conduction studies; SMA, spinal muscular atrophy.

Adapted from Crawford TO. Clinical evaluation of the floppy infant. *Pediatr Ann*. 1992;21:348–354.

Neurology and Neurosurgery

29

GUILLAIN-BARRÉ SYNDROME

1. **Definition:** acute inflammatory demyelinating polyneuropathy (AIDP)
2. **Clinical features**
   a. Commonly preceded by infection
   b. Rapid onset of weakness from distal to proximal muscles, usually symmetrical, often starting in legs
   c. Associated with pain, sensory ataxia
   d. May have facial weakness and other cranial nerve involvement, respiratory symptoms, autonomic dysfunction
   e. Clinical course: symptoms reach maximum by 4 weeks, plateau for up to 4 weeks, then recovery (weeks to months)
3. **Investigations**
   a. Blood work: CBC, alanine aminotransferase (ALT), creatinine, CK, infectious workup (including stool for enterovirus and poliovirus)
   b. CSF protein can be elevated or normal in the first week
   c. Neuroimaging: no role except to rule out spinal cord lesions
4. **Diagnostic criteria**
   a. Progressive motor weakness of more than one limb
   b. Areflexia: universal areflexia (distal areflexia and proximal hyporeflexia if other features are consistent)
   c. ↑CSF protein (more common >1 week after symptom onset)
   d. CSF white blood cell (WBC) <10/mm^3
5. **Management**
   a. Monitor respiratory and cardiac function closely (pulmonary function tests twice daily for 2–3 days), consider early critical care admission, monitor for autonomic dysfunction
   b. Intravenous immune globulin (IVIG) or plasmapheresis; no role for corticosteroids
   c. Pain management
   d. Physiotherapy: range of motion, monitoring muscle strength, ambulation
   e. If prolonged immobilization, consider deep vein thrombosis prophylaxis

> ✦ **PEARL**
>
> Doubt the diagnosis of GBS if asymmetrical weakness, fever at onset, sharp spinal cord level, acute severe localized back pain, or CSF white blood cell count >50.

FLOPPY INFANT

1. **History:** pregnancy history (TORCH infections, which includes Toxoplasmosis, Other (syphilis, varicella-zoster, parvovirus B19), Rubella, Cytomegalovirus (CMV), and Herpes infections; drug and alcohol use, fetal presentation, fetal movements), delivery, postnatal period

2. **Historical clues**
    a. History of hip subluxation, high-arched palate, or arthogryposis increases likelihood of in utero hypotonia
    b. Motor delay with normal social and language development increases likelihood of peripheral neuromuscular disease
    c. Regression increases concern for neurodegenerative disorders
    d. Feeding history revealing sucking and swallowing difficulties that "fatigue" or "get worse" with repetition may indicate diseases of the neuromuscular junction
    e. Consider infantile botulism with history of honey or corn syrup consumption and pupillary involvement

3. **Family history:** history of recurrent miscarriages, developmental disability, consanguinity, delayed motor milestones (congenital myopathy), premature death (metabolic or muscle disease)

4. **Additional important points on history**
    a. Age at onset versus age at first recognition
    b. Static versus improving versus progressive
    c. Episodic periodic worsening (note precipitating factors)

5. **Approach based on anatomic localization:** see Table 29.7

> ☀ **PEARL**
>
> Central hypotonia if floppy and strong; peripheral hypotonia if floppy and weak.

MOVEMENT DISORDERS

1. **History**
    a. Is the number of movements excessive (hyperkinetic) or diminished (hypokinetic)? If hyperkinetic, are individual movements normal or abnormal?
    b. Are movements paroxysmal (sudden onset and offset), continual (repeated again and again), or continuous (without stopping)?
    c. Are movements present at rest (body part supported against gravity), with maintained posture, with action, with approach to a target (intention), or a combination?
    d. Have the movements changed over time?
    e. Do environmental stimuli or emotional states precipitate, exacerbate, or alleviate the movements?
    f. Is the patient aware of the movements?
    g. Can the movements be suppressed voluntarily?
    h. Are the movements heralded by a premonitory sensation or urge?
    i. Do the movements abate with sleep?
    j. Are there other findings suggestive of focal neurological deficit or systemic disease?

k. Developmental history and any underlying medical conditions (seizures, medications, intoxications, trauma, attention deficit hyperactivity disorder, other CNS pathology)
l. Is there a family history of a similar or related condition?

2. **Movement types:** see Table 29.8

Table 29.8	Types of Involuntary Movements	
Type of Movement	**Description**	**Examples**
Chorea	Brief, semi-directed, irregular movements that are not repetitive or rhythmic, but appear to flow from one muscle to the next	Benign hereditary chorea Sydenham's chorea Anti-NMDAR encephalitis Wilson's disease
Athetosis	Slow, continuous, writhing movement often seen with chorea, usually affects distal body parts	Choreoathetosis Cerebral palsy due to kernicterus
Ballismus	High-amplitude, affecting proximal joints (extreme form of chorea)	Hemiballism (stroke/demyelination/ vascular lesion in the contralateral subthalamic nucleus)
Tardive dyskinesia	Complex syndrome: buccolingual mastication movements (tongue protrusion, lip smacking, puckering, chewing) and/or extremities/trunk involvement (chorea, athetosis, dystonia, or tremor)	Commonly after exposure to dopamine antagonist (neuroleptics, antiemetics)
Dystonia	Involuntary muscle contraction of agonist and antagonist muscles leading to repetitive and sustained twisting movements and/or abnormal posture	Dopa-responsive dystonia Wilson's disease Cerebral palsy Neurodegeneration with brain iron accumulation (NBIA)
Tics	Involuntary, non-rhythmic, repetitive, stereotyped movements or vocalizations that resemble voluntary actions	Persistent motor or vocal tics Tourette syndrome Wilson's disease

NMDAR, N-methyl-D-aspartate receptor.

TICS

1. **Definition:** sudden, rapid, recurrent, non-rhythmic motor movement or vocalization that is briefly suppressible; not because of medication or another condition
   a. **Motor**
      i. **Simple:** eye blinking; head or shoulder jerks; brief, sudden movements of the arms or legs
      ii. **Complex:** repeated, coordinated jerks of multiple muscle groups (e.g., touching, hitting, or jumping)

b. **Phonic**
    i. **Simple:** noises including throat clearing, grunting, sniffling
    ii. **Complex:** linguistically meaningful noises, coprolalia, echolalia
2. **Natural course:** generally occur <18 years, severity and frequency decline with age. Often have a waxing and waning course.
3. **Treatment:** reassurance; alpha-2-agonists, such as clonidine and guanfacine for Tourette syndrome

ACUTE ATAXIA

1. **Definition:** poor voluntary coordination of movement
    a. Appendicular: poor limb coordination, manifests as dysmetria and dysdiadochokinesia
    b. Gait: wide based, unsteady, difficulty with tandem gait
    c. Truncal
2. **Etiologies**
    a. **Infectious/immune related:** cerebellar disorders, such as acute cerebellar ataxia, acute disseminated encephalomyelitis (ADEM), brainstem encephalitis
    b. **Toxic ingestions:** alcohol and other drugs
    c. **Space occupying lesions:** tumors and vascular lesions
    d. **Hydrocephalus**
    e. **Trauma:** cerebellar contusion or hemorrhage
    f. **Stroke:** vertebrobasilar dissection/thromboembolism
    g. **Paraneoplastic/inflammatory:** opsoclonus-myoclonus-ataxia syndrome
    h. **Sensory ataxia:** Guillain-Barré syndrome, Miller-Fisher syndrome
    i. **Paretic ataxia:** upper or motor neuron causes of ataxia
    j. **Other:** inborn errors of metabolism (IEM), basilar migraine, benign paroxysmal vertigo, labyrinthitis, psychogenic

ACUTE (POST-INFECTIOUS) CEREBELLAR ATAXIA

1. **Clinical features:** self-limiting process that occurs in preschool children. Follows a febrile viral infection or immunization (varicella is the most common). Can occur up to 3 weeks after the systemic illness has subsided. Usually recovery is within 2 weeks.
2. **History:** recent infection, recent immunizations, headache, vomiting, vertigo, other cerebellar findings, exposure to drugs/toxins, family history of migraine or genetic/metabolic disorders
3. **Investigations:** neuroimaging primarily to rule out other etiologies (MRI is often normal or nonspecific), may consider CSF analysis, viral studies, toxicology screen, metabolic/genetic workup, urine catecholamines to rule out neuroblastoma, EEG

4. **Management:** supportive management, ensure safety from accidental self-injury

NEUROINFLAMMATORY CONDITIONS

ACUTE DISSEMINATED ENCEPHALOMYELITIS/TRANSVERSE MYELITIS
1. **Description:** immune-mediated demyelinating CNS disorder
2. **Diagnosis**
   a. First polyfocal clinical CNS event with presumed inflammatory demyelinating cause
   b. Encephalopathy
   c. Brain and/or spine MRI abnormalities consistent with demyelination during the acute phase
   d. No new clinical or MRI findings > 3 months after clinical onset
3. **Neurological manifestations**
   a. Pyramidal signs
   b. Ataxia
   c. Acute hemiparesis
   d. Optic neuritis or other cranial nerve involvement
   e. Seizures and status epileptics
   f. Spinal cord syndrome
   g. Impairment of speech
4. **Neuroimaging features**
   a. No absolute imaging criteria to differentiate ADEM from multiple sclerosis (MS)
   b. Spinal cord imaging shows large confluent lesions extending over multiple segments, sometimes associated with cord swelling
5. **CSF findings**
   a. Mild pleocytosis, elevated protein
   b. Generally negative for intrathecal oligoclonal immunoglobulin G synthesis
6. **Treatment:** IV corticosteroids, IVIG and/or plasma exchange

ANTI–N-METHYL-D-ASPARTATE RECEPTOR ENCEPHALITIS
1. **Clinical presentation**
   a. Usually present with
      i. Early: abnormal behavior (psychosis, delusions, hallucinations, agitation, aggression, catatonia)
      ii. Irritability and insomnia
      iii. Later: speech dysfunction, dyskinesias (orofacial dyskinesias, choreoathetosis, dystonia, oculogyric crisis, rigidity, opisthotonic postures), memory deficits, autonomic instability, decreased level of consciousness
      iv. Seizures can take place at any time

b. Young children more frequently present with abnormal movements or seizures

2. **CSF findings:** associated with CSF immunoglobulin G (IgG) antibodies against GluN1 subunit of the NMDA

3. **Neuroimaging features**
   a. No clear patterns of brain involvement
   b. MRI of the brain is unremarkable or may show nonspecific T2 or fluid-attenuated inversion recovery (FLAIR) signal hyperintensity within the hippocampus, cerebellar, frontobasal, insular cortex, basal ganglia, brainstem, and occasionally the spinal cord

4. **Treatment**
   a. Immunotherapy: IV corticosteroids, IVIG, plasma exchange, rituximab
   b. Teratoma detection and removal, if applicable

SPINAL CORD LESIONS

ACUTE SPINAL CORD LESIONS

1. **Clinical features:** back pain or painless, deteriorating gait, lower extremity weakness and/or altered pinprick/vibration sensation, changes in bowel and bladder function, hypotonia, hyporeflexia

2. **Etiology**
   a. **Trauma:** transection or contusion of the spinal cord
   b. **Tumors:** ependymoma, astrocytoma, neuroblastoma, lymphoma
   c. **Infections:** epidural abscesses
   d. **Neuroinflammatory disorders:** transverse myelitis, neuromyelitis optica, ADEM
   e. **Vascular:** ischemic infarction

3. **Physical examination:** look for sensory level, abdominal reflexes, bowel and bladder involvement, distribution of weakness

4. **Investigations:** urgent MRI brain/spine

5. **Management:** depends on underlying cause

SPINAL DYSRAPHISM

1. **Definition:** neural tube defects resulting from failure of normal neurulation (refers to all forms of spina bifida)

2. **Major types**
   a. **Spina bifida occulta:** midline defect of vertebral bodies; no protrusion of meninges or the spinal cord, often asymptomatic. LP not contraindicated unless another dysraphic lesion present.
   b. **Meningocele:** protrusion of meninges through a defect in the posterior vertebral bodies
   c. **Myelomeningocele:** protrusion of all tissue layers (spinal cord, nerve roots, meninges) through a defect in the posterior vertebral bodies

3. **Physical examination:** dimpling (concern if diameter >5 mm, >2.5 cm above anal verge, multiple dimples, caudal appendage, or outside sacrococcygeal region), pigmentation, hemangioma or hair tufts in the lower thoracic, lumbar, or sacral region, dermal sinus or pit, gluteal cleft anomalies. Assess distal motor paralysis, spasticity, sphincter dysfunction, musculoskeletal deformity.
4. **Investigations:** Spine ultrasound ±MRI brain/spine. May have hydrocephalus or Chiari malformation.
5. **Management:** if open defect, keep newborn prone, apply a sterile saline dressing. Urgent referral to neurosurgery. May require orthopedic and urology assessment. Otherwise, neurosurgical evaluation if any radiographic abnormality or if discharge observed or reported.

TETHERED CORD

1. **Definition:** spinal cord becomes caught or tied down during vertebral column bone growth by scar tissue, fatty mass (lipoma), or a developmental abnormality resulting in stretching of the cord. May be associated with spinal dysraphism.
2. **History:** insidious onset of progressive leg weakness, bowel and bladder incontinence, scoliosis, back pain
3. **Physical examination:** assess for cutaneous signs at base of cord and signs of acute spinal cord lesion
4. **Investigations:** MRI spine
5. **Management:** referral to neurosurgery for surgical untethering of cord if evidence of neurological symptoms or deterioration

CHIARI MALFORMATIONS

CHIARI I MALFORMATIONS

1. **Clinical manifestations:** often asymptomatic and found incidentally. Can present with headaches, occipital pain that increases with Valsalva maneuver, cerebellar symptoms, sleep apnea, feeding difficulties or dysphagia, sensory changes, pain in the shoulders, back and limbs.
2. **Imaging findings:** herniation of the cerebellar tonsils through the foramen magnum ≥5 mm
3. **Management:** surgical decompression with duroplasty relieves symptoms, conservative approach generally adopted in minimally affected patients. LP might be contraindicated depending on extent of the tonsillar descent.

CHIARI II MALFORMATIONS

1. **Clinical manifestations:** symptoms of hydrocephalus, brainstem deficits, and spinal cord paralysis

2. **Imaging findings:** herniation of cerebellum and brainstem through foramen magnum
3. **Management:** surgical repair of neural tube, CSF shunt for hydrocephalus. If deficits attributable to the Chiari II, surgery may be offered.

VENTRICULOPERITONEAL SHUNT FAILURE

1. **Etiology:** VP shunting is used to treat hydrocephalus. Shunt failure can be caused by
   a. Obstruction
   b. Infection
   c. Overdrainage
   d. Loculated ventricles
2. **History**
   a. Headaches: morning headaches, positional (worse when lying down)
   b. Vomiting at night
   c. Abdominal pain
   d. Fever
   e. Neurological changes: new weakness, sensory or cognitive changes
   f. History of previous shunt malfunctions and similar associated symptoms
3. **Investigations**
   a. Imaging
      i. Shunt series (skull x-ray, chest, and abdomen) to rule out shunt-tube disconnection
      ii. CT or MRI to compare ventricular size with previous imaging
   b. CSF sample through subcutaneous reservoirs (by neurosurgery) if suspicion of infection

Oncology

Amy Lu • Mohammed Al Nuaimi • Reena Pabari • Sumit Gupta

Also see page xviii for a list of other abbreviations used throughout this book

AFP	alpha-fetoprotein
ANC	absolute neutrophil count
ALL	acute lymphoblastic leukemia
AML	acute myeloid leukemia
APL	acute promyelocytic leukemia
ATRA	all-trans retinoic acid
βhCG	beta-human chorionic gonadotropin
BMA	bone marrow aspirate
BMT	bone marrow transplant
CHF	congestive heart failure
CMV	cytomegalovirus
DAT	direct antiglobulin test
DIC	disseminated intravascular coagulation
FDG-PET	fluorodeoxyglucose-positron emission tomography
G-CSF	granulocyte-colony stimulating factor
HL	Hodgkin lymphoma
HLA	human leukocyte antigen
HLH	hemophagocytic lymphohistiocytosis
HSCT	hematopoietic stem cell transplantation
HTLV	human T-lymphotropic virus
HVA	homovanillic acid
ICH	intracranial hemorrhage
IT	intrathecal
JIA	juvenile idiopathic arthritis
LCH	Langerhans cell histiocytosis
LN	lymph node
MAS	macrophage activation syndrome
MIBG	meta-iodobenzylguanidine
MRD	minimal residual disease
NF1	neurofibromatosis type 1
NHL	non-Hodgkin lymphoma
PET	positron emission tomography
PLT	platelet
RT	radiotherapy
SBE	subacute bacterial endocarditis
SIADH	syndrome of inappropriate antidiuretic hormone secretion
SLE	systemic lupus erythematosus
SVC	superior vena cava
TB	tuberculosis
TLS	tumor lysis syndrome
VMA	vanillylmandelic acid

Oncology

30

1. **Common presentations:** see Table 30.1
2. **Approach to clinical signs of malignancy:** see Table 30.2

Table 30.1	Common Clinical Presentations of Malignancy
Malignancy	**Signs and Symptoms**
Leukemia	Fatigue, malaise, fever, bruising, bleeding, petechiae, bone pain, hepatosplenomegaly, lymphadenopathy
	AML: skin lesions, chloromas (extramedullary disease), DIC
Lymphoma	Fever, night sweats, weight loss, fatigue, lymphadenopathy (head, neck, chest, abdomen), pruritus, recurrent respiratory symptoms
Neuroblastoma	Mass (can occur anywhere, most commonly abdominal), emesis, Horner syndrome, persistent respiratory symptoms, periorbital ecchymoses ("raccoon eyes"), blue subcutaneous nodules ("blueberry muffin"), opsoclonus-myoclonus, ataxia, sweating, hypertension, watery diarrhea
Wilms tumor	Abdominal mass or distension, hypertension, hematuria
Bone tumors	Limp, bone pain, joint pain
Brain tumors	Headache, nausea, vomiting, ataxia, irritability, seizures, focal deficits, papilledema, vision changes, proptosis, neuroendocrine deficits

AML, Acute myeloid leukemia; *DIC,* disseminated intravascular coagulation.

Oncology

30

Table 30.2

Approach to Common Oncological Presentations

Presentation	Clinical Evaluation	Red Flags	Differential Diagnosis	Investigation/Management
Lymphadenopathy	Onset, duration, progression, tenderness, location (localized vs. generalized), overlying skin changes Recent infections, travel, sick contacts, animal exposure (e.g., *Bartonella* from cat scratch), dietary exposures (e.g., brucellosis from unpasteurized milk, uncooked meats) Rash, signs of Kawasaki disease, joint symptoms, bone pain, constitutional symptoms, organomegaly	Firm, matted, rubbery, non-tender Supraclavicular ≥2 cm Persistent/rapid growth, lack of regression after 4 weeks Constitutional symptoms Abnormal CXR, blood film	Infectious - Bacterial, e.g., *Staphylococcus aureus*, group A Streptococcus, *Bartonella* - Viral, e.g., EBV, CMV - Mycobacterial - Fungal, e.g., histoplasmosis - Protozoal, e.g., toxoplasmosis Rheumatological Malignancy	If no red flags: observe up to 4 weeks, consider antibiotics if suspected infectious etiology Investigate with bloodwork, imaging ±biopsy if - Red flags - No response to antibiotics - No regression with resolution of associated acute symptoms
Splenomegaly	History of hemolytic anemia, jaundice, bleeding/bruising Constitutional symptoms, rash, bone/joint symptoms Neonatal umbilical catheter (portal vein thrombus) Petechiae/purpura, lymphadenopathy Size of spleen, liver; evidence of liver disease Signs of infectious or inflammatory disease, e.g., rash, joint changes	Almost always abnormal, re-quiring further investigation Particularly concerning if concomitant hepatomegaly, lymphadenopathy or clinical suspicion for systemic disease	Infectious, e.g., EBV, CMV, TB, SBE, malaria Hematological, e.g., sickle cell sequestration, thalassemia, spherocytosis, myeloproliferative disorder Infiltration, e.g., storage disorder, malignancy Congestive, e.g., portal hypertension, CHF Rheumatological, e.g., SLE, JIA	CBC, differential, DAT, blood smear, LFTs, viral serology Others as indicated, e.g., - ANA, complement - Abdominal US for organomegaly, lymphadenopathy - Doppler for portal vein thrombosis - BMA/biopsy if red flags

Continued

Oncology

30

| | Approach to Common Oncological Presentations—cont'd | | | |

Presentation	Clinical Evaluation	Red Flags	Differential Diagnosis	Investigation/Management
Abdominal mass	Onset, progression, associated symptoms, e.g., pain, urinary symptoms, bleeding/bruising, fatigue, unexplained fever, weight loss, night sweats Hypertension, diaphoresis, other masses (lymphadenopathy)	Systemic symptoms Abdominal mass should always be investigated further	Majority benign renal masses, e.g., hydronephrosis, poly/multicystic kidney Most common malignancies: Wilms, neuroblastoma; others include leukemia, lymphoma, hepatoblastoma Normal anatomy can be mistaken for masses, e.g., stool, especially if constipated Wide differential based on location	CBC; polycythemia in Wilms; anemia, leukocytosis, cytopenias in leukemia Extended electrolytes, urea, creatinine Urinalysis Urine HVA, VMA: elevated in neuroblastoma Tumor markers as indicated, e.g., AFP Imaging: US and/or CT
Mediastinal mass	History of cough, wheeze, dyspnea, dysphagia without clear etiology or unresponsive to conventional therapy Constitutional symptoms Examine for SVC obstruction (see Table 30.4) and Horner syndrome Lymphadenopathy (supraclavicular), organomegaly May be incidental finding on CXR	Always requires further investigation	Figure 30.1	CBC, differential, smear AFP, βhCG (germ cell tumor) Thyroid function, extended electrolytes if possible goiter CXR, CT, MRI Diagnostic biopsy BMA/biopsy May require emergency management (see Table 30.4)

Bone lesion	Pain, swelling, palpable mass	Nocturnal pain	Benign (more common)	XR
	May be incidental finding on XR	Pathological fracture	- Osteoid osteoma	CT, MRI, bone scan
		Systemic symptoms	- Osteochondroma	Biopsy
			- Unicameral/aneurysmal bone cysts	
			- LCH	
			Malignant	
			- Osteosarcoma (most common)	
			- Ewing sarcoma	
			- Other malignant infiltration, e.g., leukemia, metastases	

AFP, Alpha-fetoprotein; *ANA*, antinuclear antibody; *BMA*, bone marrow aspirate; *CBC*, complete blood count; *CHF*, congestive heart failure; *CMV*, cytomegalovirus; *CT*, computed tomography; *CXR*, chest x-ray; *DAT*, direct antiglobulin test; *EBV*, Epstein-Barr virus; *HVA*, homovanillic acid; *JIA*, juvenile idiopathic arthritis; *LCH*, Langerhans cell histiocytosis; *LFT*, liver function test; *MRI*, magnetic resonance imaging; *SBE*, subacute bacterial endocarditis; *SLE*, systemic lupus erythematosus; *SVC*, superior vena cava; *TB*, tuberculosis; *US*, ultrasound; *VMA*, vanillylmandelic acid; *βhCG*, beta-human chorionic gonadotropin.

Oncology

30

Figure 30.1 Differential Diagnosis of a Mediastinal Mass on a Lateral Chest X-Ray

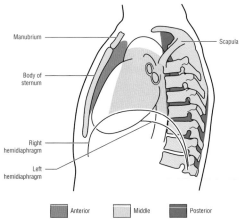

	Anterior Mediastinum	**Middle Mediastinum**	**Posterior Mediastinum**
Benign	Thymic cyst/enlargement, angioma, lipoma, ectopic thyroid tumor	Lymphadenopathy (infectious/inflammatory), bronchogenic cyst, granuloma, esophageal lesions	Meningocele, hemangioma, ganglioneuroma, neurofibroma
Malignant	Lymphoma, teratoma, T-cell leukemia	Mainly lymphoma	Neuroblastoma, pheochromocytoma, rhabdomyosarcoma

ONCOLOGICAL EMERGENCIES

TUMOR LYSIS SYNDROME

1. **Pathophysiology:** breakdown of malignant cells with release of intracellular contents; potential harmful downstream effects (arrhythmias, renal failure, etc.)
2. Most common in malignancies with high tumor burden or rapid cell proliferation, e.g., Burkitt lymphoma, leukemia; far less common in solid tumors
3. Can occur before or after initiation of therapy
4. **Clinical manifestations:** see Table 30.3
5. **Management:** see Figure 30.2

Table 30.3	Clinical Manifestations of Tumor Lysis Syndrome and Their Management	
Laboratory Derangement	**Clinical Manifestations**	**Management**
Hyperkalemia	Cardiac arrhythmias, death	See Hyperkalemia in Chapter 15 Fluids, Electrolytes, and Acid-Base for management General principles - Shift: salbutamol, insulin + dextrose - Bind: K binders - Excrete: furosemide
Hyperphosphatemia	Renal injury caused by calcium phosphate crystallization in tubules Secondary hypocalcemia	Aluminum hydroxide given at mealtimes: prevents absorption of oral phosphate intake
Hypocalcemia - Due to elevated phosphate	Hypotension, cardiac arrhythmia, tetany, seizures, renal injury from calcium phosphate	See Hypocalcemia in Chapter 14 Endocrinology for management General principles - Correct underlying hyperphosphatemia - Do not give exogenous calcium unless symptomatic or ECG changes
Hyperuricemia - Due to metabolism of nucleic acids	Renal injury from urate crystallization in tubules and crystal-independent mechanisms Causes renal vasoconstriction, activation of renin-angiotensin system	Allopurinol: prophylactic, inhibits urate production Rasburicase: if high risk; recombinant urate oxidase, removes pre-formed urate

ECG, Electrocardiogram.

Figure 30.2 General Management of Tumor Lysis Syndrome

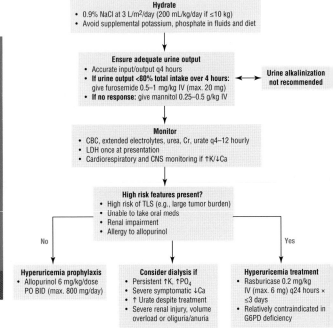

Hydrate
- 0.9% NaCl at 3 L/m^2/day (200 mL/kg/day if ≤10 kg)
- Avoid supplemental potassium, phosphate in fluids and diet

Ensure adequate urine output
- Accurate input/output q4 hours
- **If urine output <80% total intake over 4 hours:** give furosemide 0.5–1 mg/kg IV (max. 20 mg)
- **If no response:** give mannitol 0.25–0.5 g/kg IV

Urine alkalinization not recommended

Monitor
- CBC, extended electrolytes, urea, Cr, urate q4–12 hourly
- LDH once at presentation
- Cardiorespiratory and CNS monitoring if ↑K/↓Ca

High risk features present?
- High risk of TLS (e.g., large tumor burden)
- Unable to take oral meds
- Renal impairment
- Allergy to allopurinol

No

Yes

Hyperuricemia prophylaxis
- Allopurinol 6 mg/kg/dose PO BID (max. 800 mg/day)

Consider dialysis if
- Persistent ↑K, ↑PO$_4$
- Severe symptomatic ↓Ca
- ↑ Urate despite treatment
- Severe renal injury, volume overload or oliguria/anuria

Hyperuricemia treatment
- Rasburicase 0.2 mg/kg IV (max. 6 mg) q24 hours × ≤3 days
- Relatively contraindicated in G6PD deficiency

BID, Twice daily; *CBC*, complete blood count; *CNS*, central nervous system; *Cr*, creatinine; *G6PD*, glucose-6-phosphate dehydrogenase; *IV*, intravenous; *LDH*, lactate dehydrogenase; *PO*, by mouth; *TLS*, tumor lysis syndrome.

FEVER AND NEUTROPENIA

1. Risk of overwhelming sepsis; patients can deteriorate rapidly
2. Some guidelines may allow for outpatient management if patient meets specific low-risk criteria
3. **Management:** see Figure 30.3
4. **Duration of therapy:** consider discharge if cultures negative at 48 hours, patient afebrile, and clinically well
   a. If severely neutropenic (ANC $<0.1 \times 10^9$/L) and blood cultures negative: await hematological recovery (ANC $\geq0.1 \times 10^9$/L for 2 days) before discontinuing IV antibiotics
5. **Follow-up:** ensure close follow-up and clear understanding of when to return to hospital promptly
   a. Approach fever recurrence as new fever in neutropenic hosts: requires immediate re-evaluation

Figure 30.3 Management of Fever and Neutropenia

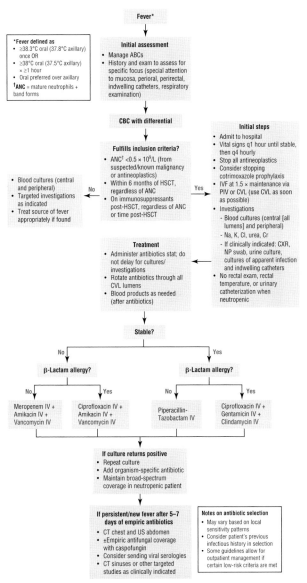

ABCs, Airway, breathing, circulation; *ANC*, absolute neutrophil count; *CT*, computerized tomography; *CVL*, central venous line; *CXR*, chest x-ray; *HSCT*, hematopoietic stem cell transplantation; *NP*, nasopharyngeal; *PIV*, peripheral intravenous; *US*, ultrasound.

OTHER ONCOLOGICAL EMERGENCIES

1. See Table 30.4

Table 30.4	Other Oncological Emergencies			
Emergency	**Etiology**	**Clinical Manifestations**	**Investigations**	**Management**
Superior vena cava/ mediastinal syndrome - Compression of SVC ± trachea	Anterior mediastinal mass: NHL, HL, germ cell tumor, ALL Thrombosis: associated with CVL, CVS surgery/catheterization, vessel compression, etc. Less common: granuloma, infection	Swelling, plethora of face, neck, and upper extremities Conjunctival suffusion Engorged collateral veins Cough, hoarseness Dyspnea, orthopnea, wheeze, stridor; worsens when supine Dysphagia Chest pain Altered mental status, syncope	CXR, CT chest (prone or decubitus); evaluate for mediastinal mass ECG, echo: assess cardiac function/anesthetic risk ± for intravascular thrombus if no mediastinal mass See Table 30.2 for workup of mediastinal mass	Anesthetic risk - Elevate head of bed >45 degrees, avoid supine position - Avoid sedation/stress as can precipitate respiratory arrest - Do not intubate unless airway compromise (challenging extubation) - Maintain IV access Critical airway compression: Empiric treatment of hematological malignancy and airway edema with prednisolone or methylprednisolone; biopsy as soon as patient stable, ideally within 24 h of steroid initiation
Spinal cord compression	Primary or metastatic tumor: sarcoma, neuroblastoma, germ cell tumor, lymphoma, leukemia, LCH, medulloblastoma	Back pain with localized tenderness (80%) Motor/sensory deficits Bowel/bladder dysfunction, e.g., incontinence, retention	XR spine: may be normal Urgent MRI with gadolinium contrast CT myelography if MRI unavailable	If neurological deficits - Dexamethasone - Urgent initiation of radiation ±chemotherapy, depending on which malignancy is suspected - Consult neurosurgery for decompression laminectomy

Hyperleukocytosis (WBC $>100 \times 10^9$/L)	Common presenting feature in ALL, AML, CML	CNS: headache, seizure, decreased LOC, delirium, focal deficits	CBC and differential: ensure manual PLT count, can be falsely elevated with high WBC	TLS prevention and treatment: see Figure 30.2
	High number of blasts → increased viscosity of blood (leukostasis) → decreased tissue oxygenation → tissue ischemia	Respiratory: cough, dyspnea, respiratory distress	Blood smear	DIC/↓ PLT
				- Aggressive correction with FFP (10 mL/kg)
		GU: oliguria, anuria	INR, PTT, D-dimer, fibrinogen	- Keep PLT $>50 \times 10^9$/L, to reduce risk of ICH
	Can cause thrombosis, secondary hemorrhage	Vascular: DIC, cerebral thrombosis, retinal vein thrombosis, retinal vein hemorrhage/thrombosis (blurred vision), renal vein thrombosis, limb ischemia, myocardial infarction, priapism	TLS monitoring, including creatinine and urea	- Avoid pRBC transfusion (worsens hyperviscosity) unless severe symptomatic anemia, CHF (then slow transfusion 3–5 mL/kg)
			Consider CT head for ICH, ischemia; caution with contrast in case of renal failure	Early start of chemotherapy ±leukapheresis, if
				- Symptomatic
				- ALL and WBC $>400 \times 10^9$/L
				- AML and WBC $>200 \times 10^9$/L

ALL, Acute lymphoblastic leukemia; *AML*, acute myeloid leukemia; *CBC*, complete blood count; *CHF*, congestive heart failure; *CML*, chronic myeloid leukemia; *CNS*, central nervous system; *CT*, computed tomography; *CVL*, central venous line; *CXR*, chest x-ray; *DIC*, disseminated intravascular coagulation; *ECG*, electrocardiogram; *FFP*, fresh frozen plasma; *GU*, genitourinary; *HL*, Hodgkin lymphoma; *ICH*, intracranial hemorrhage; *INR*, international normalized ratio; *LCH*, Langerhans cell histiocytosis; *LOC*, level of consciousness; *MRI*, magnetic resonance imaging; *NHL*, non-Hodgkin lymphoma; *PLT*, platelet; *pRBC*, packed red blood cell; *PTT*, partial thromboplastin time; *SVC*, superior vena cava; *TLS*, tumor lysis syndrome; *WBC*, white blood cell; *XR*, x-ray.

> **PEARL**
>
> In the evaluation of a child with possible leukemia, always remember
> 1. Rule out mediastinal mass (CXR)
> 2. Monitor for tumor lysis syndrome (TLS) (urate, LDH, extended lytes) and ensure adequate hydration (IV fluids)
> 3. Check for disseminated intravascular coagulation (DIC) (CBC, INR, PTT, fibrinogen, D-dimer)
> 4. Have a low threshold to start broad-spectrum antibiotics

1. Comprises 25% to 30% of all childhood cancers
2. **Acute:** 97%; acute lymphoblastic leukemia (ALL), acute myeloid leukemia (AML), mixed phenotype acute leukemia (MPAL, rare)
3. **Chronic:** 3%; chronic myeloid leukemia (CML), juvenile myelomonocytic leukemia (JMML)
4. **Comparison of ALL and AML:** see Table 30.5

Table 30.5	Comparison of Acute Lymphoblastic Leukemia and Acute Myeloid Leukemia	
	Acute Lymphoblastic Leukemia (ALL)	**Acute Myeloid Leukemia (AML)**
Epidemiology	~75% childhood leukemia	~20% childhood leukemia
	Originates in lymphoid cells in bone marrow (80% B-cell, 15%–20% T-cell lineage)	Originates in myeloid cells in bone marrow
	Peak age 2–5 years, M>F	Incidence peaks in neonatal period and adolescence
		Molecular classification provides diagnostic and prognostic information, helps guide management
Factors in risk stratification	Cell of origin: T-cell lineage confers higher risk of relapse	Cytogenetics - May be favorable, intermediate risk, or high risk - Myeloid leukemia of Down syndrome has lower risk of relapse
	Age - Standard risk: 1–9 years - High risk: <1 or ≥10 years	Response to induction treatment: MRD-positive after induction is associated with a higher risk of relapse; role in determining treatment intensity is unclear
	WBC count - Standard risk: WBC <50 × 10⁹/L - High risk: WBC ≥50 × 10⁹/L	
	Cytogenetics: may be favorable, neutral, or unfavorable	
	Response to induction treatment: induction failure (MRD >0.01%) confers high risk, intensifies therapy	
	Other - High-risk features: CNS-positive, testicular disease - Steroid pretreatment affects risk stratification	

Oncology

30

Table 30.5	**Comparison of Acute Lymphoblastic Leukemia and Acute Myeloid Leukemia—cont'd**	
	Acute Lymphoblastic Leukemia (ALL)	**Acute Myeloid Leukemia (AML)**
Clinical manifestations	Bone pain	Similar to ALL
	Anemia: fatigue, pallor	Extramedullary disease: CNS disease, leukemia cutis, myeloid sarcoma (chloromas), gingival hypertrophy
	Thrombocytopenia: bruising/bleeding, petechiae	
	Hepatosplenomegaly, lymphadenopathy	Myelofibrosis: hepatic and bone marrow
	Unexplained fevers, neutropenia	DIC
Investigations	CBC and differential, reticulocyte count, blood film, INR, PTT, G6PD	Initial investigations as in ALL
	Extended electrolytes, urea, creatinine, urate, LDH, ALT, AST, albumin, bilirubin, glucose	Echo: before starting treatment, as first day chemotherapy includes cardiotoxic medications
	Immunoglobulins; VZV, CMV, EBV, HSV serology	CT/MRI of myeloid sarcomas (chloromas)
	CXR: to rule out mediastinal mass	
	Flow cytometry on peripheral blood sample	
	BMA and biopsy for morphology, flow cytometry, cytogenetics, molecular genetics	
	LP with CSF cell count, cytospin	
	Echo: if high-risk features	
Treatment	Induction treatment usually includes - Prednisone/dexamethasone, PEG-asparaginase, vincristine, IT chemotherapy - Anthracyclines added if high risk	Common therapeutic agents: cytarabine, daunorubicin, etoposide - No maintenance chemotherapy - Length of treatment: 4–6 months
	Length of treatment: approximately 2.5 years (girls)–3.5 years (boys)	HSCT for high-risk patients: poor responders, unfavorable cytogenetics
Prognosis	Low risk: >90% overall survival High risk: >80% overall survival	Low risk: 75% overall survival High risk: <35% overall survival

ALT, Alanine aminotransferase; *AST,* aspartate aminotransferase; *BMA,* bone marrow aspirate; *CBC,* complete blood count; *CSF,* cerebrospinal fluid; *CMV,* cytomegalovirus; *CNS,* central nervous system; *CT,* computed tomography; *CXR,* chest x-ray; *DIC,* disseminated intravascular coagulation; *EBV,* Epstein-Barr virus; *G6PD,* glucose-6-phosphate dehydrogenase; *HSCT,* hematopoietic stem cell transplantation; *HSV,* herpes simplex virus; *INR,* international normalized ratio; *IT,* intrathecal; *LDH,* lactate dehydrogenase; *LP,* lumbar puncture; *MRD,* minimal residual disease; *MRI,* magnetic resonance imaging; *PEG-asparaginase,* polyethylene-glycol-conjugated asparaginase; *PTT,* partial thromboplastin time; *VZV,* varicella zoster virus; *WBC,* white blood cell.

5. **Risk factors for leukemia:** vast majority have none
   a. Exposure to ionizing radiation, chemotherapy, e.g., alkylating agents, topoisomerase II inhibitors, anthracyclines, radiotherapy
   b. Predisposition syndromes, e.g., T21, Noonan, Bloom, neurofibromatosis, ataxia telangiectasia, Li-Fraumeni, inherited marrow failure syndromes especially Fanconi anemia

> **! PITFALL**
>
> Acute promyelocytic leukemia (APL) has a high early mortality rate because of bleeding. Urgent Oncology consultation with prompt administration of ATRA and transfer to a tertiary care center is necessary.

LYMPHOMA

> **! PITFALL**
>
> Sedation can threaten airway patency in a patient with a mediastinal mass. Consult ICU/Anesthesia promptly if concern for respiratory compromise or before imaging (CT/MRI) with sedation. Keep the head of the bed elevated and avoid agitating the patient.

1. **Two major groups:** see Table 30.6

Table 30.6	Comparison of Hodgkin Lymphoma and Non-Hodgkin Lymphoma	
	Hodgkin Lymphoma (HL)	**Non-Hodgkin Lymphoma (NHL)**
Background	Common in older children, peaks at age 15–34 years, rare <5 years M = F	Common in younger children, median age 10 years F > M
Risk factors	EBV infection First-degree family member with HL	Immunodeficiency syndromes Post-transplant immunosuppression Biological therapies, e.g., infliximab Viruses, e.g., EBV, HIV, HTLV
Clinical manifestations	Painless lymphadenopathy (90%) - "Rubbery" nodes - Cervical and mediastinal most common, can include supraclavicular, axillary, and inguinal regions Pruritus B symptoms - Weight loss >10% over 6 months - Unexplained fever >3 days - Drenching night sweats Splenomegaly, hepatomegaly	Based on size and location of disease - 70% present with advanced disease, including GI, CNS, bone marrow involvement Cervical/axillary lymphadenopathy, anterior mediastinal mass Burkitt (40%) - Rapidly growing intra-abdominal mass causing obstruction, ascites, or intussusception - TLS, renal failure common

Table 30.6	Comparison of Hodgkin Lymphoma and Non-Hodgkin Lymphoma—cont'd	
	Hodgkin Lymphoma (HL)	Non-Hodgkin Lymphoma (NHL)
Investigations	CBC, liver and renal function, urate, ALP (bone, liver), ESR (active disease), ferritin, immunological profile (T-, B-cell counts, T-cell function, immunoglobulins) Staging - CXR, CT neck/chest/abdomen/pelvis, FDG-PET - BMA and biopsy (bilateral) Tissue diagnosis - Excisional or core lymph node biopsy - Avoid fine needle aspiration because of sampling error	CBC, liver and renal function, LDH, urate, PO_4, Ca LP to assess for CNS involvement Staging - CXR, CT neck/chest/abdomen, bone scan
Treatment	Combination chemotherapy ± radiotherapy Chemotherapeutic combinations include: doxorubicin, bleomycin, vincristine, etoposide, prednisone, cyclophosphamide	Chemotherapy combinations depend on diagnosis Radiation generally not used in primary treatment
Prognosis	Stages IA/B, IIA cure rate: >90% Stages IIB, IIIA/B, IV cure rate: >80% Adverse outcomes: advanced stage, B symptoms, bulky disease, extranodal extension, male sex, high ESR, Hb < 100 g/L, WBC > 11.5 × 10⁹/L	Stages I, II cure rate: >85% Stage III, IV cure rate: depends on subtype; ranges from 70% to 95%

ALP, Alkaline phosphatase; *BMA*, bone marrow aspirate; *CBC*, complete blood count; *CNS*, central nervous system; *CT*, computed tomography; *CXR*, chest x-ray; *EBV*, Epstein-Barr virus; *ESR*, erythrocyte sedimentation rate; *FDG-PET*, fluorodeoxyglucose-positron emission tomography; *GI*, gastrointestinal; *Hb*, hemoglobin; *HIV*, human immunodeficiency virus; *HTLV*, human T-lymphotropic virus; *LDH*, lactate dehydrogenase; *LP*, lumbar puncture; *TLS*, tumor lysis syndrome; *WBC*, white blood cell.

NEUROBLASTOMA AND WILMS TUMOR

. **Comparison:** see Table 30.7

Table 30.7	Comparison of Neuroblastoma and Wilms Tumor	
	Neuroblastoma	Wilms Tumor
Pathogenesis	Small round blue cell tumor of childhood Arises from primordial neural crest cells that normally develop into adrenal medulla and sympathetic ganglia	Also called nephroblastoma Derived from primitive metanephric mesoderm WT1 (11p13) mutations in 15% to 20% of tumors

Continued 845

Table 30.7	Comparison of Neuroblastoma and Wilms Tumor—cont'd	
	Neuroblastoma	**Wilms Tumor**
Epidemiology	7% of all pediatric malignancies	6% of all pediatric malignancies
	Most common extracranial solid tumor	Most common primary renal tumor
	Most common malignancy of infancy	Peak age 3–4 years
	Peak age 2 years	
Associated syndromes	Other neural crest disorders, including - Neurofibromatosis type I (NF1) - Hirschsprung disease - Congenital central hypoventilation syndrome	Denys-Drash: Wilms tumor, early renal failure with mesangial sclerosis, male pseudohermaphroditism
		WAGR: <u>W</u>ilms tumor, <u>A</u>niridia, <u>G</u>enitourinary abnormalities, <u>R</u>ange of developmental delays
		Perlman: overgrowth, developmental delay, cryptorchidism, dysmorphic facial features
		Beckwith-Wiedemann
Clinical manifestations	Early stages often asymptomatic	Often asymptomatic
	Can present anywhere along the sympathetic chain, most commonly as an adrenal mass	Palpable abdominal mass: most common presentation (60%) ± abdominal pain (often following trauma)
	Presentation varies by site - Head/neck/thoracic: neck mass, dyspnea, dysphagia, Horner syndrome - Abdominal: palpable mass, pain, vomiting, constipation, urinary retention - Paraspinal: back pain, abnormal gait, hypotonia, paraplegia, bowel/bladder dysfunction - Metastasis (detected at time of diagnosis in 75%): bone pain, periorbital ecchymoses ("raccoon eyes"), proptosis, skin nodules ("blueberry muffin"), cytopenias	Hypertension (25%)
		Hematuria (25%): usually microscopic
		Polycythemia
		Bleeding diathesis caused by acquired von Willebrand syndrome
		Associated congenital anomalies (12%–15%): commonly hamartomas, GU/MSK anomalies, hemihypertrophy, aniridia
	Paraneoplastic syndromes - Opsoclonus-myoclonus-ataxia syndrome: immune-mediated - Vasoactive intestinal peptide release: intractable watery diarrhea - Catecholamine release: sweating and hypertension	

	Neuroblastoma	**Wilms Tumor**
Investigations	Urine HVA, VMA	CBC, INR, PTT, fibrinogen
	US abdomen, CXR	LFTs (metastases), urea, creatinine
	Additional tests for diagnosis/staging - CT/MRI abdomen ± chest - MRI for paraspinal masses - Tissue biopsy - BMA and biopsy (bilateral) - MIBG; FDG-PET if not MIBG-avid	Urinalysis (hematuria)
		US abdomen, with Doppler for renal veins and IVC
		CT/MRI abdomen (evaluate both kidneys)
		CT chest (metastases)
		If other congenital anomalies: peripheral blood for chromosomal analysis
		If possible bone/brain metastases: bone scan, MRI brain
Staging	Based on - Extent of disease: localized tumor vs. involvement of nearby structures or metastases - Ability to perform complete surgical resection	Based on - Extension of tumor from kidney into the abdomen - Evidence of distant metastasis or bilateral kidney involvement - Histology: presence of anaplasia - Molecular features
Treatment	Very low risk: may be observed, as most cases spontaneously regress	Surgical excision followed by chemotherapy
	Low risk: surgical resection	Many require RT
	Intermediate risk: chemotherapy, surgery	
	High risk: chemotherapy, RT, surgery, autologous BMT, immunotherapy, cis-retinoic acid	
Prognosis	Good prognosis - Age <18 months at diagnosis - Favorable histology - Overall survival >90%	Good prognosis - Young age - Low stage - Favorable histology - Overall survival >95%
	Poor prognosis - MYC-N amplification, other chromosomal aberrations - Overall survival improving, most recent data suggest 75%–85%	Poor prognosis - Bilateral disease, large tumor size, presence of metastases - Poor histological and molecular features - Overall survival >85%

BMA, Bone marrow aspirate; *BMT*, bone marrow transplant; *CBC*, complete blood count; *CT*, computed tomography; *CXR*, chest x-ray; *FDG-PET*, fluorodeoxyglucose-positron emission tomography; *GU*, genitourinary; *HVA*, homovanillic acid; *INR*, international normalized ratio;

IVC, inferior vena cava; *LFTs,* liver function tests; *MIBG,* meta-iodobenzylguanidine; *MRI,* magnetic resonance imaging; *MSK,* musculoskeletal; *PTT,* partial thromboplastin time; *RT,* radiotherapy; *US,* ultrasound; *VMA,* vanillylmandelic acid.

Modified from Ater JL. Neuroblastoma. In: Behrman RE, Kliegman R, Jenson HB, eds. *Nelson Textbook of Pediatrics.* 17th ed. Philadelphia, PA: WB Saunders; 2004: 1709–1711; Jaffe N, Huff V. Neoplasms of the kidney. In: Behrman RE, Kliegman R, Jenson HB, eds. *Nelson Textbook of Pediatrics.* 17th ed. Philadelphia, PA: WB Saunders; 2004: 1711–1714; Neuroblastoma outcomes derived from Park Y, Kreissmann SG, London WB, Naranjo A. A phase III randomized clinical trial (RCT) of tandem myeloablative autologous stem cell transplant (ASCT) using peripheral blood stem cell (PBSC) as consolidation therapy for high-risk neuroblastoma (HR-NB): a Children's Oncology Group (COG) study [abstract]. *J Clin Oncol.* 2016;34 (suppl; abstr LBA3).

HISTIOCYTIC DISORDERS

1. Rare, diverse group of diseases characterized by excessive proliferation and accumulation of cells of the mononuclear phagocyte (including monocytes and macrophages) and/or dendritic cell system

LANGERHANS CELL HISTIOCYTOSIS (LCH)

1. Clonal proliferation of immature dendritic/myeloid precursor cells
2. Leads to accumulation of LCH cells (pathologically similar to Langerhans cells) in tissue and organs, along with eosinophils, macrophages, lymphocytes, multinucleated giant cells
3. Approximately 60% demonstrate BRAF V600E mutation
4. **Peak incidence:** 1 to 4 years of age
5. **Clinical manifestations:** see Table 30.8
   a. Varied presentation ranging from spontaneous remission to rapid progression and death
   b. **Single-system** (i.e., single organ): unifocal (single site) or multifocal (multiple sites), most often skin or bone
   c. **Multisystem** (i.e., two or more organs): high risk if hematopoietic system, liver or spleen involvement
6. **Investigations**
   a. Thorough history and physical examination: assess for hepatosplenomegaly
   b. Initial bloodwork: CBC and differential, liver function tests
   c. Targeted imaging based on clinical findings: consider US abdomen, skeletal survey, positron emission tomography (PET), MRI brain
   d. Diagnostic biopsy demonstrating characteristic cell surface markers
7. **Treatment**
   a. Local therapy for solitary lesions (e.g., skin, bone): topical steroids, radiotherapy, curettage
   b. Systemic therapy for refractory or multisystem disease: chemotherapy
8. **Prognosis:** poorer outcomes if multisystem disease with high-risk organ involvement (see clinical manifestations above) or poor response to initial therapy

Table 30.8	Common Clinical Manifestations of Langerhans Cell Histiocytosis
Organ System	**Common Manifestations and Associated Symptoms**
Bone (60%–80%)	Lytic lesions of long bones (most common) or skull: pain, fractures, mass effect (e.g., exophthalmos)
Skin	Varied; most commonly diffuse papular scaling lesions similar to seborrheic atopic dermatitis
Lung	Cystic changes, nodular infiltrates or fibrosis: tachypnea, dyspnea, cyanosis, cough, pneumothorax, pleural effusion
Liver	Hepatomegaly, liver dysfunction
Hematopoietic system	Pancytopenia secondary to hypersplenism or direct bone marrow involvement
CNS (more common in multisystem)	Pituitary involvement: diabetes insipidus (characteristic feature of systemic LCH), hyperprolactinemia, hypogonadism
	Space-occupying lesion(s): headache, seizures
	Neurodegenerative: abnormal reflexes, ataxia, intellectual impairment, variable progression to serious CNS disease
Lymph nodes	Massive cervical lymphadenopathy
Gastrointestinal	Diarrhea, malabsorption, hematochezia

CNS, Central nervous system; *LCH*, Langerhans cell histiocytosis.

HEMOPHAGOCYTIC LYMPHOHISTIOCYTOSIS (HLH)

1. Life-threatening disorder characterized by unregulated, excessive activation, and proliferation of macrophages, leading to hypercytokinemia
2. **Primary:** familial form (autosomal recessive), either sole manifestation or as part of broader inherited disorder (e.g., Chediak-Higashi)
3. **Secondary:** also known as macrophage activation syndrome (MAS); response to a trigger, such as infection (e.g., CMV, EBV), malignancy, or rheumatological disorder
4. **Clinical manifestations:** prolonged high fever, hepatosplenomegaly, cytopenias (usually affecting two cell lines), elevated serum ferritin
5. **Diagnosis:** see Box 30.1
   a. Bone marrow evaluation helpful to assess for hemophagocytosis and to rule out malignancy
6. **Treatment**
   a. **Primary:** steroids, etoposide, methotrexate, followed by hematopoietic stem cell transplant (HSCT)
   b. **Secondary:** varies; treat underlying cause, steroids, intravenous immune globulin (IVIG), may require etoposide

Box 30.1 Diagnostic Criteria for Hemophagocytic Lymphohistiocytosis

Molecular diagnosis consistent with HLH, or meeting 5/8 of the following criteria

1. Fever
2. Splenomegaly
3. Cytopenias (affecting ≥2 of 3 lineages)
   Hb < 90 g/L (<100 g/L in infants <4 weeks); PLT < 100 × 10⁹/L; neutrophils < 1 × 10⁹/L
4. Hypertriglyceridemia and/or hypofibrinogenemia
   Fasting triglycerides ≥3 mmol/L; fibrinogen ≤1.5 g/L
5. Ferritin ≥500 mcg/L
6. Low or absent NK-cell activity (per local laboratory reference)
7. Soluble CD25 (i.e., soluble IL-2 receptor) ≥2400 units/mL
8. Hemophagocytosis in bone marrow, spleen, or lymph nodes, with no evidence of malignancy

Hb, Hemoglobin; *IL*, interleukin; *NK*, natural killer; *PLT*, platelet.

Modified from Henter JI, Horne A, Aricó M, et al., for the Histiocyte Society. HLH-2004: diagnostic and therapeutic guidelines for hemophagocytic lymphohistiocytosis. *Pediatr Blood Cancer.* 2007;48:124–131.

MALIGNANT BONE TUMORS

1. ~6% of all childhood malignancies
2. **Most common types:** osteosarcoma (56%) and Ewing sarcoma (34%); see Table 30.9

Table 30.9	Comparison of Osteosarcoma and Ewing Sarcoma	
	Osteosarcoma	**Ewing Sarcoma**
Epidemiology	Bimodal age distribution: peaks in adolescence (age of highest growth velocity) and adults >60 years	Peak incidence in adolescence, uncommon in young children and adults, M > F
Presentation	Local pain and swelling, pathological fracture	Local pain and swelling, pathological fracture
		Constitutional symptoms including fever
		Pelvic/paraspinal tumors may present with symptoms of spinal cord compression
Predisposition	Familial cancer predisposition syndromes, e.g., Li-Fraumeni	None known
	Retinoblastoma (germline RB1 mutation)	
	Paget's disease	
	Radiation exposure	
	Treatment with alkylating chemotherapy	

| Table 30.9 | Comparison of Osteosarcoma and Ewing Sarcoma—cont'd |

	Osteosarcoma	Ewing Sarcoma
Site	Epiphysis/metaphysis of long bones (lower > upper) Most common sites: distal femur, proximal tibia	Diaphysis of lower extremity long bones (45%) and pelvis (20%); also axial skeleton
Investigations	CBC, ALT, AST, LDH, ALP, total bilirubin, urea, creatinine, urinalysis XR, MRI of affected bone Chest CT, bone scan, or FDG-PET/CT to assess for metastases Tissue biopsy	Bloodwork as with osteosarcoma MRI of primary site CT chest, PET (or bone scan) Bilateral BMA and biopsy Pathology: small round blue cell tumor, diagnostic molecular marker EWS/FLI1 t(11;22)
Radiographic signs	Radiating calcification ("sunburst" spiculated pattern) Sclerotic, lytic, or mixed lesions with soft tissue extension	Laminar periosteal reaction ("onion skinning") Can demonstrate similar findings as osteosarcoma
Metastasis	15%–20% have metastasis at diagnosis Most common to lungs and bone	25% have metastasis at diagnosis Lungs (50%–60%), bones (40%), bone marrow (19%)
Treatment	Neoadjuvant and adjuvant chemotherapy Local control achieved by limb-salvage surgery (endoprosthesis, rotationplasty) or amputation Surgical resection of metastatic disease if possible	Chemotherapy Surgery for primary tumor, if resectable Radiation therapy for unresectable or residual disease
Prognosis	No metastases: 60%–70% cure Poor prognosis: metastasis at diagnosis (10%–50% survival), incomplete resection, poor response to chemotherapy, axial skeleton tumor, large tumor, proximal tumor location within limb, short time to recurrence	No metastases: 60%–70% cure Poor prognosis: metastasis at diagnosis (10%–30% survival), older age, axial skeleton tumor, large tumor, high LDH, fever, anemia, aberrant molecular markers, recurrence <2 years from diagnosis

ALP, Alkaline phosphatase; *ALT,* alanine aminotransferase; *AST,* aspartate aminotransferase; *BMA,* bone marrow aspirate; *CBC,* complete blood count; *CT,* computed tomography; *FDG-PET,* fluorodeoxyglucose-positron emission tomography; *LDH,* lactate dehydrogenase; *MRI,* magnetic resonance imaging; *XR,* x-ray.

Modified from Arndt CAS. Neoplasms of bone. In: Behrman RE, Kliegman R, Jenson HB, eds. *Nelson Textbook of Pediatrics.* 17th ed. Philadelphia, PA: WB Saunders; 2004: 1717–1720; Federman N, Van Dyne EA, Bernthal N. Malignant bone tumors. In: Lanzkowsky P, Lipton JM, Fish JD, eds. *Lanzkowsky's Manual of Pediatric Hematology and Oncology.* 6th ed. Amsterdam: Elsevier Academic Press; 2016:Table 27.1, and text.

Oncology

30

1. Second most common type of childhood malignancy; most common type of pediatric solid tumor
2. Leading cause of childhood cancer-related mortality
3. **Classification:** based on molecular features, pathology, and intracranial location (supratentorial vs. infratentorial)
4. **Risk factors:** genetic conditions (e.g., NF1/2, tuberous sclerosis, Gorlin syndrome, Turcot syndrome), radiation exposure
5. **Red flags for CNS malignancy:** see Table 30.10
6. **Comparison of CNS tumors:** see Table 30.11
7. **Infratentorial tumors**
   a. **Most common:** juvenile pilocytic astrocytoma, medulloblastoma
   b. Also: cerebellar astrocytoma, ependymoma, brainstem tumor
   c. **Symptoms:** poor balance, truncal ataxia, incoordination, impaired conjugate/lateral gaze, facial nerve palsy, signs of increased intracranial pressure (ICP)

Table 30.10	Red Flags for Central Nervous System Malignancy
History	**Examination**
Early morning headache and vomiting	Large head circumference
Waking from sleep with headache	Papilledema
Diplopia	Cranial nerve VI palsy (inability to abduct)
Altered level of consciousness	Sun-setting (limited upward gaze)
Irritability, personality change	Cushing's triad (hypertension, bradycardia, abnormal respiration)
Back pain	Gait disturbance
Bowel/bladder dysfunction	Focal neurological deficits
Unexplained failure to thrive	

Table 30.11 **Comparison of Brain Tumors**

	Astrocytoma	Medulloblastoma	Ependymoma
Epidemiology	50% of CNS tumors Peak ages: 5–6 and 12–13 years	20% of CNS tumors Peak ages: 3–4 and 8–10 years 80% occur <15 years of age	9% of CNS tumors Median age: depends on subtype
Description	Glial cell origin	Embryonal tumors of the posterior fossa Divided into four molecular subtypes: Wnt, Shh, Group 3, Group 4	Arise from ependymal cells that line ventricles and spinal cord Can be separated into different biological subtypes based on molecular features
Presentation	Cerebellar, cerebral, or optic pathway tumors (seen in NF1)	Up to 40% spread beyond primary tumor at diagnosis, rarely outside CNS	Posterior fossa (70%), supratentorial or in spinal cord Clinical symptoms depend on location of tumor
Management	Low grade: surgical excision, may use chemotherapy High grade: surgical debulking, RT, chemotherapy	Gross total resection, RT, chemotherapy	Surgical excision, RT Limited role for chemotherapy
Prognosis	Low-grade cerebellar tumor - Complete excision (75%–90%): >90% survival - Incomplete resection: 70%–90% survival Low-grade cerebral tumor: prognosis related to rate of tumor growth, location High grade: 20%–30% overall survival	Outcomes depend on - Extent of residual tumor - Presence of metastases - Histology and molecular subgroup 5-year survival - >80% for standard risk - ~65% for high risk	Outcomes depend on - Molecular characteristics - Histology - Location of tumor - Degree of resection

CNS, Central nervous system; *NF1,* neurofibromatosis type 1; *RT,* radiotherapy.

Adapted with modifications from Strother DR, Pollack IF, Fisher PG, et al. Tumours of the central nervous system. In: Pizzo PA, Poplack DG, eds. and *Principles and Practice of Pediatric Oncology.* 5th ed. Philadelphia, PA: Lippincott Williams & Wilkins; 2006: 778–785, 787–791, 795–798, 801–803.

Oncology

30

8. **Supratentorial tumors**
   a. **Most common:** astrocytoma
   b. Also: ganglioglioma, ganglioneuroma, craniopharyngioma (associated pituitary dysfunction), hypothalamic hamartoma, pineal tumors (e.g., germ cell tumors)
   c. **Symptoms:** seizures, behavioral problems, upper motor neuron signs (hemiparesis, hyperreflexia, loss of sensation), signs of increased ICP, may affect optic pathway (visual field deficits, nystagmus, head tilt)
   d. **Diencephalic syndrome:** seen in hypothalamic tumors; aged 6 months to 3 years; emaciated, anorexic, but hyperalert and euphoric
   e. **Parinaud syndrome:** seen in pineal tumors; failure of upward gaze and pupillary light reaction
9. **Diagnosis**
   a. **CT:** emergent imaging or in unstable patients; also to evaluate for bony invasion, hemorrhage, necrosis, calcification
   b. **MRI ± gadolinium of brain and spine:** functional and anatomic information; differentiates cystic from solid tumors, highlights areas of blood-brain barrier breakdown, can identify mass effect and signs of increased ICP
   c. **Cerebrospinal fluid (CSF):** assess for tumor cells
   d. **Resection:** if possible for tissue diagnosis, relief of increased ICP, definitive treatment in some cases
   e. Biopsy of brainstem tumors often avoided because of high morbidity
10. **Treatment**
   a. **Surgery:** required upfront for many tumors; often a gross total resection is important for best outcome
   b. **Radiotherapy:** can have major role in treatment depending on pathology, extent of resection, patient age—avoided in young children because of adverse neurocognitive effects
   c. **Chemotherapy:** used in select primary brain tumors and often in young children

CHEMOTHERAPY

1. Mainstay of treatment for most malignancies
2. **Key principles:** use of dose-intense, combination chemotherapy; need to balance toxicity with therapeutic anti-cancer effect
3. **Common agents:** see Table 30.12

Table 30.12

Medication	Mechanism of Action	Adverse Effects
Asparaginase	Depletes asparagine, inhibiting RNA and DNA synthesis, resulting in cell apoptosis	Hypersensitivity reactions (~15%), anaphylaxis, coagulopathy, thrombosis (including CNS), pancreatitis, hyperbilirubinemia, hyperglycemia
Cisplatin	Heavy metal complex; platinates DNA-inducing cross-links, leading to apoptosis	Nephrotoxicity (azotemia, electrolyte abnormalities), ototoxicity, neurotoxicity (paresthesias, seizures), nausea, emesis, mild myelosuppression
Cyclophosphamide	Alkylating agent; inhibits DNA replication and initiates cell death	Hemorrhagic cystitis, myelosuppression, alopecia
Cytarabine	S phase-specific antimetabolite; inhibits DNA polymerase, interfering with DNA repair/replication, and resulting in cell death	Myelosuppression, nausea, emesis, fever, rash, conjunctivitis, rarely neurotoxicity (cerebellar symptoms)
Dexamethasone/Prednisone	Binds to nuclear steroid receptors, interferes with NF-kB activation and apoptotic pathways	Immunosuppression, hypertension, bradycardia, hyperglycemia, acute vascular necrosis, peptic ulcer, pancreatitis, psychosis, Cushing syndrome, adrenal suppression
Doxorubicin	Anthracycline; induces topoisomerase-mediated DNA damage	Myelosuppression, mucositis, alopecia, nausea, emesis, cardiotoxicity, hyperbilirubinemia
Etoposide	Inhibits topoisomerase II, resulting in accumulation of DNA breaks, inhibition of DNA replication and transcription, and apoptosis	Anaphylactoid reaction, peripheral neuropathy, myelosuppression, hepatotoxicity
Mercaptopurine	Affects DNA synthesis by inhibiting nucleotide interconversions and purine synthesis	Hepatotoxicity, myelosuppression, immunosuppression, hypoglycemia, hyperuricemia
Methotrexate	Antimetabolite and antifolate agent, inhibits nucleic acid synthesis	Intrathecal: neurotoxicity (seizures, episodic acute hemiparesis, encephalopathy) IV: myelosuppression, mucositis, nephrotoxicity, hepatotoxicity
Vincristine	Interferes with formation of mitotic spindle in S phase of cell cycle, thereby arresting tumor cells in metaphase	Neuropathic pain, peripheral motor and sensory neuropathy (e.g., foot drop, vocal cord paralysis, jaw pain, severe constipation), SIADH, hyperbilirubinemia

Common Chemotherapeutic Agents

CNS, Central nervous system; *DNA*, deoxyribonucleic acid; *IV*, intravenous; *NF-kB*, nuclear factor kB; *RNA*, ribonucleic acid; *SIADH*, syndrome of inappropriate antidiuretic hormone secretion.

Oncology

30

1. **Hematopoietic stem cells:** characterized by their ability to self-renew and differentiate into all mature blood lineages
2. **Hematopoietic stem cell transplantation (HSCT):** a therapeutic modality for many malignant (e.g., high-risk leukemias, some solid tumors to facilitate the administration of high-dose chemotherapy) and non-malignant (e.g., metabolic disorders, immunodeficiencies) conditions
   a. Also known as bone marrow transplant (BMT)
3. **Classification:** patient receives stem cells from a donor (allogeneic) or from themselves (autologous)

PROCEDURE

1. **Collection:** human-leukocyte antigen (HLA)-matched stem cells collected from bone marrow, peripheral blood, or umbilical cord blood
   a. Each source carries own risk and benefit profile
2. **Myeloablation:** patient receives conditioning regimen (chemotherapy ± radiation) to prepare bone marrow to receive HSCT
3. **Infusion:** stem cells administered via central line; known as Day 0
4. **Engraftment:** typically defined as neutrophils $>0.5 \times 10^9$/L for 3 days
5. **Monitoring:** patient monitored closely post-transplant for complications including graft-versus-host-disease, serious infections, long-term effects of the conditioning regimen (e.g., cardiorespiratory compromise), and relapse

NOVEL TREATMENTS

IMMUNOTHERAPIES

1. **Mechanism:** harness patient's immune system to target malignant cells
2. **Bispecific T-cell engager (BiTEs):** antibody construct linking T-cells with antigen on tumor cells (e.g., blinatumomab, linking CD19-expressing tumor cells to CD3 on T-cells)
3. **Chimeric antigen receptor T-cells (CAR T-cells):** patient's T-cells engineered to target specific antigen on cancer cells (e.g., anti-CD19 CAR T-cells used in recurrent/refractory ALL)
4. **Checkpoint inhibitors:** tumor cells can express proteins that allow them to evade detection by regulatory T-cells, such as programmed death-ligand 1 (PD-L1). Checkpoint inhibitors block these inhibitory proteins, allowing T-cells to detect and clear malignant cells (e.g., pembrolizumab, an anti–PD-L1 antibody).

TARGETED THERAPIES

1. **Antibody-drug conjugates:** monoclonal antibody specific for an antigen on tumor cell surface, linked to cytotoxic therapy (e.g., gemtuzumab ozogamicin, anti-CD33 linked to calicheamicin)

2. **Kinase inhibitors:** target constitutively activated signaling pathways that drive certain malignancies (e.g., MEK inhibitors inhibit the mitogen-activated protein kinase [MAPK] pathway)

SUPPORTIVE CARE

ANEMIA

1. Common, usually because of treatment-related myelosuppression
   a. May be related to malignant infiltration, secondary myelodysplasia, viral suppression, blood loss, hemolysis
2. **Transfusion threshold:** Hb ≤ 70 g/L in patients receiving chemotherapy and/or radiotherapy
   a. Consider transfusing at higher Hb if: symptomatic anemia, hemodynamic instability, bleeding/hemolysis, long time to expected marrow recovery
3. **Transfusion dosing:** 15 mL/kg packed red blood cells (pRBCs), expected to increase Hb by 20 to 30 g/L
4. **Irradiated blood:** reduces risk of graft-versus-host disease due to donor lymphocytes
   a. Use in: infants <6 months, history or ongoing use of intense chemotherapy (purine analogs, alemtuzumab, antithymocyte globulin), leukemia, lymphoma, HSCT
5. **Leukoreduced blood:** all Canadian blood products have white cells removed via filtration before storage
   a. Considered CMV-safe, equivalent to CMV-negative products
   b. Previously used CMV-negative blood in seronegative patients to prevent severe CMV infection if immunocompromised or previous/upcoming HSCT

THROMBOCYTOPENIA

1. Common, because of myelosuppression from chemotherapy, radiotherapy, or malignancy
2. **Transfusion dosing:** 10 mL/kg platelets (max. 300 mL), expected to increase PLT count by 50 to 100 × 10^9/L
3. **Transfusion threshold:** determined based on the clinical scenario, to minimize risk of bleeding

NEUTROPENIA

1. **Management of neutropenia with fever:** see Figure 30.3
2. **G-CSF:** indicated in certain scenarios to reduce duration of neutropenia after high-risk chemotherapy
   a. **Dosing:** 5 mcg/kg/day SC/IV once daily
   b. **Duration:** variable, often continued until ANC recovery (usually 10–14 days post-myelosuppressive chemotherapy)
   c. **Adverse effects:** bone, joint, muscle pain (common); fever, rash, nephrotoxicity (uncommon)

LATE EFFECTS IN CHILDHOOD CANCER SURVIVORS

1. Five-year overall survival for childhood cancers now >80%
2. **Treatment-related effects:** common; secondary to chemotherapy, radiation, or surgery
3. **Highest morbidity/mortality:** secondary neoplasms, followed by cardiac disease
   a. Endocrine disorders also very common
   b. See Table 30.13 for details
4. **Management:** targeted screening and follow-up to identify such late effects and facilitate early intervention

Table 30.13	Late Effects in Survivors of Childhood Cancer	
System	**Associated Treatment(s)**	**Late Effects**
Cardiac	Anthracyclines (e.g., daunorubicin, doxorubicin), chest/mantle radiotherapy	Cardiomyopathy, CHF, valvular heart disease, early onset adult coronary artery disease
CNS	Cranial irradiation, tumor resection, IT chemotherapy	Neurocognitive deficits, developmental delay, focal neurological deficits, hearing loss
Endocrine	Alkylating agents (cyclophosphamide, ifosfamide), head/body radiotherapy, surgical resection	Pituitary dysfunction (short stature, early/delayed puberty), infertility, hypothyroidism
Respiratory	Bleomycin, radiotherapy	Pulmonary fibrosis, interstitial pneumonitis, restrictive/obstructive lung disease
Psychosocial	All modalities	Mental health (depression, anxiety, PTSD), chronic pain/fatigue, marital issues, under/unemployment
Other	Radiation, chemotherapy (topoisomerase II inhibitors, alkylating agents)	Secondary malignancy

CHF, Congestive heart failure; *CNS*, central nervous system; *IT*, intrathecal; *PTSD*, post-traumatic stress disorder.

FURTHER READING

Lanzkowsky P, Lipton JM, Fish JD. *Lanzkowsky's Manual of Pediatric Hematology and Oncology.* 6th ed. Amsterdam: Elsevier Academic Press; 2016.
Orkin SH, Nathan DG, Ginsburg D, Look AT, Fisher DE, Lux SE., eds. *Nathan and Oski's Hematology of Infancy and Childhood.* 8th ed. Philadelphia, PA: Elsevier Saunders; 2015.
Pizzo PA, Poplack DG, eds. *Principles and Practice of Pediatric Oncology.* 5th ed. Philadelphia, PA: Lippincott Williams & Wilkins; 2006.

USEFUL WEBSITES

American Cancer Society. Available at: www.cancer.org
British Columbia Cancer Agency. Available at: www.bccancer.bc.ca
National Cancer Institute. Available at: www.cancer.gov

Ophthalmology

Shelby Thompson • Asim Ali

Also see page xviii for a list of other abbreviations used throughout this book

CN	cranial nerve
CPS	Canadian Pediatric Society
EOM	extraocular movement
FB	foreign body
ICP	intracranial pressure
NAI	nonaccidental injury
OD	right eye
OS	left eye
OU	both eyes
RAPD	relative afferent pupillary defect
ROP	retinopathy of prematurity

> ### ✳ PEARL
>
> Mnemonic for quick childhood eye examination: FAIR
> **F**ixation (vision)
> **A**lignment
> **I**nspection
> **R**ed reflex

PHYSICAL EXAMINATION OF THE EYE

A. Visual Acuity

Always measure visual acuity before manipulating the eye. Testing is typically performed at 6 m (20 ft) but may vary according to age and specific test. Testing is completed one eye at a time, with the suspected better eye first. Test best corrected vision (wearing glasses, or through pinhole). The highest level of the chart recognizable by the child should be used (e.g., if a child can recognize Snellen letters at 4 years of age, then use Snellen chart). In urgent cases, do crude tests, such as counting fingers, hand motion, or light perception.

1. **Infants:** Infants can face follow from 0 to 4 weeks of age and can follow a target at 2 months of age. Test the ability to fixate, follow a target (brightly colored toy, target with lights, caregiver's face).
2. **Children 3 to 5 years old:** Use schematic picture or other illiterate eye chart; HOTV chart (four letter shapes), or Lea symbols (shapes)
3. **Children over 5 years old:** Test at 6 m (20 ft) with Snellen chart (OD, OS, OU); record results as ratio (e.g., "20/50^{-2} " indicates patient read line of letters at 20 ft that a normal eye could read at 50 ft; minus 2 indicates two mistakes made)

B. Confrontation testing for visual fields

1. Test all four quadrants in one eye, while occluding the other eye (e.g., face the patient, the patient fixes their left open eye on your right open eye, test

patient's ability to see target/finger that you bring in from periphery to center, comparing with your own visual field. Repeat with patient's opposite eye).

C. Extraocular movement and ocular alignment

1. **Range of movement**: check eight cardinal gaze positions: right, left, up, down, up right, up left, down right, and down left

2. **Smooth pursuit** and **saccadic eye movements**

3. **Strabismus**

    a. **Hirschberg (corneal light reflex) test**: shine penlight onto cornea of both eyes simultaneously; light reflection should be centered symmetrically in both pupils or just nasal to center; if one eye is not aligned with the other, light reflection is displaced in the opposite direction of misalignment relative to pupil center (Figure 31.1).

    b. **Cover, uncover test**: child fixates on object approx. 6 m away. Performed by covering one eye at a time. The uncovered eye should not move. The covered eye should also not reposition when exposed. If any such movement occurs during this test, providing vision is good (fixation is well maintained) then there is an ocular misalignment (strabismus) and the child should be referred for further assessment.

Figure 31.1 Hirschberg Test

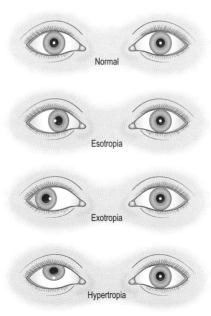

Normal

Esotropia

Exotropia

Hypertropia

Patient focuses on light source held ~2 feet away and light reflection on cornea is observed by examiner.

D. Pupillary examination
1. Assess if **equal in size** and **reaction to light and accommodation**
2. Assess for **bilateral red reflex**.

E. External examination (with or without slit lamp)
1. **General inspection**
2. **Individual examination of the following:**
    a. Lids, lashes, and lacrimal gland
    b. Sclera and conjunctiva
    c. Cornea (if necessary, consider fluorescein dye to aid in diagnosis of abrasions and ulcers)
    d. Anterior chamber: slit lamp required for assessment of depth, clarity, presence of cells
    e. Iris

F. Fundus examination
1. Using **direct ophthalmoscope** (ideally with well-dilated pupils using short acting mydriatics) examine the **optic disc** (should have clear margins, appear pink-orange in color with central pallor [cup], cup-to-disc ratio 0.3), the **macula** (oval shaped pigmented area near center of retina), and retinal **vessels** (look for dilatation or tortuosity, hemorrhage). If view of fundus is blurred, may indicate vitritis or vitreous hemorrhage.

See Table 31.1

Table 31.1	Routine Eye Screening	
Age	Screening Test	Referral to Ophthalmology Required
Premature neonates	ROP	See Chapter 27 Neonatology
Newborn– 3 months	- A complete examination of the skin and external eye structures, including the conjunctiva, cornea, iris, and pupils - An inspection of the red reflex to rule out lenticular opacities or major posterior eye disease	- Structural defects should be referred; high-risk newborns (at risk of ROP and family histories of hereditary ocular diseases) should be examined by an ophthalmologist - Absent (black/white) or asymmetric red reflex require urgent referral
6–12 months of age	- Conduct examination as described above - Ocular alignment should be observed to detect strabismus. The corneal light reflex should be central and the cover- uncover test should be normal - Fixation and following a target are observed	- As described above plus for abnormal eye movements - Strabismus (constant at any age, intermittent manifest strabismus after 4–6 months of age)
3–5 years of age	- Conduct examination as described above - Visual acuity testing should be completed with an age-appropriate tool	- As described above; ≥2 line difference between eyes on repeated vision testing, worse than 20/30 either eye before age 5 years or worse than 20/20 either eye after age 5 years
6–18 years of age	- Screen as described above whenever routine health examinations are conducted. Examine whenever complaints occur	

ROP, Retinopathy of prematurity.

EYELIDS

A. Hordeolum (stye) and chalazion
1. **Definition:** obstruction and/or inflammation of ducts of eyelid glands; on eyelid margins (**stye, hordeolum**) or within lid (**chalazion:** noninflamed, painless bump from obstruction of meibomian gland and associated with chronic granulomatous inflammation); usually sterile despite swelling/discharge but if infected most likely *Staphylococcus aureus.*
2. **Management:** daily baby shampoo eyelash scrubs with cloth; warm compresses to lids daily to bid; may add ophthalmic erythromycin or fusidic acid ointment until symptoms subside; refer if symptoms affect vision or

863

condition persists despite lid scrubs for 4 to 6 weeks. Same treatment is recommended for blepharitis (inflammation, crusting of lid margins).

B. Ptosis
1. **Definition:** drooping of eyelid (usually upper eyelid); unilateral or bilateral; congenital or acquired; isolated or associated with other ocular disorders (e.g., lid tumors, congenital fibrosis syndrome, cranial nerve [CN] III palsy, Horner syndrome) or systemic disorders (e.g., myasthenia gravis, muscular dystrophy, botulism).
2. **Pseudoptosis:** differential includes enophthalmos (after blow-out fracture), small eye (microphthalmia), eyelid lesion (e.g., chalazion/stye, tumor), eyelid swelling

ORBIT

A. Orbital cellulitis
1. See Table 31.2 for preseptal (periorbital) versus orbital cellulitis

Table 31.2	**Preseptal (Periorbital) Versus Orbital Cellulitis**	
	Preseptal Cellulitis	**Orbital Cellulitis**
Anatomy	Infection anterior to orbital septum, including lid	Serious infection posterior to orbital septum. May spread posteriorly to cavernous sinus and brain (causing cavernous sinus thrombosis or meningitis).
Possible precipitants	Infection on eyelids or face (stye/chalazion, skin trauma, insect bite, dacryocystitis)	Paranasal sinusitis, dental abscess, bacteremia; less often from preseptal cellulitis, intraocular infection or tumor
Symptoms	Pain, redness, systemically well	Pain, redness, systemically unwell
Signs		
Fever	Afebrile (but may be febrile)	Febrile
Eyelids	Red, swollen	Red, swollen
Vision	Normal	Decreased acuity; decreased visual field (if optic nerve involved)
Proptosis	None	Present
EOMs	Normal, full	Decreased, painful EOMs
Pupils	Normal, reactive	Abnormal reaction (if optic nerve involved)
Common organisms	- Nontraumatic: *Streptococcus pneumoniae*, group A streptococci, *Staphylococcus aureus*, *Haemophilus influenza* - Traumatic: *S. aureus* (including MRSA), group A streptococci	*S. aureus* (including MRSA), *strep* species, *H. influenzae*. If sinusitis must consider anaerobes

Table 31.2	Preseptal (Periorbital) Versus Orbital Cellulitis—cont'd	
	Preseptal Cellulitis	**Orbital Cellulitis**
Workup	No imaging required	CT w/contrast to look for orbital/subperiosteal abscess, or cavernous sinus thrombosis (dilated superior orbital vein)
Treatment	- PO antibiotics for mild cases (nontraumatic: cefuroxime; traumatic: cephalexin) - IV antibiotics if infection severe, worsening on antibiotics, systemically unwell, immunocompromised, or <3 months old (nontraumatic: ceftriaxone; traumatic: cefazolin or cloxacillin)	- Prompt ophthalmology and ENT consults - Inpatient IV antibiotics with aerobic and anaerobic coverage (ceftriaxone + cloxacillin + metronidazole; vancomycin only if MRSA concern) - ENT may recommend intranasal steroids, otrivin, salinex if sinusitis - Ophthalmology examination daily; consider surgical drainage if not improving or abscess is present

CT, Computed tomography; *EOM*, extraocular movement; *ENT*, ear nose and throat; *IV*, intravenous; *MRSA*, methicillin-resistant *Staphylococcus aureus*; *PO*, orally.

NASOLACRIMAL DUCT

A. Nasolacrimal duct obstruction

1. **Definition:** failure of canalization of nasolacrimal duct as it enters nose. Seen in infants <12 months old (congenital).

2. **Signs and symptoms:** recurrent mild discharge that worsens on waking with crusted lid margins, with no conjunctival injection, ± tearing that worsens outdoors and during upper respiratory infection. Rarely develops into acute infection of nasolacrimal sac (see later).

3. **Management:** massage several times per day (place index finger in sulcus between eye and side of nasal bridge and apply pressure posteriorly; discharge may be expressed onto eye surface); clean crusted lids with moist cloth; only if obvious conjunctivitis, add topical antibiotics for 1 week.

4. **Natural history:** majority resolve spontaneously by 1 year of age; if persistent, refer to ophthalmologist for duct probing.

B. Dacryocystitis

1. **Definition:** rare acute infection of nasolacrimal sac with inflammation of surrounding tissues between eye and nose; may be associated with or preceded by lacrimal sac mucocele, which can cause respiratory compromise. More common in infants <1 month old.

2. **Management:** IV antibiotics, nasolacrimal probing, as needed, by ophthalmology

A. Ophthalmia neonatorum

1. **Definition:** form of purulent conjunctivitis in infants <1 month old; discharge, eyelid edema, and conjunctival erythema and chemosis

2. **Prevention:** mothers should be screened for STIs before delivery and treated accordingly. Neonatal conjunctivitis prophylaxis strategy remains the subject of debate; CPS currently not recommending routine ocular prophylaxis with erythromycin.

3. Types of neonatal conjunctivitis:

   a. *Neisseria gonorrhoea* **conjunctivitis**
      i. Presentation: marked purulent discharge and lid edema, which manifests usually 2 to 5 days after birth; vision-threatening emergency
      ii. Investigations: conjunctival culture, stat Gram stain (shows intracellular gram-negative diplococci). If unwell, consider blood cultures and cerebrospinal fluid (CSF) cultures.
      iii. Management: one dose of ceftriaxone (IM or IV) or cefotaxime. Perform frequent ocular lavage in hospital with normal saline to reduce bacterial load. Must consult ophthalmologist as gonorrhea keratitis can rapidly result in corneal perforation.

   b. **Chlamydia conjunctivitis**
      i. Presentation: milder conjunctivitis, less discharge and lid edema compared with gonococcus and also presents later at 5 to 14 days after birth
      ii. Investigations: eye swab for rapid immunologic tests, Giemsa stain, and special tissue culture. If born to mother with untreated chlamydial infection, monitor for symptoms but routine culture for asymptomatic infants not necessary.
      iii. Management: erythromycin 50 mg/kg/day PO divided QID for 14 days (or azithromycin 20 mg/kg/day PO q24 ×3 days)

   c. **Other:** conjunctivitis in newborn can also be caused by various other bacteria and viruses (including pseudomonas, streptococcus and staphylococcus species, and other gram negative organisms)

B. Conjunctivitis beyond neonatal period

1. See Table 31.3 for common causes of conjunctivitis

Table 31.3	Clinical Comparison of Common Causes of Conjunctivitis[a]					
Feature	Bacterial (Nonchlamydial)	Viral (Nonherpetic)	Herpetic	Chlamydial	Allergic	Chemical
Discharge	Purulent	Clear or mildly purulent	Clear	Clear or mildy purulent	Clear ± stringy mucous	Rare acutely
Lid swelling	Moderate to severe	Mild to severe	Mild	Mild	Mild to severe	Mild to severe
Onset	Subacute	Subacute	Acute	Subacute or chronic	Hyperacute (exposure) or chronic (seasonal)	Acute
Injection	Severe	Moderate to severe	Moderate	Moderate	Mild to severe	Mild to severe (white eye suggests tissue necrosis)
Cornea fluorescein stain	Nonspecific	Nonspecific	Superficial punctate keratitis, dendritic ulcer	Nonspecific	None	Nonspecific
Unilateral/bilateral	Uni/bilateral	Usually bilateral (second eye affected days later)	Unilateral (bilateral may be seen if history of atopy)	Usually bilateral	Usually bilateral	Uni/bilateral
Contact history	Common	Common	No	Common (STI)	Rare	Common

Continued

Table 31.3 — Clinical Comparison of Common Causes of Conjunctivitis[a]—cont'd

Feature	Bacterial (Nonchlamydial)	Viral (Nonherpetic)	Herpetic	Chlamydial	Allergic	Chemical
Preauricular node	Common	Common	Occasional	Occasional	None	None
Other associations	- Otitis media - More common in children <5 y/o	- Otitis media, pharyngitis Viral prodrome - Burning, gritty feeling in eye.	- History of eyelid or oral lesions	- Genitourinary infection	- Chemosis, itchy, history of atopy	- Chemosis, limbal ischemia - Alkali injury worse than acid
Treatment	- Erythromycin BID-QID, Gramcidin/polymyxin B (polysporin) or polymyxin B/trimethoprim (Polytrim) q4–12h - Avoid sulfa agents, aminoglycosides, quinolones	- Symptomatic relief, cool compresses, artificial tears PRN - Hand hygiene important to prevent spread	- PO acyclovir - Consult ophthalmologist - Do NOT prescribe steroids	- Systemic treatment (azithromycin) - Consult ophthalmologist	- Avoid allergens, consider artificial tears, mast cell stabilizers, systemic antihistamines	- Irrigate eye with water ASAP - In ER: copious lavage with saline after instillation of anesthetic drops; use 2L or until pH neutral/equal to unaffected eye (~pH 7) - After lavage treat as corneal abrasion and consult ophthalmologist

[a]Not all cases of conjunctivitis are infectious or allergic in nature.

PO, Orally; *PRN*, as needed; *STI*, sexually transmitted infection.

C. Subconjunctival hemorrhage

1. **Etiology:** most commonly from trauma or elevated pressure (Valsalva maneuver, forceful coughing, vomiting). If extensive (180–360 degrees) and history of trauma, suspect ruptured globe.

2. **Management:** artificial tears for comfort; blood resorbs over few weeks

CORNEA

A. Corneal abrasion

1. **Signs and symptoms**: may include pain, tearing, photophobia, rarely decreased vision; pain improves with topical anesthetic (diagnostic and temporarily therapeutic); may have minimal symptoms

2. **Diagnosis:** absent corneal epithelium seen when fluorescein dye instilled in eye (water-soluble orange dye; becomes green when viewed under cobalt/fluorescent blue light); if vertical linear abrasion(s), suspect conjunctival FB under upper lid and perform lid eversion. Look for chalky white or yellow lesion (i.e., ulcer) on slit lamp examination (urgent referral if present). If patient is in significant pain/discomfort, can instill anesthetic drops (proparacaine 0.5% or tetracaine 0.5%) before examination (do not prescribe for home use).

3. **Management**

   a. If no ulcer, treat with ophthalmic antimicrobial (erythromycin ointment or gramicidin-polymyxin B drops or trimethoprim-polymyxin B drops); if pain severe can use cycloplegic agent (e.g., cyclopentolate HCl, tropicamide). Refer to ophthalmologist if symptomatic after 24 to 48 hours, large central abrasion, or poor healing.

   b. Topical anesthetics should not be prescribed because they delay healing and may cause an ulcer

   c. No need to patch eye (does not improve healing or pain); may patch if patient prefers

   d. Patch should **never be used for contact lens wearers**, even after contact lens has been removed (increased risk of infection) or in those who have abrasion secondary to vegetable matter in eye (e.g., tree branch).

⁂ **PEARL**

Bacterial keratitis is a serious infection of the cornea which can affect contact lens wearers. Symptoms include pain, foreign body sensation, tearing, and photophobia. Contact lenses should be removed, and urgent ophthalmology consultation sought.

ANTERIOR CHAMBER

A. Hyphema

1. **Definition:** blood in anterior chamber (behind cornea in front of iris). Usually sign of severe ocular trauma, diagnosis is made based upon history of eye trauma and examination. Slit lamp examination may be necessary to rule out microhyphema.

2. **Management:** urgent Ophthalmology consultation. Bed rest with 30-degrees elevation of head of bed, dim lighting, eye shield, topical steroids, cycloplegics, and antiglaucoma drops, and antiemetics if necessary.

3. **Complications:** recurrent hemorrhage and secondary glaucoma may occur, especially in first 3 to 5 days; daily ophthalmic follow-up during this period.

B. Uveitis and iritis

1. **Definition:** inflammation of **uvea (iris, ciliary body, and choroid)**. Anterior uveitis = iritis (most common).

2. **Etiology:** consider traumatic, inflammatory (Kawasaki disease, pauci-articular arthritides), infectious, and malignant causes

3. **Iritis signs and symptoms:** pain, ciliary flush (conjunctival injection at corneoscleral junction), photophobia, lacrimation

4. **Diagnosis:** slit lamp and funduscopic examination by ophthalmologist: cells and flare in the anterior chamber (iritis), vitritis, and chorioretinitis

5. **Management:** refer to ophthalmologist for topical cycloplegics and steroids; oral and/or IV steroids, and other immune-modulating drugs in severe cases

PUPIL AND IRIS

A. Afferent pupil defect (Marcus Gunn pupil)

1. **Definition:** a medical sign observed during the swinging-flashlight test whereupon the patient's pupils constrict less (therefore appearing to dilate) when a bright light is swung from the unaffected eye to the affected eye

2. **Etiology:** unilateral or asymmetric defects of anterior prechiasmal optic pathway (e.g., optic neuritis) or extensive retinal dysfunction (e.g., total retinal detachment); pupils should still be of equal size because of intact pupil-light reflex

B. Anisocoria

1. **Definition:** pupils of unequal size. If physiologic (approximately 20% of population) relative difference (usually 1 mm) in pupil size is same in bright or dim illumination.

2. **Diagnosis:** must ascertain which pupil is abnormal by examining under different illuminations: if anisocoria is worse in dim light, a smaller pupil is abnormal (does not dilate properly [e.g., Horner syndrome]); if anisocoria is worse in bright light, a larger pupil is abnormal (does not constrict normally [e.g., CN III palsy, traumatic, or pharmacological mydriasis])

Coloboma
Definition: inferior nasal defect in iris ("keyhole" pupil) and/or choroid. May be associated with microphthalmia (small eye) or cataract; refer to ophthalmologist.

Leukocoria
Definition: white pupillary reflex
Etiology: retinoblastoma until proven otherwise (ocular emergency). Other causes include cataracts, infection (*Toxoplasma*), retinal detachment, persistent hyperplastic primary vitreous, retinopathy of prematurity (ROP), metabolic disorders, trauma, prematurity.

Absent red reflex
Definition: absent (black) reflex
Etiology: light unable to pass because of obstruction (e.g., corneal opacity, hyphema, cataract, vitreous hemorrhage). Requires consultation with ophthalmologist. Most common cause is small pupils; no referral needed if normal red reflex after pharmacologic dilation of pupils.

ETINA

. Retinal hemorrhage
Etiology
a. Common in newborns after routine vaginal delivery; resolves within weeks
b. Most common cause after birth in <4 years is nonaccidental injury (NAI); must consider and evaluate for child maltreatment (see Chapter 9 Child Maltreatment)
c. Other rare causes include leukemia, vasculitis, meningitis, cyanotic congenital heart disease, endocarditis, sepsis, blood dyscrasia, severe life-threatening accidental head trauma (<3%)
d. Sickle cell disease, diabetes, and seizures do not cause retinal hemorrhages in first few years of life

LAUCOMA

Definition: Elevated pressure within the eye that leads to optic nerve damage and visual field loss. May be congenital, juvenile, or secondary.
Signs and symptoms: Infantile (congenital) glaucoma characterized by enlarged eyeball (buphthalmos), watery eyes, photophobia, blepharospasm. Other signs may include corneal edema/clouding, conjunctival injection. May be asymptomatic.
Management of glaucoma: Primarily surgical. Urgent Ophthalmology consultation in all cases to treat/prevent amblyopia and irreversible nerve damage.

Watery eyes and photophobia in an infant should raise suspicion for congenital glaucoma!

OPTIC NERVE

A. Clinical features of optic nerve disease

1. Reduced vision, impaired color vision (may be preserved), afferent pupil defect, visual field loss, ± pain with extraocular movements (EOMs).

B. Papilledema

1. **Definition:** swelling of optic nerve head because of increased intracranial pressure (ICP); typically bilateral. When unilateral, consider papillitis, optic nerve infiltration by malignancy, tuberculosis, sarcoidosis.
2. **Examination findings:** blurred disc margins with diminished view of vessels on disc surface; splinter hemorrhages, disc head elevation, loss of optic nerve central cup, dilation and tortuosity of retinal veins, retinal exudates, loss of spontaneous venous pulsation. Vision usually unaffected but may get transient bilateral visual blurring or loss; in chronic papilledema, fibrosis/atrophy may cause visual loss with visual field constriction. Early and severe vision loss is typical of papillitis.
3. **Etiology:** intracranial tumors, hydrocephalus, intracranial hemorrhage, meningoencephalitis, trauma with cerebral edema, metabolic disease
4. **Management:** depends on underlying cause but neurologic emergency. Brain MRI is initial neuroimaging modality of choice. See Chapter 2 Emergency Medicine for management of increased ICP.

C. Optic atrophy

1. Characterized by disc pallor (white disc): may be congenital or acquired. Requires thorough ophthalmic and neurologic investigations.

D. Optic nerve hypoplasia

1. **Etiology:** congenital anomaly characterized by smaller than normal optic nerve
2. **Symptoms:** may maintain good vision in mild cases; severe forms can cause blindness and nystagmus
3. **Diagnosis** is clinical. MRI brain and endocrine assessment recommended (rule out septooptic dysplasia or pituitary insufficiency).

E. Optic neuritis

1. **Definition:** inflammatory, demyelinating condition affecting the optic nerve
2. **Signs and symptoms:** acute, rapid progression of vision loss. Pain is often present and worsens with EOMs. Relative afferent pupillary defect

may see optic nerve inflammation (papillitis) or normal funduscopic exam. Check for signs of neuromyelitis optica and multiple sclerosis (on exam and neuroimaging).

STRABISMUS

1. **Definition:** any abnormal eye alignment
2. **Diagnosis:** assess with Hirschberg test (Figure 31.1) and cover/uncover test (described earlier). Tests are normal in **pseudostrabismus.**
3. **Etiology**
   a. Primary: idiopathic, syndrome-associated
   b. Secondary: vision deprivation (cataracts, ptosis), muscular disorders, cerebral injury (cerebral palsy, head trauma)
4. **Management:** refer child with strabismus after 3 to 4 months of age (unsteady ocular alignment may be present in normal newborns up to this age). Refer sooner if eyes extremely misaligned or not moving normally. Strabismus is only emergent when eye(s) cannot move fully in all directions (may indicate paretic muscle (e.g., CN palsy) or restriction (see blow-out fracture in Table 31.4).

AMBLYOPIA

1. **Definition:** Functional reduction in visual acuity caused by abnormal visual development early in life; most common pediatric cause of vision loss
2. **Etiology:** May result from strabismus, refractive error, or vision deprivation (ptosis, cataract). Can be unilateral or, less commonly, bilateral.
3. **Management:** Children with suspected amblyopia should be referred to an ophthalmologist

> **! PITFALL**
>
> Left untreated, amblyopia can lead to serious vision problems. It is almost completely preventable if identified before visual maturation (6–8 years).

TRAUMATIC EYE INJURIES

See Table 31.4

Table 31.4	Traumatic Ocular Injuries		
	Corneal Lacerations or Ruptured Globe	**Blow-Out Fracture**	**Retrobulbar Hemorrhage**
Preceding trauma	Blunt or penetrating	Blunt	Blunt
Eye symptoms and signs	Abnormally shaped pupil, hyphema, prolapsed iris, tissue protruding from sclera, 360 degrees subconjunctival hemorrhage, chemosis	Restricted EOMs; initially proptotic and later enophthalmic; upward gaze restriction with inferior rectus entrapment, hypoesthesia over inferior orbital skin (inferior floor fracture)	Decreased vision, proptosis
Diagnostic aids	Nonpressure techniques to gently examine: stop examination once confirmed	CT scan (axial + coronal)	Afferent pupil defect, raised intraocular pressure
Management	Eye shield; no pressure on eye; no eyedrops/patch If hyphema avoid NSAIDs, aspirin	Iced compress + elevation of bed 12–24 h ± antibiotics. Avoid blowing nose. Surgery for severe enophthalmos, diplopia in primary position especially >2 weeks, >50% fracture of orbital floor, orbital roof fracture, failed medical management	Prompt canthotomy/cantholysis to release pressure
Referral to Ophthalmology	Emergent	Urgent	Emergent

CT, Computed tomography; *EOM*, extraocular movement; *NSAID*, nonsteroidal antiinflammatory drug.

COMMON OCULAR COMPLAINTS

See Box 31.1

Box 31.1	Differential Diagnosis of Common Ocular Complaints
Red eye	Conjunctivitis, subconjunctival hemorrhage, trichiasis (lashes growing in toward the cornea), blepharitis, lagophthalmos (incomplete eyelid closure), acne rosacea, iritis (ciliary flush), episcleritis, scleritis, dacryocystitis, contact lens related, traumatic (conjunctival, corneal abrasion), foreign body (FB)
Tearing	Nasolacrimal duct obstruction (most common), FB, congenital glaucoma
Discharge	Conjunctivitis, blepharitis, corneal ulcer, endophthalmitis
Photophobia	Conjunctivitis, corneal abnormality (abrasion/FB/ulcer/contact lens related), iritis, albinism, aniridia, congenital glaucoma, drugs (dilating drops), migraine, meningitis, optic neuritis
Blurry vision	Refractive error, amblyopia, conjunctivitis, corneal, abnormality (abrasion/FB/ulcer/contact lens related) iritis, vitritis, retinal pathology (e.g., detachment, vasculitis), optic nerve pathology (papillitis, optic neuritis, papilledema), drugs

Box 31.1	Differential Diagnosis of Common Ocular Complaints—cont'd
Eyelid swelling	Traumatic, stye/chalazion, contact dermatitis, herpes simplex, lid/lacrimal gland mass, dacryocystitis, preseptal or orbital cellulitis
Proptosis	Orbital cellulitis, orbital mass, retrobulbar hemorrhage, thyroid eye disease, cavernous sinus thrombosis, carotid cavernous fistula, idiopathic orbital inflammation (pseudotumor), pseudoproptosis (e.g., contralateral enophthalmos, high myopia, congenital glaucoma)
Acute vision loss	Visual media problems: Globe injury/trauma, iritis, glaucoma, vitreous hemorrhage, etc. Retinal problems: Retinal detachment, vascular occlusion, tumors. Neurovisual pathway problems: Optic nerve pathology (e.g., papilledema (chronic) from various causes, optic neuritis), optic pathway tumors. Other: Ocular migraine, TIA, vertebrobasilar artery insufficiency
Monocular diplopia	"Double vision" in one eye only (less common): visual axis abnormalities, media opacities, corneal/pupil/lens-related problem (cataract, subluxed lens [e.g., in Marfan syndrome, homocystinuria]), or retinal pathology
Binocular diplopia	"Double vision" which resolves when one eye is covered: decompensated phoria, posttrauma/surgery, orbital inflammatory disease (pseudotumor), myasthenia gravis, thyroid eye disease, internuclear ophthalmoplegia, CN III, IV, or VI palsy, carotid cavernous fistula
Flashing lights	Flashes lasting seconds: retinal tear or detachment Flashes lasting minutes: ocular migraine Other: seizure (rare), oculodigital stimulation
Floaters	Posterior vitreous detachment, migraine, vitritis

CN, Cranial nerve; *TIA*, transient ischemic attack.

FINDINGS ON OPHTHALMOLOGIC EXAMINATION LINKED TO SYSTEMIC DISEASE

See Box 31.2

Box 31.2	Ocular Manifestations of Systemic Disease
Connective tissue disorders	1. Marfan syndrome: lens dislocation. Severe myopia, corneal flattening, iris hypoplasia, hypoplastic ciliary muscle, retinal tear, early opacity of lens or glaucoma 2. Weill-Marchesani syndrome: microspherophakia, ectopia lentis, lenticular myopia, glaucoma
Genetic diseases	1. Tay Sachs disease, Niemann Pick disease: cherry red spot 2. Ushers syndrome, Bardet Biedl syndrome: retinitis pigmentosa 3. Sjogren Larsson: retinal glistening yellow white dots that are pathognomonic

Continued

Box 31.2	Ocular Manifestations of Systemic Disease—cont'd
Metabolic disease	1. GM1 and GM2 Gangliosidoses: cherry red spot 2. Galactosemia: cherry red spot, oil droplet cataracts 3. Sialidoses: cherry red spot 4. Fabrys disease: cornea verticillata, vortex keratopathy. Retinal, conjunctival vessel tortuosity and dilatation 5. Refsums disease: night blindness 6. Gyrate atrophy: chorioretinal degeneration 7. Hurler syndrome: corneal clouding
Gastrointestinal	1. Alagille syndrome: posterior embryotoxon, iris stromal hypoplasia, microcornea, pigmentary retinopathy, optic nerve dysplasia/drusen, choroidal hypoplasia
Neurocutaneous syndromes	1. Tuberous sclerosis: retinal hamartomas 2. Neurofibromatoses: Type 1 (iris hamartomas; Lisch nodules, optic nerve glioma, congenital glaucoma, eyelid hamartoma). Type 2 (cataracts, retinal and pigment epithelial hamartomas) 3. Von Hippel Landau: capillary hemangiomas
Infectious disease	1. HIV: d/t opportunistic infections, cotton wool spots and retinal hemorrhages, optic neuropathy, dry eyes 2. Congenital Rubella: cataracts, pigmentary retinopathy, glaucoma 3. Toxoplasmosis: chorioretinitis, microphthalmos, cataracts, panuveitis, optic atrophy 4. CMV: chorioretinitis, optic atrophy, microphthalmos, keratitis
Craniofacial anomalies	1. Crouzon syndrome: exophthalmos 2. Apert syndrome: proptosis, hypertelorism 3. Goldenhar syndrome: ptosis, nasolacrimal gland obstruction, lid colobomae, epibulbar dermoid 4. Treacher Collins syndrome: lower lib colobomas, limbal dermoids, nasolacrimal duct obstruction, canthal dystopia
Muscular disorders	1. Mitochondrial myopathy: optic neuropathy, ophthalmoplegia and ptosis, pigmentary retinopathy, retro chiasmal visual loss 2. Myotonic dystrophy: ophthalmoplegia, extraocular myotonia
Rheumatologic	1. Sarcoidosis: granulomatous uveitis, iris nodules, synechiae, vitreous opacities, retinal microaneurysms, keratoconjunctivitis sicca, adnexal granulomas, keratitic precipitates 2. Behçet disease: panuveitis, conjunctivitis, episcleritis, optic neuropathy 3. Antineutrophil cytoplasmic antibody-associated vasculitidies: Wegener granulomatoses: scleritis, periorbital edema, panniculitis, myositis, dacryoadenitis, dacryocystitis/canaliculitis 4. Kawasaki disease: bilateral nonexudative conjunctivitis 5. Juvenile spondyloarthropathies: acute, unilateral nongranulomatous uveitis 6. Reactive arthritis: mucopurulent bilateral conjunctivitis
Other	1. Abeta lipoproteinemia: night blindness 2. Albinism: refractive errors, delayed visual maturation, foveal hypoplasia, Rabbit's eye reflex 3. Lipemia retinalis: retinal arteries and veins creamy white or pale pink

CMV, Cytomegalovirus; *GI*, gastrointestinal; *HIV*, human immunodeficiency virus.

Orthopedics

Allyson Shorkey • Unni Narayanan

COMMON ABBREVIATIONS

Also see page xviii for a list of other abbreviations used throughout this boo

AVN	avascular necrosis
JIA	juvenile idiopathic arthritis
NSAID	nonsteroidal antiinflammatory drug
NVS	neurovascular status
ORIF	open reduction internal fixation
ROM	range of motion
SCFE	slipped capital femoral epiphysis
LCP	Legg-Calve-Perthes disease
SLE	systemic lupus erythematosus

Orthopedics

FRACTURES

A. General considerations

1. Bones of growing children have open physes or **growth plates** and secondary ossification centers at the ends of long bones, which if not recognized, might lead one to misdiagnose a fracture when there is none, or miss a fracture through the growth plate
2. Fractures involving the growth plate are generally classified by the **Salter-Harris classification** system (Figure 32.1)

Figure 32.1 Salter-Harris Classification of Growth Plate Injuries

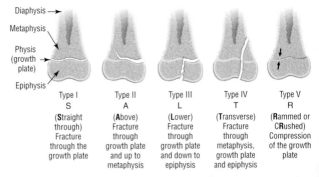

(Modified from Granadillo VA, Bachmann K. School age. In: Miller MD, Hart JA, MacKnight JM. *Essential Orthopaedics.* 2nd ed. Philadelphia, PA: Elsevier; 2020.)

3. Always examine and image the joints above and below to avoid missing associated injuries
4. Always check neurovascular status of the limb (color, warmth, and palpable pulses; pertinent sensory and motor examination)
5. Fractures involving the joint (articular surface) require anatomic alignmen which might require open reduction

6. Displaced fractures typically need reduction to improve the alignment
7. Unstable fractures need some form of internal or external fixation to maintain alignment, whereas relatively stable fractures can be managed with splints or circumferential casts (see Chapter 5 Procedures for splint application)
8. Ensure adequate pain management and splint the limb after thorough examination

> **! PITFALL**
>
> When there are open wounds around fracture sites, do not forget to consider the possibility of an open fracture (requires IV antibiotics and urgent orthopedic consultation).

> **✳ PEARL**
>
> Always consider the possibility of non-accidental trauma in pediatric patients presenting with a fracture.

B. Specific common fractures
1. See Tables 32.1 and 32.2
2. See Chapter 34 Plastic Surgery for hand trauma

Table 32.1	Upper Extremity Fractures		
Fracture Type	**Description/ Findings**	**Management**	**Complications/ Comments**
Distal radius	Typically involves metaphysis, but can involve physis	Buckle/incomplete/ undisplaced: removable splint × 3–4 weeks with primary MD f/u; Displaced: closed reduction, below elbow cast, ortho f/u within 5 days	Growth arrest possible with physeal injuries
Radius and/or ulnar shaft		Deformity requires closed reduction, above elbow cast, and ortho f/u within 5 days; Operative intervention for irreducible or unstable fractures (loss of reduction) or open fractures	Imaging must include elbow and wrist. Assess skin integrity and distal NVS. Risk of compartment syndrome.
Monteggia	Ulnar shaft fracture with dislocated radial head. Look at radial head alignment with capitellum (it is dislocated if it does not point to it)	Urgent orthopedic referral: may require closed reduction or surgical fixation	Radial head dislocation is often missed; Plastic deformity of ulna (bent not broken) can also be associated with radial head dislocation

Table 32.1 **Upper Extremity Fractures—cont'd**

Fracture Type	Description/ Findings	Management	Complications/ Comments
Radial neck	Fracture through base of radial head	Undisplaced: long arm cast, ortho f/u 1 week; Displaced/angulated: refer to ortho for reduction	
Supracondylar fracture of distal humerus	95% are extension type: displaced posteriorly and angled into extension. Fractures may be occult (only x-ray sign is presence of "fat pad"), undisplaced, or displaced	Occult or undisplaced: above elbow cast flexed to no more than 80 degrees. Ortho f/u within 5 days; Displaced: immediate ortho referral for closed reduction and pinning in the OR	Displaced fractures may be associated with neurological (median/radial/ulnar) and vascular (brachial artery) compromise. Risk of compartment syndrome. Malunion (cubitus varus) if poorly reduced or stabilized
Lateral condyle	Swelling and tenderness isolated to the lateral aspect of the elbow	Urgent ortho referral; Undisplaced: cast and ortho f/u in 5 days to rule out displacement; Mildly displaced: percutaneous pinning; Displaced: open reduction & pinning	"Undisplaced" fracture requires internal oblique x-ray to see maximal displacement. Risk of delayed or nonunion, late-presenting ulnar nerve palsy.
Medial epicondyle	Tenderness over the medial aspect of the elbow; often associated with an elbow dislocation	Urgent referral to ortho (above elbow cast vs. ORIF in some cases)	Risk of ulnar nerve stretch injury. Fracture might be missed if the fragment is trapped within the elbow joint.
Proximal humerus	Fracture of proximal humeral metaphysis, may involve physis	Sling or shoulder immobilizer in majority of cases. Refer to ortho if displaced. If not, f/u with ortho in 5 days.	Tremendous remodeling as long as >3 years growth remaining
Clavicle	Collar bone tenderness with limited shoulder ROM	Sling or collar & cuff × 6 weeks. Internal fixation only for skin tenting or open fractures	Tremendous remodeling capacity of even displaced fractures

f/u, Follow-up; *MD,* medical doctor; *NVS,* neurovascular status; *OR,* operating room; *ORIF,* open reduction, internal fixation; *ROM,* range of motion; *XR,* x-ray.

Orthopedics

32

| Table 32.2 | **Lower Extremity Fractures** | | |

Fracture Type	Description/ Findings	Management	Complications
Femoral neck	Middle or base of femoral neck (physis less common)	Immobilize with skin traction; Immediate ortho referral; Most need operative intervention	Avascular necrosis of femoral head is common complication
Femoral shaft	Fracture can be transverse, oblique, or spiral pattern based on mechanism. Multiple fragments (comminuted fracture) suggests high energy injury.	Immediate ortho referral; Smaller children (<5 years; <20 kg): closed reduction and hip spica cast under GA; Older, heavier children or open fractures need operative fixation	Common injury in children. Rule out other injuries. Consider NAI in infants (before walking age) and select cases (see Chapter 9 Child Maltreatment)
Distal femur physeal	SH I and II most common	Immediate ortho referral; Undisplaced: above knee cast; Displaced: reduction under GA and internal fixation	Risk of vascular injury in displaced fractures; High risk for premature growth arrest
	"Corner" fractures are specific physeal injuries in infants		"Corner" fractures in infants suspicious for NAI (see Chapter 9 Child Maltreatment)
Proximal tibia	Can involve the tibial spine, proximal tibial physis, the tibial tubercle, proximal tibial metaphysis	Undisplaced: ortho referral and long leg cast Displaced: urgent ortho referral; Closed or open reduction and internal fixation	Undisplaced fractures of proximal tibial metaphysis are at high risk of medial overgrowth, leading to valgus deformity. Displaced fractures of proximal tibial metaphysis and tibial tubercle are at risk for vascular injury and compartment syndrome.
Tibial shaft	Transverse, oblique, or spiral fractures	Undisplaced: above knee (long leg) cast with ortho follow-up within 1 week; Displaced: ortho referral for closed reduction and immobilization with above knee (long leg) cast; Unstable or open fractures require operative management and fixation.	High energy injuries at risk for compartment syndrome
Toddler's fracture	Nondisplaced spiral fracture through mid-distal tibia in toddler	Below knee splint/cast for 3 weeks	

Orthopedics

32

Continued

Fracture Type	Description/ Findings	Management	Complications
Distal tibial physeal fractures (ankle)	Common in children 8–15 years. SH-II; Triplane fractures (SH-IV); Tillaux fracture (SH-III through anterolateral tibia); Medial malleolus: (SH III or IV); Associated fibula fractures in all aforementioned	Urgent ortho referral; Closed reduction and below knee cast followed by CT scan to assess articular alignment if the fracture involves joint; Persistent displacement and intraarticular involvement (SH-III and IV) usually require open reduction and internal fixation	These injuries often need CT scan to define fracture pattern and displacement at joint surface and physis. Increased risk of growth arrest especially for medial malleolus (SH-III or IV) fractures
Lateral ankle injury (negative x-ray)	Often ankle sprain (undisplaced SH-I fracture of distal fibula is rare)	All can be treated as sprains: splint or air cast and weight bearing as tolerated for 3–4 weeks	
Foot	Talus and calcaneus; Midfoot; Metatarsals; Phalanges	Urgent ortho referral for fractures of hindfoot (talus and calcaneus), and for displaced or intraarticular fractures and fracture-dislocations of the foot; Undisplaced metatarsal fractures: air cast or short leg splints; Extraarticular phalangeal fractures: "buddy taping"	

CT, Computed tomography; *GA*, general anesthesia; *NAI*, non-accidental injury; *SH*, Salter-Harris; *XR*, x-ray.

C. Common fracture complications

1. **Nerve injury** caused by stretch or direct contusion; or entrapment in the fracture site
2. **Vascular injury** from stretch over, penetration from, or entrapment within fracture fragments
3. **Compartment syndrome**
   a. Edema causes pressure that exceeds capillary pressure, leading to poor perfusion of muscles and nerves within the compartment. This leads to reversible ischemia, and later to permanent necrosis, nerve injury, muscle fibrosis and contractures.
   b. Common predisposing conditions
      i. Fractures associated with a vascular injury
      ii. Crush injuries

iii. High energy or displaced fractures: supracondylar fractures of elbow, forearm (radius and ulna), two level injuries (e.g., elbow and forearm), proximal tibial metaphysis and tibial tubercle, and tibial shaft

iv. Tight circumferential casts (these should be bivalved to accommodate increased swelling)

c. Early signs and symptoms: swollen extremity tense to palpation, constant/increasing pain unrelieved by analgesics, pain exacerbated by passive extension of fingers/toes; paresthesias (tingling and numbness) and pulselessness are late signs

d. Emergent (within 4–6 hours) surgical decompression of involved compartments (fasciotomy) to minimize risk of permanent necrosis and fibrosis

4. **Loss of reduction** caused by inadequate stabilization

5. **Malunion** caused by inadequate reduction or loss of reduction, leading to visually or biomechanically unacceptable deformities

6. **Permanent damage to growth plate** leading to complete arrest (length differences) or partial arrest leading to angular deformity

APPROACH TO THE LIMPING CHILD

See Table 32.3 for a differential diagnosis of limp and Table 36.3 for differential diagnosis of limb pain

Table 32.3	Differential Diagnosis for the Limping Child
Congenital/developmental	Developmental dysplasia of the hip, Legg-Calvé-Perthes disease, leg length discrepancy, Osgood-Schlatter disease, osteochondritis dissecans
Infectious	Cellulitis, septic arthritis, osteomyelitis, viral arthritis, lyme arthritis, psoas abscess, diskitis
Postinfectious or reactive arthritis	Preceding episode of respiratory (GAS), GI (shigella, salmonella, campylobacter), or GU (chlamydia trachomatis) infection
Neoplastic	Leukemia, primary bone tumor, neuroblastoma
Musculoskeletal/trauma	Stress fracture, SCFE, lacerations/puncture wounds
Vascular/hematologic	Hemarthrosis/hemophilia, sickle cell disease
Neuromuscular	Cerebral palsy, muscular dystrophy
Autoimmune	JIA, seronegative spondyloarthropathies, SLE, Henoch-Schönlein purpura
Other	Transient synovitis, serum sickness, maltreatment, hypermobility, psychogenic, numerous abdominal and genitourinary conditions (appendicitis, testicular torsion, etc.)

GAS, Group A Streptococcus; *GI*, gastrointestinal; *GU*, genitourinary; *JIA*, juvenile idiopathic arthritis; *SCFE*, slipped capital femoral epiphysis; *SLE*, systemic lupus erythematosus.

> ✦ **PEARL**
>
> If there is a concern for bone or joint infection, initial blood work should include a WBC, ESR, CRP, and blood culture.

OSTEOMYELITIS

1. **Clinical manifestations:** fever, malaise, local pain/swelling/warmth/ erythema/point tenderness, decreased use of limb, decreased range of motion (ROM) of adjacent joint
2. **Presentation:** may be acute, subacute, or chronic
3. **Common sites:** metaphysis of long bones including the femoral neck, distal femur, proximal and distal tibia
4. **Etiology**
   a. Hematogenous spread of bacteria from other site (often history of recent infection). Direct inoculation (from trauma, surgery) is uncommon.
   b. Most common bacteria are Staphylococcal or Streptococcal species
5. **Investigations**
   a. **Laboratory tests:** CBC and differential, ESR, CRP, blood cultures
      i. Elevated WBC and neutrophilia may or may not be present
      ii. ESR (>35–40 mm/h) and CRP (>20 mg/L) almost always elevated
   b. **Radiographs:** obtain anteroposterior (AP) and lateral x-rays of the affected site (bilateral if hips). X-rays are typically normal in acute osteomyelitis. Periosteal elevation or radiolucent lesion suggests longer duration (10–14 days) of infection. In chronic osteomyelitis, x-rays show periosteal new bone formation (involucrum) walling off dead sclerotic bone (sequestrum).
   c. **Ultrasound:** to assess for subperiosteal abscess, fluid collections in adjacent soft tissue, or adjacent joint effusion
   d. **MRI:** necessary to confirm the diagnosis and determine the duration of antibiotic treatment
6. **Management** of uncomplicated acute osteomyelitis
   a. Antibiotics: IV antibiotics until clinical improvement and/or decrease in CRP, followed by equivalent oral antibiotics for total duration of 4 to 6 weeks. Use empiric antibiotics (see Chapter 24 Infectious Diseases) until specific organism and sensitivities identified.
   b. Surgery is only indicated for concomitant adjacent septic arthritis, large subperiosteal abscess, failure to respond to antibiotics
7. **Subacute and chronic osteomyelitis** may require longer duration of antibiotics, ± surgery in chronic cases

Orthopedics

32

SEPTIC ARTHRITIS

Clinical manifestations

a. Fever, malaise, localized pain, swelling, erythema, warmth, joint line tenderness, effusion in the joint

b. Antalgic positioning of the limb (e.g., hip is flexed, abducted, and externally rotated)

c. Painful and limited passive ROM of affected joint

d. Inability to bear weight

Common sites: hip, knee, ankle, elbow, shoulder

Etiology

a. Hematogenous spread of infection (commonly Staphylococcal or Streptococcal species) from another site. Direct inoculation (from trauma or surgery) is uncommon.

Investigations

a. **Laboratory tests:** CBC, differential, ESR, CRP, blood cultures
   i. Elevated WBC and neutrophilia may or may not be present
   ii. ESR ($>$35–40 mm/h) and CRP ($>$20 mg/L) almost always elevated

b. **Radiographs:** obtain AP and lateral x-rays of the affected site (bilateral if hips). X-rays are typically normal (effusion might be apparent in some joints).

c. **Ultrasound:** confirms joint effusion, especially for the hip and other joints, which are not directly palpable. The absence of a joint effusion rules out septic arthritis.

d. **Joint aspiration:** should be performed as early as possible; best done in the operating room (OR) followed by irrigation and debridement of the joint if purulent. Synovial fluid WBC count ($>$50,000 WBC suggests bacterial infection) and organism identification are critical for diagnosis.

Management

a. Urgent orthopedic consultation

b. Prompt OR drainage of the joint with copious irrigation and debridement

c. Once specimen is obtained, IV antibiotics until clinical improvement (see Chapter 24 Infectious Diseases for empiric treatment), followed by equivalent oral antibiotics for a total duration of 3 to 4 weeks (shorter courses may be used for gonococcal arthritis)

d. Delayed treatment of septic arthritis can cause permanent damage to articular cartilage (e.g., avascular necrosis [AVN] of femoral head and permanent growth arrest)

TRANSIENT SYNOVITIS

1. **Definition:** transient, self-limited inflammation of synovium leading to joint effusion. This is a diagnosis of exclusion after other causes of joint effusion, such as septic arthritis are ruled out.
2. **Common joints involved:** hip
3. **Clinical presentation**
   a. Typical features: <6 years old, afebrile or low-grade fever, recent viral infection, well-appearing, limp or some reluctance to bear weight; painful passive hip ROM typically in the terminal ranges (rather than pain throughout the arc of motion)
   b. Can appear identical to early septic arthritis
4. **Investigations:** Often a clinical diagnosis in mild cases
   a. Bloodwork: WBC may be elevated, ESR/CRP are normal or only marginally elevated
   b. Imaging
      i. X-rays are normal
      ii. Ultrasound should show an effusion, without much synovial thickening, and no echogenic debris. Joint aspiration only indicated if septic arthritis cannot be definitively ruled out.
5. **Management**
   a. NSAIDs
   b. If inflammatory markers are borderline elevated, start NSAIDs and observe over the next 12 to 24 hours. Consider septic arthritis for ongoing/worsening symptoms.

 PEARL

Presence of elevated inflammatory markers helps to differentiate septic arthritis from transient synovitis.

DISORDERS OF THE HIP

DEVELOPMENTAL DYSPLASIA OF THE HIP (DDH)

1. **Definition:** congenital condition of the hip ranging from hip subluxation (partial displacement) to dislocation. Hip(s) may be reducible or irreducible
2. **Risk factors:** family history, female, frank breech, foot deformities, torticollis, oligohydramnios
3. **Physical examination**
   a. See Figure 32.2 for examination of neonatal hips
   b. Limited abduction of the affected hip/s; asymmetric limitation of abduction if unilateral
   c. Asymmetric thigh folds/skin creases are not consistent findings

Figure 32.2 Examination of the Hip in the Newborn

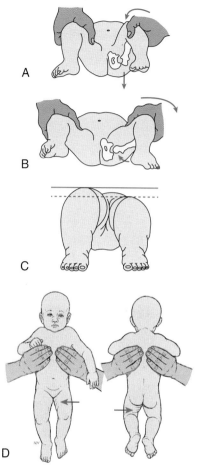

A

B

C

D

(A) Barlow's maneuver: Adduction and gentle posterior push cause dislocation ("clunk") of unstable hip. (B) Ortolani's maneuver: Abduction and ventral push over the greater trochanter leads to reduction ("clunk") of dislocated hip. (C) Galeazzi sign: With hips and knees flexed, the knee is lower on the affected side due to posterior displacement of dysplastic hip. (D) Asymmetric leg creases (inguinal, gluteal, thigh, or popliteal)

d. After 3 to 4 months of age, Barlow and Ortolani signs are seldom present. Limitation of hip abduction or a positive Galeazzi sign (if unilateral) persist.

e. At walking age, unilateral DDH is associated with a painless limp and functional difference in leg lengths. Bilateral DDH is associated with a waddling gait pattern.

4. **Investigations**
   a. For infants under 6 months, dynamic ultrasound is diagnostic
   b. Ultrasound is indicated for infants with positive physical findings; or those with more than one risk factor and/or equivocal findings of hip instability
   c. AP x-ray of the pelvis is the diagnostic imaging of choice after the appearance of the secondary ossification center of the proximal femoral epiphysis (approximately 4 months in girls and 6 months in boys). Secondary ossification is usually delayed on the affected side(s).

> **! PITFALL**
>
> If you suspect DDH after 6 months of age, x-rays (rather than ultrasound) are the diagnostic test of choice.

5. **Treatment**
   a. Refer to orthopedics. Goal is to obtain and maintain stable reduction; method is age-dependent.
      i. Pavlik harness first-line treatment for infants up to 6 months of age (>90% success with nonoperative treatment in <3 months of age)
      ii. Closed reduction followed by immobilization in a spica cast is indicated for infants who have failed to reduce with a Pavlik harness or for infants older than 6 months. Open reduction is indicated for older children who fail closed reduction.

LEGG-CALVÉ-PERTHES DISEASE

1. **Definition:** idiopathic avascular necrosis of the femoral head
2. **Epidemiology:** typically age 3 to 10 years (males > females)
3. **Clinical manifestations:** usually insidious onset, mild hip (groin) pain, and limp. No constitutional symptoms.
4. **Physical examination**
   a. Mild limp or Trendelenburg gait
   b. Decreased ROM of the affected hip, with limited abduction and internal rotation
   c. Groin pain with internal rotation of the hip
   d. Atrophy of thigh and buttock
5. **Investigations**
   a. **AP and frog-leg lateral x-ray of the pelvis** is diagnostic: changes of the femoral head, which range from sclerosis (increased density), radiolucency or fragmentation, to collapse of height and loss of sphericity (flattening)
   b. MRI is more sensitive in detecting early disease, but only indicated if x-rays are normal

6. **Treatment**
   a. NSAIDs
   b. Limitation of high impact weight-bearing activity when symptomatic
   c. Maintain ROM of the hip with physiotherapy or recreational activity (e.g., swimming or biking)
   d. Containment: keeps femoral head within the acetabulum to evenly distribute weight-bearing forces (primarily achieved by abduction ROM exercises, casting/bracing). Surgical containment may be indicated in some cases.
7. **Prognosis**
   a. Early onset (<6 years) and smaller volume of femoral head involvement is associated with a good prognosis
   b. Later onset (>8 years) and more severely involved femoral head is associated with a worse prognosis and early onset osteoarthritis

SLIPPED CAPITAL FEMORAL EPIPHYSIS

1. **Definition:** condition in which the femoral head slips posteriorly on the femoral neck through the growth plate
2. **Epidemiology**
   a. Typically 10 to 16 years. More common in males, obese, Afro-Caribbean descent.
   b. Sometimes associated with endocrinopathy (e.g., hypothyroidism, pituitary deficiencies, hypogonadism, renal osteodystrophy)
3. **Clinical presentation**
   a. Acute: <3 weeks of symptoms (only ~10% of cases). Chronic: insidious and episodic symptoms over many weeks to months, with acute exacerbations (acute on chronic) is most common
   b. Stable slip: painful limp with groin, medial thigh, or knee pain; may need crutches to walk
   c. Unstable slip: inability to bear weight and unable to walk even with crutches
   d. Bilateral in up to 40%; either presenting concurrently, sometimes with one side asymptomatic, or second slip presenting within 18 to 24 months of the first slip
4. **Physical examination**
   a. Antalgic gait if able to walk
   b. Affected leg externally rotated when upright and supine, with limitation of internal rotation of affected hip
   c. Attempted flexion of knee forces hip into abduction and external rotation
5. **Investigations**
   a. **AP and frog-leg lateral x-rays** (or cross table lateral if severe symptoms) of both hips

b. AP view may show reduction of the height of epiphysis compared with opposite side; physeal widening or irregularity may be subtle; Klein's line along the superior border of femoral neck barely intersects the femoral epiphysis (Figure 32.3)

Figure 32.3   Slipped Capital Femoral Epiphysis

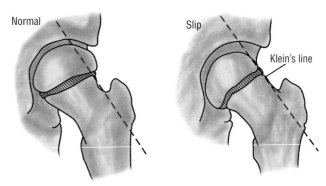

A line drawn along the superior border of the femoral neck (Klein's line) should intersect the lateral 10% to 15% of the femoral head. (From Hubbard EW. School age. In: Miller MD, Hart JA, MacKnight JM. *Essential Orthopaedics.* 2nd ed. Philadelphia, PA: Elsevier; 2020.)

6. **Treatment**
    a. Nonweight bearing (crutches) and refer immediately to orthopedics
    b. Urgent surgical screw fixation of the slipped femoral epiphysis
7. **Complications**
    a. Younger skeletal age at greater risk of contralateral slip. Must monitor for this.
    b. AVN is a devastating complication with no cure; rare in stable slips, but up to 50% in unstable slips (early diagnosis is essential!)
    c. Other: leg length difference, gait abnormality, osteoarthritis

> **! PITFALL**
>
> Diagnosis of slipped capital femoral epiphysis is often missed or delayed because pain is frequently reported only in the knee or medial thigh.

NONTRAUMATIC DISORDERS OF THE KNEE

OSGOOD-SCHLATTER DISEASE

1. **Definition:** inflammation of the tibial tubercle at the site of patellar tendon insertion caused by overuse

  Clinical presentation: painful bump where the patellar tendon inserts into the tibial tubercle. Symptoms are episodic and recurrent, usually worse with activity, better with rest.

  Epidemiology: usually in male adolescents between 10 and 15 years. May be unilateral or bilateral.

  Investigations: usually unnecessary; x-rays only to rule out other conditions

  Treatment: modification or reduction of physical activity (sports), local application of ice before and after activity, quadriceps and hamstring stretching and strengthening, NSAIDs and reassurance

  Prognosis: usually self-limiting, although symptoms may last for ≥18 months

PATELLOFEMORAL PAIN SYNDROME

  Definition: anterior knee pain along the extensor mechanism of the knee (quadriceps tendon, patellofemoral joint, patellar tendon) because of increased forces on patellofemoral joint

  Clinical presentation: classically presents with pain "around" or "under" the patella; more common in adolescent girls. Pain increases with activities that load the patellofemoral joint, such as squatting and climbing stairs. Can be associated with recurrent patellar instability (subluxation).

  Physical examination: pain reproduced by compressing patella against femur; tenderness along the patellar facets (under-surface of the patella). Assess alignment of lower limb to rule out excessive valgus (knock-knee) or varus knee movement.

  Investigations: x-ray normal; can help rule out bony lesions (tumors, infection)

  Treatment: quadriceps strengthening, hamstrings stretching exercises

  Prognosis: usually self-limiting, but can last up to 2 to 3 years

DISORDERS OF LOWER LIMB ALIGNMENT

PHYSIOLOGICAL BOWING AND KNOCK-KNEE DEFORMITY

Lower limb alignment in the frontal plane changes in the growing child (Figure 32.4). Extremes of this pattern are noticeable and cause concern. Pathological causes must be ruled out to distinguish these from physiological variants that require no treatment.

  Definitions

   a. **Physiological bowing** (varus): persistent bowed legs after 18 months. Bilateral and usually symmetric with normal growth plates. Spontaneous improvement is expected by 3 years.

   b. **Physiological knock knees** (valgus): increased valgus deformity at 3 to 6 years. Bilateral and symmetric with normal growth plates. Spontaneous improvement is expected by age 8 years.

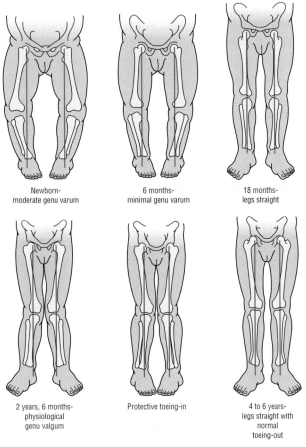

Newborn-
moderate genu varum

6 months-
minimal genu varum

18 months-
legs straight

2 years, 6 months-
physiological
genu valgum

Protective toeing-in

4 to 6 years-
legs straight with
normal
toeing-out

(Modified from Magee DJ. *Orthopedic Physical Assessment.* 6th ed. St. Louis, MO: Elsevier; 2014.)

PATHOLOGICAL VARUS KNEE (BOWED LEGS)

1. **Etiology**
   a. **Infantile tibia vara (Blount disease)**
      i. Progressive varus deformity of the tibia because of disorder of medial part of the proximal tibial growth plate causing asymmetric growth
      ii. More common in obese children, early walkers, Afro-Caribbean descent. Bilateral in >50%.

iii. X-rays reveal medial beaking with downward slope of proximal tibia metaphysis and epiphysis (x-ray changes may not appear until after 2 years)

iv. Treatment: surgical correction of alignment before the age of 4 years; delayed treatment is associated with higher rates of recurrence

b. **Rickets (metabolic bone disease)**

i. Deficient bone mineralization most commonly caused by vitamin D deficiency

ii. X-rays reveal systemic involvement of entire skeleton with poor bone density, widened growth plates and metaphyseal flaring

c. **Acquired physeal disturbance or growth arrest**

i. Partial growth arrest caused by prior trauma or infection involving the growth plate. Medial growth arrest causes varus; lateral growth arrest would cause valgus

IN-TOEING

1. **Definition:** feet point inward (toward midline) during walking (normal/typical position: feet are angled 10–15 degrees outwards)

2. **Etiology**

a. Most of these are physiological variants that self-correct with growth

b. The most common sources of in-toeing in typically developing children are: **metatarsus adductus, internal tibial torsion**, and **femoral anteversion**. See Table 32.4 for descriptions.

Table 32.4	Causes of In-Toeing		
	Clinical Presentation	**Main Features**	**Treatment**
Metatarsus adductus	Congenital <1 year Bilateral Symmetric	Medial deviation of forefoot while hindfoot remains in normal position (lateral border of foot is convex). Foot lays flat on ground. Normal Metatarsus adductus	No treatment; Spontaneous resolution by 1–2 years. Serial casting ± surgery in very rare, non-resolving cases.

| Table 32.4 | **Causes of In-Toeing—cont'd** |

	Clinical Presentation	Main Features	Treatment
Internal tibial torsion	1–4 years Bilateral Symmetric	Internal (medial) rotation of the tibia Knees pointing straight ahead	No treatment; spontaneous resolution by 10 years. Surgical correction may be indicated for nonresolving cases.
Excessive femoral anteversion	3–6 years Bilateral Symmetric	Persistence of increased infantile anteversion—the angle at which the femoral neck points anteriorly from the horizontal plane Knees pointing inward	No treatment; Spontaneous resolution by 10–12 years. Surgical correction may be indicated if it persists into adolescence or if developmental delay (cerebral palsy).

Images from From Kelly DM. Congenital anomalies of the lower extremity. In: Beaty JH, Azar FM, Canale ST (eds.), Campbell's Operative Orthopaedics, Thirteenth Edition. Elsevier; 2017; Pedro A. Sanchez-Lara, Graham JM. Smith's Recognizable Patterns of Human Deformation. 4th ed. Elsevier; 2016; Nelson SE, Miller DJ. Selected topics in orthopedics. In: Dean T, Jr., Bell LM. Nelson Pediatrics Board Review: Certification and Recertification. Elsevier; 2019; Mercier LR. Practical Orthopedics. 6th ed. Elsevier; 2008.

Idiopathic toe walking

a. **Etiology:** common physiological variant of normal development in young children

b. **Clinical manifestations:** toe walking begins at onset of walking (12–15 months); bilateral and symmetric; not associated with any functional difficulties. Normal developmental history and neurological examination.

c. **Physical examination:** reduced dorsiflexion of ankle caused by contracture of Achilles tendon (heel cords)

d. **Treatment:** heel cord stretching exercise; serial casting if persistent beyond age 5 years

e. **Natural history:** majority (about 80%) correct spontaneously by 4 to 5 years of age. Refer to orthopedics if any atypical history or physical examination findings.

Known causes or conditions associated with toe-walking: careful history and physical examination is required to rule out known causes of toe-walking

a. **Autism spectrum:** the cause is unclear. Onset is typically at 2 to 3 years. Usually not associated with functional difficulties. More refractory to treatment, as patients are less likely to tolerate serial casting.

b. **Neurological causes:** equinus gait unilateral (e.g., hemiparesis/plegia) or bilateral (diplegia) is the most common gait pattern in children with cerebral palsy. Gestational, birth, and developmental history and physical findings of upper motor neuron disorders, including hypertonia, hyperreflexia, and contractures help to establish diagnosis.

c. **Muscular dystrophy:** equinus gait might be the earliest indication of proximal muscle weakness in conditions like Duchenne muscular dystrophy (DMD), where the toe-walking is a compensatory strategy for the proximal weakness

ONGENITAL AND ACQUIRED DEFORMITIES OF THE FOOT

e Table 32.5 for diagnosis and management of various foot abnormalities

Orthopedics

32

Table 32.5	**Diagnosis and Management of Foot Deformities**		
	Etiology	**Main Features**	**Treatment**
Clubfeet (Talipes equinovarus)	Congenital idiopathic (most common); Congenital neuromuscular or syndromic conditions (spina bifida, arthrogryposis); Acquired clubfoot in neurological conditions (cerebral palsy)	1. Plantar flexed ankle (equinus); Hindfoot turned inward (varus) 2. Cavus ("high arch"): deep medial crease in the plantar aspect of midfoot 3. Adductus of the forefoot (curved lateral border)	Ponseti method of serial casting followed by percutaneous Achilles tenotomy is successful in >95% of idiopathic cases. Needs foot abduction brace up to 4 years to prevent recurrence. Recurrence usually responds to additional casting. Surgical correction often needed for neurogenic and syndromic clubfeet
Calcaneovalgus	Congenital, in-utero positional contracture	Dorsiflexion of the foot (dorsum of foot in contact with anterior tibia)	Usually corrects spontaneously within days or weeks. Gentle stretching might help expedite the correction. Serial casting usually unnecessary. If associated with bowing of tibia, calcaneovalgus still resolves spontaneously. Posteromedial bowing of tibia also tends to correct with growth, but almost always with shorter tibia leading to leg length difference that needs treatment.
Metatarsus adductus (see Table 32.4)	Congenital	Medial deviation of forefoot, convex lateral border	Usually corrects by age of 2 years. Occasionally needs casting and rarely needs surgery.

Table 32.5	Diagnosis and Management of Foot Deformities—cont'd		
	Etiology	**Main Features**	**Treatment**
Congenital vertical talus	Congenital associated with spina bifida, arthrogryposis	Hindfoot is in equinus, Midfoot is dorsi-flexed: resulting in rocker-bottom foot	Serial casting using the reverse Ponseti method, followed by surgery to obtain correction. Bracing to maintain correction
Pes planus	2+ years. Flexible flat feet: associated with physiological ligamentous laxity. Very common in young children.	The arch ligaments flatten with weight bearing, but arch reconstitutes when non-weight bearing or when on tiptoe	Reassurance and no treatment if asymptomatic. No need for orthotics.
	Rigid flat feet: can become painful and sometimes associated with tarsal coalition.		Painful/stiff flatfeet should be referred to orthopedics. Tarsal coalition is ruled out with x-ray. May need treatment if symptomatic.
Pes cavus	10+ years. Associated with neurological conditions: e.g., Charcot-Marie-Tooth disease	Fixed high arch. May be associated with clawing of toes. Cavus might also be accompanied by hindfoot varus.	Rule out neuromuscular conditions

DISORDERS OF THE SPINE

TORTICOLLIS

1. **Definition:** neck is held in lateral flexion (head tilted to one side) and neck rotation (chin pointed to the opposite side)
2. **Etiology:** multiple causes
   a. **Congenital muscular torticollis**
      i. **Clinical manifestations:** contracture of sternocleidomastoid muscle, resulting in tilting of head and neck toward side of contracture

ii. **Treatment:** treat with stretching. Surgery for late diagnosis or persistent torticollis.
b. **Acquired torticollis**
  i. **Common causes:** muscle injury/inflammation, acute head and neck infections (muscle spasm or referred pain), rotary displacement of C1 on C2 (results from ligamentous laxity from local infection/inflammation, trauma, surgery), bony abnormalities of cervical spine, benign paroxysmal torticollis, Sandifer syndrome, congenital muscular torticollis (neonate/infant), dystonic reaction
  ii. **Life threatening diagnoses to rule out:** retropharyngeal abscess, suppurative jugular thrombophlebitis, cervical spine injury, spinal epidural hematoma, CNS tumors

BACK PAIN

1. **Etiology:** see Box 32.1 for differential diagnosis

Box 32.1 Differential Diagnosis of Back Pain

- Muscular disorders: strain, overuse
- Mechanical: spondylolysis, spondylolisthesis, Scheuermann kyphosis, scoliosis, herniated nucleus pulposus
- Injury: bony contusion, fracture, dislocation
- Inflammatory: spondylitis, juvenile rheumatoid arthritis
- Infectious: osteomyelitis, discitis, spinal epidural abscess
- Tumors and tumor-like conditions: benign bony tumor, bone cyst, malignant bony tumor, leukemia, metastatic malignancy, eosinophilic granuloma (histiocytosis X)

---

2. **History:** pain location and distribution (localized or radiating), onset and duration (i.e., acute or chronic), timing (nighttime; postactivity), pain characteristics, neurological symptoms, morning stiffness, constitutional symptoms (e.g., fever, weight loss)
3. **Physical examination:** complete musculoskeletal (MSK) and neurological examination
4. **Investigations:**
   a. **Laboratory studies:** CBC, CRP, ESR, as needed
   b. **Imaging studies:** AP and lateral x-rays; advanced imaging (MRI/CT) as needed to confirm suspicion of specific problems

SPONDYLOLYSIS AND SPONDYLOLISTHESIS

1. **Definitions**
   a. **Spondylolysis:** defect or fracture of the pars interarticularis of the lumbar spine (typically L4 or L5). The pars interarticularis is the bony portion of the vertebra that connects the pedicles to the inferior facet (collar of "Scotty dog" seen on oblique x-rays of lumbar spine).

b. **Spondylolisthesis:** vertebral body above slips forward (ventral subluxation) over the vertebral body below. L5–S1 segment most commonly involved. Can be congenital (malformation L5 pars) or acquired (trauma).

2. **Clinical presentation:** common among gymnasts and wrestlers (repetitive hyperextension exercises)
   a. Spondylolysis: often asymptomatic, but may present with low back pain increasing with spine extension and activity
   b. Spondylolisthesis: same as spondylolysis. Also may have pain radiating down the legs (sciatica). Rarely may present with cauda equina syndrome.

3. **Physical examination:** limited lumbar spine flexion, positive straight leg test

4. **Imaging studies:** AP, lateral, oblique lumbosacral spine x-ray. Lateral views demonstrate grade (magnitude) of slippage or subluxation of L5 over S1 (25%–100%).

5. **Treatment**
   a. **Spondylolysis:** NSAIDs and activity modification or rest; bracing/cast might increase rate of healing; surgery for persistent symptoms to promote healing
   b. **Spondylolisthesis**
      i. Low-grade (0%–50%) asymptomatic slip: observe, no need to restrict activity
      ii. Low-grade symptomatic slip: restrict sports, physiotherapy for abdominal and back strengthening exercises (avoid extension exercises). Bracing/casting might have role to reduce symptoms.
      iii. High-grade (75%–100%) asymptomatic slip: treatment controversial; restrict contact sports and observe to skeletal maturity; or consider surgery to prevent future symptoms
      iv. High-grade symptomatic slip: restrict activity and refer to orthopedics for surgical fusion

SCOLIOSIS

1. **Definition:** a three-dimensional deformity of the spine that includes rotational component; coronal plane spinal deformity must be at least 10 degrees for diagnosis

2. **Etiology**
   a. Idiopathic scoliosis: diagnosis of exclusion, but most common (>60%)
   b. Congenital scoliosis: for example, hemivertebrae seen with VACTERL (*v*ertebral defects, *a*nal atresia, *c*ardiac defects, *t*racheoesophageal fistula, *r*enal anomalies and *l*imb abnormalities) syndromes
   c. Neuromuscular scoliosis: cerebral palsy, myelomeningocele (spina bifida), spinal muscular atrophy, Duchenne muscular dystrophy

    d. Syndromes and connective tissue disorders: neurofibromatosis (NF-1), Marfan, Ehlers-Danlos

    e. Compensatory scoliosis: attributed to a functional or true leg length difference

3. **History:** age of onset, pubertal stage, progression, family history, painful or painless, review of systems for other anomalies

4. **Physical examination**

    a. Complete MSK exam. Rib prominence, asymmetric waistline or shoulder height suggests scoliosis. Positive Adams forward bend test (Figure 32.5).

    b. Syndromic features (Marfanoid body habitus, café-au-lait spots, midline skin defects)

Figure 32.5   Adams Forward Bend Test

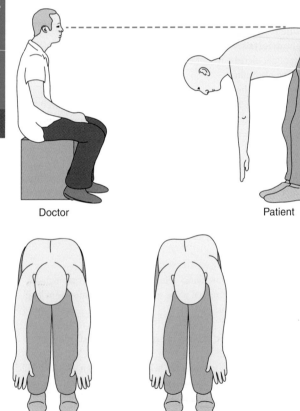

Doctor   Patient

Normal   Scoliosis

c. Thorough neurological examination

d. See Box 32.2 for red flags suggestive of an intraspinal canal problem

Imaging studies: x-ray (standing PA of full spine, sitting if unable to stand); measure Cobb angle(s), number and direction of each curve, radiographic signs of skeletal maturity

Treatment of idiopathic scoliosis

a. Clinical observation for curves <25 degrees

b. Bracing for progressive curves >25 degrees in skeletally immature patients

c. Surgery considered for curves >50 degrees or curves likely to progress after skeletal maturity

d. Early onset scoliosis: initial treatments include body casting; growing rod systems to prevent deterioration without fusing spine before adequate development of chest wall and lungs

Prognosis

a. Early onset scoliosis (age 6–7 years) may compromise lung development

b. Adolescent idiopathic scoliosis (late onset) affects body shape more than function

Complications: cosmetic deformity and psychological consequences, respiratory compromise in severe curves (>70–90 degrees), chronic back pain

BONE LESIONS

See Box 32.3. Also see Chapter 30 Oncology

Box **32.3** Bony Lesions	
Benign	**Malignant**[a]
Osteochondroma	Osteosarcoma
Unicameral bone cyst	Ewing sarcoma
Aneurysmal bone cyst	Leukemia
Osteoid osteoma	Metastatic disease
Enchondroma	
Nonossifying fibroma	

[a]Red Flags: Pain at rest, increasing pain over weeks to months, pain nonresponsive to nonsteroidal antiinflammatory drugs, systemic symptoms, osteolytic lesions, atypical soft tissue/bony swelling.

Otolaryngology

Talia Greenspoon • Sharon L. Cushing

Also see page xviii for a list of other abbreviations used throughout this book

ABR	auditory brainstem response
ABRS	acute bacterial rhinosinusitis
AOM	acute otitis media
cCMV	congenital cytomegalovirus
ET	eustachian tube
FB	foreign body
GAS	group A β-hemolytic streptococcus
IAC	internal auditory canal
ITP	immune thrombocytopenic purpura
MEE	middle ear effusion
OAE	otoacoustic emissions
OE	otitis externa
OM	otitis media
OME	otitis media with effusion
OSA	obstructive sleep apnea
PPV	positive pressure ventilation
RPA	retropharyngeal abscess
RST	rapid strep test
TEF	tracheoesophageal fistula
TM	tympanic membrane
TMJ	temporomandibular joint
URTI	upper respiratory tract infection
VRA	visual reinforcement audiometry
vWD	von Willebrand disease

Otolaryngology

33

EAR

APPROACH TO EAR EXAMINATION

A. Tips for examining ears

1. **Important to have child still or restrained** to avoid injury. Younger infants and children may sit supported and restrained on parent's lap, older children may sit alone

2. **Retract the auricle posteroinferiorly**
   See Table 33.1 and Figure 33.1

B. Ear wax (cerumen) removal

Cerumen is a protective covering in ear canal. It is usually asymptomatic and rarely causes hearing loss or discomfort but may prevent assessment of the ear canal and tympanic membrane (TM)

Table 33.1   Ear Examination by Area

External Ear	Mastoids
- Laceration, ecchymosis, hematoma, swelling - Deformity or tenderness - Erythema - Rashes - Masses, fluctuance - Lymphadenopathy (pre- and postauricular) - Frostbite or sunburn - Tragal tenderness	- Tenderness - Discoloration - Swelling
Auditory Canal	**Tympanic Membrane**
- Erythema - Swelling - Discharge - Stenosis - Cerumen - Masses - Foreign bodies - Bullae - Eczematous changes (flaking)	- Ensure adequate visualization - Anatomy: manubrium, short process - Position: neutral, retracted (OME), bulging (AOM) - Translucent vs. opaque - Color: amber (OME), white or yellow (OME or AOM), intense red (AOM), pink/injected (nonspecific: fever, crying), purple (hemotympanum, high riding jugular bulb), yellow/green (purulent effusion) - Perforations - Squamous debris - Tympanostomy tubes - Pneumatic otoscopy

AOM, Acute otitis media; *OME,* otitis media with effusion.

Figure 33.1   Tympanic Membrane: Landmarks and Pathology

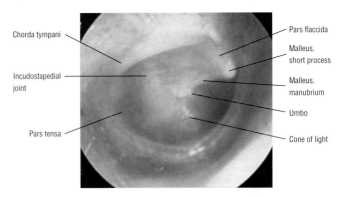

Chorda tympani — Incudostapedial joint — Pars tensa — Pars flaccida — Malleus, short process — Malleus, manubrium — Umbo — Cone of light

. **Cerumenolytic agents** (used to emulsify and lubricate cerumen to facilitate its removal)
    a. Examples: water and saline solutions, mineral oil, carbamide peroxide, docusate
    b. Instill 2 to 3 drops for no more than 3 to 5 days and follow up with otoscope examination
    c. Avoid in the setting of TM perforation or tympanostomy tubes
2. **Irrigation**
    a. Attach 16 to 18 gauge angiocatheter to a large syringe (60–200 mL)
    b. Use room temperature water or saline (may mix 1:1 with hydrogen peroxide)
    c. Insert tip of angiocatheter ~1.0 cm into auditory canal and irrigate using gentle steady pressure
    d. Contraindicated in in the setting of TM perforation or tympanostomy tubes
3. **Manual cerumen removal**
    a. Requires proper visualization
    b. Curettes, spoons, forceps, triangular applicator with cotton
    c. Suction may be performed on soft cerumen

EAR PAIN (OTALGIA)

1. **History**
    a. Age
        i. Infants and toddlers—mostly middle ear
        ii. Older children & teens—otitis externa, throat infections, TMJ disease
    b. Head trauma or barotrauma: mental status change, headache, seizures, focal neurologic deficit, nausea or vomiting, otorrhea
    c. Fever: common in minor infections but may also indicate complications
    d. Nasal congestion: acute otitis media (AOM) and otitis media with effusion (OME) usually follow recent URTI with nasal congestion
    e. Ear tenderness upon movement of the pinnae: indicates external ear disease
    f. Hearing loss
    g. Ear drainage
        i. Otitis externa (OE): minimal, thicker
        ii. Otitis media (OM) with perforation: copious, may be bloody, serosanguinous, purulent, or thin and watery
    h. Swimming: OE more likely, tube otorrhea if tubes present
    i. Environmental exposures: sun, cold, contact allergens
    j. Past medical history: prior ear infections, tubes, topical medications, immune deficiency
2. **Differential diagnosis**
    a. See Table 33.2

Table 33.2	**Differential Diagnoses of Otalgia by Region**		

Auricle	- Contusion (auricular hematoma)
	- Cellulitis
	- Herpes zoster oticus
	- Allergic angioedema
	- Polymorphous light eruption
	- Environmental injury
		Middle and inner ear	- **AOM**[a] and complications
			- **OME**[a]
			- **Otitis externa**[a]
			- Trauma
			  - Basilar skull fracture
			  - Epidural hematoma

Ear canal	- Otitis externa - Contact dermatitis - Furuncle - Foreign body - Cerumen impaction - Tumor	**Secondary otalgia** (referred pain from another source)	- Auricular lymphadenopathy or lymphadenitis - Sinusitis - Parotitis - Meningitis - Venous sinus thrombosis - Facial nerve palsy - TMJ dysfunction syndrome - Oropharyngeal infections - C-spine injury

[a]Most common diagnoses.

AOM, Acute otitis media; *OME,* otitis media with effusion, *TMJ,* temporomandibular joint.

OTITIS EXTERNA

1. **Pathophysiology**
   a. Inflammation of the skin of the external auditory canal because of infectious, allergic, or dermatologic disease
   b. Predisposing factors: swimming ("swimmer's ear"), minor trauma from cleaning
   c. Most common pathogens: *Pseudomonas aeruginosa, Staphylococcus epidermidis, Staphylococcus aureus*
2. **Signs and symptoms**
   a. Pain (ear pain and pain with tragus pressure or helix tug), pruritis
   b. Canal erythema and edema
   c. Thick discharge and debris in canal
   d. Hearing loss
3. **Treatment**
   a. If possible remove purulent discharge and epithelial debris
   b. Topical antimicrobials (ofloxacin otic drops), or topical antimicrobials containing corticosteroids (ciprodex otic drops)
   c. Systemic antibiotics only if infection spreads beyond ear canal

OTITIS MEDIA

1. **Risk factors**
   a. Young age
   b. Frequent contact with other children (e.g., daycare)
   c. Craniofacial abnormalities

d. Household crowding
e. Cigarette smoke exposure
f. Pacifier use
g. Shorter duration of breastfeeding
h. Prolonged bottle-feeding while supine (i.e., bottle propping)
i. Family history OM
j. Lack of routine childhood pneumococcal vaccinations

 PEARL

Acute otitis media is characterized by middle ear effusion and inflammation of the middle ear.
Otitis media with effusion is characterized by the presence of middle ear effusion without signs
of acute inflammation.

2. **Definitions and clinical features**
   a. See Table 33.3

Table 33.3	Acute Otitis Media and Otitis Media With Effusion	
	Acute Otitis Media	**Otitis Media With Effusion "Serous Otitis Media"**
Diagnosis	1. Acute onset of symptoms 2. MEE 3. Significant inflammation of middle ear	1. MEE 2. No signs of acute inflammation of middle ear
Pathophysiology	- Impaired mucociliary clearance in ET → reduced ventilation and fluid drainage from middle ear → pathogen colonization - *Streptococcus pneumoniae* - *Moraxella catarrhalis* - *Haemophilus influenza* - Group A strep - Many viruses including RSV	- Infection or allergy → ET dysfunction → fluid accumulation - May occur after AOM or independently
Clinical features	- Systemic symptoms - Ear tugging, pain - Tragus tenderness - **MEE:** decreased TM mobility, loss of bony landmarks, air-fluid level - **Inflammation of middle ear:** TM bulging, erythematous, yellow or cloudy, perforated TM, purulent discharge	- Mild ear pain, fullness - Decreased hearing - **MEE:** decreased TM mobility, loss of bony landmarks, air-fluid level

Continued

Table 33.3	Acute Otitis Media and Otitis Media With Effusion—cont'd	
	Acute Otitis Media	**Otitis Media With Effusion "Serous Otitis Media"**

Management	- Analgesics
	- Antibiotics (see Table 33.4)
	- May consider watchful waiting in some circumstances (see later)
		- Usually spontaneously resolving (antibiotics, decongestants, and steroids NOT recommended)
		- Chronic OME (persisting ≥3 months)
		  - Consider tympanostomy tubes
		  - Early surgical referral for at-risk children

Complications	- TM perforation - Acute mastoiditis - Facial nerve palsy - Labyrinthitis and vestibular dysfunction - Venous sinus thrombosis - Meningitis	- Cholesteatoma - Chronic OME associated with hearing loss and resultant developmental delays, specifically speech delay

AOM, Acute otitis media; *ET,* eustachian tube; *MEE,* middle ear effusion; *OME,* otitis media with effusion; *RSV,* respiratory syncytial virus; *TM,* tympanic membrane.

3. **Management**
   a. **Children <6 months of age:** AOM should be treated with antibiotics
   b. **Children >6 months of age:** See Figure 33.2 for AOM management algorithm
   c. **Duration of treatment**
      i. Children 6 months to <2 years old should be treated with a 10-day course of antibiotics
      ii. Children 2 years old or older with uncomplicated AOM may be treated with a 5-day course
   d. **Recommended antimicrobial agents** listed in Table 33.4
   e. Persistent middle ear effusion after therapy for AOM is expected and does not require retreatment

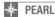 **PEARL**

"Watchful waiting" for 24–48 h may be considered in generally healthy children >6 months who are alert, have mild symptoms, fever <39°C, <48 h of symptoms, and good follow-up.

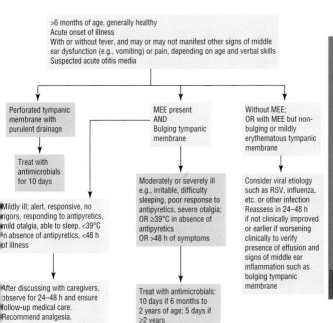

>6 months of age, generally healthy
Acute onset of illness
With or without fever, and may or may not manifest other signs of middle ear dysfunction (e.g., vomiting) or pain, depending on age and verbal skills
Suspected acute otitis media

Perforated tympanic membrane with purulent drainage

Treat with antimicrobials for 10 days

Mildly ill: alert, responsive, no rigors, responding to antipyretics, mild otalgia, able to sleep, <39°C in absence of antipyretics, <48 h of illness

After discussing with caregivers, observe for 24–48 h and ensure follow-up medical care. Recommend analgesia.

If not improved or worsening clinically, treat with antimicrobials (10 days for 6 months to 2 years of age and 5 days if ≥2 years)

MEE present AND Bulging tympanic membrane

Moderately or severely ill e.g., irritable, difficulty sleeping, poor response to antipyretics, severe otalgia; OR ≥39°C in absence of antipyretics OR >48 h of symptoms

Treat with antimicrobials: 10 days if 6 months to 2 years of age; 5 days if ≥2 years

Without MEE; OR with MEE but non-bulging or mildly erythematous tympanic membrane

Consider viral etiology such as RSV, influenza, etc. or other infection Reassess in 24–48 h if not clinically improved or earlier if worsening clinically to verify presence of effusion and signs of middle ear inflammation such as bulging tympanic membrane

MEE, Middle ear effusion; *RSV*, respiratory syncytial virus. (Modified from Le Saux N, Robinson JL, anadian Paediatric Society, Infectious Diseases and Immunization Committee. Management of cute otitis media in children six month of age and older. *Paediatr Child Health.* 2016;21(1):39–44.)

Table 33.4	Antimicrobial Agents for Acute Otitis Media
First line	- High-dose amoxicillin[a] (regular dose may be considered in other regions based on pneumococcal resistance patterns)
First line for patients with nontype I hypersensitivity to beta-lactams	- Cefuroxime - Ceftriaxone IV once daily × 3 days
First line for patients with life-threatening or type I hypersensitivity to beta-lactams	- Macrolide (clarithromycin, azithromycin)

Continued

| Table 33.4 | Antimicrobial Agents for Acute Otitis Media—cont'd |

Worsening or no symptomatic improvement by 48–72 h	- Amoxicillin/clavulanate
	- Alternative
	  - Second-generation cephalosporin (cefuroxime, cefprozil)
	  - Ceftriaxone IM/IV once daily × 3 days

Presence of otorrhea (i.e., perforated AOM, or AOM in the setting of tubes)	- AOM with perforation: CPS recommends oral antibiotics as listed earlier (otolaryngologists recommend ototopical antibiotic drops for all cases of otorrhea) - AOM in the presence of tympanostomy tubes: ototopical drops (ciprofloxacin-dexamethasone). Consider addition of oral antibiotics with severe symptoms

[a]High dose amoxicillin is 90 mg/kg/day divided TID.

Consider amoxicillin/clavulanate if the child has received amoxicillin in the last 30 days, has concurrent purulent conjunctivitis, or if coverage for beta-lactamase positive *Haemophilus influenzae* or *Moraxella catarrhalis* is desired.

AOM, Acute otitis media; *CPS*, The Canadian Paediatric Society; *IM*, intramuscular; *IV*, intravenous.

Adapted from The Hospital for Sick Children eFormulary, 2020.

4. **Recurrent AOM**
   a. Defined as ≥3 episodes of AOM in 6 months or ≥4 episodes in 12 months
   b. Prophylactic antibiotics should be used with caution because of increasing resistance
   c. Usually resolves spontaneously at 3 to 4 years old
   d. May consider referral for evaluation for myringotomy or tympanostomy tube insertion
   e. Tympanostomy tubes may be considered for children with recurrent AOM or persistent OME (>3 months), particularly for at-risk children and those with evidence of hearing loss

TRAUMATIC TYMPANIC MEMBRANE PERFORATION

1. **Assess degree of hearing loss** (clinically or with audiometry as needed)
   a. Minimal hearing loss (<40 dB) and absence of vestibular findings:
      i. Water precautions (i.e., there should be no water down the ear canal during bathing or swimming; recommend avoidance or use of ear plugs)
      ii. Ototopical ear drops (i.e., ciprodex)
      iii. Reexamination of TM by primary care provider in 4 to 6 weeks with audiometry
      iv. Otolaryngology evaluation for persistent perforation or symptoms after 4 to 6 weeks
   b. Significant hearing loss: urgent evaluation by an otolaryngologist to determine additional treatments

MASTOIDITIS

1. **Definition and etiology**
   a. Suppurative infection of mastoid air cells
   b. Extension of inflammation because of AOM beyond the middle ear into the contiguous mastoid cavity, with accumulation of purulent material, leading to destruction of bony septations between mastoid air cells
   c. May lead to abscess formation in the postauricular space
   d. Common organisms: *Streptococcus pneumoniae, Streptococcus pyogenes, S. aureus, Haemophilus influenzae, Moraxella catarrhalis,* group A β-hemolytic *Streptococcus* (GAS)

2. **Signs and symptoms**
   a. Tenderness, erythema, and swelling over mastoid bone
   b. Postauricular fluctuance or mass
   c. Protruding ear
   d. Signs of middle ear inflammation or otorrhea on otoscopy
   e. Otalgia
   f. Systemic symptoms (fever)

3. **Management**
   a. Typically a clinical diagnosis, but CT scan may be needed to determine extent of disease and guide surgical therapy
   b. Treatment
      i. IV antibiotics: cefuroxime is first line. Consider switch to oral therapy when clinically indicated
      ii. Surgical drainage of pus from middle ear with a tympanostomy tube and/or mastoid cavity with postauricular incision and drainage is sometimes required

HEARING LOSS

1. **Definition and etiology**
   a. **Hearing loss can be defined by**
      i. Degree (hearing threshold in dB)
      ii. Type (sensorineural, conductive, or mixed)
      iii. Unilateral or bilateral
      iv. Stable or progressive
   See Table 33.5 for common causes of congenital and acquired hearing loss

Table 33.5	Congenital and Acquired Causes of Hearing Loss	
Congenital	**Acquired**

- Genetic (50% of SNHL)
   - Majority related to cochlear hair cell dysfunction
   - Most are autosomal recessive
   - May be syndromic (i.e., Alport, Waardenburg, neurofibromatosis) or nonsyndromic mimickers (Usher Type 1)
- Cochleovestibular malformations
- Congenital infections (cCMV most common)
	- Obstruction (cerumen, bony growths)
	- Hyperbilirubinemia
	- Ototoxic medications
	- Infection (OM, meningitis)
	- TM perforation
	- Trauma (mechanical or noise-induced)
	- Tumors (cholesteatoma, otosclerosis)

cCMV, Congenital cytomegalovirus; *OM*, otitis media; *SNHL*, sensorineuronal hearing loss; *TM*, tympanic membrane.

2. **Management**
   a. Investigations (as needed): audiometry, electrophysiology, genetic testing, virology (i.e., congenital CMV), imaging including CT (temporal bones) or MRI (brain and internal auditory canal [IAC]), workup for extracochlear features
   b. Early accurate diagnosis and specialist referral with the goal of early, effective rehabilitation (<6 months)
   c. Late diagnosis and intervention leads to significant and irreversible effects on cortical development communication skills, cognition, literacy, and psychosocial skills
   d. Management requires a multidisciplinary team. Intervention strategies include: audiologic, medical/surgical management, educational and habilitation methods

NEWBORN HEARING LOSS AND SCREENING

Permanent hearing loss is the most common congenital disorder. Most neonatal hearing loss is sensorineural

1. **Risk factors**
   a. Family history of permanent hearing loss
   b. Craniofacial anomalies
   c. Congenital infections (i.e., cCMV) or bacterial meningitis
   d. Syndromic features
   e. NICU stay >2 days
   f. NICU stay with extracorporeal membrane oxygenation, assisted ventilation, sepsis, ototoxic drug use (i.e., aminoglycosides, diuretics), or hyperbilirubinemia requiring exchange transfusion

2. **Universal Newborn Hearing Screening (UNHS)**
   a. UNHS allows for early diagnosis but is inconsistently offered across Canada. See Figure 33.3 and Table 33.6 for diagnostic approach
   b. Currently performed with otoacoustic emissions (OAE) in the well infant and automated auditory brainstem response (AABR) in the infant who is at high risk

c. Best performed in infants over 24 hours old, at least 34 weeks corrected gestational age

Figure 33.3 Approach to Newborn Hearing Screening

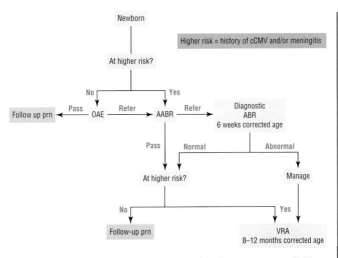

AABR, Automated auditory brainstem response; *ABR,* auditory brainstem response; *cCMV,* congenital cytomegalovirus; *OAE,* otoacoustic emission; *VRA,* visual reinforcement audiometry.

Table 33.6	Types of Newborn and Pediatric Hearing Tests and Screens
OAE	- Records emissions generated by the outer hair cells of the cochlea in response to sounds - Identifies conductive and cochlear hearing loss - Performed on well newborn infants before discharge - Results in either "pass," "refer," or "incomplete" - If "refer" or "incomplete," arrange AABR

ABR	- Records brainstem electrical activity in response to sounds
	- In addition to conductive and cochlear, identifies auditory neuropathy
	
	- AABR
	  - Technician performed, automated, computer analyzed ABR algorithm that produces a pass or refer result
	  - Performed as a screening test on high-risk newborns or if referred from OAE
	
	- Diagnostic ABR
	  - Performed and interpreted by an audiologist
	  - Produces frequency and level specific determination of hearing thresholds

VRA	- Performed on infants at a developmental age of 8–12 months - An audiologist tests hearing thresholds based on behavioral response to sounds

AABR, Automated auditory brainstem response; *ABR,* auditory brainstem response; *OAE,* otoacoustic emission; *VRA,* visual reinforcement audiometry.

EPISTAXIS

1. **Etiology**
   a. **Causes**
      i. Common: local trauma, dry mucosa (during acute URTIs and in allergic rhinitis), foreign bodies
      ii. Less common causes: injury, infection, systemic disorder (anticoagulant use or coagulopathy), tumor, septal perforation, iatrogenic, coagulopathy
   b. **Bleeding site**
      i. Anterior nosebleeds most common (arise from Kiesselbach's, or Little's area, a plexus of vessels in the anteroinferior septum)
      ii. Posterior bleeds are less common but more serious

2. **Management**
   a. **Assess severity of bleeding:** for unstable patients, ensure IV access and obtain bloodwork (CBC, blood type and match) and supplies (epistaxis tray, pRBCs)
   b. **Obtain relevant medical history:** ITP, vWD, hemophilia, transplant, oncology patient, etc.
   c. **Bedside care** (escalate to next step as needed)
      i. Direction compression: lean slightly forward and firmly pinch soft portion of nose below hard bony ridge for at least 10 minutes without release
      ii. Topical vasoconstrictors: oxymetazoline nasal spray or phenylephrine on a piece of gauze
      iii. Cautery: chemical (silver nitrate sticks) or electrical
      iv. Packing (kids >1 yo): to tamponade bleeding; may indicate a need for hospital admission
      v. OR for examination and/or treatment by an Otolaryngologist
   d. **Prevention:** apply petroleum jelly to nasal septum to moisturize and temporarily block air flow, keep nails short, use humidifier, avoid second-hand smoke, blow nose gently and avoid picking

SINUSITIS

1. **Definition and etiology**
   a. Paranasal sinus development: ethmoid and maxillary sinuses are present at birth; sphenoid sinuses begin to become aerated by age 5 years; frontal sinuses are pneumatized by 5 to 6 years
   b. Acute bacterial rhinosinusitis (ABRS): infection of paranasal sinuses because of obstruction of sinus drainage (because of mechanical obstruction or mucosal swelling, i.e., from URTI, allergic rhinitis), dysfunction of ciliary apparatus, and thickening of sinus secretions

   c. Most common organisms: *S. pneumoniae, H. influenza, M. catarrhalis,* GAS

   d. Risk factors
      i. Allergic rhinitis
      ii. Cigarette smoke exposure
      iii. Gastroesophageal reflux disease (GERD)
      iv. Anatomical abnormalities
      v. Immunodeficiency, including CF
      vi. Ciliary dyskinesia

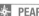 **PEARL**

Recurrent episodes of bacterial rhinosinusitis should prompt further evaluation with an allergist, cystic fibrosis (CF) test, and nasal mucosa biopsy.

2. **Signs and symptoms**
   a. Cough
   b. Nasal discharge (often purulent)/congestion
   c. Fever
   d. Other: headache, facial pain and swelling, sore throat, halitosis

3. **Diagnosis**
   a. ABRS is a **clinical diagnosis**
   b. **Imaging** (XR, CT, MRI) is **NOT necessary** to confirm the diagnosis of uncomplicated acute ABRS (symptoms <30 days)
   c. CT or MRI may be useful when complications are suspected or for recurrent or chronic (symptoms >90 days) cases
   d. Sinus aspiration is NOT routinely performed in uncomplicated ABRS

4. **Management**
   a. ABRS **usually resolves spontaneously** in 7 to 10 days; however, antibiotics can speed recovery
      i. By mouth (PO): High-dose amoxicillin or amoxicillin/clavulanate (clarithromycin for penicillin allergy)
      ii. IV: cefuroxime
      iii. Duration: 7 days after improvement of symptoms (usually a 10- to 14-day course)
   b. Nasal corticosteroid is recommended
   c. Inconsistent evidence for adjunctive therapies (antihistamines, decongestants) and may be associated with toxic effects
   d. Referral to Otolaryngology for consideration of surgical management, including obtaining a culture if unresponsive to multiple courses of antibiotics, complications, severe facial pain, or suspected sinusitis in an immunocompromised host

5. **Complications**
   a. The following findings may indicate complications: headache, vomiting, altered level of consciousness, focal neurologic deficits, stiff neck (Table 33.7)

Table 33.7	Complications of Sinusitis by Area	
Orbit	**CNS**	**Bone**
- Optic neuritis - Orbital cellulitis/abscess - Subperiosteal abscess	- Meningitis - Empyema - Abscess - Venous sinus thrombosis	- Frontal bone osteomyelitis (Pott's puffy tumor)

CNS, Central nervous system.

NASAL BONE FRACTURES

1. **Diagnosis**
   a. Complete external and internal examination of the nose including assessment of nasal obstruction, presence of septal hematoma, nasal bleeding, pain, anosmia, and cosmetic deformity
   b. Signs of nasal bone fracture: external nasal deformity, epistaxis, edema, ecchymosis, mobility
   c. Signs of septal hematoma: progressive nasal obstruction and visible swelling of the nasal mucosa (often with red or blue discoloration) that obstructs the nasal passage
   d. Assess for associated injuries to the cervical spine, central nervous system, facial bones, and teeth

2. **Investigations**
   a. XRs are generally *not helpful* in the diagnosis of nasal fractures in children (nasal bones of children are poorly visualized on plain radiographs)
   b. CT indicated when there is flattening of the nasal dorsum (possible nasoorbitoethmoid fracture), tenderness over frontal sinus (possible frontal sinus fracture), unstable palate (possible midface fracture), or suspected cerebrospinal fluid (CSF) leak

3. **Management**
   a. Children with septal hematomas and infants (obligate nose-breathers) with nasal obstruction warrant urgent Otolaryngology consultation
   b. Patients with nasal bone fracture (but no septal hematoma), may be referred to otolaryngologist within 3 to 5 days. Most nasal fractures in children with significant nasal deformity can be managed with closed reduction, which needs to occur within 2 weeks of injury. This may require general anesthesia in the pediatric population
   c. Refrain from all sport for 2 weeks and contact sports for 6 weeks

NECK MASSES

1. **Etiology** (Table 33.8 and Box 33.1)

Table 33.8	Etiologies of Neck Masses	
Congenital	**Inflammatory**	**Neoplastic**

- Branchial cleft cysts
  - Most common (20%–30%)
  - Lateral to midline
- Thyroglossal duct cysts
  - Midline
  - Acute infection after URTI
  - Malignant transformation possible
- Dermoid cysts
  - Midline
  - Do not move with swallowing
- Lymphatic malformations
  - Lateral
  - Spongy
- Laryngoceles
- Vascular malformations
- Hemangiomas
  - Rapid expansion after birth, then slowly improve
- Teratomas
- Thymic cysts
- Mucoceles
	- Reactive lymphadenopathy
	- Infectious lymphadenitis
	  - Staph and Strep most common
	  - Inflamed, large, tender
	  - Do NOT use steroids unless diagnosis confirmed
	  - May lead to abscess
	- Atypical mycobacteria
	- 5 "K's" of neck masses
	  - Kawasaki
	  - Kimura
	  - Cat scratch
	  - Castleman
	  - Kikuchi
		- Benign
		  - Pilomatrixomas
		  - Lipomas
		  - Fibromas
		  - Neurofibromas
		  - Salivary gland tumors
		- Malignant
		  - Lymphoma
		  - Rhabdomyosarcoma
		  - Neuroblastoma
		  - Thyroid carcinoma
		  - Nasopharyngeal carcinoma

URTI, Upper respiratory tract infection.

Box 33.1	Red Flags for Undiagnosed Neck Masses

- B symptoms (fever, night sweats, weight loss)
- Hard, firm or matted, rubbery
- >2 cm in size
- Supraclavicular
- Persistent, enlarging
- Absence of inflammation
- Ulceration
- Failure to respond to antibiotics
- Associated thyroid mass

Otolaryngology

33

2. **Investigations**
   a. **Laboratory tests**
      i. CBC if inflammatory or neoplastic condition suspected
      ii. Other tests as indicated: titers for Epstein-Barr virus (EBV), cat-scratch disease, CMV, human immunodeficiency virus (HIV), toxoplasmosis
   b. **Imaging studies**
      i. Ultrasound of neck region
      ii. CXR as needed
      iii. CT or MRI if suspected malignancy or deep tissue involvement
   c. **Other tests:** tuberculosis (TB) testing

OROPHARYNX

ADENOIDS AND TONSILS

1. **Anatomy**
   a. Pharyngeal tonsils (adenoids), palatine tonsils (tonsils), and lingual tonsils form ring of lymphatic tissue (Waldeyer ring) within oral cavity and nasopharynx
   b. Infection and inflammation may cause airway obstruction, which may manifest as mouthbreathing, snoring, or sleep apnea. See Table 33.9 for adenotonsillectomy indications.

Table 33.9	Considerations for Adenotonsillectomy
Indications	- Obstruction (e.g., OSA) - Infection (recurrent or chronic ear, nose, or throat infections) - Suspected malignancy
Special considerations (i.e., higher risk populations)	- Conditions that are related to velopharyngeal insufficiency (e.g., cleft palate, bifid uvula, orofacial anomalies) - Hematologic (anemia and disorders of hemostasis) - Active infection - Neuromuscular (e.g., Arnold-Chiari malformations, myotonic dystrophy, Down syndrome)
Complications	- Anesthesia-related - Respiratory compromise (airway obstruction) - Hemorrhage - Dehydration - Infection - Mortality (relates to hemorrhagic or respiratory complications)

OSA, Obstructive sleep apnea.

. Tonsillar infections (Table 33.10)

Table 33.10	Tonsillitis and Peritonsillar Abscess	
	Tonsillitis or Pharyngitis	**Peritonsillar Abscess (PTA)**
Definition	- Inflammation of palatine tonsils - Usually extends to adenoid and lingual tonsils	- Collection of pus between palatine tonsil and pharyngeal muscles; most common complication of tonsillitis
Epidemiology	- Rare <2 yo - *Strep* spp. usually 5–15 yo	- Teens or young adults
Pathophysiology	- Bacterial: GAS, *Mycoplasma pneumoniae*, *Corynebacterium diptheriae*, *Chlamydia pneumoniae*, *Neisseria gonorrhea* - Viral: EBV, CMV, HSV, adenovirus, measles virus - Fungal: *Candida* species	- Aerobes: GAS, *Staphylococcus aureus*, *Haemophilus influenzae* - Anaerobes: *Prevotella*, *Porphyromonas*, *Fusobacterium*, *Peptostreptococcus* species
Clinical features	- Fever - Sore throat - Foul breath - Dysphagia - Odynophagia - Tender cervical nodes	- Fever - Severe throat pain - Malodorous breath - Drooling - Trismus - Hot-potato voice - Neck adenopathy - Unilateral bulging of the soft palate with effacement of the tonsil on the affected side with medial displacement of uvula
Diagnosis	- Clinical (imaging not necessary) - Throat cultures if suspected GAS - Lateral neck x-ray or CT only if suspected spread to deep structures	- Clinical (imaging not typically necessary) - Throat cultures if suspected GAS - Gram stain and culture of abscess fluid - CT only if concern for spread to deeper structures
Management	- Supportive - Antibiotics ONLY for GAS (penicillin or amoxicillin). Consider tonsillectomy if recurrent	- I&D - Antibiotics (IV clindamycin)

CMV, Cytomegalovirus; *CT*, computed tomography; *EBV*, Epstein-Barr virus; *GAS*, group A β-hemolytic streptococcus; *HSV*, herpes simplex virus; *I&D*, incision and drainage; *IV*, intravenous; *spp.*, species.

RETROPHARYNGEAL ABSCESS

. Definition

  a. Suppurative deep neck infection involving the retropharyngeal space, a potential space extending from base of skull to posterior mediastinum

b. Peak incidence 2 to 4 years old (lymph nodes in the retropharyngeal space atrophy in teenage years)

2. **Etiology**
   a. Often polymicrobial: GAS, *Staphylococcus aureus*, oral anaerobes
   b. Throat swabs may not be helpful because they pick up oral flora
   c. Commonly associated with preceding URTI

3. **Signs and symptoms**
   a. May have toxic appearance
   b. Neck pain, reduced neck movement, neck swelling, neck stiffness
   c. Fever
   d. Sore throat
   e. Dysphagia, odynophagia
   f. Poor oral intake
   g. Drooling
   h. Dysphonia
   i. Respiratory distress
      See Box 33.2 for differential diagnosis

Box 33.2 Differential Diagnosis of Retropharyngeal Abscess

- Other infections: meningitis, cervical adenitis, epiglottitis, pharyngitis, peritonsillar abscess
- Trauma or foreign body in airway or esophagus
- Angioedema or anaphylaxis
- Tumors
- Musculoskeletal: torticollis or cervical spine arthritis or osteomyelitis

---

✦ PEARL

In a child <5 yo with the neck properly extended, the width of prevertebral soft tissue on lateral neck x-ray should be less than half the width of the adjacent vertebral body. It is considered widened if it is greater than a full vertebral body at C2 or C3 (or, >7 mm at C2 or >14 mm at C6/C7).

---

4. **Investigations**
   a. **Laboratory studies:** CBC, blood culture (aerobic + anaerobic)
   b. **Imaging studies**
      i. Lateral neck XR (Figure 33.4): look for prevertebral widening to support the diagnosis. Ideal XR should be taken during inspiration with neck held in normal extension
      ii. CT with contrast: Can confirm diagnosis and size/location of abscess. Indicated for those who are ill-appearing, airway compromise, or no response to IV antibiotics.

Figure 33.4 Retropharyngeal Abscess

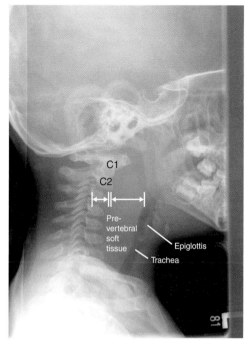

Lateral neck x-ray showing reversal of normal cervical spine curvature and widening of the prevertebral soft tissue.

5. **Management**
   a. **Antibiotics** (IV clindamycin ± cloxacillin)
   b. ± surgical incision and drainage. If no airway compromise, appropriate to trial antibiotics for 24 to 48 hours without surgical drainage
6. **Complications**
   a. Rarely, infection can spread from the retropharyngeal space to adjacent structures (aspiration pneumonia, mediastinitis, jugular vein thrombosis) and the bloodstream (sepsis).

PHARYNGITIS

1. **Etiology**
   a. **Viral pharyngitis**
      i. Most common cause of sore throat
      ii. Adenoviruses, enteroviruses, rhinovirus, parainfluenza virus, coxsackie virus, coronavirus, echovirus, CMV, EBV
   b. **Streptococcal pharyngitis:** group A Strep (*Streptococcus pyogenes*) 921

2. **Signs and symptoms**
   a. **Viral pharyngitis** often associated with sneezing, rhinorrhea, cough. Absence of pharyngeal inflammation or presence of rhinorrhea/cough increases likelihood of viral cause
   b. **Streptococcal pharyngitis**
      i. Peak prevalence 5 to 15 years
      ii. Acute onset of high fever, sore throat, tonsillar exudate, palatal petechiae, tender cervical lymphadenopathy

---

 PEARL

Children with findings suggestive of viral infection (coryza, conjunctivitis, cough, hoarseness, discrete ulcerations) should generally NOT be tested for bacterial pharyngitis with a swab.

---

3. **Investigations**
   Clinical diagnosis in most cases!
   a. **Viral pharyngitis**: in general, no studies necessary. If EBV suspected, may consider CBC with differential (atypical lymphocytes) and monospot test
   b. **Streptococcal pharyngitis**
      i. Rapid antigen detection assays
         - Highly specific (i.e., diagnostic if positive)
         - Poor sensitivity (throat culture should be sent if rapid assay negative)
      ii. Gold standard: throat culture
4. **Management**
   a. **Viral pharyngitis:** supportive care with analgesia as required
   b. **Streptococcal pharyngitis:** Amoxicillin 50 mg/kg/dose PO once daily (max 1 g/day) × 10 days to prevent development of rheumatic fever
5. **Complications of streptococcal pharyngitis**
   a. Suppurative: cervical adenitis, parapharyngeal abscess, retropharyngeal abscess, otitis media, sinusitis
   b. Nonsuppurative: rheumatic fever, glomerulonephritis

UPPER AIRWAY OBSTRUCTION

STRIDOR

1. **Definition and etiology**
   High-pitched, monophonic sound because of turbulent airflow through narrowed passageway
   a. **Inspiratory stridor:** usually *extrathoracic* obstruction; supraglottic (laryngomalacia, laryngotracheitis [croup], retropharyngeal abscess [RPA], epiglottitis)
   b. **Biphasic stridor:** associated with *fixed lesions*; mostly at vocal cords or subglottis

c. **Expiratory stridor:** usually *intrathoracic* obstruction; often congenital or enlarged nodes or tumors

---

⁕ **PEARL**

Always consider the possibility of foreign body aspiration in an infant or toddler with acute onset stridor or wheeze.

---

2. **Differential diagnosis**
   a. **Acute onset obstruction**
      i. Foreign body aspiration
      ii. Anaphylaxis (associated with respiratory distress, skin, or gastrointestinal symptoms)
      iii. Airway burns or trauma
      iv. Infections (see Table 33.11 and previous sections earlier)
         - Laryngotracheitis (croup)
         - Bacterial tracheitis
         - Epiglottitis
         - Infectious mononucleosis
         - Peritonsillar, retropharyngeal or parapharyngeal abscess
         - Submandibular/sublingual abscess (Ludwig angina)

Table 33.11	Infectious Causes of Stridor		
	Laryngotracheitis	**Bacterial Tracheitis**	**Epiglottitis**
Definition	- Inflammation of larynx and subglottic airway - Most common cause of stridor in febrile child	- Invasive exudative bacterial infection of tracheal soft tissues - Rare, life-threatening	- Inflammation of epiglottis + adjacent structures - Can rapidly obstruct airway - Rare, life threatening
Etiology	- Viral infection: Most commonly parainfluenza type 1	- Bacterial infection (typically secondary infection superimposed on viral croup): *Staphylococcus Aureus* most common, *Streptococcus pneumoniae*, Group A streptococcus, *Haemophilus influenza B*	- Bacterial infection: *Haemophilus influenza* (type B and others), *Staphylococcus aureus*, Group A streptococcus

Continued

Table 33.11	Infectious Causes of Stridor—cont'd		
	Laryngotracheitis	**Bacterial Tracheitis**	**Epiglottitis**
Clinical manifestations	- 6–36 months most common (usually <6 years) - Viral prodrome (gradual onset) - "Barking cough," inspiratory stridor, hoarseness - Rarely have signs of respiratory failure	- 3 months–6 years - Viral prodrome - Progressive stridor + cough - Rapid deterioration - High fever + respiratory distress - Prefer to lie flat	- 2–12 years - Uncomfortable and anxious - Rapid onset of distress - High temperature, muffled voice, drooling, dysphagia, stridor - Prefer "tripod position"
Imaging (NOT necessary in most cases)	- Steeple sign on CXR		- Thumbprint sign on lateral neck XR (thickened epiglottis)

Management	- *Mild cases:* Dexamethasone 0.6 mg/kg PO × 1
	- *Moderate-Severe* (stridor at rest, increased work of breathing):
	  - Dexamethasone PO and inhalational epinephrine (1:1000)
	  - If epinephrine used, observe for 2–4 h before discharge
	- *Severe airway compromise (very rare):* 100% oxygen, keep calm, PPV and intubation if necessary
		- Oxygen
		- Majority of cases require intubation; anticipate + +secretions
		- May need bronchoscopy to remove membranes in airway
		- IV Antibiotics (ceftriaxone + vancomycin)
		- Admission
			- Keep child calm; anxiety can cause worsening airway obstruction, laryngospasm, cardiac arrest
			- Oxygen, gentle PPV only if necessary
			- Typically requires intubation in controlled setting, such as OR (emergent ENT + anesthesia consult)
			- IV Antibiotics (ceftriaxone + vancomycin)
			- Admission

CXR, Chest x-ray; *ENT*, ear, nose, and throat; *IV*, intravenous; *OR*, operating room; *PO*, orally; *PPV*, positive pressure ventilation; *XR*, x-ray.

b. **Chronic or recurrent airway obstruction**
  i. Congenital anomalies (most present early in life) (Table 33.12)
  ii. Acquired conditions
      - Vocal cord dysfunction, paresis or paralysis
      - Subglottic stenosis (due to endotracheal intubation). May also be congenital.
      - Laryngeal spasm (because of hypocalcemia)
      - Neoplasms:
        - Benign: squamous papillomas (50% of mothers have a history of genital condylomas at delivery; diagnosed on laryngeal endoscopy and requires laser or mechanical resection)
        - Malignant: lymphoma, neuroblastoma, teratoma, rhabdomyosarcoma

Table 33.12	Causes of Congenital Upper Airway Obstruction			
	Nasal	**Pharyngeal**	**Laryngeal**	**Tracheal**
Etiology	- Choanal atresia: common in CHARGE syndrome (see Chapter 18 Genetics) - Nasal mass: encephalocele, glioma, dermoid cyst, lacrimal cyst - Pyriform aperture stenosis	- Retrognathia - Lingual thyroid or thyroglossal duct cyst - Relative or true macroglossia - Tonsillar hypertrophy	- Laryngomalacia: *Inspiratory stridor* worse when supine, crying, feeding, during URTI. Most cases resolve spontaneously by 1–2 years - Vocal cord immobility: may be associated with neurologic or cardiac malformations or idiopathic - Other: laryngeal cysts/webs, subglottic hemangioma, subglottic stenosis	- Tracheomalacia: *Expiratory stridor* because of abnormal flaccidity of trachea, collapse during expiration - Vascular ring: *expiratory stridor* because of external compression of trachea. May have feeding issues if esophagus also involved - Other: tracheal stenosis, TEF, lymphangioma/hemangioma
Clinical manifestations	- Cyanosis in a newborn (obligate nose breathers) relieved by crying	- Nighttime apnea, cyanosis	- Inspiratory stridor, hoarseness, weak cry	- Expiratory stridor, apneic or cyanotic spells
Diagnosis	- Inability to pass NG, flexible nasal endoscopy, CT	- Physical examination	- Endoscopy	- Bronchoscopy, airway fluoroscopy and barium swallow, MRI, echo
Treatment	- Oral airway, surgery	- Nasopharyngeal airway, surgery	- Observe, ± laser excision, medical therapy for GERD, beta-blockers for hemangioma	- Observation, tracheopexy, aortopexy

CT, Computed tomography; *GERD,* gastroesophageal reflux disease; *MRI,* magnetic resonance imaging; *NG,* nasogastric; *TEF,* tracheoesophageal fistula; *URTI,* upper respiratory tract infection.

Otolaryngology

33

Table 33.13	Approach to Foreign Body in the Ear, Nose, and Aerodigestive Tract		
	Clinical Presentation	**Approach to Removal**	**Indications for Otolaryngology Consultation**
Ear	- Ear pain - Impaired hearing - Discharge	- Irrigation with water (avoid if object likely to swell) - Grasping with forceps (soft object), cerumen loop (hard object), right-angle ball hook, or suction catheter - Acetone to dissolve Styrofoam	- Need for sedation - Canal or TM trauma - Tightly wedged or adherent to TM - Sharp - Removal attempts unsuccessful
Nose	- Pain - Unilateral, foul-smelling discharge	- Patient "blows nose" or PPV applied to mouth while other nostril obstructed - Grasping with forceps, cerumen loop, right-angle ball hook, or suction catheter - Thin, lubricated balloon-tip catheter	- Tumor or mass suspected - Edema, bony destruction or granulation tissue from chronic foreign body - Removal attempts unsuccessful
Pharynx, larynx, tracheabronchial tree	- History of ingestion - Cough, wheeze - Dysphagia - Choking or cyanotic episode - Airway distress	- Often requires endoscopic removal with sedation	- Inadequate visualization - Need for sedation - Airway compromise
Esophagus	- History of ingestion - Dysphagia - Regurgitation, vomiting, drooling - Stridor if trachea compressed	- Endoscopic removal with sedation	- Note: a button battery in any location (nose, ear, esophagus) is an emergency requiring immediate removal

PPV, Positive pressure ventilation; *TM*, tympanic membrane.

Modified from Helm SW, Maughan KL. Foreign bodies in the ear, nose, and throat. *Am Fam Phys*. 2007;76(8):1185–1189, table 1.

Plastic Surgery

Laura Kaufman • Kristen Davidge

Also see page xviii for a list of other abbreviations used throughout this book

BSA	body surface area
DIPJ	distal interphalangeal joint
FDP	flexor digitorum profundus
IPJ	interphalangeal joint
LET	lidocaine-epinephrine-tetracaine
MCPJ	metacarpophalangeal joint
PIPJ	proximal interphalangeal joint
u/o	urine output

BASICS OF WOUND CLOSURE

Also see Chapter 5 Procedures for description of suture and glue repair of wounds

A. Inspection/exploration
1. Adequate inspection may require anesthesia
2. Identify any deep tissue, nerve, artery, or tendon injuries and debride any devitalized tissues; visualize borders of the wound
3. Examine relevant range of motion and evaluate motor and sensory function
4. Consider culture as needed
5. Assess for foreign bodies; XR as indicated to assess for radioopaque material
6. XR as needed to rule out underlying fracture

B. Anesthesia
1. Use 1% or 2% lidocaine with epinephrine for local anesthesia or regional nerve block
2. Lidocaine with epinephrine should generally not be used for appendages (fingers, toes, ears, nose, penis)
3. Topical lidocaine preparations (LET) may be used to anesthetize certain small nonmucosal wounds on the face/scalp, or as an adjunct to assist with injection of local anesthesia

C. Irrigation
1. Use sterile water or saline or diluted antiseptic under increased pressures (60-mL syringe attached to 20-G catheter)
2. Wounds with heavy bacterial inoculum at time of injury and clean wounds open for >6 hours should be considered contaminated
3. Consider surgical irrigation and debridement for extensive or heavily contaminated wounds, or in those with nonviable tissue edges
4. Facial lacerations may be closed outside a 6-hour window because of healthy blood supply and cosmetic concerns

D. Primary wound closure

1. See Chapter 5 Procedures for further information on laceration repair with glue and sutures
2. See High-Risk Wounds later for description of wounds that should not be repaired via primary closure

E. Immunization Status (see Chapter 23 Immunoprophylaxis for further details)

1. Provide tetanus vaccination and tetanus immune globulin if indicated. Note that all animal bites are considered "dirty" wounds.
2. Consider rabies prophylaxis for select animal bites

HIGH-RISK WOUNDS

A. Wounds at high risk for infection where primary closure should generally not be considered:

1. Crush injuries
2. Puncture wounds
3. Human, dog, cat bites (wounds to face may be closed because of cosmetic concerns)
4. Bites involving the hands
5. Bite wounds in immunosuppressed hosts

B. Wounds which should be repaired by a plastic surgeon

1. Animal bites to cosmetically sensitive areas (face)
2. Complex facial lacerations (eyelid lacerations, lacerations crossing vermilion border, concern of injury to facial nerve or parotid duct, ear lacerations involving cartilage or with suspected hematoma, or complex/stellate lacerations)
3. Complex hand lacerations (through nail bed, partial or complete amputations, concerns about nerve/artery/tendon injury)
4. Any deep wound (extension into fascia/muscle/bone, concern about nerve/tendon/artery injury)

BITE WOUNDS

1. **Definition**
   a. High-risk wounds from an animal or human being that puncture, tear, or remove tissue
2. **Etiology**
   a. See Table 34.1 for common bites, responsible pathogens, and recommended treatment

Table 34.1	Common Bites, Organisms, and Antibiotic Therapy		
Type of Bite	**Common Organisms**	**Management**	**Comments**
Dog	- *Staphylococcus* spp. - *Streptococcus* spp. - Anaerobes (e.g., *Pasteurella canis*, *Bacteroides*)	- Role of prophylactic antibiotics uncertain - PO: amox/clav - IV pip/tazo - Penicillin allergy: ciprofloxacin + clindamycin	- 80%–90% of bites - Often crush injury
Cat[a]	- *Pasteurella multocida* - Anaerobes (e.g., *Bacteroides*)	- Prophylaxis recommended - PO: amox/clav - IV: pip/tazo - Penicillin allergy: ciprofloxacin + clindamycin	- May be associated with lymphadenopathy - Often presents infected - Treat claw punctures as bites
Human	- *Streptococcus* (α- and β-hemolytic) - *Staphylococcus aureus*, - *Eikenella corrodens*, anaerobes	- Prophylaxis recommended - PO: amox/clav - IV: penicillin + cloxacillin - Penicillin allergy: ciprofloxacin + clindamycin	- Prone to developing infection - Must consider NAI - Consider HIV/HepB, HepC prophylaxis

[a]Bites of other animals (rodents, squirrels, rabbits, guinea pigs) should be treated as cat bites.

amox/clav, Amoxillin-clavulanic acid; *HIV,* human immunodeficiency virus; *IV,* intravenous; *NAI,* non-accidental injury; *pip/tazo,* piperacillin-tazobactam; *PO,* orally.

3. **Management**
   a. Cat and human bite wounds, and delayed dog bite wounds (>6–12 hours on arm/leg and >12–24 hours on face), should generally not be sutured closed
   b. Primary closure can be considered in facial lacerations after thorough debridement and copious irrigation
   c. Delayed closure should be used for higher risk wounds (e.g., deep/large wounds, breach into oral/nasal cavity, devitalized or avulsed tissue, puncture wounds, immunocompromised patients), although evidence is controversial about whether this results in lower infection rates

 PEARL

Antibiotic prophylaxis is recommended for cat and human bites.

4. **Complications**
   a. **Infections:** identify cause (hematoma, closed space, dead tissue)

   b. **Sepsis**
- i. *Capnocytophaga canimorsus*: incubation period 1 to 7 days, malaise, abdominal pain, confusion, dyspnea, septic shock. May have petechial or purpuric rash progressing to gangrene.
- ii. *Pasteurella* sp.: necrotizing fasciitis, septic arthritis, osteomyelitis

HAND INJURIES

1. **Examination**
   a. **Inspection:** for swelling, open wounds, debris, color (pallor can suggest arterial insufficiency), deformity (consider XRs to rule out fracture)
   b. **Palpation:** tenderness, temperature, crepitus, effusion
   c. **Vascular:** pulses, capillary refill, color, tissue turgor
     i. **Allen test:** used to test for integrity of ulnar and radial arteries: patient makes fist for 30 seconds; place a finger on radial and ulnar arteries to occlude; hand should appear blanched; release finger from ulnar artery and color should return <5 seconds; repeat for radial artery

> ⭐ **PEARL**
>
> Testing sensory innervation to the hand (see Figure 34.1):
> **Median** nerve: palmar surface of index finger
> **Ulnar** nerve: ulnar side of fifth digit
> **Radial** nerve: snuffbox at base of thumb on dorsal aspect of hand

   d. **Sensory:** see Figure 34.1; assess light touch, two-point discrimination, vibration, proprioception
   e. **Motor:** if patient can open and close fist completely, likely intact. However, also important to test movement of specific muscles as follows:
     i. Median nerve: opponens pollicis; oppose thumb to touch little finger
     ii. Ulnar nerve: abductor digiti minimi; abduct little finger or finger spread against resistance
     iii. Radial nerve: wrist, finger and thumb extension ("thumb's up")
   f. **Tendons** (the following describes tests to confirm normal function)
     i. Flexor digitorum profundus: stabilize proximal interphalangeal joint (PIPJ), while patient flexes distal interphalangeal joint (DIPJ)
     ii. Flexor digitorum superficialis: patient flexes PIPJ of one digit, while examiner stabilizes all other digits
     iii. Flexor pollicis longus: patient flexes interphalangeal joint (IPJ) of thumb
     iv. Extensor tendons: patient makes fist and then extends metacarpophalangeal joint (MCPJ) and IPJ
     v. Intrinsic muscles: patient flexes MCPJ and extends IPJ

Figure 34.1 Sensory Innervation of the Hand

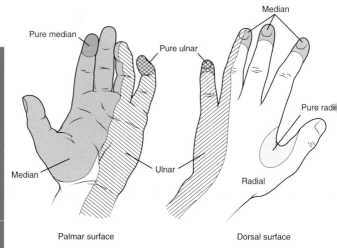

Median

Pure median

Pure ulnar

Median

Pure radial

Median

Ulnar

Radial

Palmar surface

Dorsal surface

(Modified from Trott A. *Wounds and Lacerations: Emergency Care and Closure.* 4th ed. Philadelphia, PA: Saunders; 2012.)

2. **Management**
   a. Any deep injury to flexor surface should be explored and all flexor tendon repairs done in the operating room
   b. Extensor tendons can be repaired by Plastic Surgery in the emergency room

FINGERTIP INJURIES

A. Types of injuries

1. **Laceration:** cleansing, direct repair, and dressing
2. **Nail bed hematomas**
   a. If hematoma involves <50% of nail bed, leave nail on; if >50% of nail bed, remove nail plate to repair bed (with sutures or glue) and replace nail as stent if laceration extends across eponychial fold to prevent late synechiae
   b. May use foil from suture package instead of replacing nail
   c. XR hand to rule out tuft fracture; if present may benefit from splint for comfort
3. **Crush:** cleansing, debridement, repair if possible, dressing

B. Amputation

1. XR hand (three views) and amputated part
2. Controversy regarding benefits of replacement (biologic dressing) versus secondary healing (better neurosensory recovery)
3. Young children have a better chance of amputated piece taking as a composite graft
4. Distal to DIPJ: vessels are too small to repair; revision amputation or composite graft
5. Proximal to DIPJ: place amputated part in sterile gauze in plastic bag on ice and consult Plastic Surgery for further repair as indicated

> **! PITFALL**
>
> Three-view x-rays (AP, lateral, oblique) are needed for all suspected hand or digit fractures. Many fractures can be missed if a true lateral x-ray is not performed.

HAND FRACTURES

A. Phalanx fractures

1. Examine for associated nail bed injuries and associated terminal extensor tendon injury or flexor digitorum profundus (FDP) avulsion injuries (see Hand Injury earlier; refer these to Plastic Surgery)
2. Tuft fractures and simple shaft fractures can be managed with finger splinting; intraarticular fractures should be seen by Plastic Surgery

B. Metacarpal fractures

1. Nondisplaced, well-aligned extraarticular shaft fractures can be managed with splint: ulnar gutter for fractures of fourth and fifth metacarpals, and radial gutter for first, second, third metacarpals) (Figure 34.2)
2. Acceptable angulation in shaft fractures: <10 degrees in index and middle finger, <20 degrees in ring finger, <30 degrees in little finger
3. Acceptable metacarpal neck fracture angulation: 10, 20, 30, 40 degrees in second, third, fourth, fifth digits, respectively
4. Fractures associated with malrotation, comminution, significant angulation, inadequate reduction, or shortening >5 mm should be referred to hand surgeon

> **PEARL**
>
> **Safe position for splinting:**
> A 30-degree extension at wrist, 70- to 90-degree flexion at metacarpophalangeal joints, slight flexion at distal interphalangeal and proximal interphalangeal joints, thumb abducted in opposed position.

Figure 34.2 Ulnar Guttar (A) and Radial Guttar (B) Splints

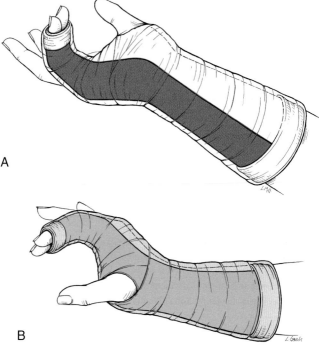

A

B

(Modified from Nguyen T, Abilez O. *Practical Guide to the Care of the Surgical Patient.* The Pocket Scalpel; and *Roberts, J. Roberts and Hedges' Clinical Procedures in Emergency Medicine.* 5th ed. Philadelphia, PA: Saunders; 2013.)

INTRAVENOUS BURNS

A. Definitions

1. **Intravenous (IV) infiltration:** fluid infuses into tissues surrounding venipuncture site
2. **Extravasation:** infiltration of a vesicant or solution
   a. **Vesicant:** can cause blistering or tissue necrosis (e.g. chemotherapeutic agents, acyclovir)
   b. **Irritant:** can cause local inflammation but no necrosis (e.g., some chemotherapeutic agents, aminophylline)

B. Management

1. **Stop infusion!** Identify what fluid was infusing and estimate volume. When possible, remove catheter.

2. **Elevate** the extremity
3. **Assess the site** for perfusion, pulses, skin discoloration, swelling, tenderness at rest and on movement, blistering (Table 34.2). Monitor for signs of compartment syndrome or tissue necrosis.

Table 34.2	Intravenous Infiltration Grades	
Grade	Appearance	Symptoms
0	No symptoms	Painless
1	Skin blanched, edema <1 inch, cool	± pain
2	Skin blanched, edema 1–6 inches any direction, cool	± pain
3	Skin blanched + translucent, edema >6 inches, cool	Pain ± numbness
4	Skin blanched + translucent, tight, discolored w bruising, edema >6 inches ± pitting edema	Moderate-severe pain

From Infusion Nurses Society. Infusion nursing standards of practice. *J Infus Nurse.* 2006;29(1 suppl): S1–S92.

4. **Determine infusate risk**
   a. If infiltrate is low volume normal saline, elevate limb and apply warm compresses
   b. Warm or cold pack compresses, or specific antidotes may be required for certain infusates and antineoplastic agents. Refer to local IV infiltration and extravasation Policies and Procedures for drug-specific guidelines, including when to consult Plastic Surgery.
5. **Wound management** (skin breakdown, blistering, necrosis) by Plastic Surgery.

CLEFT LIP AND PALATE

1. **Clinical manifestations**
   a. Variable presentation from small notch to complete separation of skin, muscle, mucosa, tooth, and bone. Unilateral cleft lip L>R is most common. Isolated cleft palate (midline) is least common. When combined can extend to hard palate ± nasal cavity.
   b. **Associated syndromes:** Van der Woude, DiGeorge, Treacher Collins, orofaciodigital syndrome. Look for ear pits, micrognathia, heart murmurs, digital abnormalities.
2. **Management**
   a. **Cleft palate team:** prompt referral to dedicated multidisciplinary team (includes surgeons, speech and language pathologists, dieticians, etc.). Lip repair at 3 months, palate repair at 1 year but individualized plan is key.

b. **Feeding:** oral feeding can be achieved with appropriate artificial nipple (Haberman bottle) and education but consider enteral tube until established

c. **Sequelae:** recurrent otitis media, dental issues, speech impairment or delay

SKULL DEFORMITIES

A. Craniosynostosis

1. **Definition:** premature fusion of one or more of the cranial sutures (sagittal [most common], coronal, metopic, lambdoid), resulting in abnormal growth of the skull (Figure 34.3)

   a. Primary (abnormal skull development) versus secondary (rickets, bone metabolic disorders, achondroplasia, prematurity, shunts)

   b. Single versus compound (multiple sutures)

   c. Syndromic (Crouzon, Apert, Pfeiffer) versus nonsyndromic

2. **Associations:** hydrocephalus, increased intracranial pressure (ICP), papilledema and optic atrophy, choanal atresia, speech and hearing deficits

Figure 34.3 Craniosynostosis

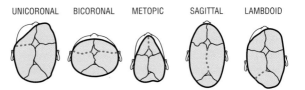

UNICORONAL BICORONAL METOPIC SAGITTAL LAMBDOID

(Modified from Polin RA, Ditmar MF. *Pediatric Secrets.* 6th ed. Philadelphia, PA: Elsevier; 2015.)

B. Positional (or deformational) plagiocephaly

> ⭐ **PEARL**
>
> The diagnosis of positional plagiocephaly is made by clinical examination. If in doubt, referral to a craniofacial specialist is the next best step.

1. **Definition:** asymmetrical head shape because of external molding related to positioning/repeated pressure on the same area of the head (cranial sutures are normal). Increased risk in congenital torticollis and developmental delay

2. **Clinical manifestations:** posterior flattening of the skull associated with anterior positioning of the ear and forehead on the ipsilateral side. Skull has the shape of a parallelogram.

3. **Management:** supervised tummy time, toys, and mirrors on opposite side, physiotherapy. Molding helmets for severe cases—most effective when started at 4 to 6 months, less effective after 12 months.

OBSTETRIC BRACHIAL PLEXUS INJURY

1. **Definition**
   a. Nerves of brachial plexus are stretched, compressed or torn during a difficult delivery, resulting in loss of motor function in upper extremity
   b. Risk factors include large birth weight, breech, shoulder dystocia, gestational diabetes, sibling with brachial plexus injury
2. **Clinical presentation**
   a. **Upper plexus palsy (Erb)** (C5–C6 ±7): most common; upper arm is adducted and internally rotated, forearm extended and pronated
   b. **Total palsy** (C5–C8 ±T1): loss of grasp and wrist movement; may have associated Horner syndrome
   c. Other clinical features: areflexive or hyporeflexive, asymmetric Moro with absent shoulder abduction and elbow flexion on involved side; if late pickup may have upper extremity size discrepancy
   d. ~5% have associated phrenic nerve paresis

3. **Management**
   a. Physiotherapy to prevent contractures
   b. Early referral (2–3 months) to Plastic Surgery essential; need/timing of surgical management depends on severity (range 2 months to 1 year of age)
   c. Better prognosis if some improvement seen in first 2 weeks of life
   d. ~1/3 require operative intervention and some degree of permanent upper limb deficits is present in patients who take longer than 1 month to recover from their injury

BURN MANAGEMENT

Also see Chapter 2 emergency medicine for resuscitation and acute management

A. Minor burn outpatient management

1. Evaluate and document burn size, location, and depth (see modified Lund Browder chart in Figure 2.9 Chapter 2 Emergency Medicine and Table 34.3)
2. Remove clothing and eliminate inciting agent using copious irrigation with water if chemical burn, cool body part, cleanse wounds with 0.9% NaCl
3. Leave intact blisters alone, debride broken blisters and loose debris
4. Apply topical antibiotics (Polysporin) then a nonadherent dressing layer (e.g. Mepitel or Bactrigras)
5. Dress with wet 0.9% NaCl gauze, followed by dry gauze, and secure with conforming gauze (Kling) bandage. Change dressing 1 to 2 × daily.
6. Review tetanus immunization status (see Chapter 23 Immunoprophylaxis)
7. Oral analgesics for pain
8. Discuss signs of infection (erythema, edema, green/violaceous discoloration, systemic signs) with caregivers and reevaluate in 2 to 5 days

Table 34.3	Severity of Burn	
Degree	**Level of Burn**	**Characteristics**
First	Epidermis	Erythema, pain for 48–72 h
Second - Superficial - Deep	Superficial dermis Deep dermis	Blisters, extreme pain, heals in 7–14 days Eschar, ±pain
Third	Subcutaneous tissue	Leathery eschar, insensate, will not heal

B. Moderate to severe burn inpatient management

See Chapter 2 Emergency Medicine Box 2.4 for criteria for hospitalizations of patients with burns

1. **Wound care**
    a. Evaluate and document burn size, location and depth (see modified Lund Browder burn chart in Figure 2.9 Chapter 2 Emergency Medicine and Table 34.3)
    b. Cleanse in burn bath (lukewarm saltwater at 38°C)
    c. Leave intact blisters alone, debride loose tissue and broken blisters
    d. Body: apply Acticoat and use a red rubber catheter to infuse water through dressing 3 times per day (which activates the silver) then apply burn gauze and cling. Acticoat will be changed in the OR every 5 to 7 days on the body.
    e. Face: Polysporin ointment; dress with gauze

. **Fluid management**
   a. If burn >15% BSA, insert urinary catheter for bladder decompression and monitor urine output (u/o) hourly
   b. Parkland formula (see Chapter 2 Emergency Medicine Box 2.3) is only a guide and fluid management should be adjusted as follows:
      i. u/o <1 mL/kg/h: consider 0.9% NaCl bolus
      ii. u/o 1 to 3 mL/kg/h: continue with Parkland formula
      iii. u/o >3 mL/kg/h: decrease fluids to 2/3 Parkland formula
      iv. For children <2 years old, give maintenance fluids in addition to Parkland formula

. **Other supportive inpatient management**
   a. Severe burns: NPO with nasogastric tube and H_2 blocker
   b. Begin enteral feeding within first 8 hours of injury and maximize feeds on second postburn day as patients will be hypermetabolic
   c. Transfuse with albumin, plasma, or blood as needed
   d. Manage pain aggressively with IV opioids as needed (see Chapter 4 Pain and Sedation)
   e. Swab for culture from nose, throat, and burn wound
   f. May require higher environmental temperature (28°C–30°C) to prevent heat loss
   g. Watch closely for sepsis
   h. Consider immediate escharotomy for deep circumferential burns with evidence of distal circulatory compromise

FURTHER READING

Romanowski KS, Palmieri TL. Pediatric burn resuscitation: past, present and future. *Burns Trauma*. 2017;5:26

Thorne CH, ed. *Grabb and Smith's Plastic Surgery*. 7th ed. Philadelphia, PA: Lippincott Williams & Wilkins; 2013.

Respirology

Tyler Groves • Wallace B. Wee • Theo J. Moraes

COMMON ABBREVIATIONS AND VARIABLES

COMMON ABBREVIATIONS

Also see page xviii for a list of other abbreviations used throughout this book

ABPA	allergic bronchopulmonary aspergillosis
AHI	apnea hypopnea index
BAL	bronchoalveolar lavage
BPD	bronchopulmonary dysplasia
CPAM	congenital pulmonary airway malformation
CCHS	congenital central hypoventilation syndrome
CF	cystic fibrosis
CFTR	cystic fibrosis transmembrane conductance regulator
CHF	congestive heart failure
CLD	chronic lung disease
CXR	chest x-ray
FEV_1	forced expiratory volume in 1 second
FVC	forced vital capacity
ICS	inhaled corticosteroid
IRT	immunoreactive trypsinogen
IVH	intraventricular hemorrhage
LVH	left ventricular hypertrophy
NO	nitric oxide
OSA	obstructive sleep apnea
PA	posterior-anterior
PEF	peak expiratory flow
PFT	pulmonary function test
PJP	*Pneumocystis jirovecii* pneumonia
PSG	polysomnography
SABA	short-acting beta agonist

RESPIRATORY VARIABLES

$PaCO_2$	arterial PCO_2
$PACO_2$	alveolar PCO_2 (approximates $PaCO_2$)
PaO_2	arterial PO_2
PAO_2	alveolar PO_2
P_{ATM}	atmospheric pressure, approximately 760 mmHg at sea level
P_{H20}	pressure of water vapor, approximately 47 mmHg
PiO_2	partial pressure of inspired O_2, approximately 150 mmHg at sea level in room air
R	respiratory quotient (CO_2 produced/O_2 consumed), approximately 0.8

RESPIRATORY INVESTIGATIONS

1. **Chest x-ray (CXR):** a systematic approach to CXR interpretation is outlined in Chapter 13 Diagnostic Imaging.
2. **Pulmonary function tests:** evaluation of pulmonary function includes:
   a. **Peak expiratory flow rate:** maximum flow rate generated during a forced expiratory maneuver. May be reduced in obstructive airway disease.
   b. **Lung volumes:** see Figure 35.1

Figure 35.1 Lung Volume Subdivisions

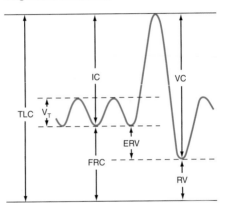

ERV, Expiratory reserve volume; *FRC,* functional residual capacity; *IC,* inspiratory capacity; *RV,* residual volume; V_T, tidal volume; *TLC,* total lung capacity; *VC,* vital capacity. (Modified from Townsend C, Beauchamp RD, Evers BM, et al. *Sabiston Textbook of Surgery: The Biological Basis of Modern Surgical Practice.* 20th ed. Elsevier; 2017.)

   c. **Spirometry**
      i. Usually reliable in those aged ≥6 years
      ii. May include bronchodilator response to assess reversibility of airway obstruction or a methacholine challenge test to assess for airway hyperreactivity
      iii. Interpretation of spirometry results shown in Table 35.1

Table 35.1	Approach to Pulmonary Function Testing Interpretation	
	Restrictive	**Obstructive**
TLC	↓	↑
RV	↓↑	↑
FVC	↓	N or ↓
FEV₁	↓	↓
FEV₁/FVC	N or ↑	↓

FEV_1, Forced expiratory volume in 1 second; FVC, forced vital capacity; RV, residual volume; TLC, total lung capacity.

Modified from Schidlow DV, Smith DS. *A Practical Guide to Pediatric Respiratory Diseases.* Philadelphia, PA: Hanley and Belfus; 1994.

3. **Overnight oximetry:** screening tool to assess patient's oxygen needs. Indications include assessment for qualification for home oxygen and as an initial screen in sleep disordered breathing.

4. **Polysomnography**
   a. To diagnose sleep disorders using electroencephalogram (EEG), oxygen saturation, heart rate, breathing, and limb movements during sleep
   b. Assesses apneas, hypopneas, respiratory effort-related arousal, hypoxemia and hypercapnia
   c. Gold standard for diagnosis of obstructive sleep apnea (OSA)
   d. Parameters that are assessed include
      i. Baseline saturation
      ii. Obstructive apnea-hypopnea index (AHI)
         i. AHI is the average number of apneas and hypopneas per hour of sleep
         ii. Scale (<13 years old, adult scale is higher):
            - Normal obstructive AHI: ≤1/h
            - Mild OSA: 2–5/h
            - Moderate OSA: 6–10/h
            - Severe OSA: >10/h

CONGENITAL LUNG DISEASE

Common congenital lung malformations are listed in Table 35.2

Table 35.2	Congenital Lung Disease			
Malformation	Etiology/Anatomy	Presentation	Diagnosis	Comments
Pulmonary sequestration	Nonfunctioning lung tissue that does not communicate with the tracheobronchial tree and receives arterial blood supply from the systemic circulation Types - Intralobar (90%) - Extralobar (10%); has own visceral pleura	Intralobar - Typically asymptomatic - Can present with neonatal heart failure or with infection Extralobar - Usually detected within first year of life - May be associated with other congenital malformations	- Prenatal US - CXR - Chest CT/MRI	
Congenital pulmonary airway malformation (CPAM)	- Abnormalities in lung branching morphogenesis - May arise anywhere in the lung - Blood supplied via pulmonary circulation	- Tachypnea - Cyanosis - Respiratory distress - Feeding difficulties - May also present with pulmonary infection	- Prenatal US - CXR - Chest CT	Prenatal complications - Polyhydramnios - Hydrops (rare) - Lung hypoplasia Postnatal complications - Recurrent lung infections - Pulmonary HTN - Malignancy Management - If asymptomatic then no treatment but may have surgical resection because of malignancy and infection risk
Bronchogenic cysts	Remnants of thin-walled bronchial tissue from early fetal airway development	- Asymptomatic or respiratory distress; depending on size and location	- CXR - Chest CT	
Congenital lobar emphysema (CLE)	Congenital overinflation of pulmonary lobe	- About 50% present within 4 weeks of age with increased WOB, tachypnea, cyanosis, FTT - Can be asymptomatic	- CXR	Cardiovascular associations in about 14% of cases

1. Acute inflammation of the lower respiratory tract with obstruction of small airways
2. Viral in etiology; respiratory syncytial virus (RSV) being most common; peak incidence in children <2 years old, and in the winter months
3. Self-limiting disease, and most recover without sequelae
4. Infants at higher risk for severe disease include premature infants (<35 weeks), <3 months of age, hemodynamically significant cardiac disease, immunodeficiency, presence of comorbidities/medically complex children
5. **Clinical features**
   a. In general preceded by coryzal symptoms, with signs and symptoms peaking 3 to 5 days into the course
   b. **Symptoms:** rhinorrhea, cough, fever, increased work breathing, poor feeding
   c. **Signs:** tachypnea, respiratory distress, wheezing, crackles, dehydration
   d. **Consideration for admission:** infants at risk of severe disease, signs of respiratory distress, supplemental O_2 requirements, dehydration or refusal to feed/poor oral intake, further assessment to rule out alternative diagnosis or significant social concerns about adequacy or safety of home management

> ## ✴ PEARL
>
> Bronchiolitis is a clinical diagnosis, based on history and examination.

6. **Management**
   a. Supportive
   b. CXR, blood tests and viral/bacterial cultures, are not recommended in typical cases
   c. Repeat clinical assessment is the most important aspect of monitoring for deteriorating respiratory status
   d. Oral and/or nasal suctioning as clinically indicated
   e. Feeding and nutrition: ensure maintenance of hydration with more frequent feeds at lower volumes (if suitable to feed), nasogastric (NG) feeds, or intravenous (IV) fluids as an alternative at clinician/family discretion

Respirology

35

f. **Respiratory therapy**
   i. Supplemental oxygen to maintain saturations based on hospital guidelines and/or with significant work of breathing
   ii. Respiratory therapy: high flow nasal cannula therapy (HFNC) may be considered with severe respiratory distress, but is not a substitute for noninvasive ventilation

> **! PITFALL**
>
> The following therapies should NOT be ordered routinely for bronchiolitis: chest physiotherapy, cool mist therapy, bronchodilator (scheduled or as needed salbutamol therapies are not recommended), antibiotics without identified bacterial focus, ribavirin, steroid therapy.

PLEURAL EFFUSION

1. **Definition**
   a. Excess fluid that accumulates in the pleural cavity, which can impair breathing by limiting the expansion of the lungs
   b. Empyema if there is evidence of intrapleural pus or an exudative parapneumonic effusion
2. **Clinical features**
   a. **Symptoms:** dyspnea, pleuritic chest pain
   b. **Signs:** decreased breath sounds and dullness to percussion on the side of the effusion
3. **Investigations**
   a. **CXR:** obliteration of the costophrenic angle and/or the "meniscus sign" (a rim of fluid ascending the lateral chest wall). On the posterior-anterior (PA) view, small effusion ≤1/4 of thorax, moderate effusion = 1/4 to 1/2 of thorax, large effusion ≥1/2 of thorax
   b. **Chest ultrasound:** indicated in moderate or large effusions to confirm the presence of fluid, determine size, nature of the effusion, and to aid in the assessment for chest tube drainage (i.e., free-flowing vs. loculated/complex)
   c. **Thoracentesis:** request cell count, flow cytometry, biochemistry (protein, glucose, pH, LDH, ± triglycerides if chylous), microbiology (Gram stain, culture, acid-fast staining, virology) and when appropriate, immunologic investigations. Interpretation is outlined in Table 35.3.

Table 35.3	Constituents of Pleural Effusions (Light's Criteria)	
Features	**Transudate**	**Exudate**
Protein	<3 g/dL	≥3 g/dL
LDH	<2/3 upper limit of normal	>2/3 upper limit of normal
Pleural-to-serum ratio, protein	<0.5	≥0.5
Pleural-to-serum ratio, LDH	<0.6	≥0.6
WBC	<1000/mm³; usually >50% lymphocyte or mononuclear cells	1000/mm³; >50% PMN (acute inflammation); >50% lymphocytes (TB, neoplasm)
pH	>7.3	<7.3 (inflammatory)
Glucose	= serum	<serum
Potential etiology	CHF, nephrotic syndrome, acute glomerulonephritis, cirrhosis, myxedema	Infection, collagen vascular disease, malignancy, pancreatitis, subdiaphragmatic abscess

CHF, Congestive heart failure; *LDH,* lactate dehydrogenase; *PMN,* polymorphonuclear neutrophils; *TB,* tuberculosis; *WBC,* white blood cell.

PULMONARY HEMORRHAGE

1. **Definition:** acute bleeding from the respiratory tract
2. **Differential diagnosis:** see Box 35.1

Box 35.1 Differential Diagnosis of Pulmonary Hemorrhage

- Infection (e.g., TB, anaerobes)
- Foreign body
- Bronchiectasis (e.g., CF, PCD) with erosion into bronchial arteries
- Congenital heart disease
- Trauma
- Infarction
- Other (rare): pulmonary renal syndromes (SLE, Wegener, Goodpasture, microscopic polyangiitis, HSP), arteriovenous malformation (e.g., hereditary hemorrhagic telangiectasia), airway hemangioma, lung tumor, coagulopathy, IPH (often diagnosis of exclusion)

CF, Cystic fibrosis; *HSP,* Henoch-Schoenlein purpura; *IPH,* idiopathic pulmonary hemorrhage; *PCD,* primary ciliary dyskinesia; *SLE,* systemic lupus erythematosus; *TB,* tuberculosis.

---

3. **Clinical features**
   a. **Acute:** cough, hemoptysis, respiratory distress, hypoxia, decreased breath sounds, crackles, wheezing, cyanosis, hemodynamic instability
   b. **Chronic:** fatigue, pallor (anemia), may have digital clubbing

4. **Investigations**
   a. **Laboratory tests:** blood gas (assess for acid-base status), complete blood count (anemia, leukocytosis). Note that hemoglobin will not change with acute hemorrhage until some volume resuscitation has occurred.
   b. **Imaging:** CXR (assess for parenchymal and alveolar opacities, cavitations, foreign bodies, etc.); chest CT if massive or recurrent to assess for lung parenchyma or anatomic abnormalities; radionuclide scan (technetium-99–labeled red blood cells [RBCs]) for active bleeding
   c. **Pulmonary function test (PFT):** may have restrictive pattern in chronic cases because of fibrosis, may have elevated carbon monoxide diffusing capacity of the lung (DLCO)
   d. **Bronchoscopy:** identify site(s) of bleeding, airway lesions; bronchoalveolar lavage (BAL) 3 to 14 days after suspected bleeding for hemosiderin-laden macrophages
   e. **Specific investigations:** directed by suspected etiology and can include TB skin test, autoantibodies, echocardiogram
5. **Management**
   a. Primary assessment and resuscitation as needed
   b. Identify and treat underlying etiology. For patients with hemoptysis more than mild (>5 mL blood) and/or of unknown cause, consultation with a respirologist advised.

ASTHMA

1. **Definition:** an inflammatory disorder of the airways, associated with reversible airflow limitation and airway hyperresponsiveness to variable stimuli (i.e., respiratory tract infections, allergens, cold air, exercise, chemical irritants, tobacco smoke)
2. **Clinical history**
   a. Symptoms of dyspnea, chest tightness, wheezing, and cough
   b. Timing of symptoms, including episodic versus persistent, daytime versus night time
   c. Precipitating factors, such as seasonal variation, exercise, cold air, occupation, night time
   d. Changes to daily routines (e.g., school absenteeism, avoiding physical activity)
   e. Prior asthma investigations—peak flow meter and pulmonary function testing
   f. Prior asthma management—reliever and preventer puffer usage, compliance, technique assessment, and response

g. Prior exacerbations—frequency, emergency department visits/hospitalizations/ICU admissions/intubations, medications (i.e., last course of systemic steroids)

h. Social: exposure to cigarette smoke, crowding at home, irritants, etc.

i. Consider alternative diagnoses, including foreign body aspiration, congenital airway malformations, cystic fibrosis (CF), bronchopulmonary dysplasia/chronic lung disease (BPD/CLD), gastroesophageal reflux, congestive heart failure (CHF), and infection

---

✦ PEARL

Red flags for poor prognosis or rapid deterioration include: frequent hospitalizations or prior intensive care unit admission, recent course of systemic steroids or multiple courses in past year, poor inhaler compliance or technique, complex medical history.

---

3. **Physical examination**
   a. Focused physical examination to estimate the functional severity of airway obstruction. Assess the use of accessory muscles, air entry in both lungs, wheezing, length of expiratory phase, level of alertness, ability to speak in full sentences and activity level.
   b. Pulse oximetry should be used in all patients
   c. Examination of the upper respiratory tract including nasal turbinates for allergic rhinitis and nasal polyps, and skin for clubbing and atopic dermatitis

---

❗ PITFALL

Beware of the "silent chest"! Severe asthma exacerbations may have significant airway obstruction or the patient is so fatigued that they are unable to generate enough airflow to wheeze.

---

4. **Investigations**
   a. Blood work, nasopharyngeal swabs, and chest imaging are not recommended for routine management of an acute asthma exacerbation, or for monitoring therapy
   b. Exceptions may include
      - Electrolytes, specifically potassium, in patients receiving frequent salbutamol ($\leq$q1h) for a prolonged period of time ($\geq$6 hours)
      - Blood gas (severe respiratory distress that is not improving with treatment)
      - Nasopharyngeal swab if high suspicion for influenza that meets treatment criteria
      - Chest radiograph: atypical or severe presentations of acute asthma, or inadequate response to treatment

5. **Diagnostic criteria:** see Figure 35.2 for diagnosis in children 1 to 5 years of age, and Table 35.4 for diagnosis in children $\geq$6 years of age

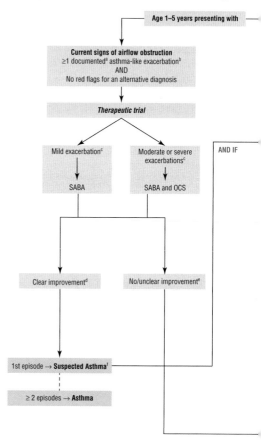

[a]Documentation by a physician or trained health care practitioner. [b]Episodes of wheezing with/without difficulty breathing. [c]Severity of an exacerbation documented by clinical assessment of signs of airflow obstruction, preferably with the addition of objective measures, such as oxygen saturation and respiratory rate, and/or validated score, such as the Pediatric Respiratory Assessment Measure (PRAM) score. [d]Based on marked improvement in signs of airflow obstruction before and after therapy or a reduction of ≥3 point on the PRAM score, recognizing the expected time response to therapy. [e]A conclusive therapeutic trial hinges on adequate dose of asthma medication, adequate inhalation technique, diligent documentation of the signs and/or symptoms, and timely medical reassessment; if these conditions are not met, conside repeating the treatment or therapeutic trial. [f]The diagnosis of asthma is based on recurrent (≥2) episodes of asthma-like exacerbations (documented signs) and/or symptoms. In case of a first occurrence of exacerbation with no previous asthma-like symptoms, the diagnostic of asthma is suspected and can be

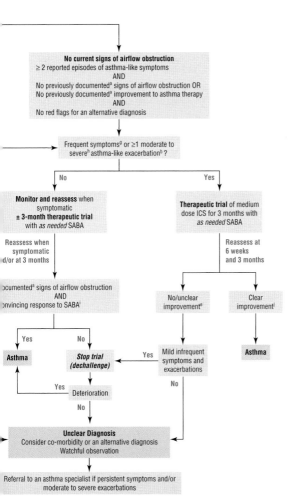

No current signs of airflow obstruction
≥ 2 reported episodes of asthma-like symptoms
AND
No previously documented[a] signs of airflow obstruction OR
No previously documented[a] improvement to asthma therapy
AND
No red flags for an alternative diagnosis

Frequent symptoms[g] or ≥1 moderate to severe[b] asthma-like exacerbation[b] ?

No → **Monitor and reassess** when symptomatic
± 3-month therapeutic trial with *as needed* SABA

Reassess when symptomatic
nd/or at 3 months

Yes → **Therapeutic trial** of medium dose ICS for 3 months with *as needed* SABA

Reassess at 6 weeks and 3 months

ocumented[a] signs of airflow obstruction
AND
onvincing response to SABA[i]

Yes → **Asthma**

No → ***Stop trial (dechallenge)***

No/unclear improvement[e]

Clear improvement[i] → **Asthma**

Mild infrequent symptoms and exacerbations

Yes → ***Stop trial (dechallenge)***

No

Deterioration

Yes → **Asthma**

No

Unclear Diagnosis
Consider co-morbidity or an alternative diagnosis
Watchful observation

Referral to an asthma specialist if persistent symptoms and/or moderate to severe exacerbations

nfirmed with reoccurrence of asthma-like symptoms or exacerbations with response to asthma therapy.
≥8 days/month with asthma-like symptoms. [h]Severe exacerbations require any of the following: systemic
roids, hospitalization; or an emergency department visit. [i]In this age group, the diagnostic accuracy of pa-
ntal report of a short-term response to as-needed SABA may be unreliable because of misperception and/or
ontaneous improvement of another condition. Documentation of airflow obstruction and reversibility
nen symptomatic, by a physician or trained healthcare practitioner, is preferred. [j]Based on 50% fewer mod-
te/severe exacerbations, shorter and milder exacerbations, and fewer, milder symptoms between episodes.
S, Inhaled corticosteroid; *OCS*, oral corticosteroid; *SABA*, short-acting beta agonist. (Modified from
ucharme FM, Dell SD, Radhakrishnan D, et al. Diagnosis and management of asthma in preschoolers: a
nadian Thoracic Society and Canadian Paediatric Society position paper (CPS Position Statement). *Can
spir J*. 2015;22(3):135–143.)

Table 35.4	Pulmonary Function Criteria for the Diagnosis of Asthma in Children ≥6 Years

Preferred: Spirometry showing reversible airway obstruction
Reduced FEV_1/FVC (<0.8–0.9) **AND** increase in FEV_1 ≥12% after a bronchodilator or after course of controller therapy

Alternative: Peak expiratory flow variability
≥20% increase after a bronchodilator or after course of controller therapy

Alternative: Positive challenge test
Methacholine challenge (PC_{20} <4 mg/mL) or exercise challenge (≥10%–15% decrease in FEV_1 post-exercise)

FEV_1, Forced expiratory volume in 1 second; FVC, forced vital capacity; PC_{20}, provocative concentration of methacholine producing a 20% fall in FEV_1.

Data from Lougheed MD, Lemiere C, Ducharme FM, et al. Canadian Thoracic Society 2012 guideline update: diagnosis and management of asthma in preschoolers, children and adults: executive summary. *Can Respir J.* 2012; 19(6):e81–e88.

6. **Management**
   a. See Acute Asthma Exacerbation in Chapter 2 Emergency Medicine for acute management
   b. If an asthma diagnosis is confirmed, see Figure 35.3 for the core components of management in the asthma management continuum
   c. If persistent symptoms and/or moderate/severe exacerbations, the mainstay of treatment is the combination of a reliever (i.e., short-acting beta-agonist [SABA]) as needed, and daily inhaled corticosteroids (ICS)
      i. 12-week trial for patients presenting with their first asthma exacerbation
      ii. Consideration of escalation in ICS dose if on prior ICS therapy
   d. Asthma education—education about inhaler and associated spacer use along with provision of a written "Asthma Action Plan" including daily medications, and plan for worsening symptoms
   e. Regular review of asthma control as outpatient
   f. Referral to asthma specialist if diagnostic uncertainty or suspicion of comorbidity, repeated (≥2) exacerbations requiring oral corticosteroids or admission to hospital despite moderate daily doses of ICS, life-threatening events (i.e., admission to pediatric intensive care unit), high maintenance medication requirements, need for allergy testing to assess the possible role of environmental allergens, and other considerations (i.e., parental anxiety, need for reassurance, and additional education)

Figure 35.3 Asthma Management Continuum

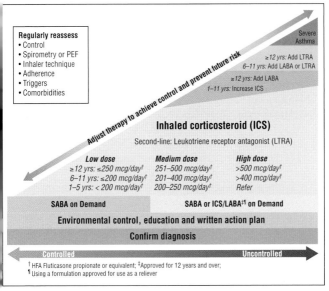

PEF, Peak expiratory flow; ICS, inhaled corticosteroids; SABA, short acting beta-agonists; LABA, long acting beta-agonists; LTRA, leukotriene receptor antagonist. (Modified from Lewis SL, Bucher L, Heitkemper MM, et al. *Medical-Surgical Nursing in Canada: Assessment and Management of Clinical Problems.* 4th Canadian Edition. Elsevier Canada; 2019.)

PNEUMOTHORAX

1. Accumulation of free air in the chest cavity. Etiology can be:
   a. Spontaneous
      i. Primary: occurs in the absence of underlying lung disease. Associated with tall stature, male gender, and genetic connective tissue disorders.
      ii. Secondary: in the presence of underlying lung disease asthma, CF, tuberculosis, and sarcoidosis
   b. Traumatic: secondary to blunt or penetrating trauma
2. **Clinical assessment**
   a. **Symptoms:** sudden-onset dyspnea, pleuritic chest pain, shoulder/back pain, respiratory distress
   b. **Signs:** may differ for nontension versus tension pneumothoraces
      i. Nontension: chest wall movement decreased on affected side, ipsilateral hyperresonance to percussion, decreased breath sounds on auscultation, subcutaneous emphysema
      ii. Tension: contralateral tracheal shift, displaced heart sounds (mediastinal shift), jugular venous distension, tachycardia, hypotension, cyanosis 953

c. **Investigations**
   i. CXR: the primary investigation; may demonstrate an absence of lung markings, radiolucent peripheral space compared with adjacent lung, and visible pleural edge
   ii. Chest computed tomography (CT) may be required to differentiate pneumothorax from blebs or other cystic formations, or to identify underlying lung pathology
   iii. May consider transillumination in neonates

3. **Management**
   a. Management is dependent on severity and suspected etiology
      i. Tension pneumothorax: medical emergency, needle decompression, or chest tube drainage
      ii. Small pneumothoraces (<15% of hemithorax transverse diameter): observation only; resorption may occur more quickly with 100% O_2
      iii. Large pneumothoraces: serial CXR to evaluate progress; chest tube drainage with underwater seal
      iv. Spontaneous, recurrent, or persistent pneumothoraces: surgical referral for possible chemical pleurodesis, open thoracotomy, pleural bleb excision

CYSTIC FIBROSIS

1. **Definition/background**
   a. Multisystem disease secondary to defective CF transmembrane regulator (CFTR) proteins causing abnormal exocrine function, and electrolyte and water transport
   b. Autosomal recessive inheritance with over 2000 known mutations, delta-F508 is the most common mutation

2. **Clinical features**
   a. Classic diagnostic triad (chronic pulmonary disease, pancreatic insufficiency, and increased sweat chloride), but clinical features can vary by age and system
   b. **General:** failure to thrive
   c. **HEENT:** chronic sinusitis, nasal polyps
   d. **Respiratory:** acute/chronic infections, chronic cough/wheezing, bronchiectasis, pneumothorax, decreased lung function
   e. **Gastrointestinal**
      i. Gastrointestinal (GI) tract: neonatal intestinal obstruction (i.e., meconium ileus), distal intestinal obstruction syndrome (DIOS), rectal prolapse, intussusception
      ii. Pancreas: CF-related diabetes (CFRD), pancreatic insufficiency
      iii. Liver: CF-related liver disease (CFRLD)
   f. **Genitourinary:** congenital absence of the vas deferens, hyperviscosity of cervical mucous
   g. **Musculoskeletal:** clubbing, salty skin

3. **Investigations**
   a. **Newborn screening and genetic testing**
      i. Involves specifically measuring the immunoreactive trypsinogen (IRT) level
      ii. If IRT level above cut-off, blood sent for genetic testing, which includes a CFTR mutation panel
      iii. IRT/DNA screening method has sensitivity of approximately 95%
      iv. Whole gene sequencing available if strong clinical suspicion, and known familial defect

> **! PITFALL**
>
> Newborn screening methods can differ among countries and provinces/states. A negative newborn screen does not rule out cystic fibrosis.

   b. **Sweat chloride:** quantitative analysis of sodium chloride content in sweat via pilocarpine iontophoresis
      i. Interpretation: sweat chloride >60 mmol/L diagnostic for CF (98% of CF patients); 30 to 60 mmol/L is borderline (repeat within 2–4 weeks); <30 mmol/L is normal
      ii. False-positive tests: untreated Addison disease, hypothyroidism, ectodermal dysplasia, some glycogen storage diseases, nephrotic syndrome, nephrogenic diabetes insipidus, glucose-6-phosphate dehydrogenase deficiency, evaporation
      iii. False-negative tests: edema of any etiology, malnutrition, overdilution of sample

   c. **Pancreatic insufficiency:** pancreatic insufficiency evaluated with 3 to 5 days fecal fat collection or stool elastase
4. **Management**
   a. Patients with CF are managed in dedicated centers by a multidisciplinary team. See "Age-Specific Care Guidelines" from the *Cystic Fibrosis Foundation* (cff.org) for more details.
   b. **Chronic pulmonary disease:** progressive course punctuated by acute exacerbations
      i. Serial clinical evaluation with PFTs and sputum samples (deep throat swabs for younger children) for microbiology. Organisms may include: *Staphylococcus aureus, Haemophilus influenzae, Pseudomonas aeruginosa, Burkhorderia cepacia,* and *Aspergillus. B. cepacia* generally seen later in life, associated with more severe disease; risk of person-to-person transmission requires avoidance of contact between infected and noninfected patients.
      ii. CFTR modulators may rescue CFTR function and either prevent or improve the organ dysfunction associated with CF. However, these drugs work in a patient-specific manner and require individual management plans.

    iii. Physiotherapy (peak expiratory pressure mask, percussion, and postural drainage) $\pm$ inhaled salbutamol

    iv. DNAse, hypertonic saline to improve secretion clearance

    v. Long-term inhaled antibiotics for those chronically colonized with *P. aeruginosa*

    vi. Nutrition management: pancreatic enzyme replacement therapy with emphasis on high-calorie, high-protein, unrestricted diet and prevention of fat-soluble vitamin deficiency.

c. **Acute pulmonary exacerbations**

    i. Characterized by fever, worsening cough and sputum, shortness of breath, fatigue, hemoptysis, anorexia, weight loss, increased work of breathing, crackles and wheezing on examination, decreased lung function (decreased forced expiratory volume in 1 second [FEV_1] by >10% from baseline)

    ii. Mild exacerbations treated with a 2- to 3-week trial of oral antibiotics based on most recent sputum cultures; close follow-up with repeated PFTs to assess response to therapy

      - First growth of *Pseudomonas species* on culture: attempt to eradicate with 1 year of inhaled antibiotics (tobramycin)

    iii. Moderate to severe exacerbations require hospitalization, IV antibiotics (usually 14 days) appropriate for sputum culture results, inhalational therapy, physiotherapy, supplemental O_2, nutritional support. If little clinical improvement, consider allergic bronchopulmonary aspergillosis (ABPA).

d. **Gastrointestinal disease**

    i. Distal intestinal obstruction syndrome: mineral oil, osmotic laxatives and/or polyethylene glycol with electrolyte solution

    ii. Meconium ileus (see Chapter 17 General Surgery)

    iii. Improved nutrition and stool quality reduces occurrence of rectal prolapse

e. **Pancreatic disease**

    i. Exocrine dysfunction

      - Some 85% of CF patients have pancreatic insufficiency and require pancreatic enzyme replacement, vitamin A, D, E, K supplementation, and a high-energy diet

      - If adequate growth not achieved with optimal pancreatic enzyme therapy, assess compliance, possible CF-related diabetes or poor intake; consider adding inhibitors of gastric acid production to improve enzyme function

    ii. Endocrine dysfunction

      - Begin annual testing for CF-related diabetes with oral glucose tolerance test (OGTT) at 10 years of age

      - May progress to becoming insulin-dependent

Outcomes

a. Current life expectancy >40 years of age

b. Predictors for poor outcome: young age of colonization with mucoid *Pseudomonas; B. cepacia, Mycobacterium abscessus;* CF-related diabetes

c. Treatment for severe advanced lung disease is lung transplant; main criteria for transplantation are FEV_1 <30% predicted, rapid decline in PFTs, and poor quality of life

SLEEP-DISORDERED BREATHING

- Sleep-disordered breathing includes OSA, central hypoventilation syndromes, and disorders of infancy (i.e., apnea of prematurity)
- Central apnea: absence of airflow secondary to absence of respiratory efforts (20 seconds in length or >3 seconds with desaturation or arousal)
- Obstructive apnea: >50% reduction in airflow with paradoxic respiratory effort, associated with desaturation or arousal
- Periodic breathing: >3 central apneas, with <20 seconds between events
- See Table 35.5 for a screening tool to identify sleep problems

Table 35.5	"BEARS" Sleep Screening Tool		
	Toddler/Preschool (2–5 Years)	**School-Aged (6–12 Years)**	**Adolescent (13–18 Years)**
1. **B**edtime problems	Does your child have any problems going to bed? Falling asleep?	Does your child have any problems at bedtime? (P) Do you have any problems going to bed? (C)	Do you have any problems falling asleep at bedtime? (C)
2. **E**xcessive daytime sleepiness	Does your child seem overtired or sleepy a lot during the day? Do they still take naps?	Does your child have difficulty waking in the morning, seem sleepy during the day or take naps? (P) Do you feel tired a lot? (C)	Do you feel sleepy a lot during the day? In school? While driving? (C)
3. **A**wakenings during the night	Does your child wake up a lot at night?	Does your child seem to wake up a lot at night? Any sleepwalking or nightmares? (P) Do you wake up a lot at night? Have trouble getting back to sleep? (C)	Do you wake up a lot at night? Have trouble getting back to sleep? (C)
4. **R**egularity and duration of sleep	Does your child have a regular bedtime and wake time? What are they?	What time does your child go to bed and get up on school days? Weekends? Do you think they are getting enough sleep? (P)	What time do you usually go to bed on school nights? Weekends? How much sleep do you usually get? (C)
5. **S**noring	Does your child snore a lot or have difficult breathing at night?	Does your child have loud or nightly snoring or any breathing difficulties at night? (P)	Does your teenager snore loudly or nightly? (P)

(C), Child-directed question; *(P)*, parent-directed question.

Modified from Owens JA, Dalzell V. Use of the "BEARS" sleep screening tool in a pediatric residents' community clinic: a pilot study. *Sleep Med.* 2005;6(1):63–69.

OBSTRUCTIVE SLEEP APNEA

1. **Predisposing factors:** adenotonsillar hypertrophy, obesity, neuromuscular conditions including muscular dystrophy, anatomic abnormalities including craniofacial abnormalities, genetic conditions (i.e., Down syndrome, Prader-Willi syndrome)

2. **Clinical features**
   a. Nocturnal symptoms of snoring, gasping, increased work of breathing or paradoxical breathing, restless sleep, witnessed apneas or mouth breathing, sleeping with neck in a hyperextended position
   b. Daytime symptoms are nonspecific and can include hyperactivity, difficulty concentrating/learning difficulties, behavioral difficulties, excessive daytime sleepiness, and moodiness

 PEARL

History and physical examination are poorly correlated with obstructive sleep apnea severity.

3. **Investigations**
   a. Overnight pulse oximetry with morning capillary gas may aid in screening, but definitive diagnosis is based on polysomnography
   b. Other investigations may include lateral soft tissue neck x-ray, and/or laryngoscopy
   c. Consider ECHO if long-standing symptoms or concerns for secondary pulmonary hypertension

4. **Management**
   a. Evaluation by ENT with adenotonsillectomy is first-line management for healthy children with OSA and significant adenotonsillar hypertrophy
   b. If significant, persistent OSA despite surgical management, strong preference for nonsurgical approach, or other associated features, consider positive airway pressure therapy (i.e., continuous positive airway pressure [CPAP] or bilevel positive airway pressure [BiPAP])
   c. Trial of nasal steroids, and/or leukotriene modifier therapy (i.e., montelukast) may benefit patients with mild OSA

CENTRAL APNEA AND HYPOVENTILATION SYNDROMES

1. Respiratory insufficiency in sleep with impaired ventilation responses and respiratory drive to hypercapnia and hypoxemia

2. **Etiology**
   a. **Primary:** congenital central hypoventilation syndrome (CCHS), late-onset central hypoventilation syndrome (CHS)
   b. **Secondary:** Arnold-Chiari type II malformations with myelomeningocele (most common), other causes of brainstem injury (i.e., trauma, encephalitis, tumor, central nervous system [CNS] infarct, elevated intracranial pressure [ICP])

3. **Investigations**
   a. Persistent evidence of sleep hypoventilation on polysomnography with $PaCO_2$ >60 mmHg, and absence of cardiac, pulmonary, or neuromuscular causes
   b. Genetic testing may support diagnosis of CCHS
4. **Management:** management of underlying cause, BiPAP, tracheostomy with mechanical ventilation

COUGH

1. Differential diagnosis of acute and chronic cough is outlined in Table 35.6. Duration of chronic cough is >4 weeks.
2. See Box 35.2 for concerning features of cough and Table 35.7 for approach to management

Table 35.6	Differential Diagnosis of Acute and Chronic Cough
Acute Cough (<2 Weeks) and Subacute (2–4 Weeks)	
Respiratory	- Infectious: URTI (e.g., croup), LRTI (e.g., bronchiolitis, pneumonia, pertussis), postinfectious - Inflammatory: asthma
Nonrespiratory	- Allergy - Foreign body aspiration - Malignancy (e.g., tumors, lymphadenopathy) - Habit
Chronic Cough (Duration >4 Weeks)	

Respiratory	- Infectious: TB, non-TB mycobacteria, postinfectious
	- Inflammatory: asthma
	- Interstitial lung disease
	- Anatomical bronchiectasis
	  - CF, PCD, immunodeficiency
	  - Structural/obstructive: tumors, lymphadenopathy

Nonrespiratory	- Medications (e.g., ACE inhibitors) - Cardiac (i.e., pulmonary edema) - Gastroesophageal reflux - Habit

ACE, Angiotensin-converting enzyme; *CF*, cystic fibrosis; *LRTI*, lower respiratory tract infection; *PCD*, primary ciliary dyskinesia; *TB*, tuberculosis; *URTI*, upper respiratory tract infection.

Box 35.2	Concerning Features of Cough

- Systemic symptoms including weight loss, night sweats, recurrent pneumonia
- Sudden onset of coughing or cough after a choking episode (suggestive of foreign body)
- Hemoptysis (can be suggestive of infection including tuberculosis, inhaled foreign body, vascular abnormalities)
- Progressive cough (can be suggestive of inhaled foreign body, an expanding intrathoracic mass, some infections—pertussis, tuberculosis)
- Difficulty feeding
- Concerning features on clinical examination: finger clubbing, barrel-shaped chest, Harrison's sulcus, features of immunodeficiency

Table 35.7	Approach to Chronic Cough in Children <14 Years

1. Is cough present daily for ≥4 weeks?

2. Identify concerning assessment and impact on the child and family

3. Spirometry for patients (>3–6 years of age) and chest x-ray

4. Specific investigations guided by red flags (i.e., pertussis testing, tuberculosis skin test, etc.)
   Refer to pediatric respirologist

5. Nonspecific cough with normal spirometry (if appropriate) and chest x-ray:
   - Consider exposures (i.e., smoke, pollutants), lifestyle management
   - Consider watchful waiting or observation for 2 weeks
   - If persistent, consider an empirical trial of therapy based on presumed diagnosis
     (i.e., inhaled corticosteroids for dry cough or antibiotics for suspected protracted bacterial bronchitis, etc.)
   - Follow-up in 2–4 weeks to assess response, discontinue to confirm/refute presumed diagnosis, and refer to pediatric respirologist if persistent/recurrent

Adapted from Kasi A, Kamerman-Kretzmer R. Cough. *Pediatr Rev.* 2019;40(4):157-167.

WHEEZING

1. Wheeze is a high-pitched sound with expiration that is often accompanied by a prolonged expiratory phase
2. Not all wheeze is asthma and a differential diagnosis is contained in Table 35.8

Table 35.8	Differential Diagnosis of Wheeze

Acute
- Infectious: bronchiolitis, other viral infections
- Inflammatory: asthma
- Foreign body aspiration
- Allergies

Chronic/Recurrent
- Anatomic: tracheomalacia/laryngomalacia, vascular compression/rings, tracheal stenosis/webs, cystic lesions/masses, tumors/lymphadenopathy, mediastinal mass
- Respiratory
  - Inflammatory: asthma
  - Cystic fibrosis
  - Recurrent aspiration
  - Primary ciliary dyskinesia
  - Bronchiolitis obliterans
  - Interstitial lung disease
- Gastrointestinal: gastroesophageal reflux
- Vocal cord dysfunction

HEMOPTYSIS

1. Most hemoptysis is mild and does not require urgent intervention
2. More than 250 mL can require intervention and prompt consideration for embolization and/or surgical intervention
3. Differentiate the source of bleeding; GI tract, upper airway (nose/mouth) versus lung. The differential diagnosis is contained in Table 35.9.
4. Management is dependent on the underlying etiology, and may include topical vasoconstrictors (i.e., epinephrine, vasopressin), selective bronchial intubation, endobronchial tamponade/embolization, or progression to lobectomy/pneumonectomy

Table 35.9	Differential Diagnosis of Hemoptysis

Infectious

- Pneumonia (i.e., bacterial, viral, fungal, parasitic)
- Lung abscess
- Tracheobronchitis
- Immunodeficiency

Trauma

- Aspiration of foreign body
- Contusion
- Iatrogenic (i.e., damage from bronchoscopy)

Bronchiectasis

- Cystic fibrosis
- Primary ciliary dyskinesia
- Post-lower respiratory tract infection

Vasculature

- Pulmonary arteriovenous malformation
- Alveolar hemorrhage syndrome (i.e., associated with renal/rheumatologic disease)
- Connective tissue disease (i.e., Goodpasture syndrome, vasculitis)
- Pulmonary thromboembolism

Neoplasm

- Bronchial adenoma
- Metastatic cancer

Rheumatology

Desmond She • Dilan Dissanayake • Shirley M.L. Tse

ANA	antinuclear antibody
ASA	acetylsalicylic acid
c-ANCA	cytoplasmic antineutrophil cytoplasmic antibody
CREST	calcinosis, Raynaud's, esophageal dysmotility, sclerodactyly, telangiectasia
CRMO	chronic recurrent multifocal osteomyelitis
CRP	C-reactive protein
DIP	distal interphalangeal
ECG	electrocardiogram
GI	gastrointestinal
IBD	inflammatory bowel disease
ILAR	International League of Associations for Rheumatology
IVIG	intravenous immunoglobulin
JDM	juvenile dermatomyositis
JIA	juvenile idiopathic arthritis
KD	Kawasaki disease
MCP	metacarpophalangeal
MCTD	mixed connective tissue disease
MMF	mycophenolate mofetil
NLE	neonatal lupus erythematosus
NSAID	nonsteroidal anti-inflammatory drug
p-ANCA	perinuclear antineutrophil cytoplasmic antibody
PIP	proximal interphalangeal
RF	rheumatoid factor
ROM	range of motion
RNP	ribonucleoprotein
SLE	systemic lupus erythematosus

Rheumatology

36

APPROACH TO THE CHILD WITH RHEUMATOLOGICAL DISEASE

1. **History**
   a. Swelling, pain (quality, night pain, radiation, aggravating/alleviating factors, timing, overlying rash/warmth), gait/movement abnormalities, morning stiffness, weakness
   b. Constitutional symptoms: fever, night pain, weight loss, fatigue
   c. Other symptoms: rash, photosensitivity, hair loss, vision problems, ulcers, gastrointestinal (GI) symptoms, dysuria, Raynaud phenomenon
   d. Impact on activities of daily life, participation, school absenteeism, sleep
   e. Family history: psoriasis, inflammatory bowel disease (IBD), joint/back problems, systemic autoimmune rheumatic disease (systemic lupus erythematosus [SLE], scleroderma, juvenile dermatomyositis

[JDM], rheumatoid arthritis), other autoimmune diseases, consanguinity, recurrent fevers

   f. Exposure: travel, specific exposure to tuberculosis (TB) or Lyme disease, trauma, sexual activity (if applicable)

   g. Treatment(s) and response: medications (pharmacological, nonpharmacological, alternative), physiotherapy

2. **Physical examination**

   a. Pediatric **G**ait **A**rms **L**egs **S**pine musculoskeletal screening exam (pGALS) (Foster HE and Jandial S. pGALS-Paediatric Gait Arms Legs and Spine: a simple examination of the musculoskeletal system. *Pediatr Rheumatol Online J.* 2013;11(1):44.)

   b. Joints: heat, swelling, erythema, active and passive range of motion (ROM), tenderness, deformity

   c. Localized bony tenderness (spine, sacroiliac, entheses [attachment of tendons to bone]), leg length, growth disturbances

   d. Gait: normal walking, walking on heels/toes

   e. Gowers test, muscle bulk, strength

3. **Possible investigations**

   a. Screening for system involvement—complete blood count (CBC) and differential, liver enzymes, creatine kinase (CK), albumin, creatinine, coagulation, urinalysis and urine protein:creatinine ratio, ophthalmological examination

   b. Screening for immune activation: erythrocyte sedimentation rate (ESR), CRP, C3, C4

   c. Autoantibodies (Table 36.1)

   d. Radiology: x-ray, ultrasound (US), magnetic resonance imaging (MRI), computed tomography (CT), bone scan as appropriate

   e. Arthrocentesis (Table 36.2)

Table 36.1	Serological Tests for Rheumatological Diseases	
Test	**Disease Entity**	**Incidence/Comments**
ANA	Nonrheumatological disease	10%–15% positive in healthy children
	Risk factor for uveitis in oligo-JIA	60%–80%
	SLE	Close to 100%, not very specific
	NLE	80%–90%
	Dermatomyositis	50%–75%
	Systemic sclerosis	90%
	Localized scleroderma	50%
	MCTD	100% very high titer
Anti-dsDNA	SLE	60%–90%

Rheumatology

Table 36.1   Serological Tests for Rheumatological Diseases—cont'd

Test	Disease Entity	Incidence/Comments
Anti-Sm(Smith)	SLE	25%–40%
Anti-RNP	SLE, MCTD	Very high titer, suggests MCTD
Anti-Ro/anti-La	SLE, NLE, Sjögren syndrome	Present in asymptomatic mothers of babies with NLE
Anti-Scl-70	Diffuse systemic sclerosis	Marker for severe disease
Anti-centromere	Limited systemic sclerosis (CREST)	Very uncommon in childhood
c-ANCA	Granulomatosis with polyangiitis	Sensitive and specific
p-ANCA	Microscopic polyangiitis	Sensitive
RF	RF-positive poly-JIA	100%
Anticardiolipin	Antiphospholipid antibody syndrome, SLE	IgG isotype most commonly associated with disease manifestations

ANA, Antinuclear antibody; *c-ANCA*, cytoplasmic antineutrophil cytoplasmic antibody; *CREST*, calcinosis, Raynaud's, esophageal dysmotility, sclerodactyly, telangiectasia; *dsDNA*, double-stranded deoxyribonucleic acid; *IgG*, immunoglobulin G; *JIA*, juvenile idiopathic arthritis; *MCTD*, mixed connective tissue disease; *NLE*, neonatal lupus erythematosus; *p-ANCA*, perinuclear antineutrophil cytoplasmic antibody; *RF*, rheumatoid factor; *RNP*, ribonucleoprotein; *SLE*, systemic lupus erythematosus.

Adapted from Laxer RM, Lee Ford-Jones E, Friedman J, Gerstle JT, eds. *The Hospital for Sick Children Atlas of Pediatrics.* Philadelphia, PA: Current Medicine LLC; 2005:450.

Table 36.2   Synovial Fluid Analysis

Measure	Normal	Noninflammatory	Inflammatory	Septic	Hemorrhagic
Clarity	Transparent	Transparent	Translucent-opaque	Opaque	Bloody
Color	Clear	Yellow	Yellow to opalescent	Yellow to green	Red
Viscosity	High	High	Low	Variable	Variable
WBC, per mm³	<200	200–2000	200–100,000	15,000–100,000	200–2000
PMNs, %	<25	<25	~50	~75	50–75
Culture	Negative	Negative	Negative	Often positive	Negative
Total protein, g/L	10–20	10–30	30–50	30–50	40–60
Glucose, mmol/L	Nearly equal to blood	Nearly equal to blood	>1.4, lower than blood	<1.4, much lower than blood	Nearly equal to blood

PMN, Polymorphonuclear cells; *WBC*, white blood cell.

LIMB PAIN

See Table 36.3

Table 36.3 — Differential Diagnosis of Limb Pain

Inflammatory

1. JIA (see Table 36.4)
2. Transient synovitis
3. Sarcoidosis
4. Systemic autoimmune rheumatic diseases (SLE, JDM, Scleroderma, MCTD, Sjögren syndrome)
5. Vasculitides (see Table 36.6)
6. Inflammatory bowel disease
7. Chronic recurrent multifocal osteomyelitis

Noninflammatory

1. Fibromyalgia
2. Reflex sympathetic dystrophy/complex regional pain syndrome
3. Hypermobility syndrome
4. Growing pains
5. Trauma
6. Nutritional deficiencies (rickets, scurvy)

Infectious

1. Primary: bacterial or viral
2. Secondary:
   a. Rheumatic fever: poststreptococcal
   b. Enteric associated: Shigella, Salmonella, Yersinia, Campylobacter
   c. Chlamydia
   d. Viral

Malignant

1. Leukemia
2. Neuroblastoma
3. Lymphoma
4. Primary bone/cartilage tumors

Hematological

1. Hemophilia
2. Sickle cell disease

Orthopedic

1. Legg-Calvé-Perthes disease
2. Osgood-Schlatter disease
3. Slipped capital femoral epiphysis

JDM, Juvenile dermatomyositis; *JIA,* juvenile idiopathic arthritis; *MCTD,* mixed connective tissue disease; *SLE,* systemic lupus erythematosus.

JUVENILE IDIOPATHIC ARTHRITIS

1. **Clinical manifestations**
   a. At least 6 weeks of arthritis with onset <16 years old
   b. Arthritis definition: joint swelling (effusion) OR ≥2 of the following: joint pain/tenderness with palpation or motion, limited ROM, joint warmth
2. **Classification:** see Table 36.4

Table 36.4	Classification of Juvenile Idiopathic Arthritis						
ILAR JIA Subtype	Systemic	Oligoarthritis	Polyarthritis (RF−)	Polyarthritis (RF+)	Enthesitis-Related Arthritis	Psoriatic Arthritis	Undifferentiated
% of patients	10%	33%–56%	11%–28%	2%–7%	3%–11%	2%–11%	11%–21%
Gender differences	F = M	F > M	F > M	F > M	M > F	F > M	—
Age at onset	Throughout childhood	Early childhood	Peaks: 2–4 years and 6–12 years	Late childhood/ early teens	Late childhood/ teens	Peaks: 2–4 years and 9–11 years	—
Joints affected	Poly- or oligo-articular	- ≤4 joints during first 6 months - Persistent: affects ≤4 joints throughout disease course - Extended: affects >4 joints after first 6 months - Large joints	- ≥5 joints in first 6 months - Symmetric - C-spine, TMJ	- ≥5 joints in first 6 months - Symmetric small/large joints - Erosive joint disease	Weight-bearing joints, especially hip	Asymmetric/ symmetric small/ large joints	—
Sacroiliitis	No	No	No	No	Yes	Rare	—
Uveitis	Rare	Common, especially if ANA+, asymptomatic	Yes	Rare	Yes, symptomatic	Yes	—

Other features	Daily fever ≥2 week + ≥1 of: rash, lymphadenopathy, hepatosplenomegaly, serositis	—	—	- Rheumatoid nodules - RF+ twice ≥3 months apart	Enthesitis, inflammatory backpain, family history HLA B27 +, arthritis onset in boys >6 years old	Nail pits, onycholysis, dactylitis, psoriasis, family history psoriasis	- Unknown cause; ≥6 weeks - Does not fulfill criteria for any or fulfills criteria for >1 category
Ultimate morbidity	- 25%–37% have severe destructive joint disease, especially hips, C-spine and TMJ - 50% remit in 1 year - Risk MAS	Ocular damage 40% progress to extended course	10%–15% severe arthritis	>50% severe arthritis	Risk of developing spondylitis in adulthood	Variable	—
RF	Negative	Negative	Negative	100% positive	Negative	Negative	—
ANA	Negative	60%–80% positive	25% positive	75% positive	Negative	Positive	—
HLA-B27	Negative	Negative	Negative	Negative	75% positive	15% positive	—

ANA, Antinuclear antibody; HLA, human leukocyte antigen; ILAR, International League of Associations for Rheumatology; JIA, juvenile idiopathic arthritis; MAS, macrophage activation syndrome; RF, rheumatoid factor; TMJ, temporomandibular joint.

SYSTEMIC LUPUS ERYTHEMATOSUS

1. Autoantibody, immune-complex mediated inflammation of blood vessels and connective tissues with female predominance
2. **Clinical evaluation**
   a. See Table 36.5 for clinical manifestations
   b. Often generalized fever, fatigue, weight loss, and nonspecific organ dysfunction

Table 36.5	Clinical Manifestations of Systemic Lupus Erythematosus
Clinical Domains	
Constitutional	Fever
Hematologic	Leukopenia Thrombocytopenia Autoimmune hemolysis
Neuropsychiatric	Delirium Psychosis Seizure
Mucocutaneous	Non-scarring alopecia Oral ulcers Subacute cutaneous OR discoid lupus Acute cutaneous lupus
Serosal	Pleural or pericardial effusion Acute pericarditis
Musculoskeletal	Joint involvement (arthritis)
Renal	Proteinuria (>0.5 g/24 h) Lupus nephritis on renal biopsy
Immunologic Domains	
Antibodies (required)	ANA ≥ 1:80
Antiphospholipid antibodies	Anti-cardiolipin OR anti-β2GP1 OR lupus anticoagulant
Complement proteins	Low C3 AND/OR low C4
SLE-specific antibodies	Anti-dsDNA OR Anti-Smith

Data from Aringer M, Costenbader K, Daikh D, et al. 2019 European League Against Rheumatism/American College of Rheumatology Classification Criteria for Systemic Lupus Erythematosus. *Arthritis Rheum.* 2019; 71(9):1400.

NEONATAL LUPUS ERYTHEMATOSUS SYNDROME

1. Passive transplacental transfer of maternal autoantibodies to fetus
2. **Clinical manifestations:** heart block, rash (typically annular), thrombocytopenia, hepatitis

Rheumatology

36

3. Investigations
   a. Neonate bloodwork (antinuclear antibody [ANA], anti-Ro and anti-La positive, cytopenias, elevated liver enzymes)
   b. Maternal bloodwork (ANA, anti-Ro, and anti-La)
   c. Electrocardiogram ([ECG], assessing for first-, second-, or third-degree heart block or signs of myocarditis) and if abnormal, echocardiogram indicated

JUVENILE DERMATOMYOSITIS

1. Capillary vasculopathy primarily affecting skin and muscle
2. **Clinical manifestations:** heliotrope rash (violaceous discoloration of upper eyelids), Gottron papules (erythematous, atrophic scaly plaques over metacarpophalangeal/proximal interphalangeal/distal interphalangeal joints and extensor aspects of elbows/knees), proximal muscle weakness, dysphonia (nasal voice), swallowing difficulties, capillary nailfold changes
3. Investigations
   a. Elevated muscle enzymes (i.e., CK, lactate dehydrogenase [LDH], liver enzymes)
   b. Muscle biopsy: perifascicular atrophy, myopathic changes (degeneration/regeneration), perivascular inflammatory infiltrate, vasculopathy, calcinosis
   c. MRI: evidence of muscle inflammation
   d. Electromyogram (rarely used): myocyte membrane irritability

SCLERODERMA

1. Sclerotic skin development and possible internal organ involvement
2. **Clinical manifestations**
   a. Localized – patchy (morphea) or linear fibrotic skin lesion
   b. Systemic
      i. Diffuse: multiorgan sclerosis including upper GI, lung, cardiac, renal; skin involvement (proximal to wrists, ankles, and trunk), anti-Scl 70 autoantibodies
      ii. Limited: CREST, anticentromere autoantibodies

MIXED CONNECTIVE TISSUE DISEASE

1. Overlap of juvenile idiopathic arthritis (JIA), SLE, JDM, scleroderma
2. High-titer ANA (speckled pattern), antibodies to U1-RNP

SJÖGREN SYNDROME

1. Multisystem autoimmune disease with lymphocytic infiltration in exocrine tissues
2. **Clinical manifestations:** dry eyes, dry mouth, parotid swelling
3. **Investigations:** anti-Ro, anti-La antibodies

APPROACH TO CHILDHOOD VASCULITIS

See Table 36.6

Table 36.6	Classification of Primary Childhood Vasculitis	
Vasculitis	**Vessels Affected**	**Characteristics**
Predominantly Large Vessel		
Takayasu arteritis	Muscular and elastic arteries; involvement of aortic arch and primary branches	Granulomatous inflammation, absent pulses, bruits, hypertension, stroke
Predominantly Medium Vessel		
Kawasaki disease	Muscular arteries (especially coronary)	Fever, conjunctivitis, oral mucosal inflammation, cervical lymphadenopathy, rash, extremity changes, coronary artery lesions
Polyarteritis nodosa	Medium and small muscular arteries, and sometimes arterioles	Fever, arthritis, myalgia, abdominal pain, renal disease, hypertension, CNS disease, peripheral neuropathy, skin (nodules, purpura, livedo reticularis, ulcers); when disease limited to skin and joints only: cutaneous polyarteritis
Predominantly Small Vessel, Nongranulomatous		
Henoch-Schönlein purpura	Arterioles and venules, often small arteries and veins	Palpable purpura, subcutaneous edema, abdominal pain, intussusception, GI bleeding, arthritis, glomerulonephritis
Hypersensitivity vasculitis	Arterioles and venules	Fever, urticaria, purpura, arthritis, precipitated by medication or other agent
Microscopic polyarteritis nodosa	Necrotizing vasculitis affecting small vessels	Pulmonary infiltrates or hemorrhage, glomerulonephritis, skin lesions, p-ANCA
Predominantly Small Vessel, Granulomatous		
Wegener granulomatosis	Small arteries and veins, occasionally larger vessels	Sinusitis, pulmonary infiltrates, nodules or hemorrhage, glomerulonephritis, c-ANCA
Churg-Strauss syndrome	Small arteries and veins, often arterioles and venules	Asthma, sinusitis, pulmonary infiltrates, mononeuritis multiplex, eosinophilia
Other Vasculitides		
Behçet syndrome	Small vessels with immune complexes	Oral and genital ulcers, uveitis, skin involvement (erythema nodosum, pseudofolliculitis, papulopustular lesions), pathergy, GI involvement

c-ANCA, Cytoplasmic antineutrophil cytoplasmic antibody; *CNS*, central nervous system; *GI*, gastrointestinal; *p-ANCA*, perinuclear antineutrophil cytoplasmic antibody.

KAWASAKI DISEASE

1. Inflammation of small/medium vessels with predilection for coronary arteries
2. Possibly triggered by viral or bacterial infection

3. **Peak:** 3 to 5 years old; incidence in Asian > Black > Caucasian
4. **Diagnosis**
   a. Complete Kawasaki disease (KD) (Box 36.1)
   b. Incomplete KD (Figure 36.1)
   c. Differential diagnosis (Box 36.2)
5. **Clinical course and management** (Table 36.7)

Box 36.1 Diagnosis of Classic Kawasaki Disease

Fever for at least 5 days, together with at least 4 of the 5 following clinical features:
1. Erythema and cracking of lips, strawberry tongue, and/or erythema of oral and pharyngeal mucosa
2. Bilateral bulbar conjunctival injection without exudate
3. Rash: maculopapular, diffuse erythroderma, or erythema multiforme-like
4. Erythema and edema of the hands and feet in acute phase and/or periungual desquamation in subacute phase
5. Cervical lymphadenopathy (≥1.5 cm diameter), usually unilateral

A careful history may reveal that ≥1 principal clinical features were present during the illness, but resolved by the time of presentation.

Data from McCrindle BW, Rowley AH, Newburger JW, et al. Diagnosis, treatment, and long-term management of Kawasaki disease, a scientific statement for health professionals from the American Heart Association. *Circulation.* 2017;135(17):e927–e999.

Figure 36.1   Incomplete Kawasaki Disease

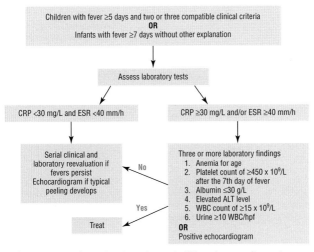

ALT, Alanine aminotransferase; CRP, C-reactive protein; ESR, erythrocyte sedimentation rate; hpf, high-power field; WBC, white blood cell. (From McCrindle BW, Rowley AH, Newburger JW, et al. Diagnosis, treatment, and long-term management of Kawasaki disease, a scientific statement for health professionals from the American Heart Association. *Circulation.* 2017;135:e927–e999.)

Box 36.2   Differential Diagnosis for Kawasaki Disease

- Measles
- Other viral infections (e.g., adenovirus, enterovirus, Epstein-Barr virus)
- Staphylococcal and streptococcal toxin-mediated diseases (e.g., scarlet fever and toxic shock syndrome)
- Drug hypersensitivity reactions, including Stevens-Johnson syndrome
- Systemic onset juvenile idiopathic arthritis
- Bacterial cervical lymphadenitis
- Mercury hypersensitivity reaction (acrodynia)
- Rocky Mountain spotted fever or other rickettsial infections (with epidemiological risk factors)
- Leptospirosis (with epidemiological risk factors)

Data from McCrindle BW, Rowley AH, Newburger JW, et al. Diagnosis, treatment, and long-term management of Kawasaki disease, a scientific statement for health professionals from the American Heart Association. *Circulation.* 2017;135(17):e927–e999.

Table 36.7	Clinical Course and Management of Kawasaki Disease	
	Clinical Course	**Management**
Acute phase	1. From onset until resolution of fever 2. Myocarditis, endocarditis, pericarditis	1. IVIG 2 g/kg (single infusion) and ASA 3–5 mg/kg/day; if persistent fever, consider additional doses of IVIG or corticosteroids 2. Investigations: ECG/echocardiography before discharge; if no coronary aneurysm, discharge on ASA 3–5 mg/kg/day until follow-up echocardiogram 3. Patients may have myocardial dysfunction—be cautious with fluid boluses 4. Reevaluate for hemolysis post-IVIG
Subacute phase	1. From resolution of fever to resolution of clinical signs 2. Associated with rise in platelets, ongoing elevation of ESR/CRP, skin peeling of hands and feet 3. Coronary aneurysm in 20% of untreated cases	1. Continue ASA 3–5 mg/kg/day until platelets normalize or indefinitely if coronary disease
Convalescent phase	1. Until normalization of inflammatory markers 2. Child appears well, but evolution/resolution of coronary artery lesions; resolution of ↑ESR/CRP and thrombocytosis	1. Echocardiography; frequency determined by cardiologist depending on initial echocardiogram finding

ASA, Acetylsalicylic acid; *CRP,* C-reactive protein; *ECG,* electrocardiogram; *ESR,* erythrocyte sedimentation rate; *IVIG,* intravenous immunoglobulin.

HENOCH-SCHÖNLEIN PURPURA

1. Most common form of systemic vasculitis in children. Often follows upper respiratory tract infection (URTI).
2. Occurs between ages 3 and 15 years; peak incidence between 4 and 5 years of age
3. Nephritis develops in ~30%
4. Favorable prognosis with 2% to 5% progressing to chronic renal failure
5. **Clinical manifestations**
   a. Nonrenal features: maculopapular rash progressing to petechiae/palpable purpura, arthritis, edema, intermittent abdominal pain, intussusception
   b. Renal features: microscopic hematuria, proteinuria, acute nephritic syndrome, nephrotic syndrome. Renal manifestations can occur up to 6 months following initial presentation, hence the importance of follow-up.
6. **Management**
   a. Supportive treatment (pain management, fluid supplementation)
   b. Corticosteroids indicated for severe abdominal pain secondary to gut vasculitis/intussusception
7. **Follow-up:** urinalysis and blood pressure monitoring (consider weekly for first month, every 2 weeks for second month, monthly for additional 3 to 6 months, and once at 12 months)
   a. Refer to nephrologist if persistent proteinuria >6 months or nephrotic syndrome
   b. Consider immunosuppressive therapy (high-dose corticosteroids, azathioprine, or cyclophosphamide) in patients with crescentic glomerulonephritis (GN) or significant proteinuria

AUTOINFLAMMATORY SYNDROMES

1. "Periodic fever syndromes"; intermittent episodes of dysregulated inflammation with no obvious autoantibodies or self-reactive T-cells; often excessive interleukin (IL)-1 production
2. Consider when ≥3 episodes of unexplained fever in 6-month period, occurring at least 1 week apart. Patients typically feel well between episodes.
3. **Differential diagnosis:** infection, malignancy, medications, other rheumatological diseases
4. See Table 36.8 for characteristic features and management

Table 36.8	Autoinflammatory Conditions							
					CRYOPYRIN-ASSOCIATED PERIODIC SYNDROMES			
Features	FMF	TRAPS	HIDS	FCAS	MWS	NOMID	PFAPA
Age of onset	<20 years	<20 years	<1 year	<1 year	Often <1 year	Birth or first few months	<5 years
Duration of attack	1–3 days	1–4 weeks	3–7 days	1–3 days	1–3 days to continuous	Hours or continuous	3–6 days
Interval of attacks	Weeks to months	Weeks to months	Weeks to months	Variable; cold-induced	Variable	Days	3–6 weeks
Skin rash	Erysipelas-like	Migratory; may be painful	Maculopapular	Cold-induced; urticarial	Urticarial	Urticarial	No
Adenopathy	No	Not typical	Common; may be generalized	Not typical	Not typical	Not typical	Yes
Oral ulcers	No	No	May occur	No	No	No	Yes
Abdominal pain	Common; peritoneal signs	Common; colicky	Often can be severe with diarrhea	May occur	May occur	May occur	May occur
MSK	Arthralgia; oligoarthritis; myalgia	Localized myalgia; arthralgia; arthritis	Symmetric oligoarthritis of large joints; arthralgia	Arthralgia	Arthralgia; arthritis; clubbing	Arthralgia; osseous overgrowth; clubbing	Arthralgia
Serositis	Peritonitis; pleuritis; pericarditis	Pleuritis; peritonitis	No	No	Pericarditis (uncommon)	Not typical	No

Amyloidosis	60% if untreated	~25% if untreated	Uncommon	May occur	~30% if untreated	May occur	No
Other	Scrotal swelling and pain	Periorbital edema; conjunctivitis; headache; testicular pain	Headache	Conjunctivitis	Conjunctivitis; episcleritis; sensorineural hearing loss	Conjunctivitis; episcleritis; papilledema; chronic meningitis; sensorineural hearing loss	None
Inheritance	AR	AD	AR	AD	AD	AD/de novo	No gene identified
Mutation							
- Chromosome	- 16p13	- 12p13	- 12q24	- 1q44	- 1q44	- 1q44	
- Gene	- *MEFV*	- *TNFRSF1A*	- *MVK*	- *NLRP3*	- *NLRP3*	- *NLRP3*	
- Protein	- Pyrin	- TNF receptor, P55	- Mevalonate kinase	- Cyropyrin	- Cyropyrin	- Cyropyrin	
Treatment	Colchicine; second-line: anakinra, canakinumab	Corticosteroids; etanercept; anti-IL-1 therapy	NSAIDs, corticosteroids; biologics (anti-TNF, anti-IL1)	Anti-IL-1 therapy (anakinra, canakinumab)			Single dose corticosteroid; tonsillectomy; cimetidine

AD, Autosomal dominant; *AR*, autosomal recessive; *FCAS*, familial cold autoinflammatory syndrome; *FMF*, familial Mediterranean fever; *HIDS*, hyperimmunoglobulin D syndrome; *IL*, interleukin; *MSK*, musculoskeletal; *MWS*, Muckle-Wells syndrome; *NOMID*, neonatal onset multisystem inflammatory disease; *NSAIDs*, nonsteroidal anti-inflammatory drugs; *PFAPA*, periodic fever aphthous stomatitis pharyngitis cervical adenitis; *TNF*, tumor necrosis factor; *TRAPS*, tumor necrosis factor receptor-associated periodic syndrome.

Modified from Laxer RM, Cellucci T, eds. *A Resident's Guide to Pediatric Rheumatology.* Rev ed. Toronto, ON: Hospital for Sick Children; 2014.

CHRONIC NONBACTERIAL OSTEOMYELITIS/CHRONIC RECURRENT MULTIFOCAL OSTEOMYELITIS

1. **Clinical manifestations**
   a. Often persistent bone pain ± fever and malaise
   b. Commonly involves clavicles, tibia, femur, tubular bone metaphyses
   c. Must exclude infection, bone malignancy (if only one lesion present), and histiocytosis
   d. Can be associated with IBD, psoriasis, acne, palmoplantar pustulosis
2. **Investigations (imaging)**
   a. X-ray: osteolytic metaphyseal bone lesions close to growth plate, sclerosis, periosteal reaction
   b. Whole body MRI: evaluates disease extent, monitor treatment response

MACROPHAGE ACTIVATION SYNDROME

1. A form of secondary hemophagocytic lymphohistiocytosis (see Chapter 21 Hematology)
2. Children with macrophage activation syndrome resulting from rheumatological disease may not fulfil standard criteria

 PEARL

Certain rheumatology patients are more at risk for MAS (SLE, systemic JIA and KD patients). In patients with persisting fever and falling blood counts, especially in context of rheumatological disease, MAS should be considered.

NONINFLAMMATORY/PAIN AMPLIFICATION SYNDROMES

Pain out of proportion with physical findings

FIBROMYALGIA

1. **Clinical manifestations:** chronic generalized pain syndrome that may be triggered by change in physical activity resulting from injury or chronic illness, as well as poor quality sleep
2. **Diagnosis**
   a. Widespread pain with symptom severity scores in
      i. Fatigue
      ii. Waking unrefreshed
      iii. Cognitive (memory or thought) problems
      iv. General physical symptoms (e.g., headaches, irritable bowel syndrome, anxiety, depression)
   b. Symptoms lasting ≥3 months
   c. Exclusion of other health problem to explain symptoms
3. **Management:** reassurance, simple analgesia, sleep hygiene, aerobic activity (30 minutes/day)

COMPLEX REGIONAL PAIN SYNDROME/REFLEX SYMPATHETIC DYSTROPHY

1. **Clinical manifestations**
   a. Chronic pain often involving peripheral extremity, which persists after inciting event of injury or immobilization
   b. Females > males
   c. Associated with psychosocial/environmental stressors
   d. Severe pain, discoloration, hypersensitivity, autonomic dysfunction (sweaty, shiny, cool skin)
2. **Management:** simple analgesics, physiotherapy, psychosocial supports

HYPERMOBILITY/OVERUSE SYNDROMES

1. **Clinical manifestations:** intermittent arthralgias/joint swelling following activity, tenosynovitis, hypermobile patella, pes planus, shin splints
2. **Diagnosis**
   a. Hypermobility (Beighton's criteria): one point given for each side (L/R): touch thumb to forearm, hyperextension of fingers parallel to forearm, hyperextension of elbows >10 degrees, hyperextension of knees >10 degrees, touch palms to floor with knees straight
   b. Score ≥6 out of 9 consistent with hypermobility
3. **Management:** simple analgesics, physiotherapy, orthotics

GROWING PAINS

1. Poorly localized pains, often lower limbs, occurs at night but never persists until morning
2. Usually between age 4 and 12 years
3. No physical/radiological signs of disability
4. Supportive management (massage, simple analgesia)

PHARMACOLOGICAL MANAGEMENT OF RHEUMATOLOGICAL DISEASE

1. **Chronic arthritis:** NSAIDs, intra-articular steroids; for uncontrolled disease activity, consider second-line agents and biologics used alone or in combination
2. **Systemic autoimmune rheumatic diseases:** systemic steroids, second-line agents, cyclophosphamide; consider biologics in refractory cases
3. See Table 36.9 for details of different pharmacological agents

Table 36.9	Anti-inflammatory/Immunomodulatory Drugs Used in Rheumatology
Drug	**Mode of Action**
First-Line Agents	
NSAIDs	Cyclooxygenase 1 and 2 inhibition, reduces prostaglandin synthesis
Steroids	Decrease activation and proliferation of immune cells, suppresses inflammatory cytokine production
Second-Line Agents	
Methotrexate	Decrease activation and proliferation of immune cells, suppresses inflammatory cytokine production
Cyclophosphamide	Depletes lymphocytes, B and T cells
Cyclosporine	Blocks transcription of T-cell genes
MMF	Inhibits B- and T-cell proliferation
Azathioprine	Inhibits T lymphocytes
Hydroxychloroquine	Inhibits phospholipid function and binds DNA
Sulfasalazine	Anti-inflammatory (5-ASA) and antibacterial (sulfapyridine) properties
Leflunomide	Decrease activation and proliferation of immune cells, suppresses inflammatory cytokine production
Biological Agents	
Anti-TNF: *etanercept (Enbrel), infliximab (Remicade), adalimumab (Humira), golimumab (Simponi), certolizumab (Cimzia)*	Blocks action of TNF (inflammation, T and B-cell signaling, and T-cell proliferation)
Anti-IL-1: *anakinra (Kineret), rilonacept (Arcalyst), canakinumab (Ilaris)*	Blocks the action of IL-1 as a receptor antagonist or antibody against IL-1
Anti-IL-6R *(IL-6 receptor): tocilizumab (Actemra)*	Blocks cell signaling by binding the IL-6 receptor
Anti-CTLA-4: *abatacept (Orencia)*	Blocks costimulation signal CTLA-4 necessary for T-cell activation
Anti-CD20: *rituximab (Rituxan)*	Depletes premature and mature B-cell numbers

5-ASA, 5-Acetylsalicylic acid; *CTLA-4,* cytotoxic T-lymphocyte-associated protein 4; *DNA,* deoxyribonucleic acid; *IL,* interleukin; *MMF,* mycophenolate mofetil; *NSAID,* nonsteroidal anti-inflamatory drug; *TNF,* tumor necrosis factor.

Adapted from Woo P, Laxer RM, Sherry DD. *Pediatric Rheumatology in Clinical Practice.* London, England: Springer-Verlag; 2007:17–18. With kind permission of Springer Science & Business Media.

Technology and Medical Complexity

Suparna Sharma • Maria Marano • Reshma Amin • Sanjay Mahant

COMMON ABBREVIATIONS

Also see page xviii for a list of other abbreviations used throughout this book

BiPAP	bilevel positive airway pressure
CPAP	continuous positive airway pressure
CMC	child with medical complexity
CVAD	central venous access device
CVL	central venous line
CXR	chest x-ray
ENT	ear, nose and throat
G tube	gastrostomy tube
GD	gastroduodenostomy
GJ	gastrojejunostomy
NG	nasogastric
NI	neurological impairment
NIPPV	noninvasive positive pressure ventilation
NJ	nasojejunal
PAP	positive airway pressure
PICC	peripherally inserted central catheter
US	ultrasound

ENTERAL FEEDING TUBES

1. **Tube types** (see Table 37.1 for examples)
   a. **Nasogastric (NG) tube:** nose into stomach
   b. **Nasojejunal (NJ) tube:** nose into jejenum
   c. **Gastrostomy (G) tube:** inserted directly into the stomach with a fluid-filled balloon or a bolster/internal bumper inside the stomach to prevent dislodgement
      i. Non-low-profile (e.g., Corflo PEG G Tube, Kangaroo G Tube) extends further out of the stomach and has a disk on the outside to keep the tube from moving too far into the stomach
      ii. Low-profile (e.g., Mic-Key G Tube) sits close to the skin and is easy to conceal
   d. **Gastrojejunostomy (GJ) tube:** inserted into the jejunum through the stomach. Jejunal feeding can be achieved by inserting an NG feeding tube into the Corflo PEG G Tube under ultrasound guidance and fluoroscopy.
   e. **Jejunostomy tube:** inserted directly into the small intestine
   f. **Combination G/GJ tube:** facilitates venting via G tube while feeding via GJ tube
2. **Indications for tube feeding**
   a. Unsafe, unable, or unwilling to take nutritional, fluid, and medication requirements needed to optimize growth, development, health, and treatment
   b. Inefficient or prolonged oral feeding
   c. NG or NJ feeding tube support >3 months

3. **Decision making:** the decision to insert an enteral feeding tube is significant
   a. Clinical decision points regarding route of enteral nutrition support (Figure 37.1)
   b. Key steps for decision making (Box 37.1)
4. **Insertion:** G, GJ, or J tubes can be inserted by interventional radiology (IR), general surgery, or gastroenterology

Table 37.1	**Examples of Enteral Feeding Tube Types**

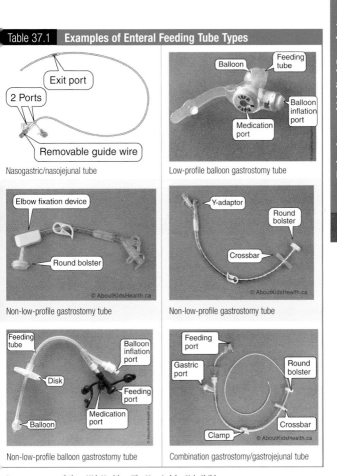

Nasogastric/nasojejunal tube

Low-profile balloon gastrostomy tube

Non-low-profile gastrostomy tube

Non-low-profile gastrostomy tube

Non-low-profile balloon gastrostomy tube

Combination gastrostomy/gastrojejunal tube

Images courtesy of AboutKidsHealth at The Hospital for Sick Children.

Figure 37.1   Algorithm for Selecting the Route of Enteral Nutrition Support

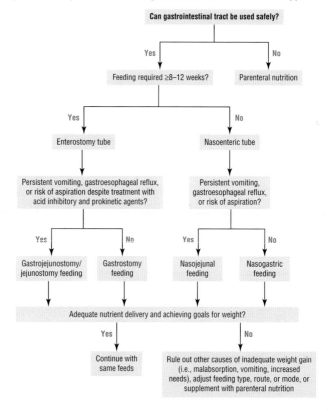

Box 37.1   Steps for Clinicians Toward Enterostomy Tube Decisions

1. Build a decision-making partnership with the family
2. Allow adequate time for repeated discussions and for families to "work through" their decision
3. Clarify the goals of enterostomy tube feeding
4. Be clear about risks and benefits, but frame the intervention in positive terms
5. Elicit family values and preferences
6. Be sensitive to family context, including culture, decision-making styles, financial resources and caregiving support at home. Involve social workers, nurses, and/or dieticians, as appropriate
7. Provide concrete examples of how enterostomy tube feeding or continued oral feeding can impact child and family life
8. Engage extended family members in discussions (when parents wish)
9. Help parents to meet and share experiences with other families who have faced this decision
10. A decision not to start enterostomy tube feeding may be appropriate. Ensure follow-up to reassess.

Adapted from Mahant S, Cohen E, Nelson KE, Rosenbaum P. Decision-making around gastrostomy tube feeding in children with neurologic impairment: engaging effectively with families. *Paediatr Child Health*. 2018;23(3):209–213.

PEARL

Tube feeding does not mean oral feeding cannot occur. Concurrent oral feeds (if safe) ± oral stimulation for development should be encouraged.

5. **Bolus and continuous tube feeding rates**
   a. Bolus/intermittent tube feeding (Table 37.2) generally given via gravity over 20 to 45 minutes as tolerated. In patients with dysmotility, intermittent feeds may be delivered more slowly over 45 to 60 minutes with the use of a feeding pump. Bolus feeds should not be given for postpyloric feeds.
   b. Continuous enteral feeds (Table 37.3) can be given through all types of feeding tubes and may be tolerated by patients who are sensitive to volume, at risk for aspiration, have severe gastroesophageal reflux, or have been on long-term parenteral nutrition and require slow initiation and advancement of feeds. Continuous feeds require a pump to control the feeding rate and are the only acceptable type of feeding for postpyloric feeds.

6. **Complications:** Table 37.4

Table 37.2	Guidelines for Initiating and Advancing Bolus or Intermittent Enteral Tube Feeds		
Patient Weight	**Initial Volume**	**Daily Increases per GI Tolerance (mL every 3–12 h)**	**Goal Volume[a]**
2–15 kg	5–75 mL every 3–4 h (5 mL/kg)	5–30 (5 mL/kg)	50–200 mL every 3–4 h
16–30 kg	15–60 mL every 4 h (5 mL/kg)	15–60	150–350 mL every 4 h
>30 kg	30–60 mL every 4 h	30–60	240–360 mL every 4 h

[a]Increase feeds as tolerated to meet total fluid intake (TFI) and estimated energy requirements and/or return to previous established feeding rate/volume, if appropriate.

GI, Gastrointestinal.

Adapted from The Hospital for Sick Children Guidelines for the Administration of Enteral and Parenteral Nutrition in Paediatrics, 2018.

Table 37.3	Guidelines for Initiating and Advancing Continuous Enteral Tube Feeds		
Patient Weight	**Initial Infusion Rate (mL/h)**	**Daily Increases per GI Tolerance (mL/h every 4–8 h)**	**Goal Rate (mL/h)[a]**
2–15 kg	1–15 (0.5–1 mL/kg/h)	1–15 (0.5–1 mL/kg/h)	15–55 or 6 mL/kg/h
16–30 kg	8–30 (0.5–1 mL/kg/h)	8–15 (0.5–1 mL/kg/h)	45–90 or 4–5 mL/kg/h
30–50 kg	15–25 (0.5 mL/kg/h)	15–25 (0.5 mL/kg/h)	70–130
>50 kg	25	10–25	90–125

[a]Increase feeds as tolerated to meet total fluid intake (TFI); estimated energy requirements and/or return to previous established feeding rate/volume, if appropriate.

GI, Gastrointestinal.

Adapted from The Hospital for Sick Children Guidelines for the Administration of Enteral and Parenteral Nutrition in Paediatrics, 2018.

Table 37.4   Complications Associated With Enteral Tubes

Peritonitis

1. Presentation: fever, irritability, pain, vomiting, peritoneal signs
2. Timing: usually within 1 week of insertion when tract not yet formed
3. Management
   a. NPO and nil by tube
   b. IV fluids and antibiotics (ampicillin, aminoglycoside, metronidazole)
   c. Consultation with interventional radiology or surgery
   d. Urgent tube check

Intussusception

1. Associated with tip of GJ tubes
2. Management
   a. Tube revision (shorter GJ tube)
   b. If severe symptoms: hold feeding ± temporary replacement of GJ with G tube.
      If recurrent: consider alternative options (GD tube, continuous G tube feeding, fundoplication)

G or GJ Migration

1. GJ tubes can migrate retrograde into stomach
2. Presentation
   a. Nonbilious or bilious emesis, vomiting, feeding intolerance, GJ formula feeds coming out of the gastric stoma or port
   b. Feeding tubes's external portion length may be different than usual
3. Investigation: G or GJ tube contrast study (under fluoroscopy)
4. Management: replacement

G or GJ Blockage

1. Etiology: administration of incompatible or inadequately dissolved medication or inadequate flushing
2. Management
   a. See Figure 37.2
   b. If aforementioned measures are unsuccessful:
      i. Tract >8 weeks from original insertion: insert a temporary Foley catheter (see Box 37.2) **OR** replacement low-profile G tube device can be reinserted by a trained caregiver, if available
      ii. Tract <8 weeks old from original insertion: discuss with team who originally inserted

G or GJ Tube Dislodgement

1. Replacement by trained caregiver, if possible, or temporary placement of Foley catheter (see Box 37.2)

Granulation Tissue

1. Description: "cauliflower-like" tissue with clear/cloudy exudates at stoma site
2. Treatment
   a. Frequent hypertonic saline soaks (up to 4 times daily)
   b. Silver nitrate (apply petroleum jelly on the healthy skin around the stoma before silver nitrate application)

G, Gastrostomy; *GJ*, gastrojejunostomy; *IV*, intravenous; *NPO*, nothing by mouth.

Figure 37.2 Blocked Enteral Tube Algorithm

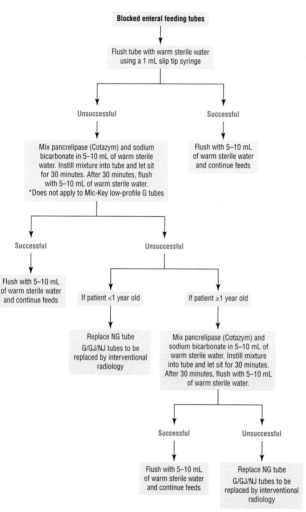

G, Gastrostomy; GJ, gastrojejunostomy; NG, nasogastric; NJ, nasojejunal. (Adapted from The Hospital for Sick Children Policy: Unblocking Enteral Feeding Tubes Using Activated Pancreatic Enzymes, 2017.)

! PITFALL

Medications which can block enteral tubes: clarithromycin suspension, ciprofloxacin suspension, magnesium oxide tablets, kayexalate, levocarnitine tablets, pyridoxine tablets.

Box 37.2   Insertion of Foley Catheter Into Enteral Tube Stoma

1. **When:** As soon as possible to maintain tract patency (e.g., posttube dislodgement)
2. **What:** Use a lubricated Foley catheter one size smaller than the G or GJ tube and secure with tape after insertion
3. **Distance:** Insert 3–4 cm if patient <3 kg or 4–6 cm if patient >3 kg
4. Following dislodgement of GJ or combination type tube, the Foley is to be placed but is NOT to be used for feeds/medication/liquid and the balloon should not be inflated. Make urgent arrangements to replace tube.
5. **Confirmation of position for use (G tube only)**
   a. **If >8 weeks of original insertion:** Confirm position by withdrawing aspirate via syringe visual inspection and check aspirate pH
      i. pH < 6.0: Inflate balloon. If safe for gastric feeding, resume feeds and medications through Foley catheter until new tube is placed. Foley can be used for as long as 1 month.
      ii. pH ≥ 6.0: Inspect aspirate fluid appearance
         - If aspirate fluid appearance appears to be gastric, inflate the balloon, give Pedialyte 5–10 mL/kg or equivalent of one feed and assess patient after 2 h. If patient is stable and tolerates feed, then resume regular feeds and medications through Foley catheter.
         - If aspirate fluid does not appear to be gastric OR if unable to obtain aspirates, confirm position radiologically (fluoroscopically)
   b. **If <8 weeks of original insertion and inserted by IR:** Do not inflate balloon or use tube for nutrition, fluids or medications. Position must be confirmed under fluoroscopic guidance prior to use (increased risk of peritoneal placement when tract is not completely formed).
   c. **If <8 weeks of original insertion and inserted by General Surgery:** Contact surgical team

G, Gastrostomy; *GJ*, gastrojejunostomy; *IR*, interventional radiology.

Adapted from The Hospital for Sick Children Policy: Management and Tube Verification of Dislodged IGT and General Surgery Placed Enteral Feeding Tubes, 2019.

RESPIRATORY TECHNOLOGY

NONINVASIVE POSITIVE AIRWAY PRESSURE

1. Main forms of noninvasive positive airway pressure (PAP)
   a. **Continuous positive airway pressure (CPAP):** delivery of a single level of continuous positive pressure support throughout the respiratory cycle
   b. **Bilevel positive airway pressure (BiPAP):** provides different pressures during inspiration and expiration to augment patient's inspiratory efforts
2. **Indications:** control of breathing abnormalities, musculoskeletal disorders, diseases affecting the upper and/or lower respiratory tract
3. **Contraindications:** hemodynamic instability, pneumothorax, facial trauma or burns, recent craniofacial, neurosurgical, upper airway or gastric surgery, loss of gag or severe bulbar palsy, uncontrolled oral secretions or gastroesophageal reflux disease (GERD), nausea, and vomiting

4. **Precautions**
   a. Fontan physiology: impact on cardiac output and venous return
   b. Risk of aspiration in children with bulbar palsy, significant sialorrhea and/or GERD
5. **Complications and associated ameliorating factors**
   a. Gastric insufflation and worsening of GERD
   b. Pneumothorax
   c. Skin breakdown, especially if use is >16 hours/day—ensure good fit of prongs or mask, use protective skin dressings at interface site, alternate different interfaces to change pressure points, use the minimal effective pressures
   d. Mid-face hypoplasia—use minimum effective pressure, maximize time off therapy as able, use a total face mask
   e. Nosebleeds and nasal congestion—humidification, nasal steroids as needed
   f. Eye irritation—artificial tears as needed, proper mask fit
6. **Considerations for home use**
   a. Ensure patient tolerance of the device before discharge home
   b. Ensure sufficient caregiver training, including cardiopulmonary resuscitation (CPR) training, if clinically indicated
   c. Safe feeding strategy while using PAP therapy
      i. Patients with G tubes receiving noninvasive respiratory support are at high risk of aspiration. G tubes should be vented with initiation of noninvasive positive pressure ventilation and concurrent feeds avoided if possible
   d. Ensure availability of home nursing and oximeters
   e. Address barriers to adherence
      i. Address financial barriers before prescribing therapy
      ii. Avoid uncomfortable or poorly fitting PAP interfaces
      iii. Use minimum effective pressure required to avoid patient discomfort, dryness of oronasal passages, and/or aerophagia
      iv. Provide patient and family education on correct and regular use of device, including how to avoid air leaks and risks of poor adherence to PAP therapy
      v. Ensure follow-up

TRACHEOSTOMY TUBES

1. Inserted into trachea via neck stoma, can be permanent or reversible
2. Indications
   a. Prolonged endotracheal intubation or multiple failed extubations
   b. Structural airway problem (upper airway obstruction)
   c. Pulmonary toileting for secretion management
   d. Need for long-term invasive ventilation at home

3. Tracheostomy tube can have two or three parts
   a. Two-part (most commonly used in children): outer cannula with neck plate (flange) and an obturator
   b. Three part: outer cannula with neck plate (flange), an inner cannula, and an obturator
   c. Tube identifiers: Box 37.3

Box 37.3   Tracheostomy Tube Identifiers

1. Brand, size, and type: located on the right flange
2. Size and length: located on the obturator
   a. Number corresponds to the diameter of the tube (which should match the one found on the right flange)
   b. The letters (NEO or PED) indicate the length of the tube
3. Inner diameter and outer diameter: located on the left flange, in millimeters

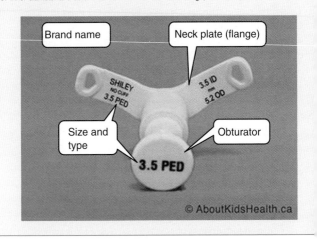

Image courtesy of AboutKidsHealth at The Hospital for Sick Children.

---

4. **Tube types**
   a. *Cuffed*
      i. Balloon gently seals the airway to prevent air or fluid from passing around the tracheostomy tube
      ii. Balloon inflates with water or air (clarify this if changing tube)
      iii. If balloon inflated, child cannot vocalize/speak and if deflated, they can
   b. *Uncuffed*: Air can pass around the tracheostomy tube, vocal cords, mouth, and nose

c. *Fenestrated:* Has holes in the outer cannula, allowing air to pass up through the vocal cords, permitting the child to vocalize/speak
5. Adjuncts that attach to the end of a tracheostomy tube include
   a. **Tracheostomy cap:** covers the opening of the tracheostomy tube, forcing the patient to breathe in and out through their nose and mouth
   b. **Heat and moisture exchanger (HME),** also referred as the *Swedish Nose:* filter-like sponge that provides humidity and moisture when the patient breathes
   c. **Speaking valve,** also referred as the *Passy-Muir Valve:* one-way valve connector that allows air to pass upwards through the vocal cords
   d. **Tracheostomy mask:** device used for administration of cold humidified air or oxygen
   e. **Heated high flow humidifier:** humidification system, allowing air to both be humidified and warmed
   f. **Ventilator:** administers positive pressure ventilation via the tracheostomy
6. **Airway complications and management:** see Figures 37.3 and 37.4

Figure 37.3 Acute Airway Concerns in a Child With Tracheostomy

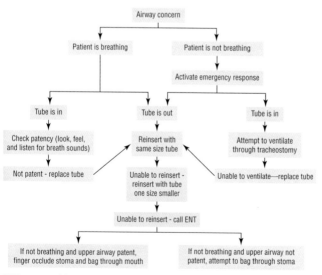

NT, Ear, nose and throat (Otolaryngology). (Modified from The Hospital for Sick Children Guide to Management of Pediatric Medical Emergencies, 2019.)

Figure 37.4 Tracheostomy Management

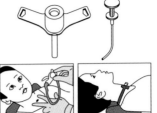

Equipment for tube replacement
- New tracheostomy tubes with ties attached
  - same size and 1 size smaller
- Blunt-nose scissors
- Towel or blanket to roll under child's shoulders
- Resuscitation bag
- Mask
- Tape
- Lubricant (optional)
- Assistant

Replacement procedure in acute setting	Check condition of tube and verify size (ensure you have one smaller size available) Attach ties before putting tube in (if patient stable) Towel under shoulders Insert obturator into new tracheostomy tube Insert by pushing back and down in arching motion Remove obturator immediately while holding tube in place with fingers Assistant fasten ties
Suctioning through tracheostomy	Ensure machine is on and working Suction depth = length of cannula (just beyond the trach tip) Check color and smell of secretions-consider sending for culture Ensure adequate humidity
Indications to consult ENT	Concerns for systemic illness? Tracheitis Significant respiratory distress Active bleeding/pink secretions or sentinel bleed Difficult changing tracheostomy Unable to replace tube Unable to ventilate Fresh tracheostomy site

Pearls

To provide effective bag-mask ventilation ensure stoma is sealed
- Use sterile gauze or gloved finger

Ensure there is adequate humidity
- May cause blocked tube by crusting or mucous plug
- Consider instillation of saline drops prior to suctioning

Ensure ties are not loose
- May cause tube to be pulled out

Pressure ventilator alarms
- High-pressure alarm = check for blocked tube or kinked connectors
- Low-pressure alarm = check ventilator connection and leaks in cuffed tube

ENT, Ear, nose, and throat (Otolaryngology). (Modified from The Hospital for Sick Children Guide to Management of Paediatric Medical Emergencies, 2019.)

7. **Approach to change in secretions**
   a. Ensure adequate hydration/fluid intake
   b. Ensure adequate amount of humidity delivered to the tracheostomy tube
   c. If infection suspected, consider tracheal aspirate, bloodwork, and/or chest x-ray (CXR)
      i. May also initiate antimicrobial therapy (consider history of previous tracheostomy colonization)
   d. If bright red blood secretions, contact Otolaryngology (ENT)

HOME INVASIVE VENTILATION

1. Mechanical device at home that provides total or partial ventilatory support of patient's own breathing via tracheostomy tube
2. Used for the management of long-term chronic respiratory failure when noninvasive ventilation is not an option
3. **Basic requirements**
   a. Access to two trained caregivers able to provide 24-hour care for the patient, 7 days a week (usually includes two family caregivers, as well as homecare nurses)
   b. Adequate housing (access to running water, electricity and heating/cooling, fire extinguishers, smoke detector, and carbon monoxide detector)
4. **Contraindications:** patient/family preference, unstable clinical condition requiring higher level of care than possible at home, unsuitable home environment, lack of adequate number of trained caregivers
5. **Complications**
   a. Disconnection from the ventilator
   b. Tracheostomy tube decannulation
   c. Tracheostomy tube blockage
   d. Infections (e.g., pneumonia, tracheobronchitis)
   e. Tracheostomy tube bleeding
   f. Stomal issues (granulation tissue, infection, false tract)
   g. Caregiver burden (e.g., financial, depression, stress, anxiety, social isolation)

> ✦ **PEARL**
>
> A child receiving home invasive ventilation must have a written emergency plan in case of device failure or acute deterioration that includes ventilator model, baseline ventilator settings and circuit details, size and make/model of tracheostomy tube, contact list of healthcare providers, and locations with access to steady power in case of power failure.

COUGH AUGMENTATION

1. Children with respiratory muscle weakness (e.g., neuromuscular disorders, spinal cord injury, paralysis) and patients with tracheostomy tubes are at risk of impaired cough
2. Consequences of ineffective cough: obstruction of the airways with secretions leading to atelectasis, predisposing to subsequent pneumonia
3. **Mechanical insufflation-exsufflation** (e.g., CoughAssist)
   a. Mechanism of action: positive pressure to inflate the lungs → rapid shift to negative pressure to shear and expectorate secretions → end expiratory pressure to prevent atelectasis
   b. Delivery options: mask, mouthpiece, endotracheal tube, or tracheostomy tube

4. **Indications:** clinical assessment consistent with impaired cough and/or peak cough flow <270 L/min for children ≥12 years of age and/or maximal expiratory pressure <60 cmH$_2$O and/or forced vital capacity <40% predicted (clinical assessment is sufficient if it is not possible to complete diagnostic testing)

5. **Contraindications:** nausea and vomiting, untreated tension pneumothorax, active hemorrhage with hemodynamic instability, C-spine and/or head injury, unrepaired tracheoesophageal fistula, uncontrolled asthma, or bronchospasm

6. **Relative contraindications:** bullous emphysema, recent lung biopsy/lobectomy, severe obstructive lung disease, evidence of increased intracranial pressure, Fontan physiology, nausea, or vomiting

7. **Complications** include pneumothorax/air leak, worsening GERD, transient oxygen desaturations because of V/Q mismatch, chest pain/muscular stretch/discomfort, bronchospasm, cardiac arrhythmias, reduced coronary artery perfusion, or cerebral perfusion

VASCULAR ACCESS

1. **Central venous access devices** include tunneled and nontunneled central venous lines (CVLs), implantable devices (subcutaneous ports), and peripherally inserted central catheters (PICCs)

2. **Indications:** see Box 37.4

Box 37.4 Indications for Central Venous Line Insertion

- Hemodialysis, plasmapheresis
- Total parenteral nutrition
- Chemotherapy, vesicant drugs
- Poor intravenous (IV) access
- IV therapy >2 weeks
- Hyperosmolar infusions
- Frequent blood sampling
- Unstable medical condition requiring inotropic support and/or multiple continuous infusions

---

3. **Complications**
   a. **Infection**
      i. Exit-site skin infection (local discharge/redness at site), tunnel infection (tracking of redness, swelling, tenderness along subcutaneous course), catheter-related bacteremia
      ii. Central-line associated bacteremia or septicemia: treat with vancomycin ± gram negative coverage (consider in immunocompromised

patients/hospital-acquired infection). Urgent line removal indicated in CVL tunnel infections and uncontrolled sepsis.

b. **Occlusion**
   i. See Table 37.5 for degree of occlusion and potential causes
   ii. CXR to check CVL tip location and breakage
   iii. See Figure 37.5 for management algorithm
   iv. Avoid high pressure or excessive force using small syringes (≤5 mL) because line may rupture
   v. PICCs smaller than 3 French cannot be reliably evaluated for patency via blood aspiration because of their small diameters

c. **Thrombosis**
   i. Investigate any patient with clinical symptoms such as head/neck swelling, respiratory distress, bluish color, collateral circulation by objective tests (ultrasound, venography, ventilation perfusion lung scans, computed tomography [CT] scan)
   ii. Lineogram: contrast study of catheter may detect tip clot or fibrin sheath formation
   iii. Venogram or Doppler US of CVL and large vessels near CVL to detect large vessel thrombus
   iv. Management of deep vein thrombosis from CVL: consult thrombosis specialist—begin anticoagulation as indicated or leave CVL in place and attempt systemic thrombolytic therapy if no contraindications

d. **Migration/dislodgement:** CXR and contrast study of catheter (lineogram) to confirm line position

e. **Fracture/breakage**
   i. External breakage: repair kits available (requires experienced personnel)
   ii. Internal breakage: exchange/retrieval (requires experienced personnel)

Table 37.5	Degree of Central Venous Access Device Occlusion and Potential Causes		
Degree or Type of Occlusion	**Ability to Infuse**	**Ability to Aspirate**	**Causes**
Partial	Sluggish flow, resistance with flushing	Resistance	Mechanical, chemical, or thrombotic occlusion
Withdrawal	Yes	No	Mechanical or thrombotic occlusion
Complete	No	No	Mechanical, chemical, or thrombotic occlusion

Adapted from The Hospital for Sick Children Policy: Assessment of Central Venous Access Device (CVAD) Patency and Management of CVAD Occlusions, 2017.

Figure 37.5 Central Venous Access Device Occlusion Algorithm

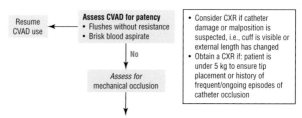

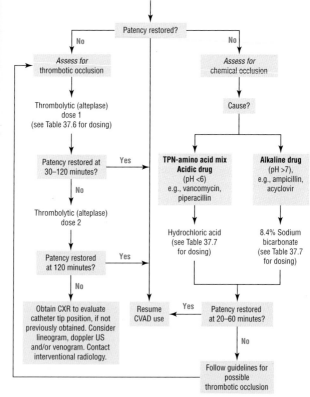

CVAD, Central venous access device; CXR, chest x-ray; TPN, total parenteral nutrition. (Adapted from The Hospital for Sick Children Policy: Assessment of Central Venous Access Device (CVAD) Patency and Management of CVAD Occlusions, 2017.)

Table 37.6	Dose Guidelines for Blood Related Occlusion (Local Installation of Alteplase)	
Type of Catheter	**Size of Patient**	**Alteplase (tPA) (1 mg/mL)**
Single lumen (CVL, PICC)	Any	Use amount required to fill volume of line, to maximum 1 mL = 1 mg
Double lumen (CVL, PICC, percutaneous CVL)	Any	Use amount required to fill volume of line, to maximum 1 mL = 1 mg per lumen. Second lumen may not need to be treated if catheter cleared.
Subcutaneous ports	<5 kg	Use amount required to fill volume of line, to maximum 1 mL = 1 mg per lumen. If double lumen port, treat one lumen at a time. Second lumen may not need to be treated if port cleared
	≥5 kg	Use amount required to fill volume of line, to maximum 2 mL = 2 mg per lumen. If double lumen port, treat one lumen at a time. Second lumen may not need to be treated if port cleared
Hemodialysis catheters	Any	Use amount required to fill volume of line, to maximum 2 mL = 2 mg. Lumen fill volumes are displayed on hemodialysis lines.

CVL, Central venous line; *PICC,* peripherally inserted central catheter.

Adapted from The Hospital for Sick Children eFormulary Antithrombotic Therapy—Blocked Central Venous Lines (CVLs), 2020.

Table 37.7	Dose Guidelines for Chemical Related Occlusion (Local Installation of Hydrochloric Acid or Sodium Bicarbonate)	
Type of Catheter	**Hydrochloric Acid 0.1 M** for Occlusions Caused by an *Acidic* Drug (pH < 6)	**8.4% Sodium Bicarbonate** for Occlusions Caused by an *Alkaline* Drug (pH > 7)
Single lumen (CVL, PICC)	Use amount required to fill volume of line, to maximum 1 mL	
Double lumen (CVL, PICC, percutaneous CVL)	Use amount required to fill volume of line, to maximum 1 mL	
Subcutaneous ports	Use amount required to fill volume of line, to maximum 2 mL	
Hemodialysis catheters (nephrology patients only, use double lumen guidelines for non-nephrology patients)	Use amount required to fill volume of line, to a maximum of 2 mL. Lumen fill volumes are displayed on hemodialysis lines	

CVL, Central venous line; *PICC,* peripherally inserted central catheter.

Adapted from The Hospital for Sick Children eFormulary Antithrombotic Therapy—Blocked Central Venous Lines (CVLs), 2020.

1. A child with medical complexity (CMC) has the following characteristics:
   a. Experiences chronic conditions which are often multiple, severe, and associated with medical fragility
   b. Functional limitations often associated with technological dependence (e.g., suctioning, tracheostomy, oxygen, tube feeding)
   c. Significant healthcare use, including multiple providers and hospital admissions
   d. Associated with significant additional need, for example, family caregiving
2. CMC experience more frequent intensive care unit (ICU) admissions, longer hospitalizations and more frequent medical error. Their care needs vary over time.
3. Coordinated programs delivering care can improve health outcomes of CMC
4. CMC have a diverse range of conditions, for example, cystic fibrosis, complex congenital heart disease. This section focuses on CMC with neurological impairment.

NUTRITION

1. Nutrition in CMC is important; when inadequate can contribute to dehydration, malnutrition, and respiratory infections (aspiration from above if unsafe to feed orally, secretions, or GERD)
2. Eating and mealtimes are more than just nutrition; they are important aspects of family life reflecting culture and communication and are integral for communication, socialization, and sensory exploration
3. See Box 37.5 for components of nutrition and feeding assessment in CMC
   a. Consider energy and growth requirements (see Chapter 19 Growth and Nutrition)
4. Children with neurological impairment can experience poor oral health (Box 37.6), ensure dental follow-up

Box 37.5 Components of a Nutrition and Feeding Assessment in the Child With Medical Complexity

1. **History**
   a. **General well-being**—history of aspiration, recurrent respiratory infections, GERD, recurrent fevers, food refusal, unexplained weight loss, potential losses (vomiting, diarrhea, drooling), constipation, oral health (see Box 37.6)
   b. **Medication and side effects**—influence taste, level of consciousness, GI motility
   c. **Dietary assessment**
      i. Detailed assessment of what the child is receiving and potential losses (vomiting, diarrhea, drooling, sweating)
      ii. Food diary documenting intake. Actual intake is frequently underreported. Consider 24-h recall or record over 3 days
      iii. Micronutrient intake
   d. **Feeding history**
      i. Time taken to feed (frequently underestimated, greater concern if time taken to complete feeds is >3 h/day)
      ii. Coughing or choking during feeding
      iii. Increased work of breathing during feeding
      iv. Behavior around feeding, e.g., interest in feed, refusing feeds
      v. Eating and drinking ability classification system (see Table 12.4 in Chapter 12 Development)
   e. **Development history**
      i. Current developmental skills including feeding skills
      ii. Activity level—many children with neurological impairment have decreased energy needs compared with healthy children
   f. **Parent and child goals**
      i. Eating and mealtimes are complex social interactions and understanding the family's current perceptions of feeding and their goals for this child and around feeding is important in planning care
2. **Physical examination** (in addition to general physical examination)
   a. Anthropometrics and centiles
3. **Investigations**
   a. **Clinical assessment** (often performed by occupational therapist or speech and language pathologist)
      i. Assessment of feeding at bedside, including observation with different food and liquid consistencies, time taken to feed, and behavior around feeding
      ii. Identification of clinical signs of impaired swallowing include coughing/choking with oral feeds, change in voice quality during oral feeds, poor secretion management, sudden, significant drop in oxygen saturation and or heart rate with oral feeds
   b. **Radiology assessment** (e.g., video fluoroscopic feeding study)
      i. Indicated if concerns identified on clinical assessment—evaluates swallow function and aspiration, and guides treatment

GERD, Gastroesophageal reflux disease; *GI*, gastrointestinal.

> **Box 37.6** Influencers on Oral Health in the Child With Medical Complexity
>
> - Prolonged bottle/sippy cup use
> - Extended eating times
> - Low fluid intake
> - Gastroesophageal reflux disease
> - Sensory issues
> - Inability or refusal to consume specific foods needed for dental mineralization
> - Limited or inconsistent dental hygiene

RESPIRATORY ISSUES

1. Sialorrhea: see www.aacpdm.org/publications/care-pathways/sialorrhea-in-cerebral-palsy for sialorrhea care pathway
2. Aspiration
   a. Aspiration is penetration of material into the lower airways
   b. Aspiration can occur
      i. From **above**
         - Aspiration of oral secretions
         - Aspiration of oral feeds: perform a nutrition and feeding assessment if CMC presents with a change in respiratory status (see Box 37.5)
      ii. From **below**
         - Aspiration of gastric contacts: see Gastroesophageal Reflux in Chapter 16 Gastroenterology and Hepatology and Figure 37.1 to determine if any changes to feeding route should be considered
   c. Aspiration pneumonia
      i. Common cause of hospitalization in CMC
      ii. Can present with or without clear history of aspiration
      iii. Treatment: see Chapter 24 Infectious Diseases

MUSCULOSKELETAL ISSUES

1. See www.aacpdm.org/publications/care-pathways/hip-surveillance-in-cerebral-palsy for hip surveillance care pathway
2. See www.aacpdm.org/publications/care-pathways/osteoporosis-in-cerebral-palsy for bone health care pathway

NEUROLOGIC ISSUES

1. See www.aacpdm.org/publications/care-pathways/dystonia-in-cerebral-palsy for dystonia care pathway

Transplantation

Lucy Duan • Jessica Woolfson • Krista Van Roestel • Vicky Ng

COMMON ABBREVIATIONS

Also see page xviii for a list of other abbreviations used throughout this book

ACR	acute cellular rejection
AMR	antibody-mediated rejection
AZA	azathioprine
CMV	cytomegalovirus
CNI	calcineurin inhibitor
GFR	glomerular filtration rate
HHV6	human herpesvirus 6
HSV	herpes simplex virus
HUS	hemolytic uremic syndrome
IS	immunosuppression
IVIG	intravenous immunoglobulin
MMF	mycophenolate mofetil
NEC	necrotizing enterocolitis
PCR	polymerase chain reaction
PFTs	pulmonary function testing
PJP	*Pneumocystis jirovecii* pneumonia
PTLD	post-transplant lymphoproliferative disease
QOL	quality of life
RSV	respiratory syncytial virus
SOT	solid organ transplant
TDM	therapeutic drug monitoring
TMP/SMX	trimethoprim-sulfamethoxazole
VZV	varicella-zoster virus

PEDIATRIC SOLID ORGAN TRANSPLANTATION

1. **Indications:** see Table 38.1
2. **Survival:** depends on organ and indication
   a. Highest rates for living donor renal transplants
   b. Lowest survival rates for lung transplant

Table 38.1	Common Indications for Pediatric Solid Organ Transplantation
Kidney	End-stage renal disease, due to - Congenital anomalies of the kidney and urinary tract - Focal segmental glomerulosclerosis - Glomerulonephritis
Liver	Biliary atresia and other cholestatic conditions
	Metabolic disease
	Fulminant hepatic failure
	Hepatoblastoma
	Others, e.g., autoimmune

Table 38.1	Common Indications for Pediatric Solid Organ Transplantation—cont'd
Heart	Congenital heart disease with no acceptable surgical option
	Cardiomyopathy with end-stage heart failure
	Myocarditis
	Malignant arrhythmias
Lung	End-stage lung disease, due to
	- Primary pulmonary hypertension
	- Cystic fibrosis
	- Pulmonary fibrosis
	- Bronchiectasis
Intestine	Intestinal failure, due to
	- Short-bowel syndrome (congenital or acquired)
	- Necrotizing enterocolitis
	- Defective intestinal motility

IMMUNOSUPPRESSION

1. **Immunosuppression (IS) medications:** see Table 38.2 for details

! PITFALL

Many medications (and foods) interact with immunosuppressive medications, causing drug levels to be high or low. Consult with a pharmacist or check for drug interactions before prescribing medications to a patient on immunosuppression post-transplant.

Table 38.2	Immunosuppressive Drugs		
Agent	**Interactions**	**Side Effects**	**Comments**
Corticosteroids	Increased bioavailability with hypoalbuminemia, liver disease	Hypertension, hyperglycemia, weight gain, growth retardation, cushingoid habitus, peptic ulceration, pancreatitis, psychosis, osteoporosis, delayed wound healing, cataracts	Stress dosing of corticosteroids required during acute illness or surgery (see section on Adrenal Insufficiency in Chapter 14 Endocrinology)
Tacrolimus (CNI)	Trough levels - Decreased by steroids, isoniazid, carbamazepine, phenobarbital, phenytoin - Increased by cyclosporine, fluconazole, erythromycin, doxycycline, calcium channel blockers, grapefruit juice	Nephrotoxicity, hypertension, post-transplant diabetes mellitus, hyperlipidemia, hyperkalemia, hypomagnesemia, seizures, tremors, HUS, pure red cell aplasia	TDM required

Continued 1003

Table 38.2	Immunosuppressive Drugs—cont'd		
Agent	**Interactions**	**Side Effects**	**Comments**
Azathioprine (AZA)		Bone marrow suppression, hepatotoxicity, pancreatitis, neoplasia	Consider monitoring CBC
Mycophenolate mofetil (MMF)		GI symptoms (mainly diarrhea), neutropenia, anemia, hepatotoxicity, nephrotoxicity, cough	TDM available; use varies by organ and institutional practice
Cyclosporine (CNI)	Trough levels - Decreased by carbamazepine, phenytoin, phenobarbital, rifampin - Increased by erythromycin, calcium channel blockers, grapefruit juice	Nephrotoxicity, hepatotoxicity, diabetes mellitus, hyperkalemia, hypertension, hirsutism, gingival hyperplasia, headache, seizures, tremors	TDM required (trough and/or 2 h post-dose level)
Sirolimus		Hyperlipidemia, nephrotoxicity, mouth ulcers, delayed wound healing, delayed graft function, pneumonitis, interstitial lung disease	TDM, lipid monitoring required; baseline PFTs recommended
Basiliximab		Hypersensitivity reactions, inflammatory rashes, neutropenia, hepatotoxicity	May have utility in patients with renal impairment
Polyclonal antithymocyte globulin (thymoglobulin)		Cytokine-release syndrome (fever, chills, hypotension), pulmonary edema, serum sickness, cytopenias	

CBC, Complete blood count; *CNI*, calcineurin inhibitor; *GI*, gastrointestinal; *HUS*, hemolytic uremic syndrome; *PFTs*, pulmonary function tests; *TDM*, therapeutic drug monitoring.

POST-TRANSPLANT COMPLICATIONS

REJECTION
1. **Risk factors**
   a. Longer time from transplantation
   b. Poor adherence to IS regime
   c. Intercurrent viral illness, e.g., CMV
2. See Table 38.3 for details of organ-specific transplant rejection

 PEARL

Live vaccines are contraindicated in post-transplant patients on immunosuppression. Killed vaccines, including seasonal influenza, are safe to give. The transplant team will arrange an accelerated immunization schedule pre-transplant.

Table 38.3

Rejection in Solid Organ Transplantation

	Kidney	Liver	Heart	Lung
Clinical	Usually asymptomatic	Usually asymptomatic	Usually asymptomatic	May be asymptomatic
	Fever, malaise, oliguria, hypertension, graft tenderness	May have unexplained fever in early post-operative period	Irritability, low-grade fever	Low-grade fever, fatigue, shortness of breath, non-productive cough
			Arrhythmia, left ventricular dysfunction	
			Gastrointestinal symptoms	
Investigations	Elevated serum creatinine	Significantly elevated AST, ALT ± rise in GGT, bilirubin	Anti-HLA antibodies if suspicious of AMR	CXR: may have perihilar infiltrates, interstitial edema, pleural effusions
			ECG	
			Echocardiogram: effusion, wall thickening, decreased function	PFTs: decreased forced expiratory volume, forced vital capacity
Diagnosis	Renal biopsy	Liver biopsy	Endomyocardial biopsy	Bronchoscopy with bronchoalveolar lavage and transbronchial biopsy
Treatment (based on type and severity)	Steroids, augmented IS regimen, antibody therapies, i.e., thymoglobulin	Most episodes responsive to pulse steroids	Steroids, augmented IS regimen, antibody-directed therapies for AMR	Most episodes resolve with medical therapy, i.e., pulse steroids, augmented IS regimen
		Refractory or recurrent rejection treated with antilymphocyte therapy, i.e., thymoglobulin or basiliximab		

AMR, Antibody-mediated rejection; *ALT*, alanine aminotransferase; *AST*, aspartate aminotransferase; *CXR*, chest x-ray; *ECG*, electrocardiogram; *GGT*, gamma-glutamyl transferase; *HLA*, human leukocyte antigen; *IS*, immunosuppression; *PFTs*, pulmonary function tests.

Transplantation

38

INFECTION

1. IS to prevent graft rejection increases susceptibility to infection, particularly opportunistic infections (see section on Immunocompromised Patients in Chapter 24 Infectious Diseases)
2. See Tables 38.4 to 38.6 for breakdown by infection, timing, and organ
3. Splenectomized and/or functionally asplenic recipients should be immunized with pneumococcal vaccine and receive appropriate prophylaxis (see section on Asplenic Patients in Chapter 23 Immunoprophylaxis)
4. **Vaccination:** pre- and post-transplant protocols available on the SickKids Transplant and Regenerative Medicine Centre website: http://www.sickkids.ca/TRMC/HCP/Resources/index.html

Table 38.4	Infectious Complications Categorized by Infection Type		
Infection	**Clinical Features**	**Prophylaxis**	**Treatment**
EBV	Spectrum from infectious mononucleosis to PTLD	Dependent on organ, presence of donor-recipient mismatch Options: ganciclovir, valganciclovir	Depends on severity, organ type and timing Options: ganciclovir, valganciclovir and/or CMV hyperimmune globulin, reduce IS
CMV	Spectrum from infectious mononucleosis-like syndrome to pneumonia, colitis, retinitis	As with EBV	As with EBV
Candida species	Spectrum from mucocutaneous to disseminated disease Oral candidiasis most common	Oral nystatin Duration varies by organ - Kidney: 3 months post-operatively - Liver/heart: until maintenance steroids discontinued - Lung: indefinitely	Oral: nystatin, fluconazole Cutaneous: topical nystatin, clotrimazole More significant disease: amphotericin, fluconazole
PJP (previously *Pneumocystis carinii* or PCP)	Fever, non-productive cough, tachypnea, dyspnea, hypoxia, respiratory failure	TMP/SMX Duration varies by organ - Kidney/heart: 6 months - Liver: 1 year - Lung: indefinitely	TMP/SMX is drug of choice Can also use pentamidine, corticosteroids (moderate-severe disease)

Table 38.4	Infectious Complications Categorized by Infection Type—cont'd		
Infection	Clinical Features	Prophylaxis	Treatment
Polyomaviruses (BK and JC virus)	Most frequent in renal and bone marrow transplant recipients Kidney: renal dysfunction; occasionally present with hemorrhagic or non-hemorrhagic cystitis Heart: can present with sudden deterioration in renal function	No prophylaxis	Reduce IS Options for therapy include cidofovir, leflunomide, IVIG
RSV	Bronchiolitis, pneumonia, exacerbation of underlying chronic lung condition	Palivizumab or RSV immunoglobulin recommended in infants <24 months with hemodynamically significant congenital heart disease at the start of RSV season (see section on RSV in Chapter 23 Immunoprophylaxis)	Supportive measures Decision to use ribavirin based on individual case

CMV, Cytomegalovirus; *EBV*, Epstein-Barr virus; *IS*, immunosuppression; *IVIG*, intravenous immunoglobulin; *PJP*, Pneumocystis jirovecii pneumonia; *PTLD*, post-transplant lymphoproliferative disease; *RSV*, respiratory syncytial virus; *TMP/SMX*, trimethoprim-sulfamethoxazole.

Table 38.5	Infectious Complications Categorized by Post-Operative Timing			
Timing	Viral	Bacterial	Fungal	Opportunistic
Early (<1 month)	HSV, RSV, influenza, parainfluenza	Surgical site infections, pneumonia, UTI, bacteremia (from indwelling catheter)	Candidal wound infections	
Intermediate (1–6 months)	CMV, EBV, adenovirus, VZV, HSV, HHV6, Hepatitis B, C	Pneumococcal	*Candida, Aspergillus* (lung transplant)	*Pneumocystis, Listeria, Cryptococcus, Nocardia, Toxoplasma, Mycobacterium*
Late (after 6 months)	Community-acquired respiratory viruses			*Pneumocystis, Listeria, Cryptococcus, Nocardia*

CMV, Cytomegalovirus; *EBV*, Epstein-Barr virus; *HHV6*, human herpesvirus 6; *HSV*, herpes simplex virus; *RSV*, respiratory syncytial virus; *UTI*, urinary tract infection, *VZV*, varicella zoster virus.

Table 38.6	Infectious Complications Categorized by Organ Transplanted	
Transplant	**Most Common Infections**	**Others**
Kidney	UTI Wound site infection Pneumonia	Polyomaviruses (BK and JC virus) can cause nephropathy, resulting in renal dysfunction; 50% risk of allograft loss
Liver	Bacterial cholangitis from biliary reconstruction Bacteremia from vascular anastomosis/central catheters	
Heart	Invasive pneumococcal disease Pneumonia Bacteremia UTI Sternotomy site infection	*Toxoplasma gondii* can be transmitted in allograft due to latency in cardiac muscle
Lung	Pneumonia (major cause of morbidity and mortality, particularly in first 90 days post-operatively) *Pseudomonas aeruginosa* and *Burkholderia cepacia* (patients with cystic fibrosis) Respiratory viruses Atypical *Mycobacteria*	Resistant bacteria Ubiquitous molds, e.g., *Aspergillus*

UTI, Urinary tract infection.

 PEARL

Transplant recipients are at increased risk of developing post-transplant lymphoproliferative disease and de novo malignancies

POST-TRANSPLANT LYMPHOPROLIFERATIVE DISEASE

1. **Heterogeneous spectrum of diseases:** reactive polyclonal lymphoid hyperplasia to monoclonal malignant lymphoma
2. **Etiology:** abnormal lymphocyte proliferation, often driven by EBV
3. **Risk factors:** type of transplant, younger age, IS regimen, EBV infection, EBV seropositive organ transplanted into seronegative recipient
4. **Presentation**
   a. **Systemic:** fever, night sweats, weight loss
   b. **Gastrointestinal:** diarrhea, GI bleeding
   c. **Respiratory:** upper respiratory tract infection with lymphadenopathy unresolved after a course of antibiotics, sinusitis, tonsillitis, tonsillar hypertrophy/snoring
   d. **CNS:** persistent headaches, neurologic symptoms

5. **Clues on investigation:** iron deficiency anemia, atypical lymphocytosis, cytopenias, hypoalbuminemia
6. **Diagnosis:** histopathology (gold standard)
7. **Treatment:** withdrawal or reduction of IS therapy $\pm$ antiviral drugs or chemotherapy

> **! PITFALL**
>
> Immunosuppressive medications have side effects on many organs, particularly nephrotoxicity, and therefore require regular monitoring

NEPHROTOXICITY

1. Chronic calcineurin inhibitor (CNI) use can lead to renal insufficiency; serial therapeutic drug monitoring (TDM) is required to maintain desired or targeted trough levels
2. **Need to manage:** elevated BP, decreasing GFR, chronic hyperkalemia and hypomagnesemia
3. **Post-transplant hypertension:** common in solid organ transplant (SOT) recipients, often caused by medications, especially steroids and CNIs
4. **Acute renal insufficiency:** SOT recipients are more vulnerable, particularly in setting of intravascular volume depletion
5. **Chronic kidney disease:** SOT recipients often have some degree (GFR <90 mL/min/1.73 m^2)
   a. Best method to determine renal function is by nuclear medicine (measured GFR)
   b. Recommend periodic screening for proteinuria
   c. If dipstick positive ($\geq 1+$), quantify with spot urine protein:creatinine and albumin:creatinine ratios (see section on Proteinuria in Chapter 28 Nephrology and Urology)
6. **Nephrotoxic medications:** use with caution or avoid if possible; require TDM, e.g., aminoglycosides

GROWTH DELAY

1. Often seen pre-transplant, as consequence of chronic illness, frequent hospitalizations, drug therapy (e.g., steroids)
2. **Nutritional prehabilitation:** aggressive pre-transplant enteral and/or parenteral nutritional therapy; may ameliorate growth failure and improve post-transplant outcomes
3. After transplant, many recipients experience significant catch-up growth
4. Human growth hormone has been used in kidney, liver, and heart transplant recipients to improve height to good effect

APPROACH TO COMMON POST-TRANSPLANT PROBLEMS

1. **Organ-specific issues:** see Table 38.7

Table 38.7	Post-transplant Organ-Specific Problems		
	Kidney	**Liver**	**All SOT**
Problem	Increased serum creatinine	Increased serum liver enzymes/bilirubin levels	Increased serum creatinine
Differential diagnosis	Rejection	Rejection	Hypovolemia
	CNI toxicity	Vascular complication	CNI toxicity
	Other drug toxicity	Biliary complication	Other drug toxicity
	UTI	ACR	BK nephropathy
	Hypovolemia	Infection	
	BK nephropathy	Drug toxicity	
	GU obstruction	Autoimmune hepatitis	
	Vascular complication	Recurrent disease	
	Recurrent disease		
Workup	All require a thorough history, including medication review, and physical examination		
	Na, K, Ca, Mg, PO$_4$, urea, creatinine, TDM	AST, ALT, ALP, GGT, bilirubin (conjugated and unconjugated), albumin, protein, CBC with differential, INR, PTT, IgG, autoantibodies, TDM	Na, K, Ca, Mg, PO$_4$, urea, creatinine, TDM
	Urinalysis and culture		Urinalysis
	Renal US (rule out obstruction and vascular complication)	US and Doppler study of liver	
	Consider graft biopsy if no improvement with treatment	Consider liver biopsy if no improvement with treatment	
Management	IV fluids	± Hold/decrease dose of medication causing toxicity	Trial of IV fluid
	Correct electrolyte abnormalities		Correct electrolyte abnormalities
	± Hold/decrease dose of medication causing toxicity		± Hold/decrease dose of medication causing toxicity
	± Antibiotics for UTI		

ACR, Acute cellular rejection; *ALP,* alkaline phosphatase; *ALT,* alanine aminotransferase; *AST,* aspartate aminotransferase; *CBC,* complete blood count; *CNI,* calcineurin inhibitor; *GGT,* gamma-glutamyl transferase; *GU,* genitourinary; *IgG,* immunoglobulin G; *INR,* international normalized ratio; *IV,* intravenous; *PTT,* partial thromboplastin time; *SOT,* solid organ transplant; *TDM,* therapeutic drug monitoring; *US,* ultrasound; *UTI,* urinary tract infection.

 PEARL

Always consider infection in a post-transplant patient with fever—have a low threshold to investigate and start empiric treatment

FEVER

1. **Definition:** single temperature reading >38.5°C or two readings 38°C to 38.5°C, 1 hour apart
2. **Assessment:** detailed history and physical examination
   a. Assess for risk factors for infection
      i. In-dwelling catheters, e.g., central venous line, peripherally inserted central catheter, drains
      ii. Previous splenectomy or functional asplenia (polyslenia or asplenia)
      iii. Opportunistic organisms
3. **Investigations:** tailor to clinical scenario
   a. CBC and differential
   b. Blood and urine cultures
   c. Viral PCRs: EBV, CMV, HSV 1 and 2
   d. Nasopharyngeal swab for respiratory viruses
   e. Chest x-ray for pulmonary infiltrates
   f. Stool for culture, virology, ova and parasites
   g. Scraping of lesions for electron microscopy
4. **Treatment:** see Chapter 24 Infectious Diseases for empiric antibiotic regimens

VOMITING AND DIARRHEA

1. **Advise to seek medical attention if**
   a. Vomiting and diarrhea persisting for >1 day, particularly in younger patients
   b. Interfering with medication administration
   c. Leading to dehydration
2. **Investigations:** as appropriate
   a. Electrolytes, urea, and creatinine if dehydrated, particularly if taking CNI
   b. *Clostridium difficile* toxin assay if taking antibiotics
   c. Diarrhea increases tacrolimus absorption and decreases cyclosporine absorption; suggest checking tacrolimus trough level before next morning dose
3. **Management**
   a. IV fluids for rehydration
   b. Vomiting while taking azathioprine (AZA) can cause elevated liver enzymes; consider holding AZA until vomiting settles

VARICELLA EXPOSURE

1. See section on Varicella in Chapter 23 Immunoprophylaxis

HERPES SIMPLEX INFECTION

1. See section on HSV in Chapter 24 Infectious Diseases

NEUROCOGNITIVE

1. Neurocognitive deficits are common post-SOT, compared with healthy population norms
   a. Rates similar to other chronic diseases
   b. Persist over time
2. Need to monitor neurocognitive development (see section on Developmental Assessment in Chapter 12 Development)
3. **Risk factors** for impaired outcomes include disease onset and severity, duration of disease, and neurotoxic medication use
4. Heart, renal, and liver transplantation: IQ within low-normal range

QUALITY OF LIFE

1. SOT recipients report lower health-related quality of life (QOL), compared with healthy population
   a. Particularly school functioning
   b. Similar to other chronic disease states
2. Disease-specific tools are available to assess health-related QOL; can complement general, validated QOL tools
3. Note the discrepancy between self- and parental proxy-reports: parents often report poorer QOL scores than recipients themselves

FURTHER READING

Fishman JA, Issa NC. Infection in organ transplantation: risk factors and evolving patterns of infection. *Infect Dis Clin North Am*. 2010;24(2):273–283.

LaRosa C, Jorge Baluarte H, Meyers KEC. Outcomes in pediatric solid-organ transplantation. *Pediatr Transplant*. 2011;15(2):128–141.

Ng VL, Feng S. Optimization of outcomes for children after solid organ transplantation. *Pediatr Clin North Am*. 2010;57(2):353–634.

USEFUL WEBSITE

SickKids Transplant and Regenerative Medicine Centre. Available at: http://www.sickkids.ca/TRMC/index.html

Transplantation

Laboratory Reference Values and Transfusion Medicine

Khosrow Adeli • Susan Richardson • En Liu • Wendy Lau • Benjamin Jung •
Victoria Higgins • Mary Kathryn Bohn

COMMON ABBREVIATIONS

Also see page xviii for a list of other abbreviations used throughout this book

BC	buffy coat platelet pool
CHF	congestive heart failure
CMV	cytomegalovirus
DDAVP	desamino-8-D-arginine vasopressin
F	factor
GABA	gamma-aminobutyric acid
Hb	hemoglobin
HLA	human leukocyte antigen
HOG	4-hydroxy-2-oxoglutarate
HUS	hemolytic uremia syndrome
IM	intramuscular
IU	international units
IVIG	intravenous immunoglobulin
JDF	Juvenile Diabetes Foundation
NMDA	N-Methyl-D-aspartic acid or N-methyl-D-aspartate
RcoF	ristocetin cofactor
SC	subcutaneous
SDP	single donor apheresis platelets
TTP	thrombotic thrombocytopenic purpura
vWF	von Willebrand factor

Laboratory Reference Values and Transfusion Medicine

39

CLINICAL BIOCHEMISTRY

Table 39.1 Clinical Biochemistry (Blood specimens unless otherwise noted)

Test Name	Age	Reference Interval/Units	Comments
α1-Acid glycoprotein (A-1-AGP) (serum)	0–<6 months	0.21–0.85 g/L	Acute phase reactant
	6 months–<5 years	0.48–2.01 g/L	Alternate test names: Orosomucoid, A-1-AGP
	5–<19 years	0.48–1.14 g/L	
Acid phosphatase, prostatic (PACP) (serum)		<2.3 mcg/L	
Acylcarnitines (plasma)			Free and total carnitine status is required for appropriate interpretation
C0 (FC)	0–<16 days	13–30 μmol/L	
	≥16 days	18–47 μmol/L	
Acetyl C2		4.65–35.39 μmol/L	
Propionyl C3		<1.08 μmol/L	
Butyryl/isobutyryl C4		<0.68 μmol/L	
Tiglyl C5:1		<0.09 μmol/L	
Isovaleryl/2methylbutyryl C5		<0.47 μmol/L	
Hexanoyl C6		<0.32 μmol/L	
OHIsoval/methylOHbutyryl C5OH		<0.14 μmol/L	
Octenoyl C8:1		<0.68 μmol/L	
Octanoyl C8		<0.3 μmol/L	
Malonyl C3DC			

Decenoyl C10:1	<0.29 μmol/L
Decanoyl C10	<0.38 μmol/L
Methylmalonyl/succinyl C4DC	<0.13 μmol/L
Glutaryl/3OHDecanoyl C5DC	<0.14 μmol/L
Dodecenoyl C12:1	<0.19 μmol/L
Dodecanoyl C12	<0.19 μmol/L
Adipyl/3meglutaryl C6DC/C53MDC	<0.14 μmol/L
3OHDodecanoyl C12OH	<0.05 μmol/L
Tetradecadienoyl C14:2	<0.09 μmol/L
Tetradecenoyl C14:1	<0.21 μmol/L
Tetradecanoyl C14	<0.11 μmol/L
3OHTetradecenoyl C14:10H	<0.05 μmol/L
3OHTetradecanoyl C14OH	<0.04 μmol/L
Palmitoleoyl C16:1	<0.09 μmol/L
Palmitoyl C16	<0.31 μmol/L
3OHPalmitoleoyl C16:10H	<0.13 μmol/L
3OHPalmitoyl C16OH	<0.05 μmol/L
Linoleoyl C18:2	<0.14 μmol/L

Continued

Table 39.1 Clinical Biochemistry (Blood specimens unless otherwise noted)—cont'd

Test Name	Age	Reference Interval/Units	Comments
Oleoyl C18:1		<0.28 µmol/L	
Stearoyl C18		<0.1 µmol/L	
3OHLinoleoyl C18:2OH		<0.03 µmol/L	
3OHOleoyl C18:1OH		<0.04 µmol/L	
Adenosine diphosphate (ADP)		46%–94%	
ADH	See *Antidiuretic hormone*		
Adrenal antibodies (serum)		Not detected	
Adrenocorticotropic hormone (ACTH) (plasma)		<17 pmol/L Morning ACTH peak falls by half through the day	Take blood at 9 a.m., cortisol should be measured in same sample
ACTH stimulation test		A normal cortisol response is indicated by a doubling of the basal value and an absolute value of >500–550 nmol/L	Measures cortisol
Alanine aminotransferase (ALT) (plasma or serum)	0–<1 year 1–<13 years ≥13 years	<40 U/L <24 U/L Female: <24 U/L Male: <29 U/L	
Albumin (plasma or serum)	0–<15 days 15 days–<1 year 1–<8 years 8–<15 years 15–<19 years	26–42 g/L 23–48 g/L 35–47 g/L 37–50 g/L Female: 35–52 g/L Male: 39–53 g/L	

Aldosterone (plasma or serum)	Upright: 111–860 pmol/L Recumbent: <444 pmol/L	- Request Na⁺ and K⁺ on same sample - Less useful than urine aldosterone, varies widely over short periods (depending on time of day, posture, Na⁺ and K⁺ intake) - To demonstrate hyperaldosteronism in hypokalemic hypertension, give K⁺ supplements until K⁺ is in normal range before aldosterone is measured - Diuretics (e.g., furosemide, spironolactone) and several other drugs (especially purgatives and licorice derivatives [e.g., carbenoxolone]) should be discontinued (if possible) for 3 weeks before assessment
Alkaline phosphatase (ALP) (plasma or serum)	0–<15 days 89–239 U/L 15 days–<1 year 125–440 U/L 1–<10 years 143–318 U/L 10–<13 years 131–393 U/L 13–<15 years Female: 66–245 U/L · Male: 119–440 U/L 15–<17 years Female: 59–120 U/L · Male: 88–315 U/L 17–<19 years Female: 55–93 U/L · Male: 64–150 U/L	Source: bone, liver, kidney, intestinal mucosa; isoenzymes exist for bone, liver, and intestine
Alkaline phosphatase isoenzymes (serum)	ALP (liver): 8–61 U/L ALP (bone): 10–64 U/L	Measures isoenzyme fractions

Continued

Table 39.1 Clinical Biochemistry (Blood specimens unless otherwise noted)—cont'd

Test Name	Age	Reference Interval/Units	Comments
Alpha fetoprotein (AFP) (serum)	0–29 days	100–10,000 mcg/L	Tumor marker, especially gonadal germ cell or primary hepatic tumor; also raised during rapid liver regeneration (e.g. acute hepatitis)
	1–<3 months	10–1359 mcg/L	
	3–<6 months	4–275 mcg/L	
	6 months–<1 year	3–148 mcg/L	
	1–<3 years	3–21 mcg/L	
	3–<19 years	1–4 mcg/L	
ALT	See *Alanine aminotransferase*		
Aluminum (plasma)		Standard: <293 nmol/L	Aluminum toxicity signs may appear in dialysis patients when aluminum >2000 nmol/L
		On aluminum antacid medication: <1100 nmol/L	
Amino acid screen (plasma)		Qualitative assessment	Screening to detect genetic-metabolic disease If screen abnormal, obtain quantitative values
Amino acids quantitative (plasma or serum)			Reference values are age dependent and should be interpreted by metabolic disease specialist
Phosphoserine		0–3 μmol/L	
Hydroxyproline	0–<7 days	28–104 μmol/L	
	7 days–<1 month	29–110 μmol/L	
	1 month–<1 year	12–59 μmol/L	
	1–<13 years	10–34 μmol/L	
	13–<19 years	1–35 μmol/L	
	≥19 years	4–25 μmol/L	

Histidine	0–<7 days	76–215 μmol/L
	7–<30 days	45–168 μmol/L
	30 days–<19 years	65–113 μmol/L
	≥19 years	50–106 μmol/L
Phosphoethanolamine	0–<7 days	0–10 μmol/L
	≥7 days	0–2 μmol/L
Asparagine	0–<19 years	38–91 μmol/L
	≥19 years	38–79 μmol/L
1-Methylhistidine	0–<7 days	0–20 μmol/L
	7 days–<1 month	0–19 μmol/L
	1 month–<19 years	1–30 μmol/L
	≥19 years	0–39 μmol/L
Taurine	0–<1 month	87–375 μmol/L
	1 month–<19 years	55–204 μmol/L
	≥19 years	31–97 μmol/L
3-Methylhistidine	0–<7 days	6–21 μmol/L
	7 days–<13 years	4–18 μmol/L
	13–<19 years	4–12 μmol/L
	≥19 years	3–10 μmol/L
Serine	0–<1 month	199–843 μmol/L
	1 month–<19 years	112–216 μmol/L
	≥19 years	60–149 μmol/L

Continued

Table 39.1 Clinical Biochemistry (Blood specimens unless otherwise noted)—cont'd

Test Name	Age	Reference Interval/Units	Comments
Glutamine	0–<7 days	451–1113 µmol/L	
	7 days–<1 year	332–789 µmol/L	
	1–<19 years	467–755 µmol/L	
	≥19 years	397–781 µmol/L	
Carnosine	0–<1 month	1–19 µmol/L	
	1 month–<19 years	2–7 µmol/L	
	≥19 years	1–13 µmol/L	
Arginine	0–<1 month	2–118 µmol/L	
	1 month–<1 year	47–138 µmol/L	
	1–<19 years	66–150 µmol/L	
	≥19 years	29–123 µmol/L	
Glycine	0–<1 month	299–782 µmol/L	
	1 month–<1 year	176–398 µmol/L	
	1–<19 years	218–407 µmol/L	
	≥19 years	141–432 µmol/L	
Anserine	0–<1 year	0–5 µmol/L	
	1–<19 years	0–2 µmol/L	
	≥19 years	0–5 µmol/L	
Ethanolamine/ars/saccharopine	0–<1 month	23–110 µmol/L	
	1 month–<1 year	9–27 µmol/L	
	1–<19 years	8–18 µmol/L	
	≥19 years	5–12 µmol/L	

Aspartate	0–<1 month	19–121 μmol/L
	1 month–<19 years	20–42 μmol/L
	≥19 years	2–19 μmol/L
Sarcosine		0–4 μmol/L
Glutamate	0–<1 month	91–401 μmol/L
	1 month–<19 years	74–266 μmol/L
	≥19 years	15–112 μmol/L
Citrulline	0–<1 year	9–44 μmol/L
	1–<13 years	16–41 μmol/L
	13–<19 years	15–36 μmol/L
	≥19 years	15–50 μmol/L
Beta-alanine	0–<13 years	3–27 μmol/L
	13–<19 years	5–20 μmol/L
	≥19 years	2–17 μmol/L
Threonine	0–<1 year	81–313 μmol/L
	1–<19 years	72–185 μmol/L
	≥19 years	54–208 μmol/L
Alanine	0–<7 days	175–427 μmol/L
	7 days–<19 years	208–588 μmol/L
	≥19 years	188–559 μmol/L
GABA/homocitrulline	0–<1 month	0–5 μmol/L
	1 month–<13 years	0–7 μmol/L
	13–<19 years	0–9 μmol/L
	≥19 years	0–3 μmol/L

Continued

Table 39.1 Clinical Biochemistry (Blood specimens unless otherwise noted)—cont'd

Test Name	Age	Reference Interval/Units	Comments
Alpha-aminoadipic acid	0–<1 month	0–4 µmol/L	
	1 month–<1 year	0–3 µmol/L	
	≥1 year	0–2 µmol/L	
Proline	0–<1 year	127–292 µmol/L	
	1–<13 years	118–372 µmol/L	
	13–<19 years	116–360 µmol/L	
	≥19 years	112–335 µmol/L	
Beta-aminoisobutyric acid	0–<1 year	0–19 µmol/L	
	1–<19 years	0–2 µmol/L	
	≥19 years	1–5 µmol/L	
Hydroxylysine 1	0–<19 years	0–1 µmol/L	
	≥19 years	0–2 µmol/L	
Hydroxylysine 2	0–<1 month	2–5 µmol/L	
	1 month–<1 year	1–4 µmol/L	
	≥1 year	0–2 µmol/L	
Alpha-amino-N-butyric acid	0–<7 days	7–42 µmol/L	
	7 days–<1 month	8–42 µmol/L	
	1 month–<19 years	8–30 µmol/L	
	≥19 years	8–38 µmol/L	
Cystathionine	0–<1 year	0–9 µmol/L	
	1–<13 years	0–2 µmol/L	
	13–<19 years	0–3 µmol/L	
	>19 years	0–2 µmol/L	

Ornithine	0–<1 month	82–365 μmol/L
	1 month–<1 year	40–132 μmol/L
	1–<19 years	34–94 μmol/L
	≥19 years	29–104 μmol/L
Cystine	0–<7 days	16–53 μmol/L
	7 days–<19 years	16–57 μmol/L
	≥19 years	20–66 μmol/L
Lysine	0–<1 month	90–319 μmol/L
	1 month–<19 years	102–259 μmol/L
	≥19 years	110–243 μmol/L
Tyrosine	0–<1 month	27–187 μmol/L
	1 month–<1 year	34–151 μmol/L
	1–<13 years	45–126 μmol/L
	13–<19 years	34–88 μmol/L
	≥19 years	28–87 μmol/L
Methionine	0–<19 years	13–44 μmol/L
	≥19 years	13–35 μmol/L
Valine	0–<1 month	87–326 μmol/L
	1 month–<13 years	128–361 μmol/L
	13–<19 years	166–301 μmol/L
	≥19 years	138–300 μmol/L
Isoleucine	0–<1 month	25–129 μmol/L
	1 month–<1 year	30–113 μmol/L
	1–<13 years	43–129 μmol/L
	13–<19 years	32–127 μmol/L
	≥19 years	37–94 μmol/L

Continued

Table 39.1 Clinical Biochemistry (Blood specimens unless otherwise noted)—cont'd

Test Name	Age	Reference Interval/Units	Comments
Alloisoleucine		0–5 μmol/L	
Leucine	0–<7 days	46–165 μmol/L	
	7 days–<1 year	55–188 μmol/L	
	1–<13 years	85–226 μmol/L	
	13–<19 years	84–227 μmol/L	
	≥19 years	74–156 μmol/L	
Phenylalanine	0–<1 month	49–107 μmol/L	
	1 month–<1 year	52–116 μmol/L	
	1–<19 years	55–100 μmol/L	
	≥19 years	40–85 μmol/L	
Tryptophan	0–<7 days	22–59 μmol/L	
	7 days–<1 month	22–62 μmol/L	
	1 month–<1 year	37–80 μmol/L	
	1–<13 years	35–76 μmol/L	
	13–<19 years	37–66 μmol/L	
	≥19 years	26–61 μmol/L	
Ammonium (plasma)	0–<1 month	<50 μmol/L	
	≥1 month	<35 μmol/L	
Amylase (plasma or serum)	0–<3 months	<30 U/L	Source: pancreas, salivary glands
	3 months–<1 year	<46 U/L	
	1–<19 years	<102 U/L	

Androstenedione (plasma or serum)	0–<14 days	0–2.5 nmol/L		- Source: ovaries, adrenals
	14 days–<1 year	0.1–2.1 nmol/L		- Can be considered "adrenal-specific" androgen until puberty in females and from 5 months to puberty in males
	1–<6 years	0.1–0.6 nmol/L		
	6–<10 years	0.2–0.9 nmol/L		
	10–<12 years	0–2.5 nmol/L		- In females, values are higher during luteal phase of cycle than during follicular phase but should still be within range shown
	12–<15 years	Female: 0.7–6 nmol/L	Male: 0.5–2 U/L	
	15–<19 years	Female: 0.5–6.5 nmol/L	Male: 0.9–3.6 U/L	
Angiotensin-converting enzyme (ACE) (plasma or serum)	0–<3 years	5–83 U/L		
	3–<8 years	8–76 U/L		
	8–<15 years	6–89 U/L		
	≥15 years	8–52 U/L		
Anticardiolipin antibody (plasma or serum)		Negative: <20 CU		Interpret in relation to plasma osmolality
Antidiuretic hormone (ADH) (arginine vasopressin) (plasma)		0.8–3.5 pmol/L		
Antimitochondrial antibody (serum)		Negative to 1:20		Alternative test name: AMA
Anti-NMDA receptor immunoglobulin G (IgG) antibody		Negative		Alternative test names: anti N-methyl-D-aspartate receptor antibodies, antiglutamate receptor antibodies
Antinuclear antibody		Negative to 1:80		Alternative test name: ANF
Antiparietal cell antibody (serum)		Negative to 1:20		Alternative test name: APCA

Continued

Table 39.1 **Clinical Biochemistry** (Blood specimens unless otherwise noted)—cont'd

Test Name	Age	Reference Interval/Units	Comments
Antistreptolysin (ASO) (plasma or serum)	0–<6 months 6 months–<1 year 1–<6 years 6–<19 years	Not established 0–30 IU/mL 0–104 IU/mL 0–331 IU/mL	- Acute and convalescent sera is required for serodiagnosis - A single ASO titer of equal to or greater than 200 IU/mL or a fourfold rise or fall in antibody titer is compatible with a recent streptococcal infection - The ASO titer reaches its peak by 3–5 weeks after infection and declines over the next 6–8 weeks - Patients with rheumatic fever have a mean ASO titer of 500 IU/mL
Antithyroglobulin antibody (Anti-Tg)		0.4–17.7 kIU/L	
Anti-TPO antibody (antithyroid peroxidase antibody) (serum)	0–<19 years	<1 IU/mL	Alternate test names: antimicrosomal antibody, antithyroid antibody
α₁-Antitrypsin (serum)	0–<19 years	1.1–1.81 g/L	
α₁-Antitrypsin phenotyping (PI typing) (serum)	0–<19 years	- PI typing: - MM, normal (89% of population) - MS, normal variant (8%) - MZ, heterozygous for deficiency (<2%) - ZZ, homozygous for deficiency	- Phenotyping may only be done if α₁-antitrypsin total is low - Positive acute phase reactant - Order only if alpha-1-trypsin is abnormal; do not order repeat protease inhibitor (PI) typing following initial confirmation

Apolipoprotein A-1 (plasma or serum)		- For clearance: falsely low values where lesion(s) in esophagus, stomach, or upper small bowel because low-pH environment degrades α_1-antitrypsin; collection must be free of urine; serum α_1-antitrypsin required (clotted blood collected during stool collection period or within 24 h after collection period)
	0–<15 days:	
	Female: 0.71–0.97 g/L Male: 0.62–0.91 g/L	
	15 days to <1 year: 0.53–1.75 g/L	
	1 to <14 years: 0.80–1.64 g/L	
	14 to <19 years: 0.72–1.54 g/L	
Apolipoprotein B (plasma or serum)	0–<15 days	0.09–0.67 g/L
	15 days–<1 year	0.19–1.23 g/L
	1–<6 years	0.41–0.93 g/L
	6–<19 years	0.31–0.84 g/L
Arginine stimulation test	Post stimulation peak Growth Hormone should exceed 5.7 mcg/L	Includes glucose, growth hormone
Arginine vasopressin (plasma)	See *Antidiuretic hormone*	
Ascorbic acid (serum)	See *Vitamin C*	
Aspartate aminotransferase (AST) (plasma or serum)	0–<15 days	<184 U/L	Source: cardiac and skeletal muscle, liver, kidney, erythrocytes
	15 days–<1 year	<77 U/L	
	1–<7 years	<52 U/L	
	7–<12 years	<43 U/L	
	12–<19 years Female: <31 U/L	Male: <41 U/L	

Continued

Laboratory Reference Values and Transfusion Medicine

39

Table 39.1 Clinical Biochemistry (Blood specimens unless otherwise noted)—cont'd

Test Name	Age	Reference Interval/Units	Comments
Bicarbonate (calculated); arterial, capillary, or venous	See *Blood gas, arterial, capillary or venous*		
β-Hydroxybutyrate	0–<14 years ≥14 years	0–0.3 mmol/L 0–0.42 mmol/L	
β₂-Microglobulin (serum)	0–<3 months 3 months–<2 years 2–<19 years	1.89–5.81 mg/L 1.31–4.54 mg/L 1.19–2.25 mg/L	
Bile acids (plasma or serum)		<6.7 µmol/L	
Bilirubin, conjugated (plasma or serum)	0–<15 days 15 days–<19 years	<10 µmol/L <1 µmol/L	
Bilirubin, delta (plasma or serum)	0–<1 year ≥1 years	<3 µmol/L <5 µmol/L	Delta bilirubin is albumin conjugated (long half-life) and associated with long-standing cholestasis
Bilirubin, total (plasma or serum)	0–<15 days 15 days–<1 year 1–<9 years 9–<12 years 12–<15 years 15–<19 years	3–284 µmol/L 1–12 µmol/L 1–7 µmol/L 1–9 µmol/L 2–12 µmol/L 2–14 µmol/L	See Chapter 27 Neonatology for interpretation and management of neonatal bilirubin

Bilirubin, unconjugated (plasma or serum)	0–<3 days	<130 µmol/L	See Chapter 27 Neonatology for interpretation and management of neonatal bilirubin
	3–<6 days	<200 µmol/L	
	6–<15 days	<109 µmol/L	
	15 days–<1 year	<11 µmol/L	
	1–<9 years	<7 µmol/L	
	9–<12 years	<9 µmol/L	
	12–<15 years	<12 µmol/L	
	15–<19 years	<14 µmol/L	
Biotinidase (plasma or serum)	0–<2 months	57–765 nmol/h/mL	
	2–<10 months	408–907 nmol/h/mL	
	10 months–<6 years	439–800 nmol/h/mL	
	6–<19 years	Female: 358–792 nmol/h/mL	Male: 480–878 nmol/h/mL
	≥19 years	369–432 nmol/h/mL	
Blood gas (arterial, capillary, venous or mixed venous)			- Blood gases (pH, pCO_2, pO_2, actual bicarbonate, base excess, and O_2 saturation calculation) - Normal values for capillary gas levels range from venous to arterial, depending on arterialization of sample site
pH (arterial)	0–<1 month	7.30–7.49	
	≥1 month	7.35–7.50	
pCO_2 (arterial)	0–<1 year	30–45 mmHg	
	≥1 year	32–45 mmHg	

Continued

Table 39.1 Clinical Biochemistry (Blood specimens unless otherwise noted)—cont'd

Test Name	Age	Reference Interval/Units	Comments
pO$_2$ (arterial)	0–<2 days	60–70 mmHg	
	2 days	70–80 mmHg	
	≥3 days	>=80 mmHg	
Bicarbonate (arterial)	0–<7 days	17–26 mmol/L	
	7–<30 days	17–27 mmol/L	
	30 days–<6 months	17–29 mmol/L	
	6 months–<1 year	18–29 mmol/L	
	≥1 year	20–31 mmol/L	
pH (capillary)		7.25–7.60	
pCO$_2$ (capillary)		20–60 mmHg	
pH (venous)		7.32–7.42	
pCO$_2$ (venous)		40–50 mmHg	
pO$_2$ (venous)		25–47 mmHg	
pH (mixed venous)		7.25–7.60	
pCO$_2$ (mixed venous)		40–50 mmHg	
Bicarbonate (mixed venous)		10–40 mmol/L	
Blood urea nitrogen	See *Urea*		
C3 complement (serum)	0–<15 days	0.5–1.21 g/L	
	15 days–<1 year	0.51–1.6 g/L	
	1–<10 years	0.82–1.52 g/L	

SI component (serum)				Comments
	0–<1 year	0.0–0.3 g/L		
	1–<19 years	0.13–0.37 g/L		
Calcitonin (serum)		Female: ≤7 ng/L	Male: ≤11 ng/L	Measured after pentagastrin stimulation
Calcium, ionized (whole blood)		1.22–1.37 mmol/L		
Calcium, total (plasma or serum)	0–<1 year	2.08–2.64 mmol/L		- Prolonged venous stasis (e.g., prolonged tourniquet use) alters result
	1–<19 years	2.22–2.54 mmol/L		- Low serum calcium levels may be normal if hypoalbuminemia present, adjusted calcium should be in normal range
				- To calculate adjusted calcium (SI units): Adjusted Ca^{2+} (mmol/L) = total calcium (mmol/L) + [40 – albumin (g/L)] × 0.025
Carbon dioxide (plasma or serum)	0–<8 days	17–26 mmol/L		Alternate test names: bicarbonate, total CO_2 (TCO_2)
	8–<30 days	17–27 mmol/L		
	30 days–<6 months	17–29 mmol/L		
	6 months–<1 year	18–29 mmol/L		
	≥1 year	22–30 mmol/L		
Carboxyhemoglobin		≤0.020		Specimen must be anaerobic
				Expressed as fraction of total hemoglobin
Carcinoembryonic antigen (CEA) (serum)		0–<7 days: 8.1–62 mcg/L		
		7 days–<2 years: <0.5–4.7 mcg/L		
		2–<19 years: <0.5–2.6 mcg/L		
Carnitine (free) (serum)	0–<16 days	12–60 µmol/L		
	≥16 days	26–60 µmol/L		

Continued

1033

Table 39.1 Clinical Biochemistry (Blood specimens unless otherwise noted)—cont'd

Test Name	Age	Reference Interval/Units		Comments
Carnitine (total) (serum)	0–<16 days	23–84 μmol/L		
	≥16 days	32–84 μmol/L		
Carotene (plasma or serum)		0.9–3.7 μmol/L		
Catecholamines (plasma)				Drugs, such as methyldopa, hydralazine (Apresoline), quinidine, epinephrine, or norepinephrine-related drugs (e.g., L-dopa) and renal function test dyes may interfere with catecholamine excretion and affect results
Epinephrine		<0.8 nmol/L		
Norepinephrine		0.8–3.4 nmol/L		
Ceruloplasmin (serum)	0–<2 month	Female: 74–237 mg/L	Male: 73–236 mg/L	Positive acute phase reactant
	2–<6 months	135–329 mg/L		
	6 months–<1 year	137–389 mg/L		
	1–<8 years	217–433 mg/L		
	8–<14 years	205–402 mg/L		
	≥14 years	Female: 208–432 mg/L	Male: 170–348 mg/L	
Chloride (plasma or serum)	0–<1 year	96–106 mmol/L		
	1–<18 years	99–111 mmol/L		
	≥18 years	98–106 mmol/L		
Chloride (sweat)	≥7 days	<30 mmol/L: negative		- If result is borderline/indeterminate, repeat test within 2–4 weeks
		30–60 mmol/L: borderline/indeterminate		- Repeat test if first result ≥60 mmol/L
		>60 mmol/L: consistent with diagnosis of cystic fibrosis (CF)		

Cholesterol, total (plasma or serum)	0–<18 years	<4.40 mmol/L	- Values based on fasting states (before feeding in babies, after 12-h fast in older children)
	≥18 years	<5.20 mmol/L	- Fasting not essential if total cholesterol requested without any other lipid determinations
Cholesterol, high-density lipoprotein (HDL, plasma or serum)	0–<18 years	>1.17 mmol/L	Take blood before feeding for neonates and infants and after 12-h fast for older children
	≥18 years	>1.04 mmol/L	
Cholesterol, low-density lipoprotein (LDL, plasma or serum)	0–<18 years	<2.85 mmol/L	Take blood before feeding for neonates and infants and after 12-h fast for older children
	≥18 years	<3.5 mmol/L	
Cholinesterase, (pseudocholinesterase) (serum)		Cholinesterase total 620–1370 U/L Dibucaine 77–83 U/L Fluoride 56–68 U/L Chloride 4–15 U/L Succinylcholine (scoline) 87–92 U/L	Cholinesterase phenotype includes chloride, cholinesterase-total, dibucaine, fluoride, scoline, and Ro 02-0683 Collect 24 h after surgery
Cholinesterase, total activity (serum)		620–1370 U/L	
Chorionic gonadotropin, β subunit (qualitative) (serum)		Negative for non-pregnant individuals	Pregnancy screen
Chorionic gonadotropin, β subunit (quantitative HCG) (serum)		<5 IU/L for pregnancy test <1 IU/L for tumor marker	
Clonidine stimulation test		Post stimulation peak Growth Hormone should exceed 5.7	Includes glucose, growth hormone
Complement	See C3 and C4 complement		

Continued

Table 39.1 Clinical Biochemistry (Blood specimens unless otherwise noted)—cont'd

Test Name	Age	Reference Interval/Units		Comments
Copper (plasma)	0–<4 months	1.4–7.2 μmol/L		
	4–<7 months	3.9–17.3 μmol/L		
	7 months–<1 year	7.9–20.5 μmol/L		
	1–<6 years	12.6–23.6 μmol/L		
	6–<10 years	13.2–21.4 μmol/L		
	10–<14 years	Female: 12.9–18.9 μmol/L	Male: 12.6–19 μmol/L	
	≥14 years	Female: 13.5–36.5 μmol/L	Male: 11.2–20.6 μmol/L	
Coproporphyrin, erythrocytes		0–45 nmol/L		
Corticosterone (plasma or serum)	0–<1 month	0.1–20 nmol/L		
	1 month–<1 year	0.3–15.4 nmol/L		
	1–<4 years	0.6–3.7 nmol/L		
	4–<6 years	1–4.1 nmol/L		
	6–<15 years	0.4–9.2 nmol/L		
	15–<19 years	0.9–15.2 nmol/L		
Cortisol (plasma or serum)	0–<15 days	13–340 nmol/L		- Result at 8 p.m. is <50% of the 8 a.m. value in 88% of cases
	15 days–<1 year	14–458 nmol/L		- Diurnal variation of cortisol may not develop until about 1 year of age
	1–<9 years	48–297 nmol/L		- In Cushing disease or syndrome, cortisol levels may be normal, but diurnal variation may be absent
	9–<14 years	61–349 nmol/L		- Other steroids produced in congenital adrenal hyperplasia or tumors may cross-react with cortisol assay; only poor diurnal variation may be evident
	14–<17 years	77–453 nmol/L		Stress or shock can elevate cortisol levels
	17–<19 years	97–506 nmol/L		

1036

Analyte	Age	Reference value	Notes
C peptide (plasma or serum)		298–2350 pmol/L	Collect after overnight fast
C-reactive protein (CRP) (serum)	0–<15 days	0.3–6.1 mg/L	
	15 days–<15 years	0.1–1 mg/L	
	15–<19 years	0.1–1.7 mg/L	
Creatine kinase (CK) (plasma or serum)	0–<11 days	Not established	- Source: skeletal and cardiac muscle, smooth muscle, brain
	11 days–<1 year	0–390 U/L	- Elevated CK levels occur after physical activity and intramuscular injections
	1–<4 years	60–305 U/L	- Bed rest for several days may drop CK levels by 20%–30%
	4–<7 years	75–230 U/L	
	7–<9 years	60–365 U/L	
	9–<11 years	Female: 80–230 U/L	Male: 55–215 U/L
	11–<14 years	Female: 50–295 U/L	Male: 60–330 U/L
	14–<16 years	Female: 50–240 U/L	Male: 60–335 U/L
	≥16 years	Female: 45–230 U/L	Male: 55–370 U/L
Creatine kinase (CK) MB mass (serum)	0–<6 years	Female: 1.44–6.05 mcg/L	Male: 1.51–9.39 mcg/L
	6–<13 years	Female: 0.88–4.37 mcg/L	Male: 1.26–5.56 mcg/L
	13–<19 years	Female: 0.46–2.04 mcg/L	Male: 0.7–4.59 mcg/L

- Sources: CK-BB, predominantly brain; CK-MB, cardiac muscle, type II skeletal muscle fibers; CK-MM, skeletal muscle, cardiac muscle
- Purpose is to help differentiate skeletal from cardiac muscle disease or trauma
- CK-MB not specific for myocardial damage in first week or month after birth; if CK-MB is borderline, consider troponin T or I

Continued

Table 39.1 Clinical Biochemistry (Blood specimens unless otherwise noted)—cont'd

Test Name	Age	Reference Interval/Units	Comments
Creatinine (plasma or serum)	0–<15 days	27–76 µmol/L	
	15 days–<2 years	8–29 µmol/L	
	2–<5 years	16–35 µmol/L	
	5–<12 years	25–50 µmol/L	
	12–<15 years	37–67 µmol/L	
	15–<19 years	Female: 40–69 µmol/L | Male: 51–89 µmol/L	
Cryoglobulin (serum)		Normally absent	
7-Dehydrocholesterol (plasma or serum)		<5 µmol/L	
Dehydroepiandrosterone sulfate (DHEA-S) (plasma or serum)	0–<2 months	28.9–40.7 µmol/L	
	2–<6 months	0.7–15.6 µmol/L	
	6 months–<1 year	0.2–4.8 µmol/L	
	1–<6 years	0.1–3.2 µmol/L	
	6–<9 years	0.1–4.1 µmol/L	
	9–<13 years	0.9–7.3 µmol/L	
	13–<16 years	1.5–12.5 µmol/L	
	16–<19 years	Female: 4–15.5 µmol/L | Male: 3.4–18.2 µmol/L	
11-Deoxycortisol (serum)	0–<1 year	0.0–5.3 nmol/L	
	1–<2 years	0.1–0.9 nmol/L	
	2–<7 years	0.1–1.1 nmol/L	
	7–<19 years	0.1–2.3 nmol/L	
Dihydropteridine reductase (blood spot)		7–22 units/n Hb	

Dihydrotestosterone			
	Female premenopausal	65–1266 pmol/L	
	Female postmenopausal	50–623 pmol/L	
	Adult male	860–3406 pmol/L	
		Pediatric ranges are not available	
Epinephrine	See *Catecholamines*		
Estradiol (plasma or serum)	0–<1 year	370 pmol/L	Reference ranges for estradiol are poorly defined in the first year of life. Levels can be elevated at birth and subsequently fall to prepubertal levels within a year.
	1 year to adrenarche	<92 pmol/L	
	Puberty	Rising to adult values	
	Adult	<165 pmol/L	
Sexual maturity rating	I	Female: <74 pmol/L	Male: <68 pmol/L
	II	Female: <96 pmol/L	Male: <67 pmol/L
	III	Female: <317 pmol/L	Male: <76 pmol/L
	IV	Female: 49–517 pmol/L	Male: <128 pmol/L
	V	Female: 69–762 pmol/L	Male: 64–126 pmol/L
Menstrual stage	Follicular phase	110–183 pmol/L	
	Luteal phase	550–845 pmol/L	
	Treated with synthetic estrogens	<165 pmol/L	
	Preovulating peak	550–1650 pmol/L	
Estradiol (high sensitivity)	0–<30 days	Female: ≤242 pmol/L	Male: ≤194 pmol/L
	30–<1 year	Female: ≤40 pmol/L	Male: ≤44 pmol/L
	1–<10 years	Female: ≤59 pmol/L	Male: ≤15 pmol/L
	10–<12 years	Female: ≤239 pmol/L	Male: ≤44 pmol/L
	12–<14 years	Female: ≤521 pmol/L	Male: ≤88 pmol/L
	14–<19 years	Female: ≤1039 pmol/L	Male: ≤114 pmol/L

Reference ranges for estradiol are poorly defined in the first year of life. Levels can be elevated at birth and subsequently fall to prepubertal levels within a year.

Laboratory Reference Values and Transfusion Medicine

39

Continued

Table 39.1 Clinical Biochemistry (Blood specimens unless otherwise noted)—cont'd

Test Name	Age	Reference Interval/Units		Comments
Estriol (unconjugated) (serum)		Female: <0.08 ng/mL	Male: <0.07 ng/mL	
Ferritin (plasma or serum)	4–<15 days	99.6–717 mcg/L		A ferritin level <10 mcg/L is critically low and should be investigated for iron deficiency. Levels >300 mcg/L are high and warrants further investigation
	15 days–<6 months	14.0–647.2 mcg/L		
	6 months–<1 year	8.4–181.9 mcg/L		
	1–<5 years	5.3–99.9 mcg/L		
	5–<14 years	13.7–78.8 mcg/L		
	14–<16 years	Female: 5.5–67.4 mcg/L	Male: 12.7–82.8 mcg/L	
	16–<19 years	Female: 5.5–67.4 mcg/L	Male: 11.1–171.9 mcg/L	
Folate (serum)	0–<5 days	Not established		
	5 days–<1 year	>23.9 nmol/L		
	1–<3 years	>25 nmol/L		
	3–<6 years	>27 nmol/L		
	6–<8 years	>29.7 nmol/L		
	8–<12 years	>25.9 nmol/L		
	12–<14 years	>27 nmol/L		
	14–<19 years	>18 nmol/L		
Follicle-stimulating hormone (FSH) (serum)	30 days–<1 year	Female: 0.4–10.4 IU/L	Male: 0.1–2.4 IU/L	
	1–<9 years	Female: 0.4–5.5 IU/L		
	9–<11 years	Female: 0.4–4.2 IU/L		
	11–<19 years	Female: 0.3–7.8 IU/L		
	1–<5 years		Male: <0.9 IU/L	
	5–<10 years		Male: <1.6 IU/L	
	10–<13 years		Male: 0.4–3.9 IU/L	
	13–<19 years		Male: 0.8–5.1 IU/L	

Test	Age/Category	Reference	Notes
Sexual maturity rating	I	Female: 0.63–4.05 IU/L	Male: <1.52 IU/L	
	II	Female: 0.27–5.76 IU/L	Male: <2.98 IU/L	
	III	Female: 0.10–7.19 IU/L	Male: <6.24 IU/L	
	IV	Female: 0.30–6.95 IU/L	Male: 0.58–5.05 IU/L	
	V	Female: 0.41–8.59 IU/L	Male: 0.79–7.19 IU/L	
Free erythrocyte porphyrin	0–<11 years	0–0.61 mmol/L	
	11–<19 years	0–1.32 mmol/L	
Galactosemia screen		Normal	- Qualitative test of red blood cell (RBC) galactose 1-phosphate uridyltransferase activity - Blood transfusion within 3 months before this test may invalidate results - Results may be falsely negative if child is not ingesting galactose-containing foods
Gases (arterial, capillary, venous or mixed venous)		See *Blood gas*	
Gastrin (plasma or serum)		13–115 ng/L	
GGT (γ-glutamyltransferase) (plasma or serum)	0–<15 days	19–196 U/L	Source: liver, pancreas
	15 days–<1 year	≤113 U/L	
	1–<11 years	≤13 U/L	
	11–<19 years	≤17 U/L	
Glucagon (plasma)		59–177 pg/mL	
Glucagon stimulation test		After stimulation, peak growth hormone should exceed 5.7 mcg/L	Includes glucose and growth hormone

Continued

Table 39.1 Clinical Biochemistry (Blood specimens unless otherwise noted)—cont'd

Test Name	Age	Reference Interval/Units	Comments
Glucose, fasting, random, 2 h pc (plasma or serum)	0–<1 month	2.7–5.5 mmol/L	
	1–<6 months	3.2–6 mmol/L	
	≥6 months	3.9–6 mmol/L	
Gonadotropins	See *Follicle-stimulating hormone (FSH) and Luteinizing hormone (LH)*		
Growth hormone (GH) (serum)	0–<3 months	0.80–33.5 mcg/L	Random samples have little diagnostic value as growth hormone levels vary throughout the day
	3 months–<2 years	0.14–6.27 mcg/L	Neonates have higher GH relative to children and adults
	2–<7 years	0.05–5.11 mcg/L	
	7–<12 years	0.02–4.76 mcg/L	
	12–<14 years	0.01–6.2 mcg/L	
	14–<19 years	Female: 0.03–5.22 mcg/L Male: 0.02–3.81 mcg/L	
Growth hormone–releasing hormone stimulation		After stimulation, peak growth hormone should exceed 5.7 mcg/L	Includes glucose and growth hormone
Haptoglobin (serum)	0–<15 days	0–0.1 g/L	
	15 days–<1 year	0.07–2.21 g/L	
	1–<12 years	0.07–1.63 g/L	
	12–<19 years	0.07–1.79 g/L	
HDL cholesterol	See *Cholesterol, HDL*		
Hemoglobin (plasma)		0–29 mg/L	Alternate test names: Hemolysis, Plasma hemoglobin, Plasma free hemoglobin

Homocysteine (plasma)	0–<1 year	2.9–10 μmol/L	
	1–<7 years	2.8–7.6 μmol/L	
	7–<12 years	3.4–8.5 μmol/L	
	12–<15 years	Female: 4.1–10.4 μmol/L	Male: 4.7–10.4 μmol/L
	15–<19 years	Female: 4.9–11.9 μmol/L	Male: 5.5–13.4 μmol/L
Human chorionic gonadotropin screen (β-HCG screen)	See *Chorionic gonadotropin, β subunit (qualitative)*		
HCG stimulation test	Normal response will have a three- to fourfold increase in testosterone when 72-h post-HCG level is compared with basal level		Measures testosterone
17-Hydroxyprogesterone (plasma or serum)	0–<14 days	0–4.8 nmol/L	Cord blood or sample taken during the first 24–48 h of life is unsatisfactory
	14 days–<1 year	0.1–3.4 nmol/L	
	1–<12 years	0.1–1.1 nmol/L	
	12–<14 years	0–2 nmol/L	
	14–<16 years	0–4.2 nmol/L	
	16–<19 years	0–3.9 nmol/L	
Very sick and stressed infants <3 months		<30 nmol/L	
Borderline for nonclassic congenital adrenal hyperplasia		6–10 nmol/L	
21-Hydroxyprogesterone (plasma or serum)	0–<1 year	0.07–0.76 nmol/L	
	1–<2 years	0.03–0.25 nmol/L	
	2–<12 year	0–0.15 nmol/L	
	12–<19 year	0–0.24 nmol/L	

Continued

Table 39.1 Clinical Biochemistry (Blood specimens unless otherwise noted)—cont'd

Test Name	Age	Reference Interval/Units	Comments
IgA (serum)	0–<1 year	0–0.3 g/L	
	1–<3 years	0–0.9 g/L	
	3–<6 years	0.3–1.5 g/L	
	6–<14 years	0.5–2.2 g/L	
	14–<19 years	0.5–2.9 g/L	
IgE (serum)	0–<7 years	≤440 IU/mL	
	7–<19 years	≤450 IU/mL	
Insulin-like growth factor 1 (IGF-1, serum)	0–<1 year	Female: 8–131 mcg/L	Male: 11–100 mcg/L
	1–<2 years	Female: 9–146 mcg/L	Male: 12–120 mcg/L
	2–<3 years	Female: 11–165 mcg/L	Male: 13–143 mcg/L
	3–<4 years	Female: 13–187 mcg/L	Male: 14–169 mcg/L
	4–<5 years	Female: 15–216 mcg/L	Male: 15–200 mcg/L
	5–<6 years	Female: 19–251 mcg/L	Male: 16–233 mcg/L
	6–<7 years	Female: 24–293 mcg/L	Male: 17–269 mcg/L
	7–<8 years	Female: 30–342 mcg/L	Male: 18–307 mcg/L
	8–<9 years	Female: 39–396 mcg/L	Male: 20–347 mcg/L
	9–<10 years	Female: 49–451 mcg/L	Male: 23–386 mcg/L
	10–<11 years	Female: 62–504 mcg/L	Male: 29–424 mcg/L
	11–<12 years	Female: 76–549 mcg/L	Male: 37–459 mcg/L
	12–<13 years	Female: 90–581 mcg/L	Male: 49–487 mcg/L
	13–<14 years	Female: 104–596 mcg/L	Male: 64–508 mcg/L
	14–<15 years	Female: 115–591 mcg/L	Male: 83–519 mcg/L
	15–<16 years	Female: 121–564 mcg/L	Male: 102–520 mcg/L
	16–<17 years	Female: 122–524 mcg/L	Male: 119–511 mcg/L
	17–<18 years	Female: 120–479 mcg/L	Male: 131–490 mcg/L
	18–<19 years	Female: 117–426 mcg/L	Male: 137–461 mcg/L

IGF-BP3 (IGF-binding protein 3) (serum)	0–<16 days	0.3–1.4 mcg/L	
	16 days–<7 months	0.7–2.9 mcg/L	
	7 month<2 years	0.7–3.7 mcg/L	
	2–<4 years	0.8–4.4 mcg/L	
	4–<7 years	1.0–5.7 mcg/L	
	7–<9 years	Female: 1.7–6.7 mcg/L	Male: 1.3–6.4 mcg/L
	9–<12 years	Female: 2.1–8.2 mcg/L	Male: 1.7–8.3 mcg/L
	12–<14 years	Female: 2.9–9.2 mcg/L	Male: 2.5–9.8 mcg/L
	14–<17 years	Female: 3.4–9.7 mcg/L	Male: 3.2–10.4 mcg/L
	17–<19 years	Female: 3.2–8.8 mcg/L	Male: 2.9–8.7 mcg/L
	19–<21 years	Female: 2.9–7.4 mcg/L	Male: 2.8–7.3 mcg/L
IgG (serum)	0–<15 days	3.2–14 g/L	
	15 days–<1 year	1.1–7 g/L	
	1–<4 years	3.2–11.5 g/L	
	4–<10 years	5.4–13.6 g/L	
	10–<19 years	6.6–15.3 g/L	
IgM (serum)	0–<15 days	0.1–0.4 g/L	
	15 days–<91 days	0.1–0.7 g/L	
	91 days–<1 year	0.2–0.9 g/L	
	1–<19 years	Female: 0.5–1.9 g/L	Male: 0.4–1.5 g/L
Insulin (plasma)			Hemolysis and insulin antibodies may lower values
Fasting	0–<1 year	7–163 pmol/L	
	1–<5 years	9–279 pmol/L	
	5–<19 years	15–345 pmol/L	

Continued

Table 39.1 Clinical Biochemistry (Blood specimens unless otherwise noted)—cont'd

Test Name	Age	Reference Interval/Units	Comments
Stimulation	30 min 1 h 2 h 3 h	170–1550 pmol/L 117–1850 pmol/L 108–1120 pmol/L 13–161 pmol/L	
Insulin antibody (plasma)		≤0.4 kU/L	
Insulin tolerance test		After stimulation, peak growth hormone should exceed 5.7 mcg/L	Includes glucose, growth hormone
Intralipid (plasma or serum)		≤0.9 g/L	
Iron (serum)	0–<14 years 14–<19 years	4.8–25.3 µmol/L Female: 5.5–31.5 µmol/L Male: 7.5–32.6 µmol/L	
Islet cell antibody (serum)		<1.25 JDF units	
Ketones (plasma or serum)		See β-Hydroxybutyrate	
Lactate (plasma)		≤2.4 mmol/L	- Used in detection of inherited causes of lactic acidemia, acidosis or sepsis - Delayed separation of serum from RBC and hemolysis both elevate result - Transport sample on ice

Lactate dehydrogenase (LDH) (plasma or serum)	0–<6 days	934–2150 U/L	- Highest concentrations in heart, liver, skeletal muscle, erythrocytes, kidney
	6 days–<4 years	500–920 U/L	- Elevated in hemolyzed samples
	4–<7 years	470–900 U/L	
	7–<10 years	420–750 U/L	
	10–<12 years	Female: 380–770 U/L	Male: 432–700 U/L
	12–<14 years	Female: 380–640 U/L	Male: 470–750 U/L
	14–<16 years	Female: 390–580 U/L	Male: 360–730 U/L
	16–<20 years	340–670 U/L	
Lactate dehydrogenase isoenzymes (total) (serum)		100–220 U/L	Rarely indicated and non-specific
LDL cholesterol	See *Cholesterol, LDL*		
Lead (whole blood)		<0.48 µmol/L	
Lipase (plasma or serum)	0–<19 years	4–39 U/L	
	≥19 years	8–78 U/L	
Luteinizing hormone (LH) (serum)	0–<3 months	Female: <2.4 IU/L	Male: 0.2–3.8 IU/L	- Ovulatory values may reach 100 IU/L
	3–<1 year	Female: <1.2 IU/L	Male: <2.9 IU/L	- Values rise through puberty to adult values
	1–<10 years	<0.3 IU/L	- LH values >7 IU/L after stimulation suggest onset of
	10–<13 years	<4.3 IU/L	puberty
	13–<15 years	Female: 0.4–6.5 IU/L	Male: <4.1 IU/L
	15–<17 years	Female: <13.1 IU/L	Male: 0.8–4.8 IU/L
	17–<19 years	Female: <8.4 IU/L	Male: 0.9–7.1 IU/L

Continued

Table 39.1 Clinical Biochemistry (Blood specimens unless otherwise noted)—cont'd

Test Name	Age	Reference Interval/Units	Comments
Sexual maturity rating	I	Female: <0.1 IU/L	Male: <1.2 IU/L
	II	Female: <2.3 IU/L	Male: <1.2 IU/L
	III	Female: <7.4 IU/L	Male: <2.3 IU/L
	IV	Female: 0.3–6.7 IU/L	Male: <4.9 IU/L
	V	Female: 0.4–21.2 IU/L	Male: 0.6–5.9 IU/L
Macroprolactin (serum)		Normal: <0.20 mcg/L	
		Borderline:	
		0.20–0.40 mcg/L	
		Abnormal:	
		>0.40 mcg/L	
Magnesium (plasma or serum)	0–<1 month	0.75–1.15 mmol/L	
	1 month–<19 years	0.7–0.95 mmol/L	
	≥19 years	0.65–1 mmol/L	
Manganese (serum)		0.017–0.053 μmol/L	
Mercury (whole blood)		0–10 nmol/L (alert value: >50 nmol/L; action value: >200 nmol/L)	
Methemoglobin (whole blood)		0%–2.9%	Must be received on ice within 60 min of collection
Norepinephrine	See *Catecholamines*		
Orosomucoid	See *α 1-Acid glycoprotein*		

Osmolality (plasma or serum)	0–<2 days	275–300 mmol/kg H_2O	
	2–<8 days	276–305 mmol/kg H_2O	
	8–<30 days	274–305 mmol/kg H_2O	
	≥30 days	282–300 mmol/kg H_2O	
Ovarian antibody (serum)		Negative	
Overnight growth hormone		Growth hormone secretion fluctuates during periods of sleep and wakefulness. No reference range for random GH sample.	
Parathyroid hormone (PTH) (serum)	0–<19 years	12–78 ng/L	Alternative test name: PTH intact
Phosphate (plasma or serum)	0–<15 days	1.89–3.53 mmol/L	
	15 days–<1 year	1.63–2.83 mmol/L	
	1–<5 years	1.46–2.29 mmol/L	
	5–<13 years	1.41–2.02 mmol/L	
	13–<16 years	Female: 1.1–1.88 mmol/L Male: 1.22–2.09 mmol/L	
	16–<19 years	1.03–1.71 mmol/L	
Porphobilinogen deaminase	≥18 years	20–43 μmol/L Erc/h	- Increased by hemolysis in sample - Alternative test names: Uroporphyrinogen 1 synthetase, HMB, Hydroxymethylbilane synthase
Potassium (plasma or serum)	0–<7 days	3.2–5.5 mmol/L	
	7–<30 days	3.4–6 mmol/L	
	30 days–<6 months	3.5–5.6 mmol/L	
	6 months–<1 year	3.5–6 mmol/L	
	1–<16 years	3.7–5 mmol/L	
	16–<19 years	3.7–4.8 mmol/L	
	≥19 years	2.5–6 mmol/L	

Continued

Table 39.1 Clinical Biochemistry (Blood specimens unless otherwise noted)—cont'd

Test Name	Age	Reference Interval/Units	Comments
Prolactin (serum)	4–<30 days	12.6–212.8 mcg/L	
	30 days–<1 year	6.3–113.7 mcg/L	
	1–<19 years	4.2–23 mcg/L	
Protein (total) (plasma or serum)	0–<15 days	54–85 g/L	
	15 days–<1 year	45–73 g/L	
	1–<6 years	62–77 g/L	
	6–<9 years	65–79 g/L	
	9–<19 years	66–83 g/L	
Protoporphyrin, erythrocytes		0–550 nmol/L	
Protoporphyrin, free erythrocyte (FEP)	0–<11 years	≤0.61 μmol/L	- Investigation of severe lead poisoning, congenital erythropoietic porphyria, erythrohepatic protoporphyria
	11–<19 years	≤1.32 μmol/L	- Increased FEP occurs in iron deficiency anemia and anemia of chronic disease
Pyruvate		0.03–0.08 mmol/L	- Lactate must be done at same time; pyruvate only analyzed if lactate is elevated - Used in detection of inherited causes of lactic acidemia
Renin, total (plasma)		9.2–86.9 μIU/mL	- Normal values vary with sodium intake, time of day, erect or supine posture, age - Ranges assume normal salt intake, 9 a.m., supine, after 1- to 12-h rest - Premature infants will have higher ranges

		Non-reactive	
Rheumatoid factor (plasma or serum)			
Selenium (plasma)	0–<1 year	0.72–1.21 μmol/L	
	1–<6 years	1.22–1.82 μmol/L	
	6–<10 years	1.28–2.04 μmol/L	
	≥10 years	1.33–2.03 μmol/L	
Sex hormone binding globulin (SHBG) (serum)		Female: 18–144 nmol/L	Male: 10–57 nmol/L
Sexual maturity rating	I	Female: 21–210 nmol/L	Male: 23–157 nmol/L
	II	Female: 30–141 nmol/L	Male: 28–133 nmol/L
	III	Female: 24–102 nmol/L	Male: 17–160 nmol/L
	IV	Female: 12–126 nmol/L	Male: 12–79 nmol/L
	V	Female: 15–93 nmol/L	Male: 8–49 nmol/L
Sodium (plasma or serum)	0–<1 year	133–142 mmol/L	Urinary sodium should be interpreted in relation to serum sodium
	1–<19 years	135–143 mmol/L	
	≥19 years	135–145 mmol/L	
Sweat chloride	See *Chloride (specimen – sweat)*		
Testosterone (serum)	4 days–<9 years	Female: <2.2 nmol/L	Male: 0.3–10.4 nmol/L
	9–<13 years	Female: <1 nmol/L	Male: <1.2 nmol/L
	13–<15 years	Female: 0.4–1.5 nmol/L	Male: <0.8 nmol/L
	15–<19 years	Female: 0.5–1.7 nmol/L	Male: <15.4 nmol/L
	4 days–<6 months		Male: 1.3–21.9 nmol/L
	6 months–<9 years		Male: 5.12–27.6 nmol/L
	9–<11 years		
	11–<14 years		
	14–<16 years		
	16–<19 years		

Continued

Table 39.1 Clinical Biochemistry (Blood specimens unless otherwise noted)—cont'd

Test Name	Age	Reference Interval/Units		Comments
Sexual maturity rating	I	<1 nmol/L		
	II	<1 nmol/L		
	III	Female: <1 nmol/L	Male: <19 nmol/L	
	IV	Female: <1 nmol/L	Male: <22 nmol/L	
	V	Female: <2 nmol/L	Male: 3–26 nmol/L	
Testosterone, bioavailable (plasma or serum)		Female: 0–0.2 nmol/L	Male: 2–8.6 nmol/L	Alternative test name: Bioavailable testosterone
Thyroglobulin (serum)		Female: 7.82–79.5 ng/mL	Male: 2.99–56 ng/mL	
	0–<2 years	6.47–34.2 ng/mL		
	2–<6 years	5.01–28.5 ng/mL		
	6–<9 years	2.5–25.8 ng/mL		
	9–<19 years			
Thyroid-stimulating hormone (TSH) (serum)	0–<6 days	3.2–19 mIU/L		
	6–<31 days	1.7–9.1 mIU/L		
	31 days–<3 months	0.5–6.3 mIU/L		
	3–<6 months	0.5–4.77 mIU/L		
	6–<1 year	0.61–4.58 mIU/L		
	1–<14 years	0.73–4.09 mIU/L		
	14–<19 years	0.47–4 mIU/L		
Thyrotropin-releasing hormone stimulation test (serum)		Normal: rises by at least 5 mIU/L to peak of 5–20 mIU/L at 20 min, decrease to 2–10 mIU/L by 60 min		Measures TSH

Thyroxine, free (free T_4) (serum)	0–<3 days	12–40.7 pmol/L
	3 days–<1 month	11–40.7 pmol/L
	1–<6 months	10–23 pmol/L
	6 months–<1 year	10–20.4 pmol/L
	1–<19 years	10–17.6 pmol/L
Thyroxine-binding globulin capacity (TBG) (serum)	0–<1 year	315–685 nmol/L
	1–<10 years	278–500 nmol/L
	≥10 years	260–575 nmol/L
Total protein (plasma or serum)	See *Protein (total)*	
Transferrin (serum)	0–<2 months	12.8–27.6 μmol/L
	2 months–<1 year	13.2–39.9 μmol/L
	1–<19 years	27.1–41.5 μmol/L
Triglyceride (plasma or serum)	0–<10 years	<0.85 mmol/L
	10–<19 years	<1.02 mmol/L
	≥19 years	<1.7 mmol/L
Triiodothyonine, free (free T_3) (serum)	4 days–<1 year	3.56–7.48 pmol/L
	1–<12 years	4.29–6.79 pmol/L
	12–<15 years	Female: 3.84–6.06 pmol/L	Male: 4.44–6.65 pmol/L
	15–<19 years	Female: 3.55–5.7 pmol/L	Male: 3.46–5.92 pmol/L
Triiodothyonine (total T_3) (serum)	4 days–<1 year	1.3–3.6 nmol/L
	1–<12 years	1.7–2.9 nmol/L
	12–<15 years	1.5–2.7 nmol/L
	15–<17 years	Female: 1.4–2.2 nmol/L	Male: 1.5–2.40 nmol/L
	17–<19 years	1.6–2.1 nmol/L

Continued

Table 39.1 Clinical Biochemistry (Blood specimens unless otherwise noted)—cont'd

Test Name	Age	Reference Interval/Units	Comments
Troponin I (high sensitivity)	0–<16 days	<968 ng/L	
	16 days–<3 months	<59 ng/L	
	3 months–<19 years	<30.9 ng/L	
Urate (uric acid) (plasma or serum)	0–<15 days	168–751 μmol/L	
	15 days–<1 year	99–377 μmol/L	
	1–<12 years	111–291 μmol/L	
	12–<19 years	Female: 157–350 μmol/L	Male: 160–453 μmol/L
Urea (plasma or serum)	0–<15 days	1.2–8.4 mmol/L	
	15 days–<1 year	1.4–6.2 mmol/L	
	1–<10 years	3.4–8.1 mmol/L	
	10–<19 years	Female: 2.8–7 mmol/L	Male: 2.8–7.7 mmol/L
Uroporphyrin (plasma)		≤35 nmol/L	
Vitamin A (retinol) (plasma or serum)	0–<1 year	0.3–1.9 μmol/L	
	1–<11 years	1–1.6 μmol/L	
	11–<16 years	0.9–1.9 μmol/L	
	16–<19 years	1–2.6 μmol/L	
Vitamin B₆ (pyridoxine) (plasma)		20–96 nmol/L	
Vitamin B₁₂ (serum)	5 days–<1 year	191–1163 pmol/L	
	1–<9 years	209–1190 pmol/L	
	9–<14 years	186–830 pmol/L	
	14–<17 years	180–655 pmol/L	
	17–<19 years	150–599 pmol/L	

Vitamin C (serum)	≥25 μmol/L	Wrap vial in foil to protect from light
Vitamin D, 1,25-hydroxy (plasma or serum)	48–190 pmol/L	
Vitamin D, 25-hydroxy (plasma or serum)	General guidelines: Toxic: >250 nmol/L Optimal: >70 nmol/L Adequate: 50–70 nmol/L Suboptimal: 35–50 nmol/L Deficient: <35 nmol/L	Ranges shown apply to summer months; reference range for winter months are slightly lower
Vitamin E (α-tocopherol) (plasma or serum)	0–<1 year 5–50 μmol/L 1–<19 years 14.5–33 μmol/L	
Xylose (plasma)	2.2–3.7 mmol/L	For investigation of intestinal absorption of xylose
Zinc (plasma)	0–<1 month 9.9–21.4 μmol/L 1–<1 year 9.9–19.9 μmol/L 1–<5 years 10.3–18.1 μmol/L 5–<9 years 11.8–16.4 μmol/L 9–<13 years Female: 12.1–18 μmol/L Male: 11.6–15.4 μmol/L ≥13 years 9.8–20.2 μmol/L	

Laboratory values taken from SickKids Guide to Lab Services and CALIPER data.

HEMATOLOGY

Table 39.2 Hematology (Blood specimen unless otherwise indicated)

Test Name	Age	Reference Interval/Units	Comments
Activated partial thromboplastin time (PTT)	0–<3 months	25–45 seconds	
	≥3 months	24–36 seconds	
Antiphospholipid screen		PNP (Lupus Sensitive aPTT): <47 seconds DRVT screen: <47 seconds DRVT ratio: <1.22	- Alternative test names: Antiphospholipid Antibody Screen, Lupus Anticoagulant Screen - PNP: platelet neutralization procedure - DRVT: Diluted Russell viper venom time
Antithrombin activity (AT III)	≥3 months	0.8–1.2 IU/mL	
Activated protein C (APC) resistance		≥120 seconds	
Complete blood cell count (CBC)			
White blood cell (leukocyte) count	0–<15 days	Female: 8.16–14.56 × 10⁹/L	Male: 8.04–15.40 × 10⁹/L	See WBC differential for reference range for differential components
	15–<30 days	Female: 8.36–14.42 × 10⁹/L	Male: 7.80–15.91 × 10⁹/L	
	31–<61 days	Female: 7.05–14.68 × 10⁹/L	Male: 8.14–14.99 × 10⁹/L	
	61 days–<6 months	Female: 6.00–13.25 × 10⁹/L	Male: 6.51–13.32 × 10⁹/L	
	6 months–<2 years	Female: 6.48–13.02 × 10⁹/L	Male: 5.98–13.51 × 10⁹/L	
	2–<6 years	Female: 4.86–13.80 × 10⁹/L	Male: 5.14–13.38 × 10⁹/L	
	6–<12 years	Female: 4.27–11.40 × 10⁹/L	Male: 4.31–11.00 × 10⁹/L	
	12–<18 years	Female: 4.19–9.43 × 10⁹/L	Male: 3.84–9.84 × 10⁹/L	
	≥18 years	Female: 4.37–9.68 × 10⁹/L	Male: 3.91–8.77 × 10⁹/L	
Hemoglobin (Hb)	0–<15 days	Female: 134–200 g/L	Male: 139–191 g/L	
	15–<31 days	Female: 108–146 g/L	Male: 100–153 g/L	
	31–<61 days	Female: 92–114 g/L	Male: 89–127 g/L	

	Age	Female	Male
	61 days–<6 months	Female: 99–124 g/L	Male: 96–124 g/L
	6 months–<2 years	Female: 102–127 g/L	Male: 101–125 g/L
	2–<6 years	Female: 102–127 g/L	Male: 102–127 g/L
	6–<12 years	Female: 106–132 g/L	Male: 107–134 g/L
	12–<18 years	Female: 108–133 g/L	Male: 110–145 g/L
	≥18 years	Female: 106–135 g/L	Male: 119–154 g/L
Platelet cell count	0–<15 days	Female: 144–449 × 10⁹/L	Male: 218–419 × 10⁹/L
	15–<31 days	Female: 279–571 × 10⁹/L	Male: 248–586 × 10⁹/L
	31–<61 days	Female: 331–597 × 10⁹/L	Male: 229–562 × 10⁹/L
	61 days–<6 months	Female: 247–580 × 10⁹/L	Male: 244–529 × 10⁹/L
	6 months–<2 years	Female: 214–459 × 10⁹/L	Male: 206–445 × 10⁹/L
	2–<6 years	Female: 189–394 × 10⁹/L	Male: 202–403 × 10⁹/L
	6–<12 years	Female: 199–367 × 10⁹/L	Male: 206–369 × 10⁹/L
	12–<18 years	Female: 194–345 × 10⁹/L	Male: 175–332 × 10⁹/L
	≥18 years	Female: 186–353 × 10⁹/L	Male: 151–304 × 10⁹/L
Hematocrit	0–<15 days	Female: 0.396–0.572 L/L	Male: 0.398–0.536 L/L
	15–<31 days	Female: 0.32–0.445 L/L	Male: 0.305–0.45 L/L
	31–<61 days	Female: 0.277–0.351 L/L	Male: 0.268–0.375 L/L
	61 days–<6 months	Female: 0.295–0.371 L/L	Male: 0.286–0.372 L/L
	6 months–<2 year	Female: 0.309–0.379 L/L	Male: 0.308–0.378 L/L
	2–<6 years	Female: 0.312–0.378 L/L	Male: 0.31–0.377 L/L
	6–<12 years	Female: 0.324–0.395 L/L	Male: 0.322–0.398 L/L
	12–<18 years	Female: 0.334–0.404 L/L	Male: 0.339–0.435 L/L
	≥18 years	Female: 0.329–0.412 L/L	Male: 0.362–0.463 L/L

Continued

Table 39.2 Hematology (Blood specimen unless otherwise indicated)—cont'd

Test Name	Age	Reference Interval/Units	Comments
Mean cell hemoglobin (MCH)	0–<15 days	Female: 31.1–35.9 pg Male: 31.3–35.6 pg	
	15–<31 days	Female: 30.4–35.3 pg Male: 29.9–34.1 pg	
	31–<61 days	Female: 28–32.5 pg Male: 27.8–32 pg	
	61 days–<6 months	Female: 24.4–29.5 pg Male: 24.4–28.9 pg	
	6 months–<2 years	Female: 23.2–27.5 pg Male: 22.7–27.2 pg	
	2–<6 years	Female: 23.7–28.6 pg Male: 23.7–28.3 pg	
	6–<12 years	Female: 24.8–29.5 pg Male: 24.9–29.2 pg	
	12–<18 years	Female: 24.8–30.2 pg Male: 25.2–30.2 pg	
	≥18 years	Female: 25.3–30.9 pg Male: 26.5–31.4 pg	
Mean cell hemoglobin concentration (MCHC)	0–<15 days	Female: 334–354 g/L Male: 330–357 g/L	
	15–<31 days	Female: 332–350 g/L Male: 327–351 g/L	
	31–<61 days	Female: 325–349 g/L Male: 323–348 g/L	
	61 days–<6 months	Female: 321–344 g/L Male: 319–344 g/L	
	6 months–<2 years	Female: 319–342 g/L Male: 316–344 g/L	
	2–<6 years	Female: 318–346 g/L Male: 320–347 g/L	
	6–<12 years	Female: 318–346 g/L Male: 322–349 g/L	
	12–<18 years	Female: 315–342 g/L Male: 318–348 g/L	
	≥18 years	Female: 310–341 g/L Male: 319–348 g/L	

Test	Age	Female	Male
Mean cell volume (MCV)	0–<15 days	Female: 92.7–106.4 fL	Male: 91.3–103.1 fL
	15–<31 days	Female: 90.1–103 fL	Male: 89.4–99.7 fL
	31–<61 days	Female: 83.4–96.4 fL	Male: 84.3–94.2 fL
	61 days–<6 months	Female: 74.8–88.3 fL	Male: 74.1–87.5 fL
	6 months–<2 years	Female: 71.3–82.6 fL	Male: 69.5–81.7 fL
	2–<6 years	Female: 72.3–85 fL	Male: 71.3–84 fL
	6–<12 years	Female: 75.9–87.6 fL	Male: 74.4–86.1 fL
	12–<18 years	Female: 76.9–90.6 fL	Male: 76.7–89.2 fL
	≥18 years	Female: 77.7–93.7 fL	Male: 80–93.6 fL
Red blood cells (RBC)	0–<15 days	Female: 4.12–5.74 ×10^{12}/L	Male: 4.1–5.55 ×10^{12}/L
	15–<31 days	Female: 3.32–4.8 ×10^{12}/L	Male: 3.16–4.63 ×10^{12}/L
	31–<61 days	Female: 2.93–3.87 ×10^{12}/L	Male: 3.02–4.22 ×10^{12}/L
	61 days–<6 months	Female: 3.45–4.75 ×10^{12}/L	Male: 3.43–4.8 ×10^{12}/L
	6 months–<2 years	Female: 3.97–5.01 ×10^{12}/L	Male: 4.03–5.07 ×10^{12}/L
	2–<6 years	Female: 3.84–4.92 ×10^{12}/L	Male: 3.89–4.97 ×10^{12}/L
	6–<12 years	Female: 3.9–4.96 ×10^{12}/L	Male: 3.96–5.03 ×10^{12}/L
	12–<18 years	Female: 3.93–4.9 ×10^{12}/L	Male: 4.03–5.29 ×10^{12}/L
	≥18 years	Female: 3.7–4.87 ×10^{12}/L	Male: 4.18–5.48 ×10^{12}/L
Red cell distribution width (RDW-CV)	0–<15 days	Female: 14.6%–17.3%	Male: 14.8%–17%
	15–<31 days	Female: 14.4%–16.2%	Male: 14.3%–16.8%
	31–<61 days	Female: 13.6%–15.8%	Male: 13.8%–16.1%
	61 days–<6 months	Female: 12.2%–14.3%	Male: 12.4%–15.3%
	6 months–2 years	Female: 12.7%–15.1%	Male: 12.9%–15.6%
	2–<6 years	Female: 12.4%–14.9%	Male: 12.5%–14.9%
	6–<12 years	Female: 12.2%–14.4%	Male: 12.3%–14.1%
	12–<18 years	Female: 12.3%–14.6%	Male: 12.4%–14.5%
	≥18 years	Female: 12.4%–15.1%	Male: 12.3%–14.3%

Continued

Table 39.2 Hematology (Blood specimen unless otherwise indicated)—cont'd

Test Name	Age	Reference Interval/Units	Comments
Red cell distribution width (RDW–SD)	0–<15 days	Female: 51.4–65.7 fL Male: 51.0–61.7 fL	
	15–<31 days	Female: 47.2–59.8 fL Male: 46.3–57.3 fL	
	31–<61 days	Female: 43.0–55.0 fL Male: 43.9–52.8 fL	
	61 days–<6 months	Female: 35.2–45.1 fL Male: 35.3–45.7 fL	
	6 months–<2 years	Female: 34.9–42.4 fL Male: 35.3–42.8 fL	
	2–<6 years	Female: 34.9–42.0 fL Male: 35.1–41.7 fL	
	6–<12 years	Female: 35.5–41.8 fL Male: 35.1–41.7 fL	
	12–<18 years	Female: 37.1–44.2 fL Male: 36.7–43.8 fL	
	≥18 years	Female: 38.4–47.7 fL Male: 37.8–46.1 fL	
Mean platelet volume (MPV)	0–<15 days	Female: 10.4–12 fL Male: 10.2–11.9 fL	
	15–<31 days	Female: 10–12.2 fL Male: 10.1–12.1 fL	
	31–<61 days	Female: 9.4–11.1 fL Male: 9.2–10.8 fL	
	61 days–<6 months	Female: 9–10.9 fL Male: 8.9–10.6 fL	
	6 months–<2 years	Female: 8.8–10.6 fL Male: 8.7–10.5 fL	
	2–<6 years	Female: 8.9–11 fL Male: 9–10.9 fL	
	6–<12 years	Female: 9.3–11.3 fL Male: 9.2–11.4 fL	
	12–<18 years	Female: 9.6–11.7 fL Male: 9.6–11.8 fL	
	≥18 years	Female: 9.6–12 fL Male: 9.7–11.9 fL	
D–Dimer, plasma	0–<4 days	≤2.5 mcg/mL FEU	Replaces fibrin degradation products
	4 days–<21 years	≤0.5 mcg/mL FEU	
Erythrocyte sedimentation rate (ESR), whole blood	0–<16 years	2–34 mm/h	
	≥16 years	Female: 2–37 mm/h Male: 2–28 mm/h	

Factor II activity	0–<4 days	0.41–0.73 IU/mL
	4 days–<21 years	0.83–1.47 IU/mL
Factor V activity	0–<4 days	0.64–1.54 IU/mL
	4 days–<21 years	0.71–1.68 IU/mL
Factor VII activity	0–<4 days	0.52–1.07 IU/mL
	4 days–<21 years	0.57–1.59 IU/mL
Factor VIII activity	0–<4 days	0.83–3.29 IU/mL
	4 days–<21 years	0.56–1.72 IU/mL
Factor VIII inhibitor	0–<21 years	<0.5 BU
Factor IX activity	0–<4 days	0.35–0.97 IU/mL
	4 days–<21 years	0.74–1.66 IU/mL
Factor IX inhibitor	0–<21 years	<0.5 BU
Factor X activity	0–<4 days	0.46–0.75 IU/mL
	4 days–<21 years	0.69–1.54 IU/mL
Factor XI activity	0–<4 days	0.07–0.79 IU/mL
	4 days–<21 years	0.63–1.52 IU/mL
Factor XII activity	0–<4 days	0.13–0.97 IU/mL
	4 days–<21 years	0.4–1.49 IU/mL
Factor XIII screen		Normal, abnormal
Factor XIII immunologic testing		0.60–1.69 IU/mL
Factor XIII, Subunit A	≥18 years	0.49–1.54 IU/mL

Continued

Table 39.2 Hematology (Blood specimen unless otherwise indicated)—cont'd

Test Name	Age	Reference Interval/Units	Comments
Fibrinogen	0–<3 months	1.6–4 g/L	
	3 months–<21 years	1.9–4.3 g/L	
Folate, erythrocytes		182–834 nmol/L	
Glucose-6-phosphate dehydrogenase (G6PD), erythrocytes	0–<2 months	7–13 U/g Hb	
	2 months–<19 years	5–11 U/g Hb	
Heinz body preparation, blood		Positive, negative	
Hematocrit (HCT)	See *Complete blood cell count (CBC)*		
Hemoglobin (Hb)	See *Complete blood cell count (CBC)*		
Hemoglobin A$_{1c}$		<6%	Abnormal or variant hemoglobins and hemoglobin F may give falsely elevated levels
Hemoglobin analysis			Tests for HbF, HbA$_2$, HbS, HbC, HbD, HbE, HbH, Hb Bart's
Hemoglobin A	0 days	8.2%–28.5%	
	1–<28 days	3.7%–45.4%	
	28–<61 days	11.8%–81.0%	
	61 days–<4 months	35.6%–98.3%	
	4–<6 months	84.4%–98.3%	
	6 months–<1 year	94.4%–98.3%	
	≥1 year	95.7%–98.3%	

Hemoglobin A$_2$	0 days	0%	
	1–<28 days	0%–0.7%	
	28–<61 days	0%–1.6%	
	61 days–<4 months	0%–2.6%	
	4–<6 months	1.5%–2.6%	
	≥6 months	1.5%–3.5%	
Hemoglobin F	0 days	71.5%–91.8%	
	1–<28 days	54.6%–96.3%	
	28–<61 days	19%–88.2%	
	61 days–<4 months	0.1%–64.4%	
	4–<6 months	0.1%–14.1%	
	6–<12 months	0.1%–4.1%	
	12–<18 months	0.1%–2.9%	
	18–<24 months	0.1%–2.6%	
	2–<3 years	0.1%–1.9%	
	3–<4 years	0.1%–1.8%	
	4–<13 years	0.1%–1.3%	
	≥13 years	0.1%–1.1%	
Hemoglobin electrophoresis	See *Hemoglobin analysis*		
Heparin, low molecular weight	0–<21 years	0.5–1 IU/mL	For Dalteparin, Enoxaprin, Tinzaparin
Heparin, standard		0.35–0.75 IU/mL	
Heparin-induced thrombocytopenia screen		Positive, negative	
International normalized ratio (INR)	0–<3 months	0.9–1.6	
	≥3 months	0.8–1.2	

Continued

Table 39.2 Hematology (Blood specimen unless otherwise indicated)—cont'd

Test Name	Age	Reference Interval/Units	Comments
Isopropanol precipitation test		Positive, negative	For unstable hemoglobin
Kleihauer test		Positive, negative	- Alternative test name: Kleihauer-Betke - To detect fetal cells or HbF-containing cells - Maternal blood is needed if test is for the detection of fetomaternal bleeding
Leukocyte count	See *Complete blood cell count (CBC) for white blood cell (leukocyte) count*		
Lymphocyte count	See *White blood cell (WBC) differential*		
Malarial antigen screen		Positive, negative	- Initial result is for malaria antigen screen and for presence or absence of malaria parasites from thin smear - Thick smear and speciation performed at public health laboratory
Mean cell hemoglobin (MCH)	See *Complete blood cell count (CBC)*		
Mean cell hemoglobin concentration (MCHC)	See *Complete blood cell count (CBC)*		
Mean cell volume (MCV)	See *Complete blood cell count (CBC)*		
Mean platelet volume (MPV)	See *Complete blood cell count (CBC)*		
Monocyte cell count	See *White blood cell (WBC) differential*		
Neutrophil cell count	See *White blood cell (WBC) differential*		

Neutrophil oxidative burst index (NOBI)		Normal: ≥32	Screens for chronic granulomatous disease
			WBC count and differential required
Nucleated cell count		per 100 WBC	See WBC differential, nucleated cells
Partial thromboplastin time (PTT)	See *Activated partial thromboplastin time*		
Platelet aggregation			
ADP (10 μM)	1 month–<21 years	56%–97%	ADP: adenosine diphosphate
ADP (4 μM)	0–<21 years	30%–88%	TRAP: thrombin receptor activated peptide
ADP (2.5 μM)	0–<21 years	25%–97%	
Arachidonic acid 1.6 mM	1 month–<21 years	57%–96%	
Collagen 2.0 mcg/mL	0–<21 years	52%–110%	
Collagen 10.0 mcg/mL	0–<21 years	66%–119%	
Ristocetin 1.5 mg/mL	1 month–<21 years	70%–102%	
Thrombin 1 Unit/mL	0–<21 years	0.29–1.93 nmoles	
TRAP 3.3 μM	0–<21 years	50%–91%	
TRAP 6.0 μM	0–<21 years	50%–91%	
U46619 2 μM	0–<21 years	69%–100%	
Platelet antibodies	See *White blood cell (WBC) antibodies*		
Platelet count	See *Complete blood cell count (CBC)*		

Continued

Table 39.2 Hematology (Blood specimen unless otherwise indicated)—cont'd

Test Name	Age	Reference Interval/Units	Comments
Protein C activity	0–<4 days	0.24–0.51 IU/mL	
	4 days–<1 year	0.28–1.24 IU/mL	
	1–<21 years	0.64–1.77 IU/mL	
Protein C antigen	0–<2 day	0.17–0.53 IU/mL	
	2–<6 days	0.20–0.64 IU/mL	
	6 days–<3 months	0.28–0.8 IU/mL	
	3–<6 months	0.37–0.81 IU/mL	
	6 months–<6 years	0.4–0.92 IU/mL	
	6–<10 years	0.45–0.93 IU/mL	
	10–<16 years	0.55–1.11 IU/mL	
	≥16 years	0.13–1.55 IU/mL	
Protein S free antigen	0–<4 days	0.28–0.67 IU/mL	
	4 days–<1 year	0.29–1.62 IU/mL	
	1–<21 years	0.67–1.94 IU/mL	
Protein S total antigen	0–<21 years	0.13–1.50 IU/mL	
Prothrombin time (PT)	See International normalized ratio (INR)		
Pyruvate kinase (PK), erythrocytes		6.7–14.3 U/g Hb	
Red blood cell count (RBC)	See Complete blood cell count (CBC)		
Reptilase time		<20 seconds	

Reticulocyte count		
	0–<4 days	3.47%–5.4%
	4–<31 days	1.06%–2.37%
	31–<61 days	2.12%–3.47%
	61 days–<6 months	1.55%–2.7%
	6 months–<2 years	0.99%–1.82%
	2–<6 years	0.82%–1.45%
	6–<12 years	0.98%–1.94%
	12–<18 years	0.9%–1.49%
	≥18 years	0.86%–1.36%
Reticulocyte cell count (absolute)		
	0–<4 days	147.5–216.4 ×10⁹/L
	4–<31 days	51.3–110.4 ×10⁹/L
	31–<61 days	51.8–77.9 ×10⁹/L
	61 days–<6 months	48.2–88.2 ×10⁹/L
	6 months–<2 years	43.5–111.1 ×10⁹/L
	2–<6 years	36.4–68.0 ×10⁹/L
	6–<12 years	42.4–70.2 ×10⁹/L
	12–<18 years	41.6–65.1 ×10⁹/L
	≥18 years	39.1–57 ×10⁹/L
Reticulocyte fraction (immature)		
	0–<4 days	30.5%–35.1%
	4–<31 days	14.5%–24.6%
	31–<61 days	19.1%–28.9%
	61 days–<6 months	13.4%–23.3%
	6 months–<2 years	11.4%–25.8%
	2–<6 years	8.4%–21.7%
	6–<12 years	8.9%–24.1%
	12–<18 years	9.0%–18.7%
	≥18 years	9.3%–17.4%

Continued

Table 39.2 Hematology (Blood specimen unless otherwise indicated)—cont'd

Test Name	Age	Reference Interval/Units	Comments
Reticulocyte hemoglobin equivalent	0–<6 months	Female: 29.2–37.5 pg	Male: 27.6–38.7 pg	- Sickle cell screen is not sensitive to low levels of Hb S in infants <6 months of age
	6–<2 years	Female: 30.1–35.7 pg	Male: 28.7–35.7 pg	- For <6 months of age, order hemoglobin analysis
	2–<6 years	Female: 29.3–37.3 pg	Male: 27.7–37.8 pg	
	6–<12 years	Female: 30.4–39.7 pg	Male: 32.4–37.6 pg	
	12–<18 years	Female: 29.9–38.4 pg	Male: 30.3–40.4 pg	
	≥18 years	Female: 30.6–40.7 pg	Male: 36–38.6 pg	
Sickle Cell screen		Positive, negative	
Thrombin time	0–<18 years	<21 seconds	
Von Willebrand factor activity	No pediatric reference ranges		
	Blood group O individuals have lower results than those of other ABO groups		
Von Willebrand factor antigen			
Blood group O		0.47–1.39 IU/mL	
Non–blood group O		0.84–1.92 IU/L	
White blood cell (WBC) differential	Also reported when applicable (×10⁹/L): blasts cell count; metamyelocyte cell count; promyelocyte cell count; atypical lymphocytes		

Test	Age	Female	Male
Neutrophil count	0–<15 days	Female: 1.73–6.75 ×10⁹/L	Male: 1.6–6.06 ×10⁹/L
	15–<31 days	Female: 1.23–4.8 ×10⁹/L	Male: 1.18–5.45 ×10⁹/L
	31–<61 days	Female: 1–4.68 ×10⁹/L	Male: 0.83–4.23 ×10⁹/L
	61 days–<6 months	Female: 1.04–7.02 ×10⁹/L	Male: 0.97–5.45 ×10⁹/L
	6 months–<2 years	Female: 1.27–7.18 ×10⁹/L	Male: 1.19–7.21 ×10⁹/L
	2–<6 year	Female: 1.6–8.29 ×10⁹/L	Male: 1.54–7.92 ×10⁹/L
	6–<12 years	Female: 1.64–7.87 ×10⁹/L	Male: 1.63–7.55 ×10⁹/L
	12–<18 years	Female: 1.82–7.47 ×10⁹/L	Male: 1.54–7.04 ×10⁹/L
	≥18 years	Female: 2–7.15 ×10⁹/L	Male: 1.82–7.42 ×10⁹/L
Lymphocyte count	0–<15 days	Female: 1.75–8 ×10⁹/L	Male: 2.07–7.53 ×10⁹/L
	15–<21 days	Female: 2.42–8.2 ×10⁹/L	Male: 2.11–8.38 ×10⁹/L
	31–<61 days	Female: 2.29–9.14 ×10⁹/L	Male: 2.47–7.95 ×10⁹/L
	61 days–<6 months	Female: 2.14–8.99 ×10⁹/L	Male: 2.45–8.89 ×10⁹/L
	6 months–<2 years	Female: 1.52–8.09 ×10⁹/L	Male: 1.56–7.83 ×10⁹/L
	2–<6 years	Female: 1.25–5.77 ×10⁹/L	Male: 1.13–5.52 ×10⁹/L
	6–<12 years	Female: 1.16–4.28 ×10⁹/L	Male: 0.97–3.96 ×10⁹/L
	12–<18 years	Female: 1.16–3.33 ×10⁹/L	Male: 0.97–3.26 ×10⁹/L
	≥18 years	Female: 1.16–3.18 ×10⁹/L	Male: 0.85–3 ×10⁹/L
Monocyte count	0–<15 days	Female: 0.57–1.72 ×10⁹/L	Male: 0.52–1.77 ×10⁹/L
	15–<31 days	Female: 0.42–1.21 ×10⁹/L	Male: 0.28–1.38 ×10⁹/L
	31–<61 days	Female: 0.28–1.21 ×10⁹/L	Male: 0.28–1.05 ×10⁹/L
	61 days–<6 months	Female: 0.24–1.17 ×10⁹/L	Male: 0.28–1.07 ×10⁹/L
	6 months–<2 years	Female: 0.26–1.08 ×10⁹/L	Male: 0.25–1.15 ×10⁹/L
	2–<6 years	Female: 0.24–0.92 ×10⁹/L	Male: 0.19–0.94 ×10⁹/L
	6–<12 years	Female: 0.19–0.81 ×10⁹/L	Male: 0.19–0.85 ×10⁹/L
	12–<18 years	Female: 0.19–0.72 ×10⁹/L	Male: 0.18–0.78 ×10⁹/L
	≥18 years	Female: 0.29–0.71 ×10⁹/L	Male: 0.19–0.77 ×10⁹/L

Continued

Table 39.2 Hematology (Blood specimen unless otherwise indicated)—cont'd

Test Name	Age	Reference Interval/Units	Comments
Eosinophil count	0–<15 days	Female: 0.09–0.64 ×10⁹/L Male: 0.12–0.66 ×10⁹/L	
	15–<31 days	Female: 0.06–0.75 ×10⁹/L Male: 0.08–0.8 ×10⁹/L	
	31–<61 days	Female: 0.04–0.63 ×10⁹/L Male: 0.05–0.57 ×10⁹/L	
	61 days–<6 months	Female: 0.02–0.74 ×10⁹/L Male: 0.03–0.61 ×10⁹/L	
	6 months–<2 years	Female: 0.02–0.58 ×10⁹/L Male: 0.02–0.82 ×10⁹/L	
	2–<6 years	Female: 0.03–0.46 ×10⁹/L Male: 0.03–0.53 ×10⁹/L	
	6–<12 years	Female: 0.03–0.47 ×10⁹/L Male: 0.03–0.52 ×10⁹/L	
	12–<18 years	Female: 0.02–0.32 ×10⁹/L Male: 0.04–0.38 ×10⁹/L	
	≥18 years	Female: 0.03–0.27 ×10⁹/L Male: 0.03–0.44 ×10⁹/L	
Basophil count	0–<15 days	0.02–0.07 ×10⁹/L 0.02–0.11 ×10⁹/L	
	15–<31 days	0.01–0.06 ×10⁹/L 0.01–0.07 ×10⁹/L	
	31–<61 days	0.01–0.05 ×10⁹/L 0.01–0.07 ×10⁹/L	
	61 days–<6 months	0.01–0.07 ×10⁹/L 0.01–0.06 ×10⁹/L	
	6 months–<6 years	0.01–0.06 ×10⁹/L 0.01–0.06 ×10⁹/L	
	6–<12 years	0.01–0.05 ×10⁹/L 0.01–0.06 ×10⁹/L	
	≥12 years	0.01–0.05 ×10⁹/L 0.01–0.05 ×10⁹/L	
Immature granulocytes (relative)	0–<2 day	0.5%–6.2%	
	2–<91 days	0.2%–4.2%	
	91 days–<6 months	0.0%–0.5%	
	6 months–<2 years	0.0%–0.9%	
	2–<6 years	0.0%–0.8%	
	6–<12 years	0.0%–0.3%	
	12–<18 years	0.0%–0.3%	
	>18 years	0.0%–0.6%	

Immature granulocytes (absolute)	0–<2 day	$0.00–1.46 \times 10^9$/L
	2–<91 days	$0.00–0.61 \times 10^9$/L
	91 days–<6 months	$0.00–0.06 \times 10^9$/L
	6 months–<2 years	$0.00–0.14 \times 10^9$/L
	2–<6 years	$0.00–0.06 \times 10^9$/L
	6–<12 years	$0.00–0.04 \times 10^9$/L
	12–<18 years	$0.00–0.03 \times 10^9$/L
	≥18 years	$0.00–0.09 \times 10^9$/L
Nucleated cell count	1–<4 days	0.1–8.3/100 WBC
	≥4 days	0/100 WBC
White blood cell (WBC) antibodies	Negative	Includes granulocytes, platelets and human leukocyte antigen (HLA) antibodies

Laboratory values taken from SickKids Guide to Lab Services and CALIPER data.

CEREBROSPINAL FLUID

Table 39.3 Cerebrospinal Fluid (CSF) Reference Values

Test Name	Age	Reference Interval/Units	Comments
Amino acids, CSF			
Histidine	0–<1 month	12–71 μmol/L	
	1 month–<7 years	10–38 μmol/L	
	7–<19 years	8–26 μmol/L	
Asparagine	0–<1 month	0–16 μmol/L	
	1 month–<19 years	6–25 μmol/L	
Taurine	0–<1 month	8–23 μmol/L	
	1 month–<5 years	5–16 μmol/L	
	5–<19 years	2–8 μmol/L	
Serine	0–<1 month	35–172 μmol/L	
	1 month–<2 years	33–111 μmol/L	
	2–<19 years	19–71 μmol/L	
Glutamine	0–<1 month	392–1953 μmol/L	
	1 month–<19 years	389–1135 μmol/L	
Arginine	0–<1 month	3–22 μmol/L	
	1 month–<19 years	11–39 μmol/L	
Glycine	0–<1 month	6–19 μmol/L	
	1 month–<5 years	4–42 μmol/L	
	5–<19 years	2–15 μmol/L	

Continued

Glutamate	0–<1 month	1–9 μmol/L
	1 month–<19 years	0–5 μmol/L
Citrulline	0–<1 month	3–9 μmol/L
	1 month–<4 years	2–10 μmol/L
	4–<19 years	0–3 μmol/L
Threonine	0–<1 month	6–19 μmol/L
	1 month–<19 years	4–20 μmol/L
Alanine	0–<1 month	23–82 μmol/L
	1 month–<19 years	15–86 μmol/L
Proline	0–<1 month	1–6 μmol/L
	1 month–<4 years	0–5 μmol/L
	4–<19 years	1–4 μmol/L
Alpha-amino-N-butyric acid	0–<19 years	1–7 μmol/L
Ornithine	0–<1 month	2–42 μmol/L
	1 month–<4 years	3–20 μmol/L
	4–<19 years	2–9 μmol/L
Cystine	0–<19 years	0–1 μmol/L
Lysine	0–<1 month	14–104 μmol/L
	1 month–<19 years	11–40 μmol/L
Tyrosine	0–<1 month	0–43 μmol/L
	1 month–<19 years	5–28 μmol/L
Methionine	0–<1 month	3–17 μmol/L
	1 month–<19 years	1–8 μmol/L

Table 39.3 Cerebrospinal Fluid (CSF) Reference Values—cont'd

Test Name	Age	Reference Interval/Units	Comments
Valine	0–<1 month	15–95 μmol/L	
	1 month–<4 years	9–39 μmol/L	
	4–<19 years	9–29 μmol/L	
Isoleucine	0–<1 month	6–33 μmol/L	
	1 month–<19 years	3–16 μmol/L	
Leucine	0–<1 month	12–51 μmol/L	
	1 month–<19 years	7–21 μmol/L	
Phenylalanine	0–<1 month	8–49 μmol/L	
	1 month–<19 years	6–33 μmol/L	
Tryptophan	0–<1 month	0–8 μmol/L	
	1 month–<4 years	1–10 μmol/L	
	4–<19 years	1–5 μmol/L	
Anti-NMDA receptor IgG antibody, CSF		Negative	Alternative test names: N-methyl-D-aspartate receptor antibodies, Antiglutamate receptor antibodies
Cell count, CSF	0–<29 days	WBC <19 × 10⁶/L	- Includes WBC, RBC, and WBC differential if WBC >10 × 10⁶/L
	29–<57 days	WBC <9 × 10⁶/L	- Bacterial meningitis: neutrophils usually 100–10,000 × 10⁶/L (but may be normal), lymphocytes usually <100 × 10⁶/L
	≥57 days	WBC ≤5 × 10⁶/L	- Viral meningitis: neutrophils usually <100 × 10⁶/L, lymphocytes 10–1000 × 10⁶/L (but may be normal)

Test	Subcategory	Value	Notes
Glucose, CSF		2.1–3.6 mmol/L	Bacterial meningitis: usually <0.4 mmol/L Viral meningitis: usually normal Take serum glucose at same time. CSF glucose should be roughly ⅔ of blood glucose
Lactate, CSF		0–2.4 mmol/L	
Oligoclonal banding, CSF			- Oligoclonal banding can be ordered for children with suspected acute demyelination of the optic nerves, brain, or spinal cord - Alternative test names: Multiple Sclerosis, IgG/Albumin Ratio, CSF IgG, CSF Albumin and CSF Electrophoresis
Albumin, CSF		0.134–0.237 g/L	
Albumin index	18–<31 years	2.7–4.7	
	31–<41 years	2.9–5.1	
	41–<51 years	3.3–5.9	
	51–<61 years	3.8–7.2	
	61–<71 years	3.9–7.3	
IgG, CSF		0.005–0.06 g/L	
IgG index		35–69	
IgG/albumin ratio		<0.250	
Protein, CSF	0–<8 days	0.4–1.2 g/L	- Bacterial meningitis: usually >1 g/L (but may be normal) - Viral meningitis: usually 0.4–1 g/L (but may be normal)
	8–<30 days	0.2–0.7 g/L	
	≥30 days	0.15–0.4 g/L	
Pyruvate, CSF		0.03–0.08 mmol/L	

RBC, Red blood cell; *WBC*, white blood cell.

Laboratory values taken from SickKids Guide to Lab Services.

URINE

Table 39.4   Urine Reference Values

Test Name	Age	Reference Interval/Units		Comments
Albumin, urine	See *Microalbumin*			
Aldosterone, urine		**Na⁺ intake (mmol/day)**	**Aldosterone (nmol/day)**	- Normal salt diet is <25 mmol/day Na⁺
		<25	47–122	- Referred out test; range subject to change
		100–200	16–69	
		>200	0–16	
Amino acids, urine				Random or timed collection
Phosphoserine	0–<3 days	0–6 mmol/mol creatinine		
	3 days–<12 years	1–8 mmol/mol creatinine		
	≥12 years	1–4 mmol/mol creatinine		
Hydroxyproline	0–<3 days	45–421 mmol/mol creatinine		
	3 days–<18 months	2–766 mmol/mol creatinine		
	18 months–<4 years	0–8 mmol/mol creatinine		
	4 years–<12 years	1–7 mmol/mol creatinine		
	≥12 years	0–5 mmol/mol creatinine		
Histidine	0–<3 days	19–144 mmol/mol creatinine		
	3 days–<15 years	40–776 mmol/mol creatinine		
	≥15 years	26–172 mmol/mol creatinine		
Phosphoethanolamine	0–<3 days	0–7 mmol/mol creatinine		
	3 days–<4 years	1–63 mmol/mol creatinine		
	4–<12 years	4–23 mmol/mol creatinine		
	≥12 years	1–11 mmol/mol creatinine		

Asparagine	0–<3 days	0–37 mmol/mol creatinine
	3 days–<13 years	2–132 mmol/mol creatinine
	≥13 years	7–35 mmol/mol creatinine
1-Methylhistidine	0–<3 days	5–85 mmol/mol creatinine
	3 days–<11 years	4–170 mmol/mol creatinine
	≥11 years	1–275 mmol/mol creatinine
Taurine	0–<3 days	330–2764 mmol/mol creatinine
	3 days–<11 years	6–2434 mmol/mol creatinine
	≥11 years	0–130 mmol/mol creatinine
3-Methylhistidine	0–<3 days	29–70 mmol/mol creatinine
	3 days–<6 years	30–107 mmol/mol creatinine
	6–<12 years	22–62 mmol/mol creatinine
	≥12 years	19–62 mmol/mol creatinine
Serine	0–<3 days	0–247 mmol/mol creatinine
	3 days–<3 years	54–723 mmol/mol creatinine
	≥3 years	10–141 mmol/mol creatinine
Glutamine	0–<3 days	0–137 mmol/mol creatinine
	3 days–<4 years	7–576 mmol/mol creatinine
	4–<12 years	47–191 mmol/mol creatinine
	≥12 years	8–116 mmol/mol creatinine
Carnosine	0–<3 days	1–176 mmol/mol creatinine
	3 days–<2 years	3–125 mmol/mol creatinine
	2–<12 years	1–26 mmol/mol creatinine
	≥12 years	1–18 mmol/mol creatinine

Continued

Table 39.4 Urine Reference Values—cont'd

Test Name	Age	Reference Interval/Units	Comments
Arginine	0–<3 days	2–36 mmol/mol creatinine	
	3 days—<2 years	3–33 mmol/mol creatinine	
	≥2 years	1–7 mmol/mol creatinine	
Glycine	0–<3 days	371–1312 mmol/mol creatinine	
	3 days—<6 months	563–2563 mmol/mol creatinine	
	6 months—<14 years	18–733 mmol/mol creatinine	
	≥14 years	23–209 mmol/mol creatinine	
Anserine	0–<3 days	10–67 mmol/mol creatinine	
	3 days—<12 years	3–102 mmol/mol creatinine	
	≥12 years	0–13 mmol/mol creatinine	
Ethanolamine/argininosuccinic acid/saccharopine	0–<3 days	178–931 mmol/mol creatinine	
	3 days—<12 years	44–260 mmol/mol creatinine	
	≥12 years	14–64 mmol/mol creatinine	
Aspartate	0–<3 days	2–49 mmol/mol creatinine	
	3 days—<12 years	1–68 mmol/mol creatinine	
	≥12 years	0–4 mmol/mol creatinine	
Sarcosine	0–<12 years	0–17 mmol/mol creatinine	
	≥12 years	0–15 mmol/mol creatinine	
Glutamate	0–<3 days	1–220 mmol/mol creatinine	
	3 days—<12 years	1–88 mmol/mol creatinine	
	≥12 years	0–21 mmol/mol creatinine	

Citrulline	0–<3 days	10–26 mmol/mol creatinine
	3 days–<3 years	1–41 mmol/mol creatinine
	≥3 years	1–3 mmol/mol creatinine
Beta-alanine	0–<3 days	1–24 mmol/mol creatinine
	3 days–<10 years	6–89 mmol/mol creatinine
	≥10 years	2–10 mmol/mol creatinine
Threonine	0–<3 days	1–388 mmol/mol creatinine
	3 days–<12 years	13–728 mmol/mol creatinine
	≥12 years	5–39 mmol/mol creatinine
Alanine	0–<3 days	48–206 mmol/mol creatinine
	3 days–<1 year	32–454 mmol/mol creatinine
	1–<12 years	27–233 mmol/mol creatinine
	≥12 years	10–90 mmol/mol creatinine
GABA/homocitrulline	0–<3 days	0–15 mmol/mol creatinine
	3 days–<5 years	1–19 mmol/mol creatinine
	≥5 years	1–10 mmol/mol creatinine
Alpha-aminoadipic acid	0–<3 days	6–49 mmol/mol creatinine
	3 days–<4 years	19–111 mmol/mol creatinine
	4–<10 years	9–43 mmol/mol creatinine
	10–<15 years	1–24 mmol/mol creatinine
	≥15 years	2–11 mmol/mol creatinine
Proline	0–<3 days	3–191 mmol/mol creatinine
	3 days–<12 years	4–269 mmol/mol creatinine
	≥12 years	1–14 mmol/mol creatinine

Continued

Table 39.4 Urine Reference Values—cont'd

Test Name	Age	Reference Interval/Units	Comments
Beta-aminoisobutyric acid	0–<3 days	2–33 mmol/mol creatinine	
	3 days–<6 years	2–317 mmol/mol creatinine	
	6–<15 years	3–136 mmol/mol creatinine	
	≥15 years	3–34 mmol/mol creatinine	
Hydroxylsine 1	0–<12 years	0–3 mmol/mol creatinine	
	≥12 years	0–4 mmol/mol creatinine	
Hydroxylsine 2	0–<3 days	6–20 mmol/mol creatinine	
	3 days–<12 years	1–65 mmol/mol creatinine	
	≥12 years	0–5 mmol/mol creatinine	
Alpha-amino-N-butyric acid	0–<3 days	3–9 mmol/mol creatinine	
	3 days–<5 years	1–35 mmol/mol creatinine	
	5–<12 years	1–8 mmol/mol creatinine	
	≥12 years	1–7 mmol/mol creatinine	
Cystathionine	0–<3 days	4–32 mmol/mol creatinine	
	3 days–<12 years	2–80 mmol/mol creatinine	
	≥12 years	0–10 mmol/mol creatinine	
Ornithine	0–<3 days	1–61 mmol/mol creatinine	
	3 days–<12 years	2–57 mmol/mol creatinine	
	≥12 years	1–2 mmol/mol creatinine	

Cystine	0–<3 days	1–85 mmol/mol creatinine
	3 days–<12 years	3–123 mmol/mol creatinine
	≥12 years	4–31 mmol/mol creatinine
Lysine	0–<3 days	0–172 mmol/mol creatinine
	3 days–<12 years	4–408 mmol/mol creatinine
	≥12 years	3–96 mmol/mol creatinine
Tyrosine	0–<3 days	3–39 mmol/mol creatinine
	3 days–<12 years	8–125 mmol/mol creatinine
	≥12 years	3–14 mmol/mol creatinine
Methionine	0–<3 days	1–36 mmol/mol creatinine
	3 days–<12 years	1–25 mmol/mol creatinine
	≥12 years	0–3 mmol/mol creatinine
Valine	0–<3 days	1–29 mmol/mol creatinine
	3 days–<10 years	5–67 mmol/mol creatinine
	≥10 years	3–11 mmol/mol creatinine
Isoleucine	0–<4 years	2–18 mmol/mol creatinine
	4–<12 years	2–6 mmol/mol creatinine
	≥12 years	1–5 mmol/mol creatinine
Alloisoleucine		Not detected
Leucine	0–<3 days	2–36 mmol/mol creatinine
	3 days–<12 years	3–51 mmol/mol creatinine
	≥12 years	2–8 mmol/mol creatinine

Continued

Table 39.4 Urine Reference Values—cont'd

Test Name	Age	Reference Interval/Units	Comments
Phenylalanine	0–<12 years	6–67 mmol/mol creatinine	
	≥12 years	3–11 mmol/mol creatinine	
Tryptophan	0–<4 years	3–10 mmol/mol creatinine	
	4–<12 years	6–64 mmol/mol creatinine	
	≥12 years	3–10 mmol/mol creatinine	
Barbiturates screen, urine		<200 mcg/L (Negative)	
β₂-Microglobulin, urine		Female: 0–212 mcg/L	Male: 0–300 mcg/L
β₂-Microglobulin/creatinine ratio, urine		0–29 mcg/mmol creatinine	
Calcium/citrate ratio (24 h collection), urine	2–<7 years	Female: 0.14–2 mmol/mmol	Male: 0.24–2.3 mmol/mmol	- Median (5%–95% reported) - Increased risk of stone formation $U_{Ca/Citr}$ ≥1.6 mmol/mmol (can apply to spot or timed collection)
	7–<13 years	Female: 0.19–2.3 mmol/mmol	Male: 0.24–2.9 mmol/mmol
	13–<18 years	Female: 0.24–2.9 mmol/mmol	Male: 0.29–3.8 mmol/mmol
Calcium/creatinine ratio (spot), urine	0–<1 year	<2.2 mmol/mmol	Values represent 95th percentile
	1–<3 years	<1.5 mmol/mmol	
	3–<5 years	<1.1 mmol/mmol	
	5–<8 years	<0.8 mmol/mmol	
	≥8 years	<0.7 mmol/mmol	
Calcium (24 h collection), urine		<0.1 mmol/kg/day	

Catecholamines, free, urine			
Norepinephrine	0–<2 years	280 (375) μmol/mol creatinine	- Values represent 95th percentile (100th centile in parentheses)
	2–<5 years	80 (150) μmol/mol creatinine	- Drugs, such as methyldopa, hydralazine (Apresoline), quinidine, and epinephrine,
	5–<10 years	60 (90) μmol/mol creatinine	norepinephrine-related drugs (e.g., L-dopa), and renal function test dyes may
	10–<20 years	55 (60) μmol/mol creatinine	interfere with catecholamine excretion and affect results
	≥20 years	76 (90) μmol/mol creatinine	- Sample not acceptable if urine pH >3.0
Epinephrine	0–<2 years	45 (150) μmol/mol creatinine	
	2–<5 years	35 (60) μmol/mol creatinine	
	5–<10 years	20 (40) μmol/mol creatinine	
	10–<20 years	20 (70) μmol/mol creatinine	
	≥20 years	14 (50) μmol/mol creatinine	
Dopamine	0–<2 years	2220 (3480) μmol/mol creatinine	
	2–<5 years	1130 (2230) μmol/mol creatinine	
	5–<10 years	770 (990) μmol/mol creatinine	
	10–<20 years	400 (510) μmol/mol creatinine	
	≥20 years	400 (580) μmol/mol creatinine	
Citrate (24 h collection, bovine serum albumin [BSA] normalization), urine	2–<7 years	Female: > 1.13 mmol/1.73 m² Male: >0.92 mmol/1.73 m²	- Values represent 5th percentile - Hypocitraturia (females): <1.3 mmol/1.73 m²/day
	7–<13 years	Female: > 1.32 mmol/1.73 m² Male: >0.84 mmol/1.73 m²	- Hypocitraturia (males): <0.94 mmol/1.73 m²/day
	13–<18 years	Female: > 1.29 mmol/1.73 m² Male: >0.68 mmol/1.73 m²	
Citrate (24 h collection, weight), urine	2–<7 years	Female: >0.027 mmol/kg Male: >0.046 mmol/kg	Values represent 5th percentile
	7–<13 years	Female: >0.026 mmol/kg Male: >0.016 mmol/kg	
	13–<18 years	Female: >0.021 mmol/kg Male: >0.011 mmol/kg	

Continued

Table 39.4 Urine Reference Values—cont'd

Test Name	Age	Reference Interval/Units	Comments
Citrate/creatinine ratio (spot, urine)	2–<7 years	Female: >0.17 mmol/mmol	Male: >0.14 mmol/mmol	- Values represent 5th percentile
	7–<13 years	Female: >0.15 mmol/mmol	Male: >0.08 mmol/mmol	- Hypocitraturia = citrate/creatinine ratio <0.1 mmol/mmol
	13–<18 years	Female: >0.13 mmol/mmol	Male: >0.053 mmol/mmol	
Copper (random), urine		0.04–0.19 µmol/L	
Copper (timed), urine		0.06–0.28 µmol/day	
Cortisol, free (24 h collection), urine	4 months–<11 years	0–73 nmol/day	
	11–<21 years	0–151 nmol/day	
	≥21 years	10–160 nmol/day	
Creatinine, urine		Reference value not applicable	Random, timed, or 24-h collection Specify specimen collection period
Creatinine clearance, urine (24 h collection)	0–<8 days	0.29–1.38 mL/s/1.73 m²	
	8–<30 days	0.92–1.38 mL/s/1.73 m²	
	30 days–<6 months	1.15–2.07 mL/s/1.73 m²	
	≥6 months	1.5–2.76 mL/s/1.73 m²	
Cystine (24 h collection, BSA normalized), urine	0–<10 years	<55 µmol/1.73 m²/day	
	10–<18 years	<200 µmol/1.73 m²/day	
	≥18 years	<250 µmol/1.73 m²/day	
Cystine (24 h collection, weight), urine	0–<10 years	6–48 µmol/day	
	10–<14 years	10–94 µmol/day	
	14–<18 years	17–102 µmol/day	
	≥18 years	24–184 µmol/day	

Cystine/creatinine ratio (spot), urine	0–<1 month	<85 mmol/mol	
	1–<7 months	<53 mmol/mol	
	≥7 months	<18 mmol/mol	
Drug screen, urine		Not detected, positive	- Drugs tested in broad spectrum urine drug screen are laboratory dependent
Eosinophil, urine		Negative, positive	
Glycerate/creatinine ratio (spot), urine	0–<6 years	<0.19 mmol/mmol	
	≥6 years	<0.123 mmol/mmol	
Glycolate/creatinine ratio (spot), urine	0–<1 year	<0.07 mmol/mmol	
	1–<5 years	<0.091 mmol/mmol	
	5–<12 years	<0.046 mmol/mmol	
	≥12 years	<0.04 mmol/mmol	
Glyoxolate (24 h collection, BSA normalized), urine		<0.5 mmol/1.73 m²/day	
HOG/creatinine ratio (spot)	Adults	<2.8 μmol/mmol	HOG: 4-hydroxy-2-oxoglutarate
Homovanillic acid (HVA), urine	0–<1 year	≤20 mmol/mol creatinine	Random or timed sample
	1–<2 years	≤17 mmol/mol creatinine	
	2–<5 years	≤14 mmol/mol creatinine	
	5–<10 years	≤9 mmol/mol creatinine	
	10–<20 years	≤8 mmol/mol creatinine	
	≥20 years	≤5 mmol/mol creatinine	

Continued

Table 39.4 Urine Reference Values—cont'd

Test Name	Age	Reference Interval/Units	Comments
Human chorionic gonadotropin screen, urine (β-HCG screen)		Negative	
5-Hydroxyindoleacetic acid		<50 µmol/day	
Iron (random), urine		0.02–0.24 µmol/L	
Iron (timed), urine		0.05–0.36 µmol/day	
Ketones, urine		Negative, positive	
Magnesium (12 hour collection), urine	5–<7 years 7–<9 years 9–<11 years 11–<13 years	<0.1 mmol/kg <0.11 mmol/kg <0.08 mmol/kg <0.07 mmol/kg	Hypermagnesuria (24 h urine): >0.2 mmol/kg/day
Magnesium/creatinine ratio (spot), urine	1 month–<1 year 1–<2 years 2–<3 years 3–<5 years 5–<7 years 7–<10 years 10–<14 years 14–<18 years	<2.2 mmol/mmol <1.7 mmol/mmol <1.6 mmol/mmol <1.3 mmol/mmol <1 mmol/mmol <0.9 mmol/mmol <0.7 mmol/mmol <0.6 mmol/mmol	
Mercury (random), urine		0–15 nmol/L	
Mercury (timed), urine		0–19.9 nmol/day	

Metanephrines, urine	0–<2 year	≤2.8 mmol/mol creatinine	
	2–<9 years	≤1.9 mmol/mol creatinine	
	9–<15 years	≤1.2 mmol/mol creatinine	
	≥15 years	≤0.6 mmol/mol creatinine	
Microalbumin (timed), urine		0–15.1 mcg/min	
Microalbumin/creatinine ratio (timed), urine		<3.5 mg/mmol	
Mucopolysaccharides screen, urine		Normal, abnormal, inconclusive	- Normal result does not rule out all mucopolysaccharidoses
Myoglobin, urine		Negative	- Reacts like hemoglobin on dipstick; confirmatory tests available
Nickel (random), urine		0–59.6 nmol/L	
Nickel (timed), urine		0–85.2 nmol/day	
Nitroprusside, urine		Negative, positive	Screen for cystinuria
Oligosaccharides, urine		Normal, abnormal, inconclusive	
Organic acids screen, urine		Normal, abnormal	
Orotic acid, urine	0–<15 days	1.4–5.3 mmol/mol creatinine	
	15 days–<1 year	1–3.2 mmol/mol creatinine	
	1–<10 years	0.5–3.3 mmol/mol creatinine	
	≥10 years	0.4–1.2 mmol/mol creatinine	

Continued

Table 39.4 Urine Reference Values—cont'd

Test Name	Age	Reference Interval/Units		Comments
Osmolality	24 h, average fluid intake	300–900 mmol/kg H$_2$O		
	Random urine depending on fluid intake	50–1200 mmol/kg H$_2$O		
Oxalate (24-h collection, BSA normalized), urine		<0.5 mmol/1.73 m²/day		24-h excretion is more accurate beyond 2 years of age
Oxalate (timed), urine	0–<17 years	161–483 μmol/day	Male: 92–564 μmol/day	
	≥17 years	Female: 46–368 μmol/day		
Oxalate/creatinine ratio (spot), urine	1–<6 months	<0.22 mmol/mmol		- Values represent 95th percentile
	6 months–<1 year	<0.17 mmol/mmol		- Oxalate/creatinine ratios are higher in premature infants than term infants
	1–<2 years	<0.13 mmol/mmol		
	2–<3 years	<0.1 mmol/mmol		
	3–<5 years	<0.08 mmol/mmol		
	5–<7 years	<0.07 mmol/mmol		
	7–<18 years	<0.06 mmol/mmol		
pH, urine		5–9		
Porphobilinogen (quantitative), urine		≤9 μmol/day		
Porphyrins, quantitative (random), urine				- Protect from light—collect in dark bottle or wrap container with foil
Coproporphyrin I		0.3–8.5 μmol/mol		- Screening tests are of value only during

Coproporphyrin III/I ratio	2.6–5.3	
Heptacarboxylic acid	≤1.3 µmol/mol	
Hexacarboxylic acid	≤0.7 µmol/mol	- Urine porphobilinogen may be increased between and during attacks of acute intermittent porphyria
Uroporphyrin I	0.4–3.9 µmol/mol	- Porphyrinuria may also occur in lead poisoning, liver disease, and conditions of increased erythropoiesis
Uroporphyrin III	≤2 µmol/mol	
Porphyrins, quantitative (timed), urine		- Specimens must be protected from light and at 4°C during the 24 h collection
Coproporphyrin I	5–90 nmol/day	
Coproporphyrin III	15–242 nmol/day	
Heptacarboxylic acid	≤16 nmol/day	
Hexacarboxylic acid	≤2 nmol/day	
Uroporphyrin III	≤20 nmol/day	
Potassium, urine	Not applicable on random urine	Depends on intake
Protein/creatinine ratio (random), urine 0–<2 years	<50 mg/mmol	Nephrotic range >200 mg/mmol
≥2 years	<20 mg/mmol	
Sodium, urine	Not applicable on random urine	Depends on intake
Specific gravity	1.005–1.035	
Sulfatides, urine	≤170 mcg/L	
Sulfocysteine (random), urine	≤15 mmol/mol creatinine	

Continued

Table 39.4   Urine Reference Values—cont'd

Test Name	Age	Reference Interval/Units	Comments
Urate/creatinine ratio (12-h collection), urine	5–<7 years	0.32–0.72 mmol/mmol	Values represent 2.5–5th percentile
	7–<9 years	0.25–0.77 mmol/mmol	
	9–<11 years	0.21–0.64 mmol/mmol	
	11–<13 years	0.17–0.51 mmol/mmol	
Urate/creatinine ratio (spot, urine)	1–<7 months	<1.6 mmol/mmol	Values represent 95th percentile
	7 months–<1 year	<1.5 mmol/mmol	
	1–<2 years	<1.4 mmol/mmol	
	2–<3 years	<1.3 mmol/mmol	
	3–<5 years	<1.1 mmol/mmol	
	5–<7 years	<0.8 mmol/mmol	
	7–<10 years	<0.56 mmol/mmol	
	10–<14 years	<0.44 mmol/mmol	
	14–<18 years	<0.4 mmol/mmol	
Urate (12-h collection, BSA normalized)	5–<7 years	0.9–2.4 mmol/1.73 m²/day	- Values represent 2.5–97.5th percentile
	7–<9 years	0.8–3 mmol/1.73 m²/day	- Hyperuricosuria: >5 mmol/1.73 m²/day (>1 year)
	9–<11 years	0.8–3.9 mmol/1.73 m²/day	
	11–<13 years	0.7–2.3 mmol/1.73 m²/day	
Urate (24-h collection), urine	3–<6 years	<0.14 mmol/kg/day	Hyperuricosuria: >0.11 mmol/kg/day
	6–<9 years	<0.07 mmol/kg/day	
	9–<12 years	<0.13 mmol/kg/day	
	12–<15 years	<0.06 mmol/kg/day	
	15–<17 years	<0.07 mmol/kg/day	

Analyte	Age	Reference value	Comments
Vanillylmandelic acid (VMA) (random), urine	0–<1 year 1–<2 years 2–<5 years 5–<20 years ≥20 years	≤14 mmol/mol creatinine ≤11 mmol/mol creatinine ≤6.5 mmol/mol creatinine ≤5 mmol/mol creatinine ≤3.5 mmol/mol creatinine	- Random collection less satisfactory than 24-h collection - For small babies, try pooling multiple and send as one random sample
Vanillylmandelic acid (VMA) (timed), urine	0–<1 year 1–<2 years 2–<5 years 5–<10 years 10–<20 years ≥20 years	≤14 µmol/day ≤12 µmol/day ≤15 µmol/day ≤18 µmol/day ≤30 µmol/day ≤34 µmol/day	Nonspecific elevations occur in fever, asthma, chronic anemia, or after surgery

Laboratory values taken from SickKids Guide to Lab Services.

STOOL

Table 39.5 Stool Reference Values

Test Name	Age/Sex	Reference Interval/Units	Comments
α_1-Antitrypsin clearance, stool and serum		<27 mL/day	
APT test (Alkali Denaturation Test), stool, gastric aspirate, vomit		Presence or absence of fetal or maternal cells	Must be bright red blood if present (fetal or maternal red blood cells [RBCs])
Calprotectin, stool		<50 mcg/g	
Fat, stool	Premature infants	<0.2	3- or 5-day stool collection required
	Term infants	<0.15	Accurate account of dietary fat necessary during period of stool collection
	≥3 months	<0.1	Regular fat study measures only amount of long chain fatty acids in stool
			Reported as fraction of intake
Fecal elastase, stool		>200 mcg/g stool	
Occult blood, stool		Negative	Qualitative study; detected when there are 4 mL whole blood per 100 g feces (i.e., 6 mg Hb/g feces)
			Alternative test name: Hemoglobin, stool

Porphyrin quantitation (random), stool	
Coproporphyrin I	<13 nmol/g
Coproporphyrin III	<12 nmol/g
Deuteroporphyrin	<14 nmol/g
Heptacarboxylic acid	<1 nmol/g
Hexacarboxylic acid	<1 nmol/g
Mesoporphyrin	<6 nmol/g
Pentacarboxylic acid	<1 nmol/g
Protoporphyrin	<38 nmol/g
Uroporphyrin I	<5 nmol/g
Uroporphyrin III	<1 nmol/g

Laboratory values taken from SickKids Guide to Lab Services.

THERAPEUTIC DRUG MONITORING

Table 39.6   Therapeutic Drug Monitoring, Blood Specimens (See Table 40.2 for information about sampling time and other considerations)

Test Name	Therapeutic Range and Critical Values	Comments
Amikacin (q8h dosing or extended dosing for renal impairment)		
Trough	Trough therapeutic range: 2.5–10 mg/L Critical for trough: >10 mg/L	
Peak	Peak therapeutic range: 20–35 mg/L Critical for peak: >35 mg/L	
Busulfan	Therapeutic range: Time/dose dependent	
Caffeine	Therapeutic range: 30–100 μmol/L	
Carbamazepine	Therapeutic range: 17–50 μmol/L Critical for trough: >63 μmol/L	Alternative name: Tegretol
Carbamazepine epoxide	Therapeutic range: 5–12 μmol/L	
Cyclosporine	Therapeutic range: Transplant Liver: 92–425 mcg/L Renal: 92–235 mcg/L Heart: 50–300 mcg/L	

Digoxin	Bone Marrow Transplant (BMT)—Malignant Related: 100–150 mcg/L Unrelated 150–200 mcg/L BMT—Nonmalignant Related: 175–200 mcg/L Unrelated: 175–200 mcg/L Critical: >500 mcg/L	
Digoxin, free	Therapeutic range: 1–2.5 nmol/L Critical: >3.5 nmol/L	
Ethosuximide	Therapeutic range: 0.8–2 nmol/L	Alternative name: Zarontin
Gentamicin (q8h dosing or extended dosing for renal impairment)	Therapeutic range: 280–710 μmol/L Critical: >1060 μmol/L	
Trough	Trough therapeutic range: 0.6–2 mg/L Critical for trough: >2 mg/L	
Peak	Peak therapeutic range: 5–10 mg/L Critical for peak: >10 mg/L	
Lithium	Therapeutic range: 0.5–1.3 mmol/L Critical: >1.5 mmol/L	
Lamotrigine	Therapeutic range: 4–39 μmol/L	Alternative name: Lamictal
Methotrexate	Protocol dependent	

Continued

Table 39.6 — Therapeutic Drug Monitoring, Blood Specimens (See Table 40.2 for information about sampling time and other considerations)—cont'd

Test Name	Therapeutic Range and Critical Values	Comments
Mycophenolic acid	Protocol dependent Critical: 10 mg/L	
Phenobarbital	Therapeutic range: 65–170 μmol/L Critical: >225 μmol/L	
Phenytoin	Therapeutic range: 40–80 μmol/L Critical: >85 μmol/L	Alternative name: Dilantin
Phenytoin, free	Therapeutic range: 4–8 μmol/L	
Primidone	Therapeutic range: 23–55 μmol/L Critical: >70 μmol/L	Alternative name: Mysoline
Sirolimus	Therapeutic range: 5–15 mcg/L Critical: >15 mcg/L	Alternative name: Rampamycin
Tacrolimus	Therapeutic range: 5–15 mcg/L Critical: >15 mcg/L	Alternative name: FK506
Theophylline	Therapeutic range: 55–110 μmol/L Critical: >110 μmol/L	
Thiopurine metabolites	Therapeutic range 6-Thioguanine (6-TG): 450–750 pmol/8 × 10⁸ red blood cell (RBC)	

Tobramycin (q8h dosing or extended dosing for renal impairment)	
Trough	Trough therapeutic range: 0.6–2 mg/L Critical for trough: >2 mg/L
Peak	Peak therapeutic range: 5–10 mg/L Critical for peak: >10 mg/L
Valproate	Therapeutic range: 350–700 μmol/L Critical: >1000 μmol/L
Valproate, free	Therapeutic range: 35–70 μmol/L
Vancomycin	
Trough	Trough therapeutic range: 5–12 mg/L Critical for trough: >20 mg/L
Peak	Peak therapeutic range: 25–40 mg/L Critical for peak: >40 mg/L
Voriconazole	Therapeutic range: 1–5 mg/L Critical: >6 mg/L

Laboratory values taken from SickKids Guide to Lab Services.

TOXICOLOGY

Table 39.7 Toxicology (Blood specimens unless otherwise indicated; Also see Chapter 3 Poisonings and Toxicology for further information)

Test Name	Toxic Cutoff/Units	Comments
Acetaminophen (plasma or serum)	Therapeutic: 66–199 μmol/L Toxic cutoff at 4 h: >1300 μmol/L Toxic cutoff at 8 h: >650 μmol/L Toxic cutoff at 12 h: >300 μmol/L	- Refer to Rumak-Matthew nomogram for toxicity levels (see Figure 3.1) - In overdose situation, draw sample anytime
Acetone (serum)	≥2 mmol/L	
Barbiturates/Sedative screen (serum)		
Amobarbital	>40 μmol/L	Also known as Amytal
Barbital	>320 μmol/L	
Butabarbital	>45 μmol/L	Also known as Butisol
Butalbital	>45 μmol/L	Also known as Fiorinal
Glutethimide	>45 μmol/L	Also known as Doriden
Meprobamate	>450 μmol/L	Also known as Miltown
Methaqualone	>20 μmol/L	Also known as Quaalude
Methyprylon	>160 μmol/L	Also known as Noludar
Pentobarbital	>40 μmol/L	Also known as Nembutal

Phenobarbital	See *Phenobarbital*	
Secobarbital	>30 μmol/L	Also known as Seconal
Benzodiazepine screen (serum, urine)	Not detected	
Diethylene glycol (serum)	>1 mmol/L	
Drug screen (serum)		- Drugs tested in broad spectrum blood drug screen are laboratory dependent - Order relevant specific drug levels individually
Drug screen (urine)		- Useful for detecting drugs in overdose situations, suicide intent, accidental poisoning and for street drugs - Drugs tested in broad spectrum urine drug screen are laboratory dependent
Ethanol (serum)	Abnormal: ≥2 mmol/L Toxic cutoff: >21 mmol/L	
Ethylene glycol (serum)	Abnormal: >2.5 mmol/L Toxic cutoff: >4.8 mmol/L	
Formic acid (serum)	Abnormal: >0.5 mmol/L Toxic cutoff: >3.3 mmol/L	Toxic metabolite of methanol
γ-Hydroxybutyrate (GHB) (serum)	Not detected, positive	
Isopropanol (plasma or serum)	Abnormal: ≥2.5 mmol/L Toxic cutoff: >6.7 mmol/L	Also known as Rubbing Alcohol
Lithium (serum)	Abnormal: >1.3 mmol/L Toxic cutoff: >1.5 mmol/L	

Continued

Table 39.7 **Toxicology** (Blood specimens unless otherwise indicated; Also see Chapter 3 Poisonings and Toxicology for further information)—cont'd

Test Name	Toxic Cutoff/Units	Comments
Methanol (serum)	Abnormal: ≥2 mmol/L Toxic cutoff: >6.2 mmol/L	Also known as Wood Alcohol, Windshield Washer fluid
Phenobarbital (serum)	Therapeutic range: 65–170 µmol/L Toxic cutoff: >225 µmol/L	Trough 0–60 min before next dose
Propylene glycol (serum)	≥2.5 mmol/L	
Salicylate (ASA, aspirin) (plasma or serum)	Therapeutic: 0.2–2 mmol/L Toxic cutoff: >2.9 mmol/L	
Trichloroethanol (TCE) (plasma or serum)	Abnormal: ≥2.5 mg/L Toxic cutoff: >40 mg/L	Metabolite of chloral hydrate
Tricyclic screen (plasma or serum)	Not detected	Identification of tricyclic antidepressants—included in the broad spectrum drug screen
Volatile screen (serum)		Includes ethanol, methanol (wood alcohol, windshield washer fluid), isopropanol (rubbing alcohol), acetone

Laboratory values taken from SickKids Guide to Lab Services.

BLOOD PRODUCTS

Table 39.8 Blood Components

Blood Components	Indications	Dosage	Description	Preparation Time	Infusion Instructions	Special Precautions
Red cell concentrate (prestorage leuko-reduced by filtration)	To correct inadequate tissue O₂ delivery. Dedicated unit for neonates birth weight <1000 g	10–15 mL/kg (increase Hb by 20–30 g/L), 10–20 mL/kg	Volume approximately 300 mL/unit	- Uncrossmatched, 5 min (physician request only) - Urgent: 45 min - Routine: average 2 h, can be 4–6 h	- Use blood filter - Transfuse within 4 h after issue	- Crossmatch required - Must be ABO compatible
FP (frozen plasma)	- Severe liver disease, coagulopathy and bleeding - DIC and bleeding - Massive and exchange transfusions	10–15 mL/kg	- Contains all coagulation factors and complement - Approximately 250–290 mL	Urgent: 30 min Routine: 1–2 h	- Use blood filter - Transfuse within 4 h after issue	Should be ABO compatible
Octaplasma/solvent/detergent (SD) treated plasma	TTP/HUS and allergic reactions to plasma	10–15 mL/kg	200 mL	Urgent: 30 min Routine: 1–2 h	- Use blood filter - Transfuse within 4 h after issue	Should be ABO compatible
Cryoprecipitate	- Hypofibrinogenemia and bleeding (fibrinogen <1 g/L) - Massive hemorrhage (fibrinogen <1.5–2.0 g/L)	- 1 unit/10 kg (raises fibrinogen 0.5 g) - Maximum 10 units/dose	- Approximate volume 5–15 mL - Contains fibrinogen (average, 200 mg/unit), F VIII, vWF, F XIII	Urgent: 30 min Routine: 1–2 h	- Use blood filter or IV push filter - Transfuse within 4 h after issue	

Continued

Table 39.8 Blood Components—cont'd

Blood Components	Indications	Dosage	Description	Preparation Time	Infusion Instructions	Special Precautions
Cryo-free FP (Cryosupernatant)	Plasma infusion or plasma exchange for TTP	10–50 mL/kg	- Plasma deficient in high-molecular-weight multimers of vWF - Approximately 270 mL	Urgent: 30 min Routine: 1–2 h	- Use blood filter - Transfuse within 4 h of issue	Should be ABO compatible
Platelet concentrates	- Bleeding from thrombocytopenia or platelet function abnormality - Prophylaxis for platelet count <10 ×10⁹/L - Prophylaxis for invasive procedures when platelet count <50 ×10⁹/L - HLA-matched SDP for patients refractory to BC because of HLA antibodies	Neonates: 10–15 mL/kg Others: 5–10 mL/kg, up to 300 mL (adult dose)	- Available as BC (300 mL), or SDP (250 mL) - One SDP product is equivalent to BC pool of 4	Urgent: 30 min Routine: 1–2 h 48 h notice usually required by issuing laboratory	- Use blood filter or IV push filter - Transfuse within 4 h of issue	- Should be ABO compatible - 5–10 mL/kg raises platelet count by 15–25 ×10⁹/L at 1 h (10–60 min) posttransfusion - Investigate for immune refractoriness if platelet increment <7.5 ×10⁹/L
Albumin	- Volume expansion/ resuscitation - Therapeutic apheresis - Hypoalbuminemia	0.5–1 g/kg/dose maximum 6 g/kg/day	Albumin 5% - 2.5 g (50 mL) - 12.5 g (250 mL) - 25 g (500 mL) Albumin 25% - 12.5 g (50 mL); 25 g (100 mL)	Issued on demand	No filter required	Order in g and mL

BC, Buffy coat; DIC, disseminated intravascular coagulation; HLA, human leukocyte antigen; HUS, hemolytic uremic syndrome; SDP, single donor platelet; TTP, thrombotic thrombocytopenic purpura ; vWF, von Willebrand factor.

Table 39.9 Factor Concentrate

Factor Concentrate	Trade Name	Indications	Source of Factor	Method of Viral Inactivation	Special Instructions
Fibrinogen	RiaSTAP (CSL Behring)	Fibrinogen deficiency	Human plasma	Pasteurized	Dose: 30–60 mg/kg
F VII	F VII concentrate (Baxalta)	Congenital F VII deficiency requiring replacement therapy	Human plasma	Steam treated	Dose (IU) = desired % increase × body weight (kg)/2, given at 12 h intervals
F VIIa	Recombinant F VIIa/NiaStase (Novo Nordisk)	- F VIII or F IX deficiency with inhibitors - Glanzmann thrombasthenia - Congenital F VII deficiency	Recombinant	DNA technology	- Vial sizes: 1000 mcg, 2000 mcg, 5000 mcg - Reconstituted with diluent (water); 1 mL = 1000 mcg - Dose: 35–90 mcg/kg, given at 2–6 h intervals - Dose: 15–30 mcg/kg, given at 4–6 h intervals
F VIII	Kovaltry (Bayer) Nuwiq (Octapharma) Xyntha (Pfizer) Obizur (porcine) (Baxalta) Koate (Grifols) Long Acting rFVIII: Eloctate (Bioverativ) Adynovate (Shire)	F VIII deficiency requiring replacement therapy	Recombinant	DNA technology	- Dose (IU) = desired % increase × body weight (kg)/2, given at 8–24 h intervals - Prophylaxis: 25–40 units/kg - Bleeding: 30–75 units/kg depending on site of bleed
Anti-inhibitor coagulant complex (F II, VII, IX, X)	FEIBA NF (Baxalta)	F VIII deficiency with inhibitors	Human plasma	Vapor heated	- Dose range: 50–100 units/kg, given at 6–12 h intervals - Daily maximum: 200 units/kg

Continued

Laboratory Reference Values and Transfusion Medicine

39

Table 39.9 Factor Concentrate—cont'd

Factor Concentrate	Trade Name	Indications	Source of Factor	Method of Viral Inactivation	Special Instructions
vWF	Humate-P (CSL Behring) Wilate (Octapharma)	von Willebrand disease, nonresponsive to DDAVP	Human plasma	Pasteurized Solvent detergent	Dose (IU vWF:RcoF) = desired % increase of vWF:RcoF (IU/dL) × body weight (kg)/1.5, given at 8–12 h intervals
F IX	BeneFix (Pfizer) Long acting: Alprolix (Biogen) Rebinyn (Novo Nordisk) Immune VH (Baxalta)	Factor IX deficiency requiring replacement therapy	Recombinant Human plasma	DNA technology	- Dose (IU) = desired % increase × body weight (kg) ×1.2 - Prophylaxis: 40–50 units/kg - Bleeding: 50–125 units/kg depending on site of bleed
F X	Factor XP Behring (CSL Behring)	Factor X deficiency requiring replacement therapy	Human plasma	Vapor heated	
F XI	Factor XI (BPL)	Factor XI deficiency requiring replacement	Human plasma	Heat treated	Dose (IU) = desired % increase × body weight (kg)/2
F XIII	Corifact (CSL Behring) Tretten (Novo Nordisk)	Congenital factor XIII deficiency requiring replacement therapy	Human plasma Recombinant	Pasteurized DNA technology	- Dose (U) = 10 units/kg, 4 week intervals - Dose (U) = 35 U/kg monthly

Prothrombin complex (F II, VII, IX, X)	Octaplex (Octapharma) Beriplex (CSL Behring)	Acquired or hereditary deficiency of factors II, VII, IX, X	Human plasma	Solvent detergent Pasteurized	Vial size: 500, 1000 IU F IX Vial size: 500 IU
AT III	Antithrombin III (Baxalta)	Congenital or acquired AT III deficiency	Human plasma	Heat treated	- Dose (IU) = desired % increase × body weight (kg) - Usual dose: ~100 IU/kg
Protein C	Ceprotin (Baxalta)	Congenital and acquired protein C deficiency	Human plasma	Vapor heated	- Vial sizes: 500, 1000 IU - Dose according to clinical response and protein C levels
C1-esterase inhibitor	Berinert P (CSL Behring) Cinryze (Shire)	Hereditary angioneurotic edema	Human plasma	Vapor heated	Dose (IU) = 20 units/kg
Fibrin sealant	Tisseel (Baxter) FloSeal (Baxter)	Achieve hemostasis, seal, or glue tissue, support wound healing	Human plasma	Vapor heated	Kit sizes: 2 mL, 4 mL, 10 mL Kit size: 5 mL

DDAVP, Desamino-8-D-arginine vasopressin; *RcoF*, ristocetin cofactor; *vWF*, von Willebrand factor.

Adapted from The Hospital for Sick Children eFormulary Transfusion Medicine—Blood and Blood Product Information, 2020.

Table 39.10 Immune Globulins

Immune Globulins	Indications/Considerations	Dose	Comments
Cytomegalovirus (CMV) immune globulin (Cytogam)	CMV prophylaxis, CMV disease	150 mg/kg/dose IV	Rate of infusion: 0.3 mL/kg/h ×30 min 0.6 mL/kg/h ×30 min Maximum rate: 1.2 mL/kg/h Maximum volume: 75 mL/h
	Epstein Barr virus disease	100–200 mg/kg/dose IV q2 days for 3 weeks, then weekly for 3 weeks	
Hepatitis B immune globulin (e.g., HyperHEP B, HepaGam B)	Infants born to HBsAg-positive women	0.5 mL IM	Administer within 12 h of birth concurrently with HepB vaccine, at a different anatomic site
	Postexposure prophylaxis	0.06 mL/kg IM	Administer as soon as possible after exposure within 7 days, when indicated. Most effective if within 48 h of exposure
Immune globulin (IM) (e.g., GamaSTAN)			
Hepatitis A	Anticipated duration of exposure <1 month	0.1 mL/kg/dose IM	
	Anticipated duration of exposure <2 months	0.2 mL/kg/dose IM	
	Anticipated duration of exposure ≥2 months	0.2 mL/kg/dose IM every 2 months	
	Postexposure prophylaxis	0.1 mL/kg/dose IM	
Measles	Postexposure prophylaxis	0.5 mL/kg/dose IM	Administer within 14 days of exposure and before manifestation of disease

			Rate of infusion
Immunoglobulin IV (IVIG) (supplied mainly as 10% solutions) (e.g., Gamunex/IGIVnex 10%, Gammagard liquid 10%, Privigen 10%, Octagam 10%, Panzyga 10%)	Fetal/neonatal alloimmune thrombocytopenia	1 g/kg/dose IV	- 0.3 mL/kg/h for 15 min (Privigen and Kawasaki patients)
	Hemolytic disease of the fetus and newborn	0.5 g/kg/dose IV over 2 h, if necessary, repeat in 12 h	- 0.6 mL/kg/h for 15 min
	Hypogammaglobulinemia	600 mg/kg/month IV	- 1.2 mL/kg/h for 15 min
	Vasculitis/macrophage activation syndrome	2 g/kg/dose IV, max: 70 g	- 2.4 mL/kg/h for 15 min
	Guillain-Barré syndrome	1 g/kg/dose IV for 2 days	- 3.6 mL/kg/h for 30 min
	Immune thrombocytopenia	0.8–1 g/kg/dose IV	- then slowly increase rate if tolerated
	Kawasaki disease	2 g/kg/dose IV max: 70 g	- Maximum rate for Kawasaki patients = 3.6 mL/kg/h
	Bone marrow transplant	400 mg/kg/dose IV when IgG level <4 g/L	- Maximum rate for other indications = 7.2 mL/kg/h
	Dermatomyositis/polymyositis	2 g/kg/dose IV once, then biweekly for 5 weeks, then monthly	
	Varicella postexposure prophylaxis	400 mg/kg/dose IV once	Administer as soon as possible within 10 days of exposure. Most effective if within 96 h of exposure.
	Measles postexposure prophylaxis	400 mg/kg/dose IV once	Within 6 days of exposure
Rho(D) immune globulin (e.g., WinRho SDF)	Treatment (Rh positive patients)	125–300 IU/kg (20–60 mcg/kg) IV	Avoid in anemia
Idiopathic thrombocytopenic purpura			

Continued

Table 39.10 Immune Globulins—cont'd

Immune Globulins	Indications/Considerations	Dose	Comments
Obstetric indications	Routine antepartum prophylaxis of Rh-negative mother	1500 IU (300 mcg) IM or IV	At week 28–30 gestation or at 12 week intervals if administered early in pregnancy
	Obstetric complications, invasive procedures during pregnancy	1500 IU (300 mcg) IM or IV	
	Postpartum prophylaxis of Rh-negative mother if newborn is Rh-positive or Rh status is unknown	600 IU (120 mcg) IM or IV	Within 72 h of birth
Tetanus immune globulin (e.g., HyperTET)	<7 years ≥7 years	4 units/kg IM 250 units IM	Administer tetanus vaccine at same time but in a different extremity with a different syringe
Varicella zoster immune globulin (e.g., VariZIG)	≤2 kg 2.1–10 kg 10.1–20 kg 20.1–30 kg 30.1–40 kg >40 kg	62.5 units IM 125 units IM 250 units IM 375 units IM 500 units IM 625 units IM	- Administer as soon as possible within 10 days of exposure. Most effective if within 96 h of exposure - See IVIG if VZIG contraindicated

Adapted from The Hospital for Sick Children eFormulary Transfusion Medicine—Blood and Blood Product Information, 2020.

Table 39.11	Recommended Interval Between Blood Product Administration and Measles, Mumps, Rubella, or Varicella Immunization	
Product	Dose	Interval[a] (Months)
Intravenous immunoglobulin (IVIG)	160 mg/kg	7
	300–400 mg/kg	8
	640 mg/kg	9
	>640–1280 mg/kg	10
	>1280–2000 mg/kg	11
Varicella immunoglobulin (VZIG)	125 units/10 kg (>40kg: 625 units)	5
Plasma-reduced red cells	N/A	3
Packed red cells	N/A	5

[a]If an outbreak of a vaccine preventable disease occurs, immunization should not be withheld regardless of the time elapsed since administration of IVIG.

Adapted from The Hospital for Sick Children eFormulary Vaccine Guidelines, 2020.

Section IV

Drug Dosing Guidelines

Drug Dosing Guidelines

Elaine Lau

COMMON ABBREVIATIONS

Also see page xviii for a list of other abbreviations used throughout this book

ac	before meals
BID	two times daily
BP	blood pressure
D10W	dextrose 10% in water
D5W	dextrose 5% in water
DDAVP	desmopressin
div	divided
EC	enteric-coated
G6PD	glucose-6-phosphate dehydrogenase
GFR	glomerular filtration rate
GI	gastrointestinal
IBW	ideal body weight
ICU	intensive care unit
IM	intramuscular
inj	injection
IO	intraosseous
IV	intravenous
MV1-12	multi-vitamin infusion without vitamin K
NG	nasogastric tube
NICU	neonatal intensive care unit
NS	normal saline (0.9% NaCl)
pc	after meals
PE	phenytoin sodium equivalents units
PJP	*Pneumocystis jirovecii* pneumonia
PN	parenteral nutrition
PO	by mouth
PR	rectal
prn	as needed
qam	every morning
qhs	at bedtime
QID	four times daily
qpm	every evening
SL	sublingual
suppos	suppository
susp	suspension
tab	tablet
TID	three times daily
TPN	total parenteral nutrition

Drug Dosing Guidelines

40

BODY SURFACE AREA

1. Body surface area (BSA) nomograms
   a. Infants (Figure 40.1)
   b. Children and adults (Figure 40.2)
   c. To use the nomogram, align ruler with the height and weight on the two lateral axes. The point at which the center line is intersected gives the corresponding value for surface area.

Figure 40.1   Body Surface Area Nomogram for Infants

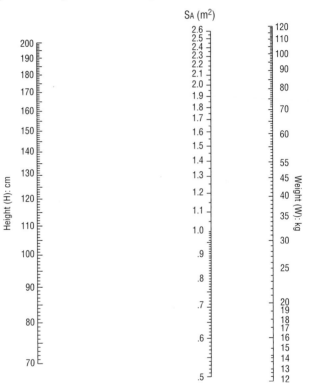

SA, Surface area. (From Haycock GB, Schwartz GJ, Wisotsky DH. Geometric method for measuring body surface area: a height–weight formula validated in infants, children, and adults. *J Pediatr.* 1978;93:62–66.)

Figure 40.2 Body Surface Area Nomogram for Children and Adults

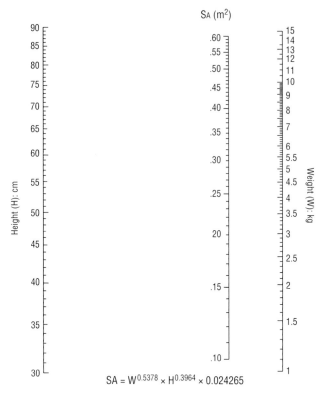

$$SA = W^{0.5378} \times H^{0.3964} \times 0.024265$$

(From Haycock GB, Schwartz GJ, Wisotsky DH. Geometric method for measuring body surface area: a height–weight formula validated in infants, children, and adults. *J Pediatr.* 1978;93:62–66.)

2. BSA calculations
   a. BSA = 0.024265 × height (cm)$^{0.3964}$ × weight (kg)$^{0.5378}$
   b. Simplified formula

   $$BSA = \sqrt{\frac{weight \times height}{3600}}$$

   weight (kg); height (cm)

IDEAL BODY WEIGHT

1. Nomogram for estimating ideal body weight (IBW) (Figure 40.3)
   a. Useful for estimation of ideal body weight in children aged 1 to 17 years; its accuracy is slightly diminished when used to estimate IBW for patients taller than 154 cm
2. Calculations
   a. IBW (kg) = 2.396 $e^{0.01863 \, (\text{height [cm]})}$
   b. Adjusted body weight (kg) = IBW + 0.4 (total body weight − IBW)

Figure 40.3 Ideal Body Weight

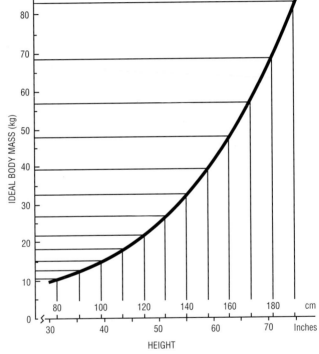

(From Traub SL, Kichen L. Estimating ideal body mass in children. *Am J Hosp Pharm.* 1983;40:107–110. Copyright 1983. American Society of Health-System Pharmacists, Inc. All rights reserved. With permission [R0317].)

 PEARL

IBW should be used for calculating dosage only if IBW is less than total body weight.

DRUG DOSAGE GUIDELINES

Table 40.1 Drug Dosage Guidelines for Neonates[a] (where specified), Infants, and Older Children

Drug[b,c]	Dose	Dose Limit	Comments
Abacavir Tab 300 mg Liquid 20 mg/mL	*INFANTS AND OLDER CHILDREN* *3 months–16 years:* 8 mg/kg/dose PO BID	600 mg/day	- If hypersensitivity rash develops, rechallenge is contraindicated
Acetaminophen Tab 325, 500 mg Chew tab 80 mg Drops/susp 80 mg/mL Rectal suppos 120, 325, 650 mg	*NEONATES* **Analgesic or antipyretic** 10–15 mg/kg/dose q4–6h *30–33 weeks:* 20 mg/kg/dose PR q12h *34–39 weeks:* 25 mg/kg/dose PR q8h *≥40 weeks:* 30 mg/kg/dose PR q6h **Patent ductus arteriosus (PDA)** 15 mg/kg/dose PO/PR q6h for 7 days *INFANTS AND OLDER CHILDREN* 10–15 mg/kg/dose PO q4–6h prn 10–20 mg/kg/dose PR q4–6h prn	*Neonates* 65 mg/kg/day PO *30–33 weeks:* 40 mg/kg/day PR *34–39 weeks:* 75 mg/kg/day PR *≥40 weeks:* 120 mg/kg/day PR *Infants and older children* 75 mg/kg/day PO or 80 mg/kg/day PR or 4 g/day if >12 years of age, whichever is less	- For doses ≤80 mg, oral drops (not susp) may be administered rectally - Single rectal loading doses of 30 mg/kg/dose (in neonates) and 40 mg/kg/dose (infants, older children) may be used for perioperative analgesia - Do not use rectal doses in <30 weeks because of limited information in this age group - Use for PDA closure after failure of 2 courses of indomethacin and/or absolute contraindications to indomethacin, including necrotizing enterocolitis, severe renal impairment, active bleeding, and refractory thrombocytopenia

Continued

Table 40.1 Drug Dosage Guidelines for Neonates[a] (Where Specified), Infants, and Older Children—cont'd

Drug[b,c]	Dose	Dose Limit	Comments
Acetazolamide Tab 250 mg Susp (HSC) 25 mg/mL Inj 500 mg/vial	***INFANTS AND OLDER CHILDREN*** **Glaucoma** *Children:* 5–10 mg/kg/dose PO/IV TID or 3.75–7.5 mg/kg/dose PO/IV QID *Adolescents:* 250–500 mg PO TID–QID; 250–500 mg IV up to QID **Epilepsy** 4–15 mg/kg/day PO in divided doses	30 mg/kg/day or 1 g/day, whichever is less	- Dose adjustment in renal impairment, moderate: q12h, severe: avoid - Use lower end of dosing range when adding to antiepileptic drug therapy
Acetylcysteine Inj 2 g/10 mL, 6 g/30 mL (20%) Liquid 200 mg/mL (20%) Liquid (HSC) 5%, 10%	***NEONATES*** **Distal intestinal obstruction syndrome (i.e., meconium ileus)** 100–250 mg (2–5 mL) of 5% liquid PO/NG q2–3 h **Prevention of PN-induced cholestasis** 75 mg/kg/day continuous IV infusion or over 18–24 h/day ***INFANTS AND OLDER CHILDREN*** **Prevention of contrast-induced nephropathy** 10 mg/kg/dose PO BID for 4 doses (starting the day before the procedure) **Acetaminophen overdose** *Standard dosing* Loading dose: 60 mg/kg/h (of 3% solution) IV over 4 h Maintenance dose: 6 mg/kg/h (of 3% solution) IV for at least 8 h until advised to stop by Poison Center	*Dose limit for patients <1.5 kg* *(to reduce the risk of aspiration):* 100 mg (2 mL) of acetylcysteine 5% solution (50 mg/mL) *Standard dosing loading dose limit:* 6000 mg/h *Standard dosing maintenance dose limit:* 600 mg/h	- For oral administration, the 20% IV solution can be diluted with water, juice, soft drinks, or chocolate milk to a final concentration of 5% and administered within the hour - To prepare 3% injection solution (30 mg/mL): - ≤20 kg: Remove 37.5 mL from 250 mL D5W bag, add 37.5 mL of 20% Acetylcysteine to 212.5 mL D5W - 21–40 kg: Remove 75 mL from 500 mL D5W bag, add 75 mL of 20% Acetylcysteine to 425 mL D5W - ≥41 kg: Remove 150 mL from 1000 mL D5W bag, add 150 mL of 20% Acetylcysteine to 850 mL D5W

	High risk dosing (used only in consultation with Poison Center based on acetaminophen levels, liver enzymes, need for dialysis, altered mental status, lactic acidosis) Loading dose: 60 mg/kg/h (of 3% solution) IV over 4 h Maintenance dose: 12 mg/kg/h (of 3% solution) IV for at least 8 h until advised to stop by Poison Center	High-risk dosing loading dose limit: 6000 mg/h High-risk dosing maintenance dose limit: 1200 mg/h	
Acetylsalicylic acid (ASA, aspirin) Chewtab 81 mg Tab 325 mg Enteric-coated tab 81, 325 mg	**INFANTS AND OLDER CHILDREN** **Pericarditis, rheumatic fever** 15–25 mg/kg/dose PO QID **Kawasaki disease** 3–5 mg/kg/dose PO qam **Antithrombotic therapy** 3–5 mg/kg/dose PO once daily	5.4 g/day 325 mg/day 325 mg/day	- Not recommended for antipyresis (risk of Reye syndrome) - Give with food; do not use enteric-coated tablets with milk, dairy products, antacids - Use extreme caution in hepatic impairment - Round dose to nearest ¼ tab - Enteric-coated tabs cannot be split
Activated charcoal Susp 25 g/112.5 mL	**INFANTS AND OLDER CHILDREN** If unknown quantity of toxin ingested, initial dose: 1 g/kg/dose PO/NG If known quantity of toxin ingested, initial dose: 10 g activated charcoal per 1 g toxin ingested		- Subsequent doses: only as advised by local Poison Control Center for particular indications

Continued

Table 40.1 Drug Dosage Guidelines for Neonates[a] (Where Specified), Infants, and Older Children—cont'd

Drug[b,c]	Dose	Dose Limit	Comments
Acyclovir Susp 40 mg/mL Tab 200, 400, 800 mg Inj 6 mg/mL (HSC)	**_NEONATES_** **Herpes simplex infections** >32 weeks PMA and ≥1200 g: 20 mg/kg/dose IV q8h for 14–21 days **_INFANTS AND OLDER CHILDREN_** _(dose on IBW if IBW less than total body weight, see Figure 40.3)_ **Herpes simplex encephalitis** _1 month–12 years:_ 20 mg/kg/dose IV q8h for 21 days _>12 years:_ 10 mg/kg/day IV q8h for 21 days **Disseminated or severe mucocutaneous HSV infections** _<12 years:_ 10 mg/kg/dose IV q8h _≥12 years:_ Disseminated HSV infection: 10 mg/kg/dose IV q8h Severe mucocutaneous HSV infection: 5–10 mg/kg/dose IV q8h PO dosing (following IV therapy): 20 mg/kg/dose PO q6h **Mild-moderate mucocutaneous HSV infections** 20 mg/kg/dose PO q6h **Herpes simplex prophylaxis** 20 mg/kg/day PO q12h **Varicella or zoster in immunocompromised hosts** _<1 year:_ 20 mg/kg/dose IV q8h _≥1 year:_ 500 mg/m²/dose IV q8h PO dosing (following IV therapy): 20 mg/kg/dose PO q6h for 5 days **Varicella in immunocompetent host** 20 mg/kg/dose PO q6h for 5 days	1.6 g/day PO (400 mg PO q6h) 800 mg/day PO (200 mg PO q6h) 1 g/day PO 3.2 g/day PO	- Dosage should be calculated based on ideal body weight if IBW is less than total body weight (Figure 40.3) - Maintain optimal hydration (1.5 × maintenance) and urine output of at least 1 mL/kg/h; measure baseline SCr; minimize use of concurrent nephrotoxins - For neonates, dose interval adjustment in renal impairment: moderate (SCr; 70–109 µmol/L), q12h; severe (SCr; 110–130 µmol/L), q24h; failure (SCr >130 µmol/L or urine output <1 mL/kg/h), 50% of dose q24–48h - For infants and older children, dose adjustment in renal impairment: moderate, q12h; severe, q24h - Oral therapy not recommended in neonates; for infants and older children, may be given PO with food - Patients receiving >30 mg/kg/day should have CBC + differential weekly

Adalimumab	**_INFANTS AND OLDER CHILDREN_** **Juvenile idiopathic arthritis (JIA) and uveitis** _≥4 years of age_ _≤30 kg_: 20 mg SC q2wk _>30 kg_: 40 mg SC q2wk **Crohn's disease** _≥40 kg_: 160 mg SC loading dose once at week 0 and 2, followed by maintenance dose of 40 mg SC q1–2 weeks starting at week 4	
Adenosine Inj 3 mg/mL	**_NEONATES_** **Supraventricular tachycardia** 0.1 mg/kg/dose IV increasing in increments of 0.05 mg/kg/dose to a maximum of 0.25 mg/kg/dose	0.25 mg/kg/dose	- Check to ensure adenosine is administered with good venous access in the upper extremity if possible. Administer by rapid IV/IO bolus over 1–2 s followed by NS flush
	INFANTS AND OLDER CHILDREN **Supraventricular tachycardia** 0.1 mg/kg/dose IV/IO; repeat q2min at 0.2 mg/kg/dose IV/IO	_First dose:_ 6 mg _Repeat dose:_ 12 mg	- Record continuous rhythm strip ECG during adenosine administration
Adrenaline	See **Epinephrine**	
Albuterol	See **Salbutamol**	

Continued

Table 40.1 Drug Dosage Guidelines for Neonates[a] (Where Specified), Infants, and Older Children—cont'd

Drug[b,c]	Dose	Dose Limit	Comments
Aldactazide Susp (HSC) Spironolactone 5 mg/mL and hydrochlorothia-zide 5 mg/mL Tab spironolactone and hydrochlorothia-zide, 25 mg each	***NEONATES, INFANTS AND OLDER CHILDREN*** 1–2 mg/kg/dose of each component PO BID	*Usual adult dose:* 2–4 tabs/day	- Give with food or milk; ineffective when GFR <30 mL/min
Allopurinol Susp (HSC) 20 mg/mL Tab 100 mg	***INFANTS AND OLDER CHILDREN*** 100–150 mg/m²/dose PO BID 6 mg/kg/dose PO BID	800 mg/day	- Maintain fluid intake: dose adjustment in renal impairment: moderate, 50%; severe, 25%–30%
Alfacalcidol Drops 2 mcg/mL Cap 0.25 mcg	***INFANTS AND OLDER CHILDREN*** Initial dose 0.02–0.04 mcg/kg/dose PO once daily		- Adjust dose according to plasma calcium and phosphate concentration (also PTH for chronic kidney disease)
Alprostadil Inj 500 mcg/vial	***NEONATES*** 0.01–0.1 mcg/kg/min IV via continuous infusion		- May cause apnea

Alteplase (tPA)

Inj 2 mg, 50 mg/vial
Inj (HSC) 1 mg/mL

INFANTS AND OLDER CHILDREN

Guidelines for blocked venous lines (see Chapter 37 Technology and Medical Complexity)

Systemic thrombolytic therapy

0.5 mg/kg/h IV for 6 h and reevaluate; use unfractionated heparin (10 units/kg/h) during infusion

Thrombolysis for hyperacute arterial ischemic stroke

≥2 years to <12 years: 0.75 mg/kg/dose IV
≥12 years: 0.9 mg/kg/dose IV
Give 10% as IV bolus dose over 5 min followed by remaining 90% as IV infusion over 1 h

Total dose limit: 75 mg/dose (Bolus dose limit: 7.5 mg, infusion dose limit: 67.5 mg)
Total dose limit (≥ 12 years): 90 mg/dose (Bolus dose limit: 9 mg, infusion dose limit: 81 mg)

- Systemic thrombolytic therapy indicated for arterial occlusions, massive pulmonary embolism, and pulmonary embolism not responding to heparin therapy; may also be indicated for acute extensive DVT and should be limited to situations in which risk of loss of life, organ, or limb because of thrombosis is present
- *Contraindications:* active bleeding, significant potential for local bleeding, general surgery within previous 10 days, neurosurgery within previous 3 weeks, hypertension, AV malformations, recent severe trauma
- *Precautions:* no IM injections; minimal manipulation of the patient; avoid concurrent use of warfarin or antiplatelet agents; no urinary catheterization, rectal temperature, or arterial punctures; take blood samples from superficial vein or indwelling catheter; maintain platelets at >100 × 10⁹/L
- Monitor INR, aPTT, fibrinogen; maintain fibrinogen at >1 g/L by infusions of cryoprecipitate

Continued

Table 40.1 Drug Dosage Guidelines for Neonates[a] (Where Specified), Infants, and Older Children—cont'd

Drug[b,c]	Dose	Dose Limit	Comments
Aluminum hydroxide Susp 64 mg/mL Chewtab 600 mg	***INFANTS AND OLDER CHILDREN*** **Antacid** *Child:* 300–900 mg pc and at bedtime *Adult:* 600–1200 mg pc and qhs **Hyperphosphatemia** *Child:* 8.3–25 mg/kg/dose PO q4h or 12.5–37.5 mg/kg/dose PO q6h; titrate to normal serum phosphate level	3600 mg/day	
Aluminum hydroxide and magnesium hydroxide (Almagel®) Aluminum hydroxide 40 mg/mL and magnesium hydroxide 40 mg/mL	**Antacid** *Infant:* 2.5–5 mL PO q1–2h *Child:* 5–15 mL PO pc and qhs *Adult:* 10–20 mL PO pc and qhs	80 mL/day	
Amantadine Liquid 10 mg/mL Cap 100 mg	***INFANTS AND OLDER CHILDREN*** **Influenza A (prophylaxis and treatment)** 2.5 mg/kg/dose PO q12h	*<10 years:* 150 mg/day *≥10 years:* 200 mg/day	- Continue prophylaxis for at least 10 days after exposure or throughout epidemic; active treatment should continue for 48 h after disappearance of symptoms; avoid alcohol - Dose adjustment in renal impairment: mild, q24h; moderate, q2d; severe, q7d

Inj 250 mg/mL Inj (HSC) 5 mg/mL	1.2–2 kg, 0–7 days: 7.5 mg/kg/dose IV/IM q12h 1.2–2 kg, >7 days: 6.7 mg/kg/dose IV/IM q8h ≥2 kg, 0–7 days: 10 mg/kg/dose IV/IM q12h ≥2 kg, >7 days: 10 mg/kg/dose IV/IM q8h		- Calculate dose according to adjusted body weight - Monitoring of serum concentrations recommended - Dose interval adjustment in renal impairment: moderate, q12h; severe, q24–48h
	INFANTS AND OLDER CHILDREN 5–10 mg/kg/dose IV/IM q8h	500 mg/dose before TDM, 1500 mg/day	
	Hematology/Oncology and HPCT patients with fever and neutropenia 2 months to <11 years: 35 mg/kg/dose IV q24h 11 to <16 years: 25 mg/kg/dose IV q24h ≥16 years: 20 mg/kg/dose IV q24h	1500 mg/day before TDM	
	Cystic Fibrosis (non-lung transplant only) 25 mg/kg/dose IV q24h	1500 mg/day before TDM	
5-Aminosalicylic acid (5-ASA)	See **Mesalamine**		
Amiodarone Inj 50 mg/mL Tab 200 mg Cap (HSC) 5 mg, 20 mg	**INFANTS AND OLDER CHILDREN** *Loading dose:* 5 mg/kg IV over 1 h, followed by infusion of 5–15 mcg/kg/min 10 mg/kg/dose PO once daily or 5 mg/kg/dose PO BID for 7–10 days *Maintenance:* 5 mg/kg/dose PO once daily	*Usual adult loading dose:* 800–1600 mg/day PO *Usual adult maintenance dose:* 200–400 mg/day PO	- Dose may require reduction in patients with liver impairment - Reduce digoxin dose by 50% during concurrent therapy - Reduce warfarin dose by 33%–50% during concurrent therapy - Will increase phenytoin concentrations (monitor for toxicity) - Monitor thyroid, liver, lung, eye function; nausea/vomiting occur frequently with loading dose

Continued

Table 40.1 Drug Dosage Guidelines for Neonates[a] (Where Specified), Infants, and Older Children—cont'd

Drug[b,c]	Dose	Dose Limit	Comments
Amlodipine Tab 5 mg, 10 mg Oral susp (HSC) 1 mg/mL	***INFANTS AND OLDER CHILDREN*** *Initial:* 0.1–0.2 mg/kg/dose PO once daily *Maintenance:* 0.1–0.3 mg/kg/dose PO once daily	15 mg/day	- Reduce initial dose in patients with liver impairment and titrate to effect - Because of long half-life, dosage adjustments should not be made more frequently than q3–5d
Amoxicillin Susp 50 mg/mL Cap 250 mg, 500 mg	***INFANTS AND OLDER CHILDREN*** 17 mg/kg/dose PO q8h **High-dose therapy—Pneumonia** 30 mg/kg/dose PO q8h **High-dose therapy—Otitis media** 45 mg/kg/dose PO q12h **Pharyngitis (Group A streptococcal infections)** 50 mg/kg/dose PO once daily ***Helicobacter pylori*–associated ulcer** *15–24 kg:* 500 mg PO BID *25–34 kg:* 750 mg PO BID *≥35 kg:* 1000 mg PO BID **Prophylaxis for asplenic patients (alternative to penicillin)** *0–5 years:* 10 mg/kg/dose PO BID *>5 years:* 250 mg PO BID	500 mg/dose 4 g/day 1 g/day	- Dose interval adjustment in renal impairment: moderate, q12h; severe, q24h - May be given with food

| Amoxicillin/clavulanic acid (Clavulin)
Susp 40 mg/mL amoxicillin and 5.7 mg/mL clavulanate (Clavulin 200), 80 mg/mL amoxicillin and 11.4 mg/mL clavulanate (Clavulin 400)
Tab 500 mg amoxicillin and 125 mg clavulanate (Clavulin 500), 875 mg amoxicillin and 125 mg clavulanate (Clavulin 875) | **INFANTS AND OLDER CHILDREN**
<3 months: 15 mg amoxicillin/kg/dose PO q12h given as 40 mg/mL susp
≥3 months, ≤38 kg: 8–15 mg amoxicillin/kg/dose PO q8h or 12.5–22.5 amoxicillin/kg/dose PO q12h, given as suspension
>38 kg: 500 mg amoxicillin PO q8–12h, given as suspension or 500 mg tablet
Bites
≥3 months, ≤38 kg: 13 mg amoxicillin/kg/dose PO q8h or 20 mg/ amoxicillin/kg/dose PO q12h, given as suspension
>38 kg: 500 mg amoxicillin PO q8h as 500 mg tablet
Otitis media
≤35 kg: 15–20 mg/kg/dose q8h, given as suspension
>35 kg: 500 mg q8h, given as 500 mg tablet or suspension
Community-acquired pneumonia
High dose: 27–30 mg amoxicillin/kg/dose PO q8h given as suspension or tablet
Treatment of intestinal bacterial overgrowth
15 mg/kg/dose PO TID or 20 mg/kg/dose PO BID (cycled with oral metronidazole or gentamicin) | *Usual adult dose:*
750–1750 mg/day amoxicillin | - Use with caution in patients with creatinine clearance <30 mL/min; adjust dose in renal failure: severe, 50%–75% of standard dose *or* adjust interval: moderate, q12h; severe, q24h
- Tabs are not recommended in children <12 years because of higher ratio of clavulanic acid to amoxicillin; tabs are not equivalent to susp; various formulations of susp exist: are not all equivalent; administer with food to reduce GI upset
- If possible, limit clavulanic acid to ~10 mg/kg/day in children to reduce GI symptoms; BID dosing may also reduce adverse GI effects, such as diarrhea |
| **Amphotericin B (conventional)**
Inj (HSC) 5 mg/mL | **NEONATES**
1 mg/kg/dose IV once daily
INFANTS AND OLDER CHILDREN
1 mg/kg/dose IV once daily | 70 mg/day or 1.5 mg/kg/dose, whichever is less | - Monitor serum potassium and renal function
- Consider premedication with meperidine, diphenhydramine
- Sodium load as tolerated |

Continued

Drug Dosing Guidelines

Table 40.1 Drug Dosage Guidelines for Neonates[a] (Where Specified), Infants, and Older Children—cont'd

Drug[b,c]	Dose	Dose Limit	Comments
Amphotericin B lipid formulations Amphotericin B liposomal (AmBisome)	**NEONATES** **CNS infection** 5 mg/kg/dose IV once daily **INFANTS AND OLDER CHILDREN** **Empiric therapy in febrile neutropenia** 3 mg/kg/dose IV once daily **Documented/suspected fungal infection** 3–5 mg/kg/dose IV once daily		- Consider in patients unable to receive conventional amphotericin because of toxicity (renal impairment, hypokalemia, infusion-related reactions) or treatment failure
Ampicillin Inj 250, 500, 1000, 2000 mg/vial	**NEONATES** **Meningitis** *0–7 days:* 67 mg/kg/dose IV q8h *>7 days:* 75 mg/kg/dose IV q6h **Clinical sepsis** *≤2 kg, 0–7 days:* 50 mg/kg/dose IV q12h *≤2 kg, >7 days:* 50 mg/kg/dose IV q8h *>2 kg, 0–7 days:* 50 mg/kg/dose IV q8h *>2 kg, >7 days:* 50 mg/kg/dose IV q6h **Other infections** *≤2 kg, 0–7 days:* 25 mg/kg/dose IV q12h *≤2 kg, >7 days:* 25 mg/kg/dose IV q8h *>2 kg, 0–7 days:* 25 mg/kg/dose IV q8h *>2 kg, >7 days:* 25 mg/kg/dose IV q6h **UTI prophylaxis** 25 mg/kg/dose IV q12h		- Dose interval adjustment in renal impairment: - Severe: q12–24h

Drug	Dosing		Comments
	INFANTS AND OLDER CHILDREN **Meningitis/severe infections** 50–100 mg/kg/dose IV q6h **Mild/moderate infections** 25–50 mg/kg/dose IV q6h	3 g/dose, 12 g/day 1 g/dose, 4 g/day	- Dose interval adjustment in renal impairment: moderate q6–12h; severe q12h
Aprepitant Cap 80 mg, 125 mg Oral suspension 20 mg/mL (HSC)	**INFANTS AND OLDER CHILDREN** **Prevention of acute chemotherapy-induced nausea and vomiting (CINV)** ≥6 months of age Day 1: 3 mg/kg/dose PO once pre-chemotherapy Day 2–3: 2 mg/kg/dose PO once daily	Day 1: 125 mg/dose Day 2–3: 80 mg/dose	- May interact with many medications; consider consulting pharmacist regarding patients taking multiple medications. - Reduce dexamethasone dose by 50% when used with aprepitant
Ascorbic acid Tablet, chewable: 500 mg Inj 250 mg/mL vial	**INFANTS AND OLDER CHILDREN** **Sepsis** 25–50 mg/kg/dose IV q6h	1.5 g/dose	- For the treatment of sepsis, IV ascorbic acid may be used with IV thiamine and IV hydrocortisone for a duration of up to 4 days
Atenolol Tab 25 mg, 50 mg	**INFANTS AND OLDER CHILDREN** ≥5 years: 0.5–1.5 mg/kg/dose PO once daily or 0.25–0.75 mg/kg/dose PO BID	2 mg/kg/day or 100 mg/day, whichever is less	- Dose interval adjustment in renal failure: - CrCl 15–35 mL/min: max 50 mg or 1 mg/kg/dose PO once daily - CrCl <15 mL/min: max 50 mg or 1 mg/kg/dose PO q2d

Continued

Table 40.1 Drug Dosage Guidelines for Neonates[a] (Where Specified), Infants, and Older Children—cont'd

Drug[b,c]	Dose	Dose Limit	Comments
Atorvastatin Tab 10 mg, 20 mg	***INFANTS AND OLDER CHILDREN*** **Hyperlipidemia, heterozygous familial hypercholesterolemia** *10–17 years:* 10 mg PO once daily, may increase to 20 mg once daily	*Children:* 20 mg *Adult:* 80 mg	- Monitor liver function tests (liver enzyme changes generally occur in first 3 months) - Rhabdomyolysis has occurred rarely (risk increased with concurrent administration of certain drugs) - In patients with impaired renal function, use lowest dose possible (max 10 mg)
Atropine Inj 0.6 mg/mL; preloaded inj 0.5 mg/5 mL	***NEONATES*** **Resuscitation** 0.01–0.02 mg/kg/dose IV/IM/SC/ETT q20min prn ***INFANTS AND OLDER CHILDREN*** **Resuscitation** 0.02 mg/kg/dose IV/IO, repeat once prn 0.04–0.06 mg/Kg ETT, repeat once prn **Pre-operative** 0.01–0.02 mg/kg/dose IM/PO 30–60 min preop **Cholinergic crisis** 0.05 mg/kg/dose IV, double dose q5min until symptoms resolve	*Minimum single dose:* 0.1 mg (0.17 mL) *Maximum single dose:* 0.5 mg (0.83 mL) *Maximum total dose:* 1 mg *Minimum:* 0.1 mg/dose *Dose limit:* 0.6 mg/dose 5 mg/dose	- ETT route to be used only if IV route not possible; dilute/follow dose by 1 mL 0.9% NaCl - Incompatible with sodium bicarbonate - Higher or repeated doses may be used with organophosphate poisoning

Atropine (ophthalmic) Ophthalmic drops: 1% (5 mL, 0.5 mL minims)	**INFANTS AND OLDER CHILDREN** **Sialorrhea (use 1% ophthalmic drops)** 1–2 drops sublingually q4–6h	
Azathioprine Susp (HSC) 50 mg/mL Tab 50 mg Inj (HSC) 10 mg/mL	**INFANTS AND OLDER CHILDREN** **Transplantation** *Heart:* 2 mg/kg/dose IV/PO once daily *Lung:* 1.5 mg/kg/dose IV/PO once daily	- May cause elevated blood pressure if systemically absorbed or photophobia/ blurred vision - Adjust dose in renal impairment: moderate: q36h or give 75% of standard dose; severe: q48h or give 50% of standard dose - Give PO dose with food
Azithromycin Tab 250 mg Susp:40 mg/mL	**NEONATES** **General dosing for a susceptible infection** 10–20 mg/kg/dose PO once daily **Pertussis treatment and postexposure prophylaxis** 10 mg/kg/dose PO q24h (usual duration 5 days) ***Chlamydia* (conjunctivitis or pneumonia)** 20 mg/kg/dose PO q24h (usual duration 3 days)	- Clearance of other drugs, including tacrolimus, cyclosporine, and phenytoin, may be decreased
	INFANTS AND OLDER CHILDREN **Pneumonia** 10 mg/kg/dose PO once on day 1, followed by 5 mg/kg/dose PO once daily on days 2–5 **Acute otitis media** *Single dose regimen:* 30 mg/kg/dose PO as a single dose *3 day regimen:* 10 mg/kg/dose PO once daily *5 day regimen:* 10 mg/kg/dose PO on day 1, then 5 mg/kg/dose PO once daily on days 2–5	500 mg/dose (day 1), 250 mg/ dose (days 2–5) 1500 mg/dose 500 mg/dose 500 mg/dose (day 1), 250 mg/ dose (days 2–5)

Continued

Table 40.1 Drug Dosage Guidelines for Neonates[a] (Where Specified), Infants, and Older Children—cont'd

Drug[b,c]	Dose	Dose Limit	Comments
Azithromycin—cont'd	**Group A streptococci (GAS) pharyngitis** 12 mg/kg/dose PO once daily for 5 days	500 mg/dose	
	Pertussis, treatment and postexposure prophylaxis *1–6 months:* 10 mg/kg/dose PO q24h for 5 days *>6 months:* 10 mg/kg/dose PO on day 1, then 5 mg/kg/dose once daily on days 2–5	500 mg/dose (day 1), 250 mg/dose (days 2–5)	
	Chlamydial urethritis, cervicitis *≥16 years:* 1 g PO stat		
	Uncomplicated gonococcal infection (add ceftriaxone, cefixime or spectinomycin) *<9 years or ≤45 kg:* 20 mg/kg PO once *≥9 years or >45 kg:* 1000 mg PO once	1000 mg/dose	
Baclofen Tab 10 mg Liquid (HSC) 5 mg/mL	***INFANTS AND OLDER CHILDREN*** *2–7 years:* 3–5 mg/dose PO TID; titrate dose q3d in increments of 5–15 mg/day PO *≥8 years:* titrate dose as earlier to maximum of 60 mg/day PO	*2–7 years:* 40 mg/day PO *≥8 years:* 60 mg/day PO *Adult max:* 80 mg/day PO	- Avoid abrupt withdrawal of drug; use with caution in patients with seizure disorder, impaired renal function
Benztropine Inj 2 mg/2 mL Tab 2 mg	***INFANTS AND OLDER CHILDREN*** **Drug-induced extrapyramidal symptoms** *≥3 years:* 0.02–0.05 mg/kg/dose PO/IM/IV 1–2 times daily	*Usual:* 2 mg/day (may increase to 6 mg/day if needed)	- IV route should be reserved for situations when oral or IM are not appropriate

Betamethasone valerate (topical) Cream 0.05%, 0.1% Lotion 0.05%, 0.1% Ointment 0.05%, 0.1%	***INFANTS AND OLDER CHILDREN*** Apply 0.05%–0.1% ointment to affected body area 2–3 times/day Apply 0.1% lotion to affected scalp area 2 times/day	
Bisacodyl Tab 5 mg Suppos 5 mg, 10 mg	***INFANTS AND OLDER CHILDREN*** *Oral:* 0.3 mg/kg/dose PO 6–12 h before desired effect *Rectal:* ≤ 6 years: 5–10 mg PR 15–60 min before desired effect >6 years: 10 mg PR 15–60 min before desired effect	15 mg PO	- Do not divide or chew tabs - Do not administer PO with dairy products or antacid
Budesonide (inhalation) Susp for inhalation 0.25 mg/2 mL, 0.5 mg/ 2 mL, 1 mg/2 mL	***NEONATES*** 0.25–0.5 mg BID via nebulizer **Acute distress** 0.5–1 mg BID via nebulizer ***INFANTS AND OLDER CHILDREN*** **Severe acute asthma** *Children:* 0.5–1 mg BID via nebulizer *Adults:* 1–2 mg BID via nebulizer **Maintenance therapy for asthma** *Children:* 0.25–0.5 mg BID via nebulizer *Adults:* 0.5–1 mg via nebulizer **Eosinophilic esophagitis** <10 years: 1 mg PO/ET once daily ≥10 years: 2 mg PO/ET once daily		- Dilute to a total of 3 mL with 0.9% NaCl if required; may be mixed with salbuta-mol, ipratropium, or tobramycin solutions immediately before use - Mix each nebule with 5 g (5 packets) of sucralose (Splenda) to create a volume of 8–12 mL for immediate administration

Continued

Table 40.1 Drug Dosage Guidelines for Neonates^a (Where Specified), Infants, and Older Children—cont'd

Drug^{b,c}	Dose	Dose Limit	Comments
Budesonide (systemic) Oral cap 3 mg	**Crohn's disease** 0.45 mg/kg/dose PO qam ac breakfast for 8–16 weeks, then taper over 2–4 weeks in 3 mg increments	9 mg/day	
Caffeine citrate Inj 10 mg base/mL	*NEONATES* *Loading:* 10 mg base/kg/dose IV/PO *Maintenance:* 3–5 mg base/kg/dose IV/PO once daily, starting 24 h after loading dose	15 mg base/kg/day	- Injection may be given PO - Dose expressed as caffeine base: 2 mg caffeine citrate = 1 mg caffeine base
Calcitriol (1,25-dihydroxycholecalciferol) Cap 0.25 mg, 0.5 mcg Inj 1 mcg/mL	**Hypoparathyroidism, vitamin D resistant rickets, dialysis** *Initial:* 0.0075–0.0125 mcg/kg/dose PO BID *Maintenance:* Increase prm gradually to 0.5–1 mcg/day PO		- Adjust dose according to plasma calcium concentration
Calcium Inj 100 mg/mL calcium gluconate (10%) = 9.3 mg elemental calcium/mL = 0.23 mmol elemental calcium/mL Inj 100 mg/mL calcium chloride (10%) = 27 mg elemental calcium/mL = 0.68 mmol elemental calcium/mL	*NEONATES* **Resuscitation or hyperkalemia/myocardial stabilizer** 0.5–1 mL/kg/dose of 10% calcium **gluconate** solution IV q10–20min prn (50–100 mg/kg/dose of calcium gluconate) **Hypocalcemia** *Initial:* 0.12–0.23 mmol/kg/dose of elemental calcium IV over 30 min (50–100 mg/kg/dose calcium **gluconate**) *Maintenance:* 0.02–0.08 mmol/kg/h elemental calcium IV (8.3–33.3 mg/kg/h calcium **gluconate IV)** 12.5–37.5 mg elemental calcium/kg/dose PO QID		- Avoid extravasation; central line - Oral calcium preparations are hyperosmolar—administer with feedings

calcium carbonate = 80 mg elemental calcium/mL = 2 mmol elemental calcium/mL Tab 625 mg calcium carbonate = 250 mg elemental calcium = 6.25 mmol elemental calcium	**Resuscitation (calcium chloride)** 20 mg/kg/dose calcium chloride IV/IO q10–20min prn (0.2 mL/kg/dose of 10% calcium **chloride**) **Calcium deficiency, initial dose for phosphate binding in chronic renal failure patients** *Infants:* 125 mg elemental calcium/dose PO TID (3.1 mmol elemental calcium/dose PO TID) *Children:* 250 mg elemental calcium/dose PO TID (6.25 mmol elemental calcium/dose PO TID) **Hypocalcemia** *Intermittent infusion (calcium **gluconate**)* 0.1–0.2 mmol elemental calcium/kg/h IV (3.8–7.8 mg/kg/h elemental calcium IV, 40–85 mg/kg/h calcium **gluconate** IV); adjust IV rate q4h according to plasma calcium concentration *Continuous infusion (calcium **gluconate**)* 0.025–0.075 mmol/kg/h elemental calcium IV (0.96–2.9 mg/kg/h elemental calcium IV, 10–31.6 mg/kg/h calcium **gluconate** IV) **Bolus dosing for symptomatic hypocalcemia/hyperkalemia (may repeat q4–6h)** *Calcium **chloride** (intensive care settings)* 0.07 mmol/kg/dose elemental calcium IV via CVL (0.1 mL/kg/dose calcium **chloride** IV, 10 mg/kg/dose calcium **chloride** IV) *Calcium **gluconate*** 0.23–0.46 mmol/kg/dose elemental calcium IV (1–2 mL/kg/dose calcium **gluconate** IV, 100–200 mg/kg/dose calcium **gluconate**)	*Maximum single dose:* 2 g (20 mL) 7 mmol/dose elemental calcium (1 g/dose calcium **chloride**) *Usual adult dose:* 2.3–4.6 mmol/dose elemental calcium (10–20 mL/dose calcium **gluconate** IV, 1–2 g/dose calcium **gluconate** IV)	- Administer slowly - Titrate dose according to serum PO_4^- or to corrected serum Ca^{2+} - Avoid extravasation; central line preferred

Continued

Table 40.1   Drug Dosage Guidelines for Neonates[a] (Where Specified), Infants, and Older Children—cont'd

Drug[b,c]	Dose	Dose Limit	Comments
Calcium polystyrene sulfonate (Resonium Calcium) Powder	**INFANTS AND OLDER CHILDREN** Initial: 1 g/kg/day PO/PR in divided doses Maintenance: 0.5 g/kg/day PO/PR in divided doses		- Contains 8% w/w calcium (1.6–2.4 mmol/g) - Use in patients with hyperkalemia and restricted sodium intake
Captopril Tab 6.25 mg, 12.5 mg, 25 mg, 50 mg Solution: dissolve 'n' dose system	**NEONATES** **Hypertension, CHF** Initial: 0.01–0.05 mg/kg/dose PO q8–12h **INFANTS AND OLDER CHILDREN** **Hypertension** Initial: 0.1–0.3 mg/kg/dose PO q8h Maintenance: 0.1–1.3 mg/kg/dose PO q8h **CHF** Initial: 0.1 mg/kg/dose PO q8h Maintenance: 0.5–2 mg/kg/dose PO q8h or 0.75–3 mg/kg/dose PO q12h	6 mg/kg/day or 200 mg/day	- Dose adjustment in renal impairment: moderate, 75%; severe, 50%
Carbamazepine Susp 20 mg/mL Tab 200 mg Tab CR 200 mg, 400 mg Chewtab 100 mg	**INFANTS AND OLDER CHILDREN** Initial: 10 mg/kg/day PO divided BID–TID Maintenance: up to 20–30 mg/kg/day PO divided BID–QID; increase dose gradually over 2–4 weeks	<6 years: 35 mg/kg/day 6–15 years: 1000 mg/day >15 years: 1200 mg/day Adults: 1600 mg/day	- Chewable tabs must be thoroughly chewed and not swallowed whole - Controlled release tabs may be split - Give with food or milk; dose may require reduction in liver impairment - Tabs (immediate release, chewtabs), suspension: dose TID–QID - Controlled release tabs: dose BID–TID

Drug	Dose		Comments
Carvediol Tab 3.125 mg, 6.25 mg, 12.5 mg Susp (HSC) 1.67 mg/mL	***INFANTS AND OLDER CHILDREN*** **CHF** *<4 years:* Initial: 0.03 mg/kg/dose PO q8h or 0.05 mg/kg/dose PO q12h Target: 0.27–0.33 mg/kg/dose PO q8h or 0.4–0.5 mg/kg/dose PO q12h *≥4 years:* 0.05–0.5 mg/kg/dose PO q12h	50 mg PO BID	- Reduce digoxin dose by 25% when carvediol is added to therapy
Caspofungin Inj 70 mg/vial Inj (HSC) 7 mg/mL	***INFANTS AND OLDER CHILDREN*** *≥1–3 months:* 25 mg/m²/dose IV once daily *≥3 months–18 years:* loading dose 70 mg/m²/dose IV once daily on day 1, then 50 mg/m²/dose IV once daily *≥18 years:* loading dose 70 mg IV once daily on day 1, then 50 mg IV once daily	70 mg loading dose, 50 mg maintenance dose	- Reduce dose in renal impairment
Cefazolin Inj 500 mg, 1 g, 10 g/vial	***NEONATES*** *<2 kg:* 25 mg/kg/dose IV/IM q12h *≥2 kg, 0–7 days:* 25 mg/kg/dose IV/IM q12h *≥2 kg, >7 days:* 25 mg/kg/dose IV/IM q8h ***INFANTS AND OLDER CHILDREN*** **Mild to moderate infections** 17–35 mg/kg/dose IV/IM q8h **Severe infections** 35–50 mg/kg/dose IV/IM q8h	1 g/dose, 3 g/day 2 g/dose, 6 g/day	- Dose interval adjustment in renal impairment: moderate, q12h; severe, q24h

Continued

Table 40.1 Drug Dosage Guidelines for Neonates[a] (Where Specified), Infants, and Older Children—cont'd

Drug[b,c]	Dose	Dose Limit	Comments
Cefixime Susp 20 mg/mL Tab 400 mg	***INFANTS AND OLDER CHILDREN*** 8 mg/kg/dose PO once daily or 4 mg/kg/dose PO q12h **Uncomplicated gonococcal infection (add azithromycin)** *<9 years or ≤45 kg:* 8 mg/kg/dose PO BID for 2 doses *≥9 years or >45 kg:* 800 mg PO once	400 mg/dose	- Dose adjustment in renal impairment: moderate, 75% standard dose; severe, 50% standard dose - Not first line for gonorrhea. Patients should optimally be treated with combination gonorrhea infection therapy in response to increased resistance
Cefotaxime Inj 1 g/vial, 2 g/vial Inj (HSC) 250 mg/mL	***NEONATES*** *<1200 g,* 50 mg/kg/dose IV/IM q12h *1200–2000 g, ≤7 days:* 50 mg/kg/dose IV/IM q12h *1200–2000 g, >7 days:* 50 mg/kg/dose IV/IM q8h *>2000 g, ≤7 days:* 50 mg/kg/dose IV/IM q8–12h *>2000 g, >7 days:* 50 mg/kg/dose IV/IM q6–8h ***INFANTS AND OLDER CHILDREN*** **Mild to moderate infections** 35 mg/kg/dose IV/IM q8h		- Reduce dose in renal impairment: severe, q12–24h
	Severe infections 50 mg/kg/dose IV/IM q6–8h	2 g/dose, 6 g/day	
	Meningitis 50 mg/kg/dose IV/IM q6h	4 g/dose, 12 g/day	
	Sickle cell disease (meningitis not suspected) 50 mg/kg/dose IV q6h or 67 mg/kg/dose IV q8h	12 g/day	- Dose interval adjustment in renal impairment: moderate, q8–12h; severe, q12–24h
		12 g/day	

Cefoxitin Inj 1 g/vial, 2 g/vial Inj (HSC) 200 mg/mL	**INFANTS AND OLDER CHILDREN** **Mild to moderate infections** 20–25 mg/kg/dose IV/IM q6h or 27–35 mg/kg/dose IV/IM q8h	2 g/dose, 8 g/day	- Dose interval adjustment in renal impairment: moderate, q8–12h; severe, q24–48h
	Severe infections 17–27 mg/kg/dose IV/IM q4h or 25–40 mg/kg/dose IV/IM q6h	12 g/day	
	Pelvic inflammatory disease (add doxycycline, ± metronidazole for outpatient therapy)		
	Inpatient (parenteral) therapy: 25 mg/kg/dose IV q6h	2 g/dose	
	Outpatient therapy: 2 g IM plus probenecid 1 g PO as a single dose, concurrently		
	NEONATES < 1.2 kg: 50 mg/kg/dose IV/IM q12h 1.2–2 kg, 0–7 days: 50 mg/kg/dose IV/IM q12h 1.2–2 kg, > 7 days: 50 mg/kg/dose IV/IM q8h ≥ 2 kg, 0–7 days: 50 mg/kg/dose IV/IM q8–12h ≥ 2 kg, > 7 days: 50 mg/kg/dose IV/IM q8h		
Ceftazidime Inj 1 g/vial, 2 g/vial, 6 g/vial Inj (HSC) 250 mg/mL	**INFANTS AND OLDER CHILDREN** **Mild to moderate infections** 35 mg/kg/dose IV/IM q8h	1 g/dose, 3 g/day	- Reduce dose in renal impairment - Dose interval adjustment in renal impairment: mild, q12h; moderate, q24h; severe, q48h
	Severe infections 40–50 mg/kg/dose IV/IM q8h	2 g/dose, 6 g/day	
	CF patients 50 mg/kg/dose IV/IM q6h	6 g/day	

Continued

Table 40.1 Drug Dosage Guidelines for Neonates[a] (Where Specified), Infants, and Older Children—cont'd

Drug[b,c]	Dose	Dose Limit	Comments
Ceftriaxone Inj 2 g/vial	***INFANTS AND OLDER CHILDREN*** **Meningitis in children ≥1 month**		- For meningitis, administration of dexa-methasone before first dose of ceftriaxone may be considered
	100 mg/kg/dose IV at 0, 12, and 24 h, then 100 mg/kg/dose IV q24h or 50 mg/kg/dose IV q12h	2 g/dose, 4 g/day	- In neonates, may induce hyperbilirubinemia
	Otitis media treatment failure		- Fatal cases of calcium-ceftriaxone precipi-tation have been reported (avoid concur-
	50 mg/kg/dose IM daily for 3 days	1 g/day	rent administration with calcium-containing products)
	Community-acquired pneumonia (non-severe), peritonitis, arthritis, bacteremia		
	50 mg/kg/dose IV/IM q24h	1 g/day	
	Sepsis, severe pneumonia in ICU patients, sickle cell disease, endocarditis, osteomyelitis, and other severe infections		
	100 mg/kg/dose IV/IM q24h	2 g/day	
	Appendicitis (perforated)		
	50 mg/kg/dose IV q24h, in combination with metronidazole	2 g/day	
	Uncomplicated gonococcal infection (add azithromycin)		
	<9 years or ≤45 kg: 50 mg/kg/dose IM once	250 mg/dose	
	≥9 years or >45 kg: 250 mg/dose IM once		
	Pelvic inflammatory disease		
	Outpatient therapy: 250 mg IM as a single dose with doxycycline ± metronidazole		

Cefuroxime Inj 750 mg/vial, 1500 mg/vial	**INFANTS AND OLDER CHILDREN** 25–50 mg/kg/dose IV/IM q8h	2 g/dose, 6 g/day	- Not to be used for the treatment of meningitis - Dose interval adjustment in renal impairment: moderate, q12h; severe, q24h
Cefuroxime axetil Susp 25 mg/mL Tab 250, 500 mg	**Otitis media, pneumonia, sickle cell patients with fever** 15 mg/kg/dose PO BID as suspension or ≥12 years: 250–500 mg PO BID as tabs	1 g/day	- Dose interval adjustment in severe renal impairment, q24h - Dosages for liquid and tabs are not interchangeable
	URTI (e.g., sinusitis, pharyngitis) 10 mg/kg/dose PO BID as suspension **Other infections (≥12 years)** *Mild to moderate:* 125–250 mg PO BID as tabs *Moderate to severe:* 250–500 mg PO BID as tabs	500 mg/day	- Give with food, milk, or formula. Suspension may be mixed with small amount of orange/grape juice or chocolate milk immediately before administration - Do not crush tabs (taste is very bitter)
Cephalexin Susp 50 mg/mL Tab 250 mg, 500 mg	**NEONATES** *≤6 days:* 25 mg/kg/dose PO q12h *7–20 days:* 25 mg/kg/dose PO q8h *21–28 days:* 25 mg/kg/dose PO q6h	250 mg/day 375 mg/day 50 mg/day	- Reserve for PO stepdown treatment in neonates with uncomplicated UTI or skin/soft tissue infections
	INFANTS AND OLDER CHILDREN 6–12 mg/kg/dose PO q6h or 8–17 mg/kg/dose PO q8h **Osteomyelitis and septic arthritis (after IV therapy)** 25–38 mg/kg/dose PO q6h or 35–50 mg/kg/dose PO q8h	1 g/dose, 4 g/day 4 g/day	- Dose interval adjustment in renal impairment: moderate, q8–12h; severe, q12–24h

Continued

Table 40.1   Drug Dosage Guidelines for Neonates[a] (Where Specified), Infants, and Older Children—cont'd

Drug[b,c]	Dose	Dose Limit	Comments
Cetirizine Tab 10 mg	***INFANTS AND OLDER CHILDREN*** *6 months to <2 years:* 2.5 mg PO daily *2–5 years:* 2.5–5 mg PO once daily or 1.25–2.5 mg PO BID *>5 years:* 5–10 mg PO once daily or 2.5–5 mg PO BID	20 mg/day	
Charcoal, activated	See **Activated charcoal**		
Chloral hydrate Syrup 100 mg/mL	***NEONATES*** 10–50 mg/kg/dose PO/PR 3 or 4 times daily **Sedation preprocedure** 25–50 mg/kg/dose PO/PR ***INFANTS AND OLDER CHILDREN*** **Hypnotic** 50 mg/kg/dose PO/PR 20–45 min before examination 25 mg/kg/dose PO/PR qhs prn **Sedation** 80–100 mg/kg/dose PO/PR 20–45 min before procedure, may repeat with 40 mg/kg/dose in 1 h	1 g/dose 2 g/dose	- Not recommended for <34 weeks GA - Reduce dose in patients with CNS, renal or liver impairment - May cause gastric irritation; if possible, dilute dose or administer after feeding

Chloramphenicol sodium succinate Inj 1 g (base)/vial	**INFANTS AND OLDER CHILDREN** **Meningitis** 20–25 mg/kg/dose IV q6h **Other** 12.5–20 mg/kg/dose IV q6h	4 g/day	- Reduce dose in renal impairment; avoid in liver impairment
Chloroquine Tab 250 mg chloroquine phosphate = 155 mg base Susp (HSC) 15 mg/mL chloroquine phosphate (= 9.3 mg base/mL)	**INFANTS AND OLDER CHILDREN** **Malaria prophylaxis** 8.1 mg chloroquine phosphate/kg/dose PO given once weekly, beginning 1–2 weeks before entering malaria zone, and continuing for 4 weeks after leaving malarial area **Malaria treatment** *Day 1:* 16.1 mg chloroquine phosphate/kg/dose PO once *Day 2:* 16.1 mg chloroquine phosphate/kg/dose PO once *Day 3:* 8.1 mg chloroquine phosphate/kg/dose PO once **Systemic Lupus Erythematosus** 2–3 mg chloroquine phosphate/kg/dose once daily	500 mg chloroquine phosphate/dose *First dose:* 1000 mg chloroquine phosphate *Subsequent doses:* 500 mg chloroquine phosphate 250 mg chloroquine phosphate/dose	- Give PO with food or milk; drug extremely bitter; tabs may be crushed and mixed with cereal, jam, or chocolate syrup; widely available as syrup in malaria-endemic countries
Cidofovir Inj 375 mg/5 mL	**INFANTS AND OLDER CHILDREN** **Adenovirus infections post-HSCT** 1 mg/kg/dose IV three times per week or 5 mg/kg/dose once weekly **CMV infections post-HSCT** 5 mg/kg/dose IV once weekly, then 3–5 mg/kg/dose IV q2wk		- Dose interval adjustment in renal impairment: moderate to severe, avoid use

Continued

Table 40.1 Drug Dosage Guidelines for Neonates[a] (Where Specified), Infants, and Older Children—cont'd

Drug[b,c]	Dose	Dose Limit	Comments
Ciprofloxacin Inj 2 mg/mL (HSC) Tab 250 mg, 500 mg, 750 mg Susp 100 mg/mL	*NEONATES* **Severe infection (e.g., sepsis)** 10 mg/kg/dose IV q12h *INFANTS AND OLDER CHILDREN* **Cystic fibrosis** 20 mg/kg/dose PO BID 10 mg/kg/dose IV q8h **Fever/neutropenia** 10 mg/kg/dose IV q12h **Other indications** 15 mg/kg/dose PO BID 10 mg/kg/dose IV q12h **Urinary tract infections** 10–15 mg/kg/dose PO BID 7.5–10 mg/kg/dose IV BID **Treatment of intestinal bacterial overgrowth** 10–20 mg/kg/dose PO BID **Crohn's disease exacerbation** 10 mg/kg/dose PO/IV BID	 750 mg/dose PO, 1500 mg/day PO 400 mg/dose IV, 1200 mg/day IV 400 mg/dose IV, 800 mg/day IV 750 mg/dose PO, 1500 mg/day PO 400 mg/dose IV, 800 mg/day IV 500 mg/dose PO, 1000 mg/day PO 400 mg/dose IV, 800 mg/day IV	- Dose interval adjustment in renal impairment: moderate to severe, q18–24h - Avoid concurrent administration with antacids, iron; may decrease clearance of warfarin, tacrolimus, cyclosporine, and other drugs - Use with caution in patients with seizure disorders

Tab 10 mg Cap (HSC) 0.5 mg, 1 mg	*INFANTS AND OLDER CHILDREN* 0.2 mg/kg/dose PO TID–QID *Usual adult dose:* 5–10 mg/dose up to QID	0.8 mg/kg/day or 40 mg/day, whichever is less	- Need to assess risk for QT interval prolongation before prescribing; reduce dose in renal or liver impairment - Many potential drug interactions; may alter absorption of other drugs
Citalopram Tab 20 mg, 40 mg	*INFANTS AND OLDER CHILDREN* ≤11 years: 5–10 mg PO once daily; increase dose slowly by 5 mg/day q2wk if necessary ≥12 years: 10–20 mg PO daily; increase dose slowly by 10 mg/day q2wk as necessary	*Usual range:* 20–40 mg/day *Dose limit:* 40 mg/day	- An increased risk of suicidal thinking and behavior has been reported with the use of antidepressants in children, adolescents, and young adults. Monitor carefully for suicidal ideation, self-harm, or hostility
Clarithromycin Tab 250 mg, 500 mg Susp 25 mg/mL	*INFANTS AND OLDER CHILDREN* 7.5 mg/kg/dose PO q12h ***Mycobacterium avium* complex** 7.5–15 mg/kg/dose PO q12h ***Helicobacter pylori*-associated ulcer** (for 14 days with PPI, amoxicillin, and metronidazole) 15–24 kg: 250 mg PO BID 25–34 kg: 500 mg PO qam, 250 mg PO qpm ≥35 kg: 500 mg PO BID	500 mg/dose, 1 g/day	- Dose reduction in renal impairment: severe, 50%, give 1–2 doses - May decrease clearance of tacrolimus, cyclosporine, other drugs
Clavulin	See **Amoxicillin/clavulanic acid**		
Clindamycin Oral solution (as palmitate) 15 mg base/mL Cap 150 mg base Inj 900 mg base/vial	*NEONATES* <1.2 kg: 5 mg/kg/dose IV q12h 1.2–2 kg, 0–7 days: 5 mg/kg/dose IV q12h 1.2–2 kg, >7 days: 5 mg/kg/dose IV q8h ≥2 kg, 0–7 days: 5 mg/kg/dose IV q8h ≥2 kg, >7 days: 5–7.5 mg/kg/dose IV q6h		- Do not administer enterally to neonates <7 days old; use clindamycin injection in neonates ≥7 days old for enteral doses

Continued

Drug Dosing Guidelines

40

Table 40.1 Drug Dosage Guidelines for Neonates[a] (Where Specified), Infants, and Older Children—cont'd

Drug[b,c]	Dose	Dose Limit	Comments
Clindamycin—cont'd Tab 10 mg Susp (HSC) 1 mg/mL	*INFANTS AND OLDER CHILDREN* **Mild to moderate infections** 5–7.5 mg/kg/dose PO/IV q6h or 7–10 mg/kg/dose PO/IV q8h **Severe infections** 7.5–10 mg/kg/dose IV q6h or 10–13 mg/kg/dose IV q8h **Piperacillin-allergic neutropenic patient with fever** 10 mg/kg/dose IV q8h **Chloroquine-resistant *Falciparum* malaria** *IV therapy:* 10 mg/kg/dose IV for 1 dose, followed by 5 mg/kg/dose IV q8h for 7 days *PO therapy:* 5 mg/kg/dose PO q6h for 7 days or 6.7 mg/kg/dose PO q8h for 7 days	1.8 g/day PO, 2.7 g/day IV 3.6 g/day IV 600 mg/dose IV 2.7 g/day PO	- Give cap PO with food or full glass of water to avoid-esophageal ulceration - Use with quinine for chloroquine-resistant malaria only if patient is unable to take doxycycline or tetracycline
Clobazam Tab 10 mg Susp (HSC) 1 mg/mL	*INFANTS AND OLDER CHILDREN* *Initial dose:* 0.25 mg/kg/dose PO qhs or 0.125 mg/kg/dose PO BID: increase gradually to 0.25 mg/kg/dose PO BID or 0.17 mg/kg/dose PO TID	*Initial dose:* 10 mg *Max dose:* 1 mg/kg/day or 80 mg/day	- Sound-alike/look-alike drug alert: **Clonazepam**
Clonazepam Susp (HSC) 0.1 mg/mL Tab 0.5 mg, 2 mg	*INFANTS AND OLDER CHILDREN* ≤30 kg: *Initial dose:* 0.005–0.025 mg/kg/dose PO BID or 0.003–0.017 mg/kg/dose PO TID increasing by 0.05 mg/kg/day every 3 days pm up to 0.2 mg/kg/day >30 kg: *Initial dose:* 0.5 mg PO TID increasing by 0.5–1 mg/day every 3 days up to 7 mg PO TID	20 mg/day	- Reduce dose in liver impairment - Sound-alike/look-alike drug alert: **Clobazam**

Clonidine Tab 0.1 mg (100 mcg) Susp (HSC) 0.01 mg/mL (10 mcg/mL)	*NEONATES* **Neonatal Abstinence Syndrome** 0.5–1 mcg/kg/dose PO q4–6h		
	Sedation and opioid withdrawal management (intensive care setting)		
	2–4 mcg/kg/dose PO q4–6h	4 mcg/kg/dose	
	INFANTS AND OLDER CHILDREN **Growth hormone stimulation test (≥10 kg)**	150 mcg/dose	
	BSA (surface area) *<0.5 m²:* 50 mcg/dose *0.5–0.67 m²:* 75 mcg/dose *0.68–0.82 m²:* 100 mcg/dose *0.83–0.99 m²:* 125 mcg/dose *≥1 m²:* 150 mcg/dose		
	Preoperative dose 4 mcg/kg/dose PO 90 min before operation	200 mcg/dose	
	Hypertension *Initial:* 1.7–3.3 mcg/kg/dose PO q8h or 2.5–5 mcg/kg/dose PO q12h; increase gradually as needed; usual dose range: 1.25–6.25 mcg/kg/ dose PO q6h	2400 mcg/day	
	Sedation/opioid withdrawal (intensive care setting) 2–4 mcg/kg/dose PO q4–6h	4 mcg/kg/dose, 100 mcg/dose	
Clopidogrel Tab 75 mg Susp (HSC) 5 mg/mL	*INFANTS AND OLDER CHILDREN* **Cardiac patients with stents** *Initial:* 1 mg/kg/dose PO once daily	*Usual adult dose:* 75 mg/day	- Use with caution in liver impairment - Proton-pump inhibitors may reduce antiplatelet effects of clopidogrel. Avoid combination
	Stroke 1 mg/kg/dose PO once daily	75 mg/day	

Continued

Drug Dosing Guidelines

Table 40.1 Drug Dosage Guidelines for Neonates[a] (Where Specified), Infants, and Older Children—cont'd

Drug[b,c]	Dose	Dose Limit	Comments
Cloxacillin Susp 25 mg/mL Cap 250 mg, 500 mg Inj 0.5 g/vial, 1 g/vial, 2 g/vial	***NEONATES*** **Meningitis** *<2 kg, 0–7 days:* 50 mg/kg/dose IV q12h *<2 kg, >7 days:* 50 mg/kg/dose IV q8h *≥2 kg, 0–7 days:* 50 mg/kg/dose IV q8h *≥2 kg, >7 days:* 50 mg/kg/dose IV q6h **Other infections** *<2 kg, 0–7 days:* 25 mg/kg/dose IV/PO q12h *<2 kg, >7 days:* 25 mg/kg/dose IV/PO q8h *≥2 kg, 0–7 days:* 25 mg/kg/dose IV/PO q8h *≥2 kg, >7 days:* 25 mg/kg/dose IV/PO q6h ***INFANTS AND OLDER CHILDREN*** **Mild to moderate infections** 12.5–37.5 mg/kg/dose PO/IV/IM q6h **Severe infections** 25–35 mg/kg/dose IV/IM q4h or 37.5–50 mg/kg/dose IV/IM q6h	*Usual adult dose:* 500 mg/dose PO 1 g/dose IV/IM/PO	- Give PO on empty stomach (1 h ac or 2 h pc)
Colistin Inj 150 mg sodium colistimethate/vial (75 mg colistin base/mL)	*Dose on ideal body mass* 75 mg base/dose inhaled BID 0.8–1.6 mg base/kg/dose IV q8h ***INFANTS AND OLDER CHILDREN***	2 g/dose, 12 g/day IV/IM 100 mg base/dose IV	Dose adjustment in renal impairment: - Mild: 1.25–1.9 mg base/kg/dose IV q12h - Moderate: 1.25 mg base/kg/dose IV q12h or 2.5 mg base/kg/dose IV q24h - Severe: 1.5 mg base/kg/dose IV q36h
Cotrimoxazole	See **Sulfamethoxazole and trimethoprim**		

Cromolyn
Nasal drops 2%
Ophthalmic drops 2%

Cyclosporine
Regular (Sandimmune)
Inj 50 mg/mL
Microemulsion (Neoral)
liquid 100 mg/mL
Cap 10 mg, 25 mg,
50 mg, 100 mg

INFANTS AND OLDER CHILDREN
Nasal drops: 1–2 drops into each nostril up to 6 times/day
Ophthalmic drops: 2 drops each eye QID

INFANTS AND OLDER CHILDREN
(Initial dose before TDM)
Hematopoietic progenitor cell transplant
Underlying malignancy, match related donor: 1.5 mg/kg/dose IV q12h
Underlying malignancy, match unrelated donor: 65 mg/m²/dose IV q12h
No underlying malignancy: 65 mg/m²/dose IV q12h
SCID
1.5 mg/kg/dose IV q12h
Lung/renal transplantation
5 mg/kg/dose PO q12h
Cardiac transplantation
1 mg/kg/day IV as a continuous infusion or 1.5 mg/kg/dose IV q12h
Juvenile idiopathic arthritis
1.25 mg/kg/dose PO q12h
Other autoimmune diseases
0.5–1.5 mg/kg/dose PO q12h

- Monitoring of serum drug concentration recommended—measure initial trough concentration within 48 h, and adjust dose as necessary
- Maintenance doses must be individualized, based on factors such as disease state or type of transplant/time since transplantation
- Reduce dose in liver impairment
- Oral to IV dose conversion as follows
  - Solid organ transplant: 3:1
  - BMT: 2.3:1
- Microemulsion may be taken with or without food as long as this is done consistently; it should always be taken with the same beverage (not grapefruit juice)
- Interacts with many other medications

Continued

Table 40.1 **Drug Dosage Guidelines for Neonates[a] (Where Specified), Infants, and Older Children—cont'd**

Drug[b,c]	Dose	Dose Limit	Comments
Danaparoid Inj 750 units/0.6 mL	***INFANTS AND OLDER CHILDREN*** 30 units/kg IV loading dose, then 1.2–2.0 units/kg/h continuous IV infusion 18 units/kg/dose SC q12h (36 units/kg/day)		- Monitor antifactor Xa activity immediately after bolus dose, then q4h until steady state has been achieved, then daily to maintain therapeutic level of 0.2–0.8 units/mL - Contraindicated in severe renal impairment - Warfarin considered contraindicated by some experts
Dapsone Tab 100 mg Susp (HSC) 2 mg/mL	***INFANTS AND OLDER CHILDREN*** **Pneumocystis pneumonia prophylaxis** *Daily dose:* 2 mg/kg/dose PO once daily *Weekly dose:* 4 mg/kg/dose PO once weekly	100 mg/day 200 mg/dose	- Caution in patients with G6PD deficiency, hypersensitivity to sulfonamides - May cause photosensitivity - Do not administer with antacids
Darbepoetin Alfa 10 mcg/0.4 mL, 20 mcg/ 0.5 mL, 30 mcg/0.3 mL, 40 mcg/0.4 mL, 50 mcg/ 0.5 mL, 60 mcg/0.3 mL, 80 mcg/0.4 mL, 100 mcg/0.5 mL, 150 mcg/0.3 mL, 500 mcg/1 mL	***INFANTS AND OLDER CHILDREN*** **Anemia of chronic renal failure** *Initial dose:* 0.45 mcg/kg/dose IV/SC weekly		- Titrate dose according to hemoglobin level - In some patients the dose interval may be extended and the dose adjusted proportionally

Desmopressin	***INFANTS AND OLDER CHILDREN***		- Consider PO route for patients with diabetes insipidus who are unable to tolerate intranasal administration; start with low dose and titrate to effect
Intranasal spray 0.25 mg/2.5 mL (10 mcg/spray)	**Diabetes insipidus**		
	Nasal: 5–20 mcg/dose intranasally once daily or 2.5–10 mcg/dose intranasally BID		
Inj 4 mcg/mL, 15 mcg/mL,	*Oral tablet:* 50–100 mcg/dose PO once daily to TID	1200 mcg/day	- Dose conversion: 100 mcg oral tablet is equivalent to 60 mcg sublingual tablet (DDAVP melt)
Oral tab 100 mcg, 200 mcg	*Sublingual tablet (DDAVP melt):* 60–120 mcg/dose SL once daily to TID	720 mcg/day	
Oral disintegrating tablet: 60 mcg, 120 mcg	*Subcutaneous:* Test dose: 0.005 mcg/kg/dose; titrate up by 50% increments until clinical response achieved		- Risk of severe hyponatremia. Restrict fluid intake and monitor fluid balance and serum electrolytes closely
	Usual starting dose range:		- Use in children <3 years is generally contraindicated
	2–5 years: 0.05–0.1 mcg SC		
	6–12 years: 0.1–0.2 mcg SC		
	13–18 years: 0.2–0.4 mcg SC		
	Coagulopathy		
	0.3 mcg/kg/dose IV/SC; may repeat dose after >12 h if necessary	20 mcg/dose	
	Enuresis		
	Oral tablet	*Oral tablet:* 600 mcg/day	
	Initial dose: 200 mcg PO qhs for 3 days		
	May increase by 200 mcg increments up to 600 mcg PO qhs		
	Sublingual tablet (DDAVP melt)	*Sublingual tablet (DDAVP melt):* 360 mcg/day	
	Initial dose: 120 mcg PO qhs for 3 days		
	May increase by 120 mcg increments up to 360 mcg PO qhs		

Continued

Table 40.1. Drug Dosage Guidelines for Neonates[a] (Where Specified), Infants, and Older Children—cont'd

Drug[b,c]	Dose	Dose Limit	Comments
Dexamethasone Susp (HSC) 1 mg/mL Tab 0.5 mg, 2 mg, 4 mg Inj 4 mg/mL	***NEONATES*** **Chronic lung disease** ≥ 7 days postnatal age: 0.075 mg/kg/dose PO/IV q12h for 3 days; 0.05 mg/kg/dose PO/IV q12h for 3 days; 0.025 mg/kg/dose PO/IV q12h for 2 days; 0.01 mg/kg/dose PO/IV q12h for 2 days		- Avoid in children with peptic ulcer disease; give PO with food or milk - To discontinue in patients receiving therapy for ≥10 days, reduce dose by 50% q48h until 0.3 ± 0.1 mg/m²/day achieved, then reduce dose by 50% q10–14days
	Subglottic edema 0.5–1 mg/kg/dose PO/IV BID (12–24 h pre-extubation and 12–48 h post-extubation, then reassess)		- In meningitis, administer first dose before antibiotics
	INFANTS AND OLDER CHILDREN **Extubation (if previous difficulties with extubation)** 0.25–0.5 mg/kg/dose PO/IV/IM q6h beginning before extubation and may continue 24–48 h afterwards	20 mg/dose	- Dexamethasone may be contraindicated if the antineoplastic protocol prohibits its use as an antiemetic or in patients receiving treatment for brain tumors; this contraindication may be reevaluated based on patient response
	Increased ICP 0.2–0.4 mg/kg/dose IV, then 0.075 mg/kg/dose IV/IM q6h; may be useful in cerebral tumors and malaria but not in head injuries	*Initial dose:* 10 mg	
	Croup 0.6 mg/kg/dose IV/PO once	20 mg/dose	
	Acute asthma 0.6 mg/kg/dose PO given once daily for 1–2 days or 0.3 mg/kg/dose PO given once daily for 5 days	20 mg/dose	

Meningitis		
0.15 mg/kg/dose IV q6h for 4 days	20 mg/dose	
Antiemetic for antineoplastic regimens		- Reduce dose to half when giving aprepitant concurrently
Highly emetogenic regimen		
6 mg/m²/dose IV/PO q12h (consider q24h for adolescents and q8h for children <12 years of age)	20 mg/day	
Moderately emetogenic regimen		
≤0.6 m²: 2 mg/dose IV/PO q12h		
>0.6 m²: 4 mg/dose IV/PO q12h		
Delayed phase chemotherapy induced nausea and vomiting		
4.5 mg/m²/dose PO q12h	8 mg/dose	
NEONATES		
Dexmedetomidine Inj 200 mcg/2 mL	**Sedation in patients receiving therapeutic hypothermia**		- For use beyond 96 h, consider decreasing by 0.05 mcg/kg/h daily to twice daily based on patient response (hypertension, tachycardia, and increased agitation)
	Initial dose: 0.05 mcg/kg/h IV; increase by 0.05 mcg/kg/h every 6 h as needed. Continue until the 72-h cooling period has ended or further sedation is not necessary	0.3 mcg/kg/h	
	Sedation in NICU (infants not receiving therapeutic hypothermia)		
	Initial dose: 0.05 mcg/kg/h IV; increase by 0.05 mcg/kg/h every 3–6 h as needed. Close vital sign monitoring required (e.g., respiratory rate, blood pressure, and heart rate) before and after each dose titration due to the risk of hypotension and bradycardia	0.5 mcg/kg/h	
	Continuous sedation (ICU)		
	Loading dose: 0.5 mcg/kg/dose IV over 10–20 min		
	Maintenance dose: start at 0.5 mcg/kg/h IV and increase by 0.1 mcg/kg/h every 30–60 min as needed	2.5 mcg/kg/h	

Continued

Table 40.1 — Drug Dosage Guidelines for Neonates[a] (Where Specified), Infants, and Older Children—cont'd

Drug[b,c]	Dose	Dose Limit	Comments
Dexmedetomidine—cont'd	**Pre-procedural sedation or anxiolysis** *Intranasal* Initial: 2–3 mcg/kg/dose intranasally via mucosal atomization device 30–60 min prior to procedure. May repeat dose 45 minutes after initial dose to a maximum of 4 mcg/kg total ***INFANTS AND OLDER CHILDREN*** **Continuous sedation (ICU)** *Loading dose:* 0.5 mcg/kg/dose IV over 10–20 min *Maintenance dose:* Start at 0.5 mcg/kg/h IV and increase by 0.1 mcg/kg/h every 30–60 min as needed **Pre-procedural sedation or anxiolysis** *IV* *Loading dose:* 0.5–2 mcg/kg/dose IV over 10 min *Maintenance dose:* 0.2–2 mcg/kg/h IV *Intranasal* Initial: 2–3 mcg/kg/dose intranasally via mucosal atomization device 30–60 min before procedure May repeat dose 45 min after initial dose to a maximum of 4 mcg/kg total *Buccal* 2–3 mcg/kg/dose buccally 30–60 min prior to procedure (using injection solution) *Oral* 5 mcg/kg/dose PO 30–60 min prior to procedure (using injection solution)	4 mcg/kg/dose intranasally or 0.5 mL/nostril 2.5 mcg/kg/h 2 mcg/kg/h IV 4 mcg/kg/dose intranasally or 1 mL/nostril (children/adults), 0.5 mL/nostril (infants)	

Dextromethorphan Liquid 3 mg/mL	***INFANTS AND OLDER CHILDREN*** 0.25 mg/kg/dose PO q6h or 0.3 mg/kg/dose PO q8h	1 mg/kg/day (*usual adult dose:* 10–20 mg PO q4h prn)
Dextrose Inj 100 mg/mL (10%) Inj preloaded 500 mg/mL (50%) Oral gel: 40% dextrose, 31 g tube	***NEONATES*** **Hypoglycemia** (using dextrose 10%) *Bolus dose:* 2–4 mL/kg IV of D10W (provides 0.2–0.4 g/kg of glucose) *Maintenance dose:* 80–100 mL/kg/day IV of D10W (provides 5–7 mg/kg/min of glucose) **Hypoglycemia** (using dextrose 40% oral gel) GA ≥35 weeks: 0.5 mL/kg/dose buccally; may be repeated up to 6 doses over 48 h. Repeat dose if still hypoglycemic or if hypoglycemia recurs after 30 min	- Dilute to 25% for infants and young children; follow bolus dose by a continu- ous dextrose infusion; except in emer- gency, administer solutions >15% via central line
	INFANTS AND OLDER CHILDREN **Hypoglycemia** (using dextrose 50%) *Bolus dose:* 1–2 mL/kg/dose IV (0.5–1 g/kg/dose) *Continuous infusion:* 3–5 mg/kg/min IV	*Usual adult dose:* 10–25 g	- Dilute to 25% for infants and young children - Follow bolus dose by a continuous dextrose infusion. Except in emergency, administer solutions >15% dextrose via central line
Diazepam Tab 0.5 mg, 1 mg, 2 mg, 5 mg Cap (HSC) 0.1 mg Inj 5 mg/mL	***NEONATES*** **Sedation** *Initial:* 0.1 mg/kg/dose IV/PO q4–6h prn or scheduled regularly. Titrate to response as needed.	0.2 mg/kg/dose	
	INFANTS AND OLDER CHILDREN 0.025–0.2 mg/kg/dose PO q6h	2–10 mg/dose PO BID–QID	- May cause hypotension and apnea when given IV

Continued

Table 40.1 Drug Dosage Guidelines for Neonates[a] (Where Specified), Infants, and Older Children—cont'd

Drug[b,c]	Dose	Dose Limit	Comments
Diazepam—cont'd	**Status epilepticus**		- For rectal doses, administer diazepam injection, undiluted
	0.3 mg/kg/dose IV q10min for 2 doses or 0.5 mg/kg/dose PR once	*<5 years:* 5 mg/dose IV	- Reduce dose in liver impairment
		≥5 years: 10 mg/dose IV	- Tablets may be crushed and mixed with food or beverage, or disintegrated in 5–10 mL of water if needed. Tablets may be disintegrated in water for NG tube administration
		20 mg/dose PR	
	Preoperative		
	0.1–0.5 mg/kg/dose PO 30–90 min before surgery	20 mg/dose PO	
	Sedation		
	0.1 mg/kg/dose IV	5–10 mg/dose IV	
	0.2 mg/kg/dose PO given 45–60 min before procedure	20 mg/dose PO	
Didanosine Susp 10 mg/mL EC caps: 200 mg, 250 mg, 400 mg	***INFANTS AND OLDER CHILDREN***		- Reduce dose in renal impairment; use with caution in hepatic impairment
	Suspension	*Adult usual dose:*	- May cause pancreatitis, peripheral neuropathy, headache, diarrhea
	<8 months: 100 mg/m²/dose PO BID	*<60 kg:* 250 mg/day	- Give higher doses if risk of CNS disease, especially in developmental delay
	>8 months:	*≥60 kg:* 400 mg/day	
	Treatment naive: 240 mg/m²/day PO as a single daily dose		
	Treatment experienced (or in selected treatment naive patients): 120 mg/m²/dose PO BID (range: 90–150 mg/m²/dose PO BID)		
	EC caps		
	20–<25 kg: 200 mg PO once daily		
	25–<60 kg: 250 mg PO once daily		
	≥60 kg: 400 mg PO once daily		

Digoxin	NEONATES, INFANTS AND OLDER CHILDREN		- Do not administer IM
Elixir 50 mcg/mL	**Digitalization (or loading) dose:** (3 doses: first stat, second in 6 h, third in another 6 h)		- Reduce dose in renal and hepatic impairment
Tab 62.5 mcg, 125 mcg, 250 mcg	*<37 weeks PCA*		- Digitalization (or loading) dose adjustment in renal impairment: severe, 50%–65%; maintenance dose adjustment in renal impairment: moderate, 25%–75%; severe, 10%–25%
Inj (HSC) 20 mcg/mL	7 mcg/kg/dose PO	*Total digitalization dose:*	
	5 mcg/kg/dose IV	1500 mcg PO, 1000 mcg IV	
	≥37 weeks PCA–2 years		- Dose reduction for drug interactions: amiodarone, propafenone, quinidine—50%; carvedilol—25%; many other drugs may interact with digoxin; once-daily dosing may be satisfactory, especially in patients >2 years
	17 mcg/kg/dose PO		
	12 mcg/kg/dose IV		
	>2 years		
	13 mcg/kg/dose PO		- Dose conversion:
	10 mcg/kg/dose IV		- IV dose = oral dose × 0.7
	Maintenance dose		- Oral dose = IV dose × 1.4
	<37 weeks PCA		- Digoxin antibody (Digibind) is available to treat potentially life-threatening digoxin toxicity
	2 mcg/kg/dose PO q12h	*Maintenance dose:* 500 mcg/day	
	1.5 mcg/kg/dose IV q12h	PO, 400 mcg/day IV	- Dose on IBW if IBW less than total body weight
	≥37 weeks PCA–2 years		
	5 mcg/kg/dose PO q12h		
	3.5 mcg/kg/dose IV q12h		
	>2 years		
	8 mcg/kg/dose PO once daily or 4 mcg/kg/dose PO q12h (once daily dosing may be satisfactory especially in patients >2 years of age)		
	2.8 mcg/kg/dose IV q12h		

Continued

Table 40.1 Drug Dosage Guidelines for Neonates[a] (Where Specified), Infants, and Older Children—cont'd

Drug[b,c]	Dose	Dose Limit	Comments
Dimenhydrinate Liquid 3 mg/mL Tab 50 mg Chew tab 15 mg Suppos 25 mg, 50 mg Inj 50 mg/mL	***INFANTS AND OLDER CHILDREN*** **Antiemetic** *<12 years:* 0.5–1.25 mg/kg/dose PO/IV/IM/PR q6–8h prn *≥12 years* *Usual dose:* 50 mg PO/IV/IM q4–6h prn 50–100 mg PR q6–8h prn	50 mg/dose 150 mg/day 100 mg/dose, 400 mg/day	- Sound-alike/look-alike drug alert: **diphenhydramine**
Diphenhydramine Elixir 2.5 mg/mL Tab 25 mg, 50 mg Inj 50 mg/mL	***INFANTS AND OLDER CHILDREN*** **Antihistamine** 1.25 mg/kg/dose PO/IV/IM q6h prn **Anaphylaxis** 1–2 mg/kg/dose IV	50 mg/dose, 300 mg/day	- Sound-alike/look-alike drug alert: **dimenhydrinate**
Dipyridamole Susp (HSC) 10 mg/mL Tab 25 mg, 50 mg Inj 5 mg/mL	***INFANTS AND OLDER CHILDREN*** 1.7 mg/kg/dose PO TID	400 mg/day	- Give on an empty stomach (1 h ac or 2 h pc)
Dobutamine Inj 250 mg/vial	***NEONATES*** 5–20 mcg/kg/min IV/IO ***INFANTS AND OLDER CHILDREN*** 2–30 mcg/kg/min IV	40 mcg/kg/min	- Avoid extravasation; administer via central line, whenever possible
Docusate Liquid 4 mg/mL Cap 100 mg	***INFANTS AND OLDER CHILDREN*** 5 mg/kg/dose PO once daily or 2.5 mg/kg/dose PO q12h	*Usual adult dose:* 100–200 mg/day	- Dilute liquid in milk or juice - Onset of action. 24–72 h

Drug	Dose	Comments
Domperidone Tab 10 mg Susp (HSC) 5 mg/mL	**NEONATES, INFANTS AND OLDER CHILDREN** 0.4–0.8 mg/kg/dose PO TID or 0.3–0.6 mg/kg/dose PO QID 30 mg/day *Usual adult dose:* 10 mg TID–QID	- Dose adjustment in renal impairment: extend interval to once or twice daily; consider dose reduction in more severe impairment; use with caution in patients with hepatic impairment - May prolong QT$_c$ interval - **Contraindicated** in patients with long QT syndrome or baseline QT prolongation - Close clinical and ECG monitoring required for patients at high risk of QT prolongation and Torsade de Pointes (TdP). Monitor ECG at baseline and 48 h after starting domperidone in patients with one or more of the following risk factors: heart rate or rhythm disorders, structural heart abnormalities, hypokalemia, on CYP3A4 inhibitors (e.g., macrolide antibiotics, azole antifungals) or potassium depleting diuretics, or domperidone doses exceeding 30 mg/day
Dopamine Inj 200 mg/250mL (800 mcg/mL), 800 mg/250mL (3200 mcg/mL)	**NEONATES, INFANTS AND OLDER CHILDREN** 5–20 mcg/kg/min via continuous IV/IO infusion 20 mcg/kg/min	- Neonates may be less sensitive to dopamine than older infants and children - Avoid dopamine >10 mcg/kg/min in neonates with PPHN - Avoid extravasation; administer via central venous line whenever possible - Do not dilute premixed bags

Continued

Table 40.1 Drug Dosage Guidelines for Neonates[a] (Where Specified), Infants, and Older Children—cont'd

Drug[b,c]	Dose	Dose Limit	Comments
Dornase alfa Inj 1 mg/mL	***INFANTS AND OLDER CHILDREN*** 2.5 mg via nebulizer once daily (twice daily dosing may be used for forced vital capacity over 85%)		- Administer undiluted - Do not mix with other drugs in nebulizer
Doxazosin Tab 1 mg, 2 mg, 4 mg	***INFANTS AND OLDER CHILDREN*** *Initial:* 1 mg PO as single daily dose *Maintenance:* 1–4 mg PO daily	*Adult max dose:* 16 mg/day	- Dose should be titrated q2wk until adequate blood pressure is achieved or dose-limiting side effects appear - Monitor for syncope and postural hypotension with first dose
Doxycycline Susp (HSC) 5 mg/mL Cap 100 mg	***INFANTS AND OLDER CHILDREN*** **Skin and soft tissue infections caused by MSSA or MRSA** 2 mg/kg/dose PO q12h for 5–10 days depending on severity **Lyme Disease** 2 mg/kg/dose PO q12h for 14 days **Lyme Disease Post-Exposure Prophylaxis** 4.4 mg/kg/dose PO once as a single dose, initiate within 72 h of tick removal **Chloroquine-resistant *Falciparum* malaria** *Treatment:* 2 mg/kg/dose PO BID for 7 days *Prophylaxis:* 2 mg/kg/dose PO as single daily dose **Pelvic inflammatory disease** ≥8 *years:* 100 mg PO BID for 14 days with Ceftriaxone (outpatient therapy) or Cefoxitin (inpatient or outpatient therapy), ± metronidazole (outpatient therapy)	100 mg/dose 100 mg/dose 200 mg/dose 200 mg/day 100 mg/day	- May be given with food - Not recommended for children <8 years

EMLA (lidocaine-prilocaine) Cream 5 g, 30 g Patch 1 g (25 mg/g lidocaine, 25 mg/g prilocaine)	**NEONATES** PNA >14 days, CGA <37 weeks: 0.5 g once (To obtain a dose of 0.5 g, cover half of the 1 g patch with adhesive bandage, and apply the remaining (exposed) half of the patch to skin) PNA >14 days, CGA ≥37 weeks: 1 g once		*Maximum application time:* 1 h	- Methemoglobinemia risk If dose limit is exceeded; do not give to children 0–12 months of age who are receiving other methemoglobin-inducing agents - Contraindicated in G6PD deficiency - Apply only to intact skin
	INFANTS AND OLDER CHILDREN		**Reference for max skin area**	
	Age	**Max skin area (cm²)**	Size of a two-dollar coin	
	>1–3 months	10	Size of a credit card	
	>3–12 months and >5 kg	20		
			Dose	Size of two credit cards	
	1–6 years and >10 kg	100	1 g/h	Size of a standard postcard	
	7–12 years and >20 kg	200	2 g/4 h		
			10 g/4 h		
			20 g/4 h		
Enalapril Tab 2.5 mg, 5 mg Susp (HSC) 1 mg/mL	***INFANTS AND OLDER CHILDREN*** **Hypertension, CHF** *Initial:* 0.1 mg/kg/dose PO once daily or 0.05 mg/kg/dose PO BID *Maintenance:* 0.1–0.5 mg/kg/dose PO once daily or 0.05–0.25 mg/kg/dose PO BID		40 mg/day	- Dose adjustment in renal impairment: moderate, 75%–100% of standard dose; severe, 50% of standard dose - Use lower initial doses in patients with hyponatremia or hypovolemia or in patients receiving concurrent diuretics
Enalaprilat Inj 2.5 mg/2 mL	***INFANTS AND OLDER CHILDREN*** 5–10 mcg/kg/dose IV q8–24h			- Monitor blood pressure and renal function - IV (enalaprilat) and PO (enalapril) doses are *not* equivalent

Continued

Table 40.1 Drug Dosage Guidelines for Neonates[a] (Where Specified), Infants, and Older Children—cont'd

Drug[b,c]	Dose	Dose Limit	Comments
Enoxaparin Inj 100 mg/mL	**NEONATES, INFANTS AND OLDER CHILDREN** ≤2 months *Initial treatment dose:* 1.75 mg/kg/dose SC q12h *Initial prophylactic dose:* 0.75 mg/kg/dose SC q12h OR 1.5 mg/kg/dose SC once daily >2 months–18 years *Initial treatment dose:* 1 mg/kg/dose SC q12h *Initial prophylactic dose:* 0.5 mg/kg/dose SC q12h OR 1 mg/kg/dose SC once daily	*Age ≤2 months:* 3 mg/kg/dose SC q12h *Age >2 months:* maximum treatment dose 2 mg/kg/dose q12h SC, maximum prophylaxis dose 30 mg SC q12h or 40 mg SC once daily	- See protocol for adjusting low molecular weight heparin (LMWH) therapy (see Table 21.13) - Hold for 2 doses before invasive procedures, such as lumbar puncture and measure antifactor Xa (LMWH level) - Enoxaparin is administered using insulin syringes where 1 mg of enoxaparin corresponds to 1 unit on an insulin syringe - Do not administer in areas where skin is damaged or edematous - Monitoring of LMWH antifactor Xa levels for prophylaxis is not required unless renal failure is present. Consult the Thrombosis Service
Epinephrine Inj 0.1 mg/mL (1:10,000), 1 mg/mL (1:1000)	**NEONATES** **Resuscitation** 0.01 mg/kg/dose (0.1 mL/kg/dose of 1:10,000 solution) IV or 0.05–0.1 mg/kg/dose (0.5–1 mL/kg/dose of 1:10,000 solution) ETT q3–5min prn **Continuous infusion** 0.05–1 mcg/kg/min IV **Inhalation** (1:1000) 1 mg/mL solution <5 kg: 0.5 mg/dose ≥5 kg: 2.5–5 mg/dose		- Verify concentration of solution before use - Incompatible with sodium bicarbonate - Administer via central venous line, whenever possible

INFANTS AND OLDER CHILDREN **Anaphylaxis** 0.01 mg/kg/dose (0.01 mL of 1:1000 solution/kg/dose) IM/SC q10–20min prn 0.1–1 mcg/kg/min via continuous IV infusion **Resuscitation** 0.01 mg/kg/dose (0.1 mL/kg/dose of 1:10,000 solution) IV/IO q3–5min prn 0.1 mg/kg/dose (0.1 mL/kg/dose of 1:1000 solution) ETT q3min prn **Vasopressor support for hypotension/shock (intensive care setting)** 0.01–1 mcg/kg/min via continuous IV infusion **Inhalation (1:1000, 1 mg/mL solution)** *<5 kg:* 0.5 mg/kg/dose *≥5 kg:* 2.5–5 mg/dose Dilute dose to 2.5 or 3 mL in 0.9% NaCl, give via nebulizer prn to max q1h	*Maximum:* 0.5 mg/dose 1 mg (10 mL) IV/IO 10 mg (10 mL) ETT	
Epoetin alfa Inj preloaded 1000, 2000, 3000, 4000, 10,000 units Inj 20,000 units/vial	**INFANTS AND OLDER CHILDREN** **Anemia of chronic renal failure** *Initial dose:* 50 units/kg/day IV/SC 3 times weekly	– Titrate dose according to hemoglobin
Epoprostenol Inj 0.5 mg, 1.5 mg vial	**NEONATES, INFANTS AND OLDER CHILDREN** *Initial starting dose:* 5 nanogram/kg/min IV *Usual dose range:* 5–12 nanogram/kg/min IV	– Titrate according to response or adverse effects – (15 × wt [kg]) mcg in 50 mL "diluent for Flolan" at 1 mL/h = 5 nanogram/kg/min – Monitor BP and heart rate (can cause hypotension, tachycardia) – Use with caution in patients receiving concomitant anticoagulants; may increase risk of bleeding

– IM route preferred

Continued

Table 40.1 Drug Dosage Guidelines for Neonates[a] (Where Specified), Infants, and Older Children—cont'd

Drug[b,c]	Dose	Dose Limit	Comments
Ergocalciferol Liquid 8280 unit/mL Inj 600,000 unit/1.5 mL	***INFANTS AND OLDER CHILDREN*** **Treatment of vitamin D deficiency in intestinal malabsorption or chronic liver disease** *Regular dose* *1–12 years:* 10,000–25,000 units PO/IM daily *>12 years:* 10,000–40,000 units PO/IM daily *High dose:* 60,000 to 150,000 units IM qmonthly to q6mo		- Dose adjusted according to vitamin D (25-OH-D) levels
Ertapenem Inj 1 g/vial	***INFANTS AND OLDER CHILDREN*** *3 months–11 years:* 15 mg/kg/dose IV q12h *≥12 years:* 1 g IV q24h	500 mg/dose 1 g/ose	- Not recommended for CNS infections - Dose limit in renal impairment: 500 mg/day if CrCl ≤30 mL/min
Erythromycin Base: tab 250 mg Lactobionate: inj 0.5, 1 g/vial	***NEONATES*** ***Chlamydia* conjunctivitis and pneumonia** 5–10 mg/kg/dose IV q6h **Pertussis postexposure prophylaxis and treatment** *0–7 days:* 10 mg/kg/dose PO q12h *>7 days, <2 kg:* 10 mg/kg/dose PO q8h *>7 days, ≥2 kg:* 10–13 mg/kg/dose PO q8h ***INFANTS AND OLDER CHILDREN*** *Base:* 7.5–12.5 mg/kg/dose PO q6h *Lactobionate:* 5–12.5 mg/kg/dose IV q6h	2 g/day PO 4 g/day IV	- Assess risk/benefit in full-term infants <14 days of age because of association with infantile hypertrophic pyloric stenosis - Dose reduction in renal impairment: severe, 50%–75% of dose - Clearance of drugs including cyclosporine, tacrolimus, and carbamazepine will be decreased - Give PO on empty stomach (1 h ac or 2 h pc) unless GI upset occurs

Esmolol Inj 10 mg/mL	***NEONATES*** **Supraventricular tachycardia** 50 mcg/kg/min IV as a continuous infusion, titrate dose by 50–100 mcg/kg/min every 5–20 min	500 mcg/kg/min	- Max concentration for PIV administration: 10 mg/mL; for concentrations >10 mg/mL, administer via central venous line
	INFANTS AND OLDER CHILDREN *Bolus/loading dose:* 100–500 mcg/kg IV over 1 min *Maintenance:* 100–300 mcg/kg/min IV as continuous infusion		
Ethambutol Tab 100 mg, 400 mg	***INFANTS AND OLDER CHILDREN*** **Tuberculosis** 15 mg/kg/dose PO once daily or 50 mg/kg/dose PO twice weekly	2.5 g/dose	- Regimens for treatment and prophylaxis vary - Give with food if GI upset occurs - Dose interval adjustment in renal impairment: CrCl 10–50 mL/min: q24–36h; CrCl <10 mL/min: q48h and/or reduce dose - 15 mg/kg/day is the preferred dosage as there is less risk of optic neuritis. At this dose, ethambutol is bacteriostatic, but will help prevent the development of resistance. It is bactericidal at a dose of 25 mg/kg/day - Regular ophthalmic examinations recommended in patients receiving >15 mg/kg/day. Use with caution in children in whom visual acuity cannot be monitored (generally <5 years of age)
Ethosuximide Syrup 50 mg/mL Cap 250 mg	***INFANTS AND OLDER CHILDREN*** *Initial dose:* 15 mg/kg/dose PO once daily or 7.5 mg/kg/dose PO BID, increase gradually q3d prn to max dose *Usual maintenance dose:* 7.5–20 mg/kg/dose PO BID	1.5 g/day or 40 mg/kg/day, whichever is less	- Reduce dose in liver impairment - Monitoring of serum drug concentration recommended - Give with food or milk

Continued

1166

Table 40.1 Drug Dosage Guidelines for Neonates[a] (Where Specified), Infants, and Older Children—cont'd

Drug[b,c]	Dose	Dose Limit	Comments
Fentanyl Inj 50 mcg/mL Transdermal patch: 12 mcg/h, 25 mcg/h, 50 mcg/h, 75 mcg/h, 100 mcg/h	***NEONATES*** **Sedation/analgesia** 1 mcg/kg/dose IV, followed by continuous infusion: 0.5–2 mcg/kg/h IV infusion; titrate upward **Rapid sequence intubation** 2 mcg/kg/dose IV **Intranasal** *Initial dose:* 1.5 mcg/kg/dose: repeat q5min prn for total of 3 doses *Maintenance dose:* may repeat initial dose q30–60min after the last dose **Sublingual** 1 mcg/kg/dose SL q30min to q4h; titrate to effect ***INFANTS AND OLDER CHILDREN*** *Intermittent dosing (patient not on a continuous infusion):* 0.5–2 mcg/kg/dose IV/SC q10min prn *Intermittent dosing (patient ON a continuous infusion):* 0.5–1 mcg/kg/dose IV/SC q30min prn *Continuous IV infusion:* 0.5–1 mcg/kg IV/kg loading dose, then 0.5–2 mcg/kg/h IV/SC continuous infusion **Procedural Sedation (intensive care setting)** 2–4 mcg/kg/dose IV, titrated to effect (may require up to 10–30 mcg/kg/dose) **Patch** *> 12 years:* initial: 25 mcg/h **Intranasal** *Initial:* 1.5 mcg/kg/dose; repeat q5min prn for total of 3 doses *Maintenance:* May repeat initial dose q30–60min after the last dose	Mean required dose *GA <34 weeks:* 0.64 mcg/kg/h *GA ≥34 weeks:* 0.75 mcg/kg/h 2 mcg/kg/dose IV/SC *Usual adult dose:* 1000 mcg/dose IV	- Reduce dose in renal or hepatic failure - Patch is not for acute pain; use only for established pain and in patients with stable opioid requirements - Adverse effects: respiratory depression, apnea, chest wall rigidity - Administer intermittent dose over at least 60 s - Administer injection solution intranasally using mucosal atomization device. Maximum volume: 0.5 mL/nostril in infants or 1 mL/nostril in children/adults. Larger volumes should be divided between both nostrils. - Injection may be given sublingually, undiluted

Ferrous sulfate/ferrous fumarate	See **Iron**		
Filgrastim (G-CSF) Inj 300 mcg/mL	***INFANTS AND OLDER CHILDREN*** **Antineoplastic-induced neutropenia** 5 mcg/kg/day SC/IV as single daily dose If response marginal after a cycle of chemotherapy, increase dose to 10 mcg/kg/day SC/IV as single daily dose after next and subsequent cycles	10 mcg/kg/day	
Flecainide Susp (HSC) 20 mg/mL Tab 100 mg	***NEONATES*** **Supraventricular tachycardia** *Initial dose:* 1 mg/kg/dose PO q12h ***INFANTS AND OLDER CHILDREN*** **Supraventricular tachycardia** *Initial dose:* 0.33–1 mg/kg/dose PO q12h or 5.7–11 mg/m^2/dose PO q8h	8 mg/kg/day	8 mg/kg/day or 200 mg/m^2/day	- Dose adjustment in renal impairment: CrCl <20 mL/min/1.73 m^2, give 50%– 75% of usual dose - Use with caution in patients with underly- ing structural heart disease - Avoid concurrent administration with milk or milk-based formulas; use caution when diet changes to decreased consumption of milk or milk-based formulas as increased absorption may occur
Fluconazole Susp 10 mg/mL Tab 50 mg, 100 mg Inj 200 mg/vial	***NEONATES*** **Treatment of systemic candidiasis** 12 mg/kg/dose IV/PO q24h **Oropharyngeal candidiasis** 6 mg/kg/dose PO for one dose followed by 3 mg/kg/dose PO once daily			- Use with caution in patients with liver impairment; interval adjustment in renal impairment: moderate: q48h or adjust dose (not interval) 50%; severe: q72h or adjust dose (not interval) 25%

Continued

Table 40.1 Drug Dosage Guidelines for Neonates[a] (Where Specified), Infants, and Older Children—cont'd

Drug[b,c]	Dose	Dose Limit	Comments
Fluconazole—cont'd	***INFANTS AND OLDER CHILDREN***		- May decrease clearance of tacrolimus, cyclosporine, phenytoin, and other medications; monitor carefully in patients also taking warfarin
	3–12 mg/kg/dose PO/IV q24h	400 mg/day (800 mg/day for CNS or severe infections)	
	Oropharyngeal candidiasis		
	3 mg/kg/dose PO once daily	200 mg/day PO	
	Esophageal candidiasis		
	6–12 mg/kg/dose PO once daily	400 mg/day PO	
	Secondary prophylaxis of candidiasis in HIV-infected patients		
	3–6 mg/kg/dose PO once daily	400 mg/day PO	
	BMT prophylaxis		
	10 mg/kg/day PO/IV once daily beginning day 0 and continuing until neutrophil engraftment	400 mg/day	
Fludrocortisone Tab 0.1 mg	***INFANTS AND OLDER CHILDREN***		- Give with food or milk
	Salt-losing hypoadrenalism		- Monitor BP, serum electrolytes
	0.025–0.1 mg/dose PO q12h		- Dosage must be individualized; infants have relatively higher dosage requirements
Flumazenil Inj 0.5 mg/5 mL	***INFANTS AND OLDER CHILDREN***		- If resedation occurs, doses may be repeated every 20 min, or the effective dose may be given as an hourly infusion
	Benzodiazepine antagonist		
	≤20 kg: 0.01 mg/kg IV over 15 s	1000 mcg/dose; total dose: 3000 mcg	
	May repeat at 1–3 min intervals as necessary to a maximum of 5 doses		
	>20 kg: 0.2 mg IV over 15 s		
	May repeat at 1 min intervals to maximum of 5 doses		

Fluticasone Inhalation 50 mcg/puff, 125 mcg/puff, 250 mcg/puff	***INFANTS AND OLDER CHILDREN*** *Moderate dose:* 100–125 mcg/dose inhaled BID *High dose:* >250 mcg/dose inhaled BID	- High doses not recommended beyond 14 days unless under the care of an asthma specialist because of risk of adrenal insufficiency - Monitor for signs of systemic corticoste- roid adverse effects
Fluoxetine Cap: 10 mg, 20 mg Liq: 4 mg/mL	***INFANTS AND OLDER CHILDREN*** *≥ 6 years* *Depression:* 10–20 mg/day *OCD, Bulimia:* Initial dose 10–20 mg/day, increase dose every few weeks to desired effect or maximum of 80 mg/day	- Increased risk of suicidal thinking and behavior has been reported with the use of SSRIs in children and adolescents. Monitor closely for suicidal ideation, self-harm or hostility
Fomepizole Inj 1000 mg/mL	***INFANTS AND OLDER CHILDREN*** *Loading dose:* 15 mg/kg IV *Maintenance dose:* 10 mg/kg/dose IV q12h for 4 doses, then 15 mg/kg/ dose IV q12h	- Consult toxicologists or poison center for management of patients with methanol or ethylene glycol intoxication - Dose adjustment required for dialysis patients - Must be diluted for administration
Fosphenytoin Inj 50 mg PE/mL	***NEONATES*** **Status epilepticus** *Loading dose:* 15–20 mg PE/kg IV/IM once **Maintenance dose** 2–4 mg PE/kg/dose IV/IM q12h	- Calculate loading dose using adjusted body weight

Continued

Table 40.1   Drug Dosage Guidelines for Neonates[a] (Where Specified), Infants, and Older Children—cont'd

Drug[b,c]	Dose	Dose Limit	Comments
Fosphenytoin—cont'd	***INFANTS AND OLDER CHILDREN*** *Status epilepticus* *Loading dose:* 15–20 mg PE/kg IV/IM once **Maintenance** *0.5–3 years:* 2.7–3.3 mg PE/kg/dose IV/IM q8h or 4–5 mg PE/kg/dose IV/IM q12h *4–6 years:* 2.5–3 mg PE/kg/dose IV/IM q8h or 3.8–4.5 mg PE/kg/dose IV/IM q12h *7–9 years:* 2.3–2.6 mg PE/kg/dose IV/IM q8h or 3.5–4 mg PE/kg/dose IV/IM q12h *10–16 years:* 2–2.3 mg PE/kg/dose IV/IM q8h or 3–3.5 mg PE/kg/dose IV/IM q12h *>16 years:* 1.3–2 mg PE/kg/dose IV/IM q8h or 2–3 mg PE/kg/dose IV/IM q12h	*<50 kg:* 1 g PE/dose *≥50 kg:* 1.5 g PE/dose	- Fosphenytoin should be prescribed in phenytoin sodium equivalent units (PE); fosphenytoin sodium 1.5 mg = phenytoin 1 mg = fosphenytoin 1 mg PE - Reduce dose in liver failure - Monitoring of serum drug concentration recommended - To minimize risk of hypotension, administer at a rate not to exceed 3 mg PE/kg/min or 150 mg PE/min, whichever is less
Furosemide Liquid 10 mg/mL Tab 20 mg, 40 mg Inj 10 mg/mL	***NEONATES*** *PMA <31 weeks:* 1 mg/kg/dose IV/PO q24h *PMA ≥31 weeks:* 1 mg/kg/dose IV/PO q12h *Continuous infusion (intensive care setting):* 0.25–0.5 mg/kg/h IV ***INFANTS AND OLDER CHILDREN*** 1–2 mg/kg/dose PO once daily. May increase by 1–2 mg/kg/dose PO q6–12h prn 0.5–2 mg/kg/dose IV/IM q6–12h *Continuous infusion (intensive care setting):* 0.25–0.5 mg/kg/h IV	Dose may be titrated based on fluid status up to a maximum of 3–4 mg/kg/day IV/PO div q6–8h 6 mg/kg/dose PO, 80 mg/dose PO/IM/IV	- Use with caution in patients with hypokalemia, hypovolemia - Monitor fluid balance and serum electrolytes, especially potassium - May displace bilirubin in neonates

Gabapentin Cap 100 mg, 300 mg, 400 mg Susp (HSC) 100 mg/mL Tab 600 mg	***INFANTS AND OLDER CHILDREN*** *Initial dose:* 7–10 mg/kg/dose PO TID; increase dose gradually over 3–7 days *Maintenance dose:* 7–17 mg/kg/dose PO TID ***Adolescents, adults*** *Initial dose:* 300 mg PO once on day 1, 300 mg PO BID on day 2, 300 mg PO TID on day 3 *Maintenance dose:* 900–1800 mg/day PO div TID	3600 mg/day (short-term) 2400 mg/day (long-term)	- Dose adjustment in renal impairment: mild, 50% standard dose; moderate, 25% standard dose; severe, 12.5% standard dose
Ganciclovir Inj 50 mg/mL	***NEONATES*** **Congenital CMV infection (symptomatic, CNS-disease)** 6 mg/kg/dose IV q12h ***INFANTS AND OLDER CHILDREN*** **Congenital CMV infection** 6 mg/kg/dose IV q12h **CMV infection** *Treatment:* 5 mg/kg/dose IV q12h *Maintenance:* 5 mg/kg/dose IV q24h **Solid organ transplant prophylaxis** *EBV/CMV high risk:* 5 mg/kg/dose IV q12h for 14 days then 5 mg/kg/ dose IV q24h for 10 weeks *CMV low risk:* 5 mg/kg/dose IV once daily for 12 weeks		- Handle as a biohazard - Consult product monograph for dose and interval adjustment in impaired renal function

Continued

Table 40.1 Drug Dosage Guidelines for Neonates[a] (Where Specified), Infants, and Older Children—cont'd

Drug[b,c]	Dose	Dose Limit	Comments
Gentamicin Inj 10 mg/mL, 40 mg/mL	**NEONATES** *0–7 days, <34 weeks PMA:* 3 mg/kg/dose IV q24h *0–7 days, ≥34 weeks PMA:* 3 mg/kg/dose IV q18h *>7 days, ≤1 kg:* 3.5 mg/kg/dose IV q24h *>7 days, >1 kg, <37 weeks PMA:* 2.5 mg/kg/dose IV q12h *>7 days, >1 kg, ≥37 weeks PMA:* 2.5 mg/kg/dose IV q8h **Intestinal bacterial overgrowth** 5 mg/kg/dose PO q8h **INFANTS AND OLDER CHILDREN** **Once-daily dosing** 9 mg/kg/dose IV q24h **Traditional (q8h) dosing** 2.5 mg/kg/dose IV/IM q8h **Fever and neutropenia (oncology or BMT patients)** *1 month–<6 years:* 10.5 mg/kg/dose IV q24h *≥6 years:* *Females:* 9.5 mg/kg/dose IV q24h *Males:* 7.5 mg/kg/dose IV q24h **Synergy with beta-lactams for gram positive infections** 1 mg/kg/dose IV/IM q8h **Intestinal bacterial overgrowth** 5 mg/kg/dose PO q8h	 800 mg/dose before TDM 120 mg/dose before TDM 800 mg/dose before TDM	- Monitoring of serum drug concentration recommended - Use IV formulation for PO administration. No TDM required for oral use - Once-daily dosing is *preferred* over (q8h) dosing or extended dosing intervals unless patient meets exclusion criteria (<5 kg, renal failure, gentamicin being used for synergy with beta-lactams, hearing impairment or family history of hearing impairment, specific types of transplant patients). For cystic fibrosis, oncology or severe combined immunodeficiency patients, use specific guidelines. - Dose interval adjustment in renal impairment for infants and older children: mild–moderate, q12h; severe, q24–48h - Calculate dose according to adjusted body weight

Glucagon Inj 1 mg/vial	***NEONATES*** 0.01–0.02 mg/kg/h IV via continuous infusion (if IV access not available, may give 0.1 mg/kg/dose IM q3–4h to max total dose of 1.5 mg/day) ***INFANTS AND OLDER CHILDREN*** **Hypoglycemia**	- For neonates, dilute in D5W or D10W to 24 mL
	≤20 kg: 0.02–0.03 mg/kg/dose IM/IV/SC once *>20 kg:* 1 mg/dose IM/IV/SC once	*≤20 kg:* maximum 0.5 mg	- Monitor glucose level in 15–20 min. May repeat in 20 min as needed
Glycopyrrolate Inj 0.2 mg/mL Liquid 0.2 mg/mL	***INFANTS AND OLDER CHILDREN*** **Control of secretions** 40–100 mcg/kg/dose PO TID or QID 4–10 mcg/kg/dose IV/IM q3–4h	3000 mcg/dose PO 200 mcg/dose IV/IM	
GoLYTELY	See PEG electrolyte		
Granisetron Inj 1 mg/mL Tab 1 mg Susp (HSC) 0.05 mg/mL	***INFANTS AND OLDER CHILDREN*** **Highly emetogenic antineoplastic therapy** 0.04 mg/kg/dose IV as a single daily dose **Moderately emetogenic or low emetogenic antineoplastic therapy** 0.04 mg/kg/dose IV as a single daily dose OR 0.04 mg/kg/dose PO q12h		- Use with caution in hepatic impairment
Growth hormone 5 mg/vial	***INFANTS AND OLDER CHILDREN*** **Growth hormone deficiency** 0.03–0.05 mg/kg/dose IM/SC given on 3 alternate days/week or 6 times weekly **Prader-Willi syndrome** 1 mg/m²/dose IM/SC once daily		

Continued

Table 40.1   Drug Dosage Guidelines for Neonates[a] (Where Specified), Infants, and Older Children—cont'd

Drug[b,c]	Dose	Dose Limit	Comments
Haloperidol Solution 2 mg/mL Tab 0.5 mg, 1 mg, 2 mg, 5 mg Inj 5 mg/mL	***INFANTS AND OLDER CHILDREN*** **Agitation and hyperactivity** *Oral:* 0.025–0.038 mg/kg/dose PO BID or 0.017–0.025 mg/kg/dose PO TID, increase by 0.5 mg/day every 5–7 days to therapeutic effect *IM (preferred parenteral route), IV:* 0.05–0.10 mg/kg/dose IM/IV q6h	0.15 mg/kg/day or 30 mg/day	- Use with caution in cardiac disease because of hypotension and in patients with epilepsy (lowers seizure threshold) - Extrapyramidal side effects in patients 6–12 years; switch to oral therapy as soon as able - With IV administration: increased risk of Torsades de Pointes and QT. Physician must be present during administration and ECG monitoring is recommended. Avoid IV use in patients with risk factors for electrolyte abnormalities, familial long QT syndrome, concomitant medications which may augment QT prolongation, hypothyroidism, underlying cardiac abnormality
Heparin Inj 100 units/mL, 1000 units/mL, 10,000 units/mL	***NEONATES*** **Maintaining patency of indwelling lines** ≤1800 g: 0.5 units/mL of 0.45% NaCl at a rate of 0.1–1 mL/h >1800 g: 1 unit/mL of 0.45% NaCl at a rate of 0.1–1 mL/h **Thrombosis** *Maintenance:* 28 units/kg/h IV via continuous infusion (do not give bolus in neonates)		- See Unfractionated Heparin in Chapter 21 Hematology for further information Monitor PTT and/or anti-factor Xa and titrate infusion rate accordingly. Measure platelet counts daily for the first 10 days, then every 3–5 days thereafter. If the platelet counts drops by >50% from baseline, there is the possibility of heparin-induced thrombocytopenia

	INFANTS AND OLDER CHILDREN	- Avoid concurrent use of ASA or other antiplatelet drugs
	Maintaining patency of indwelling lines 2 unit/mL	- Where possible, avoid IM injections and arterial punctures during anticoagulation therapy
	Thrombosis	
	Loading dose: 75 units/kg IV over 10 min (do not give loading dose if stroke or when the risk of bleeding is high)	- Antidote: protamine sulfate
	Initial maintenance dose	
	≤1 year: 28 units/kg/h IV	
	>1 year: 20 units/kg/h IV	
Hydralazine	***NEONATES***	- Interval adjustment in renal impairment: mild to moderate, q8h; severe, q8–24h
Inj 20 mg/mL	0.3–0.6 mg/kg/dose IV q4h or 0.4–0.9 mg/kg/dose IV q6h	
Oral solution (HSC) 1 mg/mL	0.2–1.3 mg/kg/dose PO q6h	- Associated with development of drug-induced lupus
Tab 10 mg, 25 mg, 50 mg	***INFANTS AND OLDER CHILDREN***	
	Initial dose	
	Intermittent: 0.15–0.8 mg/kg/dose IV q4–6h or	20 mg/dose IV
	Continuous: 1.5 mcg/kg/min IV	
	Maintenance	7 mg/kg/day PO or 200 mg/day PO, whichever is less
	0.19–1.75 mg/kg/dose PO q6h	
Hydrochlorothiazide	***INFANTS AND OLDER CHILDREN***	- Ineffective when GFR <30 mL/min
Susp (HSC) 5 mg/mL	1–2 mg/kg/dose PO q12h	*Usual adult dose:* 25–100 mg/dose PO as single daily dose, BID or q2days
Tab 25 mg, 50 mg		

Continued

Table 40.1   Drug Dosage Guidelines for Neonates[a] (Where Specified), Infants, and Older Children—cont'd

Drug[b,c]	Dose	Dose Limit	Comments

Hydrocortisone
Susp (HSC) 1 mg/mL
Tab 10 mg, 20 mg
Hydrocortisone sodium succinate inj 100 mg/vial, 250 mg/vial, 500 mg/vial, 1000 mg/vial
	NEONATES
	Hypotension secondary to adrenal insufficiency
	Initial dose: 2 mg/kg/dose (25 mg/m²/dose) IV
	Maintenance dose: 0.5–1 mg/kg/dose (6.25–12.5 mg/m²/dose) IV q6h
	Vasopressor refractory shock (intensive care setting)
	Loading dose: 2 mg/kg/dose IV
	Maintenance dose: 1 mg/kg/dose IV q6h
	INFANTS AND OLDER CHILDREN
	Acute asthma
	4–6 mg/kg/dose IV q4–6h
	Anaphylaxis
	5–10 mg/kg/dose IV
	
	Hypoadrenalism (normal endogenous production = 10 ± 3 mg/m²/day)
	Maintenance dose (to be given IV/PO div q6–8h)
	  Central adrenal insufficiency: 6–8 mg/m²/day
	  Primary adrenal insufficiency (Addison disease): 8–12 mg/m²/day
	  Congenital adrenal hyperplasia: 10–15 mg/m²/day
	Stress dose
	  Febrile or severe illness: 10 mg/m²/dose IV/PO q6h or 13 mg/m²/dose IV/PO q8h
	  Preop: 100 mg/m² IV once preop, then 25 mg/m²/dose IV q6h
	Acute adrenal crisis
	100 mg/m² IV once, then 25 mg/m²/dose IV q6h
		≤ 12 years: 100 mg/dose
		> 12 years: 200 mg/dose
			- Consider tapering the dose in patients receiving therapy for ≥10 days as follows: reduce dose by 50% q48h until <1 mg/kg/day (10 ± 3 mg/m²/day) achieved. Then reduce dose by 50% q10–14days
			- In congenital adrenal hyperplasia (CAH), administer ½ daily dose at bedtime to suppress morning surge of ACTH
			- Give PO with food or milk

Hydrocortisone (topical) Cream: 0.5%, 1% Ointment: 0.5%, 1% Lotion: 1%	**Vasopressor refractory shock (intensive care setting)** *Loading dose:* 2 mg/kg/dose IV *Maintenance dose:* 1 mg/kg/dose IV q6h **INFANTS AND OLDER CHILDREN** Apply 1% ointment to affected face or groin area 2–3 times/day	100/mg/dose 50 mg/dose
Hydromorphone Inj 2 mg/mL, 10 mg/mL Syrup: 1 mg/mL Tab 2 mg, 4 mg, 8 mg Cap CR 3 mg, 6 mg, 12 mg, 18 mg, 24 mg, 30 mg	**INFANTS AND OLDER CHILDREN** **Continuous infusion** 0.01–0.02 mg/kg IV/SC loading dose, then 2–8 mcg/kg/h IV/SC infusion **Intermittent IV/SC (with continuous infusion)** 0.002–0.008 mg/kg/dose (2–8 mcg/kg/dose) IV q2h prn **Intermittent IV/SC (without continuous infusion or in intensive care setting with continuous infusion)** 0.01–0.02 mg/kg/dose IV/SC q2–4h prn **Intermittent PO** *≤50 kg:* 0.04–0.08 mg/kg/dose PO q3–4h prn *>50 kg:* 2–4 mg/dose PO q3–4h prn (patients with prior opiate exposure may tolerate higher doses)	 1 mg/dose IV/SC 4 mg/dose PO (up to 8 mg/dose PO has been used)	- Dosing guidelines reflect *initial* dosing in opioid naive patients. Doses may be adjusted based on patient response (i.e., analgesic effect, presence of side effects) - Reduce dose in renal or hepatic impairment - Administer with or after food to decrease GI upset - If oral liquid spills on skin, remove contaminated clothing and rinse area with cool water

Continued

1177

Table 40.1 Drug Dosing Guidelines for Neonates[a] (Where Specified), Infants, and Older Children—cont'd

Drug[b,c]	Dose	Dose Limit	Comments
Hydroxyurea Cap 500 mg Solution (HSC) dissolve 'n' dose system	***INFANTS AND OLDER CHILDREN*** **Sickle cell anemia (>9 months)** 10–20 mg/kg/dose PO once daily, rounded to the nearest 500 mg. Increase dose by 5–10 mg/kg/day every 2–3 months until the maximum dose is reached or clinical efficacy is achieved	35 mg/kg/day	- Monitor CBC with differential and reticulocytes and hemoglobin F levels periodically throughout therapy
Hydroxyzine Syrup 2 mg/mL Cap 10 mg, 25 mg	***INFANTS AND OLDER CHILDREN*** **Chronic urticaria** 0.7 mg/kg/dose PO TID or 0.5 mg/kg/dose PO QID	≤40 kg: 2 mg/kg/day >40 kg: 100 mg/day	
Ibuprofen Susp 40 mg/mL Tab 200 mg, 300 mg, 400 mg, 600 mg	***NEONATES*** **Patent ductus arteriosus** *PMA <28 weeks or PNA <7 days:* 10 mg/kg/dose IV/PO once, then 5 mg/kg/dose IV/PO at 24 and 48 h after the initial dose *PMA ≥28 weeks and PNA ≥7 days:* 20 mg/kg/dose IV/PO once, then 10 mg/kg/dose IV/PO at 24 and 48 h after the initial dose If anuria or marked oliguria (urine output <0.6 mL/kg/h) is evident at the scheduled time of the second or third dose, hold dose until renal function returns to normal ***INFANTS AND OLDER CHILDREN*** *<6 months:* 5 mg/kg/dose PO q8h *6 months–12 years:* 5–10 mg/kg/dose PO q6–8h *>12 years:* 200–400 mg PO q4–6h OR 400–600 mg PO q6–8h **Anti-inflammatory (Rheumatology)** 7–12 mg/kg/dose PO TID or 5–10 mg/kg/dose PO QID	40 mg/kg/day *Maximum adult dose:* 2400 mg/day	- Consider indomethacin instead of ibuprofen for PDA in neonates <28 weeks GA and ≥8 days PNA and in those with hyperbilirubinemia or pulmonary hypertension - Do not use in patients with renal impairment; use with caution in patients with hepatic impairment, compromised cardiac function, or hypertension (may cause fluid retention, edema), or history of GI bleeding or ulcers - May inhibit platelet aggregation (duration of effect, ~5–10 h); monitor closely patients who may be adversely affected by prolonged bleeding times; give with food to minimize GI upset

Immune globulin (human, IV) Inj 10%	*NEONATES* **Hemolytic disease of the newborn, neonatal alloimmune thrombocytopenia** 0.5–1 g/kg IV once (repeat in 12 h prn)		- May increase serum concentrations of digoxin, methotrexate, lithium - Recommended as antipyretic for children with fever unresponsive to maximal doses of acetaminophen or in children intolerant to acetaminophen
	INFANTS AND OLDER CHILDREN **Hypogammaglobulinemia** 600 mg/kg/dose IV once monthly		- Rate of infusion for neonates: 0.6 mL/kg/h × 15 min, 1.2 mL/kg/h × 15 min, 2.4 mL/kg/h × 15 min, 3.6 mL/kg/h × 30 min, then slowly increase rate if tolerated
	BMT 400 mg/kg/dose IV when IgG level <4 g/L		- Rate of infusion for infants and older children: 0.3 mL/kg/h × 15 min, 0.6 mL/kg/h × 15 min, 1.2 mL/kg/h × 15 min, 2.4 mL/kg/h × 15 min, 3.6 mL/kg/h × 30 min, 4.8 mL/kg/h × 30 min, 7.2 mL/kg/h until completed. Maximum rate for Kawasaki disease: 3.6 mL/kg/h. Maximum rate for other indications: 7.2 mL/kg/h.
	Idiopathic thrombocytopenic purpura 0.8–1 g/kg/dose IV once and reassess in 24–48 h		
	Kawasaki disease 2 g/kg IV as single dose	70 g	- Side effects: minor (often related to infusion rate)—headache, chills, fever, malaise, anxiety, chest pain, nausea, pruritus, and rash. Severe—hemolysis, aseptic meningitis, anaphylaxis, viral transmission, transfusion-related acute lung injury and thromboembolic events
	Polymyositis, dermatomyositis 2 g/kg × 1 day biweekly for 5 weeks, then monthly	70 g	
	Guillain-Barré syndrome 1 g/kg/dose IV once daily for 2 days		

Continued

Table 40.1	Drug Dosage Guidelines for Neonates[a] (Where Specified), Infants, and Older Children—cont'd		
Drug[b,c]	Dose	Dose Limit	Comments
Indomethacin Susp (HSC) 5 mg/mL Cap 25 mg, 50 mg Inj 1 mg/vial	***NEONATES*** **Patent ductus arteriosus closure** 0.2 mg/kg/dose IV q12h for 3 doses		- In neonates with renal impairment, dose at 0.1 mg/kg/dose IV q24h for 5–6 doses - Reduce doses of aminoglycosides and digoxin to half until good urine output returns
	INFANTS AND OLDER CHILDREN 0.5–1 mg/kg/dose PO TID with meals	200 mg/day PO	- Infuse over 20 min - Give with food or milk (if enteral)
Infliximab Inj 100 mg/vial	***INFANTS AND OLDER CHILDREN*** **Active or refractory Crohn's disease (with or without fistulas)** 5 mg/kg IV given as an induction at 0, 2, and 6 weeks followed with maintenance doses of 5 mg/kg every 8 weeks If incomplete response, dose can be increased to 10 mg/kg		- Infuse over 2–3 h to prevent acute infusion reactions
Insulin Regular Inj 100 units/mL Inj 10 units/mL (HSC)	***NEONATES*** **Hyperglycemia** 0.01–0.02 unit/kg/h IV via continuous infusion **Hyperkalemia** *Bolus:* 0.1 units/kg **diluted** Humulin® R insulin (10 units/mL) IV plus 0.5 g glucose/kg IV over 30 min *Maintenance:* 0.1 units/kg/h **diluted** Humulin® R insulin (10 units/mL) IV plus 0.5 g glucose/kg/h IV		- Titrate infusion according to blood glucose; use regular insulin only for infusions
	INFANTS AND OLDER CHILDREN **Hyperkalemia** *Bolus:* 0.1 units/kg **diluted** Humulin® R insulin (10 units/mL) IV with 5 mL/kg/dose D10W over 30 min		

Iodine	**INFANTS AND OLDER CHILDREN** **Radiation protection**		Dilute in 1 glassful of water, juice, or milk, give with food or milk
Lugol solution 126 mg elemental iodine/mL (as 100 mg potassium iodide, 50 mg/mL iodine) Tablets: 50 mg elemental iodine (as 65 mg potassium iodide)	30 mg elemental iodine/day PO as a single daily dose **MIBG Scan** *<3 years:* 30 mg elemental iodine PO as single daily dose *3–13 years:* 50 mg elemental iodine PO as a single daily dose *>13 years:* 100 mg elemental iodine PO as a single daily dose Given the day before injection of radiopharmaceutical (¹²³I MIBG) and PO once daily for 2 days after	100 mg elemental iodine/day	- Duration of treatment depends on type of radiation exposure
Ipratropium Metered-dose aerosol (HFA) 20 mcg/puff Inhalation solution 250 mcg/mL	**NEONATES** 125 mcg (0.5 mL)/dose TID–QID prn via nebulizer **INFANTS AND OLDER CHILDREN** **Acute asthma** *Metered-dose inhaler:* 4 puffs (80 mcg) q15–20min for 3 doses *Inhalation solution via nebulizer:* 250 mcg in 3 mL NS given q20min **Maintenance therapy for asthma** *Metered dose inhaler:* 1–2 puffs (20–40 mcg) TID–QID *Inhalation solution via nebulizer:* 250 mcg in 3 mL NS given TID–QID prn **Sialorrhea** *Metered dose inhaler* *<6 years:* 20 mcg (1 puff) SL TID *6–12 years:* 20–40 mcg (1–2 puffs) SL TID *Inhalation solution* *<5 years:* 125–250 mcg SL q4–6h prn *≥5 years:* 250 mcg SL q4–6h prn	Usual adult dose: *Metered dose inhaler:* 240 mcg/day *Nebulizer:* 250–500 mcg/dose in 3 mL NS q4–6h prn	- Dilute to a total of 3 mL with normal saline if required - May be mixed with salbutamol and/or budesonide solutions immediately before administration - Metered dose inhalers are preferred method of administration over nebulizers

Continued

Table 40.1   Drug Dosage Guidelines for Neonates[a] (Where Specified), Infants, and Older Children—cont'd

Drug[b,c]	Dose	Dose Limit	Comments
Iron Susp 60 mg/mL ferrous fumarate (20 mg elemental iron/mL) Cap 300 mg ferrous fumarate (100 mg elemental iron) Tab 300 mg ferrous gluconate (35 mg elemental iron) Oral drops 75 mg/mL ferrous sulphate (15 mg elemental iron/mL)	*NEONATES* **Supplementation (prematurity, long-term PN)** *Birth weight <1000 g:* 3–4 mg elemental iron/kg PO as single daily dose *Birth weight ≥1000 g:* 2–3 mg elemental iron/kg PO as single daily dose *INFANTS AND OLDER CHILDREN* **Treatment** 6 mg elemental iron/kg/dose PO once daily or 3 mg elemental iron/kg/dose PO BID or 2 mg elemental iron/kg/dose PO TID **Prophylaxis** 0.5–2 mg elemental iron/kg/dose PO once daily or 0.25–1 mg elemental iron/kg/dose PO BID or 0.17–0.67 mg elemental iron/kg/dose PO TID	100 mg elemental iron/dose, 200 mg elemental iron/day	- Supplementation for preterm infants usually begins at 6–8 weeks PNA - Iron-fortified formula (instead of iron drops/syrup) is recommended for bottle-fed infants - Some TPN solutions do not contain iron, and patients on long-term PN may require supplementation - Before administration, dilute suspension in glass of juice or water and mix thoroughly; administer caps with ½–1 glass water or juice; administer 1 h before or 2 h after dairy products, eggs, tea, or whole-grain bread or cereal
Iron sucrose Inj 100 mg/5mL (20 mg elemental iron/mL)	*INFANTS AND OLDER CHILDREN* **Hemodialysis** If TSAT 20%–50% and ferritin is 100–800 mcg/L, 2 mg/kg/dose once weekly If TSAT <20% or if ferritin <100 mcg/L, 7 mg/kg/dose once weekly for 1 week, followed by 2 mg/kg/dose once weekly If TSAT >50% or ferritin >800 mcg/L, discontinue iron sucrose and restart when one of the above criteria is met **Non-hemodialysis** 7 mg/kg/dose once weekly	100 mg/dose 200 mg/dose 500 mg/dose	- TSAT (transferrin saturation) = iron/ (2 × transferrin) - Oral iron absorption decreased with iron sucrose; wait at least 5 days after IV iron therapy before initiating PO iron

Isoniazid
Syrup 10 mg/mL
Tab 300 mg

INFANTS AND OLDER CHILDREN
Tuberculosis (regimens for treatment and prophylaxis vary)
Daily regimen: 15 mg/kg/dose PO daily or 7.5 mg/kg/dose PO q12h
Twice weekly regimen: 20–30 mg/kg/dose PO twice weekly

Daily regimen: 300 mg/day
Twice-weekly regimen: 900 mg/day

- Pyridoxine supplementation recommended in adolescents, children with nutritional deficiencies, breastfed infants, and pregnant or lactating women
- Give on an empty stomach (1 h ac or 2 h pc) unless GI upset occurs
- Monitor liver function tests periodically

Isoproterenol
Inj 0.2 mg/mL

NEONATES
0.05–1 mcg/kg/min IV via continuous infusion

INFANTS AND OLDER CHILDREN
0.025–1 mcg/kg/min IV via continuous infusion

- In neonates, stop or slow infusion if heart rate >200/min

Itraconazole
Cap 100 mg
Liquid 10 mg/mL

INFANTS AND OLDER CHILDREN
Oropharyngeal candidiasis treatment, or secondary prophylaxis
5 mg/kg/dose PO once daily
Other fungal infections
5–10 mg/kg/dose PO once daily or 2.5–5 mg/kg/dose PO BID

400 mg/day

- Caution regarding drug interactions, including cisapride, cyclosporine, tacrolimus
- May cause hepatic dysfunction; reduce dose in liver impairment
- Oral solution and caps are not interchangeable; oral solution should be administered on an empty stomach; caps must be swallowed whole and given after a full meal; avoid giving within 2 h of antacids
- In patients with achlorhydria or taking acid-suppressing agents, administer with a cola beverage

Continued

Drug Dosing Guidelines

40

1183

Table 40.1 Drug Dosage Guidelines for Neonates^a (Where Specified), Infants, and Older Children—cont'd

Drug^{b,c}	Dose	Dose Limit	Comments
Ivabradine Tab 5 mg Cap 0.15 mg (HSC)	***INFANTS AND OLDER CHILDREN*** **Junctional ectopic tachycardia/atrial ectopic tachycardia/ postural orthostatic tachycardia syndrome** *<40 kg:* Initial: 0.05 mg/kg/dose PO BID *≥40 kg:* Initial: 2.5 mg PO BID **Congestive heart failure** *<12 months:* Initial: 0.02 mg/kg/dose PO BID *≥12 months, <40 kg:* Initial: 0.05 mg/kg/dose PO BID *≥12 months, >40 kg:* Initial: 2.5 mg PO BID	0.2 mg/kg/dose PO BID 15 mg PO BID 0.2 mg/kg/dose PO BID 0.3 mg/kg/dose PO BID 15 mg PO BID	- Titrate doses based on patient response (e.g., symptoms, HR, ECG) - Preferably given with food - Tablets may be split, chewed, or crushed. Capsules may be opened and mixed with water
Kaletra (lopinavir/ ritonavir) Tab 200 mg lopinavir + 50 mg ritonavir, 100 mg lopinavir + 25 mg ritonavir Solution 80 mg/mL lopinavir + 20 mg/mL ritonavir	***INFANTS AND OLDER CHILDREN*** **Postexposure prophylaxis or treatment of HIV infection, in combination therapy** *<6 months:* 300 mg lopinavir/m²/dose PO BID *6 months–12 years:* 230–300 mg lopinavir/m²/dose PO BID *>12 years or ≥35 kg:* 400 mg lopinavir/dose PO BID	800 mg lopinavir/day	- Plasma levels may be increased in patients with hepatic impairment - Oral solution contains 42.4% v/v alcohol - Many potential drug interactions; give with food - Absorption enhanced with high-fat meal
Kayexalate	See **Sodium polystyrene sulfonate**		

Ketamine
Inj 200 mg/20 mL,
500 mg/10 mL
	INFANTS AND OLDER CHILDREN
	Induction of anesthesia
	1–2 mg/kg/dose IV
	4–10 mg/kg/dose IM
	Procedural Sedation
	0.5–1.5 mg/kg IV, administer slowly over 1–2 min; may repeat
	0.5 mg/kg in 10 min
	4 mg/kg IM; may repeat half the total dose in 10 min
	Pre-Procedural anxiolysis
	2–5 mg/kg PO
		100 mg IV/dose	- Presence of personnel skilled in airway
			  management is required
			- Give 30 min before procedure
			- IV solution may be mixed in a suitable
			  beverage for oral administration
			- Contraindicated in infants <3 months of
			  age

Ketoconazole
Susp (HSC) 20 mg/mL
Tab 200 mg
	INFANTS AND OLDER CHILDREN
	3.3–6.6 mg/kg/dose PO once daily
		400 mg/day	- Give with food
			- May interact with many other medications
			  including cisapride, cyclosporine, tacroli-
			  mus, sirolimus
			- Avoid giving within 2 h of antacids
			- In patients with achlorhydria or taking
			  acid-suppressing agents, administer with
			  a carbonated beverage

**Ketorolac
tromethamine**
Inj 30 mg/mL
	INFANTS AND OLDER CHILDREN
	Postoperative pain
	0.5 mg/kg/dose IV q6–8h prn
		15 mg/dose	- Maximum duration of IV therapy is 2 days
			- Do not use in tonsillectomy patients be-
			  cause of increased risk of bleeding, do
			  not use in patients with impaired renal
			  function, avoid in heart transplant patients

Continued

Table 40.1   Drug Dosage Guidelines for Neonates[a] (Where Specified), Infants, and Older Children—cont'd

Drug[b,c]	Dose	Dose Limit	Comments
Labetalol Inj 5 mg/mL	***INFANTS AND OLDER CHILDREN*** **Hypertension** 1 mg/kg/h by continuous IV infusion **Acute hypertension** 1–3 mg/kg/dose IV	3 mg/kg/h	- Reduce dose in liver impairment
Lacosamide Tab 50 mg, 100 mg, 150 mg, 200 mg Inj 10 mg/mL	***INFANTS AND OLDER CHILDREN*** *Loading dose:* 10 mg/kg/dose IV × 1 *1–16 years (adjunctive therapy)* *Initial:* 0.5 mg/kg/dose PO/IV BID May be titrated by 1 mg/kg/day on a weekly basis to 2.5–5 mg/kg/dose BID	400 mg/dose 400 mg/day (300 mg/day if CrCl ≤30 mL/min or mild to moderate hepatic impairment)	- Adjust dose in renal and hepatic impairment. Not recommended in severe hepatic impairment
Lactulose Syrup 667 mg/mL	***INFANTS AND OLDER CHILDREN*** **Constipation** *Initial dose:* 5–10 mL/day PO once daily; double daily dose until stool is produced **Hepatic encephalopathy** *<1 year:* 2.5 mL PO TID–QID *Older children and adolescents:* 10–30 mL PO TID	*Usual adult dose:* 15–30 mL/day (constipation)	- For hepatic encephalopathy: decrease/discontinue if severe diarrhea develops; treatment is effective if stool is soft with pH <5.5; hypernatremia and/or hypokalemia may occur
Lamivudine Tab 150 mg Liquid 10 mg/mL	***NEONATES*** **Perinatal HIV exposure and treatment of HIV infection** *Gestational age ≥ 32 weeks:* 2 mg/kg/dose PO q12h, increase to 4 mg/kg/dose PO q12h at 4 weeks of age	150 mg/dose	- Reduce dose in renal impairment; may cause pancreatitis, peripheral neuropathy - Oral solution contains sugar - May cause pancreatitis; peripheral neuropathy

INFANTS AND OLDER CHILDREN
Postexposure prophylaxis or treatment of HIV infection, in combination therapy

Liquid
> *1 month to 16 years:* 4 mg/kg/dose PO BID
Tablet
14–19.9 kg: 75 mg PO BID
20–24.9 kg: 75 mg PO qam, 150 mg PO qhs
≥25 kg or >12 years: 150 mg PO BID

Lamotrigine
Tab 25 mg, 100 mg, 150 mg
Chew/disperse tab 2 mg, 5 mg

INFANTS AND OLDER CHILDREN
2–12 years taking valproic acid (VPA) with or without enzyme-inducing agents

Weeks 1 & 2: 0.15 mg/kg/dose PO once daily or 0.075 mg/kg/dose PO BID

Weeks 3 & 4: 0.3 mg/kg/dose PO once daily or 0.15 mg/kg/dose PO BID
To achieve maintenance dose, increase by 0.3 mg/kg every 1–2 weeks

Usual maintenance dose:
1–5 mg/kg/dose PO once daily or 0.5–2.5 mg/kg/dose PO BID
Maximum dose: 200 mg/day

2–12 years taking enzyme-inducing agents but NOT valproic acid

Weeks 1 & 2: 0.3 mg/kg/dose PO BID
Weeks 3 & 4: 0.6 mg/kg/dose PO BID
To achieve maintenance dose, increase by 1.2 mg/kg every 1–2 weeks

Usual maintenance dose:
2.5–7.5 mg/kg/dose PO BID
Maximum dose: 400 mg/day

2–12 years taking antiepileptic drugs (AEDs) other than enzyme-inducing agents or valproic acid

Weeks 1 & 2: 0.3 mg/kg/dose PO once daily or 0.15 mg/kg/dose PO BID
Weeks 3 & 4: 0.3 mg/kg/dose PO BID
To achieve maintenance dose, increase by 0.6 mg/kg every 1–2 weeks

Usual maintenance dose: 2.25–3.75 mg/kg/dose PO BID
Maximum dose: 300 mg/day

- Use with caution in patients with impaired renal or hepatic function and patients taking VPA
- Monitor for rash (may be sign of serious toxicity)

Continued

Table 40.1 Drug Dosage Guidelines for Neonates[a] (Where Specified), Infants, and Older Children—cont'd

Drug[b,c]	Dose	Dose Limit	Comments
Lamotrigine—cont'd	**>12 years taking enzyme-inducing agents but NOT valproic acid** *Initial dose:* 25 mg PO BID for 2 weeks, then increase to 50 mg PO BID for 2 weeks, then titrate dose	*Usual maintenance dose:* 150–250 mg/dose PO BID *Maximum dose:* 500 mg/day	
	>12 years taking enzyme-inducing agents with valproic acid *Initial dose:* 25 mg PO as a single daily dose for 2 weeks, then increase dose by 25–50 mg/day every 1–2 weeks	*Usual maintenance dose:* 50–100 mg/dose PO BID *Maximum dose:* 200 mg/day	
	>12 years taking valproic acid but NOT enzyme-inducing agents *Initial dose:* 25 mg PO as a single dose every other day for 2 weeks, then increase to 25 mg PO as a single daily dose for 2 weeks, then titrate dose	*Usual maintenance dose:* 50–100 mg/dose PO BID *Maximum dose:* 200 mg/day	
	>12 years taking AEDs other than enzyme-inducing agents or valproic acid *Initial dose:* 25 mg PO as a single daily dose for 2 weeks, then increase to 50 mg PO as a single daily dose for 2 weeks, then titrate dose	*Usual maintenance dose:* 112.5–187.5 mg/dose PO BID *Maximum dose:* 375 mg/day	
Lansoprazole Cap 15 mg, 30 mg Tab ODT 15 mg, 30 mg	***INFANTS AND OLDER CHILDREN*** *<10 kg:* 7.5 mg PO once daily *10–30 kg:* 15 mg PO once daily *≥30 kg:* 30 mg PO once daily	1.6 mg/kg/day or 30 mg/day, whichever is less	- Administer before food - For oral use, give caps whole, whenever possible - Consult pharmacy for administration for patients who cannot take caps or ODT tabs

Levetiracetam Tab 250 mg, 500 mg Susp 50 mg/mL (HSC) Inj 100 mg/mL	***NEONATES*** *Loading dose:* 60 mg/kg/dose PO/NG/IV once *Initial maintenance dose:* 5–10 mg/kg/dose PO/NG/IV BID May titrate dose by 10 mg/kg/day up to effective dose at the discretion of Neurology. Dose increases may be done daily if tolerated	60 mg/kg/day
	INFANTS AND OLDER CHILDREN *Loading dose:* 60 mg/kg/dose PO/IV once *Initial maintenance dose:* 5–10 mg/kg/dose PO/IV once daily or 2.5–5 mg/kg/dose PO/IV BID May increase dose q1–2wk to 20–30 mg/kg/dose PO/IV BID	60 mg/kg/dose or 4500 mg/dose 100 mg/kg/day or 3000 mg/day, whichever is less
Levocarnitine (carnitine, L-carnitine) Inj 200 mg/mL Liquid 100 mg/mL Tab 330 mg	***INFANTS AND OLDER CHILDREN*** **Metabolic crisis** Give loading dose 50–300 mg/kg IV then give same dose IV over next 24 h div q4h **Maintenance** 50–100 mg/kg/day PO/IV div q4–6h	*Usual adult dose:* 4 g/day PO div BID–TID
Levofloxacin Inj 5 mg/mL Tab 250 mg, 500 mg, 750 mg	***INFANTS AND OLDER CHILDREN*** ≥ 6 months to <5 years: 10 mg/kg/dose IV/PO q12h ≥ 5 years: 10 mg/kg/dose IV/PO q24h **Pelvic inflammatory disease** *Outpatient therapy, if beta-lactam allergy* 500 mg PO daily for 14 days ± metronidazole	750 mg/dose

- Dose adjustment in renal impairment:
  mild, 70%; moderate, 50%; severe, 30%

- Dose adjustment in renal impairment:
  moderate, 50% of dose q24h; severe,
  50% of dose q48h
- Round levofloxacin doses to nearest tablet
  (250 mg, 500 mg) or half tablet. Tablets
  may be crushed but will have a bitter
  taste when crushed

Continued

Table 40.1 Drug Dosage Guidelines for Neonates[a] (Where Specified), Infants, and Older Children—cont'd

Drug[b,c]	Dose	Dose Limit	Comments
Levothyroxine Tab 25 mcg, 50 mcg, 75 mcg, 88 mcg, 100 mcg, 112 mcg, 125 mcg, 150 mcg, 175 mcg, 200 mcg Solution, oral: dissolve 'n' dose system	***NEONATES*** 10–12 mcg/kg/day PO *≤2.5 kg:* 25 mcg *2.6–3.4 kg:* 37.5 mcg *3.5–4.4 kg:* 44 mcg *≥4.5 kg:* 50 mcg ***INFANTS AND OLDER CHILDREN*** *0–6 months:* 8–15 mcg/kg/day (usual dose: 25–50 mcg/day) *6–12 months:* 7–10 mcg/kg/day (usual dose: 50–75 mcg/day) *1–5 years:* 5–7 mcg/kg/day (usual dose: 50–100 mcg/day) *5–10 years:* 3–5 mcg/kg/day (usual dose: 100–150 mcg/day) *>10–12 years:* 2–4 mcg/kg/day (usual dose: 100–200 mcg/day)		- In neonates, measure TSH and free T₄ 2 weeks after initiation of therapy and then at 2, 3, 6, 9, and 12 months of age. Titrate dose to normalize TSH and free T4 with follow-up measurements of TSH, free T4 at 4–6 weeks after any dose adjustment. - In infants and older children, if TSH >100 start with half the dose for 4–8 weeks - Measure TSH, free T4 q6–12wk and ti- trate dose to normalize TSH and free T4
Lidocaine Cream: 5 g Inj 100 mg/5 mL ampoule (2%) Local Inj 10 mg/mL (1%), 20 mg/mL (2%) Jelly, 2% (600 mg/30 mL) Jelly, prefilled syringe: 2% (200 mg/10 mL) Ointment, topical: 5% (1.75 g/35 g)	***NEONATES*** **Arrhythmia** *Loading dose:* 0.5–1 mg/kg IV once. May repeat q10min as necessary to control arrhythmia *Maintenance:* 10–50 mcg/kg/min IV continuous infusion **Infiltration for local anesthesia** Up to 4.5 mg/kg/dose per 2-h period (= 0.9 mL/kg of lidocaine 0.5% or 0.45 mL/kg of lidocaine 1%)		

	INFANTS AND OLDER CHILDREN	
	Resuscitation	
	IV/IO: 1–2 mg/kg/dose IV/IO (0.05–0.1 mL/kg/dose) over at least 2 min. May repeat up to a max total dose of 3 mg/kg (0.15 mL/kg)	*Maximum single dose:* 100 mg (5 mL)
	Endotracheal tube: 2–3 mg/kg/dose ETT (0.1–0.15 mL/kg/dose)	*Maximum total dose:* 3 mg/kg (0.15 mL/kg)
	Infusion: 20–50 mcg/kg/min IV as continuous infusion	
Loperamide	**NEONATES**	
Solution 0.2 mg/mL	**Chronic diarrhea**	
Tab 2 mg	0.04–0.12 mg/kg/dose PO BID or 0.03–0.08 mg/kg/dose PO TID	
	Short bowel syndrome	
	0.07–0.33 mg/kg/dose PO q8h	
	INFANTS AND OLDER CHILDREN	
	Acute diarrhea (initial dose in first 24 h)	- For infants and older children, after initial dosing, 0.1 mg/kg/dose after each loose stool, not exceeding initial dose
	2–5 years: 1 mg/dose PO TID	
	6–8 years: 2 mg/dose PO BID	
	8–12 years: 2 mg/dose PO TID	
	Chronic diarrhea	
	0.04–0.12 mg/kg/dose PO BID or 0.03–0.08 mg/kg/dose PO TID	2 mg/dose
	Short bowel syndrome	
	0.27–0.33 mg/kg/dose PO q8h	

Continued

1191

Table 40.1 Drug Dosing Guidelines for Neonates[a] (Where Specified), Infants, and Older Children—cont'd

Drug[b,c]	Dose	Dose Limit	Comments
Loratadine Tab 10 mg Liquid 1 mg/mL	***INFANTS AND OLDER CHILDREN*** *2–9 years and/or <30 kg:* 5 mg PO daily *≥10 years and/or ≥30 kg:* 10 mg PO daily		- For PR administration, dilute injection according to IV instructions
Lorazepam Sublingual tab 0.5 mg, 1 mg, 2 mg Inj 2 mg/mL	***NEONATES*** **Seizures** 0.1 mg/kg/dose IV/PR; may repeat q2min once prn for ongoing seizures		
	Sedation (intensive care setting) 0.05–0.1 mg/kg/dose IV q2–4h prn		
	Agitation (intensive care setting) 0.05–0.1 mg/kg/dose IV/SL/PO/buccal/PR q4–6h prn	4 mg/day	
	INFANTS AND OLDER CHILDREN **Preoperative/procedural sedation** 0.05 mg/kg/dose SL 0.03–0.05 mg/kg/dose IV	4 mg/dose; 12 mg/12 h or 0.3 mg/kg/12 h, whichever is less	- May give SL tablets PO; for sublingual/ buccal administration, dry saliva in region to ensure tab dissolves and is absorbed in mucous membrane - Do not administer IM olanzapine within 24 h of IM/IV benzodiazepine
	Anxiety/agitation 0.03–0.05 mg/kg/dose PO/IV/IM q4–8h prn	2 mg/dose	
	Status epilepticus 0.1 mg/kg/dose IV/buccal/SL/PR, may repeat q5min once prn for ongoing seizures	4 mg/dose	
	Anticipatory chemotherapy-induced nausea and vomiting *5–10 years:* 0.5 mg/dose PO *>10 years:* 1 mg/dose PO Give doses the night before chemotherapy and/or the morning of chemotherapy		

Breakthrough chemotherapy-induced nausea and vomiting or failure of prophylaxis in the acute phase		
	0.025 mg/kg/dose IV/PO/SL q6h prn	2 mg/dose
Losartan Tab 25 mg, 50 mg, 100 mg Susp (HSC) 2.5 mg/mL	***INFANTS AND OLDER CHILDREN*** **Hypertension, proteinuria** *Initial:* 0.5–1 mg/kg/day PO once daily	1.5 mg/kg/day up to 100 mg/day	– Monitor serum potassium and renal function (especially when patients are on combined ACE inhibitor and losartan)
Loxapine Inj 50 mg/mL Tab 2.5 mg, 10 mg, 25 mg	***INFANTS AND OLDER CHILDREN*** **Acute agitation and aggression** 5–25 mg IM/PO q1–6h prn **Acute agitation and aggression (Code White)** 12.5 mg IM or 10 mg PO STAT **Maintenance therapy** 2.5–5 mg PO BID and increase gradually by 10 mg/day. *Usual dose:* 25–50 mg PO BID	150 mg/day 100 mg/day	– Contraindicated in patients with current diagnosis or history of asthma – May cause anticholinergic effects (constipation, xerostomia, blurred vision, urinary retention) – Do not combine loxapine with opiates or dopamine agonists – Dystonic reactions (i.e., dyskinesias) are characterized by intermittent spasmodic or sustained involuntary contractions of muscles in the face, neck, trunk, pelvis, extremities, and even the larynx. Dystonia can occur in minutes to hours of neuroleptic (e.g., Loxapine) administration. Serious symptoms include: tongue swelling, jaw locking, oculogyric crisis, and laryngospasms. Treatment: benztropine

Continued

Table 40.1 Drug Dosing Guidelines for Neonates[a] (Where Specified), Infants, and Older Children—cont'd

Drug[b,c]	Dose	Dose Limit	Comments
Magnesium Solution: 100 mg/mL magnesium glucoheptonate = 5 mg elemental magnesium/mL = 0.21 mmol elemental magnesium/mL 15 g/ 300 mL magnesium citrate Susp: 80 mg/mL magnesium hydroxide = 33 mg elemental magnesium/mL = 1.4 mmol elemental magnesium/mL Tab: 420 mg magnesium oxide = 252 mg elemental magnesium = 10.6 mmol elemental magnesium Inj: 500 mg/mL magnesium sulfate (50%) = 50 mg elemental magnesium/mL = 2 mmol elemental	**NEONATES** **Hypomagnesemia** *Initial:* Initial dose given by IV infusion over 30–60 min q8–12h for 2–3 doses 0.1–0.4 mmol/kg/dose (2.5–10 mg elemental magnesium/kg/dose, 25–100 mg magnesium sulfate/kg/dose) *Continuous infusion IV:* 0.005–0.01 mmol/kg/h (0.125–0.25 mg elemental magnesium/kg/h, 1.25–2.5 mg magnesium sulfate/kg/h) **INFANTS AND OLDER CHILDREN** **Hypomagnesemia** *Oral therapy:* 6.7–13.3 mg elemental magnesium/kg/dose PO TID (0.26–0.53 mmol magnesium/kg/dose PO TID) *IV therapy* *Initial dose:* 0.21–0.42 mmol magnesium/kg/dose (5–10 mg elemental magnesium/kg/dose, 50–100 mg magnesium sulfate/kg/dose) *Continuous infusion:* 0.005–0.01 mmol magnesium/kg/h (0.125–0.25 mg elemental magnesium/kg/h, 1.25–2.5 mg magnesium sulfate/kg/h) **Cathartic** *Magnesium citrate:* 4 mL/kg/dose PO *Magnesium hydroxide:* 0.5 mL/kg/dose PO	10 mmol magnesium/dose (250 mg elemental magnesium/dose, 2500 mg magnesium sulfate/dose) *Citrate:* 300 mL/dose *Hydroxide:* usual adult dose: 30–60 mL	- 1 mmol = 25 mg elemental magnesium = 250 mg magnesium sulfate - Injection must be diluted before administration - Titrate dose according to serum magnesium level - Use with caution in renal impairment - Large doses of oral magnesium may cause diarrhea - Magnesium hydroxide tabs may be swallowed whole, chewed, or dispersed in water for administration; magnesium oxide tabs must not be given by G tube

	Bronchodilation (adjunctive treatment in moderate to severe asthma)	
	25–50 mg magnesium sulfate/kg/dose IV once over 20–30 min (2.5–5 mg elemental magnesium/kg/dose IV once, 0.1–0.2 mmol magnesium/kg/dose IV once)	2.5 g magnesium sulfate/dose (250 mg elemental magnesium/dose, 10 mmol magnesium/dose)
Malarone (atovaquone/ proguanil) Adult tab: atovaquone 250 mg + proguanil base 85.6 mg (100 mg proguanil HCl) Pediatric (ped) tab: atovaquone 62.5 mg + proguanil base 21.8 mg (25 mg proguanil HCl)	***INFANTS AND OLDER CHILDREN*** **Prophylaxis** (start 1–2 days before entering malaria-endemic area, continue daily during stay and for 7 days after leaving area) *5–8 kg:* ½ ped tab PO daily *9–10 kg:* ¾ ped tab PO daily *11–20 kg:* 1 ped tab PO daily *21–30 kg:* 2 ped tabs PO daily *31–40 kg:* 3 ped tabs PO daily *>40 kg:* 1 adult tab PO daily **Treatment of resistant *Falciparum* malaria** *5–8 kg:* 2 ped tabs PO daily for 3 days *9–10 kg:* 3 ped tabs PO daily for 3 days *11–20 kg:* 1 adult tab PO daily for 3 days *21–30 kg:* 2 adult tab PO daily for 3 days *31–40 kg:* 3 adult tabs PO daily for 3 days *>40 kg (adult dose):* 4 adult tabs PO daily for 3 days	*Adult dose:* 4 tabs PO daily for 3 days	- Dose should be administered as single daily dose - Give with food or milk; if vomiting occurs within 1 h of dosing, repeat the dose

Continued

Table 40.1   Drug Dosage Guidelines for Neonates[a] (Where Specified), Infants, and Older Children—cont'd

Drug[b,c]	Dose	Dose Limit	Comments
Mannitol Inj 20% (100 g/ 500 mL), 25% (12.5 g/50 mL)	***NEONATES*** 1 g/kg/dose IV (5 mL of 20% solution/kg/dose) ***INFANTS AND OLDER CHILDREN*** **Acute symptomatic hyponatremia** 1 g/kg/dose IV rapidly **Diuresis, reduction of intracranial pressure, reduction of intraocular** **pressure** 0.2–2 g/kg/dose IV push or as an IV infusion over up to 6 h **Test for oliguria** 0.2 g/kg IV over 10 min once	*Test dose:* 12.5 g/dose	- Contraindicated in patients with anuria or impaired renal function who do not respond to test dose with adequate urine output; monitor fluid and electrolyte balance
Mebendazole Tab 100 mg	***INFANTS AND OLDER CHILDREN*** Pinworm 100 mg PO × 1 dose; repeat in 2 weeks **Other nematodes (with exception of capillariasis)** 100 mg/dose PO BID for 3 to 10 days		- Do not use for children <2 years
Mefloquine Tab 250 mg	***INFANTS AND OLDER CHILDREN*** **Prophylaxis** (start prophylaxis 1 week before travel, continue once weekly during travel and for 4 weeks after leaving the area) *5–20 kg:* 62.5 mg (¼ tab) PO once weekly *20–30 kg:* 125 mg (½ tab) PO once weekly *30–45 kg:* 187.5 mg (¾ tab) PO once weekly *>45 kg:* 250 mg (1 tab) PO once weekly		- Plasma concentrations may be increased in patients with impaired hepatic function - Do not administer quinine and mefloquine concurrently because of risk for cardiac arrhythmias - May cause various disturbances of peripheral nervous system and CNS. Use with caution in patients with cardiac or

Treatment dose for non-immune patients (total treatment dose may be divided into 2–3 doses given 6–8 h apart, give larger portion [½ to ¾ total] as first dose)

<20 kg: 20–25 mg/kg
20–30 kg: 500–750 mg
30–45 kg: 750–1000 mg
45–60 kg: 1250 mg
>60 kg: 1500 mg

- Pediatric experience limited in children <3 months and/or <5 kg-
  Administer with food and at least 240 mL liquid; tabs may be crushed and mixed with small amount of liquid or swallowed whole
- Repeated dose recommended if patient vomits <30 min after administration; repeated ½ dose recommended if patient vomits 30–60 min after administration

---

Meperidine
Tab 50 mg
Inj 50 mg/mL, 100 mg/mL

INFANTS AND OLDER CHILDREN
Analgesic
1–1.5 mg/kg/dose IV/SC/PO q3–4h prn
Preoperatively
1–2 mg/kg/dose IM/SC/PO 60 min preop
Continuous infusion
Loading dose: 0.5–1 mg/kg IV followed by initial rate 0.3 mg/kg/h, may require 0.5–0.7 mg/kg/h IV

2 mg/kg/dose or 100 mg/dose (whichever is less) IV/SC
4 mg/kg/dose or 150 mg/dose (whichever is less) PO

- Dosage adjustment required in renal or hepatic impairment; avoid in severe renal impairment
- May cause constipation, respiratory or CNS depression; dose is cumulative; metabolite may cause seizures
- IM route not recommended for analgesia
- Infusion only used in select cases
- Skin reactions and itching often respond to antihistamines and usually do not imply allergy

Continued

Table 40.1 Drug Dosage Guidelines for Neonates[a] (Where Specified), Infants, and Older Children—cont'd

Drug[b,c]	Dose	Dose Limit	Comments
Meropenem Inj 500 mg, 1 g/vial	***NEONATES*** **Meningitis** 40 mg/kg/dose IV q12h **Other indications** *0–7 days:* 20 mg/kg/dose IV q12h *>7 days:* 20 mg/kg/dose IV q8h ***INFANTS AND OLDER CHILDREN*** **Meningitis, lower respiratory tract infections in patients with cystic fibrosis** 40 mg/kg/dose IV q8h **Fever/neutropenia** 20 mg/kg/dose IV q8h **Other indications** 20 mg/kg/dose IV q8h	 2 g/dose, 6 g/day 1 g/dose, 3 g/day 1 g/dose, 3 g/day	- Dose and interval adjustment in renal impairment: mild, usual dose q12h; moderate, 50% dose q12h; severe, 50% dose q24h; dose after dialysis - Meropenem will decrease valproic acid plasma levels. Monitor valproic acid levels and consider alternate anticonvulsants
Mesalamine (5-ASA, 5-aminosalicylic acid) Tab (enteric-coated) 400 mg (Asacol®), 500 mg (Pentasa®) Rectal susp 4 g/60 g	***INFANTS AND OLDER CHILDREN*** **Ulcerative colitis, Crohn's disease** *Children:* 30–50 mg/kg/day PO div BID–QID *Adolescents, adults:* 2400–4800 mg/day PO div TID–QID (Asacol®) or 2000–4000 mg/day PO div QID (Pentasa®), then reduce to lowest possible maintenance dose *Rectal suspension:* 1–4 g PR qhs × 3–6 weeks, then reduce to lowest possible dose and frequency for maintenance	4.8 g/day (Asacol®), 4 g/day (Pentasa®) 4 g/day PR	- For best results, rectal suspension should be retained for as long as possible - Asacol® 400 mg tablets and Pentasa® 500 mg tablets are not interchangeable - Pentasa® 500 mg tablet may be dispersed in water to ease swallowing. Pentasa® 500 mg tablet may be split along score line

Metformin Tab 500 mg	***INFANTS AND OLDER CHILDREN*** *Adolescents:* 500 mg/dose PO daily	1000 mg PO BID	- Contraindicated in liver impairment
Methadone Solution 1 mg/mL Tab 1 mg, 10 mg	***INFANTS AND OLDER CHILDREN*** **Opioid-naive patients ≥2 years** 0.1–0.2 mg/kg/dose PO BID or 0.07–0.13 mg/kg/dose PO TID, titrated to effect **Opioid-tolerant patients ≥2 years** Use a fixed dose equivalent to 1/10 of the total 24-h PO morphine dose administered orally as required but not more frequently than q3h, to a maximum of 30 mg/dose On day 6, the total amount of methadone taken over previous 2 days is calculated and averaged per day and converted to a q12h regimen If prn medication is still required, increase the dose of methadone by 1/3 q4–6d	*Initial dose limit in opioid-tolerant patient:* 30 mg/dose	- Dose adjustment in renal impairment: CrCl <10 mL/min, 50%–75% - Dose and frequency should be reduced with repeated use because of the cumulative effects of methadone - Discontinuation of chronic therapy with opioids should be carried out gradually to avoid precipitating withdrawal symptoms
Methimazole Tab 5 mg	***INFANTS AND OLDER CHILDREN*** *Initial dose:* 0.4–0.7 mg/kg/day PO div q8–12h; increase up to 1.5 mg/kg/day if no improvement within 2–3 weeks *Maintenance:* 0.2 mg/kg/day PO div q8–12h or once daily	*Initial:* 60 mg/day *Maintenance:* 30 mg/day	- Give at same time in relation to meals every day - Reduce dose in liver impairment - May cause agranulocytosis
Methotrexate Tab 2.5 mg Inj 25 mg/mL	***INFANTS AND OLDER CHILDREN*** **Rheumatological disorders** 10–15 mg/m²/dose PO/SC given once weekly May increase by 1 mg/kg/week to maximum 25 mg/week	*Initial:* 10–15 mg/week *Maintenance:* 25 mg/week	- Reduce dose in renal impairment - Handle as a biohazard - Give folic acid (usual dose, 1 mg/day) - Avoid concurrent use with cotrimoxazole - High-dose penicillins may inhibit renal clearance of methotrexate. Monitor for increased methotrexate toxicity

Continued

Table 40.1 Drug Dosage Guidelines for Neonates[a] (Where Specified), Infants, and Older Children—cont'd

Drug[b,c]	Dose	Dose Limit	Comments
Methylprednisolone Inj 40 mg/vial, 125 mg/vial, 500 mg/vial, 1000 mg/vial	*INFANTS AND OLDER CHILDREN* **Acute asthma** 0.5–1 mg/kg/dose IV q6h **Pulse therapy (Rheumatology, Immunology)** 10–30 mg/kg/dose IV over 1 h **Pulse therapy (CNS inflammation)** 20–30 mg/kg/dose IV daily for 3–5 days **Idiopathic thrombocytopenic purpura** 30 mg/kg/dose IV daily for 1–3 days	 60 mg/dose, 240 mg/day 1 g/dose 1 g/dose 1 g/dose	- Consider use of oral prednisone in less severe cases
Metoclopramide Liquid 1 mg/mL Tab 5 mg, 10 mg Inj 5 mg/mL	*NEONATES* **GI motility disorders** *Initial:* 0.03 mg/kg/dose IV q8h *INFANTS AND OLDER CHILDREN* **Small-bowel intubation** 0.1 mg/kg/dose PO/IM/IV **GERD** 0.1–0.15 mg/kg/dose PO/IM/IV QID **Breakthrough chemotherapy-induced nausea and vomiting or failure of prophylaxis in the acute phase** ≥ *1 year:* 1 mg/kg/dose IV pretherapy once then 0.0375 mg/kg/dose PO q6h **Delayed phase chemotherapy-induced nausea and vomiting** ≥ *1 year:* 0.1–0.2 mg/kg/dose PO/IV q6h	0.5 mg/kg/day *Adult dose:* 10–15 mg QID 0.5 mg/kg/day	- May be used in neonates for GI motility disorders after careful screening for contraindications (e.g., seizure disorders) and ongoing safety monitoring for neurological adverse effects including extrapyramidal symptoms - Doses greater than 0.5 mg/kg/day may increase risk of adverse neurological effects - Extrapyramidal side effects may be reversed with diphenhydramine 1 mg/kg/dose IV - High-dose or long-term use (>3 months) may cause tardive dyskinesia - May alter absorption of other drugs - When used as antiemetic, consider the concurrent use of diphenhydramine or benztropine to prevent extrapyramidal effects

Metolazone Tab 2.5 mg Susp (HSC) 1 mg/mL	**INFANTS AND OLDER CHILDREN** 0.2–0.4 mg/kg/dose PO q24h or 0.1–0.2 mg/kg/dose PO q12h	10 mg/dose	
Metoprolol Tab 50 mg Susp (HSC) 10 mg/mL	**INFANTS AND OLDER CHILDREN** 0.5–2.5 mg/kg/dose PO BID	400 mg/day	
Metronidazole Susp (HSC) 15 mg/mL Tab 250 mg Inj 5 mg/mL	**NEONATES** *<1.2 kg:* 7.5 mg/kg/dose IV q48h *1.2–2 kg, 0–7 days:* 7.5 mg/kg/dose q24h *1.2–2 kg, >7 days:* 7.5 mg/kg/dose q12h *>2 kg, 0–7 days:* 7.5 mg/kg/dose q12h *>2 kg, >7 days:* 15 mg/kg/dose q12h **Intestinal bacterial overgrowth** (use IV formulation for PO) 10 mg/kg/dose PO TID		- Dose adjustment in renal impairment: severe, 50% of standard dose; dose *after* dialysis; reduce dose in liver impairment - Give PO with food or milk; avoid alcohol; suspension is chocolate-cherry flavored but very bitter tasting
	INFANTS AND OLDER CHILDREN **Anaerobes** 10 mg/kg/dose PO TID 10 mg/kg/dose IV q8h or 7.5 mg/kg/dose IV q6h	2 g/day PO 4 g/day IV	
	Clostridium difficile 7.5–10 mg/kg/dose IV/PO TID to QID for 10 to 14 days	2 g/day PO/IV	
	Giardiasis 5 mg/kg/dose PO TID for 5 days or single daily dose as follows *<25 kg:* 35 mg/kg/dose PO once daily for 3 days *25–40 kg:* 50 mg/kg/dose PO once daily for 3 days *>40 kg:* 2 g/dose PO once daily for 3 days	750 mg/day (if TID)	

Continued

Table 40.1 Drug Dosage Guidelines for Neonates[a] (Where Specified), Infants, and Older Children—cont'd

Drug[b,c]	Dose	Dose Limit	Comments
Metronidazole—cont'd	**Amebiasis**	2.25 g/day	- For *T. vaginalis*, partner must also be treated
	12–17 mg/kg/dose PO TID for 5–10 days		
	Trichomonas vaginalis		
	>13 years: 2 g PO stat		
	Gut sterilization		
	10 mg/kg/dose PO at 1300 h, 1400 h, and 2300 h, starting day before surgery		
	Treatment of intestinal bacterial overgrowth		
	10 mg/kg/dose PO BID–TID		
	Ulcerative colitis, Crohn's disease		
	3.3–6.7 mg/kg/dose IV TID		
	3.3–6.7 mg/kg/dose PO TID pc or 5–10 mg/kg/dose PO BID pc		
	***Helicobacter pylori*–associated ulcer**	1.5 g/day	- In combination with Amoxicillin + PPI + bismuth subsalicylate if <8 years, Tetracycline + PPI + bismuth subsalicylate if ≥8 years
	15–24 kg: 250 mg PO BID		
	25–34 kg: 500 mg PO qam, 250 mg PO qpm		
	≥35 kg: 500 mg PO BID		
	Perforated appendicitis	≤80 kg: 1 g/dose	
	30 mg/kg IV once daily, in combination with ceftriaxone	>80 kg: 1.5 g/dose	
	Pelvic inflammatory disease (outpatient therapy, with ceftriaxone or cefoxitin plus doxycycline OR with levofloxacin)		
	500 mg PO BID for 14 days		
Mexiletine	***INFANTS AND OLDER CHILDREN***	*Loading dose:* 1200 mg/day	- Reduce dose in renal impairment: severe 50%–75% of standard dose; reduce dose in hepatic impairment
Cap 100 mg, 200 mg	*Loading dose:* 6–8 mg/kg PO	*Usual adult dose:* 200 mg/day	
Solution (HSC) 10 mg/mL	*Maintenance:* 2–5.3 mg/kg/dose PO TID or 1.5–4 mg/kg/dose PO QID		- Give with food, milk, or antacids

Midazolam Inj 5 mg/mL Syrup (HSC) 3 mg/mL	**NEONATES** **Sedation** *Loading dose:* 0.05–0.1 mg/kg/dose IV (over 5 min) *Maintenance dose:* 0.16–1 mcg/kg/min IV via continuous infusion *Intermittent dose:* 0.05–0.1 mg/kg/dose IV q2–4h prn		- Use with caution in patients with hepatic or renal impairment, CHF, pulmonary disease; adjust doses of both drugs when used in combination with other CNS depressants
	Intranasal 0.1–0.2 mg/kg/dose	0.5 mL (2.5 mg) per nostril	- Do not discontinue abruptly in patients receiving prolonged midazolam infusions
	Status epilepticus (refractory seizures) 0.15 mg/kg/dose IV bolus, then 2 mcg/kg/min IV via continuous infusion. Increase as needed by 2 mcg/kg/min q10min for ongoing seizures. Bolus 0.15 mg/kg with each increase in the infusion rate.	24 mcg/kg/min	- Calculate dose according to ideal body weight - Administer injection solution intranasally using mucosal atomization device (MAD) - Give 0.1 mL overfill to accommodate MAD dead-space volume
	INFANTS AND OLDER CHILDREN **Sedation** *PO*		- Injection solution may be given orally
	<20 kg: 0.5–0.75 mg/kg/dose PO *≥20 kg:* 0.3–0.5 mg/kg/dose PO administered 15–30 min before procedure or surgery	20 mg/dose PO	
	IV 0.05 mg/kg/dose IV for sedation; repeat once prn 0.1–0.2 mg/kg/dose IV preoperatively	0.15 mg/kg/dose IV	
	Intranasal 0.2–0.5 mg/kg/dose intranasally for sedation; may repeat dose q5–15min to a maximum of 0.5 mg/kg total	*Infants:* 0.5 mL (2.5 mg) per nostril *Older children:* 1 mL (5 mg) per nostril (10 mg total)	

Continued

Table 40.1   Drug Dosage Guidelines for Neonates[a] (Where Specified), Infants, and Older Children—cont'd

Drug[b,c]	Dose	Dose Limit	Comments
Midazolam—cont'd	SC		
	Sedation in palliative care patients: 0.5–4 mcg/kg/min SC infusion		
	Intensive care setting		
	Initial: 0.1–0.2 mg/kg/dose IV q2–4h prn, titrate to response as needed	5 mg/dose	
	Continuous infusion: 1–6 mcg/kg/min IV		
	Status epilepticus (initial doses)		
	Intranasal: 0.2 mg/kg/dose	5 mg per nostril, 10 mg/dose	
	IM: 0.3 mg/kg/dose	10 mg/dose	
	Buccal: 0.5 mg/kg/dose	10 mg/dose	
	Status epilepticus (refractory seizures)		
	0.15 mg/kg/dose IV bolus, then 2 mcg/kg/min IV via continuous infusion. Increase as needed by 2 mcg/kg/min q5min. Bolus 0.15 mg/kg with each increase in the infusion rate	24 mcg/kg/min	
Milrinone Inj 1 mg/mL	***NEONATES***		- Reduce dose in renal impairment; half-life may be prolonged in patients with CHF and renal impairment
	<30 weeks GA		
	Loading dose: 0.75 mcg/kg/min continuous IV infusion over 3 h		
	Maintenance dose: 0.25 mcg/kg/min continuous IV infusion		
	≥30 weeks GA		
	Loading dose: 0.05 mg/kg IV over 1 h, given undiluted or in appropriate diluent		
	Maintenance dose: 0.3–0.75 mcg/kg/min continuous IV infusion		
	INFANTS AND OLDER CHILDREN		
	Loading dose: 0.05 mg/kg IV over ≥10 min, given undiluted or in appropriate diluent	1.13 mg/kg/day	
	Maintenance dose: 0.375–0.75 mcg/kg/min continuous IV infusion	1.13 mg/kg/day	

| Mineral oil (heavy) | INFANTS AND OLDER CHILDREN | Usual adult dose: 15–45 mL PO as single dose | - Because of risk of aspiration, avoid in children <1 year and children with difficulty swallowing |
| Liquid | 1 mL/kg/dose PO qhs | | |

Montelukast	INFANTS AND OLDER CHILDREN		- Administer in the evening
Chew tabs 4 mg, 5 mg, 10 mg	1–5 years: 4 mg/day		- Chew tabs contain phenylalanine: use with caution in patients with phenylketonuria
	6–14 years: 5 mg/day		
	>14 years: 10 mg/day		

Morphine	NEONATES		- Reduce dose in renal impairment: moderate, 75% of dose; severe, 50% of dose; reduce dose in liver impairment
Syrup 1 mg/mL	Loading dose: 0.05–0.1 mg/kg IV		- Injection may be given sublingually or buccally, undiluted
Tab 5 mg, 10 mg	Maintenance: 5–40 mcg/kg/h IV via continuous infusion		- Caps may be opened and contents sprinkled on soft food; pellets should not be chewed
Tab SR 15 mg, 30 mg, 60 mg, 100 mg	0.1–0.5 mg/kg/dose PO q4–6h		- IM route should not be used for analgesia
Cap SR 10 mg, 15 mg, 30 mg, 100 mg	0.05–0.1 mg/kg/dose SL/buccal q3–4h		- Continuous IV/SC infusion is preferred to intermittent dosing for management of prolonged pain requiring frequent or high-dose morphine administration
Suppos 2.5 mg, 5 mg, 10 mg	INFANTS AND OLDER CHILDREN		- Do not adjust maintenance infusion dose until current dose has been running for at least 8 h; if a maintenance dose of >100 mcg/kg/h or additional boluses seem to be required, consider consulting pain management service
Inj 2 mg/mL, 10 mg/mL, 50 mg/mL	Moderate sedation		
Inj epidural 5 mg/ 10 mL	0.05–0.1 mg/kg IV may repeat once in 15 min prn		
	0.3 mg/kg PO, 30–60 min before procedure (with syrup or immediate release tablets)		
	Preoperative sedation		
	0.05–0.2 mg/kg/dose IM 30–60 min preop		

Continued

Table 40.1   Drug Dosage Guidelines for Neonates[a] (Where Specified), Infants, and Older Children—cont'd

Drug[b,c]	Dose	Dose Limit	Comments
Morphine—cont'd	**Analgesia—intermittent dosing**		- A patient's opioid requirements should be established using immediate release for-mulations first. Conversion to sustained release products should be individualized. Doses higher than these initial dosages for sustained release dosage forms should be reserved for use in opioid-tolerant patients
	IV/SC	5 mg/dose IV/SC	
	Without continuous infusion (or intensive care patients with a continuous infusion): 0.05–0.1 mg/kg/dose IV/SC q2–4h. Start at 0.05 mg/kg/dose IV/SC q2h, and titrate as needed		
	With continuous infusion: 0.01–0.04 mg/kg/dose IV/SC q2h prn for breakthrough pain (can give q20min for palliative care)		
	PO/PR (immediate-release dosage forms)	15 mg/dose PO (no dose limit for palliative care)	
	≤50 kg: 0.2–0.5 mg/kg/dose PO/PR q4–6h (PO dose using syrup or immediate-release tablets)		
	>50 kg: 10–15 mg/dose PO/PR q4h (PO dose using syrup or immediate-release tablets)		
	SL/Buccal (using injection solution undiluted): 0.05–0.1 mg/kg/dose SL/buccal q3–4h		
	PO dosing (sustained-release dosage forms)		
	Initial dose: 0.5–1 mg/kg/dose PO q12h		
	Analgesia—continuous infusion		
	0.05–0.1 mg/kg IV/SC loading dose, THEN 10–40 mcg/kg/h IV/SC infusion. Increase infusion rate q8h prn in increments ≤25% of previous infusion rate		
	Acute painful episodes (vasoocclusive crisis) in sickle cell disease		
	Loading dose: 0.1 mg/kg IV over 5 min	*Loading dose:* 7.5 mg	
	Maintenance: 40 mcg/kg/h IV; increase dose q8h prn in increments of 20 mcg/kg/h	*Maintenance:* 100 mcg/kg/h	

Mycophenolate mofetil
Susp 200 mg/mL
Cap 250 g
Tab 500 g
Inj (HSC) 6 mg/mL
	INFANTS AND OLDER CHILDREN
	Renal transplantation
	300–600 mg/m²/dose PO q12h
	GVHD in BMT patients
	Initial dose: 450 mg/m²/dose IV q6h or 600 mg/m²/dose IV q8h
		3 g/day	- Initial dose may be lower or dose may be divided TID to allow for tolerance to GI irritation
			- Oral to IV conversion as follows
			  - BMT: 1.25:1
			  - Other patients: 1:1

Nabilone Cap 0.25 mg, 0.5 mg, 1 mg	***INFANTS AND OLDER CHILDREN*** **Prevention of acute chemotherapy-induced nausea and vomiting** *9 to <18 kg:* 0.25 mg/dose PO BID *18 to <34 kg:* 0.5 mg/dose PO BID *34 to <50 kg:* 1 mg/dose PO BID *≥50 kg:* 1 mg/dose PO TID	0.06 mg/kg/day	- Reduce dose in liver impairment
Nadolol Susp (HSC) 10 mg/mL Tab 40 mg, 80 mg	***INFANTS AND OLDER CHILDREN*** **Hypertension** 1 mg/kg/dose PO once daily or 0.5 mg/kg/dose PO BID; increase dose by 1 mg/kg/day q3–4days prn	4 mg/kg/day or 320 mg/day, whichever is less	- Reduce dose in renal impairment: moderate, 50% of dose; severe, 25% of dose

Continued

Table 40.1 Drug Dosage Guidelines for Neonates[a] (Where Specified), Infants, and Older Children—cont'd

Drug[b,c]	Dose	Dose Limit	Comments
Naloxone Inj 0.4 mg/mL	***NEONATES*** **Resuscitation** 0.1 mg/kg/dose IV/ETT; repeat prn **Management of adverse opioid-related effects** 0.001–0.005 mg/kg IV (IM, SC, ETT routes may be used if IV route unavailable). Repeat at 2–3 min intervals as needed	*Maximum total dose:* 0.1 mg/kg	- Whenever possible, titration of naloxone dose is more desirable; in sedated patients, administration of naloxone should be reserved for emergency use (i.e., severe obtundation and respiratory depression)
	INFANTS AND OLDER CHILDREN **Resuscitation** Titrate to effect with 0.01 mg/kg/dose IV/ETT increments or 0.1 mg/kg/dose IV/ETT, repeat prn **Partial opioid reversal for sedated patients** 0.001–0.01 mg/kg/dose IV prn	2 mg/dose	- Following administration of naloxone, patients must be cared for in a constant care setting and discharged only when fully awake and a minimum 3 h has elapsed
	Management of adverse opioid effects *Intermittent dosing:* 0.001–0.01 mg/kg/dose; observe and repeat q10min prn *Continuous infusion:* 0.5–1 mcg/kg/h starting dose (range: 0.25–2 mcg/kg/h)	*Maximum total dose:* 0.1 mg/kg	
Naproxen Susp 25 mg/mL, Tab 125 mg, 250 mg, 375 mg Suppos 500 mg	***INFANTS AND OLDER CHILDREN*** 5–10 mg/kg/dose PO BID *25–49 kg:* 250 mg/dose PR ≥*50 kg:* 500 mg/dose PR	1 g/day	- Reduce dose in liver impairment; use with caution and monitor closely in patients with impaired renal function; avoid in patients with severe renal impairment
Nelfinavir Tab 250 mg, 625 mg	***INFANTS AND OLDER CHILDREN*** *2–13 years:* 45–55 mg/kg/dose PO BID >*13 years:* 1250 mg PO BID	*Adult dose:* 2500 mg/day	- Reduce dose in liver impairment - Administer with meal or light snack; tabs may be dissolved in small amount of

Neostigmine Inj 0.5 mg/mL	**INFANTS AND OLDER CHILDREN** **Supraventricular tachycardia** 0.01–0.04 mg/kg/dose IV **Curare antagonism** 0.02–0.08 mg/kg/dose IV **Myasthenia gravis** 0.01–0.04 mg/kg/dose IV/IM/SC q2–4h	2.5 mg/dose 2.5 mg/dose (10 mg/24 h) 375 mg/day	– Have atropine at hand
Nevirapine Susp 10 mg/mL Tab 200 mg	**NEONATES** **Prevention of perinatal HIV transmission** *<34 weeks PMA:* 100 mg/m²/dose once daily PO for first 2 weeks, then 100 mg/m²/dose q12h PO for 2 weeks *≥34 weeks PMA:* 150 mg/m²/dose once daily PO for first 2 weeks, then 150 mg/m²/dose q12h PO for 2 weeks **INFANTS AND OLDER CHILDREN** *1 month to <8 years:* 200 mg/m²/dose PO as a single daily dose for 14 days, then 200 mg/m²/dose PO q12h *≥8 years:* 150 mg/m²/dose PO as a single daily dose for 14 days, then 150 mg/m²/dose PO q12h	200 mg/dose, 400 mg/day	– For HIV prophylaxis in neonates, initial measurement of nevirapine trough level is recommended on Day 7. Additional nevi- rapine trough level on Day 14 is recom- mended if Day 7 level is out of range, ad- dition or discontinuation of an interacting drug (e.g. fluconazole, phenobarbital), and/or hepatic impairment

Continued

Table 40.1   Drug Dosing Guidelines for Neonates[a] (Where Specified), Infants, and Older Children—cont'd

Drug[b,c]	Dose	Dose Limit	Comments
Nifedipine Cap 5 mg, 10 mg	**INFANTS AND OLDER CHILDREN** **Hypertension (chronic)** *Initial dose:* 0.17 mg/kg/dose PO q8h (minimum: 1.25 mg/dose) (use immediate-release capsules). Increase gradually prn to 1–1.5 mg/kg/day PO **Acute prn dosing** 0.125–0.25 mg/kg/dose PO q4h prn (use immediate-release capsules)	*Usual adult dose:* 10–30 mg/dose *prn dose:* 10 mg/dose, 2 mg/kg/day	- Do not use in neonates - Extended-release (XL) tablets may be given once a day. Do not crush or split XL tablets - For more rapid action, direct patient to bite and swallow immediate-release capsules - Use short-acting capsules with caution in patients with coronary artery disease or vascular disease of the head and neck vessels (e.g. Takayasu, Moya Moya) where a sudden drop in BP could cause stroke or MI
Nitrazepam Susp (HSC) 1 mg/mL Tab 5 mg	**INFANTS AND OLDER CHILDREN** *Initial dose:* 0.25 mg/kg PO once daily or 0.08 mg/kg/dose PO TID. Increase gradually prn to 1.2 mg/kg/day PO		- Reduce dose in liver impairment - Give with food or milk
Nitrofurantoin Macrocrystals, cap 50 mg, 100 mg Susp (HSC) 10 mg/mL	**INFANTS AND OLDER CHILDREN** **Treatment** 1.25–1.75 mg/kg/dose PO q6h **UTI prophylaxis** 1–2 mg/kg/dose PO once daily	400 mg/day or 10 mg/kg/day, whichever is less *Usual adult dose:* 50–100 mg qhs	- Give with food or milk - Do not give to infants <1 month - Avoid if GFR is <50 mL/min - May discolor urine rust-yellow to brown - Has also been given on an alternate-day schedule

Nitroglycerin Inj 5 mg/mL	***NEONATES*** *Initial:* 0.1–0.5 mcg/kg/min via continuous IV infusion *Usual:* 1–3 mcg/kg/min via continuous IV infusion	*Usual maximum dose:* 5 mcg/kg/min via continuous IV infusion	- May enhance the effects of inhaled nitric oxide when administered concomitantly. - Closely monitor systemic blood pressure and signs of methemoglobinemia (e.g., cyanosis, hypoxia)
	INFANTS AND OLDER CHILDREN 0.5–10 mcg/kg/min via continuous IV infusion		
Nitroprusside Inj 50 mg/2 mL	***NEONATES*** 0.2–0.5 mcg/kg/min via continuous IV infusion	2 mcg/kg/min via continuous IV infusion	- May enhance the effects of inhaled nitric oxide when administered concomitantly. - Closely monitor systemic blood pressure and signs of methemoglobinemia (e.g., cyanosis, hypoxia)
	INFANTS AND OLDER CHILDREN 0.5–10 mcg/kg/min via continuous infusion	2.5 mg/kg/day cumulative dose	- Caution regarding cyanide toxicity
Norepinephrine Inj 2 mg/mL norepinephrine bitartrate = 1 mg/mL norepinephrine base	***NEONATES*** *Initial:* 0.01–0.1 mcg/kg/min via continuous IV infusion (as norepinephrine base)	2 mcg/kg/min	- Avoid extravasation - Administer via central line, when possible
	INFANTS AND OLDER CHILDREN 0.02–0.1 mcg/kg/min via continuous IV infusion (as norepinephrine base)		
Nystatin Drops 100,000 units/mL	***NEONATES:*** **Oral candidiasis treatment** 100,000–200,000 units/dose PO QID		
	INFANTS AND OLDER CHILDREN **Oral candidiasis prophylaxis and treatment** 100,000–600,000 units/dose PO QID		

Continued

Table 40.1 Drug Dosage Guidelines for Neonates[a] (Where Specified), Infants, and Older Children—cont'd

Drug[b,c]	Dose	Dose Limit	Comments
Octreotide Inj 50 mcg/mL, 500 mcg/mL, 1000 mcg/mL	**INFANTS AND OLDER CHILDREN** **Chylothorax** *Intermittent dosing:* 5 mcg/kg/dose IV/SC q8h for 3 doses, then 10 mcg/kg/dose IV/SC q8h for 3 doses, then 13.3 mcg/kg/dose IV/SC q8h for 5 days. Wean by 25% q24h as follows: 10 mcg/kg/dose IV/SC q8h for 3 doses, then 6.7 mcg/kg/dose IV/SC q8h for 3 doses, then 3.3 mcg/kg/dose IV/SC q8h for 3 doses, then stop *Continuous infusion:* Start at 0.5 mcg/kg/h, then double the dose q24h until 4 mcg/kg/h. Usual duration of therapy: 5 days **Portal hypertensive GI bleeding** *Continuous Infusion:* 1–2 mcg/kg IV bolus followed by 1–2 mcg/kg/h IV infusion	10 mcg/kg/h	- Reduce dose in renal impairment - Regular monitoring for glucose tolerance, biliary tract abnormalities, and hypothyroidism is required
Olanzapine Tab 2.5 mg, 10 mg Tab (ODT) 5 mg	**INFANTS AND OLDER CHILDREN** 2.5–5 mg/dose PO once daily. Titrate weekly by 2.5 or 5 mg/week	*Usual target dose:* 15–20 mg/day	- Consider dose adjustment in renal or hepatic impairment
Omeprazole Delayed-release tab 10 mg, 20 mg Susp (HSC) 2 mg/mL	**NEONATES** 0.5–1.5 mg/kg/dose PO once daily **INFANTS AND OLDER CHILDREN** **Erosive esophagitis, gastroesophageal reflux disease** *1 month–2 years:* 1–3 mg/kg/dose PO once daily or 0.5–1.5 mg/kg/dose PO BID *>2 years:* 0.7–2.5 mg/kg/dose PO once daily or 0.35–1.25 mg/kg/dose PO BID	3.5 mg/kg/day, or 80 mg/day, whichever is less *Usual adult dose for initial therapy:* 20–40 mg PO daily	- Reduce dose in liver impairment - Recommend giving omeprazole at least 1 h before feeds or at least 1 h after feeds (does not apply to postpyloric feeds)

Helicobacter pylori–associated ulcer

15–24 kg: 20 mg PO BID
25–34 kg: 30 mg PO BID
≥35 kg: 40 mg PO BID

INFANTS AND OLDER CHILDREN

Antiemetic with antineoplastics

Highly emetogenic regimens: 5 mg/m²/dose (0.15 mg/kg/dose) IV/PO pre-therapy ×1, then q8h

Moderately emetogenic regimens: 5 mg/m²/dose (0.15 mg/kg/dose) IV/ PO pre-therapy ×1, then q12h — 8 mg/dose

Low emetogenic regimens: 10 mg/m²/dose (0.3 mg/kg/dose) IV/PO pretherapy once — 16 mg/dose

Postoperative nausea and vomiting

Prophylaxis: 0.1 mg/kg IV once preoperatively or intraoperatively — *Usual adult dose:* 4 mg/dose IV or 8 mg/dose PO

Rescue therapy: 0.1 mg/kg/dose PO/IV q8h prn — *Maximum dose:* 0.15 mg/kg/dose or 8 mg/dose

Nausea and vomiting because of gastroenteritis

0.15 mg/kg/dose IV once
8 to ≤15 kg: 2 mg PO once (ODT)
15 to ≤30 kg: 4 mg PO once (ODT)
>30 kg: 8 mg PO once (ODT)

Cyclic vomiting syndrome

0.3–0.4 mg/kg/dose IV q4–6h — 16 mg/dose

Ondansetron
Tab 4 mg, 8 mg
Tab ODT 4 mg, 8 mg
Inj 2 mg/mL
Liquid 0.8 mg/mL

- May prolong QTc interval. Avoid in patients with congenital long QT syndrome

Continued

Table 40.1	Drug Dosage Guidelines for Neonates[a] (Where Specified), Infants, and Older Children—cont'd		
Drug[b,c]	Dose	Dose Limit	Comments
Oseltamivir Cap 30 mg, 45 mg, 75 mg Susp 6 mg/mL	**INFANTS AND OLDER CHILDREN** **Treatment (5 days)** <1 year: 3 mg/kg/dose PO BID ≥1 year, ≤15 kg: 30 mg PO BID ≥1 year, 15 to ≤23 kg: 45 mg PO BID 23 to ≤40 kg: 60 mg PO BID >40 kg: 75 mg PO BID **Prophylaxis (10 days)** ≥3 months–1 year: 3 mg/kg/dose PO daily ≥1 year, ≤15 kg: 30 mg PO once daily ≥1 year, 15 to ≤23 kg: 45 mg PO daily 23 to ≤40 kg: 60 mg PO once daily >40 kg: 75 mg PO once daily	*Usual adult dose:* 75 mg PO BID for 5 days (treatment); 75 mg PO daily for 10 days (prophylaxis)	- Dose interval adjustment in renal impairment: moderate, q24h (treatment), q48h (prophylaxis); no recommendation available for end-stage renal disease - Capsules may be opened and the contents mixed with sweetened liquids, such as regular or sugar-free chocolate syrup
Oxcarbazepine Tab 150 mg, 300 mg, 600 mg Susp 60 mg/mL	**INFANTS AND OLDER CHILDREN** **Adjunctive therapy** *1 month–4 years:* Initiate at 5 mg/kg/dose PO BID, increase by 10 mg/kg/day every 5 days up to usual maintenance dose of 15–20 mg/kg/dose BID **Maintenance (>4 years)** 20–29 kg: 450 mg/dose PO BID 29.1–39 kg: 600 mg/dose PO BID >39 kg: 900 mg/dose PO BID	60 mg/kg/day	- Dose adjustment in renal impairment: CrCl <30 mL/min, start at 300 mg/day and titrate slowly - Cross-sensitivity with carbamazepine in 25%–30% of patients

		Monotherapy
		20–24 kg: 300–450 mg/dose PO BID
		25–34 kg: 450–600 mg/dose PO BID
		35–44 kg: 450–750 mg/dose PO BID
		45–49 kg: 600–750 mg/dose PO BID
		50–59 kg: 600–900 mg/dose PO BID

Oxybutynin
Syrup 1 mg/mL
Tab 5 mg

INFANTS AND OLDER CHILDREN
Neurogenic bladder
1–<5 years: 0.2 mg/kg/dose PO BID–QID
≥5 years: 5 mg/dose PO BID, up to 5 mg/dose PO QID

Usual adult monotherapy dose:
2400 mg/day

Oxycodone
Tab (immediate-release)
5 mg, 10 mg, 20 mg

INFANTS AND OLDER CHILDREN
0.05–0.15 mg/kg/dose PO q4–6h prn

5–10 mg/dose in opioid naïve patients

Palonosetron
Inj 0.25 mg/5 mL
Cap 0.5 mg

INFANTS AND OLDER CHILDREN
Antiemetic for antineoplastics and/or radiotherapy
1 month to <17 years: 0.02 mg/kg IV once prechemo
≥12 years: 0.5 mg PO once prechemo
≥17 years: 0.25 mg IV or 0.5 mg PO once prechemo

1.5 mg/dose IV

- Children receiving multiple day therapy may receive palonosetron q48h during the acute phase
- Consider oral administration for children ≥12 years of age

Pamidronate
Inj 30 mg/10 mL

INFANTS AND OLDER CHILDREN
Hypercalcemia
0.5–1 mg/kg/dose; may repeat in 1 week
Osteogenesis imperfecta, McCune–Albright syndrome
<2 years: 0.5 mg/kg/day IV over 3–4 h × 3 days q2mo
2.1–3 years: 0.75 mg/kg/day IV over 3–4 h × 3 days q2mo
>3 years: 1 mg/kg/day IV over 3–4 h × 3 days q2mo
Reduce the first dose (day 1, cycle 1) by 50%

- Use with caution in renal impairment
- Maintain hydration and urine output during treatment
- Monitor electrolytes. May cause ↓ Ca^{2+}, ↓ Mg^{2+}, ↓ K$^+$, ↓ phosphate

Continued

Table 40.1 Drug Dosage Guidelines for Neonates[a] (Where Specified), Infants, and Older Children—cont'd

Drug[b,c]	Dose	Dose Limit	Comments
Pancrelipase Cap: lipase 10,000 USP units, amylase 40,000 USP units, protease 35,000 USP units ECS Enteric coated capsule-10: lipase 10,000 USP units, amylase 33,200 USP units, protease 37,500 USP units	***INFANTS AND OLDER CHILDREN*** *Infants:* 1 Cotazym® regular capsule/120 mL formula *Children and Adolescents: Creon 10®* (*enteric coated capsule*) *1–4 years:* 2–3/meal, 1–2/snack *5–12 years:* 3–5/meal, 1–3/snack *>12 years:* 5–8/meal, 2–3/snack **Blocked enteral feeding tube** Open 1 Cotazym® regular capsule and combine with 1 crushed tablet of sodium bicarbonate 325 mg. Dissolve in 5–10 mL of sterile water before instilling into clogged tube	4000 USP units lipase/g fat or 10,000 USP units lipase/kg/day	- Do not chew or crush cap contents; titrate dose to stool fat content - See Figure 37.2 for unblocking enteral feeding tube algorithm
Pantoprazole Inj 40 mg/vial	***NEONATES*** **GERD, acid suppression, postresection hypergastrinemia** 1–1.5 mg/kg/dose IV once daily or 0.5–0.75 mg/kg/dose IV q12h ***INFANTS AND OLDER CHILDREN*** **GERD, acid suppression requiring a PPI and oral PPI is not feasible** 1–1.5 mg/kg/dose IV once daily or 0.5–0.75 mg/kg/dose IV q12h **Upper GI bleeding** *5–15 kg:* 2 mg/kg/dose IV once and then 0.2 mg/kg/h IV *>15–40 kg:* 1.8 mg/kg/dose IV once and then 0.18 mg/kg/h IV *>40 kg:* 80 mg/dose IV once and then 8 mg/h IV	40 mg/dose *Bolus:* 80 mg/dose *Max rate:* 8 mg/h *Max infusion duration:* 72 h	- May divide q12h if trough gastric pH <5 - For upper GI bleeding, gastric pH should be monitored to maintain pH >6 - For indications other than GI bleeding, gastric pH may be monitored as clinically necessary

PEG 3350 Oral powder	***INFANTS AND OLDER CHILDREN*** **Maintenance therapy for chronic constipation** 0.5–1 g/kg/dose PO once daily **Acute treatment of encopresis or disimpaction** 1–1.5 g/kg/day for 3–6 days	*Maintenance:* 17–34 g/day. May increase to a maximum dose of 100 g/day in children weighing >34 kg who have failed to respond to lower doses *Acute treatment:* 100 g/day	- Mix in approximately 120–240 mL of suitable beverage (water, juice, tea, coffee or soda)
PEG electrolyte liquid (GoLYTELY, PegLyte) Oral powder	***INFANTS AND OLDER CHILDREN*** 100 mL/year of age/h PO/NG until rectal effluent is clear *Adolescents* 240 mL PO q10min until rectal effluent is clear	1 L/h, 4 L total	- Use with caution in patients with renal insufficiency - For PO administration, product is more palatable when chilled
Penicillin G Benzathine Inj 1.2 million units/ syringe	***INFANTS AND OLDER CHILDREN*** **Prophylaxis to prevent recurrence of rheumatic fever** ≤27 kg: 600,000 units IM every 3–4 weeks >27 kg: 1.2 million units IM every 3–4 weeks		- For intramuscular use only. Do not administer IV.

Continued

Table 40.1 Drug Dosage Guidelines for Neonates[a] (Where Specified), Infants, and Older Children—cont'd

Drug[b,c]	Dose	Dose Limit	Comments
Penicillin G Na (parenteral/aqueous) Inj 5 million units/vial, 10 million units/vial	***NEONATES*** **Meningitis** *0–7 days:* 80,000–150,000 units/kg/dose IV/IM q8h *>7 days:* 112,000 units/kg/dose IV/IM q6h **Other infection** *0–7 days, <2 kg:* 25,000 units/kg/dose IV/IM q12h *0–7 days, ≥2 kg:* 25,000 units/kg/dose IV/IM q8h *>7 days, <1.2 kg:* 25,000 units/kg/dose IV/IM q12h *>7 days, 1.2–2 kg:* 25,000 units/kg/dose IV/IM q8h *>7 days, ≥2 kg:* 25,000 units/kg/dose IV/IM q6h **Congenital syphilis** *0–7 days:* 50,000 units/kg/dose IV/IM q12h *>7 days:* 50,000 units/kg/dose IV/IM q8h ***INFANTS AND OLDER CHILDREN*** **Mild to moderate infections** 25,000–37,500 units/kg/dose IM/IV q6h **Severe infections** 41,500–66,500 units/kg/dose IM/IV q4h **Meningitis** 66,500 units/kg/dose IM/IV q4h **Congenital syphilis** 50,000 units/kg/dose IV q4–6h for 10 days	4 million units/dose, 20 million units/day 4 million units/dose, 24 million units/day 4 million units/dose, 24 million units/day	- Contains 1.68 mmol Na$^+$/million units - 600 mg = 1 million units - Reduce dose interval in renal impairment: moderate q8–12h, severe q12–18h

| Penicillin VK
Tab 300 mg | INFANTS AND OLDER CHILDREN
GAS pharyngitis
50 mg/kg PO once daily
Streptococcal infection (mild to moderate infections)
12.5–25 mg/kg/dose PO BID for 10 days
Other infections
12.5–25 mg/kg/dose PO q6h or 17–33 mg/kg/dose PO q8h
Rheumatic fever treatment
≤27 kg: 300 mg PO BID for 10 days
>27 kg: 600 mg PO BID for 10 days
Rheumatic fever prophylaxis
>5 years: 300 mg PO BID
Prophylaxis in asplenic patients
3 months–5 years: 150 mg PO BID
>5 years: 300 mg PO BID | 500 mg/dose, 1.5 g/day

3 g/day | - Reduce dose in renal impairment: moderate, 75% of dose; severe, 25%–50% of dose
- May be given with food
- 300 mg = 480,000 units |
| Pentamidine
isethionate
Inj 300 mg/vial | INFANTS AND OLDER CHILDREN
Pneumocystis pneumonia
Treatment: 4 mg/kg/day IM/IV as a single daily dose for 14–21 days
Prophylaxis: 4 mg/kg/dose IV q2wk OR 300 mg/dose by inhalation monthly | | - Dose interval adjustment in renal impairment: moderate, q24–36h; severe, q48h
- IV preferred over IM administration
- Dose of inhaled pentamidine should be individualized for younger uncooperative children (600 mg/dose) |

Continued

Table 40.1 Drug Dosage Guidelines for Neonates[a] (Where Specified), Infants, and Older Children—cont'd

Drug[b,c]	Dose	Dose Limit	Comments
Phenobarbital Elixir 5 mg/mL Tab 15 mg, 30 mg, 100 mg Inj 30 mg/mL, 120 mg/mL	*NEONATES* **Status epilepticus** *Loading dose:* 20 mg/kg IV, may repeat 5–10 mg/kg IV up to maximum total dose of 40 mg/kg **Maintenance** 4–6 mg/kg/day IV/PO once daily	*Total:* 40 mg/kg	- Reduce dose in liver impairment - Administer IV undiluted at a rate not to exceed 2 mg/kg/min or 60 mg/min, whichever is less - Monitoring of serum drug concentration recommended
	INFANTS AND OLDER CHILDREN **Status epilepticus** 20 mg/kg IV for 1	1 g/dose	
	Maintenance <3 months: 5–6 mg/kg/dose PO/IV once daily or 2.5–3 mg/kg/dose PO/IV BID ≥3 months: 3–5 mg/kg/dose PO/IV once daily or 1.5–2.5 mg/kg/dose PO/IV BID *Adolescents:* 2–4 mg/kg/dose PO/IV once daily or 1–2 mg/kg/dose PO/IV BID	*Maintenance dose:* 200 mg/day	
Phentolamine Inj 10 mg/mL	*NEONATES* **Treatment of extravasation of vasoactive drug** (e.g., dopamine) Prepare solution of 5 mg in 10 mL NS (0.5 mg/mL) and give 0.2 mL SC to infiltrate area of extravasation. Up to 2 doses may be given.	2.5 mg total	
	INFANTS AND OLDER CHILDREN **Treatment of extravasation of vasoactive drug** (e.g., dopamine) Prepare solution of 5 mg in 10 mL NS and use SC to infiltrate area of extravasation	5 mg	

Phenylephrine Inj 10 mg/mL	***INFANTS AND OLDER CHILDREN*** **Supraventricular tachycardia** 0.01 mg/kg/dose IV; increase in increments of 0.01 mg/kg up to 0.1 mg/kg/total dose **Tetralogy of Fallot spell** 5 mcg/kg/dose IV followed by continuous IV infusion of 0.1–4 mcg/kg/min		- For SVT and Tetralogy of Fallot spells, the final dose should be based on a successful result or a 50% increase in BP over baseline - Should only be given by physicians who are experienced with using phenylephrine for SVT or tetralogy spell
Phenytoin Susp 25 mg/mL Chewtab 50 mg Cap 30 mg, 100 mg Inj 50 mg/mL	***NEONATES*** *Loading:* 20 mg/kg IV, may repeat with 10 mg/kg (total 30 mg/kg) *Maintenance:* 2–4 mg/kg/dose IV/PO BID or 1.3–2.7 mg/kg/dose IV/PO q8h	*Total:* 30 mg/kg	- Administer IV at a rate not to exceed 1 mg/kg/min or 50 mg/min, whichever is less - Compatible only in NS or Ringer's lactate; incompatible with dextrose-containing solutions
	INFANTS AND OLDER CHILDREN **Status epilepticus** *Loading dose:* 20 mg/kg IV once		- Poorly absorbed after oral administration in infants <6 months - Reduce dose in liver impairment
	Antiepileptic (maintenance dose) *<3 years:* 2.7–3.3 mg/kg/dose PO/IV q8h or 4–5 mg/kg/dose PO/IV q12h *≥3–6 years:* 2.5–3 mg/kg/dose PO/IV q8h or 3.75–4.5 mg/kg/dose PO/IV q12h *7–9 years:* 2.3–2.7 mg/kg/dose PO/IV q8h or 3.5–4 mg/kg/dose PO/IV q12h *10–16 years:* 2–2.3 mg/kg/dose PO/IV q8h or 3–3.5 mg/kg/dose PO/IV q12h *≥16 years:* 1.3–2 mg/kg/dose PO/IV q8h or 2–3 mg/kg/dose PO/IV q12h	*Loading dose* *<50 kg:* 1 g/dose *≥50 kg:* 1.5 g/dose	- Monitoring of serum drug concentration recommended - Calculate loading dose according to adjusted body weight - Injection and caps are the sodium salt form of phenytoin (equivalent to 92% phenytoin)
	Arrhythmia *Loading dose:* 15 mg/kg/dose IV over 1 h. Simultaneously, Option 1: give 3 mg/kg/dose PO once, then 6 h later give 2 mg/kg/dose PO hour; start maintenance 6 h later, OR Option 2: 5 mg/kg/dose PO q6h for 4 doses, OR Option 2: 5 mg/kg/dose PO q6h for 4 doses, then 2.5 mg/kg/dose PO q6h for 4 doses *Maintenance:* 1.7–2 mg/kg/dose PO q8h or 2.5–3 mg/kg/dose PO q12h		

Continued

Table 40.1 Drug Dosage Guidelines for Neonates[a] (Where Specified), Infants, and Older Children—cont'd

Drug[b,c]	Dose	Dose Limit	Comments
Phosphate Inj sodium phosphate 3 mmol phosphate/mL (4 mmol sodium/mL) Inj potassium phosphate 3 mmol phosphate/mL (4.4 mmol potassium/mL) Oral solution sodium phosphate USP 4.2 mmol elemental phosphate/mL (4.8 mmol elemental sodium/mL) Effervescent tab (Phosphate Novartis) 500 mg elemental phosphate (16 mmol phosphate) Rectal (enema) solution (Fleet®) *Pediatric:* sodium biphosphate 3.9 g and sodium phosphate 10.4 g and sodium biphosphate 20.8 g and sodium phosphate 7.8 g/130 mL unit. *Adult:* Sodium phosphate 3.9 g/65 mL unit.	***INFANTS AND OLDER CHILDREN*** **Hypophosphatemia** (moderate) *Oral therapy:* 1–2 mmol/kg/day PO div BID–QID **Hypophosphatemic rickets** 1–3 mmol/kg/day PO div QID **Hypophosphatemia** (moderate to severe) *IV therapy:* 1–2 mmol phosphate/kg/day IV or 0.042–0.083 mmol phosphate/kg/h IV as a continuous infusion **Constipation** ≥2 years: 1 enema PR once daily as needed	*Max rate of infusion:* 0.125 mmol/kg/h *Maximum:* 1 enema every 24 h	- Monitor serum phosphate, sodium and calcium. Maintain adequate hydration and monitor renal function - Risk of severe dehydration, electrolyte abnormalities (e.g., hyperphosphatemia, hypocalcemia, hypernatremia), acute kidney injury and arrhythmias with use of oral or rectal products to treat constipation. Caution in children less than 5 years of age, patients with dehydration, renal impairment, bowel inflammation or obstruction, and heart failure. Caution in patients who are also taking diuretics, ACE inhibitors, ARBs and NSAIDs

Phytonadione (Vitamin K₁)

Inj 1 mg/0.5 mL, 10 mg/mL

Tab 5 mg

NEONATES

Hemorrhagic disease of the newborn

Prophylaxis: 0.5–1 mg IM/SC at birth

Treatment: 1 mg/dose IM/IV

Routine INR reversal (intensive care settings)

0.1–0.2 mg/kg/dose IV over 30–60 min

INFANTS AND OLDER CHILDREN

Warfarin antidote

No bleeding, future need for warfarin: 0.5–2 mg/dose PO

No bleeding, no future need for warfarin, OR significant bleeding, not life threatening: 2–5 mg/dose PO or IV

Significant bleeding, life threatening: 5 mg/dose IV over 10–20 min

Acute fulminant hepatic failure

Infants: 1–2 mg/dose IV

Children: 5–10 mg/dose IV

Malabsorption

2.5–5 mg/dose PO, given 1–7 days/week (titrate dose and frequency to effect) or 1–2 mg/dose IV — 25 mg/dose PO

Routine INR reversal (intensive care settings)

0.1–0.2 mg/kg/dose IV over 30–60 min — 10 mg/dose IV

- Severe anaphylactoid reactions have occurred with IV administration; use caution during IV administration. Give IV in emergency situations only.
- Injection may be given by mouth, undiluted
- Oral tabs available for long-term patients

Continued

Table 40.1 Drug Dosage Guidelines for Neonates[a] (Where Specified), Infants, and Older Children—cont'd

Drug[b,c]	Dose	Dose Limit	Comments
Piperacillin and tazobactam Inj 3.375 g (piperacillin 3g + tazobactam 0.375 g) 4.5 g (piperacillin 4 g + tazobactam 0.5 g)	***NEONATES*** *<1.2 kg:* 50–100 mg/kg/dose IV q12h *1.2–2 kg, 0–14 days:* 50–100 mg/kg/dose IV q12h *1.2–2 kg, >14 days:* 50–100 mg/kg/dose IV q8h *>2 kg, 0–7 days:* 50–100 mg/kg/dose IV q12h *>2 kg, >7 days:* 50–100 mg/kg/dose IV q8h ***INFANTS AND OLDER CHILDREN*** *1—<6 months:* 80 mg piperacillin/kg/dose IV q6h (infused over 30 min) *≥6 months:* 100 mg piperacillin/kg/dose IV q6h (infused over 30 min)	100 mg piperacillin/kg/dose or 4 g piperacillin/dose, whichever is less	- Dose and interval adjustment in renal impairment: severe, decrease dose by 30% and give q8h
Polyethylene glycol (PEG) 3350	See **PEG 3350**		
Polyethylene glycol-electrolyte solution	See **PEG electrolyte liquid**		
Potassium chloride Solution 1.33 mmol/mL Cap SR 600 mg (8 mmol) Inj 2 mmol/mL	***NEONATES*** **Maintenance** 0.5–1 mmol/kg/dose IV/PO once daily or 0.25–0.5 mmol/kg/dose IV/PO q12h. Adjust based on serum potassium concentrations **Treatment of hypokalemia** 0.7–1.7 mmol/kg/dose IV/PO q8h or 0.5–1.25 mmol/kg/dose IV/PO q6h **High KCl infusion** (intensive care settings, CVL only) 0.25 mmol/kg/h IV, with ECG monitoring	Usual range: 2–4 mmol/kg/day IV/PO in divided doses 2 mmol/kg/dose 0.5 mmol/kg/h IV	- Give PO with food; dilute oral solution in water or juice and give over 5–10 min; cap may be opened and contents sprinkled on soft food for administration (pellets should not be chewed)

	INFANTS AND OLDER CHILDREN		
	Prevention of hypokalemia during diuretic therapy		
	1–2 mmol/kg/dose PO once daily or 0.5–1 mmol/kg/dose PO BID	*Usual adult maximum:*	
		Maximum PO: 80 mmol/day	
		Maximum IV: 400 mmol/day	
	Treatment of hypokalemia		
	0.7–1.7 mmol/kg/dose IV/PO q8h or 0.5–1.25 mmol/kg/dose IV/PO q6h		
Prednisolone, prednisone	***INFANTS AND OLDER CHILDREN***		- See Table 40.3 for steroid equivalents
Prednisolone liquid 1 mg base/mL	**Asthma**		- Give with food or milk
Prednisone	1–2 mg/kg/day PO as a single daily dose for 5 days	60 mg/day	- To discontinue in patients receiving therapy for ≥10 days, reduce dose by 50% q48h until 2.5 ± 0.8 mg/m²/day is achieved, then reduce dose by 50% q10–14d (except in pneumocystic pneumonia)
Susp (HSC) 5 mg/mL	**Nephrotic syndrome**		
Tab 1 mg, 5 mg, 50 mg (1 mg prednisolone base = 1 mg prednisone)	*Initial*: 60 mg/m²/day PO as single daily dose or in divided doses	60 mg/day	
	Juvenile idiopathic arthritis (JIA)		
	Initial: 2 mg/kg/day PO daily or in divided doses	60 mg/day	- For patients requiring prednisone oral liquid (which is very bitter), consider prednisolone liquid (commercially available as Pediapred 1 mg base/mL)
	Pneumocystis pneumonia		
	0.8 mg/kg/day PO BID for 5 days, then 0.8 mg/kg/day as a single daily dose for 5 days, then 0.4 mg/kg/day as a single daily dose for 11 days	40 mg PO BID for 5 days, then 40 mg PO daily for 5 days, then 20 mg PO daily for 11 days	
	Idiopathic Thrombocytopenic Purpura (ITP)		- ITP: for life-threatening bleeding, consider IV methylprednisolone if patient unable to tolerate oral therapy
	4 mg/kg/day PO div BID to QID for 4 days (no taper)	150 mg/day	

Continued

Table 40.1	Drug Dosage Guidelines for Neonates[a] (Where Specified), Infants, and Older Children—cont'd		
Drug[b,c]	Dose	Dose Limit	Comments
Primaquine phosphate 15 mg base/tab	***INFANTS AND OLDER CHILDREN*** ***Plasmodium vivax* or *Plasmodium ovale* (prevention of relapse)** *Patients ≥6 months with intermediate or normal G6PD levels (≥3 units/g Hb):* 0.5 mg base/kg/dose PO once daily for 14 days *Patients ≥6 months with deficient G6PD levels (<3 units/g Hb):* 0.75 mg base/kg/dose PO once weekly for 8 weeks (**Note:** Chloroquine is preferred over primaquine in this population)	*Adult dose:* 30 mg base/day *Adult dose:* 45 mg base/week	- Dosed as base: 26.3 mg primaquine phosphate = 15 mg primaquine base - Check G6PD level before use
Primidone Tab 125 mg, 250 mg	***INFANTS AND OLDER CHILDREN*** *≤ 8 years:* Starting dose: 125 mg PO qhs, then increase on day 7 to 125 mg PO BID, then increase on day 14 to 125 mg PO TID, then increase on day 21 to 10–25 mg/kg/day PO div TID or QID *> 8 years:* Starting dose: 250 mg PO qhs, then increase on day 7 to 250 mg PO BID, then increase on day 14 to 250 mg PO TID, then increase on day 21 to 750–1500 mg/day PO div TID or QID		- Dose interval adjustment in renal impairment: moderate, q8–12h; severe, q12–24h; reduce dose in liver impairment - Monitor serum concentrations of primidone and phenobarbital
Procainamide Inj 100 mg/mL	***INFANTS AND OLDER CHILDREN*** *Loading dose* ≤1 year: 3–7 mg/kg/dose IV over 30–60 min >1 year: 7–15 mg/kg/dose IV over 30–60 min *Maintenance dose* 20–80 mcg/kg/min via continuous IV infusion	1 g/dose IV, 2 g/day IV	- Dose interval adjustment in renal impairment: moderate: q6–12h; severe, q8–24h - IV loading dose should be switched to maintenance infusion rate before completion

Propafenone Tab 10 mg, 150 mg, 300 mg Inj 3.5 mg/mL	**INFANTS AND OLDER CHILDREN** 67–200 mg/m²/dose PO TID or 50–150 mg/m²/dose PO QID	900 mg/day *Usual adult dose:* 150–200 mg/ dose PO q8h or 225–300 mg/ day PO q12h	- Reduce dose in renal or liver impairment - Give with food or milk - Reduce digoxin dose by 50% when initiating concurrent propafenone therapy
Propofol Inj 10 mg/mL	**INFANTS AND OLDER CHILDREN** *Induction:* 2–5 mg/kg/dose IV *Maintenance:* 30–160 mcg/kg/min IV *Rapid sequence intubation:* 1–4 mg/kg/dose IV (dose depends on hemodynamic state of patient)		- Expertise and experience required for use - Titrate against response. Caution: hypotension/bradycardia - Not approved for long-term sedation (maximum duration 12 h)
Propranolol Susp (HSC) 5 mg/mL Tab 10 mg, 40 mg Inj 1 mg/mL	**NEONATES** **Resuscitation** 0.01–0.1 mg/kg/dose IV **Arrhythmia** *Initial:* 0.5–0.75 mg/kg/dose PO q6h or 0.67–1 mg/kg/dose PO q8h **Other** 0.125–0.25 mg/kg/dose PO q6h 0.01–0.15 mg/kg/dose IV q6–8h, titrate dose slowly		- Reduce dose in liver impairment - Give IV propranolol only under ECG monitoring, undiluted over 2–10 min, at a rate not exceeding 1 mg/min - Use caution when converting between oral and IV routes of administration. Oral to IV conversion is 10:1

Continued

Table 40.1 Drug Dosage Guidelines for Neonates[a] (Where Specified), Infants, and Older Children—cont'd

Drug[b,c]	Dose	Dose Limit	Comments
Propranolol—cont'd	***INFANTS AND OLDER CHILDREN***		
	Arrhythmia	3 mg/dose IV	
	0.01–0.15 mg/kg/dose IV q6–8h prn		
	0.5–0.75 mg/kg/dose PO q6h or 0.67–1 mg/kg/dose PO q8h		
	Antihypertensive		
	0.17–1.3 mg/kg/dose PO TID or 0.125–1 mg/kg/dose PO QID		
	Tetralogy of Fallot spells		
	0.05–0.1 mg/kg/dose IV over 10 min		
	Maintenance: 0.3–2 mg/kg/dose PO TID or 0.25–1.5 mg/kg/dose PO QID		
	Wolff-Parkinson-White syndrome		
	0.67–3.3 mg/kg/dose PO TID or 0.5–2.5 mg/kg/dose PO QID		
Propylthiouracil Tab 50 mg Oral susp (HSC) 5 mg/mL	***INFANTS AND OLDER CHILDREN*** *Initial dose:* 50 mg/m²/dose PO q8h or 3.3 mg/kg/dose PO q8h	Initial dose *6–10 years:* 150 mg/day *>10 years:* 300 mg/day (higher doses can be used when necessary)	- Reduce dose in liver impairment - Give at same time in relation to meals every day - Once patient is euthyroid, reduce dose to minimum required (usually ⅓–½ of initial dose) - May cause agranulocytosis or hepatic dysfunction
Prostaglandin E₁	See Alprostadil		

Protamine sulfate Inj 10 mg/mL	***INFANTS AND OLDER CHILDREN*** **Unfractionated heparin antidote** *Time from last dose* *<30 min:* 1 mg/100 units of unfractionated heparin *30–60 min:* 0.5–0.75 mg/100 units of unfractionated heparin *61–120 min:* 0.375–0.5 mg/100 units of unfractionated heparin *>120 min:* 0.25–0.375 mg/100 units of unfractionated heparin	50/dose (regardless of the amount of unfractionated heparin received)	- Protamine sulfate should be administered in a concentration of 10 mg/mL at a rate not to exceed 5 mg/min. If administered too quickly may cause cardiovascular collapse - Hypersensitivity risk in those with fish allergy, those who received protamine-containing insulin, or previous protamine therapy - Obtain blood for aPTT/ heparin antifactor Xa level, INR 15 min after the administration of protamine
Pseudoephedrine Syrup 6 mg/mL Tab 60 mg	***INFANTS AND OLDER CHILDREN*** *<2 years:* 1 mg/kg/dose PO q6h prn *2–5 years:* 15 mg/dose PO q6h prn *6–12 years:* 30 mg/dose PO q6h prn **Priapism (sickle cell disease)** 0.5 mg/kg/dose PO qhs prn	*Usual adult dose:* 60 mg/dose PO q4–6h prn 30 mg/dose	- Use with caution in hypertensive patients and children <2 year - Dose combination products according to pseudoephedrine content
Pyrazinamide Tab 500 mg Susp (HSC) 100 mg/mL	***INFANTS AND OLDER CHILDREN*** **Tuberculosis** (regimens for treatment and prophylaxis vary) 35 mg/kg/dose PO daily or 17.5 mg/kg/dose PO q12h 50–70 mg/kg/dose PO twice weekly	2 g/day	- Dose reduction may be required in hepatic impairment; dose reduction in severe renal impairment: 50%–100%

Continued

Table 40.1 Drug Dosage Guidelines for Neonates[a] (Where Specified), Infants, and Older Children—cont'd

Drug[b,c]	Dose	Dose Limit	Comments
Pyridoxine (Vitamin B₆) Inj 100 mg/mL Solution (HSC) 1 mg/mL Tab 25 mg, 100 mg, 250 mg	**NEONATES, INFANTS, AND OLDER CHILDREN** **Pyridoxine-dependent seizures** *Initial:* 10–100 mg/dose IV/PO *Maintenance:* 50–100 mg/day PO **Drug-induced neuritis** *Treatment:* 10–50 mg/day PO *Prophylaxis:* 1–2 mg/kg/day PO		- Monitor EEG concurrently
Quetiapine Tab 25, 100, 200 mg	**INFANTS AND OLDER CHILDREN** Children *(initial dose):* 12.5 mg/dose PO once daily or BID Adolescents *(initial dose):* 25 mg/dose PO once daily or BID	*Usual adult target dose:* 300–600 mg/day	- Reduce dose in liver impairment - To achieve maintenance dose, increase by 25–50 mg q2d
Quinine Cap, as sulfate (83% quinine base): 200 mg sulfate (166 mg base) 300 mg sulfate (249 mg base) Inj, as dihydrochloride 300 mg/mL (245 mg/mL quinine)	**INFANTS AND OLDER CHILDREN** **Severe plasmodium (all types)** 20 mg/kg (of quinine dihydrochloride) IV loading dose over 4 h, followed by 10 mg/kg IV over 2–4 h q8h until oral therapy can be started **Uncomplicated *Falciparum* or sequential oral therapy** 9 mg (of quinine sulfate)/kg/dose PO TID (duration dependent on geographic area)	1.8 g (dihydrochloride), or 1.5 g (base)/day	- If more than 48 h of parenteral treatment is required, the quinine dose should be reduced by one-third to one-half - Give with food or milk - Chloroquine-resistant strains generally require a total of 7 days treatment with quinine or quinidine and a second drug - If persistent acute kidney injury or no clinical improvement in 48 h: 10 mg (of quinine dihydrochloride)/Kg IV q12h - Do not administer quinine and mefloquine concurrently because of risk of cardiac arrhythmias. If both agents are necessary to treat severe malaria, delay mefloquine ad-

Raltegravir Chew tab 25 mg, 100 mg	***INFANTS AND OLDER CHILDREN*** **Postexposure prophylaxis or treatment of HIV infection** **in combination therapy** *<12 years* *11 to <13.9 kg:* 75 mg PO BID *14 to <19.9 kg:* 100 mg PO BID *20 to <27.9 kg:* 150 mg PO BID *28 to <39.9 kg:* 200 mg PO BID *≥40 kg:* 300 mg PO BID *≥12 years:* 400 mg PO BID	
Ranitidine Solution 15 mg/mL Tab 75 mg, 150 mg	***NEONATES*** 2 mg/kg/dose PO q8h ***INFANTS AND OLDER CHILDREN*** **Peptic ulcer, GERD** *Treatment:* 1.7–3.3 mg/kg/dose PO q8h or 2.5–5 mg/kg/dose PO q12h for 8 weeks *Maintenance:* 2.5–5 mg/kg/dose PO once daily or 1.25–2.5 mg/kg/dose PO q12h	*Usual adult dose:* 300 mg/day PO as a single hs dose or div q12h 300 mg PO BID	- Reduce dose in renal impairment, moderate: 75% usual dose; severe: 50% usual dose - Monitor gastric pH predose and titrate dose based on gastric pH (target minimum pH 4–5) and monitor gastric pH in patients requiring IV therapy
Rasburicase Inj (HSC) 1.5 mg/mL	***INFANTS AND OLDER CHILDREN*** 0.2 mg/kg/dose IV over 30 min q24h	1.5 mg/dose	- Contraindicated in G6PD deficiency - Do not give for longer than 7 days

Continued

Table 40.1 Drug Dosage Guidelines for Neonates[a] (Where Specified), Infants, and Older Children—cont'd

Drug[b,c]	Dose	Dose Limit	Comments
Rifampin Susp (HSC) 25 mg/mL Cap 150 mg, 300 mg Inj 600 mg/vial	**NEONATES** 10–20 mg/kg/dose IV once daily or 5–10 mg/kg/dose IV BID 10 mg/kg/dose PO q12h **INFANTS AND OLDER CHILDREN** **Tuberculosis** (regimens for treatment and prophylaxis vary) 15 mg/kg/dose PO/IV once daily or 7.5 mg/kg/dose PO/IV q12h 10–20 mg/kg/dose PO twice weekly **Meningococcal prophylaxis** 10 mg/kg/dose PO q12h for 2 days **Haemophilus influenzae prophylaxis** 20 mg/kg/dose PO once daily for 4 days **Cholestatic pruritus** 5 mg/kg/dose PO BID, may be titrated up every 2–4 weeks or more quickly as inpatients	600 mg/day 1200 mg/day 600 mg/day 20 mg/kg/day or 600 mg/day	- Reduce dose in liver impairment; may discolor urine, sweat, saliva, tears; give on an empty stomach (1 h ac or 2 h pc) unless GI upset occurs; monitor liver function tests periodically; may reduce serum concentration of many other medications, including anticoagulants, tacrolimus, cyclosporine, and oral contraceptives
Rifaximin Tab 550 mg	**INFANTS AND OLDER CHILDREN** **Hepatic encephalopathy** 10–15 mg/kg/dose PO BID (oral suspension) *7.5–15 kg:* 137.5 mg PO BID *>15–30 kg:* 275 mg PO BID *>30 kg:* 550 mg PO BID	550 mg/dose, 1100 mg/day	- Tablets may be split, chewed, or crushed. - Preferably given without food (may be given with food in patients without severe hepatic impairment)

Small intestinal bacterial overgrowth		
10–15 mg/kg/dose PO BID–TID for 7–10 days	550 mg/dose, 1650 mg/day	- Reduce dose in renal or liver impairment
7.5–15 kg: 137.5 mg PO BID–TID for 7–10 days		- To achieve maintenance dose, increase by
>15–30 kg: 275 mg PO BID–TID for 7–10 days		0.5–1 mg q3–4d
>30 kg: 550 mg PO BID–TID for 7–10 days		
Risperidone	***INFANTS AND OLDER CHILDREN***	
Liquid 1 mg/mL	*Children, initial dose:* 0.25–0.5 mg/dose PO once daily or 0.25 mg/dose	
Tab 0.25 mg, 1 mg, 2 mg	PO BID	
	Adolescents, initial dose: 1 mg/dose PO once daily or 0.5–1 mg/dose	
	PO BID	
	Titrate dose upward based on clinical response	
Risperidone	***INFANTS AND OLDER CHILDREN***	*Usual adult target dose:*
		4–6 mg/day
Rituximab	***INFANTS AND OLDER CHILDREN***	375 mg/m²/dose	- Premedication with acetaminophen, di-
Inj 100 mg/10 mL	*Standard dose:* 375 mg/m²/dose IV weekly	1000 mg/dose	phenhydramine, and IV methylpredniso-
	Other: 500 mg/m²/dose IV		lone is recommended
Rizatriptan	***INFANTS AND OLDER CHILDREN***		
Oral disintegrating tabs	*≥6 years*		
5 mg, 10 mg	<40 kg: 5 mg PO as a single dose		
	≥40 kg: 10 mg PO as a single dose		
	Dosage adjustment with concomitant propranolol use		
	<40 kg: Do not use rizatriptan		
	≥40 kg: 5 mg PO as a single dose		

Continued

Table 40.1   Drug Dosage Guidelines for Neonates[a] (Where Specified), Infants, and Older Children—cont'd

Drug[b,c]	Dose	Dose Limit	Comments
Rocuronium Inj 50 mg/5 mL	**_NEONATES_** _Tracheal intubation:_ 0.3–0.6 mg/kg/dose IV q30min to q2h prn _Facilitating mechanical ventilation:_ 0.3 mg/kg/dose IV q30min to q2h prn _Maintenance:_ 4–10 mcg/kg/min IV (i.e., 0.24–0.6 mg/kg/h) **_INFANTS AND OLDER CHILDREN_** **Intensive care settings** _Tracheal intubation:_ 1 mg/kg/dose IV _Maintenance:_ 0.5 mg/kg/dose IV prn		- Monitor blood pressure and heart rate closely - The target response is variable depending on indication (e.g., to maintain minimal movement in a sedated patient or to facilitate mechanical ventilation). When using to facilitate mechanical ventilation, the target response should be respiratory suppression—not paralysis of arm or leg. Mandatory evaluation is required at least every 24 h
Rufinamide Tab 100 mg, 200 mg, 400 mg	**_INFANTS AND OLDER CHILDREN_** _<30 kg:_ 100 mg PO BID _≥30 kg:_ 200 mg PO BID Increase by 5 mg/kg/day q2wk based on response	_<30 kg:_ 1300 mg/day _30–50 kg:_ 1800 mg/day _>50–70 kg:_ 2400 mg/day _≥70 kg:_ 3200 mg/day	- Use of rufinamide with other antiepileptic drugs can alter each other's concentrations. Initiate rufinamide at the lowest dose and titrate slowly when the patient is taking other antiepileptic drugs. Monitor serum levels of concomitant antiepileptic drugs
Salbutamol Inhalation solution 5 mg/mL Metered-dose inhaler (MDI) 100 mcg/puff Inj 1 mg/mL Tab 2 mg, 4 mg	**_NEONATES_** 0.25 mL/dose via nebulizer q4–12h prn, up to q2h maximum **_INFANTS AND OLDER CHILDREN_** **Acute asthma** _MDI_ _<20 kg:_ 4 puffs (400 mcg) q20min for 3 doses, then q1–4h and q1h pm _≥20 kg:_ 8 puffs (800 mcg) q20min for 3 doses, then q1–4h and q1h pm		- MDIs are preferred method of administration over nebulizers - Monitor for tachycardia, hypokalemia - May cause hypokalemia. Consider checking serum potassium in patients who are receiving salbutamol q1h or less for 6 h or for a prolonged period of time

Inhalation solution via nebulizer (intermittent dosing)
<20 kg: 0.5 mL (2.5 mg) in 3 mL NS via nebulizer q1–4h prn
≥20 kg: 1 mL (5 mg) in 3 mL NS via nebulizer q1–4h prn
Continuous nebulization (intensive care setting only)
10–20 kg: 10–15 mg (5–7.5 mL)/h continuous nebulization
>20 kg: 15–20 mg (7.5–10 mL)/h continuous nebulization
IV Infusion (intensive care setting only): Initial rate: 1 mcg/kg/min IV; increase by 1 mcg/kg/min q15min prn up to max of 10 mcg/kg/min

Minimum: 0.5 mL/dose
Maximum: 1 mL/dose

<12 years: usual 5 mcg/kg/min, caution for doses up to 10 mcg/kg/min.
≥12 years: doses up to 4 mcg/kg/min may be considered based on clinical need. Usual adult limit 20 mcg/min.

Maintenance therapy for asthma
1–2 puffs (100–200 micrograms) q4h prn (MDI)
0.5–1 mL (2.5–5 mg) in 3 mL NS via nebulizer q4h prn

Maximum nebulizations 4 times/day

Hyperkalemia
4 mcg/kg IV over 20 min

Senna
Syrup 1.7 mg/mL
Tab 8.6 mg

INFANTS AND OLDER CHILDREN
Liquid
2–5 years: 3–5 mL/dose PO qhs
6–12 years: 5–10 mL/dose PO qhs
Tablet
6–12 years: 1–2 tabs/dose PO qhs

Usual adult dose: 2–4 tabs qhs

- Have patient drink plenty of fluids
- Effects occur within 6–24 h after PO dosing; avoid prolonged use

Continued

Table 40.1 Drug Dosage Guidelines for Neonates[a] (Where Specified), Infants, and Older Children—cont'd

Drug[b,c]	Dose	Dose Limit	Comments
Sertraline Cap 25 mg, 50 mg, 100 mg	***INFANTS AND OLDER CHILDREN*** ***Depression and anxiety disorders*** *6–12 years:* 12.5–25 mg PO once daily; titrate dose upwards by 25–50 mg/day increments at intervals of at least 1 week if necessary *> 12–17 years:* 25–50 mg PO once daily; titrate dose upwards by 50 mg/day increments at intervals of at least 1 week if necessary	200 mg/day	- An increased risk of suicidal thinking and behavior has been reported with the use of antidepressants in children, adolescents, and young adults. Monitor carefully for suicidal ideation, self-harm, or hostility
Sevelamer Tab 800 mg	***INFANTS AND OLDER CHILDREN*** *Initial:* 400 mg PO BID; titrate dose to serum phosphorus *Usual dose:* 800–1600 mg PO TID with meals. Additional doses may be required with snacks		- Tabs should not be split or chewed - Separate administration from that of other medications whenever possible, administering them at least 1 h before or 3 h after sevelamer - If calcium supplements required, give sevelamer qhs; monitor serum calcium and phosphate at least q1–3wk until target concentrations are achieved
Sildenafil Inj 0.8 mg/mL Oral suspension 2.5 mg/mL Tablet 25 mg, 50 mg, 100 mg	***NEONATES, INFANTS AND OLDER CHILDREN*** *Oral: Initial starting dose:* 0.25–0.5 mg/kg/dose PO every 4–8 h Titrate according to response *IV:* Bolus: 0.1 mg/kg IV over 30 min, followed by continuous infusion of 0.03 mg/kg/h IV	2 mg/kg/dose PO q4h	- Monitor BP (can cause hypotension)
Simethicone Oral drops 40 mg/mL	***INFANTS AND OLDER CHILDREN*** *<2 years:* 20 mg PO QID *2–12 years:* 40 mg PO QID *>12 years:* 40–250 mg PO QID	500 mg/day	- Administer after meals and at bedtime - May be mixed with water or other liquids

Sirolimus Liquid 1 mg/mL Tab 1 mg	**INFANTS AND OLDER CHILDREN** *Loading dose (de novo transplant recipient):* 0.42 mg/kg/day PO *Initial maintenance dose:* 0.14 mg/kg/day PO once daily	15 mg/dose	- Reduce dose in liver impairment - Maintenance dose individualized based on disease state, type of transplant, and time since transplant - Tabs should not be cut or crushed; liquid must be further diluted with water or orange juice (not grapefruit juice) - Sirolimus may interact with many other medications
Sodium bicarbonate Inj 4.2% (0.5 mmol/mL), 8.4% (1 mmol/mL) Oral solution (HSC) 1 mmol/mL Tab 325 mg (3.9 mmol); 500 mg (6 mmol)	**NEONATES** **Correction of metabolic acidosis/hyperkalemia with cardiac instability** 1–2 mmol/kg/dose IV over 2–5 min as 4.2% (0.5 mmol/mL) concentration; may repeat every 10 min as needed **Correction of metabolic acidosis** *Half correction:* IV dose (mmol HCO_3) = (0.3 × weight [kg] × HCO_3 deficit [mmol/L])/2 Administer half correction, then assess need for additional half correction **INFANTS AND OLDER CHILDREN** **Correction of metabolic acidosis/hyperkalemia with cardiac instability** *<2 years:* 1–2 mmol/kg/dose IV over 2–5 min as 4.2% (0.5 mmol/mL) concentration; may repeat every 10 min as needed *≥2 years:* 1–2 mmol/kg/dose IV over 1–2 min as 8.4% (1 mmol/mL) concentration; may repeat every 10 min as needed **Correction of metabolic acidosis** 2–5 mmol/kg IV infusion over 4–8 h; subsequent doses should be based on patient's acid-base status **Blocked enteral feeding tube** 325 mg (see Figure 37.2 for unblocking enteral feeding tube algorithm)		- *Neonates:* 0.3 represents the estimated volume of distribution for bicarbonate - Dilute the 8.4% strength 1:1 with sterile water or use the 4.2% strength undiluted - Incompatible with epinephrine, calcium, atropine - Administer slowly; make sure that the patient is effectively ventilated

Continued

Table 40.1 Drug Dosage Guidelines for Neonates[a] (Where Specified), Infants, and Older Children—cont'd

Drug[b,c]	Dose	Dose Limit	Comments
Sodium picosulfate, magnesium oxide, and citric acid (Pico-Salax®) Sachet: sodium picosulfate 10 mg, magnesium oxide 3.5 g, and citric acid 12 g	**INFANTS AND OLDER CHILDREN** **Preprocedural** (2 doses given 6–8 h apart on the day before the procedure) *1–6 years:* 1/4 sachet am, 1/4 sachet pm *6–12 years:* 1/2 sachet am, 1/2 sachet pm *>12 years:* 1 sachet am, 1 sachet pm		- Empty contents of sachet into glass of cold water (approx. 150 mL or 5 oz for 1 sachet, 60–90 mL or 2–3 oz for 1/2 or 1/4 sachet. Stir frequently for 2–3 min until dissolved. Drink the prepared solution. *Caution:* solution may become hot - It is important to drink plenty of clear fluids throughout the treatment until the bowel movements have ceased. In general, patients should drink about 250 mL of clear fluid (including a balanced electrolyte solution) every hour while they feel the effects of Pico-Salax®. Do not drink just water alone
Sodium polystyrene sulfonate (Kayexalate) Powder Susp 250 mg/mL Enema 30 g/120mL	**NEONATES** 1 g/Kg/dose in water or D5W PO/PR (PR is preferred over PO) **INFANTS AND OLDER CHILDREN** 1 g/Kg/dose PO q6h prn 1 g/Kg/dose PR q2–6h prn	*Usual adult oral dose:* 15 g/dose *Usual adult rectal dose:* 30–50 g/dose	- Exchanges approximately 1 mmol K⁺/g of resin - Administer rectally in appropriate volume of tap water, D10W, or equal parts tap water and 2% methylcellulose; moisten resin with honey or jam for PO use. Do not administer orally to neonates with reduced gut motility.
Somatropin	See **Growth Hormone**		

Sorbitol Syrup 70% Liquid 3% (HSC)	**INFANTS AND OLDER CHILDREN** **Cathartic** 1.5–2 mL/kg/dose PO	150 mL/dose
Sotalol Susp (HSC) 5 mg/mL Tab 80 mg, 160 mg	**INFANTS AND OLDER CHILDREN** **Arrhythmias** *Infants:* 0.67–1.7 mg/kg/dose PO q8h *Older children:* 0.67–1.7 mg/kg/dose PO q8h or 1–2.5 mg/kg/dose PO q12h	*Usual adult dose:* 160 mg/dose PO BID *Maximum dose:* 480 mg/day	- Dose reduction in renal impairment: moderate, 30% standard dose; severe, 15%–30% standard dose; reduce dose in hepatic impairment
Spironolactone Susp (HSC) 5 mg/mL Tab 25 mg, 100 mg	**NEONATES** 1–2 mg/kg/dose PO q12h **INFANTS AND OLDER CHILDREN** 1–4 mg/kg/day PO given once daily–QID	*Usual adult dose:* 25–200 mg/day PO	- Avoid when creatinine clearance <10 mL/min - For spironolactone combined with hydrochlorothiazide, see **Aldactazide**
Succinylcholine Inj 200 mg/10 mL	**NEONATES** **Rapid sequence intubation** 2 mg/kg/dose IV **INFANTS AND OLDER CHILDREN** **Intubation** 1–2 mg/kg/dose IV (give single dose and avoid giving repeated dosing)		- DO NOT USE in patients with renal insufficiency, hyperkalemia, burns, crush injuries and multitrauma, myopathies, extensive denervation of skeletal muscle or upper motor neuron injury, positive personal or family history of malignant hyperthermia. *Caution:* Unidentified, undiagnosed, or unexplained neurodevelopmentally delay or muscular illness - Physicians administering succinylcholine must be experienced with airway management, ventilation and resuscitation, and be familiar with the treatment of hyperkalemic cardiac arrest

Continued

Drug Dosing Guidelines

40

Table 40.1 Drug Dosage Guidelines for Neonates[a] (Where Specified), Infants, and Older Children—cont'd

Drug[b,c]	Dose	Dose Limit	Comments
Sucralfate Susp 200 mg/mL Tab 1 g	***INFANTS AND OLDER CHILDREN*** *≤10 kg:* 250 mg/dose PO q6h *>10–20 kg:* 500 mg/dose PO q6h *>20 kg:* 1 g/dose PO q6h	*Adult dose:* 4 g/day PO div QID (1 h ac +qhs)	
Sucrose Oral solution 24%	***NEONATES AND INFANTS <18 MONTHS OF AGE*** 0.1 mL PO 2 min before painful procedure		- Dose may be repeated at 5-min intervals for prolonged procedures - Contraindicated in short-bowel syndrome, carbohydrate intolerance, unconscious or heavily sedated with absent gag reflex
Sulfamethoxazole and Trimethoprim (TMP) Susp trimethoprim 8 mg/mL + sulfa-methoxazole 40 mg/mL Pediatric tab trimethoprim 20 mg + sulfamethox-azole 100 mg Adult tab trimethoprim 80 mg + sulfa-methoxazole 400 mg Inj trimethoprim 16 mg/mL + sulfamethoxazole	***INFANTS AND OLDER CHILDREN*** **Bacterial infection (treatment)** 4–6 mg trimethoprim/kg/dose PO/IV q12h (includes 20–30 mg/kg/dose sulfamethoxazole) **Urinary tract infection (prophylaxis)** 2–5 mg trimethoprim/kg/dose PO once daily **Treatment of intestinal bacterial overgrowth** 5 mg trimethoprim/kg/dose PO BID (available only as tablets in increments of 10 mg TMP) ***Pneumocystis jiroveci* (carinii) treatment** 5 mg trimethoprim/kg/dose IV/PO q6h (includes 25 mg/kg/dose sulfamethoxazole)	160 mg TMP/dose, 320 mg TMP/day	- Maintain fluid intake; may be given with food; dose interval adjustment in renal impairment: moderate, q18h; severe, q24h - Use with caution in patients with G6PD deficiency - Do not give to infants <1-month-old

PJP prophylaxis, Hematology/Oncology		
	150 mg trimethoprim/m²/day PO or 5 mg/kg/day PO given as a single daily dose or div BID on 3 consecutive days/week	320 mg TMP/day for 3x/weekly regimen
	PJP prophylaxis, HIV-infected/exposed children	
	5 mg trimethoprim/kg/dose PO once daily or 2.5 mg trimethoprim/kg/dose PO q12h, given 3 times weekly or 7 days per week	160 mg TMP/day
	PJP prophylaxis, other immunocompromised children	
	2.5–5 mg trimethoprim/kg/dose PO once daily, given 3 times weekly	160 mg TMP/day
Sulfasalazine Susp (HSC) 100 mg/mL Tab 500 mg EC tab 500 mg	***INFANTS AND OLDER CHILDREN*** **Juvenile idiopathic arthritis (JIA)** 40–60 mg/kg/day PO div BID-QID **Ulcerative colitis** *Acute:* 40–70 mg/kg/day PO div TID-QID pc *Maintenance:* 20–50 mg/kg/day PO div BID-QID	 6 g/day 2 g/day	- Give with food - Reduce dose in renal impairment - Maintain fluid intake - May discolor skin, tears, and urine orange yellow - Monitor for blood dyscrasias - Caution in patients with hypersensitivity to salicylates or sulfonamides and in patients with G6PD deficiency - For JIA: begin with ⅓ recommended dose and increase q2d to maximum required dose
Surfactant (BLES) 3, 5 mL vial	***NEONATES*** 5 mL/kg/dose; may be repeated q2–6h for 2 doses	
Sumatriptan Solution, nasal spray 5 mg, 20 mg	***INFANTS AND OLDER CHILDREN*** *20–39 kg:* 5–10 mg intranasal once *≥40 kg or >12 years:* 20 mg intranasal once May repeat dose once after 2 h if headache returns or if only partial response to first dose	40 mg/24 h

Continued

Table 40.1 Drug Dosage Guidelines for Neonates[a] (Where Specified), Infants, and Older Children—cont'd

Drug[b,c]	Dose	Dose Limit	Comments
Tacrolimus Inj 5 mg/mL Cap 0.5 mg, 1 mg, 5 mg Susp (HSC) 0.5 mg/mL	***INFANTS AND OLDER CHILDREN*** **Initial dose before TDM** *Cardiac transplantation:* 0.01 mg/kg/day IV as a continuous infusion or 0.1 mg/kg/dose PO/NG q12h *Liver transplantation:* 0.1 mg/kg/dose PO/NG q12h *Renal transplantation:* 0.1 mg/kg/dose PO/NG q12h *Various indications:* 0.025–0.15 mg/kg/dose PO q12h, adjust by TDM		- Maintenance dose should be individualized based on factors, such as disease state, type of transplant, and time since transplantation - Measure initial trough concentration within 48 h and adjust dose as necessary - To switch from cyclosporine to tacrolimus, discontinue cyclosporine and start tacrolimus 24 h later - Tacrolimus may interact with many other medications - Tacrolimus should always be taken with the same beverage (not grapefruit juice) - Cap should be used in patients with short gut
Tamsulosin Cap, SR 0.4 mg	***INFANTS AND OLDER CHILDREN*** 0.2 mg PO once daily, increase by 0.2 mg/day based on response	*Usual dose:* 0.4 mg/day *Maximum dose:* 0.8 mg/day	- Capsules may be opened and the contents mixed with food (e.g., yogurt or pudding) or juice. Do not administer capsule contents via enteral feeding tubes because of risk of blockage

Drug	Dosing	Max dose	Comments
Tetracycline Cap 250 mg	***INFANTS AND OLDER CHILDREN*** 6.25–12.5 mg/kg/dose PO q6h **Alternative agent for *Helicobacter pylori* eradication** 25 mg/kg/dose PO BID or 12.5 mg/kg/dose PO QID	3 g/day 1 g BID	- Dose interval adjustment in renal impairment: moderate, q12–24h; avoid in severe renal impairment; use with caution in patients with hepatic insufficiency - Do not use in children ≤8 years as may cause permanent discoloration of teeth, enamel hypoplasia, and (usually reversible) retardation of skeletal development - Give on an empty stomach; do not administer with dairy products, milk formulas, antacids, bismuth, or iron products - Enhances effects of warfarin - May cause photosensitivity
Thiamine Inj 1 g/10 mL Tab 100 mg	***INFANTS AND OLDER CHILDREN*** **Refractory septic shock in critically ill patients** *Infants and children:* 25–50 mg IV once, then 10 mg IV q24h *Adolescents:* 200 mg IV q12h **Wernicke's encephalopathy** 100 mg IV daily × 7 days In older children or those who do not respond to lower dose, may consider adult dosing: 500 mg IV TID × 2–3 days followed by 250 mg IV daily × 2–3 days **Seizures/encephalopathy (for basal ganglia disease)** 7.5–10 mg/kg/dose PO/NG BID	20 mg/kg/day or 900 mg/day, whichever is less	- For the treatment of sepsis, IV thiamine may be used with IV ascorbic acid and IV hydrocortisone for a duration of up to 4 days - For the treatment of seizures/encephalopathy for basal ganglia disease, high dose enteral thiamine is used in combination with high dose biotin

Continued

Table 40.1 Drug Dosage Guidelines for Neonates[a] (Where Specified), Infants, and Older Children—cont'd

Drug[b,c]	Dose	Dose Limit	Comments
Tobramycin Inj 10 mg/mL, 40 mg/mL	***NEONATES*** *0–7 days, <34 week PMA:* 3 mg/kg/dose IV q24h *0–7 days, ≥34 week PMA:* 3 mg/kg/dose IV q18h *>7 days, ≤1 kg:* 3.5 mg/kg/dose IV q24h *>7 days, >1 kg, <37 week PMA:* 2.5 mg/kg/dose IV q12h *>7 days, >1 kg, ≥37 weeks PMA:* 2.5 mg/kg/dose IV q8h		- Calculate dose according to adjusted body weight - In neonates, reduce dose in renal impairment; for infants and older children, adjust dose interval in renal impairment: moderate, q12h; severe, q24–48h - Monitoring of serum drug concentration recommended - Peripheral venous sampling to be done in patients on concurrent inhaled and IV tobramycin
	INFANTS AND OLDER CHILDREN **Once-daily dosing (excluding CF, Hematology/Oncology, and HPCT patients)** 9 mg/kg/dose IV q24h	800 mg/dose before TDM	
	Traditional (q8h dosing) or extended dosing intervals for renal impairment 2.5 mg/kg/dose IV/IM q8h	120 mg/dose before TDM	
	Hematology/Oncology and HPCT patients with fever and neutropenia *1 month to <6 years:* 10.5 mg/kg/dose IV q24h *Females ≥6 years:* 9.5 mg/kg/dose IV q24h *Males ≥6 years:* 7.5 mg/kg/dose IV q24h	800 mg/dose before TDM	
	CF patients (non-lung transplant patients) *Females <7 years:* 11 mg/kg/dose IV q24h *Females ≥7 years:* 9 mg/kg/dose IV q24h *Males <16 years:* 11 mg/kg/dose IV q24h *Males ≥16 years:* 9 mg/kg/dose IV q24h 80 mg BID to TID via inhalation	*CF:* no maximum single dose	

Tocilizumab Inj 20 mg/mL	**INFANTS AND OLDER CHILDREN** **Polyarticular JIA** <*30 kg*: 10 mg/kg/dose IV q4wk ≥*30 kg*: 8 mg/kg/dose IV q4wk **Systemic JIA** <*30 kg*: 12 mg/kg/dose IV q2wk ≥*30 kg*: 8 mg/kg/dose IV q2wk **Cytokine release syndrome** <*30 kg*: 12 mg/kg/dose once ≥*30 kg*: 8 mg/kg/dose once Dose may be repeated as needed, based on response and chemotherapy protocol	800 mg	
Topiramate Tabs: 25 mg, 100 mg Sprinkle caps: 15 mg, 25 mg	**INFANTS AND OLDER CHILDREN** ≥*2–16 years* *Initial dose:* 1–3 mg/kg/day PO as a single daily dose at night or div BID. Increase dose at 1–2 week intervals by 1–3 mg/kg/day div BID *Maintenance dose:* 5–9 mg/kg/day PO div BID ≥*17 years* *Initial dose:* 50 mg PO daily. Increase dose at weekly intervals by 50 mg/day div BID *Maintenance dose:* 200–400 mg/day PO div BID	*Initial dose:* 25 mg *Maximum increase:* 50 mg *Maximum maintenance dose:* 600 mg/day	- Dose or interval adjustment in renal impairment: moderate, q36h or give 75% of standard dose; severe, q48h or give 50% of standard dose - Give PO dose with food; tabs may be split. Sprinkle caps may be opened, sprinkled on small amount (5 mL) of soft food and swallowed (not chewed)

Continued

Table 40.1   Drug Dosage Guidelines for Neonates[a] (Where Specified), Infants, and Older Children—cont'd

Drug[b,c]	Dose	Dose Limit	Comments
Tranexamic acid Inj 100 mg/mL Tab 500 mg Mouth rinse (HSC) 4.8 mg/mL	**INFANTS AND OLDER CHILDREN** **Before procedures or dental surgery in patients with coagulopathy** 7–10 mg/kg/dose IV preprocedure and TID–QID afterward until able to take PO medications 25 mg/kg/dose PO TID–QID, beginning 1 day before procedure and for up to 6–8 days afterward **Trauma dosing for critically bleeding patients** (within 3 h since time of injury only) *<12 years:* 15 mg/kg IV over 10 min, then 2 mg/kg/h IV for 8 h or until bleeding stops *≥12 years:* 1 g IV over 10 min, then 1 g IV infusion over 8 h	1 g/dose	- Adjust interval in renal impairment: mild, q12h; moderate, q24h; severe, q48h or adjust dose: mild, 50% usual dose; moderate, 25% usual dose; severe, 10% usual dose - May give injection undiluted over at least 5 min or at maximum rate of 100 mg/min; faster infusion may cause hypotension - Contraindicated in patients with history or risk of thrombosis unless also receiving anticoagulation - Ophthalmic assessment recommended before and during chronic therapy (e.g., treatment several weeks in duration)
Trazodone Tab 50 mg, 100 mg	**INFANTS AND OLDER CHILDREN** **Agitation/aggression** *≥5 years:* 12.5 mg PO BID to TID; titrate to effect (usual target dose: 1.6 mg/kg/dose PO BID–TID) **Insomnia** *≥5 years:* 0.75–1 mg/kg/dose or 25–50 mg PO qhs	200 mg/day 100 mg/day	

Trimethoprim Susp (HSC) 10 mg/mL Tab 100 mg	***NEONATES*** **UTI prophylaxis** 2–3 mg/kg/dose PO once daily OR 1–1.5 mg/kg/dose PO BID ***INFANTS AND OLDER CHILDREN*** **Treatment** 2–3 mg/kg/dose PO q12h **UTI prophylaxis** 2–3 mg/kg/dose PO once daily or 1–1.5 mg/kg/dose PO BID	*Usual adult dose:* 200 mg/day (treatment) *Maximum dose:* 100 mg/day (prophylaxis)	- Interval adjustment in renal impairment: moderate, q18h; severe, avoid - May be given with food
Ursodiol Tab 250 mg Susp (HSC) 50 mg/mL	***INFANTS AND OLDER CHILDREN*** 5–10 mg/kg/dose PO BID or 3.3–6.7 mg/kg/dose PO TID	45 mg/kg/day	
Valacyclovir Tab 500 mg	***INFANTS AND OLDER CHILDREN*** **Orolabial HSV (initial or recurrent episode)** *3 months to 11 years* *6 to <15 kg:* 250 mg PO BID for 3 days *15 to <30 kg:* 500 mg PO BID for 3 days *30 to 36 kg:* 750 mg PO BID for 3 days *>36 kg:* 1000 mg PO BID for 3 days *≥12 years:* 2000 mg PO BID for 1 day **Genital HSV (initial episode)** *≥12 years:* 1000 mg PO div BID for 10 days **Recurrent genital HSV (episodic treatment)** *≥12 years:* 1000 mg PO daily or BID for 3 days		- Dose adjustment in renal impairment: - Recurrent orolabial HSV, episodic treatment (moderate: 50% usual dose; severe: 25% usual dose; ESRD: 25% usual dose and give q24h) - Recurrent genital HSV, episodic treat- ment (severe/ESRD: 50% usual dose) - Recurrent genital HSV, daily suppres- sive treatment (severe/ESRD: 50% usual dose) - Varicella or Zoster (moderate/severe: give q24h; ESRD: 50% usual dose and give q24h)

Continued

Table 40.1　Drug Dosage Guidelines for Neonates[a] (Where Specified), Infants, and Older Children—cont'd

Drug[b,c]	Dose	Dose Limit	Comments
Valacyclovir—cont'd	**Recurrent HSV (daily suppressive therapy)** *≥12 years:* 500–1000 mg PO daily. Reassess after 1 year. **Varicella or zoster** *2–17 years* 　*6 to <15 kg:* 250 mg PO TID for 5 days 　*15 to <30 kg:* 500 mg PO TID for 5 days 　*30–36 kg:* 750 mg PO TID for 5 days 　*≥36 kg:* 1000 mg PO TID for 5 days		
Valganciclovir Oral solution 50 mg/mL Tab 450 mg	***NEONATES*** **Treatment of congenital CMV infection** 16 mg/kg/dose PO BID ***INFANTS AND OLDER CHILDREN*** **Treatment** *Induction:* 900 mg PO BID for 7–14 days *Maintenance:* 900 mg PO once daily		

Valproic acid Syrup 50 mg/mL Cap 250 mg Tab (divalproex) 125 mg, 250 mg, 500 mg Inj 100 mg/mL	**INFANTS AND OLDER CHILDREN** **Seizures (chronic dosing)** 15 mg/kg/day PO once daily or div q8–12h. Increase dose weekly prn by 5–10 mg/kg/day up 30–60 mg/kg/day PO div TID or QID **Status epilepticus** *Loading dose:* 30 mg/kg/dose IV diluted 1:1 in normal saline over 2–5 min; give additional loading dose of 10 mg/kg if status not controlled within 10 min *IV maintenance:* 10 mg/kg/dose IV q8h	60 mg/kg/day	- Reduce dose in liver impairment - Monitoring of serum drug concentration recommended - Dose conversion from PO to IV is 1:1; whereas total daily IV dose equals total daily PO dose, IV dose should be divided q6h
Vancomycin Cap 125 mg Liquid (HSC) 25 mg/mL Inj 500 mg; 1 g/vial, 5 g/vial, 10 g/vial	**NEONATES** **CNS infections** *<27 weeks PMA:* 24 mg/kg/dose IV q24h *27–36 weeks PMA:* 18 mg/kg/dose IV q8h *≥37 weeks PMA:* 15 mg/kg/dose IV q6h **Other infections** *<27 weeks PMA:* 24 mg/kg/dose IV q24h *27–36 weeks PMA:* 18 mg/kg/dose IV q12h *≥37 weeks PMA:* 22.5 mg/kg/dose IV q12h		- Monitoring of serum drug concentration recommended - Dose interval adjustment in renal impairment: - Neonates: 15 mg/kg/dose once, check serum drug concentrations at 12–24 h postdose and adjust dose accordingly - Infants and children: mild, q8–12h; moderate, q18–48h; severe, q3–7d - IV formulation may be used for oral/ enteral dosing in cases where the compounded oral liquid is not suitable (e.g., ketogenic diet, short bowel syndrome). Capsules not suitable for administration through enteral feeding tubes - Calculate doses according to adjusted body weight
	INFANTS AND OLDER CHILDREN **Usual dosing** 10 mg/kg/dose IV q6h	500 mg/dose before TDM	
	Severe infections (i.e., meningitis, unstable neutropenic patients with fever, sickle cell disease, MRSA infections) 15 mg/kg/dose IV q6h	1 g/dose before TDM	
	***Clostridium difficile* colitis** 10 mg/kg/dose PO q6h	125 mg/dose PO, 500 mg/day	

_Continued

Drug Dosing Guidelines

Table 40.1 Drug Dosage Guidelines for Neonates[a] (Where Specified), Infants, and Older Children—cont'd

Drug[b,c]	Dose	Dose Limit	Comments
Verapamil Susp (HSC) 8 mg/mL Tab 80 mg, 120 mg Inj 2.5 mg/mL	***INFANTS AND OLDER CHILDREN*** *2–15 years:* 0.1–0.3 mg/kg/dose IV; may repeat once in 30 min prn *Maintenance:* 4–10 mg/kg/day PO div TID or QID	*Repeat dose:* 10 mg/dose IV *Usual adult dose:* 240–480 mg/day	- Administer IV under ECG monitoring - Avoid use in early postcardiosurgical period, in severe CHF, or in presence of beta-blockers
Vigabatrin Tab 500 mg Powder (sachet): 500 mg Solution (HSC) dissolve 'n' dose system	***INFANTS AND OLDER CHILDREN*** **Infantile spasms** *Day 1:* 25 mg/kg/dose PO BID *Day 2:* 50 mg/kg/dose PO BID *Day 3:* 62.5 mg/kg/dose PO BID *Day 4 and onward:* 75 mg/kg/dose PO BID		- Reduce dose in renal impairment - May be given with food - Concurrent use of vigabatrin may decrease serum phenytoin levels - Regular ophthalmological monitoring required
Vitamin B₁	See Thiamine		
Vitamin B₆	See Pyridoxine		
Vitamin C	See Ascorbic acid		
Vitamin K₁	See Phytonadione		
Voriconazole Inj 200 mg/vial Oral suspension 40 mg/mL Tab 50 mg, 200 mg	***INFANTS AND OLDER CHILDREN*** *IV dosing* *2–12 years:* 9 mg/kg/dose IV q12h *>12 years:* 6 mg/kg/dose IV q12h for 2 doses, then 4 mg/kg/dose IV q12h	350 mg/dose IV	- May interact with many medications; consider consulting pharmacist regarding patients taking multiple medications - Oral tablets have improved absorption if given at least 1 h before or 1 h after a meal

	Oral dosing (following IV therapy) *2–12 years:* 9 mg/kg/dose PO q12h *>12 years, <40 kg:* 200 mg PO q12h for 2 doses, then 100 mg PO q12h *>12 years, ≥40 kg:* 400 mg PO q12h for 2 doses, then 200 mg PO q12h	- Measurement of voriconazole serum concentrations are recommended for invasive fungal infections - Caution when using IV voriconazole in patients with renal impairment. Monitor renal function closely and if significant changes occur, consider changing to oral voriconazole therapy, if clinically appropriate - Visual changes, such as blurred vision, photophobia, changes in visual acuity and color have been reported
Warfarin Tab 1 mg, 2 mg, 2.5 mg, 5 mg	***INFANTS AND OLDER CHILDREN*** *Loading dose:* 0.2 mg/kg/dose PO as single daily dose For dosing guidelines, see Warfarin in Chapter 21 Hematology	5 mg/dose	- Avoid in infants less than 12 months of age except in infants with mechanical valves - Loading period is approximately 3–5 days for most patients before a stable maintenance phase is achieved - May interact with many medications; consider consulting pharmacist regarding patients taking multiple medications - Patients on warfarin and TPN should be ordered 10 mL of MVI-12 which does not contain any phytonadione (vitamin K)

Continued

Table 40.1   Drug Dosage Guidelines for Neonates[a] (Where Specified), Infants, and Older Children—cont'd

Drug[b,c]	Dose	Dose Limit	Comments
Zidovudine Liquid 10 mg/mL Cap 100 mg Combination tab (Combivir): 300 mg zidovudine + 150 mg lamivudine Inj 200 mg/20 mL	***NEONATES*** **Perinatal HIV exposure and treatment of HIV infection** *Gestational age <30 weeks* 2 mg/kg/dose PO q12h, increase to 3 mg/kg/dose PO q12h at 4 weeks of age 1.5 mg/kg/dose IV q12h, increase to 2.3 mg/kg/dose IV q12h at 4 weeks of age *Gestational age ≥30 to <35 weeks* 2 mg/kg/dose PO q12h, increase to 3 mg/kg/dose PO q12h at 2 weeks of age 1.5 mg/kg/dose IV q12h, increase to 2.3 mg/kg/dose IV q12h at 2 weeks of age *Gestational age ≥35 weeks* 4 mg/kg/dose PO q12h 3 mg/kg/dose IV q12h ***INFANTS AND OLDER CHILDREN*** **Postexposure prophylaxis or treatment of HIV infection,** **in combination therapy** *6 weeks to 12 years:* 240 mg/m²/dose PO BID *>12 years or ≥30 kg:* 300 mg PO BID	600 mg/day	- Reduce dose in renal or liver impairment - Start perinatal dosing 6–12 h after birth and continue for 6 weeks

Zinc sulfate	**INFANTS AND OLDER CHILDREN**		- Give with food to reduce GI irritation
Solution (HSC) 10 mg/mL elemental zinc as zinc sulfate	**Supplementation**		
	0.5–1 mg elemental zinc/kg/day PO div BID–TID	30 mg elemental zinc/day	
	Acrodermatitis enteropathica		
Inj 10 mg elemental zinc/10 mL	1–2 mg elemental zinc/kg/day PO div BID–TID	45 mg elemental zinc/day	
Zoledronic acid	**INFANTS AND OLDER CHILDREN**		- Before infusion, ensure patient has eGFR >90 mL/min/1.73 m², sufficient vitamin D level, dental review, serum total calcium >2 mmol/L
Inj 4 mg/5 mL	**Osteogenesis imperfecta, hypercalcemia (total calcium >3 mmol/L)**		
	First dose: 0.0125 mg/kg/dose IV	4 mg/dose	- Dose limit adjustment in renal impairment:
	Maintenance: 0.0125–0.05 mg/kg/dose IV q6mo		- CrCl 50–60 mL/min: 3.5 mg
			- CrCl 40–49 mL/min: 3.3 mg
			- CrCl 30–39 mL/min: 3 mg
			- Post infusion, check serum calcium and give calcitriol for 4 days
Zolmitriptan	**INFANTS AND OLDER CHILDREN**		
Nasal spray 5 mg	*>12 years:* 5 mg intranasally once. May repeat dose once after 2 h if headache returns or if only a partial response to first dose	10 mg/day	
Zopiclone	**INFANTS AND OLDER CHILDREN**		
Tab 5 mg, 7.5 mg	2.5–7.5 mg/dose PO 30–45 min before bedtime	7.5 mg/day	

[a]Neonates: guidelines apply to all neonates until a postmenstrual age (PMA) of >44 weeks and a postnatal age (PNA) of >4 weeks have been achieved.

[b]Drug dosage forms listed may be used as a guide only and are not reflective of all dosage forms available.

[c]Liquids and suspensions noted with "HSC" (Hospital for Sick Children, Toronto, Ontario, Canada) are manufactured preparations; most formulations can be found at http://www.sickkids.ca/pharmacy/.

Adapted from The Hospital for Sick Children eFormulary, 2021.

Drug Dosing Guidelines

40

THERAPEUTIC DRUG MONITORING

Table 40.2 Therapeutic Drug Monitoring

Drug	Time for First TDM[a]	Ideal Sampling Time[b]	Optimal Concentration Range	Comments
Acetaminophen		≥4 h after ingestion		- Toxicology only; see nomogram, Figure 3.1
Amikacin q8h dosing or extended intervals for renal impairment (such as q12h, q24h, etc.)	On day 4 of therapy (or in selected patients,[c] after the third or fourth dose)	*Trough:* 0–30 min before dose *Peak:* (IV) 30–60 min after end of infusion	*Trough:* 2.5–10 mg/L *Peak:* 20–35 mg/L	- Half-life may be prolonged in patients with renal dysfunction - Both clearance and volume of distribution may be increased in cystic fibrosis
Amikacin Once-daily dosing	"Special" concentrations 3 h and 6 h after the first dose		*Peak:* 60–80 mg/L (Hematology/Oncology), 60–100 mg/L (cystic fibrosis) Drug-free interval (where concentration <4 mg/L) of at least 4 h	- Restricted to febrile neutropenia in Hematology/Oncology/ hematopoietic progenitor cell transplant (bone marrow transplant) and cystic fibrosis patients
Aminophylline Theophylline level	*Loading:* no restrictions *Continuous IV infusion:* after 12–24 h *Intermittent IV:* *Neonates:* 48–72 h; *Infants and Older Children:* 24–48 h	*Loading:* at least 1 h post load *Continuous IV infusion:* no restrictions *Intermittent IV:* *Trough:* 0–30 min before dose *Peak:* 1–2 h post dose	*Apnea of prematurity:* 28–67 µmol/L *Bronchodilation, diuresis:* 55–110 µmol/L	

Drug			
Carbamazepine	*Initial dose:* 1 week (then twice/week until stable) *Dose change:* 3 days	*Trough:* 0–1 h before dose	17–50 µmol/L	- Because of enzyme autoinduction, half-life during chronic dosing may be considerably shorter than after first dose; consequently, within first 2–4 week of therapy, dose may need to be increased
Carbamazepine-10, 11 epoxide		*Trough:* 0–1 h before dose	5–12 µmol/L	
Cyclosporine	*Continuous infusion:* 2 days *Intermittent (IV or PO):* 2 days	*Continuous infusion:* no restrictions *Intermittent: Trough:* 0–60 min before dose	ªSee comments	- Monitoring considered mandatory to avoid extremely low or high levels that may precipitate therapeutic failure or nephrotoxicity
Digoxin	*After load:* 24 h *Maintenance:* 5 days (2 days if risk factors: poor therapeutic re-sponse, symptoms of toxicity, renal or hepatic impairment, drug interactions [e.g., amiodarone, propafenone])	*Trough:* 0–60 min before dose (or at least 8 h after last dose)	1–2.5 nmol/L	- Half-life may be prolonged in renal impairment - In infants and children, concentration–effect relationship somewhat imprecise; if level normal on day 5 without clinical problems, repeat level on weekly basis as inpatient and every 3 months as outpatient
Enoxaparin Treatment dosing	Day 1 and/or day 2, a blood sample should be drawn 4 h after the SC administration		*LMWH Antifactor Xa Level:* 0.5–1 units/mL	- Monitoring of LMWH Antifactor Xa levels for prophylaxis is not required unless renal failure is present
Ethosuximide	7 days	*Trough:* 0–60 min before dose	280–710 µmol/L	- Selected patients may tolerate and benefit from levels that are higher than recommended max level
Fosphenytoin	see Phenytoin			

Continued

Drug Dosing Guidelines

40

Table 40.2 Therapeutic Drug Monitoring—cont'd

Drug	Time for First TDM[a]	Ideal Sampling Time[b]	Optimal Concentration Range	Comments
Gentamicin q8h dosing or extended intervals for renal impairment (such as q12h, q24h, etc.)	On day 4 of therapy (or in selected patients,[c] after the third or fourth dose)	*Trough:* 0–30 min before dose *Peak:* 30–60 min after end of infusion	*Trough:* 0.6–2 mg/L *Peak:* 5–10 mg/L	- Target peak concentration for indication (for q8h or extended interval dosing) - *UTI:* 3–5 mg/L - *Pyelonephritis, cellulitis:* 5–7 mg/L - *Pneumonia, wound infection:* 6–8 mg/L - *Positive culture with neutropenia:* 7–9 mg/L - Risk factors should prompt closer monitoring (neutropenia, positive cultures, persistent fever, concurrent therapy with a nephrotoxic agent, unstable renal function or fluid imbalance, abnormal cardiac status, prematurity, severe burns) - Frequency of continued monitoring depends on clinical status and renal function; however, in stable patients, creatinine and trough concentrations are usually obtained approximately every 7 days; consult pharmacist regarding monitoring in dialysis patients
Gentamicin Once daily dosing	"Special" concentrations 3 h and 6 h after the first dose if intended course is >72 hours		*Peak (Non-Hematology/ Oncology patients):* 16–25 mg/L *Peak (Hematology/ Oncology patients with fever and neutropenia):* 20–25 mg/L *Drug-free interval (where concentration <2 mg/L):* at least 4 h	

Heparin	Obtain blood for aPTT and/or heparin Antifactor Xa (standard heparin assay) 4 h after the bolus dose was administered and followed by heparin infusion, or 6 h after start of infusion if no bolus was given	Heparin Antifactor Xa level: 0.35–0.75 units/mL aPTT 60–85 s	- Draw heparin Antifactor Xa level in first 24 h to check for correlation with aPTT. If aPTT and heparin Antifactor Xa level correlate (and child greater than 12 months of age) use the aPTT to continue to monitor unfractionated heparin therapy.
Lithium	*Trough:* 12 h after dose	0.5–1.5 mmol/L	
Methotrexate (high dose)	Dependent on treatment protocol	*See comments	- Concentrations elevated by impairment of renal filtration or secretion
Mycophenolic acid (MPA) MMF metabolite	*Trough:* 0–60 min before dose		
Phenobarbital	*IV loading:* at least 1 h after load *Maintenance: Trough:* 0–60 min before dose	65–170 μmol/L	- Specific patients tolerate and may benefit from serum levels that are significantly higher than "recommended maximum limit"
Phenytoin	*IV loading:* at least 1 h after load *Maintenance: Trough:* 0–1 h before dose	40–80 μmol/L	- Simultaneous monitoring of free phenytoin levels not routine but may be of assistance
Phenytoin (free)	*Trough:* 0–1 h before next dose	*Free:* 4–8 μmol/L	
Salicylate, ASA Toxicology	At least 6 h after ingestion	*Overdose:* see Table 3.6	- Time to peak varies and is prolonged with enteric-coated product
Salicylate, ASA Therapeutic dose	*Trough:* 0–1 h before dose	*JIA:* 1.1–2.2 mmol/L *Kawasaki disease, pericarditis:* <2.2 mmol/L	

Duration to steady state / restrictions (second column group):

Drug	
Lithium	4–6 days
Mycophenolic acid (MPA)	3 days
Phenobarbital	*IV loading:* no restrictions *Maintenance:* 4 days (7 days for steady state)
Phenytoin	*IV loading:* no restrictions *Maintenance:* 3 days (then twice/ week until stable)
Phenytoin (free)	3 days
Salicylate, ASA Toxicology	No restrictions
Salicylate, ASA Therapeutic dose	3 days

Continued

Table 40.2 Therapeutic Drug Monitoring—cont'd

Drug	Time for First TDM[a]	Ideal Sampling Time[b]	Optimal Concentration Range	Comments
Sirolimus	5 days	*Trough:* 0–30 min before dose	5–15 mcg/L[d]	
Tacrolimus	3 days	*Trough:* 0–30 min before dose	5–15 mcg/L[d]	
Theophylline Intermittent PO	24–48 h	*Trough:* 0–30 min before dose *Peak:* 1–2 h after immediate-release preparations or 3–7 h after sustained-release preparations	55–110 µmol/L	
Tinzaparin	See Enoxaparin			
Tobramycin q8h dosing or extended intervals for renal impairment (such as q12h, q24h, etc.)	On day 4 of therapy (or in selected patients,[c] after the third or fourth dose)	*Trough:* 0–30 min before dose *Peak:* 30–60 min after end of infusion	*Trough:* 0.6–2 mg/L *Peak:* 5–10 mg/L	- See comments for gentamicin
Tobramycin Once daily dosing	"Special" concentrations 3 h and 6 h after the first dose if intended course is >72 hours		*Peak (cystic fibrosis patients):* 25–35 mg/L *Peak (noncystic fibrosis patients):* 16–25 mg/L *Drug-free interval (where concentration <2 mg/L):* at least 4 h	
Valproic acid	2 days	*Trough:* 0–1 h before dose	350–700 µmol/L	- Half-life may be prolonged in patients with hepatic disease and may be shortened in patients receiving other anticonvulsant drugs

Vancomycin	Fourth dose (earlier if significant renal impairment or dosing intervals ≥q12h)	*Trough*: 0–30 min before dose	*CNS infections*: 10–15 mg/L *Other infections*: 5–12 mg/L	Peak routinely determined *only* for patients who may have altered pharmacokinetics (febrile neutropenic patients, burn patients, neonates); peak concentrations are of no utility when drug is infused for >1 h and do not correlate with toxicity or effectiveness; additional trough monitoring required for dosage adjustment, treatment >7 days in duration, addition of nephrotoxic drugs, high minimum inhibitory concentration (MIC) isolate, renal insufficiency/failure
Voriconazole	3 days	*Trough*: 0–30 min before dose	*Trough*: 1–5 mg/L	For subtherapeutic/low trough level on day 3 of initial therapy, special levels during dose interval (e.g., 8 h postdose) can be drawn for assessment of shorter dose interval

Under certain circumstances, it may be necessary to collect samples for monitoring at times that do not coincide with normal "peak" and "trough" assessment; such samples are referred to as "*special*" concentrations. Special drug concentrations may have to be obtained when:

- patients are receiving peritoneal dialysis, hemodialysis, or CVVH
- patients have unstable or poor renal function
- therapy has been stopped after previous high drug concentration

[a]Time for first therapeutic drug monitoring; refers to first routine opportunity for sampling after new order or order change; normally represents attainment of steady state. Routine drug levels should not be measured before attainment of steady-state conditions unless failure of therapeutic response or onset of toxicity suspected.

[b]Ideal sampling time permits direct comparison with optimal concentration range; results of tests conducted on samples collected at other than ideal times must be interpreted cautiously.

[c]Renal impairment, premature infants, term infants <7 days, documented infections where therapy continues >72 h, therapy >7 days, concurrent nephrotoxic drugs (e.g., amphotericin, cyclosporine), patients with severe burns.

[d]Optimal concentration range is dependent upon clinical status of the patient, type of transplant, and time since transplant and assay matrix.

aPTT, Activated partial thromboplastin time; *CNS*, central nervous system; *CVVH*, continuous venovenous hemofiltration; *IV*, intravenous; *JIA*, juvenile idiopathic arthritis; *LMWH*, low-molecular-weight heparin; *MMF*, mycophenolate mofetil; *PO*, per os (by mouth); *TDM*, therapeutic drug monitoring; *UTI*, urinary tract infection.

Adapted from The Hospital for Sick Children eFormulary Therapeutic Drug Monitoring, 2021.

Drug Dosing Guidelines

40

DOSE EQUIVALENTS OF COMMONLY USED STEROIDS

Table 40.3	Dose Equivalents of Commonly Used Steroids	
Drug	**Glucocorticoid Effect Equivalent to Cortisol 100 mg PO**	**Mineralocorticoid Effect Equivalent to Fludrocortisone Acetate (Florinef) 0.1 mg[a]**
Cortisone	125	20
Hydrocortisone	100	20
Prednisone	25	50
Prednisolone	20–25	50
Methylprednisone	15–20	No effect
Triamcinolone	10–20	No effect
9-alpha-Fluorocortisol	6.5	0.1
Dexamethasone	1.5–3.75	No effect

[a] Total physiological replacement for salt retention is usually 0.1 mg fludrocortisone acetate (Florinef) regardless of patient's size.

ENDOCARDITIS PROPHYLAXIS

Box 40.1 Cardiac Conditions in Which Prophylaxis is Reasonable (High-Risk Conditions)

1. Based on the balance of risk versus benefit, antibiotic prophylaxis is no longer recommended for dental procedures based solely on an increased lifetime risk of infective endocarditis (IE). Prophylaxis is reasonable only for patients with underlying cardiac conditions associated with the highest risk of adverse outcome from IE.
2. Cardiac conditions in which prophylaxis is reasonable (high-risk conditions)
   a. Prosthetic cardiac valves, including bioprosthetic and homograft valves or prosthetic material used for cardiac valve repair
   b. Previous bacterial endocarditis
   c. Congenital heart disease (CHD)
      i. Unrepaired cyanotic CHD, including palliative shunts and conduits
      ii. Completely repaired congenital heart defect with prosthetic material or device, whether placed by surgery or catheter intervention during the first 6 months after the procedure
      iii. Repaired CHD with residual defects at the site or adjacent to the site of a prosthetic patch or prosthetic device
   d. Cardiac transplant recipients who develop cardiac valvulopathy
   e. Rheumatic heart disease with significant residual valvular disease
3. Cardiac conditions in which prophylaxis is **NO LONGER** recommended (moderate to low risk conditions)
   a. Mitral valve prolapse
   b. Hypertrophic cardiomyopathy
   c. Other congenital cardiac malformations (other than those listed in high-risk category earlier)

Adapted from The Hospital for Sick Children eFormulary Antimicrobial Guidelines - Endocarditis Prophylaxis, 2019.

Box 40.2 Dental Procedures Requiring Subacute Bacterial Endocarditis Prophylaxis

Dental procedures in which endocarditis prophylaxis is reasonable (prophylaxis is recommended only for patients with the high-risk cardiac conditions listed in Box 40.1):

All dental procedures involving the manipulation of gingival tissue or the periapical region of the teeth or perforation of the oral mucosa including tooth extraction, biopsies, suture removal, and placement of orthodontic bands.

Adapted from The Hospital for Sick Children eFormulary Antimicrobial Guidelines - Endocarditis Prophylaxis, 2019.

Box 40.3 Other (Non-dental) Procedures Requiring Subacute Bacterial Endocarditis Prophylaxis

1. Antibiotic prophylaxis is not necessary for the sole purpose of preventing infective endocarditis (IE) in nondental procedures. Various nondental procedures reportedly cause transient bacteremia and have been anecdotally associated with endocarditis. Listed subsequently are some examples of procedures for which IE prophylaxis can be considered:
   a. *Oral or respiratory tract procedures* (invasive procedures of the respiratory tract that involve incision or biopsy of the respiratory mucosa)
      i. Tonsillectomy/adenoidectomy
      ii. Surgical procedures on the upper respiratory tract
      iii. Nasal packing and nasal intubation
      iv. Cosmetic piercing of the tongue or involving oral mucosa
   b. *Gastrointestinal/genitourinary procedures*
      i. Sclerotherapy for esophageal dilatation
      ii. Esophageal stricture dilatation
      iii. Endoscopic retrograde cholangiopancreatography
      iv. Hepatic/biliary operations
      v. Surgical operations involving intestinal mucosa
      vi. Cystoscopy
      vii. Urethral dilatation
2. Antibiotic prophylaxis is only recommended <u>at the time of insertion</u> of nonvalvular devices, including central venous catheters, to prevent surgical site infection. Antibiotic prophylaxis is NOT required for dental procedures in patients who have indwelling central lines.
3. In patients who would normally receive standard perioperative antibiotic prophylaxis or in patients with an established infection at the procedure site, the antibiotic regimen should be modified to include an agent active against the most common causes of IE in the procedure
   a. Viridans group streptococci for oral or respiratory tract procedures (Table 40.4)
   b. Enterococci for gastrointestinal, hepatic/biliary, or genitourinary procedures (e.g., ampicillin, piperacillin, or vancomycin, ± low-dose gentamicin for synergy)
   c. Staphylococci and beta-hemolytic streptococci for procedures on infected skin, skin structure, or musculoskeletal tissue (e.g., cephalexin, cefazolin, clindamycin, or vancomycin ± low-dose gentamicin for synergy)

Adapted from The Hospital for Sick Children eFormulary Antimicrobial Guidelines - Endocarditis Prophylaxis, 2019.

Table 40.4	Recommended Prophylactic Regimens for Dental Procedures	
Situation	**First-Line Agent**	**Alternative Agent(s)**
Standard general prophylaxis	Amoxicillin 50 mg/kg (max 2 g) PO 1 h before procedure	
Unable to take oral medications	Ampicillin 50 mg/kg (max 2 g) IM/IV 30 min before procedure	Cefazolin or ceftriaxone 50 mg/kg (max 1 g) IM/IV 30 min before procedure
Allergic to penicillins	Clarithromycin or azithromycin 15 mg/kg (max 500 mg) PO 1 h before procedure	Clindamycin 20 mg/kg (max 600 mg) PO 1 h before procedure
Allergic to penicillin and unable to take oral medications	Clindamycin 20 mg/kg (max 600 mg) IM/IV 30 min before procedure	

Additional Considerations

If patients are already receiving long-term therapy with an antibiotic that is also recommended for infective endocarditis (IE) prophylaxis, it is likely they would have developed some underlying resistance to that antibiotic. In such cases, a different antibiotic should be selected for IE prophylaxis. In the case of long-term therapy with penicillins, cephalosporins should be avoided for IE prophylaxis because of potential cross-resistance. If possible, it would be preferable to delay a dental procedure for at least 10 days after completion of the antibiotic therapy to allow the usual oral flora to be reestablished.

Adapted from The Hospital for Sick Children eFormulary Antimicrobial Guidelines - Endocarditis Prophylaxis, 2019.

ALTERNATIVE MEDICINE INTERACTIONS

Table 40.5	Interactions Between Commonly Used Alternative Medications and Commonly Prescribed Medications
Alternative Medication	**Drug Interactions**
Alfalfa	- Cyclosporine/steroids: may have immune stimulating effects - Hypoglycemic medications: may cause further hypoglycemia - Warfarin: ↑↓INR (may contain warfarin constituents or ↓ effect because of vitamin K content in herb)
Aloe	- Digoxin, thiazide diuretics: ↑ cardiac toxicity because of electrolyte imbalance
Anise	- MAOIs: herb may ↑ risk of hypertensive crisis - Warfarin: ↑INR (may contain warfarin constituents)
Bitter melon	- Additive hypoglycemic effects in combination with antidiabetic agents, such as insulin or oral hypoglycemics
Bitter orange (synephrine)	- Caution with QT interval–prolonging drugs (amiodarone, procainamide, quinidine, sotalol, thioridazine) - Increases levels and adverse effects of midazolam - MAOIs: increased blood pressure, hypertensive crisis - CNS stimulants: increased risk of hypertension and adverse cardiovascular effects

Alternative Medication	Drug Interactions
Capsicum	- MAOIs: ↑ risk of hypertensive crisis - ACE inhibitor: may ↑ cough - Theophylline: oral administration of capsicum may ↑ theophylline absorption
Cascara	- Various medications: ↓ absorption because of increased GI transit time - Digoxin/thiazides/steroids: may potentiate hypokalemia
Chamomile	- Warfarin: ↑INR (may contain warfarin constituents) - Iron: contains tannic acids that may ↓ iron absorption
Chromium picolinate	- Nephrotoxic drugs: may ↑ renal failure and rhabdomyolysis - Hypoglycemics: may cause hypoglycemia
Coenzyme Q10 (ubiquinone)	- β-Blockers: may counteract negative inotropic effects - Antihypertensive drugs: may have additive blood pressure–lowering effects - Warfarin: ↓INR (may decrease effect of warfarin)
Dandelion	- Diuretics and lithium: may ↑ diuretic effect and ↑ lithium toxicity - Warfarin: ↓INR (↓ effect because of vitamin K content in the herb)
Echinacea	- Immunosuppressant drugs (e.g., corticosteroids, cyclosporine): echinacea has immunostimulant effects that may interfere with these drugs - Hepatotoxic drugs (e.g., ketoconazole, isoniazid, methotrexate, terbinafine): herb may have additive hepatotoxicity if used for >8 weeks - Hypoglycemic drugs: may cause hypo/hyperglycemia - Midazolam (IV): reduced levels and effect - Warfarin: ↑INR
Feverfew	- Antiplatelets: increased risk of bleeding
Flaxseed	- Warfarin: ↑INR (may ↑ bleeding time)
Garlic	- Antiplatelet and anticoagulant drugs (e.g., aspirin, NSAIDs, clopidogrel, dipyridamole, warfarin, heparin, low molecular weight heparins): increased risk of bleeding - Isoniazid, saquinavir: reduced plasma levels with garlic - May reduce levels and effects of the following drugs by ↑ metabolism (P450 3A4 inducer): azole antifungals (ketoconazole, itraconazole), calcium channel blockers, chemotherapy drugs (etoposide, paclitaxel, vinblastine, vincristine, vindesine), cyclosporine, HIV protease inhibitors and NNRTIs (nevirapine, efavirenz), midazolam, oral contraceptives
Ginger	- Antihypertensives: may ↑ or ↓ effect with these medications - Hypoglycemics: may cause hypoglycemia - Antiplatelet and anticoagulant drugs: excessive amounts of ginger could increase bleeding risk

Continued

Table 40.5	Interactions Between Commonly Used Alternative Medications and Commonly Prescribed Medications—cont'd
Alternative Medication	**Drug Interactions**
Ginkgo	- Anticonvulsant drugs: may lower seizure threshold - Antiplatelet and anticoagulant drugs (e.g., aspirin, NSAIDs, clopidogrel, dipyridamole, warfarin, heparin, low molecular weight heparins): increased risk of bleeding
Ginseng	- Corticosteroids: may affect steroid concentrations - Cardiac and antihypertensive medications: have negative chronotropic and inotropic activity and may cause possible ↓ blood pressure - Estrogens/corticosteroids: may have possible additive effects - Furosemide: may reduce effect of furosemide - Hypoglycemics: may have additive hypoglycemic effect - MAOIs, mood stabilizers: ↑ tremor/mania - Warfarin: ↑ ↓INR
Glucosamine	- Hypoglycemics/insulin: may cause insulin resistance - Doxorubicin and etoposide: may cause resistance to these drugs
Goldenseal	- Cardiac and antihypertensive medications: can have variable effects on the heart and blood pressure - Heparin: can counteract effect of heparin - Sedatives: may have additive sedative effects
Hawthorn	- Digoxin and antihypertensives: may interfere with these medications - MAOIs: may contain tyramine: ↑ risk of hypertensive crisis
Horse chestnut	- Warfarin: ↑INR
Licorice	- Antihypertensives/digoxin/diuretics: may cause hypokalemia and sodium and fluid retention which can ↑ blood pressure (i.e., pseudoaldosteronism) - Corticosteroids: may ↑ systemic and topical steroid effects - Digoxin: herb may interfere with effect of digoxin - Hypoglycemics: may cause ↓ glucose tolerance - Oral contraceptives: may lead to hypertension, edema, and ↓ potassium - Warfarin: herb may inhibit platelet activity
Melatonin	- Anticonvulsant medications: may lower seizure threshold - Drugs affecting metabolism of melatonin through CYP1A2 may alter its effects (*increased effect:* amiodarone, ciprofloxacin, fluoxetine, fluvoxamine; *decreased effect:* carbamazepine, phenobarbital, phenytoin, rifampin, ritonavir) - Hypoglycemic medications: may have ↓ effect - Nifedipine: ↑ blood pressure and heart rate with melatonin - Other antihypertensive drugs: additive effects - Warfarin: ↑ ↓INR
Milk thistle	- Hypoglycemics: herb may have additive hypoglycemic effect

Table 40.5

Alternative Medication	Drug Interactions
Nettle	- Contains tannic acids that may ↓ iron absorption - Warfarin: ↓INR (may contain vitamin K)
Passionflower	- MAOIs/SSRIs/TCAs: may ↑ risk of serotonin syndrome - Warfarin ↑INR: herb may contain warfarin constituents
Royal jelly	- Asthma medications: may cause bronchospasm
Senna	- Digoxin/thiazides/steroids: may potentiate hypokalemia - Various medications: ↓ absorption because of increased GI transit time
St. John wort (SJW)	- Reduces levels and effects of the following drugs by ↑ metabolism (P450 3A4 inducer): azole antifungals (ketoconazole, itraconazole), calcium channel blockers, chemotherapy drugs (etoposide, imatinib, irinotecan, paclitaxel, vinblastine, vincristine, vindesine), cyclosporine, digoxin, HIV protease inhibitors, midazolam, nevirapine, omeprazole, oral contraceptives, phenobarbital, phenytoin, sumatriptan, theophylline, warfarin - Increases activity of clopidogrel - SSRIs, TCAs, MAOIs, meperidine, sumatriptan: increased risk of serotonin syndrome
Valerian	- Sedatives: may have additive sedative effects

ACE, Angiotensin-converting enzyme; *CNS,* central nervous system; *GI,* gastrointestinal; *HIV,* human immunodeficiency virus; *INR,* international normalized ratio; *IV,* intravenous; *MAOI,* monoamine oxidase inhibitor; *NNRTI,* nonnucleoside reverse transcriptase inhibitors; *NSAID,* nonsteroidal antiinflammatory drug; *SSRI,* selective serotonin reuptake inhibitor; *TCA,* tricyclic antidepressant.

DRUG INFUSION CALCULATIONS

Table 40.6 Drug Infusion Calculations

Desired Concentration	Dose (mg) in 50 mL
0.33 mcg/kg/min = 1 mL/h	$1 \times$ wt (kg)
1 mcg/kg/min = 1 mL/h	$3 \times$ wt (kg)
10 mcg/kg/h = 1 mL/h	$0.5 \times$ wt (kg)
0.25 mg/kg/h = 1mL/h	$12.5 \times$ wt (kg)
1 mg/kg/day = 1 mL/h	$2 \times$ wt (kg)
	Dose (units) in 50 mL
0.0001 unit/kg/min = 1 mL/h	$0.3 \times$ wt (kg)
10 units/kg/h = 1 mL/h	$10 \times 50 \times$ wt (kg)

INDEX

Page numbers followed by *b* indicate boxes; *f*, figures; *t*, tables.

Index

Index

Index

Index

Index

Index

1313

Index

Index